ENCYCLOPAEDIA OF AIDS

ENCYCLOPAEDIA
OF
AIDS

(In 7 Volumes)

(Volume 1)

Editor

Dr. G.C. Satpathy

PUBLICATIONS

KALPAZ PUBLICATIONS

DELHI - 110052

ENCYCLOPAEDIA OF AIDS
(*Health, Reference*)

Rs. 7000 (Set)
Rs. 1000 (each volume)

ISBN: 81-7835-112-9 (Set)
ISBN: 81-7835-132-3 (Vol. 1)

Published in 2003 in India by
Kalpaz Publications
C-30, Satyawati Nagar
Delhi-110052
e-mail: kalpaz@hotmail.com

Laser Typeset at: Alphabet, Delhi
Printed at: Mehra Offset Press, Delhi

Contents

PART-VI: AIDS, WOMEN AND HUMAN RIGHTS

PART-VII: AIDS AND ETHICS

Preface

The later half of the twentieth century will be remembered in the history of medicine for two remarkable events, one good, that is the eradication of smallpox, and the other one bad, when the world was alerted to the first case AIDS in 1981, now running in a pandemic proportion. In a little over two decades it is estimated that over 36 million people are now infected with HIV/AIDS with 5.3 million being infected every year. India alone has about 4 million HIV/AIDS patients, the second highest number among all nations. Now it is well perceived as a serious threat to humanity, and the control of this epidemic lies not only in the hands of physicians alone but the entire society must involve to the task. No cure or vaccine is yet in sight. So the only mode of controlling it is prevention. The key to prevention lies in information, education and communication.

Twenty years of observation and study of the syndrome has generated profound interest among all branches of medicine, social activists, research workers, public health issues, health and sex education strategies, with innumerable clinical and pharmacological research being conducted on it all over the world. It is not possible to compile the whole saga of AIDS, which is unique in many ways and not yet fully understood. We have tried to accumulate as much information as possible in this seven-volume encyclopaedia, probably the first such attempt made ever. Since the process of acquiring information is never-ending, we hope to provide more and more information in future.

It has been a herculean task to compile the huge materials systematically, besides being an unique experience. In spite of the best efforts for accuracy and perfection, there may be shortcomings, which may be excused. It will be a success story for us if by this work the society to which the work is dedicated is benefited at large. The study does not end here. It shall be a continuous series in future with comprehensive details having a deep bearing on the subject.

Guwahati-23
Rathyatra-2002

Dr. G.C. Satpathy
MD, IPM

Acknowledgements

During the course of this research work, I happened to visit several academic fora which willingly afforded their support and facilitated my work. These are the Ministry of Health, Govt. of India, World Health Organisation, health departments of the States and academic institutions of higher learning. I have used the material from published works including scholarly journals and magazines to fill up the gaps in these volumes.

I have also taken academic support from several sources, which include universities, institutes, centres for higher learning, Acts passed in this direction, Statistical Year Book (UNESCO), voluntary organisations, legal luminaries, social activists, prison management, legal issues of AIDS, Legislation Enquiry Commission on HIV Law, Sri Lanka, Prevention of Brothels Act, Myanmar, Laws of HIV/AIDS in Pakistan, Documents in sub-Saharan, Africa, European Council Recommendations, UNESCO Courier, Philippines Overseas Employment Agency, Foreign Exchange Regulations Deptt., Central Bank of the Philippines, National Advisory Committee on AIDS in Singapore, Vietnamese National AIDS Committee, National Blood Transfusion Centre in Cambodia, Infectious Diseases Act, Thailand, AIDS Prevention Act in Korea, Labour Protection Law, Thailand, Social Security Act, Thailand, Homosexual Law Reform Act, 1986, Universities of Nairobi, Manitola (in Canada) and Washington, Institute of Systemic Therapy, Harare, Zimbabwe, The AIDS Service Organisation, Kampala, Uganda, Health Economics and HIV/ AIDS Research Division, University of Natal, Durban, School of

Public Health, University of Natal, South Africa Institute for Medical Research, Johannesburg, Centre for African Family Studies, Nairobi, Kenya, Malwai Institute of Management, Malwai.

I feel much grateful to these institutions and learned authors whose writings have proved useful in the texts of these seven volumes.

The publisher and myself feel much beholden to the panel of highly qualified and experienced advisers who are distinguished in their respective fields, for their valuable and timely guidelines, contributions and encouragement in making this work an epoch-making one.

I am grateful to several other research institutes and NGOs etc., scholars whose writings have been used in these volumes.

I am extremely grateful to my wife, son Anurag and daughter Anamika for their consistent encouragement to me during this stupendous research work.

Dr. G.C. Satpathy

Our Distinguished Panel of Advisers

1. Dr. A.K. Das, MD, MNAMS, Ph.D., FICA	Dean and Director-Prof. Dept. of Medicine, JIMPER, Pondicherry
2. Mr. D.K. Arya IPS (Retd.)	Former Director General, BSF
3. Dr. K.V. Dakhina Murty MD, DM, DNB, FISN	Prof. & Head, Deptt. of Nephrology, Nizam's Instt. of Medical Sciences, Panjagutta, Hyderabad
4. Maj. Gen. K.K. Ganguly	VSM (Retd.)
5. Col. M.K. Bhandari MD, FICA	Asso. Prof. of Medicine, Armed Forces Medical College, Pune
6. Dr. M.C. Dash	Vice Chancellor, Sambalpur University, P.O.: Jyoti Vihar, Orissa
7. Dr. N.C. Borah MD, DM	C.M.D. GNRC Hospitals Ltd. Dispur, Guwahati
8. Dr. P.C. Bhattacharya MD	Sr. Consultant, downtown hospital Dispur, Guwahati
9. Dr. S.B. Gupta MD	Physician and Cardiologist Central Railway Hospital, Mumbai

Introduction

The second half of the twentieth century witnessed the outbreak of an awfully dangerous pandemic, called the 'AIDS'. Like an epidemic, people gave enough heed to the discovery of this new human killer and much hue and cry was made by the well-aware lots of people in the world. But, even that much of hue and cry fell short to express the magnitude of the danger which this disease possessed for the mankind. Large numbers of medical experts poured in their efforts to find out everything about AIDS, but they were surprised with every new finding about it. The world was shocked to know that it is not like other epidemics like plague, malaria or cholera, but, instead, it remains hidden for years inside the body of the patient, and by the time he feels himself having received infection, he has already reached a very advanced stage of the disease. This is the reason why AIDS has been termed as the 'Silent Killer'. To their surprise, scientists came to know that they do not have any potent weapons (medicines) to kill this human killer. Over two decades have passed since the first report came on AIDS, but we still far away from a workable formula for the proper cure of AIDS patients.

The most worrying fact about AIDS is that, unlike other epidemics or potent human killers, it is not a disease in itself, but the destroyer of human body's resistance to *any* disease. Once an Human Immunodeficiency Virus (HIV) completes its job in a human body, even a petty ailment becomes difficult to be treated because the body of the patient gives no response to any medicine. Thus, once the immune system of a man is destroyed, which is done by the HIV in an AIDS patient, a man falls an inescapable prone to many diseases. Since no medicine brings favourable results in such a body, the man has no option but to wait haplessly for a slow and painful death.

Man has always been fighting many challenges posed for its survival by the nature. It has been overcoming almost all of them too, and that is why the man is flourishing to this day and leads a comfortable life despite so many natural calamities harming him in many ways. But, in the form of AIDS, the nature seems to be in a different mood, not to let the man overcome this severe threat to his very survival.

The fight is on, and though we have not become successful in curing those who have fallen victims to this disease, yet, we have developed the ways which can surely keep us unharmed against this dreaded human killer. Till now, awareness has been considered as our most important weapon against this enemy. An aware person can take enough measures to remain untouched by this disease while an unknown person has many chances of falling prey to it. No Vaccine yet in sight.

Keeping this in view, the present series is presented. Almost every aspect has been taken into account while preparing this series on AIDS. The present book provides the basic information about the AIDS to the readers. It, nevertheless, provides him with the wide purview in which this pandemic should be seen.

The book contains seventeen chapters divided into Seven different parts.

The first chapter gives the early cases of the AIDS reported in the different parts of the world. It presents the early history of AIDS as also the early reaction of the people to the outbreak of the new disease. The knowledge of the nature of the causing agent, the HIV, and its survival are also discussed in this chapter. Then, the theories of the origin of the AIDS which came soon after its breakout have also been given herein. The connection of AIDS with Haiti has been described, as also the blaming of the Haitians by the world for the origin and spread of the AIDS.

Chapter 2 deals with the Human Immunodeficiency Virus (HIV), the infection of HIV and the disease called AIDS. It brings out the significant features of the nature of HIV. Another variant of HIV, which caused enough problems to be recognised by the medical experts, and later came to be known as HIV-2 is also described in this chapter. The significant fact about the AIDS, that it is not a single disease, but the root cause, which paves the way for even the slightest of ailment to make human body its permanent home, finds place in this chapter. The mechanism how HIV is harmful to our Immune System has been given herein.

Chapter 3 deals with the different modes of transmission of the AIDS virus. As is well known, HIV is transmitted mainly through the sexual intercourse between two persons. If a healthy (uninfected) person makes sexual relations with an infected person without using a condom, the HIV gets transmitted from the infected body to the healthy one. In another mode of transmission, HIV is transmitted through the transfusion of the blood. When a healthy person receives the blood from an infected person, he gets infected with HIV which is present in the blood of the infected person. The third mode of the transmission is from mother to her child. It is well known that the child is but a part of the mother's body for about nine months before he or she is born. Thus, the HIV finds an easy way into the body of the child from the mother when the child is in mother's womb.

This chapter also discusses the worldwide HIV infections as well as some groundless fears about the transmission of HIV.

Chapter 4 describes AIDS as a global epidemic. The World Health Organisation (WHO) has estimated the number of total AIDS victims as well as the number of infected persons in different parts of the world.

Chapter 5 deals with a very serious effect of AIDS on our society. It takes up the issue of children who lose their mothers due to AIDS. A separate section of this chapter is devoted to Africa's motherless children. A realistic picture has been presented of the crippling cost of the treatment of AIDS, which goes all in vain leaving the family almost starving in poverty. It is a matter of grave concern that most of the AIDS victims come from the lesser-income group of the society. On the other hand, the treatments, howsoever, efficacious they are, drain so heavily on the resources of patient's family that it is left struggling for bread and butter even. The chapter also deals with the impact of the deaths caused by AIDS.

Chapter 6 informs the reader how different parts of the world blamed each other for origin and spread of AIDS. It also shows how different groups of people were affected with the imposition of blame on themselves. The effect of blame on Nigeria, was very significant. Also, every African student was thought to be a carrier of AIDS, and they were required to go through either voluntary or forced screening to remain and study in India and some other parts of the world. It also shows that how, after the confirmation of infection in some Africans, which was greatly due to careless screening, other African students denied to go through screening. Many foreign groups of people were restricted to enter many parts of the world due to the fear of spread of AIDS. The effect of AIDS on tourism in Kenya is given in this chapter. Also a list of countries which went for screening of foreigners is given herein.

Chapter 7 deals with the awareness programme about AIDS. It has been realised that the awareness is the most important preventive measure for AIDS. The more aware are the people, the more are the chances of their staying away from the disease. Again, making more and more people aware of the various aspects of this disease would result in the lesser people being infected with HIV.

Chapter 8 is given to caring for the victims. With the rapid spread of AIDS in the world, more and more people are getting patients who need not only the medicines, but also love and care of others. A person infected with HIV is considered by many people as a heap of lose HIVs, the touching of and going near to whom would make them too infected with the same virus. Therefore, only a few, those who are aware of reality, go to care the miserable. The poor patients are left alone even by their family members in many cases. This chapter throws light on this particular issue. This chapter also shows how women are organising themselves to help each other in bad time.

Besides, a section of the chapter also discusses the problem of children's future in families of AIDS patients.

Chapter 9 deals with the struggle of man against AIDS. This suggests a number of ways for the prevention of this dreaded disease. The National AIDS programmes are a significant umbrella against the killing rain of AIDS. Mobilising whole of the nations against AIDS can be made possible through these programmes. Comprehensive prevention is also discussed in this chapter. The importance of the local activists has been emphasised under the head, 'Grass-Roots Players'. A light has been thrown on the possible ways for the prevention of AIDS are hinted at under the head, 'Better tools in store?' Vaccination has been our prime weapon against the spread of many epidemics in the past. So, we must attempt to develop vaccines against AIDS. But, this process is not an easy and a short one. It will take a long time to experiment different ways to prepare a vaccine for AIDS.

The conventional sexually transmitted diseases (STDs) are discussed in a new context. They are studied herein in special relation to AIDS. Women are told some protective methods which they can adopt to save themselves from AIDS. Also a section deals with the head 'Societies under the Microscope'.

Tenth Chapter deals with a very important issue. We all know that one of the modes of transmission of HIV is through the injections. The needles and syringes used by an infected person comes to have HIV and, when an uninfected person used such a syringe or needle, the virus enters his body easily. We also know that drug injectors use a single injection equipment for all members in a group. Thus, a single infected needle can cause AIDS to whole of the group. This chapter describes two successful experiments for the prevention of AIDS among drug injectors in Glasgrow and Thailand. The value of personal experience in this campaign is of great importance, according to this chapter.

Chapter 11 deals with the common preventive method of AIDS. It advocates and explains the use of condoms to keep away the AIDS. Condoms are made up of thin elastic material, which does not let the body fluids enter each other's body parts during copulation. So, both the partners remain safe if any of them is infected. In fact, a large number of prostitutes became easy victims of AIDS just because they did not use condoms and happened to have sex with an infected person unknowingly. These prostitutes, after becoming infected, became a medium of spread for AIDS as other persons having sex with them without condoms also became infected with HIV. Thus, the use of condoms makes the sex safer for both men and women. This chapter underlines this simple method of prevention.

Chapter 12 underlines the rights, duties and liabilities of

health care practitioners in a changed atmosphere. The issues of due awareness, treatment, counselling, confidentiality and the warning as also the problem of an HIV-infected health care practitioner—all are explained in detail in this chapter. It is in deed very important to make our health care practitioner aware of their changed role in a new social set-up, with many AIDS patients.

The next chapter, Chapter 13, takes up the issue of AIDS and insurance. It is, again, a matter of great importance that the person infected with HIV gets a security of finances. As mentioned earlier (in Chapter 5) the mountainous costs of the AIDS treatment leave a family almost nowhere. And, when a person dies after exhausting all the resources of the family, the family is almost ruined. Thus it is very essential that AIDS victims are provided an insurance.

This chapter deals with two kinds of insurance—the health and the life insurance. Both of these insurance are discussed with particular references of the U.S.A., British isles, Africa, Asia, Australia and New Zealand, Europe and Canada.

Other matters like contracting HIV, death futures, insurance of coverage of tort actions of HIV, blood transfusion, etc. are also discussed herein.

The conclusion gives the real situation and an ideal way for the problem.

Chapter 14 provides for the role of non-governmental organisations (NGOs). The author sees a great role for the NGOs in bringing the National response to the AIDS. In this chapter, it has also been made clear that NGOs, like elsewhere, lead the governmental efforts in this field too.

Chapter 15 deals with the real problems facing our present society. Many legal issues are raised when doctors and other workers perform their duty to save people from AIDS. There are a lot of human rights like the right to privacy and to found a family which are armed during the anti-AIDS programmes. This chapter brings out an analysis of this problem in detail.

Chapter 16 deals with the problem of ethics in the modern society confronting a disease like AIDS. Many people say some measures to be unethical, but non-adoption of such measures leads to unabated spread of the killing disease. This problem is underlined sincerely in this chapter.

Chapter 17, or the last chapter of the book takes up the ethical issues at the time of HIV screening. This unveils the real problems which the anti-AIDS workers face while conducting their campaigns.

Thus, the present book contains almost every aspect of AIDS and provides valuable stuff in a very systematised way. Members of the medical profession, Researchers, Social and Voluntary Organisations are requested to take full advantage of it, in promoting the three basic mantras of prevention of AIDS, i.e., Information, Education and Communication.

G.C. Satpathy

Part I

Origin and Causes

One

Origin of AIDS

The appearance of a new and deadly disease naturally makes the people curious about the origin and spread of such disease. As far as the AIDS is concerned, we do not know the origin of the HIV virus, which causes the AIDS.

A large number of scientific efforts have been devoted to solve this question. Unfortunately, the debate about the origin of AIDS has become hopelessly mixed with the questions like: which country, which race, should be blamed for starting the epidemic.

As we know that how HIV is transmitted, it is usually possible to work out the possibility of each AIDS patient, its way of infection, or it would be, if everyone was willing to be completely frank about their past sexual intercourses, which rarely few people are.

Primary Cases: The US, Africa, Europe and Haiti

Theoretically it could be possible to find out, when and where the first case of AIDS occurred. But practically, it is not a easy task. The medical condition which was later to be known as AIDS began to be noticed in the late 1970s and early 1980s in many widely separated locations, including France, Haiti, Belgium, the United States, Zambia and Zaire.

As the researchers in the United States and elsewhere learnt to diagnose AIDS, and in an effort to better understand that what they were up against, they began to look backwards in time, in search of the "first case" of the new disease. Step by step, this quest led as far back as 1959, where the trail, for the present at least, runs cold.

The primary medical reports of the syndrome soon to be named as AIDS were published in the United States in June 1981. After the publication of these reports, a small but increasing number of homosexual men and their physicians in New York City, Los Angeles and San Francisco came to notice some rare or unusual disease symptoms like that of pneumonia, Kaposi's sarcoma in young men and a host of infections not found in otherwise healthy people. These ailments seemed to be related to inexplicable deterioration in the immune system of the human beings.

The doctors were helpless to help such patients, or even to explain what had gone wrong with their bodies' defences. Now, they began to suspect the existence of a new, sexually transmitted infection. Some doctors at the US Centres for Disease Control (CDC) in Georgia, Atlanta also began to suspect the blood transmission to be a factor. They also noticed similar symptoms among intravenous drug users. By the end of 1981, disease had claimed the lives of 248 people in the United States.

By the beginning of 1982, doctors in the Zairean city started to document dozens of cases where the patients' multiple infections seemed to relate to the collapse of the body's immune system. The appearance of a new and more aggressive form of Kaposi's sarcoma in Zambia prompted a physician working there to observe the similarity between the symptoms of Zambian patients and those studied among American homosexuals.

With the backward tracking by the medical professionals through the 1970s, it became clear that some of the earliest known cases of AIDS had been seen by Belgian doctors in Africans. The first case seems to be a 34 year old Zairean airline secretary, who flew to Belgium with her child in 1977, to find out reasons for their persistent respiratory and intestinal infections.

In early 1981 some doctors at a Parisian clinic were perplexed by the cases of *pneumocystis* pneumonia reported in a Portuguese man recently arrived from Angola, in a Zairean and a French woman who had recently lived in Zaire. Out of the first 200 patients affected by this new disease in Europe, 42 were African.

The tell-tale combination of uncontrollable opportunistic infections and Kaposi's sarcoma seems, first to have appeared in 1978 in Haiti coincides with the earliest cases of Kaposi's sarcoma in homosexual men in the United States, and the arrival of first African patients with a new disease in Europe. The number of

Haitian refugees with immuno-deficiency disease increased significantly in New York City and Miami during 1980-81. By mid-1982 the CDC had registered 34 such cases. By October 1982 researchers had diagnosed as many as 61 cases in Haiti.

The investigators went through the medical histories of past patients, and found a small number of probable cases of AIDS going back nearly 30 years on three continents. In doing so, they found AIDS-like symptoms in patients as early as 1959:

1. 1959—a 45 year old US man born in Haiti died;
2. 1959—a British sailor with Kaposi's sarcoma and pneumocystis died in Manchester;
3. 1969—a 15 year old black US boy died with Kaposi's sarcoma and opportunistic infections in St. Louis;
4. 1975—a previously healthy seven-month old black infant was found to have pneumocystis in New York City;
5. 1977—a 47 year old Danish surgeon who had worked in rural Zaire, died in Denmark;
6. 1977—a 34 year old Zairean woman who sought treatment in Belgium died in Kinshasa in 1978;
7. 1977—a 27 year old Rwandan mother developed the novel immuno-deficiency symptoms;
8. 1979—a 44 year old homosexual man died with Kaposi's sarcoma in New York City.

In some of these cases, the retrospective diagnoses of AIDS have now been supported by positive blood tests for HIV. However, most cases have been identified as the possible early cases of AIDS on the basis of symptoms alone. The research goes on, and it is possible that eventually earlier possible cases will be found somewhere.

The medical detective work of the past extends more uncertain the retrospective diagnoses tend to become. People do not die of AIDS itself, for AIDS is not really a disease but a syndrome of opportunistic infections which strike when one's immune system gets impaired by HIV. Hence, to determine retrospectively, whether the infections that killed the patient were actually related to the syndrome is guesswork at the best.

Testing of Samples of Old Blood

If the patients had been dying since 1959 from what is now called AIDS, they must have become infected by the virus known as HIV some time before the death. In the mid-1980s medical researchers started to test old samples of blood which had originally been taken for some other purposes and stored for years in laboratory freezers.

At this time, it was widely assumed by the medical professionals that AIDS was originated in Africa. This was thought because the early European cases had African links, and unlikely that such an unusual disease could have gone unnoticed for long in the United States. Therefore, much of the early blood research was directed at Africa, though the results were highly controversial.

The US scientists tested the first batches of stored African blood samples by using a type of test which was much less reliable than many of those available today. The results, which were discredited later claimed to show the presence of HIV antibodies in more than 50 per cent of stored blood samples which had been taken in Kenya and Uganda in the 1960s and 1970s. Some other scientists who carried out tests on stored blood samples in Africa found no evidence of such early infection of HIV. No sample taken from elderly people during these decades in the West Nile district of Uganda, tested positive for HIV.

As the first erroneous results claimed that AIDS was endemic in central Africa, they received widespread attention in the media. The blood surveys carried out on a large scale around the same time showed much lower levels of infection. Using a different type of test than that employed by the US researchers another group found that out of 1000 blood samples taken in Kinshasa in 1970, only 2 per cent were seropositive. This finding was announced at the first international conference on AIDS in Brussels in June 1985 but failed to attract the same extensive attention of the media. Similar researches on stored blood samples taken from North Americans and Europeans in the 1960s and 1970s could have been performed, since these samples were available for this purpose.

Testing of Blood in the Tropics

The early fictitious results, stored blood samples contributed to many confusions and misunderstandings about the history of AIDS. Though more improved tests are now available which help to minimise confusion, it remains the case that some types of tests are more appropriate than others for use in the tropics, where hot climate makes unintentional bacterial contamination of blood samples. Such contaminated samples are prone to give fictitious results. Moreover, in some rural tropical areas where people commonly suffer from multiple parasitic infections, problems of interpretation can make the accurate reading of HIV antibody tests very difficult. The immune system of such multiply-infected people remains in a chronically activated state, the HIV antibody test can be confounded by excessive number of antibodies.

The problem of ensuring accurate readings, when testing contaminated blood samples, has been approached in different ways. A US technique is to subject the blood samples, which appear on the first test to contain HIV antibodies to a second confirmatory test usually known as the Western Blot. The samples which the presence show the presence of HIV antibodies by Western Blot are considered to be truly positive. The second technique has been put forwarded by British researchers. Their contradiction with the US method is that it employs two tests which are too similar to rule out false positive results on tricky blood samples, particularly in the tropics. The British researchers employ two types of test which are very different from one another, so that any omission in the first test is compensated by the second one.

The testing of blood samples for the presence of antibodies to the AIDS virus is a complicated process and like any form of screening or diagnostic test, the results are not infallible. Nevertheless, during the past three years in which HIV antibody detection tests have been in use, great improvements have been made in their sensitivity and specificity.

Unfortunately, the accurate results cannot erase the legacy of early inaccurate results which led to the labelling of Africa as the "AIDS continent". Dr. Richard Tedder, who participated in the development of a successful British test said, "Bad results in the early days of testing muddied the waters and this is what many people tend to remember. They level the accusation that 'you scientists got it once wrong, why should we believe that your results are any better now?' Explaining that there are many types of tests and some of these are better than others, is not always convincing for people who have become suspicious. It is understandable but unfortunate that some Africans believe that any and all serological results are questionable."

Back-Tracking the AIDS Virus

The presence of antibodies to HIV has recently been recognised in the stored blood of the New Orleans teenager who died in 1969 in the US. These samples had been preserved because the doctors who treated him said that they were so puzzled by his symptoms that they stored specimens for future research which might help to explain his illness. The earliest known blood sample registering seropositive by means of a number of different antibody tests was taken in 1959 in Kinshasa, Zaire.

The history of AIDS was also investigated by going back to the earliest North American cases and interrogating the friends of AIDS patients about their sex lives. One unproved suggestion was that all US cases go back to a homosexual Air Canada steward who infected a large number of people across North America. No body knows where this man caught the disease or if the suggestion was true. There is little scientific evidence for this back-tracking because the key witnesses are now dead. Even if true, it does not help to solve the question of how the AIDS virus came to exist in the first case.

Neither medical nor journalistic enquiry helped to trace HIV infection further back than 1959, when the HIV trail had been traced in Africa and the United States. What could have accounted for the sudden existence of this deadly virus?

HIV: Survival of the Virus

At present, as we know the history of AIDS or HIV infection is not older than 1959. Thus, the HIV virus which causes AIDS could have been around before 1959. Where and how did it emerge?

There were only a handful of human viruses known at the

end of World War II. Hundreds more have been discovered since as a result of advanced techniques for culturing them in the laboratory. Viruses are parasitic and infect almost every form of life, from single-celled bacteria up to human beings.

In scientific terms, the host and virus populations engage in fighting, which most often results in the elimination of the viral infection by the host's immune system. Influenza, polio and measles are examples of viral diseases which our bodies combat successfully, rendering us immune to further infection by the same virus. These diseases are of short incubation periods of days or weeks, and their symptoms are generally short-lived. To maintain its existence within the host population , the virus must pass from infected to uninfected individuals within this short period, or risk of being eliminated as an increasing number of hosts develop protective immunity. In this case virus requires a very large host population in order to survive.

In some other types of diseases, however, the virus employs a different survival strategy. After infecting the host and triggering an initial acute bout of symptoms, viruses stop producing any obvious sickness and become latent. Hence, they continue to live unnoticed in the host's cells for months or years until conditions are favourable for triggering off of another acute outburst of symptoms. Latent viruses can survive in small host populations infecting their hosts periodically only during the acute phase of the illness.

The another viral survival strategy features the aspects of above approaches. The infectivity which lasts for much of the duration of the illness with persistence in the host's body long after the appearance of first symptoms, the viruses like those of Hepatitis B and AIDS seem to cause lifelong infections. In these cases the host is capable of transmitting the virus to others as well.

Persistent viral infections can be retained for long periods of time in small host populations. Theoretically they can be spread to a new and uninfected host population by a single carrier. When the disease caused breaks out months or years later, with deceptive suddenness, it becomes impossible to trace out how or when the infection was first introduced. This persistency explains why the exact case which marks the beginning of an AIDS epidemic in a given population can so rarely be identified, but it does not enable us to explain where the AIDS virus came from in the first case.

Reporting Scientific Contemplation

The scientific views about the origin of HIV have molded many times, as a new evidence has been revealed, evaluated and refined. In the consequence, each new twist raised almost as many questions as it answered. Determining the cause and origin of any new infectious disease is a complex investigative task. This requires co-operation among many branches of biological, medical and social science. It takes a long time to finally draw the accurate conclusions.

The scientific discussions taken on the way to such conclusions are largely preliminary suppositions or guesses, rather than the statements of fact. Media reporting of latest scientific thoughts, without full consideration of the background, may disfigure the distinction between what is known and what is only suspected.

The media's task in reporting the origin of the AIDS virus has been much difficult, and the international media have not always precisely distinguished between evidence and speculation. At times, the scientists themselves have also been careless, some perhaps influenced by the race for profitable AIDS research contracts, available in some developed countries. In the field of research, the prizes sometimes seem to go to those whose ideas on the origin of AIDS are the most dramatic and well reported.

Epidemic Diseases: The Origin of Syphilis

The origin of the HIV virus may never be discovered, just as we still do not know the origin of a virulent epidemic 'syphilis' which appeared in Europe in the 1490s, and outraged for much of the next century. Still now, science is uncertain where and how this disease originated. Until the widespread use of antibiotics in the 1940s, syphilis was feared almost as much as AIDS is today.

The new outbreak of syphilis seems, on the first hand, to have appeared in Italy. By 1495, it spread over France, Germany and Switzerland; it reached Holland and Greece in 1496. It invaded England and Scotland in 1497, and Hungary and Russia in 1499.

Then, there was furious debate on the origin of this new disease, like is today with AIDS. The foreigners were usually blamed. So the Russians blamed the Poles, and both the English and the Turks called it to be a French disease. The French called it the Italian and the Italians called it the Spanish disease. And finally, the Spanish called it the sıckness of Hispaniola, believing it to have come from Haiti with Columbus return from his voyage to the America.

The scientists still argue about the origin of the syphilis, and with the discovery that it leaves tell-tale signs in bones. The story has gone further and further back in time. There arises some significant questions about the origin of syphilis, like—Did European explorers bring syphilis to the New World, or did New World peoples gifted it to the European colonisers? Did mankind become infected with syphilis in Asia 5,000 years ago with the colonial development, or in Africa 100,000 years ago, or have humans had syphilis since their evolution from their ancestors?

The Theories of AIDS Origin

The main theories to explain the origin of the HIV virus are that it has developed from an old human disease unknown to science; that it has developed from a natural viral disease of some other species, most probably of apes; and that it was accidentally manufactured in a laboratory.

The first theory states that HIV has been around among humans for a very long time unnoticed, perhaps because it has been confined to very few people, or perhaps because it has recently become more virulent. Another possibility is that the disease came from a small and isolated ethnic group, which had acquired immunity against it so that it rarely caused death. When this disease spread outside this immune group, and reached the people who had no such immunity, it became an epidemic.

This theory seems to be true because the diseases familiar in one part of the world, when carried to a new area, have often proved a mortal danger to the freshly exposed population. European diseases like measles and smallpox virtually wiped out some North American Indian peoples in the eighteenth and nineteenth centuries. This theory is important for a key reason that if this were the origin of HIV virus, the isolated group's immunity might enable a vaccine to be developed to protect the rest of the population.

There may be a part of completely isolated population left in the world, mainly in the rainforests of New Guinea, Amazonia and, perhaps, the Central Africa. Since one of the early grounds of AIDS was Central Africa, much emphasis was focused on this possibility. Though, this theory is very difficult to disprove, but there exists some evidences which argue against it.

The second theory states that HIV existed long time ago as an animal disease, and managed to infect and trigger an epidemic in humans recently. There are other examples of diseases which were transferred from animals to mankind. Since a virus similar to HIV has been found in a species of monkey, this possibility received considerable attention. In 1988, the scientists who earlier announced that they had isolated a virus similar to HIV, from the wild African green monkey, declared that they had made a mistake.

The third theory states that HIV is a man-made virus, which accidentally originated in a germ warfare laboratory. Unlike the above described theories, this is not a scientific theory posed in terms which are open to experimental confirmation and presented for critical investigation in scientific journals. It has been transmitted like a rumour campaign with various versions picked up and published in different newspapers and magazines all over the world.

As Dr. Kenneth Kaunda, the President of Zambia has said, it is necessary to know where AIDS is going than where it has originated from, and the debate about HIV's origin is largely irrelevant to immediate action against the epidemic. The linkages of its origin and blame constitute a persistent 'infection' of the global dialogue and action which is important to combat the spread of AIDS, and creates conflict and delay.

Whenever, a complete explanation for the origin of AIDS is revealed, it may help efforts to control it. But the World Health Organization as well as most of the specialists in this field agree that the prevention of AIDS is independent of such explanations.

The Connection with Haiti

The two countries of the developing world, Africa and Haiti have received global publicity as the possible birthplace of AIDS. Haiti, the Caribbean country whose most population is racially of African descent, was pointed out first.

In 1982, the US Centres for Disease Control (the federal public health laboratory) published a new article on the fatal disease which had already killed about 100 homosexual men in US and infected about 200 more. In a period of one year, five US states reported 34 cases of the AIDS in Haitian patients. Thirty out of the 34 were men, who denied homosexual relationship and drug use. This incident was a new clue to the nature of the disease. After this event, CDC alerted the doctors attending to Haitian patients to "be aware that such opportunistic infections may occur in this population too." CDC soon classified the Haitians, along with homosexual men, haemophiliacs, and intravenous drug users, as a 'high-risk' group for AIDS. By 1983, this concept was under attacked by Haitian physicians, who were working in the United States. Since Haitians constituted only 6 per cent of the 1,220 AIDS cases, and any other US ethnic group could have constituted a similar or greater percentage of the total, why were Haitians being pointed out, the Haitian asked?

The CDC explained that Haitian AIDS patients were indeed a high risk group as they had no other significant risk factors. But as the Haitian doctors admitted, it was only because Haitian men were normally reluctant to accept homosexual relationship or intravenous drug use. The lack of other risk factors was not a problem but the unfamiliarity of non-Haitian American researchers with Haitian attitudes toward these matters. A US doctor who worked in Haiti quoted in the UK medical journal *the Lancet*: "To admit one's homosexuality is difficult enough in America, in a country like Haiti homosexuality or homosexual prostitution will remain a deeply hidden secret".

The Haitian doctors said that more sensitive discussions with patients could have revealed the true risk factors involved. The Vice-President of the Association of Haitian Physicians Abroad and co-chairman of the Haitian Coalition on AIDS Dr. Jean Claude Compas told a US congressional committee, "Most of the data used by the CDC and other health authorities were collected by hospital-based physicians who had no knowledge of French or Creole".

The grouping of Haitians, with homosexuals and drug users in a separate "risk group" was, according to Dr. Jean Pape, "a serious error in interpretation of the epidemiological data. The CDC never wondered why 88 per cent of the early Haitian AIDS cases in US were reported in males. In 1983, our group identified risk factors, bisexuality and blood transfusion, in 79 per cent of Haitian AIDS patients".

Whether or not CDC's decision was justified by the very limited evidences available at that time, it became accepted by the US medical professionals that Haitians were indeed at risk from AIDS, and more or less scientific speculation started as to why it might be so. Thus, it became a common assumption that the AIDS might have originated in Haiti, and spread to the United States.

Some of the US researchers supposed that AIDS began with an outbreak of African swine fever in Haitian pigs, and that the swine virus had been passed to humans. While others suggested that a Haitian may have taken the swine virus with undercooked pork, and then passed it on to homosexual partners from the United States. Another thought was that animal sacrifice and other voodoo rituals could explain the occurrence of human infection. Others also proposed that Haitians may have contracted the virus from monkeys as part of bizarre sexual practice in Haitian brothels.

There was no or a little evidence for these ideas, but these were widely repeated in the United States and international media. By July 1983 the Haitian doctors' arguments started to have some impact within the public health profession, and the New York City Health Commission excluded Haitians from its list of risk groups for AIDS.

But until May 1985, nearly three years after its initial statement, CDC did not withdraw its view officially. Even then, Haitians still felt that they were being officially victimised by the US authorities. "When the CDC excluded Haitians from its list of risk groups, it refused to admit that it had made an error," says Dr. Pape. "Even now, the CDC continues to stigmatise Haitians by preventing them from donating their blood in the United States".

Blaming the Haitians

By the year 1985, the popular view that being a Haitian automatically put one at "high risk" of AIDS had caused much harm to Haitians in the United States as well as in Haiti. The CDC's low key report of 1982, and the more lurid speculations on why Haitians were at "high risk", was quickly transformed into news stories linking Haitians in the US with the spread of the mysterious gay disease. The growing number of AIDS cases in Haiti itself received widespread US publicity.

About 100,000 to 300,000 Haitians refugees, fleeing the economic stagnation and political repression of the Duvalier dictatorship, had reached the United States in the year 1980. At least 50 per cent of these refugees were living in the US illegally, because Haitian boat people were not generally welcome, and many US immigration officials did not regard Haitians, the political refugees. Unlike, the thousands of Cubans making a similar claim, the Haitians were fleeing the regime supported by the US Government and not a communist one.

By the year 1982, all these immigrants found themselves officially grouped as a "risk group" for the AIDS. The head of a Roman Catholic Haitian refugee centre in New York City, told the *New York Times*, "Those who did not like Haitian, have found a new element. They are saying that they do not want Haitians here because they are AIDS carriers".

It was reported in the United States that in some areas the unemployment rate for Haitians was twice that of other black workers, a situation they felt was directly related to AIDS. According to the AIDS Discrimination Unit of the New York City Commission on Human Rights: "Haitian students are beaten in school, Haitian businessmen have gone bankrupt, and Haitian families have been evicted from their homes".

Unfortunately, Haiti became the first country to be singled out by international publicity as the possible centre for the origin of AIDS. Its own AIDS epidemic was focused in the international spotlight.

Haitian tourism, the country's second largest source of foreign earnings before 1982, fell from 70,000 visitors in the winter of 1981-82 to 10,000 visitors the following year. Some hotels were closed, while some were facing financial trouble. The tourism, which was once the second largest source of foreign income for the country, has never recovered.

Haitian tourism had indirectly supported about 25,000 jobs in an economy plagued by unemployment. As the visitors were chiefly from the upper end of the market, the revenue was substantial. "The negative impact on our already perplexed economy has been awful", wrote the Haitian ambassador to the United States in a letter to the *New England Journal of Medicine* in September 1983.

Although the political climate in Haiti certainly bore a considerable share of responsibility, the intellectual Haitian commentators believed that the AIDS scare and not the politics killed off the tourism industry.

The new medical opinion has totally abandoned the view that AIDS originated in Haiti. While it seems likely that some homosexual visitors from the United States picked up the virus by having sex in Haiti, it seems equally probable that some others took AIDS to Haiti.

Battle of the Blood Tests: An Old African Disease?

During the year 1983, at about the same time when the CDC put Haitians on the AIDS 'risk group' list. Belgian and French physicians were noticing the increasing numbers of immuno-deficient Central African patients who reached Europe in search of treatment of their unusual sickness, soon to be identified as AIDS. The doctors suspected that AIDS might have existed for many years, unnoticed, in the tropical Africa. This was a reasonable speculation, as rare tropical diseases may sometimes be carried back to developed countries. The views of the medical profession were picked up and amplified by the media. The author of an article published in the *British Medical Journal* in August 1984, suggested that ".....the infectious agent causing AIDS, whatever its nature, is endemic and unrecognised in some parts of sub-Saharan Africa from where it got scattered into external populations." In the same context a CDC virologist, Dr. Donald Francis, told the *New York Times*: "I think AIDS is an old African disease which was introduced somewhere into an amplification system—for example, the indiscriminate segment of the homosexual community".

By the end of year 1985, some circumstantial evidences supporting such beliefs seemed at hand. Results, newly-developed blood tests which could identify antibodies to the HIV virus were published by US researchers working on African blood samples. These samples were collected from groups of patients in Kenya and Uganda in the 1960s and 1970s and stored for research purposes. When American virologists tested these samples for antibodies to the AIDS virus they found a very high percentage of positive results. In samples collected between 1980 and 1984 from the Turkana people of Kenya, for example, seemed to show that 59 per cent were seropositive. Blood samples collected from Ugandan children during 1972-73 showed 66 per cent to be seropositive.

Such "false positive" results were thought to certify that AIDS had been existing for generations, and possibly centuries, in the Central Africa. These reports received widespread publicity, it has since become clear that the testing technique was faulty and better tests, employing different techniques, have since been developed. Some researchers drew false conclusion that HIV infection had been widespread in Africa long before appearing in the United States or Europe. "I believe that the virus was present in Central Africa for a long period of time", Dr. Robert Gallo, co-discoverer of the AIDS virus, told the *Los Angeles Times* in 1985.

The implication was that the AIDS had been present in Africa for a long time, unnoticed and undiagnosed by the African physicians. It was considered insulting by African physicians, and does not accord with the known facts. When cases of AIDS began to appear in African hospitals, the physicians quickly diagnosed, it to be a new disease, and tried to identify it. The African doctors' anger was increased by the way that some of the early blood samples removed from African hospitals, and tested in the United States and Europe with little or no consultation with African doctors.

Nowadays there is a strong opinion among scientists that the AIDS is new to the African continent as it is to the rest of the world. A large number of serological studies using sensitive and specific blood tests, have failed to find high prevalence of the AIDS virus in Africa before the mid-1970s, exactly same as in the United States and Europe. The oldest African blood sample known to show HIV antibodies was collected from Kinshasa, Zaire, in 1959.

On the basis of the evidences available to date, the opinion that AIDS as a disease was any more widespread in Africa than it was in the United States and Europe before the 1980s, seems to be a premature conclusion drawn on the basis of faulty blood-tests. The political effects of this mistake marked Central Africa as the birthplace of AIDS, leading to the second great epidemic of blame and counter-blame.

Two

The HIV, the Infection, and the AIDS

HIV: A Slow-acting Virus

Most viruses produce their major impact or symptoms in a period of days or weeks. The influenza virus, for example, produces flu within one week, and hepatitis A virus takes about four weeks to develop after its infection.

The case of HIV is different. Except for a generally mild illness, i.e., fever, sore throat and rash etc., that about 70 per cent of infected people experience a few weeks after initial infection with this virus. Most HIV-infected people have no clear symptoms for the first five or so years. They look in good health and feel well—although right from the beginning they are able to transmit the virus to others. Once infected, people are infected for their whole life because scientists have not as yet found a way of curing them, or making them non-infectious to others. The recent evidence suggest that, in the absence of other causes of death, almost all HIV-infected people will finally die of AIDS.

Soon after a person gets infected with HIV, his or her immune system produces antibodies to neutralize the virus. As the antibodies to HIV are much easier to detect than the virus itself, their presence or absence in the blood is the basis for the most widely used test of HIV antibodies is said to be HIV-positive or seropositive, which means that he or she is infected with HIV.

HIV antibodies usually take about two weeks to three months to appear in the blood, though they have been known to take longer. The period before antibodies are produced is known as "window period" during which—although the infected person is particularly infectious due to the high concentration of virus in the blood—the person will test negative on the standard antibody blood tests.

However, the body's immune system reacts against the invasion of HIV by producing antibodies, these do not inactivate the virus in the usual way. Actually, the virus attacks the particular key cells in the immune system and causes a gradual break-down in the body's defence system against other infections.

HIV-2

In the early years of 1980s, a large number of cases showing all the characteristics of AIDS—but turned out not to be caused by HIV—were noticed in people from parts of west Africa. One patient was a Portuguese man who had passed all his life on the Cape Verde islands, 800 km far from the coast of Senegal. In the year 1982 he developed symptoms of AIDS, for which he eventually sought treatment in Paris. In the year 1985 scientists successfully isolated the virus that was causing the man's illness when viewed under electron microscope, it had an appearance unlike HIV, but further investigations revealed that it was a variant of the first human immuno-deficiency virus. It was later called HIV-2.

HIV-2 appears to be somewhat different in genetic make-up from what has been known as HIV-1. This virus attacks the immune system in the same way, and infects the people who are vulnerable to the same opportunistic infections, though the researches have suggested that people infected with HIV-2 progress more slowly towards AIDS. However, most AIDS cases resulted from HIV-2 have been noticed in people living in west Africa, but some cases have also been found on other continents.

AIDS: Not a Single Disease

It is widely known that AIDS stands for Acquired Immuno-deficiency Syndrome. It is not a single disease. It is the end stage of HIV infection, characterised by a group—or "syndrome"—of life-threatening illnesses. Although, people with AIDS can be helped with medicines, there is as yet no cure, and most patients die within one to three years after diagnosis of the syndrome.

In some cases the period between infection with HIV and the development of the symptoms of AIDS is few years, but in others may be it may be 10 years or more. Intensive research is being conducted to find out the possible reasons for these variations.

Scientists believe that these variations could be due to differences in the aggressivity (virulence) of various HIV strains, or in genetic make-up of the individuals or immune response; or due to the presence of some other diseases that might accelerate the infectious process. Disease progression is especially swift in infants and young children—around 80 per cent become seriously ill or die before their fifth year of age.

Most HIV patients suffer intermittent bouts of illness which increase in severity as their immune systems collapse. Various pathogenic micro-organisms break through the immune system at different stages. Doctors can explain approximately the state of the immune system from the symptoms reported in their HIV-infected patients. The number of CD4+ cells in the blood can also provide some indication of immune status.

The process of HIV infection can be divided into several stages—only the last of these stages is called AIDS. In the earliest stage, an HIV-infected person may be having no symptoms except for swollen lymph nodes in the neck, armpits and groin which do not make the person feel ill but may prompt a visit to the doctor.

As the infection proceeds the individual may suffer a variety of conditions including persistent cough and fever, intense fatigue profuse sweating at night, skin rashes, diarrhoea and sudden loss of weight, mouth ulcers and oral thrush, herpes infections including shingles, and a normally rare condition called oral hairy leukoplakia in which patches of white warts appear on the side of the tongue and inner side of the cheeks.

The individuals with a healthy immune system usually have more than 950 CD4+ cells in each microlitre sample of blood, although a few people never have more than 500 CD4+ cells per microlitre and remain healthy.

The number of CD4+ cells normally falls over the course of HIV infection. People with HIV infection usually have a CD4+ count below 200 cells per microlitre of blood.

A number of opportunistic diseases collectively occur at this last stage of HIV infection known as AIDS. Tuberculosis and Kaposi sarcoma, a tumour characterised by purple patches on the skin and internally, are usually observed relatively early, when the CD4+ count is still above 100. Some severe fungal infections like *Candida* oesphagitis, *Cryptococcus* meningitis, and penicillosis; and parasitic infections like *Pneumocystis carinii* pneumonia or *Toxoplasma gondii* encephalitis, etc. tend to occur when the CD4+ count is around 100. People whose counts are below 50 have the late opportunistic infections such as cytomegaloviral retinitis.

A large number of AIDS patients get affected by a wasting syndrome that is known, especially in Africa, as "slim disease". It is characterised chronic diarrhoea and severe weight loss. Another condition observed worldwide is AIDS encephalopathy or AIDS dementia, which is caused by HIV crossing the so-called "blood-brain barrier", which normally prevents the foreign agents from reaching the brain. In its later stages, AIDS encephalopathy resembles senile dementia or Alzheimer's disease. AIDS dementia appears to result not from opportunistic infection but from the viral action itself.

HIV and the Immune System

The body cells that are the prime targets of HIV are T-lymphocytes and monocytes, which turn into macrophages when they leave the bloodstream to enter a body organ. In the immune system of a healthy person, the monocytes/macrophages defend the body by seeking out and eliminating foreign particles (antigens) and dead or infected cells. The body also defends itself by manufacturing some special proteins called antibodies to render foreign bodies (antigens) harmless. HIV infection interferes with both these processes, and gradually weaken the immune system of the body.

The cells which manufacture antibodies are a type of lymphocyte (WBCs) known as B-cells. These cells produce antibodies specific to the antigen they seek to destroy, and some retain a memory of the antigen they have encountered. This memory enables the immune system to react swiftly if the antigen reappears even years later.

Another important type of lymphocytes in the immune system are the T-lymphocytes, which circulate in the bloodstream and concentrate at the sites of invasion by a foreign body (antigen). Besides serving as specialized killers and helping B-cells to produce antibodies, the T-lymphocytes coordinate the immune system's response to an antigen and switch the system off when danger is overcome. Some T-lymphocytes, too, retain the memory of antigens encountered.

The T-lymphocytes that regulate and coordinate the other cells are called T-helper cells. These are the main target of HIV. The virus breaks into the cells and throws the whole immune system into chaos by sidelining all the other cells dependent on the T-helper cells. (The T-helper cells—whose full name is CD4 + T-lymphocyte—also commonly known as CD4+ cells) HIV again outwits the immune system by changing continuously and becoming unidentifiable to antibodies produced against it.

On entering the CD4+ cell, HIV uses the cell's machinery to reproduce rapidly and massively. The new generation viruses form buds on the surface of the host cell before bursting into the bloodstream to invade other fresh cells. A very low count of CD4+ cells in the blood indicates an impaired immune system, which means a person is unable to overcome diseases or infections that would normally pose little threat.

HIV also attacks the monocytes/macrophages but it does not destroy them in the same way as it does the CD4+ cells. Instead, it hides in them and is carried to the different parts of the body, particularly the lymph nodes.

Part II

Spread of AIDS

Three

Modes of HIV Transmission

Today, the modes of HIV transmission are quite clear. The HIV spreads primarily through sexual intercourse, which makes HIV infection basically a sexually transmitted disease (STD). Like many other STDs, HIV may also be transmitted through infected blood, blood products, and transplanted organs and tissues (including sperm), and from a infected mother to her children.

Sexual Transmission

"Epidemics are not accidents", said Dr. Nathan Clumek of St. Pierre Hospital, Brussels, who was one of the first physicians to describe AIDS in heterosexuals. "A new pathogen enters a community only when the conditions are ripe for it."

In the world where an estimated 250 million people yearly acquire an STD, including syphilis, chancroid, genital warts (papilloma), gonorrhoea, and genital herpes, it will readily be accepted that there is enough opportunity for HIV to spread. In many countries, HIV infections have appeared first among people with more than one sex partners, although it is only a matter of time before the virus finds its way outside these circles. Sexual transmission alone accounts for approximately 75 per cent of all HIV infections worldwide.

Worldwide HIV Infections

Mode of Transmission	*Percentage*
Sexual intercourse	70-80
Needle-sharing by drug users	5-10
Mother to child	5-10
Blood transfusion	3-5
Accidental needle-sticks to Health care workers	less than 0.01

As per 1993 data.

Every single attempt of unprotected sexual intercourse with an HIV-infected person exposes the healthy partner to the risk of infection. The size of the risk depends upon a number of factors, including the presence of other STDs, the sex and age of the healthy partner, the type of sexual act, the stage of illness of the infected partner, and the virulence of the HIV strain involved.

A study of 565 European heterosexual couples in which only one partner was infected, at the beginning, suggested that transmission from male to female was about twice as likely as from female to male. Normally, women are more vulnerable to HIV infection because a larger surface is exposed in comparison to men. Moreover, seminal fluid contains a far higher concentration of HIV than vaginal and cervical fluids.

The anal intercourse carries a higher risk of transmission than vaginal intercourse because it is more likely to injure the tissues of the receptive partner. Further, as for vaginal sex, the female partner is at greater risk than the male partner.

Though, both seminal and vaginal fluid contain HIV, there is a theoretical risk of HIV transmission through oral sex—both cunnilingus and fellatio. The real risk is difficult to measure scientifically, few people engage in oral sex only, and if they become infected, the route of transmission is unclear. Oral sex, however, poses far less risk of HIV transmission than vaginal or anal intercourses. This enables us to explain the rarity of HIV transmission through sex between women. For all types of sex, the risk of HIV transmission is greater where the abrasions of the skin or mucous membrane are involved. For oral and vaginal sex, the risk is greater in a case when the woman is menstruating.

The age acts as a factor in the susceptibility of women. Women are more vulnerable to HIV infection in their teens and again over the age of 45 years. In adolescent women the immature cervix is thought to be a less efficient barrier against HIV than the mature genital tract of older women. The thinning and drying of the vaginal mucosa after the menopause is believed to lessen the barrier effect for women who have reached this stage of life. The production of mucus in the genital tract of adolescent girls and postmenopausal women is not as generative as in a reproductive women, and this condition may also enhance their susceptibility to the infection of HIV.

As far as HIV-infected people are concerned, they are more infectious to others in the very earlier stages, i.e., before antibody production, and when infection is well advanced, because the concentration of virus in the blood is higher than that of at other times.

Another important biological factor affecting the probability of HIV transmission is the presence of some other sexually transmitted disease. The presence of any STD in either the HIV-positive or the HIV-negative partner facilitates the transmission of HIV.

- If an STD, for example syphilis, herpes, etc., causes ulceration in the genital or perineal area of the healthy partner, it becomes far easier for HIV to pass into his or her tissues. Medical studies suggest that the risk of infection increases many-fold.
- For a person with a non-ulcerative STD such as gonorrhea or chlamydial infection, there is also an increased risk.
- STD causes inflammation: The lymphocytes and monocytes/macrophages, sent to check the infection, accumulate in the genital area. In persons already infected with HIV, some of these key cells will be carrying the virus, which increases the risk of transmission of virus to the healthy partner.

Transmission through Blood Transfusion

The contaminated blood is much infective when introduced directly into the bloodstream. The risk of getting HIV infection from blood transfusion of a unit of infected blood is estimated to be over 95 per cent. HIV can readily be transmitted through infected blood products, like untreated factor VIII, administered to people with haemophilia.

Intact skin acts as an effective barrier against the Pathogens. When it is pierced by needles or other invasive instruments that have been contaminated with HIV, infection may take place if the strength of virus is sufficient. A small possibility arises that blood-borne virus might enter the body through mucous membrane, for example, by blood spurting into the eyes during surgery. There is a less theoretical risk of infection from a contaminated razor blade, but transmission of HIV through this route has not yet been reported.

Since the possibility of HIV transmission through contaminated blood depends on the strength of virus injected, the risk of getting infected through a contaminated needle, syringe or any other invasive instrument is very less than with blood transfusion. Nevertheless, among drug users who inject drugs with needles, this route of transmission is significant because exposure is repeated so often—in some cases, many times a day. Moreover, needle-sharing by drug users is a major cause of HIV transmission in many countries, both developed and developing, and in some of them it is the predominant cause.

Transmission from Mother-to-Child

The virus of AIDS may pass from an infected woman to her child, or to her infant during delivery or breast-feeding. This is called mother-to-child transmission, and approximately one-third of the children of HIV-infected mothers worldwide get infection through this route.

The medical studies have suggested that the risk of HIV transmission from mother to infant is more if the mother is newly infected or she has already developed AIDS, than if she has an established HIV infection without any symptoms. Worldwide, about 5-10 per cent of the total HIV infections in 1993 were thought to have been transmitted through this route. Though infants and children progress much rapidly to AIDS, however, they already account for about 20 per cent of total AIDS cases to date.

Some Groundless Fears

The lack of knowledge about how the HIV is transmitted together with the fatal nature of AIDS and its association with condemned behaviour, has resulted in a cruel mixture of prejudice and discrimination. The AIDS epidemic abounds with stories not only of sick, wasted people and orphan children, but also of infected people finding their belongings on the street and deprived of their homes; of workers fired, children expelled from school, and many lesser insults and indignities. Thus, establishing how the virus is not transmitted is as important as establishing how it is.

In laboratory, scientists have successfully isolated HIV in tears, sweat, urine and saliva, but only blood, semen, vaginal fluid and breast-milk have been found to contain high enough concentration of HIV to be infective. Furthermore, HIV must come into direct contact with a mucous membrane or blood for infection to take place. Hence doorknobs, toilet seats, towels, swimming pools and drinking fountains cannot transmit HIV. There is no danger in riding on a bus, sharing a meal or holding hands with people infected with HIV.

Studies have shown that HIV does not transmit through casual, everyday contact. For example, scientists in the US studied 206 offsprings, siblings, parents and friends sharing the home of someone infected with HIV. Most lived in overcrowded conditions especially conducive to the spread of infection. Yet even after close contact over a period of 23 months, not a single person tested got infected with HIV.

There were a number of days on which someone drank out of the same glass as the infected person, and hundreds of occasions on which household members hugged, kissed, and shared baths and even beds (without sexual intercourse), but not becoming infected.

There are suspicions that some blood-sucking insects might transmit HIV in much the same way as malaria, dengue and yellow fever. But such fears have now been laid to rest. Epidemiological studies and laboratory work provide clear evidence that insects do not transmit HIV.

For example, if mosquitoes were agents for HIV transmission, we would expect to find HIV spread evenly throughout the population, irrespective of age groups. The epidemiological pattern of HIV infection is totally different. Cases of HIV infection are rarely found in people who are generally sexually inactive, i.e., youngsters under 15 years of age (except for those infected through their mothers) and very old people. The rates of HIV infection tend to be lower in rural areas than in urban, though in many countries mosquitoes are more abundantly found in the countryside.

Four

AIDS: A Global Epidemic

Presently, as the WHO's conservative estimates show, more than 12 million people are infected with HIV—the virus which causes AIDS. By the end of 1992, over 600,000 cases of AIDS were reported to WHO, however, estimates are that this figure is closer to 2.5 million. The mismatch between reported and estimated cases can be understood via underreporting, reporting delays and misdiagnosis.

In the Asia and Pacific regions, WHO estimated that more than 40,000 people had developed AIDS since the start of the epidemic. But it must be remembered that AIDS takes about 10 years on an average to develop from the time of infection with the HIV. Thus, these cases reflect infections which probably occurred before a decade or more.

According to the estimates of WHO, out of the 12 million HIV infections, more than one and a half million have been reported in the Asian and Pacific regions. Although, 1.5 million is an enormous figure, it may not sound frighteningly large in comparison to other parts of the world. Moreover, sub-Saharan Africa has more than 7 million cumulative infections. Unlike Africa, Asia is at the beginning stage of the epidemic. The virus is spreading at a very fast rate. In the first half of year 1992, WHO estimated that one million new infections occurred worldwide. Over 30 per cent infections occurred in Asia alone.

The problem of AIDS in the Asia and Pacific region can be illustrated with the help of some examples. The number of HIV infections has grown explosively among injecting drug users. In India's north-east states, prevalence rose from less that 1 per cent to 50 per cent in just a period of one year. Drug injectors in Yunnan Province of China had infection rates ranging from 10 to over 50 per cent in 1990, and those in Myanmar it was about 72 per cent in

1991. The transmission of HIV due to drug injection has become an alarming problem in Malaysia, where prevalence in a sample of 9,000 injecting drug users, in a rehabilitation centre, was found to be 11 per cent in 1991. In the first quarter of 1993, about 10 per cent of injecting drug users in Ho Chi Minh City, Vietnam were found to be HIV-positive. The surveys done in the Philippines, Japan and Singapore however, have not revealed HIV infection among injecting drug users.

Among the persons having sexually transmitted diseases (STD), the rate of HIV infection in Thailand have grown from zero in mid-1989 to 6 per cent in mid-1992, and in Myanmar from 2 to 9 per cent between 1990 and 1991. However, in some countries of Asia and Pacific region, HIV infection among STD clients remains at low levels, less than 1 per cent, except Cambodia where a recent survey found that about 4.2 per cent of 72 persons were infected.

The high rates of seroprevalence are now being reported among female commercial sex workers (CSWs) in some parts of Asia. The first HIV infection among female CSWs was documented in Thailand in 1989, when the first national survey detected a prevalence rate of 44 per cent among "lower class" brothel sex workers in Chiang Mai. In India, the HIV prevalence in female CSWs has also grown rapidly. The prevalence has been estimated at 30-50 per cent in Mumbai, while in Delhi it has been found to be over 30 per cent among female CSWs.

In some other parts of Asia, the spread of HIV has not yet occurred to the same extent as in Thailand and India. The highest prevalence among female CSWs to date has been documented in Cambodia. Some surveys have seen infection rates of 12-15 per cent. There has been a gradual increase in prevalence among female CSWs in Malaysia.

During 1980s, the prevalence among female CSWs in the Philippines was reported between 1 per cent and 2.5 per cent. Surprisingly, recent surveys in parts of the country, including Cebu City, reported no infection among the 800 CSWs tested, though the testing bias cannot be excluded. A very low level of infection has been found in Korea and Vietnam while no infection has been reported recently among female CSWs in Singapore, Japan, Hong Kong and Australia.

The surveys carried out among homosexual men have reported relatively high levels of infection, for example, up to 30 per cent in Sydney and 11 per cent among foreign homosexual/bisexual men in Japan. However, the surveys in Singapore, Philippines and Taiwan revealed a low level of HIV infection.

The seroprevalence among the general population has reached up to 4 per cent in Thailand and 7 per cent in Myanmar. In India, cumulative infections counted half a million at the end of 1991 and reached more than one million by the end of 1992.

Such type of statistical data tells us several important things. Firstly, Asia and the Pacific have the same mix of transmission modes as we have seen in elsewhere in the world. The same risk behaviours exist here as in other parts of the world. In Asia and the Pacific, the number of HIV infections has tripled in the last two years. And, by the end of the century, WHO predicted that in Asia and the Pacific, over one million adults would become infected with HIV each year.

The epidemic of AIDS would follow this great epidemic of HIV infection. By the year 2000, close to 2 million adults in this region were thought to have died of AIDS. During that year alone, some half a million HIV-infected people would have developed AIDS and require care, according to the estimates of WHO.

Worldwide, by the end of the century, as per the WHO projections there should be a cumulative total of 30-40 million HIV infections in men, women and children, of which 90 per cent should be in developing countries. The projected cumulative total of adult AIDS cases should be close to 10 million, of which 90 per cent in developing countries. And there should be 10 million or more children less than 10 years of age orphaned as a result of AIDS, primarily in the developing world.

Still there are facts and confusions about HIV that seem not to be fully understood by the public. Until they are, the epidemic will continue to grow out of control. Getting these facts known and accepted, and the confusions removed, are some big challenges which the Asian and Pacific countries are facing.

Moreover, HIV is not casually contagious. Fortunately for us, HIV is not one of the viruses that spread through air or water, through saliva, urine or faeces. It spreads via blood, semen, vaginal fluids and breast milk. There is need to understand that we cannot catch HIV by eating food with an HIV-infected person, or by sharing toilet or bathing tubs or through sneezing, shaking hands or hugging.

The health care workers need to be careful while handling the body fluids, particularly blood, of all patients as it is always a potential source of HIV. It should also be understood that there is no reason to isolate HIV-infected people from society, test hospital patients for HIV or isolate them in special hospitals or wards.

The most important thing that people need to know is how to prevent the transmission of HIV from an infected person to another person. People need to know that unprotected sexual intercourse can lead to HIV infection, sharing drug injecting equipments can lead to HIV infection, and that HIV-infected mothers can infect their children during pregnancy, delivery or through breastfeeding.

The people need to know how to reduce their risk of getting HIV infected, i.e., methods of safe sexual intercourse, use of disposable injecting equipments and options for infected mothers. They must know that HIV infection is lifelong and a person with HIV infection is infectious throughout the life.

On the basis of these statistical data a bleak picture has been created. The estimates used here are conservative. In the light of this picture, strong links must be built between the legal and human rights communities and the existing AIDS prevention institutions and organisations, to help overcome discrimination against people with AIDS. The interests of stigmatised groups like commercial sex workers and homosexuals should be defended and protected. The status of women must be improved. Those seeking to bring about true community development must be supported.

The HIV infection is preventible for the estimated 9 million people in Asia and the Pacific who will become infected with HIV in the coming years.

Part III

Effects of AIDS

Five

The Effect of AIDS

Tum is a little child whose mother was young, single and HIV-positive woman. When she went to the maternity hospital to give birth a child; she was checked in under a false name and address and slipped out of the hospital when her baby was only a few hours old. With his big eyes and delicate features Tum is immensely appealing. But until now, no one has provided him a home or family.

HIV-infected women who abandon their babies are generally already sick themselves and face an early death. Few can dare to watching their children struggle through a short life should they have passed on the virus during pregnancy.

Though the overwhelming majority of infected mothers do not abandon their babies. Such babies are an increasingly common feature of the AIDS epidemic almost everywhere. But they are part of a far larger phenomenon that is turning out to be one of the most serious social consequences of the epidemic—the phenomenon of AIDS orphans. According to WHO, by the end of this decade, the mothers of some 5-10 million children under 10 years of age worldwide will be died in the epidemic, leaving their child to survive alone or in the care of relatives or friends who are often ill-equipped to take on the tough task of raising some one else's children.

AIDS orphans, like the abandoned babies, present a far-reaching effects of the epidemic. In this chapter we will try to find out how this disease, like a stone dropped into a pool, sends out ripples to the very edge of society, affecting first the family, then the community, and then the nation.

Africa's Motherless Children

By the end of this century, the vast majority of the children orphaned by AIDS has been in sub-Saharan Africa region, where formerly the extended family could always be relied upon to take in the dependents of those who died. But today the traditional social security system—which has proved itself resilient to so many social changes—is buckling under the unprecedented strain of AIDS.

In the Kagera region of the United Republic of Tanzania, the closest and most senior male relative automatically assume the responsibility for the wife and children of a man who died. Today, there are too many stranded dependents for any system to cope with. The traditional family has almost totally disappeared in the region, which has been hit simultaneously with blight and pests sweeping through the banana plantations, decimating the staple food crop.

No one knows exactly how many children are involved. But it is estimated that in east and central Africa alone, between 3.1 and 5.5 million children—that is, 5-10 per cent of all children under 15—lost their mothers to AIDS during the 1990s. In these countries there are already a number of households composed of the young and the old left to fend for themselves after the death of the breadwinners.

"In the developing country, social security does not mean a government check, but having enough able-bodied people in your family to rely on for food and shelter," Dr. Michael Merson, Director of WHO's Global Programme on AIDS, told the US Congress in 1992. "AIDS is cutting vast holes in this ancient safety net, and millions of people are falling into it. Besides the children who are orphaned, there are huge numbers of elderly people who, having lost their adult children to AIDS, live out their last few years impoverished and alone."

The Odetas from Kagera are an example of a family still struggling to survive after the death of all its young children. Today, six children live with their grandfather, who often drinks to excess, and their grandmother who, since the death of her only son, Dominic, in 1988, became broken-hearted and ill. They live at the end of a narrow track through tall trees in a house whose cracked walls let in wind, rain and broken shafts of sunlight. But there is no money to repair the houses or even for new clothes. Nor is anyone big enough or strong enough to farm the small *shamba*. The family is bound to depend on charity and the goodwill of neighbours for everything from labour and food, to school uniforms for the youngsters.

Their mother, who died in 1991, deliberately knew how hard life would be for the old folk and the children when she died. Working ceaselessly, she dug and weeded the *shamba*, and started to build a house for the family. But before she could finish the house she lose her strength and today she lives beside its roofless walls in a grave next to her husband's, marked with a wooden cross.

Johannsen Johanna is headmaster of the nearby primary school where more than one in ten of his pupils have lost their parent in the epidemic. Most of the orphans, he says, are not in a position to afford their fees; they come to school without pencils and exercise books, too. But unlike other headmasters who refuse to admit children in his school who cannot pay the fees, Mr. Johanna cannot turn away his orphans. Their shame at being different from the others as they sit at their desks without equipment or decent uniforms is obvious to see, and frequently their ability to learn is blocked by emotional problems.

"Sometimes kids come to school without eating" said Prudencia Rweyemera, one of the teachers. "Due to weaknesses they fall asleep on their desks, and I become compel to take them back to my home to give them a meal."

Many who cannot bear the hardship and humiliation simply drop out of school, and some end up in very young, unskilled and full of frustration on the streets of nearby towns. "Places like Mwanza and Bukoba [on the shores of Lake Victoria] never had problems with street children before," said a nurse-educator working in Kagera. "But now there are little gangs of orphaned kids who have run away from their villages and who live by robbing people."

Without a family background and school life they may never be able to play a constructive role in society. "AIDS orphans will undoubtedly pose one of the greatest problems to economic development in Africa in recent history," says Elizabeth Preble, former AIDS advisor for UNICEF.

The Crippling Cost of Illness

By the time parents die, their children and elderly dependents are often awfully impoverished because of the costs in time and money of caring for someone with AIDS. In Zaire, a single admission to Kingshasa's main hospital, Mama Yemo, for a child suffering from AIDS costs the equivalent of several months of an average salary, and funerals cost the equivalent of nearly one year's salary. And in Thailand, lifetime treatment costs per person with AIDS are estimated at a minimum of US$1000, which is about 30-50 per cent of the annual income of the average Thai family.

The struggle at family level to carry the burden of AIDS is reflected at the national level. In the United Republic of Tanzania the national health budget is US$5 per head—less than the cost of a single blood test for AIDS.

Mentioning the crisis facing the health services in Ethiopia in 1992, Dr. Bona Hora said: "We have a total of 11000 hospital beds, and by the end of this year we are expecting to have nearly 26000 adult cases of AIDS, and perhaps 12000 paediatric cases." In many of the large hospitals of Central and East Africa, 20-40 per cent of beds are already occupied by people with AIDS, and rates in some others are still higher.

In developed countries also, the epidemic is making significant demands on health services, and these demands will increase as those already infected with HIV develop AIDS. The cost of caring for an AIDS patient from diagnosis to death in the USA, for example, has been calculated at around $50000-$60000, and by 1991 such patients were expected to account for twice as many hospital bed—days per year as lung cancer—one of the nation's leading causes of death.

According to an estimate in 1992, the cost of medical care for some half a million people with AIDS was close to US$5000 million. Industrialised countries accounted for over 90 per cent of these costs although they accounted for only 22 per cent of the cases. But almost 80 per cent of the world's new infections are now occurring in the developing countries. The burden on these countries, including some of the poorest countries in the world, can only increase. In the time to come, the developing countries will spend over US$ 1000 million on health care for AIDS victims.

The Impact of AIDS Deaths

Using special modelling techniques, WHO and the World Bank have provided with a picture of the likely demographic impact of AIDS deaths on a hypothetical sub-Saharan country with a current high prevalence of HIV. Between 1985 and 1990 in this country, the death rate has increased by 0.3 per 1000 population as a result of AIDS deaths, and a further increase of 1.1 per 1000 population has been expected by the mid-1990s. In the absence of AIDS, death rates would have been expected to begin declining from 1985.

Because a number of factors that might affect the picture are not known or unpredictable, there are inherent limitations in such projections. However, the model indicates the following:

- Life expectancy for a person born in this hypothetical country will subside from about 50 years in 1985 to 47 in the year 2010. In the absence of AIDS, life expectancy would have increased by more than 11 years.
- Between 1985 and 1990, AIDS added an average of 10 per cent to the annual death rate for people age ranged from 15-49; by the mid-1990s, it will enhance adult death rates by more than 40 per cent. These projections are for the country as a whole: in the worst-affected urban areas, adult deaths are expected to double or triple.
- By the mid-1990s, infant mortality is expected to be 4 per cent higher than it would be in the absence of AIDS. By this time, too, AIDS deaths in children will start to reverse the progress made over the past two decades in child survival through programmes such as immunization and oral dehydration of children with diarrhoea.
- The increasing rate of deaths in children under 5 and those aged 15-44 is not expected to result in an actual decline in the size of the population in this hypothetical country, nor in any sub-Saharan African country. It will solely slow down the population's growth rate. The population, which grew by about 3.4 per cent in 1990, would be increasing by 2.4 per cent a year by 2010, instead of by around 3 per cent, as it would in the absence of AIDS.

Thus, the most dramatic demographic effect will be not on the size of the population, but on its age structure. As young and middle-aged adults are picked off by AIDS, there will be disproportionate numbers of old people and, especially, children in the population, skewing the "population age pyramid".

It thus ensures that the economic effects of the epidemic will be felt far beyond the health sector, for countries will lose their most productive members, the men and women on whom the economy depends. In several countries, their loss will undermine the development process itself.

There have been relatively some detailed studies of overall economic impact in developing countries, but some data from Thailand are instructive. These reveal that the direct health care costs of AIDS—around $1000 a year per patient—are dwarfed by the indirect costs of the premature illness and death of adults in very young which the Thai economists estimate at $22000 per death (equal to approximately 14 times the 1991 gross national product per capita).

Their study also reveals that, in aggregate, these costs are enormous. Health care costs plus the value of lost income and other indirect costs to the nation will increase from $100 million in 1991 to a maximum of $2200 million by the year 2000 (or a minimum of $1800 million, in the best-case scenario). In another way, during the 1990s, between $7300 million and $8700 million will have been lost to the Thai economy as a result of AIDS illness and death.

Indicating the economic impact in Africa, WHO has calculated that AIDS deaths in Uganda will triple the number of potentially productive years lost in the 20-50 age group. And researchers at Harvard University predicted that economic losses for want of AIDS in five badly affected central African countries would exceed the total supply of foreign aid to those countries by 1991.

The economic effect on industrialized countries will also be substantial but it will not be overwhelming as these countries are rich. The developing countries will suffer immeasurably harder both because their baseline economies are so much weaker and because they cover 90 per cent of the world's HIV infections by the year 2000.

It is easier to predict the explosive impact of the AIDS epidemic than to foresee how the pieces will fall. Societies and economies are moveable, and the good news from past epidemics is that people and institutions are flexible and can accommodate considerable change. However, societies will be not in a position to make the most of their potential flexibility unless they take the epidemic seriously and start now to analyse, sector by sector, what AIDS will mean for the economy.

As a special panel set up by the US National Research Council stresses, "Difficult though it might be to predict the future import of the present impact of the HIV/AIDS epidemic, one should not shrink from the task, especially when one must plan for the future".

Six

AIDS: The Blame Game

For hundreds of years, the reflex response to plague and pestilence has been to bar strangers from the city gates. Today blood tests for antibodies to HIV replace barricades but fear of contagion and its consequences remain the same. Press clippings, interviews and other documentary material from every continent display that the appearance of AIDS in any community has almost inevitably been accompanied by the urge to point the finger at someone else. The kinds of AIDS blaming are as numerous, and often as ill-judged, as the prejudices which existed before them.

Blame Goes Round the World

Though African countries have been incessant in their criticism of the United States and Europe over AIDS, Africans have also sometimes blamed ethnic minorities in their own, or in a neighbouring countries.

"During the rule of the white man we had all the different kinds of medicines to cure all the diseases", said Lute, a Zambian woman to a Zambian reporter in Lusaka. "But now the Indian doctors in our hospitals say that this disease cannot be cured. The government has mounted the AIDS campaign to hide the inefficiency of the Indian doctors."

Kenya has sometimes accused neighbouring Uganda. A May 1987 editorial in the *Kenya Times*, for example, accused Uganda of "trying to pass the buck, and the bug, elsewhere".

Uganda had the largest number of AIDS cases in Africa, said the *Kenya Times*, the newspaper of Kenya's ruling party, and this might be linked to the fact that Ugandans were lax in matters of sexual morality. "As our Ugandan brothers and sisters are well aware a number of the people over there who occasionally fall victim to venereal diseases usually joke about their ill-luck, saying they are suffering from a fever of sorts." The editorial urged Ugandans to pay much attention to the advice contained in a pastoral letter written by Kenya's Catholic bishops, who warned that "nature has its own law of retribution".

Apartheid and AIDS

In South Africa, AIDS is sometimes discussed in such a way as if there were two separate viruses: white HIV and black HIV. The national health authorities, who by early 1988 had reported 65 cases of AIDS in white homosexuals since 1982, have only recently corroborated the presence of the virus in the black community. Blood test surveys have recognised HIV antibodies in over 1,000 black South Africans, and doctors in South Africa's blood transfusion service estimate that as many as 15,000 blacks and 5,000 whites might now be carrying the virus. A less alarming picture is given by the chairman of the AIDS Advisory Committee, who estimates the number of black carriers at 3,000.

When information that HIV had appeared among blacks became public in July 1987, the mass-market *Sunday Star* ran the headline: "Experts fear spread of African AIDS". In opposite to the AIDS already present among whites, "African AIDS" was the "heterosexual variant of the killer disease" which had "entered South Africa from the North". Migrant mine workers from African neighbouring countries had carried the virus into South Africa with them, charged the *Sunday Star*, spreading it to the black South African women with whom they made sexual relations.

"There is no doubt that an epidemic of African AIDS is coming", a University of Cape Town virologist is quoted as saying, while a blood specialist is said to have remarked that "It is essential that we will have cases of African AIDS". The government's own AIDS advisory group of medical experts publicly rejected suggestions that there is such a thing as "African AIDS", but the distinction between "African" and "European" AIDS was maintained in some newspapers.

Disbelief: A Reaction to Blame

The perception that blame has been cast can have negative results, whether or not the perception is itself accurate. A sea-change in Nigerian public opinion on AIDS—from open mindedness to suspicion and disbelief—surfaced after Western scientists focused the attention of an international AIDS conference on AIDS in Africa and the possible African origins of the AIDS virus. Nigerian science journalist Seun Ogunseitan watched these events closely. He concluded that Nigerians' perception of blame was a serious set-back for Nigerian AIDS information and participation in international AIDS prevention efforts, is explained in the article which follows.

Nigeria: Publicity Put the Clock Back

In the beginning of December 1985 I reported in the *Guardian* that doctors in one of Nigeria's leading medical institutions might have diagnosed the country's first AIDS cases. Some of my colleagues were not happy with my having "put Nigeria on the AIDS map".

About six months before I wrote that first story, Nigerians had wanted to know as much as possible about AIDS. Few of them were concerned about the origin of the disease. The population was so receptive to information then that individuals who could not find reasons for weight loss, but knew it was a symptom of AIDS, were writing to newspapers anxious to know more about the disease.

The enthusiasm with which Nigerians sought information on AIDS probably exceeded the interest in the disease of average Americans; but the fear and paranoia common in Europe and the United States were largely absent. Nigerians considered themselves as part of a global community under common threat. Unprompted, they related AIDS to men and women of "easy virtue", and wondered about the activities of suspected bisexuals.

A single event marked the transformation from this atmosphere of unselfconscious inquiry. In mid-1985 an international congress was held in Brussels under the title "Conference on African AIDS". This was a major mistake. African delegates—including Nigerians—raised objection publicly against the title, but the rest of the researchers present failed to respond coherently to this criticism. It was at this point that the international community of AIDS researchers lost their credibility with Nigerians and other Africans. The suggestion that AIDS originated in Africa and the implication that it is a disease of blacks made ordinary citizens begin to doubt the claims of these researchers.

One immediate after-effect of the Brussels conference was the maintenance of secrecy by health authorities in Africa, who would otherwise have approached AIDS as a serious health issue which should not be concealed. Whereas most Nigerians believed that the disease was killing tens of people every week in East and Central Africa, once it was suggested that it originated in Africa, they started to suspect the truth of Western media reports on the epidemic.

Before the "origins" question became an issue, the average Nigerian would have thought thrice about statistics, which said that up to 68 per cent of adult groups in some African communities were carrying the AIDS virus; now the figures were regarded with unveiled scepticism.

In such climate of opinion my report of the arrival of AIDS in Nigeria was interpreted as "joining them in the preposterous assertion that the disease originated in Africa". Several reasons were found to show why AIDS should not be reported as being present in Nigeria. Discussion about the severity of the problem was alternately a "gimmick to gain more funds for research", or "all Western propaganda".

However, a number of Nigerians suspected that "the West has finally found a good ploy to force Africans to accept the use of condoms. It claims that condoms should now be used for protection against AIDS, but its main aim is to further its long-term population control plan for Africa."

At the end of 1985 several governments, particularly in Africa, were unwilling to accept the presence of AIDS or even the likelihood of its presence among their citizenry. This dangerous silence was also true in Lagos, and many Nigerians wanted to keep it that way. Nigerian press reports were erroneously suggesting that AIDS was just one more dangerous sexually transmitted disease said to be ravaging communities of homosexuals and intravenous drug users in Europe and America.

Only with reluctance did the Nigerian media carry the first reports of what is now a recognised AIDS epidemic in East and

Central Africa. To most Nigerians in 1985, AIDS was someone else's problem. It was not their disease, was not present in Nigeria—and nobody should suggest the contrary.

In writing my story I had expected to influence the government to adopt a more open approach towards AIDS. But following the charges of racism, which followed the Brussels meeting the import of the story was lost on several Nigerians. With the issue of the origins of the disease festering in the public mind it was not possible to make any headway in reporting how the epidemic was spreading. Even people with symptoms of the disease met hostility because of the public link between AIDS and racism.

In the meantime, the information carried in thousands of reports on AIDS in the international press were lost on the now-biased Nigerian public. Some of the Nigerian scientists were vilified by the government and, to a lesser extent, the public for "joining them in confirming the existence of AIDS in the country".

There is no doubt that the opportunity for extensive Nigerian co-operation in the international fight against AIDS in the early part of the recent pandemic was lost. The damage was done when Western researchers and the media highlighted their opinions on the origins of AIDS too early, and without taking sufficient pains to make distinction between opinion and fact. On highly sensitive issues such as this, opinions should be stated for what they are and not granted the authority of science before incontrovertible proof to support them can be found.

Blame on the Students

In Europe, African students have been generally blamed for AIDS. In 1987, Belgium ordered compulsory HIV tests for all foreign students on government grants, many of whom came from Africa, especially Zaire. Soon, a new slogan—"Black AIDS" –began to appear on metro walls. "Why only Third World students?" asked Ekanga Shungu, Zairean editor of a monthly African magazine in Belgium, explaining that AIDS had become such a stigma that Zaireans were now afraid to talk about it.

Little has appeared in the West about attitudes to AIDS in the Soviet Union and Eastern Europe, as very few cases have so far been reported. But an African student in Moscow reported in August 1987 that while "they used to refer to us as monkeys now they point and say the word for AIDS". In the same month it was reported that a group of Soviet graduate medical students had written to the Academy of Medical Sciences in Moscow, vowing that as practising doctors they would block any cure for AIDS because it was a "noble disease" which would eliminate "drug addicts, homosexuals and prostitutes".

"African AIDS deadly threat to Britain" was the headline of the front-page story of the British *Sunday Telegraph* on 21 September 1986, in a classic instance of Europeans blaming Africa for AIDS. The article had claimed that an investigation into the potential risks to Britain posed by AIDS in Africa, ordered by the British foreign secretary, had resulted in "a series of alarming reports" from British embassies in Tanzania, Uganda and Zambia. British diplomats, the story said, warned that African visitors to Britain" could be a main source of infection and they should be bound to compulsory tests".

The UK Foreign Office accepted receiving a report, but said that no immediate action would be taken. But the *Sunday Telegraph* made its position explicit. "It would be monstrous if ministers were to hold back from action lest they be accused of racial discrimination. For in this example there is a positive duty to discriminate. In the matter of AIDS", it asserted, "Black Africa does have a typically bad record". Within some weeks, the United Kingdom let it be known that there were no plans to screen Zambians, after strong behind-the-scenes pressure from the UK health department and from its medical advisors. From a public health stand point, to test a few score black Zambians a year, and not to test hundreds of thousands of white US tourists who tend to visit Britain annually, was seen by many British AIDS workers as absurd and racist.

Blame Hinders AIDS Campaigns

But the damage had been done, Zambia's minister of health reacted soon to the suggestion that Zambians, notably students, should be screened for the AIDS virus on entering Britain: "We will make intense study of the situation, and we may reciprocate in the same way if Britain goes ahead. After all, AIDS is a capitalist disease which is not only common in Zambia but across the world".

The screening explicitly contemplated by the British Government was seen as a political insult in Zambia, where a number of British physicians and researchers had been working in collaboration with Zambian colleagues on AIDS-related projects. An immediate result was some delay in plans to screen Zambian blood supplies: while health officials were rigid to do this, political support for action on AIDS was still confined, and the UK testing row undermined it.

Various other AIDS projects were disrupted following the British story and reaction to it, at a moment when time was critical in Zambia's battle to contain the spread of the AIDS virus. A few months before the Sunday Telegraph story, a medical symposium in Lusaka had been told that 17 per cent of healthy people coming into the city's hospital for medical check-ups were HIV-positive, and that Zambia might have 6,000 babies and infants with AIDS by 1987.

On the economic side, Zambian officials were concerned about the results on tourism of the *Sunday Telegraph's* story, particularly since the majority of tourists were European. The year 1986 had been marked as an all-time low for the Zambian tourist trade, with revenues down nearly 25 per cent from 1985. Although the political instability in southern Africa and international currency fluctuations contributed a lot to this decline, Zambian officials were of the view that an important factor was "negative publicity campaigns in our traditional tourist markets".

The fear of bad publicity about AIDS was all the more acute because Zambia has been struggling for its economic life. Declining revenue from copper, its principal export, has initiated a downward spiral which has seen per capita income fall by two-thirds since 1980. Zambia expects tourism will offset the loss of copper earnings, by bringing in hard currency and creating even more employment than the 30,000 plus jobs which have sprung up as a result of foreign visitors.

After the publication of the *Sunday Telegraph* story, British researchers received a letter from a Zambian official which read in part: "I regret to inform you that the mass media in recent weeks have highlighted problems which, require questions to be asked as to whether collaboration should be continued with outside researchers. I am afraid that we are in a political world, and such matters, as they are reported in the British press, make it difficult to continue".

Zambia is not the only country to reconsider joint AIDS efforts due to media coverage judged to be unfavourable. African sensitivities to Western research on AIDS were increased by the enthusiasm of Western scientists to carry out "parachute" research: dropping in to collect blood samples, data or clinical observations, and just as quickly taking off again, to write up their findings for a (Western) scientific journal. African officials would find themselves in the position of first reading about the "latest" AIDS statistics from their country in such a journal or, worse, in a sensationalised account in the international press.

Undoubtedly, political tensions over AIDS have sometimes damaged the campaign to contain the disease. But not all Western researchers drop into and out of the African countries they are studying. Very often there is no clear-cut differences between the work of expatriate researchers and that of their African counterparts. In Kenya, Rwanda, Tanzania, Uganda, Zambia, Zaire, Senegal and other African countries, foreign and African experts have been working sincerely together on a range of AIDS research and control projects, some of several years' duration. Without this international collaboration, much of the progress on AIDS control would have not been possible.

Blame on African Students in India

The conspicuous willingness of some British diplomats to blame AIDS on Zambian students was followed six months later by a similar differences in India, again about students from Africa.

Upheaval in India

In February 1987, the Indian Government took a decision to enforce strictly the screening of all foreign students for AIDS, and began deporting those found HIV-positive. Africans, who are average 85 per cent of the foreign student population, were incensed at what they percepted to be a "racist and unscientific" policy. Their nationwide protest brought AIDS to the centre of a political controversy and India, a champion of anti-apartheid, was drawn into a diplomatic difference with friendly, African nations over an apparently non-political issue.

A chance finding of AIDS antibodies in a Tanzanian student in Madras in June 1986 led the government to focus on foreign students, Africans in particular. Earlier that year, 22 of 130 prostitutes tested in Madras had been found HIV-positive by one of the surveillance centres being run by the Indian Council of Medical Research (ICMR). Swayed by press reports about high prevalence of AIDS in Africa, ICMR casually screened a few African students in Madras. One of them turned out to be carrying the HIV.

The result scared away the rest of the African students in Madras and they refused to volunteer for the test. On the one hand, ICMR was worried about the potential threat from African students, and on the other it was sensitive to the likely political results of revealing its find. It therefore kept its discovery away from the press and recommended to the Health Ministry that foreign students be compulsorily tested for AIDS. The decision was informed to the Department of Education in the Ministry of Human Resources and Development, which then informed heads of all universities that all foreign students must be tested for AIDS and those found positive should be expelled.

The circular was issued on 12 August 1986, but the university authorities paid scant attention to it until receiving a reminder on 23 January 1987. Foreign students were directed to nearest medical centres for the AIDS test, at which point demonstrations broke out. In Delhi, about 1,000 African students held a six-hour solidarity meeting and hold a procession waving banners that said "Down with Medical Apartheid" and "We are prepared to go home rather than be humiliated", before confronting with the police. In Bombay, the 500-odd African students boycotted the medical examination. Reactions elsewhere were similar.

Fear, social ostracism and psychological trauma put the educational career of African students in danger. The African Students Association alleged that the AIDS test had reached such absurd lengths that the district collector of Jabalpur ordered burning of the personal effects of an African student suspected of AIDS. This led to the local population started avoiding shops and hotels being run by Africans; there was effective segregation within and outside the university. According to Salek Osoro, a Delhi University student: "We are shocked by our erstwhile friends in the university, and in the private houses where we live. We are treated as untouchables."

African diplomats were upset by the press publicity-identifying students by name and nationality, and some vehemently criticised the government's stand. The Ugandan high commissioner in India, Dr. S.C. Chebrot, said he was distressed at the "discriminatory test started against the African students." The Kenyan health minister, Mr Peter Nyakiamo, who was on a 10-day tour of India in February, said his countrymen on return that "the smear campaign was exacting a devastating psychological toll on Kenyan students." Verbal protests were organised to Indian heads of mission in African countries. The AIDS tests dominated the meetings between India's External Affairs Minister, Mr N.D. Tiwari, and the Kenyan President, Mr Daniel Arap Moi, in course of the former's visit to Kenya, where two dailies frontpaged stories of how two Kenyan students were "kicked out" of India because of AIDS.

Off the record, an Indian Government official said the whole matter was mishandled by authorities of educational institutions. "Their approach was clandestine and crude and they failed to explain to students the purpose of the test." Throughout the controversy, the Indian press in general had been sympathetic to the plight of the African students. Describing the government's decision as "an example of unwisdom," an editorial in the *Chandigarh Tribune* wrote: "The Government must remove the feeling from the minds of the African students that the AIDS test is aimed at them." *The Hindustan Times* said the decision was in hastle and a "panic reaction". It added that by singling out students from Africa and Asia "the government in a way is casting a slur on their sexual habits." *The Times of India* wrote the government action was "ill thought out, insensitive and brazenly discriminatory."

The African agitation raised an uproar in the Parliament. Several opposition members wanted the AIDS test stopped because it will not be good for India's relations with African countries. However, Mr P.V. Narasimha Rao, Minister for Human Resources Development, said the tests would continue because "AIDS is very serious a matter to be daunted by protests." All foreign students would be tested, not just Africans. The Communist Party Secretary, Mr. R.C. Rajeswara Rao, said the test "is humiliating to say the least" because, in effect, "it is being enforced on Aricans who constitute the majority of foreign students."

The government's decision to go ahead with the screening of foreign students collapsed when the African students decided to launch fresh protests. To avoid political embarrassment, the Indian Government ceded to the Africans' demand that the AIDS test would be mandatory only for fresh students.

Although India's policy has now changed to ensure anonymity of testing and the testing of all tourists staying in the country longer than a year, many students feel there is still some partiality. "Why are diplomats and diplomatic staff exempted?" asked John Mageto of Delhi University. Raid Ibrahim, a student from Kuwait, asked: "Why only foreigners? Why not Indians returning from abroad?" A Palestinian pointed out that the new policy discriminates even today because it exempts the high-risk "freak-looking tourists" coming for a short stay while "attention continues to be focused on students".

Kenya: AIDS and Tourism

At about the same time as Kenyan diplomats were defending their students in India, another AIDS row was growing in Nairobi and London. On 3 February 1987 the United Kingdom's *Guardian* newspaper published a report that British soldiers on exercise in Kenya had been instructed to stay out of Nairobi after 6 p.m. because of the threat of contracting AIDS and other sexually transmitted diseases. This was said with a view to follow an earlier decision by the UK military making the port of Mombasa, and the resort town of Malindi, off-limits for British troops. Soldiers who were returning from Kenya were "strongly advised" to have a test for the AIDS virus on their arrival in Britain. Of those who did so, none were found to be HIV carriers, although press reports in March indicated that a number had contracted other STDs.

The British troops report caused embarrassment for Kenya for a number of reasons. Kenya normally plays down the yearly arrival of British troops for manoeuvrers. And, like Zambia, it also relies substantially on its tourist industry. With more and more nations competing for the tourist dollar, and tourists easily switching from one destination to another, the responsible Kenyan officials viewed any stories about AIDS as a threat to their expansion plans. Over 650,000 visitors injected more than US$250 million into the Kenyan economy in 1986, and the tourism ministry predicted a million tourists annually by the year 2000.

The Kenya Government was already concerned about AIDS stories. In November 1985 it had banned an issue of the *International Herald Tribune* that discussed AIDS among prostitutes in Nairobi. And a 1987 international conference of air traffic controllers was almost aborted when the Austrian controllers' association became aware at reports that mosquitoes might be responsible for spreading the AIDS virus in Africa. The Austrian association wanted a change of venue "to another city, not located on the African continent" not wishing, they said, "to expose our families to such a danger."

The conference had gone ahead, but Kenyan authorities had been shaken. When the *Guardian's* troops story came into light in February 1987, the Kenyan minister of foreign affairs said it was part of a "definite overseas smear campaign" against Kenya. The health minister said there was "no scientific ground for the hysterical and alarmist media presentation", and the minister for works and housing expressing his disappointment with the "holier than thou" attitude of European countries. "The promotion of tourism in our country", wrote the Kenyan *Standard,*" constitute a major part of our development strategy. Many Western tourists choose Kenya not only because of the natural attractions the country has to offer, but equally because of the country's political stability and high moral standards for which have earned Kenyans worldwide respect."

The Kenyan minister of tourism denied rumours of widespread cancellations of hotel bookings. But a magazine specialising in African affairs later said that huge cancellations had ensued, and the Kenyan *Daily Nation* quoted a Kenyan travel firm as losing over US$3 million in contracts with British travel agencies after the publication of first reports of AIDS in the country surfaced in the international press.

Blame on the Foreigners

In several countries—Panos has got reports from the Middle East, China, India, Japan, Malaysia, the Philippines, Sri Lanka, Colombia, Costa Rica, Cuba, Ecuador, Mexico, Nicaragua, Venezuela, the USSR and Eastern Europe—a common target has been the "degenerate" West.

When in the beginning of 1987 a Japanese prostitute from the city of Kobe was diagnosed as having died from AIDS, the assumption that she had been infected during sexual contact with a foreigner was reached overnight. "Her death", as one Japanese newspaper published, "was the result of an infatuation with Europe". Japanese health officials told journalists that the government was exploring the ways to prevent HIV-positive foreigners entering the country, since they considered that all cases of AIDS in Japan were the result of foreign contact.

This measure soon became confused with the desire to exclude all non-Japanese. In the red-light district of Tokyo warning signs suddenly appeared: "*Gaijin* [foreigners] off limits". There was no discouragement of Japanese customers who had recently been abroad.

In a survey of school teachers, Professor Bin Takeda of Chiba University turned up deep-seated fears of coming into contact with foreigners. He concluded that 85 per cent of the teachers are of the view that AIDS could not be contracted from swimming pools or from Western-style toilet seats (traditional Japanese toilets are the squat variety). But 45 per cent still said they didnt like using swimming pools or toilets in places frequented by foreigners. A number of Japanese think foreigner equals AIDS carrier," commented Dr Masayoshi Negishi, who treats AIDS patients at Tokyo's Komagome Hospital.

Blame on the United States

The United States has been widely blamed for AIDS. When Filipina journalist Erlinda Bolido, who is an employee of the Press Foundation of Asia, conducted an informal poll in mid-1987 for

Panos on the streets of Manila, several of the people she questioned said they believed the United States is responsible for starting the AIDS epidemic. The AIDS problem started "when some people indulged [in sex] beyond God-ordained limits," said 25-year-old secretary Tess Martelino, adding that American and other homosexuals were responsible. Nineteen-year-old Anna May Sanga knew the disease is the result of a virus. "I think it comes from a virus which was originally found in an African ape," she said. But Arsenio Alano, a retired accountant aged 73, was less sure. "I read somewhere that AIDS originated in Africa, but I always thought that like most things good or bad, Americans are responsible too." Added Sanga: "people who have sexual intercourse with homosexuals, with those Americans in the military bases and with call girls" are likely to catch the disease. Erlinda Bolido reports that Americans are commonly identified as being responsible for introducing the HIV virus into the Philippines, and fear of AIDS has become an additional argument for those who demand that the bases be dismantled.

In many countries, US military and naval personnel have been blamed for spreading AIDS. In August 1987 the Turkish magazine *Islam* carried a rumour which soon became prevalent in the Middle East. US soldiers in Vietnam had contracted the AIDS virus by making sex with monkeys, the magazine claimed, and then carried it back to the United States, where they spread it to others. Variants of this rumour gained momentum in Latin America,claiming that a US sailor had first spread AIDS around the world. Public concern about AIDS in Japan in 1986 led to calls for a ban on the US fleet, while in 1987 Costa Rica turned away a US warship due for a routine visit when the US Navy could not guarantee that all the seamen were HIV-negative.

"Hospitality women" in the Philippines, feared of contracting the disease from US servicemen, continue to demand that the soldiers be tested for AIDS. The Filipina women have levelled charges that "AIDS from US military bases poses the danger of genocide". They demanded that the Philippine Government deny entry to any US serviceman not certified AIDS-free. The feasibility of HIV infection brought to the Philippines by US servicemen is, in the women's opinion, sufficient to justify the cancellation of the

US-Philippines military bases agreement before its current term of effect runs out in 1991. In February 1988 the Philippine Government acceded. All foreign seamen are now required to be screened for HIV-antibodies.

Some US foreign policy experts are of the view that "access for American ships, aircraft and other military forces to foreign bases or normal ports-of-call could become a serious security problem".

The claim that the HIV virus came from a US germ warfare laboratory has been widely believed in some Central and South American countries, and as AIDS spreads fastly in Latin America and the Caribbean, placards linking AIDS to the United States have appeared during anti-US political demonstrations. At a 1987 meeting of the Pan American Health Organization in Quito, Ecuador, participants passed a resolution which recommended that the superpowers recognise the magnitude of the threat posed by AIDS to the security of all nations, agree to arms limitations, and should allocate the resources saved to an international AIDS prevention and control fund which stressed the needs of developing countries.

The Quito meeting also highlighted one of the important aspects of AIDS which touches on racial and ethnic divisions: that of the discriminations in treatment available to people with AIDS depending on their economic, social and geographic conditions. AZT, the only drug proven to be effective in extending the lifespan of certain categories of AIDS patients is much expensive that many US AIDS patients, especially those from poor backgrounds in inner city black of ethnic minority neighbourhoods, do not receive it. Outside the United States and Europe, the use of AZT has met opposition by Mexican health officials on the grounds that it is prohibitively expensive. "Why should we tend to pay hard-earned dollars to an American company for a drug to treat a disease exported to us from the US, a country that already takes many millions from us in interest payments on our debt, to diagnose AIDS patients, who are unlikely to survive very long in any case?", asked a Mexican participant in the Quito conference. "It is sad, but the hard facts are that for that money we could save many more lives in other health programmes."

Barring the Foreigners

Confronted with a new disease whose infectious carriers may look outwardly healthy for years, and with medical authorities recommending politically-controversial countermeasures like sex education in schools, condoms in prisons and free one-time needles for intravenous drug users, several governments have decided to impose blood tests on suspect groups of foreigners.

Only a few governments have yet taken seriously the suggestion of essential testing all their own citizens. There are two problems: practical and theoretical. The practical difficulty is that the test is relatively expensive and requires many trained technicians. The theoretical problem is what a government then does about people who test HIV-positive. Are they to be quarantined at government expense? Encouraged not to have sex? Issued with recognising armbands? Public health officials in most countries have spoken out strongly against any form of compulsory mass blood tests; they afraid that the discrimination against carriers would setback the public education campaigns which are the main weapon against the epidemics in existing period.

But these problems do not apply to foreigners. They can be made to pay for the tests themselves, or simply be required to produce a certificate saying they are HIV-negative. And there is no difficulty about what to do with foreign HIV-positives: keep them out of the country, and let their own government sort out what to do with them.

Probably most importantly, screening foreigners is usually politically popular. The general wish to blame AIDS on other people is satisfied; the requirement for politically controversial action against the disease at home can be avoided or postponed; the government will be seen as acting with determination. Many governments have to a greater or lesser extent given in to the epidemic of blaming others.

By March 1988, 18 countries (list given ahead) were known to have taken decision to adopt screening for at least some groups of foreigners. The World Health Organization's suggestion against testing tourists has so far been generally accepted. According to WHO, screening tourists is epidemiologically ineffective (because people can be carriers of the virus but still show up HIV-negative in blood tests for up to six months after being infected), and it turns attention from measures (such as screening blood supplies and educating the public at home) more likely to slow down the epidemics.

WHO's remit does not extend to making recommendations about another categories of travellers, such as students, immigrants and guest workers, who are strictly national responsibilities. Within these categories restrictive measures have been taken and continue to be imposed, as listed below. For whatever reasons, the countries mentioned above have decided that the benefits of restricting other types of visitors outweigh the costs.

This list of countries is based on information available to the Panos Institute in March 1988. It may not be totally accurate, although Panos has made efforts to confirm the measures with the health or immigration authorities in each country. Those planning travel to abroad should check with officials of the country of destination for up-to-date information on current regulations.

List of Countries Testing Foreigners for AIDS

Belgium	Foreign students getting scholarships from the Ministry of Foreign Affairs are tested for HIV-antibodies.
Bulgaria	All foreigners staying longer than one month, and all Bulgarians returning from working abroad, are being tested for HIV-antibodies.
China	All foreigners staying longer than one year must be tested for HIV-antibodies. Although visitors staying for less than this time are not routinely tested, those discovered to be carrying the virus are placed in isolation and deported.
Costarica	All foreign students and all applicants for residence are being tested for HIV-antibodies.
Cuba	Foreigners (but not tourists) and Cubans returning from AIDS-endemic areas are required to be tested on

	arrival for HIV-antibodies. If the result is negative, the test is repeated six months later. Cuba is in the process of screening all its own citizens, and seropositive individuals are quarantined.
Czechoslovakia	Foreign students are being tested for HIV-antibodies.
West Germany	All students getting a scholarship from the Ministry of Economic Co-operation are tested for HIV-antibodies. In the state of Bavaria, all foreigners applying for a residence permit, excepting nationals of the European Community and all other western European countries, must undergo a test for HIV-antibodies.
India	All foreigners staying longer than a year are being tested for HIV-antibodies.
Iraq	All foreigners entering Iraq and staying more than five days (and all Iraqis returning from abroad) are bound to undergo testing.
Kuwait	A number of reports indicate that all foreigners applying for a work permit are tested although the Embassy in London denies this.
Philippines	Foreigners applying to stay more than six months and all foreign seamen must present "AIDS-Clearance certificate" approved by the Philippine Government.
Qatar	Applications for work permits are tested.
Saudi Arabia	Applicants for work permits for more than one month are required to prove they are HIV-antibodies-free.

South Africa	Applicants for work permits are being tested. All citizens and foreigners may be tested on demand for HIV-antibodies with foreigners subject to deportation if found positive.
Soviet Union	Foreign students are automatically got tested for HIV-antibodies. Other foreigners (and Soviet citizens) may be tested on demand.
Syria	Foreign students and applicants for work permits are being tested for HIV-antibodies. Syrian scholarship students returning from abroad are tested.
United Arab Emirates	Press reports indicate that all foreigners applying for a work permit are being tested, although the embassy in London denies this.
United States	All applicants for immigrant visas are being tested for HIV-antibodies.

A number of other countries have made legislations to allow exclusion of foreigners with HIV or AIDS, without requiring of specific groups. These comprised Indonesia and Thailand, who prohibit non-citizens with AIDS from entering the country, and Sri Lanka and South Yemen, who have been known to expel individuals with HIV or AIDS.

Several countries have been reported to be considering restrictions on some or all foreign visitors. Among them are Israel, Jamaica, Japan, Libya, the Republic of Korea, Papua New Guinea and Turkey.

The Irrationality of Controls

A frequent characteristic of the controls is their inconsistency and arbitrariness, suggesting that they are indeed often motivated largely by the gut reaction of blaming others than by logic or public health. Thus, students and other young people are often tested, as are applicants (especially relatively unskilled applicants) for work permits: various countries can afford to exclude them.

Governments have been less interested to shut out other categories of visitor: diplomats and airline personnel are not tested; businessmen and tourists are rarely tested.

The travel restrictions have so far hurt Africans the most particularly several hundred students who have been expelled from countries requiring them to undergo AIDS blood tests. Many African countries rely heavily on foreign universities to train their students in the professional disciplines needed to advance their economic, technological and social development. Closing the way to higher education to those who are HIV-positive may prove a serious setback. Few African governments can afford to retaliate by discouraging foreign tourists or investment.

The United States has taken decision to screen all potential immigrants; the USSR and South Africa give health authorities discretionary powers to screen all visitors. The US legislation prompted Nigerian officials to speak of possible retaliatory measures, while the USSR's move caused British authorities to request that UK citizens in the Soviet Union be excluded from testing unless certified sterile needles and syringes—sometimes in short supply in Russia—could be made available.

Seen as a quick response to the blaming others syndrome, the controls are perhaps unsurprising. But from a public health perspective they have resulted in a number of absurdities.

The new US regulations, for example, mean that immigrants at present residing illegally in the United States face a test for the AIDS virus before they can legalise their status. Many of these immigrants—no one knows how many—will have contracted the virus in the United States, and then be expelled when they apply for legal residence and are found to be HIV-positive. A measure introduced on the grounds that the United States does not intend to import AIDS cases from the rest of the world will mean that the United States is effectively exporting AIDS.

Belgium only screens foreign students, many from Africa, receiving scholarships from the ministry; are non-scholarship students taken less likely to have been exposed to the virus?

Cuba screens nationals returning from AIDS-endemic regions, and all foreigners except tourists and the Philippines screens foreign seamen but not tourists. Does the hard currency which accompanies the tourists prevent them from picking up or passing on HIV?

India screens foreign students, though not its own students, who may have travelled to different countries and exposed themselves to the virus in the very countries from which the foreign students originate.

A country with no or very few cases of AIDS is prominently most likely to become infected from abroad. And rigorous exclusion of potential carriers certainly *sounds* as if it should be a useful countermeasure against a domestic AIDS epidemic ever starting. But to be really effective it would have to involve quarantining visitors (and making sure they had no access to unsafe sex) for six months, since it can take this long before an HIV-carrier shows a positive blood test. Likewise measures would also have to be imposed on domestic citizens returning from abroad, and also on both domestic and foreign airline crews, seamen, truck drivers, tourists and businessmen.

Such kinds of strict policy would probably be politically, administratively and economically not possible. So the grounds for screening have often tended to be political rather than medical: intentionally or unintentionally giving official help to the concept that AIDS should be blamed on foreigners.

Part IV

AIDS: Awareness and Prevention

Seven

Spreading Awareness About AIDS

In a street busy with shoppers and office workers emerging into the warm evening air, Semon C. Naron waits for his taxi to fill with passengers. Naron has been a taxi driver for 15 years, covering the route through the rice fields and small villages.

Some years ago he heard that taxi drivers were invited to attend an AIDS information course at the local community hospital. "I did't really believe then that AIDS existed," Naron says. "I thought it was a government policy to eliminate brothels. But I went along anyway, and ended up as one of 20 drivers asked to become volunteer educators."

Since then, five of Naron's regular passengers have died of AIDS. He has witnessed the distress of their families as mourners at the funerals have refused to touch the rice prepared, hurried away after the ceremony, and shunned them ever since. As a volunteer educator, with training and support from the health services, he regularly supplied AIDS information leaflets to stuck into the containers in his passenger cab, stickers with catchy messages about AIDS, and condoms to offer to the passenger riding beside him if the opportunity should arise.

Naron says that practically all his passengers take up a leaflet, and that today they are very ready to discuss AIDS as people they know begin to fall sick. An elderly relative in Naron's own family recently died of AIDS. "No one wanted to touch him, or touched only with gloves on," he said. "But I knew from my training that there was nothing to fear to touch and I should not keep away from him."

"Our thought was that taxi drivers could be used very effectively as agents for change as they remain in contact with so many people a day, and often ferry customers to the brothels," says Dr. Surasing a dentist in the office of the Provincial Medical Officer and the man behind the volunteer educator campaign. The team of around 80 taxi drivers in five districts is part of a larger campaign to reach out to people at the grass roots. The network of volunteer educators includes hairdressers like Mrs Prathum, whose small, neat saloon is running on a busy main road. She took up the work after frightened and ignorant people started whispering that having a haircut posed a danger of infection with HIV.

As she trims and curls and brushes, she engages her customers in conversation about AIDS, gently challenging denial, removing misconceptions, and handing out leaflets they can take home. Mrs. Prathum—married to a school teacher and mother of two daughters—a mission to protect people by giving them the knowledge she has gained about AIDS. Her saloon has a reputation for rigorous hygiene and she proudly displays a notice in her window stating that she passed her training with the health department and is one of their star educators.

Brothel managers, prostitutes, Buddhist monks and "tuk-tuk" drivers, whose nippy, three-wheeled open vehicles are the most popular public transport in cities snarled with cars have been included in the network of campaign. Dr. Surasing and his team have written a series of radio scripts. The team also produces calendars for the general public—"There's a different AIDS message on each page, and it has thirty days to sink in," says Dr. Surasing—and videos for showing on the air-conditioned, long-haul buses running daily. These feature ordinary citizens who tell how they became infected with HIV, in an effort to dispel the belief that AIDS is always someone else's problem.

To evaluate the effectiveness of such an education campaign is extremely difficult, says Dr. Surasing, but it is very significant that the rate of new STD infections in the city has slowed and that the incidence of HIV infection among sex workers seems to be stabilizing.

The reason behind the success of the campaign is the fact that it uses "peer educators", people of the same background and same social standing as their target audiences, who speak the same language, share the same values and know better how to communicate with them. "A major principle of good communication is to start from where people are, not where you think they are," says Dr. Herbett Friedman, head of WHO's Adolescent Health Programme. "This is very much difficult if education comes from professionals in ivory towers." It is the principle that has been widely recognized and applied in the fight against AIDS.

Peer educators are being used extensively in youth programmes. It has been assumed that young people not only know best how to communicate with each other; they will also be trusted by their peers not to have a hidden agenda. Youngsters are often imaginative, using currently fashionable styles of music, theatre and art as powerful vehicles for knowledge about it.

For example, Teens for AIDS Prevention (TAP), a project based in Washington, DC, emphasis to include secondary school pupils to become peer educators, and intensive training is being given to them for two weeks at lunch time and during free time between lessons. Giving knowledge about the basic facts of AIDS is the quickest and easiest part of the training. To give youngsters a deep appreciation of what AIDS means, training also includes long discussion periods, role play (often based on newspaper cuttings collected by recruits), and meetings with people with AIDS. The peer educators then devise their own campaigns for use among their fellow students. One outcome has been a catchy song about AIDS called "Stupid Cupid".

However, the imparting knowledge to young people about sex and AIDS has been a subject of controversy. Many parents and school authorities are feared that sex education might give approval—and even encouragement—to early sexual activity. "We adults deny adolescent sexuality hoping that if we don't think about it, it won't happen," says Dr. Mariella Baldo, a youth expert in WHO's Global Programme on AIDS. "But there is a great evidence that youngsters become sexually active far earlier than many adults are prepared to recognize." It is also evident from a number of surveys that sex education does *not* lead to early intercourse. If anything, it encourages responsibility: youngsters who have had sex education tend either to postpone intercourse or, if they do decide to have sex, use contraceptives.

"But it has come to know that giving information is not

enough on its own," says Dr Baldo. "If sex and AIDS education in schools is to be effective, young people must have access to condoms and to family planning and STD services. And they must learn the more and more knowledge that are so crucial in sexual relationships.

"Giving young women decision-making and negotiating skills means, among other things, teaching them to recognize the outcome of their actions so that they can withdraw from a potentially compromising situation before it goes too far," she explains.

If peer education becomes useful with young people, it is even more crucial for groups of people who are stigmatized and harassed by mainstream society, and therefore suspicious of actions from outside.

One such groups are of sex workers, whose business has been declared illegal in many countries, though often openly practised. An AIDS education campaign among female prostitutes in Accra, Ghana, was started in 1987 with the training of six women who were articulate, had leadership qualities, and were recognised by their fellow prostitutes.

They worked with the project organizers to develop educational materials which they then distributed, along with free condoms and spermicide tablets, among their co-workers in Accra nightclubs. Each woman sought out of ten of her colleagues to work with, informing them about the risks of HIV infection and encouraging them to use the condoms and/or spermicides.

The result was remarkable. Before the project started only 13 per cent of the prostitutes reported ever using condoms or spermicides. Three months into the project, a survey found that of 268 sexual contacts reported, 94 per cent were protected by either condoms or spermicides or both.

When the project was evaluated after some months, proportionately fewer of the women who had taken part tested positive for HIV than did prostitutes outside the project.

The AIDS Council of Southern Australia financially assisted an effective peer group project organized by the Prostitutes Collective of Victoria, Melbourne. Those female sex workers were involved in the project, whose trade had been driven underground by oppressive laws and police action, had been considered particularly hard to reach through other strategies. A dynamic peer educator, trained by a health centre and the Family Planning Association, consulted many prostitutes working secretly from their home, giving them information and advice about HIV/AIDS, and low-cost condoms. The Collective also published a bimonthly news-letter called *Working Girl*, with articles written by prostitutes about many aspects of their work, consisting of those related to AIDS, STD, and prevention of violence. The Collective has also been involved in negotiations with the government for changing the law.

In Ethiopia in 1989, a nurse-counsellor called Aster Wolde Kidane started a peer education project in Addis Ababa after a serosurvey revealed that many of the city's sex workers were HIV-positive. She started to encourage as a group of women working at the poorest end of the sex trade, operating out of their own tiny, back-street rooms, to organize themselves into a mutual support group.

Sister Aster supervises weekly meetings in a room behind the local community clinic. Sister Aster trains the literate women to teach the others about AIDS using colourful pictorial flip charts to stimulate discussion. The meetings have become a springboard for other activities, too. The group has started saving money with the hope of opening their own café or handicraft stall. Each week there are women spinning cotton, deftly rolling the spindle along their thighs, as one of their colleagues leads the discussion on AIDS and hands out condom supplies.

According to the women, the main advantage they derive from the group is the feeling of control and the enhanced self-respect it gives them Malfuz for example, felt very frightened and helpless when she first heard about AIDS over the grapevine. But now, she says, she now knows the means to protect herself, and finds little opposition from clients to condom use because everyone is becoming aware. "Before when we got sick there was no one to take care of us. Now we try to look after our health, and we look after each other. Sister Aster has become a real friend to us, and the group is like having a family."

Some projects have effectively used non-peer educators to reach people living on the fringes of society. In the *Pegacao* project in Rio de Janeiro, Brazil, a team consisted mainly of young psychologists provides education, counselling and condoms to young male prostitutes, particularly aged between 11 to 23 years, who hang out in the Copacabana area looking for clients.

Pegacao, which is a slang expression meaning "to cruise", started in 1989 after a survey disclosed that 43 per cent of the male prostitutes tested were HIV-positive.

The project team for the first time visited the areas where the young men operate and talked to them about their lives and concerns. "We found that to survive was much more important than to live well or to have any kind of personal care", says Paulo Henrique Longo, *Pegacao's* coordinator. AIDS was not a priority; their lives were already endangered by hunger, fear and violence. Because many did not consider themselves homosexual and indeed had wives or girl friends (who knew nothing of their activity). They did not consider AIDS messages addressed to homosexuals to have anything to do with them. Many do not even understand the written materials because they were illiterate, while others were not interested to carry leaflets for fear of police harassment or arrest.

The team realized that most of the young men were less interested and had low self-esteem. The first task was therefore to win their trust by being regularly available and showing concern for all their problems; only then would they be interested to AIDS information. Team members have become familiar faces in the area. The regular meetings are held at bars and cafes in town where discussion is encouraged and safer sex practices are explored through games. The team also works with the young men to create AIDS information materials that are useful to their lives. The objective is to build self-esteem at the same time as creating awareness. "It is very important to listen to the men rather than to talk at them," said Mr Longo, "because the factors that prompt behaviour change are different with each individual."

Pegacao's results have been remarkable. Within six months of its starting, the proportion of young men of condoms users increased from 15 per cent to 65 per cent—a figure which had gone up to 80 per cent by the end of the first year. The proportion of not condom users fell from 77 per cent to 7 per cent. The great majority of newcomers are introduced to the programme by other male prostitutes who have already benefited. *Pegacao* has been elected to represent community-based organizations on the State Commission which is accountable for AIDS policy in Rio de Janeiro.

However, the project has had little success in one area—improving the men's access to health care. This is in part because of laws that make essential minors to have an adult authorize their treatment, and in part because of the less interest of health workers to treat prostitutes.

Another programme similar to *Pegacao* operates among men who have sex with men in Australia. Called the "Sydney Beats Outreach Project", it makes contact with men in the Sydney area who are not part of the organized gay community, by going to the places where they find out sex partners. Known as "beats", these include beaches, public toilets and parks, and roadside rest-stops. The project was organized because of sociological research which revealed that although considerable behaviour change had occurred within organized gay communities, largely through community-level efforts, there were many homosexually active men who were not being reached by any of these interventions because of their social and geographical isolation.

In Scotland, a gay "outreach" project being run by Scottish AIDS Monitor (SAM) propagates AIDS information and safer sex messages in the places in Edinburgh and Glasgow where homosexually active men meet. "We have a problem here in that some of the younger men entering the gay scene see AIDS as an 'older man's problem' that does't really concern them," says Paul Trainer of SAM. Furthermore, he says, male prostitution is increasing in Scotland's large cities, much of it related to maintaining a drug or alcohol habit, and the causes of violence against homosexuals, directly related to the commercial sex scene, is rising. "However, because of AIDS, these controversial issues like poverty, drug use, sexuality, which had finished one time are being looked at again and debated."

Besides seeking out their target audience in the popular cruising spots and bars, SAM's workers try to cast their net more widely with their "Safer Sex Roadshow".

Issues of Credibility

The credibility of "messenger" is very important in growing AIDS awareness campaigns, and people with personal experience of HIV infection or AIDS are some of the most believable messengers around. "PWAs [people with AIDS] have crossed a certain threshold. They already have the disease which has feared them a lot. They've had to learn to live with that fear and many of them have transcended it. We can help people to learn to lessen the fear which blinds them to realities of AIDS," said Richard Rector, a member of WHO's Advisory Council on AIDS.

Rector is one of a growing number of people with AIDS in many countries who are active in the campaign to halt the epidemic. Besides lending their hard-earned expertise to the planning of campaigns and creation of educational material, many go personally to address groups in factories, colleges, schools. By doing so they give facts and figures, and substance to the threat, which helps break down the belief that "AIDS could never happen to me".

Their invaluable contribution has been recognized by the then Secretary General of the United Nations, Dr BoutrosBoutros-Ghali, who paid special tribute to people with AIDS during an address to the United Nations General Assembly in New York in 1992. Appealing to others to speak out, Dr Boutros-Ghali said: "It is thanks to them, thanks to their speeches that the authorities in the communities where they live should be liable to take initiatives. And these initiatives will be beneficial not only for the community of the sick; will also be very useful as a means of prevention."

Given the level of discrimination against them, it takes commitment, vision and tremendous courage for people with HIV infection or AIDS to reveal their condition. However, the benefit flows both ways: for such individuals to be active campaigners rather than passive recipients of care, pity and prejudice is life-affirming and, some are of the view that helps to keep physical illness at bay. "When you have AIDS so much is taken from you. But speaking to young people gives me back something," said Sukona Ferona. "I'm not a person with AIDS waiting to dies. I'm a person fighting for my life, fighting for understanding and fighting to educate others that yes, this *could* happen to them."

Robert Mugemana, from Rwanda and one of the first people to suffer with AIDS in Africa to commit himself openly to AIDS prevention, said: "I had no one to talk to, no shoulder to lean on when I was struck with HIV. I don't want anyone to go through that nightmare. This is the only way I can hit back at the disease which turned my entire life upside down". Mugemana died in 1992.

In the war against ignorance, imagination is the key to reaching people. However, creating awareness is not sufficient in itself to stop the spread of the virus of AIDS. Our long experiences have taught that there is no direct connection between knowledge and behaviour change. As the following chapters will show, information and education are just one part of an interdependent package of preventive measures that are truly effective only if applied together.

Eight

Caring for the Victims

The epidemic of disease is increasing everywhere like a tidal wave that has been gathering force. Nothing that is done in the field of prevention can stop the wave from breaking, as the millions who are already suffering with HIV go on to develop AIDS. In the communities where the virus started spreading first, and where AIDS has already become part of everyday life, the need for care—often over a period of years—has given a challenge to families, friends and health care systems. This chapter will describe how a few of these communities are coping with the challenge.

Caring for the People

In the Kagera Region of the United Republic of Tanzania, on the western shore of Lake Victoria, nearly sixty per cent of all hospital beds are filled up with AIDS patients. In remote areas of the land, many more people are suffering and dying of AIDS at home, without any contact with the health services. In 1990, staff at Rubya Hospital, tucked away in a hilly rural area of the region and serving many villages near about, decided to provide clinical care to AIDS patients in their own homes as a way to ease pressure on the hospital and reach those who never came for treatment. Soon a small volunteer team including two nurses and a clinician were walking on foot or go by bicycle to see patients in the villages during their off-duty hours.

But the team soon realized that simple clinical care was not enough: patients and their families also needed some kind of counselling, their fears of death, and their anxieties about their children's future. So they appealed to WAMATA, a self-help organization for people with HIV/AIDS, to counsel them. WAMATA which had been established in Dar es Salaam had recently started a branch in the Rubya area.

Under the guiding principles of WAMATA, Rubya Hospital's home-based care project got the support of an international donor, becoming, in June 1991, the country's first pilot project for home-based care.

Today, the team consists of a paid administrator and assistant, besides the health professionals, who continue to render their services free of cost. Every village in the project area has two or three village health workers (VHWs), all of them people with HIV infection or AIDS, who have been trained in basic health care, AIDS education and counselling skills. The project's eyes and ears at village level, the VHWs do what they can for people with AIDS and the problem to the professional volunteers. Patients too sick are admitted for home care to hospital, sometimes accompanied by a family member who is then taught how to care for the patient when discharged home.

Odelia Rwenyagira, a nurse-educator spends much of her time with the team in teaching home care to families and people in the community. She stresses good nutrition, the avoidance of opportunistic infections, and the number of resources to support those families struggling with sickness and poverty. "We found that a number of patients were dying not only because of infections but also they were starving," says Mr Protase Karani, the project's administrator. "After prolonged illness when they couldn't work, they had nothing to subsist on. We talked to the community and got them to see that, rather than all contributing to the burial fund as is the tradition, they should contribute to looking after people suffering from AIDS while they are still alive."

Besides the VHWs, some people who are suffering from AIDS are also involved in the project as counsellors. "They are valued easily by fellow patients because they have the same problems, and that's a big advantage in counselling," says Karani. "But working for the project helps the people suffering from AIDS too. They get a small regular income; they get supplies from the project's small farm to keep up their strength; and because they are always in contact with us, they get early treatment whenever they have a health problem."

One problem the project has identified is denial, even in the presence of debilitating symptoms.

The woman had nursed her older sister—an AIDS patient—in Dar es Salaam until she died, only to return home sick herself. However, she would not acknowledge that she, too, had AIDS. One should easily accept his condition of suffering from AIDS. "As long as they continue to deny their condition they are very hard to help," said Odelia. "Acceptance is one of the most important helping elements in treatment. But we do not force them. Perhaps after two or three visits this young woman will automatically start trust us and open up."

Rubya's home-based care programme has answered a real need. "If WAMATA had not been there I would already be dead. I had lost the will to live," says Dominic France, a father of seven who suffered tuberculosis and now works as a peer counsellor when he is not troubled by swollen legs. His testimony is echoed by many in the hills near Rubya, where people who were wasting away from lack of care, hunger and despair have been thrown a lifeline.

However, there are a number of people who live beyond the scope of the programme. Thirty-eight villages were originally involved in the home-based care scheme, but when it was chosen as a pilot project to be funded by foreign aid, the donor agency would not cover all of the villages. "Being left out of the pilot study was a terrible blow to those communities," says nurse Odelia. "People became badly demoralized and most have gradually given up the struggle to organize self-help."

The mushrooming workload on the now tiny programme imposes a heavy strain, says Protase Karani. Having started with only 23 patients, the project had registered 227 people on its books within 18 months. The demand for counselling is such that patients want the project team at the hospital should be visited if they need to talk, rather than wait for their visit. The strains are exacerbated by the deepening poverty of the community, as more people become ill and die, leaving fewer and fewer resources on which to draw.

"The village government wants to pay the VHWs. But the village does not have money, so the project is paying a small honorarium to prevent them from becoming demoralized," says Karani. "WAMATA also has a revolving loan scheme and VHWs are given priority in recognition of their work. We are also planning to provide them with bicycles because they often have a long way to travel."

The model's reliance on low-paid or voluntary work, though unavoidable in most countries may be one of its chief drawbacks. A social worker in the regional capital, Bukoba, tried to sell the idea of home-based care to a gathering of "Ten Cell" leaders—officials of the lowest tier of the Tanzanian government who are responsible for ten households each. One man, who had been listening carefully, asked: "Who is going to run this thing? This is 1992, times are hard, who can afford to work for nothing?" He sat down to a round of applause from his fellow officials, who looked expectantly at the social worker for an answer.

But despite scepticism from some quarters, home-based care programmes— reliant on volunteers from the communities served—run successfully in a number of African countries including Kenya, Zambia, Zimbabwe and, most notably, Uganda, where The AIDS Service Organisation (TASO) was the pioneer in the field. The appeal of home-based care is that it uses the traditional care network in rural Africa, the extended family, while providing professional support to help families shoulder the extra burden of AIDS. The burden falls mainly on women, who are the family's traditional care-givers.

Dr Roland Swai, head of the Tanzanian national AIDS programme, says the government is aware that hospitals could not cope alone with the burden of AIDS. "Treating chronically ill people gets cheaper the closer to the community you can deliver care," he said. "And with AIDS, care in the community is feasible. Families can do a lot if they are supported."

Women Organise to Help Themselves

In the developed world, the majority of people suffering from AIDS still look to mainstream health services for treatment. But the need for psychological and emotional support is increasingly being given by organizations outside the system—by support groups, hospices, and AIDS agencies set up at grass-roots level.

London's "Positively Women" is one such organization,

started in 1987 by a woman who found herself completely isolated after learning that she was HIV-positive. This was the only AIDS organizations in existence at that time had been set up by gay men; their perspective on the epidemic and the services they provided were naturally based on the experiences and needs of gay men. Women who came for help to this organisation were frustrated by the lack of understanding of their circumstances. Some, for example, were mothers, anxious that their children would be taken away from them or subjected to discrimination at school.

There was also a great deal of denial in the developed countries that HIV was even a threat to women. Health personnel believed to be unsympathetic towards women who wanted to be tested for HIV, and sometimes incredibly insensitive when giving them their test results.

"I was told that I was hysterical woman wasting National Health Service resources. After all 'women do not get AIDS, do they?,'' recalls Kate Thomson, a founder member of Positively Women. A former drug user, she had gone for an HIV test with the expectation that her long history of drug-taking had left no lasting mark. "When the result came back positive, the doctor just said: 'You'd better not get pregnant because we've found antibodies to HIV in your blood'." Searching the shelves of bookshops for help and enlightenment, Thomson could find no women's faces in the literature on AIDS, so she answered an advertisement in the personal column of a feminist magazine for contact with seropositive women.

Most of Positively Women's early members had been infected through drug infections, and the organization found it hard to get taken seriously or to attract funds because of prejudice about women drug users and concerns about their little work experience. But as the group became more effective, it received handsome financial support from the British Government. In 1990 it was able to move from cramped spare rooms to its own spacious premises.

The old house in a remote area of London has been renovated by using glass, wood, bright paint, and lots of green plants to create an environment that is restful and uplifting to enter. "We realised it was important for people suffering with their own problems to have somewhere nice to come to, rather than some grimy basement," says Thomson. "One thing that also comes up again and again is the importance of having a safe space, a place where a person doesn't have to hide her true identity or feelings, a place where women no longer have to live a lie." So, from the outside, the house is just one of the row with nothing to indicate its purpose.

Positively Women's clients come from different social backgrounds and circumstances. They include university students, women in advertising, housewives, journalists, nurses, teachers and sex workers. Their joint struggle with HIV and prejudice tends to bring social barriers down, but due to the diverse needs of people there are a number of diverse support groups to choose from. For example, there is a special group for African women who intend to discuss experiences particularly to their communities. One-to-one peer support is available for those women who are not ready to face a group, or for times of particular crisis.

The project provides a telephone help-line and make the best effort to reach out to socially isolated women, for example, minority or immigrant women, or those in prison. Clients are given information and advice about welfare and benefits, and housing problems. And the organization gives professional massage to satisfy the deep need of HIV-positive people for physical contact. Support for women at national and international level is another aspect of the group's work; members are often called on to speak in public or to supply technical assistance to other agencies.

An organization like this must have a clear idea of what it wants to achieve and why, says Kate Thomson. "You must decide how much you can handle because staff who take too much responsibility on their shoulders soon burn out. It's very important that there are mechanisms for staff support in place, because the work is emotionally very draining—helping people through sickness and death and facing the anger of their families."

Future of Children

In London, as elsewhere, women with HIV infection are in deep concern, about who will take care about their children when they get sick or die. The problem is most acute for single women.

"Positive Options" was set up in August 1991 by Barnardos, one of the UK's oldest and biggest children's charities. Research had revealed that some family issues were being neglected by existing AIDS organizations. "Generally speaking, we found a dearth of awareness about child-care issues among specialist HIV/AIDS workers, while child-care workers had very little knowledge about the issues surrounding AIDS," says Joan Fratter. Even when volunteers looked after children for sick parents, it tended to be an temporary arrangement, with few if any safeguards for the children's welfare.

Positive Options has launched a scheme which sends child-care specialists on two-year assignments to work in existing AIDS organizations for the children in AIDS-affected families. One such specialist is working with Positively Women; another is with Turning Point, a drugs and AIDS project; and a third works with families affected by haemophilia and AIDS.

A second scheme is the Planning Scheme, which operates out of the organization's own premises. A specially trained child-care officer helps parents with HIV infection to ensure the long-term future of their children. It also includes who will care for them when the parent is sick or hospitalized, or simply in need of a break.

The best for the children is to be cared for by a relative when the parents die, says Joan Fratter. But the stigma of AIDS and the incessant fear of rejection make it difficult for parents to explore these issues with anyone. Most of the people have kept their status secret even from their families, and some are inhibited from talking to them because of the financial result of taking on extra dependants. Dealing with these crippling inhibitions is often the first task of Positive Options.

Other options include fostering and adoption, and here all kinds of issues need discussions says Fratter. "For example, one of our clients was a single mother with a very young child. She knows that she had another two years of life ahead and she intends to meet and get to know the family who would adopt her child. This is unusual but not unique. It means that a child can be helped by someone who cares and who has shared memories of the parent. Some continuity in life is preserved."

However, it is all not very easy. Because it is not just a matter of who will take up the burden of care. There is also the question of how to prepare children for bereavement, and child-care officers say the parents to make some personal record of their lives, and of their times with their children they spent. Some parents have made video and audio recordings for their children, others have compiled photo albums or books of memories, and some have gathered objects of sentimental value into a box.

"Children generally want to know about themselves like what time they were born, the first words they spoke and when they took their first step. And they also want to know about the history of their families," said Fratter. "We try to make parents aware of these needs of their children. But it can be a painful process and we let parents work through these things at their own pace."

Because of the expanding need for such a service and the pressure of work on the small staff, Positive Options sees its role as complementing the other kinds of long-term support given to people with AIDS by counsellors, social workers and doctors.

Undoubtedly, the availability of funds is an important factor when it comes to the care and support of people with HIV infection and AIDS. But as these few examples show, it is not the solely factor. Some of the most humane and caring systems have been established in the world's poorest countries, while some of the worst physical and psychological suffering has been allowed to occur in developed countries to spare. For effective programmes to be put in place, what seems most necessary is the determination to fight the stigma of AIDS that, in many places, still hides ordinary human faces and terrible human suffering.

Nine

Fighting AIDS

Unlike other epidemic diseases such as cholera or measles, HIV infection does not cause sudden death, but remains hidden for many years after it begins to spread. This characteristic, coupled with the fact that AIDS involves behaviour that many societies condemn, has been a great hurdle in setting up programmes to challenge the epidemic. In the early days, too, the general debate about AIDS was mired in confusion, blame, prejudice and fear that it tended to paralyse governments.

However, with strong support from individuals and groups across the globe—and assistance from WHO and other international agencies—virtually every country now has launched an AIDS programme. (See tables in Annex for information on and from national programmes). Most are complied by the objectives and principles of the global AIDS strategy (23).

National AIDS Programmes: The Umbrella

There is threefold task of a national AIDS programme:

— to formulate the policies, information campaigns, and health and social services that people need to protect themselves from HIV infection (see panel, next page);

— to meet the gradually widening need for care as those who are infected with HIV go on to develop AIDS.

— to plan for and cope with the adversel effects of AIDS.

Besides, the national programme ensures coordination and a technical support structure for all those who are working in the field. These include government officials from the health and other different sectors (see Annex, Table 4) like blood bank staff, nurses in primary health care clinics, members of the media and business communities, private individuals, and a wealth of non-governmental organizations—some of them are international, most at the grass roots of their own countries.

The umbrella today is working on a wide range of activities, like poverty, political instability and war. A good example of what is happening in many developing countries is provided by Malawi. One of the world's poorest nations, Malawi is host to hundreds of thousands of refugees from war-ravaged Mozambique, and is in the grip of one of the worst AIDS epidemics in Africa.

Here, the AIDS programme works with and through many different social and community organizations to impart information, care and support to people at the grass roots. Women's groups and young people belonging to the Malawi Young Pioneers have received AIDS information and training in peer education. Muslim leaders are also being trained in workshops on AIDS prevention and on the counselling of people with HIV infection or AIDS, and the subject is also discussed at every Friday mosque meetings. Paramedics have been taught about AIDS prevention and enlisted to distribute condoms. And the business community has also been drawing into the network with training courses in AIDS prevention and condom promotion.

The Mass-medias also play an important role. Newspapers and radio programmes cover AIDS issues, emphasis particular efforts to address fears and correct misconceptions; local choirs take part in AIDS song contests; popular musicians write and record music with AIDS themes; drama groups perform AIDS plays; and AIDS comics are produced for kids.

Most of the countries are showing trivial interest as far as the prevention and controlling of AIDS is concerned. In Swaziland, for example, an organization "Mantalk" efforts its best to make the dialogue between men and women on sexual matters. In Ethiopia, where a short while ago unmarried women were denied access to contraception, condoms are now available in a wide variety of outlets from bars and street kiosks to petrol stations. And in parts of Thailand, agreements is being made in discussions between the AIDS programme and policemen that drug users can attend treatment clinics without fear of arrest. Thus users are not forced underground where they are cut off from information and other HIV prevention services.

AIDS prevention is still very much a journey through uncharted territory, and programmes are changing and adapting in the light of experience all the time. For example, a number of countries—including Australia, Brazil and the United Kingdom—tried honestly to instil fear as a way of encouraging people to change their behaviour. Posters and newspaper advertisements showed coffins being lowered into the ground, for example, or depicted death in the shape of the "Grim Reaper". But this has left adverse impact on the infected people rather than encouraging them. Besides, it had led to increasing anxiety in people who had little power to protect themselves.

Thailand, too, used fear in early campaigns to try to change behaviour. Posters showed close-up shots of some of the more explicit and distressing opportunistic infections. But the focus changed in the light of experience. "Thailand's AIDS programme is very active, very dynamic, and very quick to learn and adapt as necessary," says Steve Kraus, GPA technical officer stationed in Bangkok. "It has become something like a university for the study of AIDS prevention in the region. Practically every country sends its representatives here to observe how the Thai programme operates. The reason everyone knows about AIDS in Thailand is that the society is very open here in comparison to others region.

Comprehensive Prevention

In the early days of the epidemic, national AIDS programmes and community groups attempting to stem the tide of HIV spread had no choice but to experiment. There was no way to know with certainty what prevention approaches would work best, especially for convincing people to change their sexual or drug-taking behaviour. And there was no guarantee that promoting condoms, say, or giving drug users clean injection equipment, would not somehow rebound and result in more rather than less unsafe behaviour.

Today, based on a decade of experience, we know that some prevention approaches work and others do not. What does not work is making people unduly fearful, or harassing them, or alienating them with threats of compulsory testing. What does work is to create a supportive social environment in which people can be informed about the whole range of options for safer behaviour, encouraged to assume responsibility for their own behaviour, and given the necessary social and health services support.

The current consensus is that a basic HIV prevention package includes at least the following:

- Condom social marketing; that is, the promotion and distribution of condoms in the general population
- Treatment of the conventional STDs, because of their role in facilitating HIV transmission.
- AIDS education in schools to slow transmission to young people, who now account for about half of all HIV infections.
- AIDS information through the mass media, aimed at the general population.
- Promotion of condom use by prostitutes and their clients.
- Maintenance of a safe blood supply
- Neele-exchange programmes for injecting drug users.

There is now solid evidence that these prevention approaches reduce HIV transmission without encouraging risk behaviour. What is more, they can work in a matter of months, not the years or even decades once believed necessary for changing human behaviour.

Grass-roots Players

As already has been stated, a vital—and, in some places, a dominant—role in national action against AIDS is played by non-governmental organizations (NGOs). In number of cases, they were first to respond to the distress of communities.

"It is hard for a Ministry or for civil servants to work with so vast populations which do not officially exist," says Dr Hakima Himmich, professor of medicine at the University of Casablanca, Morocco, who founded the first non-governmental AIDS organization in the Maghreb.

Professor Himmich, who was a member of the national AIDS programme, started the Moroccan Association Against AIDS (*Association marocaine de Lutte contre le SIDA, ALCS*) when she came to know about the cultural and religious constraints on the government programme. "There were certain aspects of AIDS prevention that could on no account be done by the Ministry of Health—in particular the work among female sex workers or among homosexuals. None of the groups with risk behaviour could be touched by a Ministry," she said. "For example, it has not yet been admitted in Morocco that prostitution exists. People *know* it takes place, but its existence has not been admitted officially."

She recognized, too, that stigmatized people are feared of government authorities and reject any programme with an official stamp. She started ALCS in 1988 to disseminate information, encourage behaviour change, and offer care and support to people with HIV/AIDS. The organization is in particular committed to the protection of human rights and dignity and fighting discrimination.

Among its many activities, ALCS produces leaflets, runs an AIDS helpline and runs free, anonymous testing centres. It has also launched safer-sex programmes (including condom distribution) among female sex workers and gay and bisexual men. By showing respect for society's feelings and traditions, it has broken down some barriers to the prevention of AIDS in Morocco. Today, the Minister of Health is Honorary President of the association.

While this community initiative has been recognised by the Moroccan Ministry of Health, some non-governmental organizations run in an atmosphere of official suspicion or indifference. But GPA's Deputy Director, Dr Dorothy Blake, emphasis that close collaboration between national programmes and NGOs is essential for a strong campaign. "The two have complementary strengths. While governments have overall authority and can provide leadership and sometimes funds, NGOs are more in close contact with communities at grassroots level," she says.

Above all, many NGOs work in remote areas, so they are well aware of the gaps and shortcomings in the provision of services. It also makes good sense to pool rather than to duplicate resources and effort." GPA promotes what it considers an invaluable partnership by encouraging national AIDS programmes to devote at leat 15 per cent of their budget to NGO activities.

Better Tools in Store?

Encouragement of behaviour change, condom promotion, STD care, the technology for HIV prevention is limited. And the medicines available for people who are already infected are inadequate. AIDS is still an incurable, fatal disease. Can we expect to science for better tools for prevention and care?

When the first case of AIDS was recognized in 1981 the medical world was mystified. Yet within four years scientists had established that they were dealing with an infectious disease; they had isolated the casual virus, developed tests capable of detecting infection, and established the main routes of transmission. Never before has so much been learned about a new disease in so short span of time.

An unprecedented effort continues to be made by biomedical researchers to uncover more of HIV's secrets, and to find a preventive vaccine and a cure. Meanwhile, social scientists are working to improve methods for helping people to achieve and sustain behaviour change in the difficult areas of sex and drug use.

Preparing for Vaccine Trials

While virus infections are not easy to cure, they have traditionally been good candidates for prevention with the help of vaccines. Small-pox, eradicated thanks to a vaccine, was a virus infection, and so are measles and polio—fatal diseases against which most of the world's children are now immunized.

But early aspirations of developing an HIV vaccine gave way to deepening doubts as scientists felt they were up against an extremely complicated virus, which changes incessantly and varies strikingly from one part of the world to the next.

"Smallpox is very stable; there is only one type of the virus, so the vaccine developed against it was effective everywhere in the world," says Dr Jose Esparza, chief of vaccine development at GPA. "Influenza is not durable. The virus often changes every year, which means that a vaccine effective in one epidemic period is not essentially effective in the next. But though influenza changes over time, it's basically the same virus across the globe. HIV is much more complicated because it varies both temporally and geographically. So we have many different virus strains—all of them evolving—in various parts of the world."

Development of an HIV vaccine has also been stymied by the unusual immune system reaction to infection with this virus and the dearth of a good animal model in which to test candidate vaccines. Chimpanzees—to date, the only animals of potential use in HIV vaccine development—are a rare and expensive species, and their use in scientific research is controversial.

Despite these hindrances, a number of candidate vaccines have passed the preclinical phase of trials, consisting of studies of their safety in animals, and have entered small clinical trials in humans. Only large-scale efficacy trials, including several hundreds or thousands of volunteers, will show if these vaccines really protect people against HIV infection.

Following the great variability in HIV strains, vaccine trials will have to be conducted not only in industrialized countries but in the developing world also. Steps are being taken in cooperation with WHO to ensure that at least four countries—Brazil, Rwanda, Thailand and Uganda—are ready to join the global vaccine development compaign and begin large-scale trials just as soon as safe and appropriate candidate vaccines are available. These sites were chosen by an international committee of experts who were seeking:

- Study populations with a high incidence of HIV infection, who have the most to gain from successful vaccine development.
- Relatively settled populations, due to the need for regular and long-term follow up of trial participants;
- Populations with comparatively well-developed health and laboratory facilities;
- Locations where there would be popular and political support for trails.

To ensure that the chosen locations will be able to cope with the vaccine trials, WHO has embarked upon to strengthen their infrastructure, by upgrading health and research facilities and training local scientists as essential. A worldwide network of laboratories has also been established to isolate local HIV strains for use in vaccine and drug research. Trials conducted at these sites will have to conform to the highest ethical standards, respecting volunteers' individual rights and community traditions. Elaborate health education, including the distribution of condoms, will continue throughout the trials—even though this may cause slow down of research findings.

But it is not wise to expect a quick end to the HIV epidemic with a vaccine. Even if efficacy trials are launched by the mid-1990s, a vaccine cannot even deliberately be on the market before the year 2000. And at best a vaccine will only complement other prevention methods. For one thing, vaccine programmes take a prolonged time to approach most or all of the target population. It took national immunization programmes close to two decades to receive global coverage rates of 80 per cent with BCG and vaccines against diphtheria, whooping cough, tetanus and measles—and, unlike an HIV vaccine, these did not have to be developed from scratch. Another issue is that no HIV vaccine can be 100 per cent effective. As AIDS is a fatal disease, vaccinated people will probably want and need to use other means of protection as well.

In other words, there is no getting round the fact that prevention endeavours will have to continue to rely on safer sex (through behaviour change and the use of condoms and other barriers to HIV) and prompt, substantial treatment for conventional STDs.

New Light on Old STDs

The now clear link between the rapid spread of HIV infection and the presence of other STDs (see Chapter 3) has focused attention on a badly neglected public health problem. Every year, at least 250 million infections other than HIV are transmitted through unprotected sexual contact, yet the control of STDs carries a low priority in most of the world. Treatment facilities are often not adequate and unwelcoming, and the stigma connected with STD makes many people reluctant to acknowledge symptoms and seek treatment. This is particularly true in case of women, even though their complications tend to be more severe in comparison to men—pelvic inflammatory disease, infertility, and ectopic pregnancy, which can be fatal.

In addition to many STDs—again, especially in women—are

relatively symptom-free in the early stages, so that people are unaware they are infected.

While the conventional STDs make easy the transmission of HIV, HIV can make these STDs harder to treat following immune suppression. So it is urgent to the task of controlling STDs. Fortunately, several measures aimed at prevention—education and information, promotion of condoms and other safer sex practices—are the same for both HIV and the conventional STDs. And the target audiences are similar. WHO is therefore encouraging STD programmes and AIDS prevention programmes to cooperate, or even merge in some cases.

There are still major obstacles, including making STD services more user-friendly, and motivating people to get early treatment. But one problem may now be solved. "Up to now it was said that you needed laboratory tests to diagnose STDs in women. But there are many countries where there is not a single laboratory which can do that," says Dr Peter Piot, GPA's Associate Director who is in charge of STDs. "So we have found out a method for diagnosis based on just asking a few questions and doing some examination. For instance, a recent change of sex partner raises an individual's risk of infection immensely. By eliciting information which gives you a risk profile, and by doing a simple examination, you can get a properly accurate diagnosis."

Protection Methods for Women

Experience of the last five to ten years has made it clear that women are less able than men to protect themselves from the sexual transmission of HIV because condom use requires —at the very least—cooperation from men.

Proper STD care should go some way towards reducing women's vulnerability, but science keeps other hopes as well. Endeavours are under way to develop "barrier methods" that can be used by women when they are not in a position to get their partner to use a condom, or when they otherwise wish to control the prevention process.

The "female condom"—essentially a pouch that women insert into the vagina before intercourse—is now on the market in some developed countries. Initial studies suggest that it is acceptable in some settings to women at high risk of HIV infection, like prostitutes. Though the female condom has been developed and recommended for contraception, studies will soon be began to determine its efficiencies in preventing STDs. Another issue is that the female condom is expensive and has been approved for single use only. Research is under way to find out if it continues to be effective if washed and reused.

A further drawback of the female condom is its visibility. There is an urgent need to find barrier methods that women can apply, if necessary, without their partner's knowledge.

Spermicides are one feasibility. Intravaginal spermicides have been used as a female-controlled method of contraception for the past few decades. As they also have antimicrobial properties, these products likewise decrease the risk of acquiring some STDs and they have been shown, at least in test-tubes, to inactivate HIV. Its drawback is that spermicides, especially when used many times a day (as in sex work), have been found to cause vaginal irritation, and this might actually increase the risk of HIV transmission. The WHO is giving top priority to determining the safety and protective efficacy of existing spermicides, and developing a non-irritating product that will protect against HIV infection and other STDs—perhaps even one without spermicidal activity, for women who wish to conceive a child.

Societies Under the Microscope

With prevention riding above all on behaviour change, social scientists are conducting research to find out the best ways of achieving this.

"In the early days of the epidemic, we were severely handicapped in absence of basic information about patterns of sexual behaviour and patterns of injecting drug use, but great deal has been learned since then," says Dr. Peter Aggleton, chief of social and behavioural studies for GPA. "In a way, AIDS made it legitimate to study sexuality and sexual behaviour. A great experience has been gained in only a few years. We now know that sexual behaviour is considerably more divergent than was imagined before. Homosexual as well as heterosexual behaviour, for example, is present in every societies and is part of the normal repertoire of human sexual expression. By adopting and using this diversity as our starting point, we can plan more effective interventions."

Behavioural research has also examined the ways in which individuals understand themselves—as opposed to how society might define them. For example, in several parts of the world it is general to receive gifts and perhaps money in exchange for sex, yet only sometimes do the women and men concerned consider themselves prostitutes. More commonly, to receive such favours is simply a way of life. Prevention strategies that make erroneous assumptions about how people see themselves will be confined in their effectiveness.

So will prevention strategies that fail to take account of "commonsense" beliefs about health, illness and disease. It is often believed that there is a direct link between knowledge and behaviour: once people are provided with the medical and scientific facts, they change their behviour. Such simplistic beliefs are now known to be untrue. Everyday beliefs about diseases such as AIDS, which can distort the impact of health education messages, need to be taken into consideration –"creatively", says Dr. Aggleton—in public information campaigns, peer education, and counselling.

Research is under way, in WHO and elsewhere, into the ways in which households and communities have responded to AIDS. Information from this work will throw light on how best to support affected families and communities. It may lead, too, to an explicit understanding of how to combat prejudice and discrimination against infected individuals and against groups popularly supposed to be at risk.

But social scientists have to work regularly in an atmosphere of suspicion and mistrust. Governments often fear that the information turned up by researchers may paint a less than favourable picture of how a society really operates. In some places, endeavours have even been made to limit or prevent social and behavioural research. This is a challenge that has been taken up by WHO and others. If social scientists are permitted to carry out their research, the AIDS prevention activities they help design are bound to gain in effectiveness.

Ten

AIDS Prevention Among Drug Injectors

The attempt to control the spread of HIV among people who inject drugs is greatly complicated by the fact that the taking of drugs, other than tobacco and (in most countries) alcohol, is almost globally condemned. In a number of countries, strict and harsh laws and diligent policing drive drug users beyond the reach of health and social services into a twilight world of secrecy and fear, largely neglected by the rest of society.

AIDS necessitated a new urgency to the debate about how best to deal with drugs, highlighting the age-old controversies and moral dilemmas surrounding this issue. But, Jo Kittelsen, a Norwegian specialist in programmes for injecting drug users, says, "the good news is that drug injectors are able and willing to change their practices to lessen the risk of HIV infections if they get the right support."

Today, more than a decade into the epidemic, there is substantial evidence that several different approaches work, all of them based on a non-judgmental approach towards drug users and practical support to help them avoid getting infected with HIV through contaminated injection equipment. For instance, programmes for the distribution of clean needles and syringes have been used quite successfully in several countries including Australia, Canada, the Netherlands, New Zealand, Sweden, and the United Kingdom; while bleach distribution is more popular in those places where needles and syringes are too costly to give away.

There has been strong political opposition to these harm-reduction programmes in several countries on the grounds that they supply the "wrong message" to drug users and undermine the war on drugs. However, the police often tolerate unofficial syringe exchanges, such as those in Tacoma, Washington, and San Francisco in the USA. Most important, the evidence contradicts the claim that such programmes result in increased drug use. In Amsterdam, for example, neither the total number of drug injectors, nor the frequency with which individuals inject, has increased since syringe exchanges were opened.

The first syringe exchange in the United Kingdom was set up in 1986. Since 1987, when the government gave its approval to the strategy, more than 200 syringe exchanges were established. A triumph of pragmatism over prejudice, the exchanges have become the cornerstone of the endeavour to arrest the spread of HIV among injecting drug users in Britain. The fact is that AIDS is a deadlier threat than drug use. Exchanges do not overlook the use of drugs, says Gerry Stimson, Director of the London-based Centre for Research on Drugs and Health Behaviour, but they identify the need to work with people who continue to inject drugs with a view to reduce HIV transmission.

Syringe exchanges are not always readily accepted by the local community, however, so they require to be carefully planned and tailored to meet the needs of both the target audiences and the neighbourhoods in which they live.

Trial and Error Successful in Glasgow

"Our first effort at operating a syringe exchange was not a success," says John Cameron, coordinator of Glasgow's programme. "The places were picketed for six months by local residents who believed that crime would increase, that their streets would be littered with used needles, and that people would be dealing and injecting outside. Resultant, injecting drug users were a rare species at that first exchange."

After 18 months, the project was still seeing only 15 to 25 people a week out of a drug injecting population estimated at between 8000 and 12000. One mistake was committed that the syringe exchange was housed in an unattractive building that maintained very little privacy to visitors because it was exposed; furthermore, it was inaccessible to several parts of the city. So the first place was closed and the programme moved to the heart of the communities where it was most required. There, it got swift success. Within three months of opening its doors, one exchange had more than 150 clients, most of whom were local people who used it continuously. Moreover, it had a return rate of used equipment of more than 100 per cent as clients started bringing in for safe disposal syringes they had bought at pharmacies.

By the end of 1991 there were six syringe exchanges in Glasgow, with others planned. The number of attendance at the exchanges that year was around 21000, during which some 190000 syringes were handed out, with a return rate of 130 per cent.

"It's important to prepare the ground carefully before starting a project," says John Cameron. "I start by visiting and talking to everyone, from members of parliament and the local council to the community groups." Receiving the confidence of the community is particularly important, he says, because drug injectors naturally fear that such a project will expose them to the police (drug use is illegal) or to social workers, who might evict them from their homes.

One of Britain's earliest exchanges setup in Easterhouse, a grey high-rise estate sandwiched between motorways on the outskirts of Glasgow, where a number of unemployed young people stand on exposed street corners. "The drug problem here is all lie with hopelessness and helplessness. Half the people on this estate have no jobs to do" said John Cameron, leaning against a table in the brightly lit community exchange one April evening, while a steady stream of clients passed through.

Opening plastic carrier bags before the health worker seated at a big table, clients showed what used equipment they had brought back before dropping the package into the big bin. They asked the workers what kind of clean needles they like, how many condoms, and whether they wanted bleach to clean their needles in an emergency. And for those who were worried about their health or other worries, there were specialist staff—including a community nurse and psychiatric nurses—available down the hall.

"My belief is that the problem exists, you can't neglect it, and it's my duty to try to prevent people harming themselves," said a nurse who has special insight into the community in which she works because she grew up there herself. "One lad I saw tonight had an abscess and a mottled leg he was in danger of losing. But some people just like to have someone taking care of them and showing them respect."

John—a thin, nervous, blond-haired man age around twenty one who said he had been injecting drugs for 10 years—came in with two friends. The three were enthusiastic clients of the exchange. "Before the opening of this place the life was really dangerous," said John. "You could't get variety of equipment you wanted, so you used to share, and to use a needle until it was like an old nail and your veins collapsed." He shook his head at the memory. "Now I can get new needles and special plastic containers that keep them safely out of the reach of my kids."

Like John, several drug users are family people, and the fear that their children will be taken away is one of the things that keeps them away from drug programmes.

At Easterhouse there is a security guard at the door to ensure that no drug dealing could be possible on nearby—a situation which would undermine public support for the project—and clients are not allowed to inject on the premises. "We took these decisions because we can't be liable for clients harming themselves or overdosing. You know what rules are necessary as you go along," says Cameron.

Effectiveness of Syringe Exchanges

Syringe exchanges in the United Kingdom have now been operating long enough for the strengths and weaknesses of the strategy to be clear. According to Gerry Stimson and his colleagues from the Centre for Research on Drugs and Health Behaviour who have kept an eagle eye on the UK programme, syringe exchanges have been particularly effective at reaching people not approached by more conventional drugs services. Around 60 per cent of new clients at syringe exchanges say they have had no prior contact with any other drug project.

Exchanges answer a real need because the majority of clients are worried about scarcity of needles and syringes, and are not in favour of sharing because of fear of AIDS. They have also proved to be effective entry-points to other services, providing previously isolated drug users a place to receive help and advice with a number of other concerns, from health care to housing, finance and the law.

By 1991, levels of needle-sharing in the United Kingdom had felled to between a half and a third of the level found before the syringe exchange programme was introduced. Furthermore, needle-sharing levels are lower than those in countries, such as the USA, which do not have official syringe exchange schemes.

On the minus side, syringe exchanges in the United Kingdom are not working to capacity, and they have failed in particular to attract younger people, women, ethnic minorities, and those who have recently started injecting. Furthermore, they are having little success in encouraging safer sexual behaviour, largely because the people who staff the exchanges, like their clients, find the subject of sex hard to bring up.

In the final analysis, syringe exchanges are only part of the answer to a highly complex problem, and in the United Kingdom there is a range of services and education initiatives. The stress on these programmes is to minimize the harm done by drug injecting—particularly the threat of HIV infection, but also such injection-related problems as abscesses, hepatitis B and endocarditis, all of which have sharply lowered with the decline in the re-use of dirty needles.

As a first step to harm reduction there requires to be a shift away from emphasis on law enforcement, and towards making treatment and health and social services more available.

Scope of Comprehensive Prevention

We now know what works when it comes to preventing HIV infections: a basic package consisting of condom social marketing, STD treatment, AIDS information and education in schools and through the mass media, condom promotion for prostitutes and clients, safe blood supply, and needle-exchange programmes for drug users, all conducted within a supportive social environment. But what impact can prevention be expected to have?

AIDS prevention in a sense is more powerful than, say, cancer prevention. Preventing one HIV infection now will not simply prevent one death from AIDS, as preventing one incurable cancer would prevent one cancer death. Preventing an HIV infection now will help break the chain of epidemic transmission, averting the risk that the infected person will unknowingly pass the virus on to others who in turn might infect a still wider circle of people in the familiar "epidemic snowball".

This is the reason the impact of a basic HIV prevention package would be very large indeed. WHO has calculated that if comprehensive prevention were applied in all developing countries beginning in 1993, it could *halve the number of new adult infections* during the rest of this decade. This means saving the lives of almost 10 million people—over 4 million in Africa, over 4 million in Asia, and about 1 million in Latin America. But the ultimate saving in human lives would be even bigger because the main impact of reducing the epidemic snowball would be seen later, well into the twenty-first century.

Thailand Tackling Drug Problem

After more than a decade of having working with people dependent on drugs, the Health Bureau of Bangkok Metropolitan Administration (BMA) is really aware of how difficult it is for recovering drug users to bring them to a social environment in which they face all the pressures, frustrations and hopelessness that led to their drug dependence in the first place. There are three out of four people who complete detoxification courses at the BMA's narcotics clinics are back on drugs within months, a pattern that is fairly consistent worldwide.

Since 1985, both the BMA and a number of non-governmental organizations have been continuing programmes for ex-drug users to help them find employment or to give them skills training that will allow them to work for themselves. Developing such efforts became a matter of urgency when it became clear that drug-related AIDS was a serious problem.

Between 50,000 and 100,000 of Bangkok's 8 million people are dependent on drugs. The great majority inject heroin. The BMA established 17 narcotics clinics after the extent of drug use became apparent in the 1970s—a period of sharp social and technological change that, Thai experts say, alienated many ordinary people. In 1988, serosurveys among clients of the clinics showed that HIV was spreading through the drug injecting population at a phenomenal rate. The first survey, got practised in January-March 1988, showed a seroprevalence of 15.6 per cent—a figure that increased to 42.7 per cent by the time of the second serosurvey, just six months later.

These alarming figures prompted the BMA to make available special courses on AIDS to all clinic staff, and today AIDS programmes among injecting drug users consist of regular peer group counselling sessions for those who attend the clinics of their own accord—an average of 2000-3000 people a day—as well as outreach into the community to make contact with those not yet motivated to seek help.

"Rather than just giving instructions, we try to make group discussions to talk about their own concerns and to discuss the problem of AIDS themselves. That way we can know about their habits and the best ways of helping them to change," said a social worker at one downtown clinic.

Adorned with a colourful flip chart giving the facts about HIV/AIDS, packets of bleach and a supply of condoms, she was organising a session with six young men and women. All watched interestingly as she showed how to mix bleach in the suitable proportions and clean needles and syringes. Then came the discussion of safer sex. Smiles lit their faces as the social worker unrolled a condom and demonstrated how to put one on.

Among their peers, the clinic clients appear very ready to discuss their behaviour, the need for change, and how hard it is to alter one's lifestyle fundamentally. Here, too, the staff realise the need to minimize the harm of drug use, in the face of AIDS, and not to insist on abstinence. The clinics now give a number of treatment options ranging from a 45-day detoxification course based on replacing heroin with methadone in gradually diminishing doses, to developing safer ways of administering heroin (e.g., by smoking), to meditation to slash the need for a chemical high. "Addiction is a symptom of many causes, so there must be many responses," says Dr Suphak Vanichseni, Deputy Director of the BMA's health department. "We're making research to determine the best forms of treatment. But addiction is not like malaria, which we can diagnose with one kind of pill."

Staff at the clinics take great pains to find the programme that is best suited to each client, and to involve families in counselling too. In the meantime, clients are encouraged to avoid needle-sharing or at least to inject more safely, after cleaning their equipment with bleach. "We believe there is not too much reliance today on the 'shooting galleries' where dealers inject drugs for their clients practising the same equipment on many people", says the Director of the BMA's Health Department, Dr N. Choopanya.

The success of the clinic-based programme depends largely on an agreement with the police that they will not arrest clients visiting the clinic—a fear that prevents several drug-takers from coming forward. This is not something that can be agreed once and for all, but a subject that required constant negotiation with the police, says Dr Choopanya.

Community health workers, and a group of peer educators with personal knowledge of the drug scene, contact drug injectors who do not come themselves for treatment, providing them with information, bleach and condoms. Mrs. Boouma Sua Wong, who runs a bakery in the working-class district of Suan Oy, has been a village health volunteer for over five years. Her face is known in the small, slatted wooden houses and narrow streets of the suburb where her task has been to encourage pregnant women to go for antenatal care, to weigh babies, advise on feeding, and remind their mothers to have them immunized. She provides first aid, too, from the short supply of plasters and pills provided by the health centre. But over current years Mrs. Sua Wong has been most preoccupied with spreading awareness of AIDS.

Besides her first aid kit she carries information leaflets, packets of condoms, and bleach, as she accumulates people around her at any opportunity to talk, demonstrate, and hand out supplies. Does she know of any people who take drugs in her area? She nods her head vigorously. "I encourage them to attend the narcotics clinic," she says. "But if they're not interested, I show them myself how to use bleach and send them away with some packets. I usually provide for them extra bleach and ask them to show their friends, because there are many drug users here who won't show their faces."

Mrs. Sua Wong thinks her work does have an impact in her

small corner of Bangkok. "People are very worried about AIDS now and they hear what I say, though they didn't believe it at first. But not many people come to ask for condoms, so I go outside to visit people I think are at risk in their homes," she says.

Measuring the overall impact of the BMA's AIDS prevention programme among injecting drug users is extremely difficult, but serosurveys hint that the prevalence of HIV among clients of the narcotics clinics has stabilized at around 40 per cent.

However, the programme has had little achievements with peer education than anticipated. By 1991, several hundred former drug users had been trained in health education workshops and given a small stipend for finding out hidden drug users to provide them with AIDS information, condoms and bleach. They were supposed to inform each month to the clinic staff, but many failed to turn up after a few months of work. "The drop-out rate is about 50 per cent," says Dr Suphak Vanichseni. One problem lying, in fact, is that many get involved in taking drugs again when they come in contact with other users, a problem that drug outreach projects in various countries have faced.

Another programme found it hard to recruit former drug users for outreach as such people did not want others to know they had used drugs, and they did not want reminders of their previous situation.

Personal Experience: A Valuable Commodity

In spite of the problems highlighted by Thailand's experiences, people who have themselves taken drugs play vital and valuable role in the fight against AIDS in many countries. They work as expert consultants to organizations framing out programmes and information materials, and as peer educators and outreach workers where their own experience makes them more readily accepted and respected than anyone from outside the drug-taking community. But the collective experience of such projects in a number of countries suggests that strong support, close supervision, and realistic expectations are very important to success.

"An important lesson we've learnt is that ex-users and current drug users are often willing to take on this accountability because they see AIDS as a serious problem. But getting a project off the ground can be a difficult process," says Jo Kittelsen. "People who are active users or who have just come off drugs are often very sensitive people, and they're not used to being in control or to interacting with public or health officials on an equal footing. On the other hand, having a new source of income and a structure to life can sometimes help people reduce their dependence on drugs."

There are grounds for hope. Some studies have revealed high levels of AIDS awareness among drug users, an increased demand for sterile equipment, involving an increased use of bleach, and a reduction in the sharing of needles and syringes. There is proof, too, of changes in the social etiquette of drug taking in some countries so as needle-sharing is no longer seen as normal behaviour, but as an exceptional response to any emergency.

But in spite of all that has been learnt about successful strategies for prevention, the stigma tagged to drug taking continues to frustrate efforts to control the drug-related spread of HIV. In various countries, politicians continue to stress criminal prosecution over social support, driving drug users underground and out of the reach of AIDS prevention programmes. Until they know that drug taking is a social problem, rather than simply a legal and policing one, and until tried and tested methods of prevention stressing harm reduction are used, vulnerable people—drug users and their partners, and their partners in turn—will continue to die.

Eleven

Promoting Safer Sex

The rules of the game have changed with the development of AIDS. Communities are under threat from such a fatal disease which have suddenly become deadly, such as unprotected casual sex.

But encouraging safer sexual practices means negotiating a path through the minefield of taboos, prejudices and prohibitions that surround sexual activity in almost every society — a task made more tough by the problems associated with the condom, at present the only mechanical barrier to the sexual transmission of HIV.

The male condom has a long history both as a contraceptive and as a barrier against disease. Ancient Egyptians used sheaths of animal membrane to stop pregnancy, and in 16th century Italy the anatomist Fallopius designed a linen sheath to protect against syphilis. The measure itself is said to derive its name from a Dr. Condom who made sheaths for King Charles II of England in the 17th century.

Today, in the absence of either a vaccine or cure, latex condoms have a potent role in the fight against AIDS. It is important to give people the full range of substitutes for preventing sexual transmission: abstinence, mutual fidelity, non-penetrative sex, and intercourse protected by a condom. The knowledge of national AIDS programmes in past ten years shows that condom use is often the method selected.

Unfortunately, condoms have a serious image problem. In different parts of the world, they are particularly associated with prostitution, casual affairs, and STD prevention. People believe condoms reduce intimacy and impair sensation. For instance, sex with a condom has been compared to eating a sweet with the wrapper on.

In developed countries, the sheath's popularity declined sharply with the advent of the contraceptive pill and intrauterine device (IUD). Barring Japan, where 45 per cent of all couples—69 per cent of family planning users—depend on condoms, their use by married couples in the developed world has declined to between 5 per cent and 15 per cent. In developing countries, only 4 per cent of married couples use condoms, and in sub-Saharan Africa the figure is often below 1 per cent.

There are also cultural hindrances to the condom's use. "In sub-Saharan Africa, we have an expression: skin to skin", says Dr Faustin Yao of GPA's Youth and General Public unit. "A condom interferes with the traditional 'mystical' meaning of sexual intercourse as it blocks skin contact and prevents the man's sperm from being deposited in the woman. Interestingly", he adds, "women appear more prepared than men to get rid of this contact and use a condom if it means avoiding a fatal disease—perhaps because they are the ones who care for the sick and dying, and death for them is more vivid, more real."

Technical problems serve to undermine confidence further. In various countries people say that condoms tear—especially those purchased from open-air markets, where they have been exposed to sunlight, tropical humidity and pollution. The risk of damage to a condom is greater in anal intercourse than in vaginal or oral sex. And when condoms are applied as contraceptives they have a failure rate of about 12 per cent in the first year, before couples become experienced. It must be emphasised, however, that the effectiveness of a condom depends on how consistently it is used: *the most common cause for its failure as a contraceptive is the couple's failure to use it every time they have intercourse.*

In several countries, family planning associations have taken up the challenge of developing the condom's image, promoting it as a device that has no side-effects, is safe for young people to use, and requires no medical supervision. In Colombia, the Profamilia organization planned to increase condom sales by 50 per cent through an intensive advertising campaign. Elsewhere, too, family planning associations have launched imaginative programmes to promote condoms. Some have set aside "male hours" at their clinics; some have established AIDS telephone hotlines (particularly popular with young people); and some have developed special projects catering for the counselling and condom requirements of men who have sex with men.

Some, like the Planned Parenthood Association of Ghana, made a collaboration with trade-unions and business management to provide regular training sessions and disseminate condoms in the workplace. The Association has also established special clubs for men in some rural areas. The clubs are mainly recreational, but they use the regular evening gatherings to discuss health and sex and to give condoms. They also encourage fathers to talk to their sons about sex and advise them on how to reach the subject.

However, it would not be wise to put the responsibility for condom promotion on family planning programmes alone. Some family planning staff are not interested to take on AIDS work, or worry that the association with disease might affect the image of family planning. Without extra staff, specialist training, transport, equipment and outreach, family planning programmes could not possibly integrate AIDS prevention into their normal work.

Condoms as a Commodity

One most effective way of getting condoms to those who need them is through "social marketing": the application of commercial sales and marketing techniques to a public health problem. "Using the private sector and its distribution networks makes condoms easily available to people in ways that public health programmes usually cannot," explained Carlos Ferreros, who has directed condom social marketing programmes in various countries. "You can buy Coca-Cola, beer, cigarettes just about anywhere. No matter how bad the roads are, no matter how rural the village, there's always some villager getting goods out there".

Successful social marketing largely depends on having the right product at the right price in the right place, with the right promotion. It has been used for decades to promote family planning, oral dehydration for diarrhoea, STD treatment and other public health views. With the advent of AIDS, social marketing has moved condoms into some of the remotest corners of the world, particularly in Africa. In Zaire, where 35 million people are widely scattered across a land with very poor communications, condom distribution increased from less than half a million in 1987 to 8 million in 1990 and 18 million in 1991 as a small army of salesmen working on commission basis took boats, trains, trucks, and, where necessary, walked to reach remote villages with their products.

In Ethiopia, condoms are distributed almost exclusively through family planning clinics, which served married couples mainly. Condoms were one of the less popular methods of contraception: in 1987, only about 20,000 were distributed across the nation. But in 1991, just one year after Ethiopia's social marketing programme was launched, sales of condoms shot up to 6 million. In spite of logistic problems caused by the civil war, condoms were available in near about 100 towns and villages. And soldiers from the army of Mengistu Haile Mariam, the former Ethiopian ruler, got a take-home pack of AIDS information and condoms on demobilization.

Some years ago, you couldn't mention the word condom," says Teshome Wakene, an enthusiastic young marketing representative with Population Services International (PSI-Ethiopia), which runs the country's social marketing programme. "At first, people were hesitating about asking for them at street kiosks, pharmacies and such places. But I tell them that condoms are just like medicines; they save us from disease and save our lives. And now no one would be shy about asking for medicine if they needed it. Now everyone talks about them".

Teshome spends most of his working day on the road, making the rounds of small shops, bars, hotels and even petrol stations, which he has considered as good places to reach the long-distance lorry drivers whose way of life makes them specially vulnerable to HIV infection. Along the narrow streets of the *mercato*—one of the biggest and busiest markets in Africa—he ducks into the small rooms of prostitutes. With friendly greetings, he opens his blue suitcase to hand out packets of "Hiwot" condoms, (the word means "life" in Amharic), AIDS information material, and a key-ring/condom holder with the Hiwot logo, as a free gift for his customer.

Teshome and his fellow marketing representatives sell the condoms at 25 US cents for a packet of four, and their customers re-sell those condoms for 30 cents. The small profit made by the retailers gives them an incentive to stock the product.

One of Teshome's best customers is Mrs Askala Tekale, owner of the Blue Nile Bar in a square in central Addis Ababa. A large, friendly woman, she sits in the bar's backyard under a washing-line of lacy underwear and tells why she is so devoted to condoms. As a housewife, she purchased the bar in the early 1980s to make some extra money. But, she chuckles, selling beer without sex is not very profitable, so she engaged a number of young women to sell drinks and started renting out rooms behind the bar to customers. When she found that pregnancy among the bar-girls became a big problem, she started promoting condoms.

"Mrs Tekale already had stickers on her walls saying 'no sex without condoms' when we first came to have discussion our selling campaign with her," says Teshome. Today she talks about AIDS with her customers, who are generally teachers, students and office workers. She has put Hiwot dispensers beside the bar and in the public toilets and says that opposition to their use has all but vanished as awareness of the epidemic has grown.

PSI-Ethiopia also has launched a high-school programme. Operating through the different special-interest students' clubs, it reaches around 120,000 young people in 27 schools with AIDS information and condoms. A student representative at each school takes supply of condoms from PSI and pays the programme back from the proceeds of previous sales. According to Zenebework Bissrat, the programme officer, at first there was some opposition to the idea of giving AIDS information in schools, as parents and education authorities chose to avoid the evidence that young unmarried people are sexually active. "Virginity is much prized," she says, "and adults were blinding themselves to the fact that teenage pregnancy is on the increase in Ethiopia and youngsters are contracting HIV."

The job of PSI-Ethiopia's sales force is helped largely by the national AIDS programme, whose imaginative "Fight AIDS Together" campaign trains representatives from a whole range of grass-roots organizations—from community and church groups to professional associations and government departments—to act as peer educators. The information campaign also take the help of mass media and popular culture such as drama, songs and poetry to educate and inform the people. The result is high levels of awareness about HIV/AIDS, particularly in urban areas, and high demand for condoms. The national AIDS programme has also organized several campaigns targeted at sex workers in some of the busier towns.

The chief problem for Ethiopia's social marketing programme has been keeping up with condom demand and ensuring continued supplies to customers even when political instability obstruct the marketing network. In the busy market town of Nazareth, an effective peer education and condom supply programme for sex workers almost waned in late 1991 when civil war reached the town, community health posts were destructed and looted of equipment, and peer educators fled home to their villages.

Targeting the Most Vulnerable

Constrained by lack of money, bad roads, lack of transport, and short supplies, some countries decided to concentrate their attention on condom promotion among people thought to be most vulnerable to HIV infection, rather than to cover the whole population. One such country is the United Republic of Tanzania where, in September 1989, the African Medical and Research Foundation (AMREF) launched a project focussing on long-distance truckers and their sex partners.

Christopher Mwaijonga, a Health and Behaviour Officer with AMREF, visits the truck stops along the busy highways connecting the Tanzanian capital, Dar es Salaam, to neighbouring countries. Many truck stops have become satellite communities by drawing people from remote villages to trade, catch transport, or provide services to the passing traffic. Truck drivers and their crews spend their leisure hours here resting in the myriad brightly lit bars and small hotels with such names as "The Just Imagine Hotel", "The Paris Centre" and the "Welcome Good Time Shop". Drink, companionship and casual sex are abundantly on offer.

"We faced some opposition at first from church leaders who thought promoting condoms would also promote promiscuity," says Mwaijonga. "But I told them that the time would come when priests would see only empty benches on Sundays if we didn't recognize reality and take the steps required to control the spread of HIV."

Mwaijonga is liable for recruiting candidates from among the bar girls and bar proprietor to be trained as peer educators, and for supervising and supporting them after training. To be effective, candidates must have to seek the approval and support not just of their co-workers, but the hotel proprietors and local community leaders also. And, once they are trained, they need recognition as valued and expert members of the AMREF team, for their job is not easy and stressful. "Some of the girls I work with are very resistant to my messages," says Siasa, leaning against a bar stool in the sticky heat of a Tanzanian summer night. "Their approach is that they know me well, they grew up with me, and what can I teach them?" But Siasa, one of the most committed of the project's 20 peer educators, knows her colleagues take in what she says about AIDS because she has seen the demand for condoms rise steadily.

When women go into bars to talk about AIDS they sometimes meet with bitter hostility, even violence, from truckers, who resent being singled out by the AIDS campaign. "I don't think we have done our best to avoid discrimination against truckers," says Dr. Ulrich Laukamm-Josten, Director of AMREF in the United Republic of Tanzania. "We have talked with a number of truckers about their role played in spreading HIV infection in Africa without due regard to their sensibilities. The life of a trucker is full of frustrations, and at night when they stop they drink and want to have sex as a way of compensating for all this. They are understandably hostile if they think someone has stigmatized their way of life and is trying to interfere with it."

But over the years, the kindly, non-judgmental manner of Christopher Mawijonga and his colleagues has earned respect and softened opposition. Many of the trucks have AIDS and condom stickers displayed on cabin windows. And today, education sessions in the bars are generally crowded, lively occasions for discussion and questioning. "We have a rule that educators mustn't give just any answer to a query. If they don't know something they must say so, and tell the inquirer they'll find out," says Mwaijonga.

Distribution of condoms at the truck stops increased from 60,000 between September and December 1989 to almost 700,000 between January and April 1991. Besides, the proportion of women at the truck stops who reported using condoms rose from 50 per cent to 90 per cent over the 16-month period to mid-1991. For men, the reported rise was from 54 per cent to 74 per cent. Guest house proprietors report greater demand for condoms and say that truckers sometimes ask about the availability of condoms before get booking a room.

Laukamm-Josten believes the project will prove effective far beyond the highway out of Dar es Salaam. "When truckers return back to their village, they take along new ideas. If they've been using condoms they'll take some back home and word will get around that they're using such things. This will leave a profound impact on their peers," he says. "Eventually they'll run out of condoms and not be able to get any at the village store. So, because they know that unprotected sex is dangerous, they will reduce their sexual activity for a while until they get more supplies or leave again for work. Gradually a pattern of using condoms or saying 'no' to sex will be established. We have no proof that this is happening, but a lot of anecdotal evidence. This is the kind of behaviour change that is going to be required to stop the epidemic."

An evaluation of AMREF's truckers project found that a number of the women were reportedly unable to insist on condom use with reluctant customers, some of whom offer extra money or threaten violence to get unprotected sex. This is a common and global problem that consistently undermines the effort to contain AIDS. AMREF is an effort to provide special training to help the women stand up for themselves.

Redressing the Balance of Power

At a massage parlour in an Asian resort, a woman in a short dress and fishnet tights stands up and turns to face her colleagues who was sitting in broad light on the dance-floor combing their hair, appraising their make-up with tiny hand-mirrors, or laughing softly with their friends. Sex Worker Number 236, as a card was pinned to her dress with this number she is about to demonstrate how a condom packet can be opened with long finger-nails without tearing it, and how to put it on a customer in a pleasurable way. She bents her head and giggles at the peal of laughter from the floor as she strokes the condom onto an outstretched finger with exaggerated movements.

But the lesson being taught to the young women on the dance-floor is being undermined by the bar owner, who sits watching the demonstration with a small group of customers. "What goes on between the girl and the customer is their own business," she says. "The management doesn't insist on condoms or interfere with the transaction even if a customer gets rough with a girl. There's very competition in this town."

It was to change working practices like these, and to generate an environment supportive of safer sex, that Thailand's national AIDS programme conceived the "100 per cent condom campaign". The principle is that all sex establishments in an area should follow a "no sex without a condom" policy simultaneously, so that customers cannot threaten to go to the brothel next door to avoid condoms.

The campaign is managed by local governments, which are liable for convincing the owners of all sex establishments in their area of the AIDS threat and explaining the scheme. Brothel owners are told that the women will be checked properly for STDs, and that there will be penalties, ranging from fines to closure of the premises, for non-compliance with the condom rule. Besides the prostitutes and their clients, key players in the campaign are the health sector, which provides STD services, health education and condoms, and is accountable for monitoring the incidence of STDs; and the police, who act on information from STD clinics to penalize establishments whose workers continue to contract such diseases—evidence that condom use is less than 100 per cent.

Brothel owners also have an interest in keeping to the rules, says Dr Surasing, an enthusiastic advocate of the campaign. "Having several of your girls off work because of STDs costs money and gives the brothel a bad name. Those kinds of problems could be avoided if condoms are always used."

The campaign has had its problems. Initially, for example, too little efforts were made to inform the sex workers about the campaign, or to involve them in decision making about how to implement it—both of which would have ensured better cooperation from these key players.

After some of these problems were solved, the campaign was expanded and by early 1992 it was operating in 66 of Thailand's 73 provinces. Surveys started to assess its effectiveness have found that STD prevalence has delined sharply, from 13 per cent to less than 0.5 per cent among sex workers in Samut Sakhon, for example, where lot of condoms distributed in brothels increased almost fourfold within a month of the campaign's introduction. In Chiang Mai, Thailand's northern province which has been particularly adversely affected by AIDS, condom use among sex workers is reported to have rose by 50-60 per cent since the start of the campaign.

Thailand's "100 per cent condom campaign" has been an initiative from the top. "In various countries, the first to recognize the need for condom use and to take decisive steps to authorise women have been women themselves," says Priscilla Alexander, an expert on prostitution. In many countries as Australia, Ethiopia, and the Philippines, to name just afew, sex workers have formed collectives based on reciprocal support, and followed community-based policies whereby condoms are compulsory and customers who resist are not served. Such organizations also give heavily stigmatized and marginalized sex workers a way to raise their concerns and press for their rights—notably an end to oppressive laws and law enforcement practices. Such laws drive prostitution underground and thereby make every aspect of HIV/AIDS prevention more difficult—from holding educational gatherings, for creating information materials targeted at sex workers, to carrying condoms. For example, if Mrs Tekale or the sex workers of Ethiopia's *mercato* feared arrest or prosecution, they would not be really willing to cooperate with PSI's social marketing campaign, which draws attention to their activities.

The most successful "safer sex" projects among prostitutes include those that do not focus just on AIDS but also concern themselves with the other problems of their daily lives, like discrimination against their children, police harassment and violence by clients.

"It is important for funding bodies and educators alike to

understand that AIDS cannot be treated only as a single and separate issue in the sex industry," says Andi Sebastian of the Prostitutes Collective of Victoria. "AIDS is one risk in a series of risks. It is one cause to be terrified amongst many causes to be terrified. It is one problem to deal with amongst many. AIDS is an occupational health and safety issue, it is an economic factor, it is a personal concern and it is one of an infinite kind of factors which marginalise sex workers in the community".

This is a message that holds true beyond the world of commercial sex, too. Until AIDS prevention projects are based on a full understanding of the reality of people's lives and the driving forces behind their behaviour, they have not very good chance of success.

Part V

The Challenges

Twelve

Health Care Practitioners: Rights, Duties and Liabilities

This framework of the legal rights, duties and liabilities of health care practitioners related to the risk of HIV infection and AIDS is based on experiences that have evolved in the Common law jurisprudence of a developed country. The jurisprudence and legal institutions of other legal systems, consisting of those based on Civil law, Roman-Dutch law, and religious law, may require the principles addressed here to be applied somewhat differently. Similarly, the chapter may reflect circumstances of health care professional licensure, discipline, supply and funding that differ among countries. It definitely reflects experiences of legislation, litigation in courts and access to lawyers' services that depart from perceptions in other settings. Its purpose is to focus on issues that are likely to arise in different legal and health care cultures, and to recognise a number of key legal questions that are likely to be asked, rather than to present uniform answers. It is expected that the parts that are not relevant to any particular jurisdiction are balanced by parts that are, and that the discussion will help to understanding through comparisons and contrasts that readers can make with the legal and health care systems with which they are most familiar.

Health Care Practitioners

In conventional western analysis, the primary health care practitioners are physicians, consisting of specialists in such areas, for example, as virology and urology, and general practitioners, who may include family practitioners in areas where family practice is not considered a speciality. Nurses are an obvious parallel cadre of health care practitioners, and, evolving from their traditional role as handmaidens to physicians, public health nurses and nurse practitioners are achieving status in some areas as independent professionals in health care. They have powers to prescribe medications derived from the right to make clinical diagnoses. Similarly, midwives are emerging from the supervision of physicians and the nursing profession in few areas to be valued as professionals who practise under independent licensure. Psychiatric and other social workers, lacking any basis in medical sciences as such, are also health care practitioners, in that their services help to patients' and families' health in the sense in which the World Health Organization characterizes health, namely as "a state of complete physical, mental and social well-being and not only the absence of disease or infirmity."

Traditional healers and, for example, birth attendants significantly practice health care in many areas. They often serve where western-recognized practitioners are not found, but also practise as substitute health professionals where the latter are available, sometimes practising with them as reciprocally respectful colleagues. A legal differences remains, however, between academically qualified, professionally licensed health care practitioners such as physicians and nurses, and practitioners who have got no training that complied with widely recognized standards, who accept allegiance to no enforceable code of ethical practice, and whom the law would not hold to higher standards of knowledge, proficiency and care than are expected of a layperson. The legal rights, duties and liabilities of those who bear health care services differ, depending on their status and the expectations they reasonably create of the availability and ability of the services they offer.

Where HIV infection is concerned, important health care services may be performed, neglected or repudiated by professionals who are not health care practitioners. School teachers deserve to inform pupils of dangers of infectious diseases in general, consisting of their modes of transmission, and HIV and other sexually transmitted diseases in particular. Ministers of religion may also give preventive health care information, not just in moralistic condemnation of sex outside marriage but for example by reinforcing the moral imperative of practising safer sex, in marriage and outside, where risk of HIV infection arises. Similarly, industrial personnel and concerned staff training officers dealing, for example, with adolescent and slightly older recruits to a workforce coming from rural areas may inform and alert newcomers to the dangers of HIV infection, mainly from sexual interactions and drug use. Such practitioners fall outside the analysis of this chapter, although the ethics of their actions in promoting, failing to promote and hindering promotion of HIV prevention programmes are amenable to evaluation comparable to that applied to health care professionals.

Health care practitioners who are not routinely trained to face unusual dangers from HIV infection. Dentists, for example, may be exposed to patients' blood, and if their equipment is not properly sterilize they may transmit infection between one patient and another. Laboratory technicians, clinic waste disposal personnel and staff who clean operating theatres after surgery who are not exposed to patients as such are in contact with their body fluids that may be a cause of infection, to themselves or to others their employing institutions have legal liabilities to protect.

Accordingly, there are some if any health care practitioners whom the risk of HIV transmission does not affect, in doing their professional or work-related activities, or in protection of their personal health or of that of their family members. Self-interest and the interests of other dependent on them require them to maintain vigilance and skill, and to be aware of developing knowledge and experience of HIV spread and prevention.

Due Awareness

The legal duty to maintain professional awareness in good repair has a direct and an indirect component. The direct component concerns those to whom health care professionals owe legally enforceable duties of care, notably their patients and patients' family members but also their colleagues and staff members. Duties to the former, who suffer means of self-protection against unknown risks, are somewhat greater than duties to the latter, who may be hoped to take due precautions and therefore may help to any injury they suffer. The indirect component concerns professional liability to maintain educational and technical fitness to practise as a condition of continuing or renewed licensure, and liability to licensing authorities' disciplinary charges of misconduct and unprofessional behaviour arising from lack of relevant knowledge of HIV infection and prevention.

Even where professional licensing authorities do not make obligation on licensees to attend at continuing professional education courses as a condition of licensure, professionals are expected by the courts and by their own professional associations to keep abreast of the literature and developing perceptions and standards of performance in their field. For example, the Australian Medical Association's June 1991 policy on AIDS says that "medical practitioners have an ethical and professional obligation to inform themselves about all conditions they care for and to behave in a scientifically accountable manner" (Art. 1.2) and that "Both this tradition and this obligation must be maintained throughout the AIDS epidemic" (Art. 1.3).

Where professionals charge fees for services, an implied term of the fee-for-service contract is that professionals maintain the standards of awareness and proficiency that encourage patients to place their health care in such professionals' hands. Like fee-for-service practitioners, salaried health care professionals and others with no contractual links to the patients they treat are bound by the law of torts or delict, since the duty of care that must be observed under the law of negligence is made by courts as a matter of policy and of keeping faith with popular expectations.

How widely professionals should inform themselves of matter pertinent to their practise, and how promptly they should include new understanding and awareness into their clinical or public health care practise, are more complex matters. Not every new experience is sound and scientifically established, and not every prevailing practice that a study shows ineffective or counter-therapeutic need be abandoned. There is a legal view that a practice supported by a "responsible body" or "respected minority" of practitioners of a health care profession satisfies the standard of care set in negligence law. The responsible or respected minority rule allows maintenance of a traditional therapy that most practitioners have discontinued for persuasive reasons, and also, at the other end of the evolutionary spectrum, adoption of a promising new procedure not incorporated into general patient care. Accordingly, prevailing understanding, for example, of the safety of a procedure, need not yield instantly to reasoned criticism based, for example, on the evident liability to transmit HIV infection. Equally, a reasonable belief that a new practice is effective to resist viral transmission may be held in preference to a management of proven efficacy, even though later evidence and clinical experience may discredit the innovation. It is ultimately in the hands of the courts to determine if a practice, whether old or new, majority or minority, satisfies legal standards of competence, and ineffective or harmful practices will quickly be found unsatisfactory.

Awareness is central to clinical diagnosis of HIV infection, public health care concerning, for example, safety of the blood supply for transfusion, and to implementation of clinical and community health protection practices. Unawareness that, by good fortune, does not result in HIV infection to a patient or compromise community health will usually escape legal liability in a direct sense. Liability for negligence requires proof that failure to meet the legal standard of care caused calculable injury. Responsibility for breach of contract could arise without proof of resulting injury, but an award of damages is usually related to material loss and calculable pain and suffering. However, indirect legal responsibility may arise when a health professional's licensing authority finds a degree of unawareness that constitutes professional misconduct or improperness to practise. The mandate of governmental licensing authorities is usually protection of the public, and such authorities are not limited to acting *ex post facto*. They have authority and ethically bound to take preventive action in reasonable anticipation of the individual or community health disaster that a practitioner's lack of due awareness threatens.

Popular political, religious and other hindrances to awareness of the risks of HIV infection are not usually amenable to correction by the legal system. Health professionals' standards of practice are legally checked up at the clinical level by litigation and at the level of public protection by professional regulatory authorities appointed under legislation and acting according to due process of law, and they are thereby held to higher standards than non-professionals. Beyond the risks implicit in their own practices, they are legally bound to be aware both of risks implicit in patients' known and reasonably interpretable circumstances and lifestyles, and of the incidence of HIV infection among different categories of the populations they treat. Practice based on crude mischaracterization of AIDS and HIV infection as disorders of only homosexual and bisexual men, commercial sex workers and people who use drugs by injection, will fail to satisfy legal standards where viral infection is prominent among the heterosexual population, and the epidemic prevalent among women of adolescent or older reproductive age. Not every country or region supplies accurate data of HIV prevalence from reliable screening programmes, but global, national and regional data provide a basis of relevant awareness. The law requires professionally competent responses to the knowledge that exists, and incorporation of that knowledge into practice, even if that knowledge later proves imprecise, inaccurate or inadequate.

The Diagnosis

HIV infection is diagnosable by laboratory detection of properties of body tissue samples, specially antibodies to the human immunodeficiency virus, but AIDS itself is not a disease. It is a syndrome that explains various manifestations of individuals suffering compromised immune systems due to viral infection. Suspicion of a patient's suffering from AIDS can be confirmed or refuted by testing for HIV infection, but a health care professional may be legally obliged to recognize a patient's symptoms as feasibly being AIDS related. Some conditions may be strongly indicative of dangerous HIV related disease, but other conditions such as unexplained wasting of body tissues should serve to put health care professionals on notice that a patient may be infected with HIV. The repeated linking in the literature of such situations as Kaposi's sarcoma and *Pneumocystis curinii* pneumonia with HIV infection, particularly when such conditions are recurrent, should also alert health care professionals to the need to consider the HIV diagnosis. Whether pulmonary or extra-pulmonary tuberculosis, invasive cervical cancer or, for instance, cytomegalo virus retinitis should sound the same alarm will depend on its general prevalence in the patient's community or relevant sub-population, and whether a diagnosis of HIV infection can reasonably be discounted. A high possibility of familial cervical cancer, for instance, may explain a woman's condition in detail to make HIV infection a less probable diagnosis.

The legal duty of competent diagnosis is chiefly owed to the patient, but the relationship between physicians and patients, and courts may find between other health care professionals and their patients or clients, is legally considered particular. The law recognizes that, in such a special relationship, a duty is owed to whoever the health professional actually foresees, or reasonably should foresee, would be responsible to be injured by his or her act or omission. Accordingly, if a professional should perceive that a patient may be HIV infected and is responsible to infect another person such as a sexual partner, the professional owes a legal duty to both the patient and also the partner at risk of infection to offer the patient diagnosis, due counselling and advice. If the patient refuses diagnosis and related services, the health professional's duty to the partner maybe satisfied, but the professional may nevertheless have a power, if not a duty itself, to warn the partner of the suspected risk (see 8, below). No duty may arise, however, when a woman patient who has been completely informed takes the risk of transmitting HIV infection to a child *in utero*, if the only preventive means is non-conception or abortion, due to general legal policies not to punish voluntary conception and not to compel advice or performance of abortion. Others to whom health care professionals owe duties are those at risk of infection by professionals' use of unsterilized or inadequately sterilized equipment, and those who may foreseeably be exposed, perhaps inadvertently, to patients' body fluids when they could be a source of HIV infection.

Health care practitioners have diverse degrees of familiarity with those they treat. Some know well patients' family histories, personal characteristics and lifestyles, while others have only a transitory and nominal interaction with them. General or family practitioners of medicine may have a depth of personal knowledge of patients that specialist consultants do not achieve, and, for example, hospital emergency room personnel may know nothing beyond the immediately presenting conditions of those for whose care they suddenly become liable. In several cases, however, professionals can ask questions of patients, and interpret the significance of their answers. This is potent in diagnosis of HIV infection because, when a clinical diagnosis is not available, or negative, a social or lifestyle diagnosis may be relevant. During the incubation period due to infection, a patient may prove negative when tested for viral antibodies, but nevertheless be capable of transmitting the infection to others. The risk of transmission may be perceived by a health care professional who has knowledge of a patient's lifestyle.

Epidemiological data reveal the risks of HIV infection in different segments of societies, including for instance adolescent girls from rural areas who take employment in large cities and are subject to sexual inducements and depredations by more worldly men. Similarly, married men may have sexual encounters when on business or other travel, and acquire HIV and other sexually-transmitted infections they transmit to their wives. Accordingly, a health care professional should be aware of the many ways in which HIV can be acquired and transmitted, and want information from patients that may indicate HIV infection as a possible diagnosis of the conditions they present.

Universal Precautions and Due Care

Because many patients may have to be treated before a diagnosis of HIV infection can be made, and infected patients in the beginning stages of incubation may not have developed the antibodies that tests detect and therefore provide a negative test result although they may transmit infection, health care practitioners cannot await an HIV positive test result before they take adequate precautions against infection. These are often explained as "universal precautions". They are "universal" in the sense that they need to be taken in connection with every patient and every other person to whose body fluids a health professional may become exposed. They are not essentially uniform, however, but may be calibrated to the degree of risk of exposure. The risk of a surgical patient's spurting blood, for example, requires more precaution than moving a sealed sample container. The former includes use of eye protection as well as protective cover of exposed facial and other skin, while the latter requires little if anything more than routine gloves and use, if available, of shatter-proof containers that open without spilling contents.

Hospital emergency room personnel and health care professionals who go to treat trauma patients where accidents take place should ideally be educated, trained, equipped and mandated to exercise universal precautions, but a number of professionals will be exposed to the risk of infection in circumstances that are less than fully secure against risk of HIV infection. For example, women giving birth and newborn babies infected *in utero* may present irreducible minimum risks of viral transmission to health care and related attendants. The goal of professionals' self-protection must always be to minimize infection risk without prejudicing patients' care. Similarly, employers of health care practitioners often have legal obligations, as terms of contracts of employment and/or under occupational health and safety legislation, to make available employees with a safe work environment and with secure conditions of employment. Education, training and equipment may have to be made available as part of this obligation, although staff who refuse or fail to accept them may alone assume the risk of suffering infection.

In several examples, courts will have to decide whether the precautionary services available to practitioners satisfy legal standards of care. The ways in which inadequate resources are allocated and priorized among limitless demands of, for example, patient care, community preventive education programmes, institutional, clinical and out-patient services, staff training and provision of staff equipment may be called into question. Courts are often disposed to defer to governmental or other public agencies on the level of protective services that should be available with a view to determine legal standards of care owed to staff, so that what level of precautions should be given to health care practitioners will be influenced by what public authorities actually provide. If this is woefully inadequate, however, or where courts are prepared to bound public agencies to reallocate budgets as judges indicate, courts may be prescriptive in establishing the extent to which health care practitioners must be facilitated to take universal precautions. At a minimum, courts may expect some guidelines to contain the spread of hepatitis from patients to health facility staff to be observed and enforced.

Precautions are also important for protection of patients, health facility employees who do not attend patients directly, and others at risk of so-called "nosocomial" or institutionally spread HIV infection, such as through use of unsterilized or inadequately sterilized equipment. Improper sterilization of medical apparatus and instruments may pose obvious dangers of spread of HIV infection, and equally obvious areas of potential legal responsibility for negligence. More problematic is infection through contamination of the supply of blood for transfusion, since no system can guarantee safety from infection. Lack of any effective screening of donors may create legal liability, but when a system exists, no liability will arise for its unavoidable imperfections.

The problem of multiple use of single-use or "disposable" medical devices is becoming commonplace as health care practitioners and institutions, even in relatively wealthy areas, cannot afford to use precious or scarce devices on only a single patient when the devices remain physically capable of re-use, particularly following sterilization. The use of devices in such a way that contradict or depart from their manufacturers' instructions raises legal questions, specially under the laws of liability for negligence and of product liability. Due care must be taken, for instance, against excessive dilution of solvents employed in sterilization, operator error in the sterilization process and damage to the safe and proper use of devices caused for instance by solvents, and surface scratching of materials that causes crevices in which contaminated debris may lodge. Courts may be called on to set the standard of care that warrant reuse of devices that manufacturers and suppliers describe as designed or intended for single use, when reuse may cause spread of HIV infection from one patient to another. When scarcity of essential devices compels reuse, however, health care practitioners and facilities may invoke the law of necessity to excuse their risk-taking in use of the only means available to them to treat patients in emergency. Outside cases of emergency, the law of consent may make essential that prospective patients for whose care reuse of devices supplied for single use is proposed be so informed, so that they can exercise choice in terms of the convenience, immediacy and risk of the care they accept.

Treatment

In several countries, health care practitioners in general have not proven better informed or more enlightened than members of the lay public about the sources and spread of HIV infection, and have shared the dysfunctional misperceptions and negative stereotypes that prevail among the general population. One result has been a denial by some practitioners to treat those they know are HIV infected, or who they think, for example from their lifestyle, may be HIV infected. A refusal by health care practitioners to take care to people in need of their services on the ground that such people may be sick seems perverse, and a negation of the conscientious commitment to their calling that health care practitioners often profess and that justifies public esteem. Disregard of the ethical duty to treat the sick gives rise to legal responsibility in different circumstances. Practitioners employed in a contractual relationship with a health care facility, for example, may violate terms of their contracts by failure or denial to render care to those eligible to receive it from them, provided that facilities have observed mutual duties to provide an adequately safe work environment. It is explicit from the nature of their functions that health care facilities cannot provide those they engage with work settings free from the risk of infection, and the undertaking of minimization of risk is not an assurance of its elimination.

The legal claims of those wrongly refused health care depend on their circumstances. A tendency exists, not least among health care practitioners, to describe those eligible to receive treatment as "patients", but a vital legal difference is drawn between those who are patients in law and those who are seeking to become patients. Where a diagnostic or therapeutic relationship exists between a health care practitioner and a person, that person is a patient, and a refusal or failure to render appropriate care exposes the practitioner to legal liability for negligence, abandonment and/ or breach of contract. Similar responsibilities may arise where the patient's legal relationship is not with one or more particular practitioners but with a special hospital or other health care facility. Patients cannot make demand every or any special treatment even when the costs of treatment can be met, since practitioners and facilities may exercise judgment about what treatment is indicated by patients' circumstances and what treatment is contraindicated in patients' best interests or would be futile. Nevertheless, they are legally obliged to provide care that is indicated, and to refer patients elsewhere for indicated care that they lack the specialization to provide. The standard of care that patients are entitled to be offered is finally determinable by a court, as an implied term of the contract of care and/or as an element of the law of negligence. Some courts are reinforcing patients' rights to appropriate care by invoking the concept of fiduciary duty, which binds health care practitioners to conscientious duties to keep faith with the appropriate expectations of persons in need whom they have agreed to assist through their superior knowledge.

Where no prior relationship exists between a person who wants to become a patient and a special health care practitioner or facility, no duty binds the practitioner or facility to enter such a relationship. Some facilities may in emergency treat persons they do not accept as patients, and must then conform to a legally determined standard of care, but the legal status of facility outpatients differs among jurisdictions and must be studied in detail to determine whether or not they are patients like those legally recognised as such. Some health facilities and practitioners have legally binding funding or other agreements with governmental or other public or private agencies, consisting of religious and charitable foundations, that require them to admit designated people, such as residents of specified areas or people in evident need of emergency treatment, as patients. Denial or failure to treat such eligible people will violate those agreements, but it is a matter of law in each jurisdiction whether such third party beneficiaries of agreements get legal rights to enforce them and to sue upon their breach.

Several licensing authorities of health care practitioners and professional associations, health care facilities and health service funding agencies put obligations of non-discrimination that preclude practitioners and facilities from declining to accept and treat persons on the bases, among others, of any physical or mental disability they may have. Further, jurisdictions at municipal, state or provincial and federal or central levels of government may have legally enforceable human rights codes that do not permit discrimination on grounds not only of race, sex and religion, but also of physical or mental disability. These are inspired by international human rights treaties that give legal force to the United Nations' Universal Declaration of Human Rights of 1948. For example, the International Convention on Economic, Social and Cultural Rights recognizes rights to the highest attainable standard of physical and mental health and to the benefits of scientific progress on the basis of non-discrimination, and the International Covenant on Civil and Political Rights apparently includes rights to non-discrimination on the basis, for example, of sexual orientation. Similarly, the Convention on the Rights of the Child recognizes children's rights to health care.

Practitioners and facilities that refuse to accept people as patients on the grounds of their actual or presumed HIV infection may be in breach of laws that give effect to countries' domestic implementation of these international commitments. Action may be taken by persons denied services, but alternatively they may complain to police or other public authorities, which may consider the matter to transcend a private wrong between the person and practitioner or facility, but to affect the public interest. Public prosecutors may feel obliged to become involved, and in some jurisdictions actions may be taken, for civil or criminal remedies, by an officer as high as an Attorney General or Minister of Justice. At stake is not just the denied right to proper health services of the person requesting care, but the integrity of the country's commitment to principles of non-discrimination against disabled persons, and the interest of its commitment to its international human rights duties. Indeed, a state's failure to work against private acts of discrimination may lead a violation of the country's obligation under international law to give effect to its human rights obligations. Even when no legislation or public law enforcement authorities give importance to human rights principles of non-discrimination, however, private law may be invoked. Health care practitioners who are the members of professional associations whose ethical codes require non-discrimination, and/or who are entitled to practise subject to their observance of a code of professional practice, may face expulsion and loss or suspension of licensure, and may violate contractual obligations of employment that require their compliance with ethical codes and rules of licensure. Thus, both public law and private law may be applied against discriminatory act.

The legal measures pointed out above that might enforce the duty to treat persons who are HIV infected supposes that refusal to treat properly to HIV infection amounts in law to discrimination on grounds of physical or mental disability. AIDS-related dementia affects many persons in developed stages of sickness, but, at the other end of the spectrum of infection, several people who are HIV infected are asymptomatic and doing function well. They may require medical care, however, for conditions not concerned to infection, or indeed to illness; they might, for instance, break limbs in accidents or be pregnant and preparing for childbirth. The legal issue is whether refusal of services to them following their HIV status is illegal discrimination on a ground of disability, when they are neither mentally nor pathologically impaired.

An effective decision of the United States Supreme Court was given in the *Arline* case. This did not directly relate AIDS or HIV positivity, and actually reserved whether it was applicable to HIV infection, but is widely considered relevant. The Court held that if others refused to work or otherwise deal with a person because of that person's infectious or other medical condition, even when the person was mentally and physically capable of discharging routine functions, they were discriminating on the basis of disability. The person affected was not able to work, because the interactions with others on which normal ability to function depends was refused by those others. The person was not medically disabled, but disabled from working in social, employment, economic or other ways that anti-discrimination legislation also addresses and prohibits. Thus, health care practitioners who avoid or fail to accept or treat a person as a patient on the basis of the person being HIV infected, even when the person shows no symptoms, disable that person, and face responsibility for discrimination on grounds of the disability that person suffers that they have caused.

It does not follow, however, that HIV infected persons can therefore legally postulate any health service from any practitioner or facility. Practitioners are entitled and often legally obliged by licensing authorities to refuse to act beyond their trained skills, but must refer applicants for care to practitioners or facilities able to give it. There is no duty to treat beyond the ability to treat, but rather a duty not to treat so. Further, when a person who is HIV infected or who is responsibly considered responsible to be infected seeks health care from a practitioner or facility capable of giving it, a refusal would be legally justifiable, and consistent with human rights and antidiscrimination law, if an accessible alternative centre had been established to provide care to such persons. A practitioner or facility may refer to an alternative regional source of care available to the HIV infected person where the regional resource has personnel trained, equipped and experienced to treat such patients.

A local facility or practitioner may justifiably refuse to deliver treatment that is offered elsewhere that is as convenient to the person seeking care, or that presents no significantly greater inconvenience, when, for example, the agency first approached is the principal health resource for a major population but lacks the means, such as sterilization equipment or operatives, to protect other patients against spread of HIV infection. Treatment is not discriminatory in law simply because it is available in specially designated facilities, provided that there is no substantive disadvantage or stigma appended to receiving care there. Accordingly, the duty to treat HIV infected persons is discharged by referring them to accessible facilities that are best suited to give care, including appropriate counselling. Specialized facilities may attract practitioners specially sympathetic to those with HIV infection. Facilities that do not recognise such persons but refer them to specialized alternative facilities may attract practitioners fearful of suffering infection or averse to those whose behaviour displays high risk of infection, but the law is not effective to address the bias and prejudice that health care practitioners feel, but at best only the discrimination they exhibit.

In routine medical management of patients, therapeutic treatment is usually different from research, and although therapeutic innovation often has an experimental aspect, it is usually considered to be a category of treatment. However, since no cures exist for AIDS or HIV infection, infected persons may demand that they be given unproven medical and other products in the hope that improved care and even a cure will be achieved. It has been observed concerning management of HIV infected patients that "experimentation and research come to look more and more like treatment." The duty of health care professionals to begin research is ethical rather than legal. Professionals may incur research duties to institutions that employ them, but they owe no legal duty to patients for whose care they are liable to propose research on them. Any research that is undertaken, even at patients' insistence, must similar requirements of ethical approval by institutional review boards, and the law on research subjects' consent. Further, research results must be carefully monitored, on both legal and ethical grounds, to assess their implications for treatment. This is an element of health care practitioners' legal duty to be aware of scientific developments in their field.

Underlying the duty to treat is the capacity to treat. Those bound by the duty must employ resources reasonably available to them for this purpose, but management of HIV infection and AIDS in various regions of the world is surrounded by unavailability of indicated means. The cost of such drugs as AZT, which can, for example, significantly reduce the risk of a mother transmitting HIV to her baby, may be beyond the sources of national health services and individual patients to pay. The law does not require that the impossible be accomplished, and unless indicated treatments are reasonably available there is no legal duty to employ them or to reveal them as options that patients may want to pursue by their own means and expenditures. Indeed, tantalizing desperate patients by giving information that means of relief exist to which they have no real feasibility of access may be adverse to their well-being, and hostile to their care. Information that impresses patients with their powerlessness, isolation, poverty or subjection to misfortunes they cannot restrain or escape may justifiably be omitted from discussions about their care.

The Counselling

Counselling of patients regarding HIV infection and testing cannot be adequately undertaken by health care practitioners whose own understanding of the infection, its transmission and epidemiology is not adequate. Practitioners who are able to counsel should be able to offer counselling regarding whether HIV testing is indicated because of a patient's symptoms or high risk behaviour or experience, in terms of implications of a positive and a negative test result, and the medical, social, moral, and perhaps legal implications of a patient declining an indicated test. Counselling on the appropriateness of taking an HIV test is in some ways the most difficult due to mixed social messages about HIV infection and AIDS. As awareness grows of the risks of infection and rising statistics of HIV infection and AIDS-related deaths, patients can be panicked into believing they should be tested, consisting of those patients whose behaviour places them in a low risk category for infection. As against this, since the virus does not survive long in air and is transmissible primarily through intimate exchanges of body fluids, chiefly in sexual relations, needle-sharing injection of drugs and transfusion of unscreened or contaminated blood, the virus do not casually spread. People who engage in high risk behaviour may accordingly feel justified in believing in their immunity, specially when they recognize no symptoms of infection. Counsellors, therefore, face the double challenge of comforting the inappropriately troubled, and troubling the inappropriately comfortable.

A patient whose HIV test proves negative must be asked about earlier conduct, and counselled about the incubation period during which negative outcomes will be shown in tests on recently infected persons who are capable of transmitting the virus to partners. That is, patients must be counselled that a negative test result must be interpreted in the perspective of preceding and subsequent behaviours before it can be taken to show the negation of infection. If a health care practitioner does not properly counsel a patient whose test is negative but who later infects another due to a belief that there was no need, for example, to take sexual precautions, the practitioner is at risk of legal responsibility, particularly if that other was induce to rely on the practitioner's implied assurance that the patient was not HIV infected.

Legislation in several jurisdictions proposes containment of the spread of contagious and infectious diseases, containing sexually transmitted diseases, by mandating that health care practitioners who learn of such disorders must notify a public health officer. The officer will make effort to detain an infected person or otherwise subside risk of spread of infection, learn identities of the person's associates at risk and undertake partner notification and contact tracing, as far as possible, to *** partners and contacts that they may have been exposed to infection. This legislation speaks of the coercive or policing power of the state to protect public safety and welfare, and is not dependent on infected persons' consent. Whatever its practical effect may be, its legal effect is to protect the health care practitioner whose HIV infected patient does not obey advice given in counselling aimed at protection of third parties against infection by a patient. The practitioner's report to be designated public health officer may discharge any duties owed to patients' partners at risk of infection.

Whether legislation mandates reporting of patients a health care practitioner finds not to have AIDS but believes may be HIV infected when they refuse to be tested depends upon its particular wording. However, when reporting is not essential, practitioners usually have a legitimate discretion to report any person they believe believable and in good faith may be a danger to public health by being a potential source of infection to others. Under such conditions, there will be no illegal violation of the patient's confidentiality if the belief of infectivity is right, nor actionable defamation if it is incorrect because exposure will be covered by the law of qualified privilege. Practitioners themselves do not need to know a person's HIV status in giving treatment, since they should take wide precautions, including in treating persons who test HIV negative. Whether practitioners can legally withdraw from treatment of patients who refuse to be HIV tested depends on the law of contract and rejectment, and on anti-discrimination law, but proposed withdrawal make essential the practitioner to provide counselling on both the patient's protection of others and on how to maintain his or her health and secure appropriate services from other practitioners.

Counselling should also explain differences between

compulsory, mandatory, routine and voluntary HIV testing, where relevant to a patient's conduct. The terms are not always used seriously, but compulsory testing is usually taken to mean involuntary testing compelled by legislative or judicial authority, such as testing of persons convicted or accused of sexual assault, perhaps in violation of human rights principles such as the presumption of innocence. Compulsory testing makes submission to testing a condition of exercise of otherwise voluntary choices. For example, patients who seek treatment for HIV infection may reasonably be expected to permit testing to establish that they are infected, plaintiffs who sue defendants they claim infected them may be required to give evidence that they are actually HIV infected, and persons who want to serve as blood donors, sperm or organs must expect that the donated materials will be tested for protection of potential recipients. Patients do not have to take treatment, plaintiffs do not have to sue and persons do not have to donate, but if they want to move forward with their plans to be patients, plaintiffs or donors it is mandated that they submit to relevant tests, and have test results made appropriately available.

Routine testing is based on implied consent. When a patient gives a blood or other tissue sample to be tested, it is in the perspective of a particular diagnosis or circumstance, such as monitoring of therapy. The patient knows well the overall purpose of testing, but not essentially each of the individual characteristics or properties of the sample it will be tested to detect. Some centres and health care practitioners are of the view that samples should routinely be tested for HIV infection, such as by detection of antibodies to the virus, and that patients need not specifically be asked to consent to this, or be explicitly informed that this test will be performed. Other authorities find this highly objectionable, and prohibit HIV testing without explicit consent.

Patients should be counselled that what is presented to them as routine testing may contain an HIV test, however, and that they may take an initiative to ask about this test and to object to it if they are interested. An ethical view that prevails in many health care settings to which courts of law may be sympathetic is that an HIV test is not just a test like various others, because of the severe stigmatization and prejudice that may follow if the test proves positive. Accordingly, an HIV test should be performed only because of a person's adequately informed and freely given consent. Courts may determine in each case whether an HIV test may legitimately be inserted in routine testing on the ground of implied consent, but if the sample was taken for any legal purpose its taking does not become an assault merely because a test to which no legal consent was given is conducted. That is, illegal testing of the sample for HIV antibodies is not an assault on the patient provided that the sample was taken for another, legitimate purpose. A patient will, therefore, have to seek a legal device on other grounds such as breach of privacy or confidentiality, if such grounds are available.

Confidentiality and the Warning

The stigmatization and prejudice generally directed against persons with HIV infection provide reasons why HIV infected patients' confidentiality should be preserved. The implied terms of a contract, the law of negligence, the law on breach of fiduciary duty and, in some jurisdictions, the law on privacy may reinforce the duty of confidentiality. The countervailing consideration, however, is that timely exposure of a risk of HIV infection may be prevented, preserve a persons' health and prolong a life. Health care practitioners may accordingly confront the dilemma of preserving a patient's confidentiality but emerging complicit in an innocent persons' suffering and premature death, or of prioritizing the welfare of a non-patient over that of a patient by betraying the patient's trust. The dilemma of a health care practitioner is aggravated when the person at risk of HIV infection is also the practitioner's patient, such as a patient's spouse, other family member or companion for whose welfare the practitioner is also liable.

The legal dilemma of preservation of confidentiality can be eased, if only in an analytical sense, by an observation of the Supreme Court of California in 1976 that has achieved considerable importance. In the much discussed *Tarasoff* case, where health care practitioners were held civilly responsible for not giving due warning to an identified person at risk of a grave danger they rightly anticipated would be caused by a patient, the Court identified the special nature of the therapist-patient relation, held that this imposed a duty towards the person at risk to protect from foreseen harm, and observed that "the protective privilege [of confidentiality] ends where the public peril begins". Exposure was thereby analysed not to be a breach of confidentiality, because what the Court described as "the privilege" of confidentiality did not extend so far as to preclude exposure where an individual was considered to be in grave peril. This confirms that, while confidentiality is potent value in the relation between a health care practitioner and a patient, it is not the only value, nor necessarily the highest. The Court prioritized a duty to warn of anticipated grave peril, limiting the scope of confidentiality. As confidentiality is not necessarily absolute, courts may give further impetus to anti-discrimination legislation.

The legal duty under the *Tarasoff* principle is not to make correct predictions of risk, but only to act properly in light of the prediction actually made, so that a competently reached assessment that there is no or small risk will be an excusable fault if it proves incorrect. In *Tarasoff*, the potential victim was identifiable, and the predicted crisis was great. The same may be the case when a patient who is HIV infected has a heterosexual or same-sex partner. Where local legislation makes essential to reporting the identities of HIV infected persons to a public health officer, a health care practitioner should inform the patient of the reporting duty and of prospective contact tracing, but in any event should counsel the patient about risk of transmission to the partner. Unless the practitioner is assured that the partner is or will be properly notified of the risk and afforded protection, for instance by the patient and/or the local public health officer, the practitioner may have to be proactive.

The practitioner may, for instance, ask the patient to have the identified partner contact the practitioner, inform the patient that the practitioner will directly contact the partner or, for instance if the practitioner is not a physician but knows a physician responsible for the partner's health care, contact that physician. If the patient reveal no identifiable partner at risk, the practitioner has no duty of investigation, but may discharge legal duties to unidentified others by informing a responsible public health officer of the patient's HIV status. Whether such officers work under legislative authority or not, they are legally obliged to afford due confidentiality to the identities of persons of whose health status they learn, and are usually expected not to reveal identities of their informants.

If local jurisprudence does not recognise the *Tarasoff* rationale that confidentiality does not negate duties to warn, but recognizes instead the priority in principle of confidentiality, a practitioner who percepts morally obliged to notify an identified person at apparent risk of infection may invoke the legal principle of necessity to protect human life. In law, there are mandatory, justifiable, excusable and culpable disclosures. Mandatory disclosure arises, for example, under public health legislation and the *Tarasoff* principle, and justified disclosure would arise with patients' assent and if patients fail to object when adequately notified of intended future disclosures. The law on necessity provides that, although it does not justify unauthorized exposure, which is therefore unlawful, it may excuse from culpability a person who discounts other legal duties when a considerably more important value is at stake. The law concerning the confidentiality of HIV status protects patients against social stigmatization and prejudice in search of various interests, but a court may find that protection of an unaware person against avoidable HIV infection and its consequences to health and life is a more important value.

The consent to provide such protection may accordingly be held excusable so as to exempt a health care practitioner from punishment or culpability for the illegal act of unauthorized disclosure.

Lawyers may find it not easy to advise health care practitioners to act in reliance on necessity, however, because a court may not recognize the priority of the claimed necessity, and in any event the conduct would be illegal, even if considered not punishable or culpable by a court of law. A professional disciplinary authority may be able to impose sanctions for professional misconduct for behaviour that is illegal, even when a court finds it excusable. Accordingly, lawyers may advise health care practitioners about their legal obligations of confidentiality, and that if they tend to violate them with a view to warn others of the risk of infection that patients present, the breach of confidentiality may be found excusable and so not punishable or compensable. However, lawyers are unlikely positively to advise health care practitioners to act illegally and to expect the courts will excuse them. Courts may not, and even if they do, professional disciplinary authorities may not. Further, legal professional disciplinary authorities usually will not allow lawyers to give advice that the law may be broken, even if courts find particular breaches to be excusable. Necessity may provide an *ex post facto* defence, but not a prospective basis of legal advice to disregard the law of confidentiality, where the *Tarasoff* principle does not constrained the legal scope of confidentiality in the face of public peril.

When a patient requests a health care practitioner to send a copy of the patient's medical record to a third party, the practitioner is bound to do so. Even though the record may be contained on materials owned and possessed by a health care facility or the practitioner, courts increasingly recognize that the information itself belongs to the patient and that the practitioner, as trustee of the information, must provide it and give copies of it in accordance with the patient's directions. Nevertheless, since patients often do not know the full contents of their medical records or appreciate the way information contained there may be understood and used by others, health care practitioners are legally bound to give patients counselling about foreseeable consequences of their compliance with patients' requests to reveal confidential medical information.

Patients seeking, for example, employment or insurance may not appreciate that their medical records may include information that motivates prospective employers or insurers not to accept them, and to give honest or contrived causes for denial influenced by local anti-discrimination laws. Health care professionals cannot advise or be parties to deception of those with whom their patients may interact, but must ensure that patients are afforded means to exercise properly informed consent in exposing their confidential health information to others. When patients' information requires to be shared with other health care practitioners, however, practitioners are entitled and usually bound to make revelation to them of information relevant to serve the patients' interests. Even when patients are unaware of such sharing of information, it is a part of legitimate practice to enhance patients' interests to which they impliedly consent, and no breach of confidentiality arises. Recipients of such shared information owe patients the same duties of confidentiality as the practitioners who make it available.

Testing of identifiable patients raises confidentiality concerns, but testing is not similar like screening. Population screening studies are epidemiological surveys to determine, for example, the prevalence of HIV infection in a target group. The group is composed, of course, of individuals, but data are accumulated to learn not about the individuals as such but about the incidence of infection in the group as a whole. Screening studies may use personally identifying health records or, for example, unlinked anonymous data gathered from individual records or from aggregated data sources. Legal concerns about individual confidentiality are occasionally invoked to prevent or regulate screening studies designed to establish HIV prevalence in a given population, but this seems a misapplication of clinical values to the detriment of public health systems. Individuals' health is endangered where public health authorities lack information of the incidence of diseases, and therefore cannot take effective preventive or remedial action or develop and locate treatment resources properly. Those who conduct HIV prevalence screening programmes may on occasion learn personally identified health information, but they are usually legally bound to observe confidentiality. Often, however, no individual confidences are violated by screening studies. Some are authorized by public health legislation that conspicuously supersedes or confines individual confidentiality. Since such studies are directed to the welfare of individuals as a public health measure, they may be taken to have views given at a communal or macroethical level, and not to violate the ordinary legal obligations to preserve confidentiality of individual health information.

Death certificates are frequently public documents. In law, duties such as of confidentiality are not usually owed to people due to their deaths, but forms of certification can implicate the HIV status of living persons such as companions and family members of those who have died, including their young children.

Where death is certified as AIDS-concerned, no confidence of the deceased is legally violated, but interests of living persons may be endangered. Local law governs how clear and comprehensive death certification is, but unless legislation or regulations expressly provide otherwise, physicians have the right to certify death as due only to its immediately precipitating causes, like carcinoma, pneumonia or tuberculosis, or to add that the causes were AIDS-related.

The HIV Infected Health Care Practitioner

The danger of patients being exposed to health care practitioners' HIV infected body fluids has seemed so low that some have claimed the problem to be non-existent. However, surgeons or dentists may cut themselves through their protective gloves, specially in undertaking procedures in which they do not have sight of their hands, and they may then bleed into patients' bodies before it is surgically or otherwise appropriate for them to remove their hands. There are few if any proven examples of an HIV infected health care practitioner infecting a patient, but were a practitioner to do so, a court would deliberately assess liability by strict criteria because the practitioner would be held to a higher standard of care than a layperson. This is not to say that HIV infected health care personnel cannot practise as such; in fact, they may be peculiarly suited and perhaps willing to attend certain HIV infected patients. In countries where HIV infection is regular occurring and health care practitioners scarce, there may be no alternative to infected practitioners remaining in practice. They would be expected however, to maintain a high degree of vigilance and care to protect patients against any threat they might pose. If an HIV vaccine is developed and practitioners decide to take it for protective purposes, their HIV status will become positive because they will be responsible to develop antibodies to the virus, but they will pose little, if any, risk to patients.

Infected practitioners might be expected to remove themselves from all but the irreducible minimum risk of exposing patients to their body fluids. For example, HIV positive surgeons might limit their practice to external procedures, and get rid of undertaking any in which they would not have full sight of their hands at all times. They might also be expected, for example, not to work in emergency or trauma centres. They might be required to explain to health facility department or unit heads why they are not suited to particular styles of practice. All infected health care practitioners should seek specialist advice and monitoring on their professional practice, because compromised immune systems might leave them specially susceptible to contract infections from patients, and to spread such infections other than HIV itself. Their stamina might also decline, although they might well become incapable of practice some time before susceptible to AIDS-related dementia.

Health care practitioners who treat or otherwise learn of a colleague's HIV infection have a duty to inform responsible institutional, or licensing authorities if they believe that advice to protect patients is not being followed and that the colleague's fitness to practice may be impaired. Proper warning protects both patients and the colleagues from havoc, and may facilitate the colleague's appropriate care. Those who learn of a colleague's HIV infection must observe confidentiality in the ordinary way, but selective exposure to protect patients and also the colleague would not constitute a breach of confidentiality, since colleagues are hoped to monitor and ensure each other's professional capacity to practice. It must be remembered that, where legislation makes essential that a designated public health officer be notified that a patient has been diagnosed with AIDS or HIV infection, the duty to notify applies no less to patients who are health care practitioners than to others. A number of health care professions have specified practitioners' duties to protect patients on suspicion of their own HIV infection in ethical codes, and it has been seen that ethical codes may be not illegally enforced through licensing authorities' and others' disciplinary powers to contain professional misconduct. As against this, a practitioner's dismissal from employment or refusal of the right to practice on account of HIV infection alone raises legal issues under anti-discrimination laws, including whether non-infection is a bona fide employment requirement for the tasks the practitioner seeks to undertake.

Local law will condition whether HIV infected practitioners must inform patients of their status before undertaking invasive or other procedures on them. If patients inquire about practitioners' HIV status, they must be answered honestly. In principle, however, there seems to be no requirement to volunteer disclosure keeping in view the relatively low risk of practitioners infecting patients, and of analogies with the more easily infectious conditions practitioners might transmit to patients that they are not required to reveal. Information that patients are generally entitled to receive centres on what is material to the choices they have to make, and risks that are so low as to be almost less important do not have to be disclosed, unless patients show that they consider them significant by asking about them.

Some patients, in the United States who were treated by health care practitioners they did not know were HIV infected, were not infected themselves, but despite all these brought legal proceedings claiming that, once they learned of their practitioners' HIV status, they became afraid of the risk of infection and had to undergo invasive testing to determine their own HIV status. The ground of the claims was deliberate or negligent infliction of emotional distress. It will have to be seen whether such "AIDS phobia" claims will become influential in a country's jurisprudence. Fearing responsibility, health facilities may bar surgeons, dentists, and possibly other health care practitioners from performing certain and perhaps any procedures on patients who have not given prior consent to receive services from practitioners who may be HIV infected. Alternatively, facilities may outline the protective devices they take, and say that persons not willing to receive care under those measures should not become patients there. Neither strategy would cover emergency care, however, which may justify the exclusion of HIV infected practitioners from taking such care except when life is in immediate danger and no alternative practitioners are available. A counter-argument, however, is that the universal precautions that health care practitioners take to protect themselves against HIV infection from patients also protect patients against infection spread by practitioners, and that their exclusion from routine emergency services would be unlawful discrimination on the basis of their HIV-based disability. Health care practitioners remain members of the general community protected by human rights laws against discrimination.

Thirteen

HIV and Insurance

Insurance is a potent necessity, particularly in a free market, industrialized society. To HIV seropositive individuals, insurance is decisive, not only in order to obtain medical care, but also to pay one's debts after death and provide for spouses and children. This chapter compares the problem of insurance concerned to the HIV seropositive primarily in the United States, Europe, and certain African and Asian countries. Hopefully, by comparing diverse systems one may learn to resolve the HIV seropositive insurance issue better in one's own country.

The insurance industry in the United States is necessarily a risk allocation contract where the policy holder "transfers particular risks of loss to another, the insurer, for a monetary consideration." "It is axiomatic that insurance does not cover known losses. Insurance covers the risk of loss." The industry is generally heavily regulated only by the state unless a particular aspect of insurance is pre-empted by federal law.

Health Insurance

1. United States of America

Following the high risk of private health insurance, it is essential that employees, particularly those with HIV, belong to some workplace health plan. While many states have protected HIV seropositive employees from insurance workplace discrimination, it was not possible to predict that the Employee Retirement Income Security Act of 1974 (ERISA), a law formulated to protect employee benefits, could be judicially interpreted to virtually eliminate HIV seropositive insurance protection. Whether the Americans with Disabilities Act (ADA) will restore such protection is still not certain, although the federal administrative

agency implementing the ADA has clearly indicated that discrimination based on HIV is not only a violation of the ADA, but will result in financial penalties against the entity accountable for such discrimination.

Within the United States, private health insurance costs are extremely expensive. Approximately 83 per cent of all private health insurance is given through the workplace, with the employer often paying a major portion of premiums. It is undisputed that the more employees in a business, the more likely the company will have a health plan. For instance, 90 per cent of the firms with twenty-five to forty-nine employees have a health plan compared to 54 per cent of those with five to nine workers and 26 per cent of firms with under four employees.

2. *Self-funding*

In the United States, lifetime medical costs for HIV are estimated at $119,000. Following cost and other barriers for health insurance, HIV seropositive persons have sought work at those companies that have large group insurance policies—these companies put little conditions to obtain health insurance. Some employers have concluded that economic necessity should mandate a reduction for HIV benefits, a measure which would result in violation of several state anti-discrimination laws.

Rarely, very rarely, do corporations exclude HIV seropositive coverage following HIV problems resulting from "personal lifestyle decisions". Circle K Corporation, the second largest operator of convenience stores in the United States, excluded HIV coverage for claims of gays and drug users, but not for claims resulting from blood transfusions. Public pressure forced Circle K to drop its HIV exclusion. Galaxy Carpet Mill (Ga.) imposed a lifetime $10,000 cap on health advantage on "voluntarily contracted HIV" and other sexually transmitted diseases. As in Circle K, the cap was dropped as a consequence of public pressure.

Increasingly, however, companies are turning to self-funded insurance programmes regulated by ERISA, which pre-empted state regulations. In fact, by 1995, "over 65 per cent of (US) workers who are given health advantage .... are in self-insured plans.

This federal law was passed long before HIV was an issue,

and its objective was partly to protect employees' pensions and health benefits granted by an employer. While ERISA created substantive regulations covering pension plans, it did not generate the same for welfare plans. It has come under judicial criticism, especially when applied to health care plans and HIV.

Judicial decisions under ERISA have generally been unfavourable to persons with AIDS (PWA). In *Phelps v. Field Real Estate Co.*, plaintiff, hired in 1985, learned he was HIV seropositive in 1986, but did not reveal his condition. In 1988, he informed his employer that he had a fatal disease which he had kept secret out of fear of losing his job and health insurance. In 1989, after being removed for poor work performance and for company reorganization, the plaintiff filed an ERISA complaint, alleging that his removal was the result of fear of catastrophic benefit cost increase. The Court of Appeals affirmed the trial court verdict for the defendant because the latter did not base any part of its removal verdict on saving benefit costs. The plaintiff was furthermore unable to show that it was more probable than not that his medical condition motivated his employer to remove his employment.

Under ERISA, there is no specification as to what the standard of review should be concerning the determination by an administrator in self-funded plans. In *Kennedy v. System One Holdings*, the HIV seropositive former employee claimed that he was deliberately misled by the employer and plan administrator as to the permitted time to recover long-term disability advantage under the company welfare plan. One factor in granting the defendant summary judgment was that courts will defer to the plan administrator's factual determination unless there is an abuse of discretion.

Courts will generally defer to the decision of an insurance plan administrator related to benefits and will uphold his decision as long as it is not arbitrary and capricious. In *Florence Nightingale Nursing Service v. Blue Cross & Blue Shield of America*, the patient's employer provided medical advantages through a plan administered by the defendant. The plan provided reasonable charges only for medically essential private-duty nursing. In the first month, the provider billed the defendant for at-home intravenous care for an HIV seropositive patient. In the second month, the defendant was billed for at-home care notwithstanding that the patient was no longer receiving IV treatment. Blue Cross paid less than half the cost of the first month and nothing for the second month as it said that the patient's family could have given post-IV treatment care.

The court refused to defer to the claims administrator's expertise since Blue Cross had in this matter a potential conflict of interest, given that it had to follow the sponsoring employer's emphasis upon containing costs. The court then examined the matter de novo and arrived at a conclusion that medical costs were reasonable by comparing them to other home nursing services that cared for HIV seropositive patients, and because HIV seropositive patients were a special case. The trial court hold the view that "recruit(ing) nurses for treating AIDS victims must be like recruiting kamikaze pilots. It takes a special breed."

When many employers in self-insurance plans realized that they, in lieu of the insurer, had to pay medical costs, they then introduced caps on HIV payments for all employees, while leaving intact medical advantages for other illnesses. In two instances, federal appellate courts upheld employer caps on HIV in self-funded plans.

In *McGann v. H & H Music Co.*, the company changed from a group insurance plan to a self-insurance plan and subsided lifetime maximum health benefits from $1 million to $5,000 only for HIV. This had disastrous results for plaintiff McGann, who had been diagnosed HIV seropositive seven months (December 1987) before the policy changed. When McGann sued, alleging a violation of Section 510 of ERISA, the court granted the defendant summary judgement as the plaintiff had not shown discriminatory intent on the employer's part, despite all these the plaintiff being the only affected employee. H & H Music had also reserved the right to modify the plan which prevented the defendant from successfully alleging interference with any inherent right. In dicta, the Court of Appeals stated that there would have been no ERISA violations "even though the employer's decision...may stem from some 'prejudice' against AIDS or its victims generally..."

A similar result was reached in *Owens v. Storehouse, Inc.*, where the employer, with a view to obtain stop-loss insurance, switched to a self-insurance plan that reduced lifetime benefits from $1 million to $25,000. *Owens*, in following *McGann*, came to conclusion that ERISA pre-empted state law and that "absent proof of retaliation or interference with the attainment of an entitled right..., ERISA provides no right to regular health insurance with immutable terms." As in *McGann*, the plaintiff furthermore failed to show that his former employer deliberately interfered with any vested right of the plaintiff.

3. The Americans with Disabilities Act

The Americans with Disabilities Act (ADA) of 1990 extended some anti-discrimination provisions of the 1964 Civil Rights Act to disabled persons. In 1991, a protected individual pursuant to a graduated damages provision could get a maximum award of $300,000. The ADA became effective for all employers with 25 or more employees on 25 July, 1992, and for employers with 15 to 24 employees on 26 July, 1994. While the ADA does not mention HIV, its congressional history and court decisions have concluded that even asymptomatic HIV seropositive has protection under the ADA. The Equal Employment Opportunity Commission (EEOC) is the federal administrative agency liable for the implementation of much of the ADA, and its regulations are generally given valuable deference by federal courts. Should the EEOC determine that an employer's HIV benefits policy is in violation of the ADA, it may receive relief only through litigation in a federal court if settlement attempts fail.

The ADA makes essential for an employer to make reasonable accommodations and prevents discrimination against "a qualified individual with a disability" unless such accommodations would create undue hardship. Concerning insurance programmes, the ADA prevents an employer from using insurance risk classifications "as a subterfuge to evade (the statutes) purposes." The employer may neither ask about medical conditions nor require a blood test before offering employment. When an offer is accepted, an employer may reject an applicant for employment only if the physical examination demonstrates it is physically not possible for the applicant to work.

The "plain language" of the ADA "provides no specific guidance" whether HIV is included. Therefore, "substantial deference" is given to the interpretation of its provisions by the EEOC. The EEOC has issued "some guidelines" which would make caps on HIV reimbursement all but not feasible for an employer to defend. When various companies enacted caps pertaining to HIV reimbursement, the EEOC issued determination letters claiming that such caps were in violation of the ADA.

In accordance with EPA-guidelines, if there is a disability based distinction, then the burden of proof transfers to the employer to show that the distinction is not a subterfuge to evade the ADA. The employer may rebut this subterfuge allegation by showing disparate treatment is either based on sound actuarial data, accepted standards for fiscal soundness (under-writing risks), or to prohibit a drastic reduction in coverage for other employees.

The ADA does not protect gay employees, but does protect an employee fired for cause of HIV. In *Doe v. Cooper Investments*, a terminated employee alleged he was fired two weeks after he revealed that he was HIV seropositive. The judge ordered the employer either to obtain continuing insurance for the employee or to absorb his medical expenses. In Arizona, a gay HIV seropositive employee was fired soon after filing an insurance claim for HIV illness. The company alleged it was the employee's poor work performance, and the judge informed the jury that if the dismissal was based "solely" on the plaintiff's sexual orientation, it should find for the defendant.

4. Caps

There have been frequent attempts made by companies to set caps on AIDS-related illnesses, but they generally have been withdrawn after objection raised by the EEOC. The following examples are typical: In *Mason Tenders District Council Welfare Fund v. Donaghey*, a self-insured labour management health trust fund (the construction union fund) in 1991 had cut off medical facilities for Donaghey and three other HIV seropositive workers. When the EEOC arrived at conclusion that *Mason Tenders* had violated the ADA, the fund then sought a declaratory judgment claiming that the fund was only covered by ERISA and not the ADA, as it did not employ Donaghey and the other claimants.

The fund was most adamant about not conceding or settling until a federal judge refused the fund's motion for summary judgment and also insisted that at a subsequent trial the fund would have to show an actuarial basis for HIV cap. In September 1994, the US Attorney filed a RICO (racketeering) complaint, claiming that organized crime controlled the fund and had skimmed "benefit funds", containing that which excluded HIV coverage. It was not easy for the fund to argue lack of money for HIV coverage while simultaneously defending charges that organized crime had pilfered its funds.

In *Estate of Kadinger v. IBEW, Local 110*, an agreement was made between the EEOC and the plaintiff with the union and its benefit reimbursement plan. In 1987, the plan imposed a $50,000 lifetime cap for HIV costs while maintaining a $500,000 cap for other illnesses. Kadinger was diagnosed HIV seropositive after the enforcement of the cap, but before the ADA became effective. In the consent decree, the fund agreed to remove the cap retroactive to 26 July, 1992 and pay $100,000 to Kadinger's estate, which would reimburse Kadinger's hospital costs and pay $2,500 to the Minnesota AIDS project.

In other settlements, the EEOC made an agreement with Connecticut Refining Company to remove a $10,000 cap for HIV while retaining a $1 million cap for other illnesses. In February 1992, the company instituted this cap retroactive to November 1991 when Collimore, the plaintiff, was diagnosed with HIV, but left intact the $1 million cap for other illnesses. In February 1993, the EEOC arrived at a conclusion that the defendant had violated the ADA. In March 1994, the parties signed a conciliation agreement whereby the defendant eliminated the $10,000 cap retroactive to 26 July 1992, and agreed to pay $35,000 to Collimore for pain and suffering.

It is important to emphasize that the settlements were made with no admission of responsibility and often only in order to avoid protracted litigation. In *Anderson v. Gus Mayer Boston Store of Delaware*, the plaintiff alleged that the employer changed its group health insurance carrier following the plaintiff's HIV seropositive condition and that it knew the new carrier would reject the plaintiff; and therefore, this would result in lower premiums. The EEOC determined that the defendants had violated the ADA and made what defendants considered to be "a gun to the head, offer of conciliation" requiring the defendant to pay $100,000."

5. Jurisdiction

It seems that self-funded plans are jurisdictionally subject to the ADA. In Carparts Distri. Ctr. v. Automotive Wholesaler's, the Court concluded that the ADA did cover a self-funded medical reimbursement plan. The plaintiff, who also was the sole shareholder of Carparts Inc., had enrolled in 1987 in the plan of Automotive Wholesale Association of New England, Inc., which patronised a self-funded health benefit plan. The plaintiff was diagnosed HIV seropositive in 1986, but a lifetime cap of $25,000 for HIV was established effective from 1991, which left $1 million for other illnesses. The District Court gave the decision that the defendant was neither an employer nor a public accommodation within the meaning of the ADA. The Court reversed by giving decision that the plan had the authority to determine the level of benefits and this was an "employer" subject to Title 1 of the ADA, and that the plaintiff might have a feasibility of showing that the defendant is a public accommodation, and, therefore, subject to Title III of the ADA.

6. If No Insurance Workplace Coverage

While two-thirds of US employees are covered by an employment insurance plan, the remainder must either get a private plan or do without one. In 1991, it was estimated that 29 per cent of those with HIV had private health insurance. Forty per cent were covered by Medicaid, 2 per cent by Medicare, and 29 per cent had no health insurance.

Private medical plans regulated completely by states predictably will exclude pre-existing conditions, but often courts will interpret state statutes liberally in favour of the insured. In *Gonzales v. Associates Life Ins. Co.*, the Court of Appeals overturned the summary judgment in favour of the defendant. The plaintiff, who sought reimbursement from the medical policy for HIV, was denied coverage due to the AIDS/ARC conditions limitation. The appellate court concluded that the AIDS exclusion clause was not disclosed in explicit manner as required by Florida statute. While the AIDS exclusion was visibly legible and not buried in fine print, it was unenforceable.

Approximately 27 states have established risk pools which require insurers to share in underwriting policies for persons otherwise uninsurable. Generally, the state will form an association of all health insurance companies doing business within that state. One company would then be selected to formulate the plan pursuant to guidelines on premiums, deductibles, and other matters. The plan would often provide for prescription costs and skilled nursing care. The premiums, however, are generally 125 to 200 per cent higher than non-risk policies and exclude pre-existing conditions. Very few states have set up subsidies for indigent persons.

Should an HIV seropositive person lose his job, he would have a right to convert his health plan to private coverage pursuant to the Consolidated Omnibus Budget Reconciliation Act (COBRA). COBRA, which is an amendment to ERISA, mandates that employers of minimum 20 employees allow terminated employees, except for gross misconduct, to pay privately for group insurance plans up to 18 months. This is specifically important for an HIV seropositive employee because COBRA, unlike a new insurance policy, may not exclude pre-existing conditions.

While COBRA limits premiums to 102 per cent of the cost of insurance, the payment may be very difficult for a PWA. The Ryan White Care Act (The Comprehensive AIDS Resources Emergency Act) permits states to use federal funds to help PWA continue private health insurance coverage. COBRA also may not protect a former employee from a cap on health benefits. In *Gonzales v. Garner Fast Foods Inc.*, plaintiff was removed once the employer discovered his HIV seropositive status when he submitted a medical claim through the company's self-funded health programme. Although the plaintiff exercised his COBRA rights, the company, six months later (October 1991), enacted an HIV cap of $40,000, down from $1 million lifetime. The judge granted the defendant's motion to dismiss because the cap was enacted before July 26, 1992, the effective date of the ADA.

Should an HIV seropositive worker lose his job and benefits, he will be compelled to seek financial help, but only at the point of bankruptcy will he be eligible for Medicaid. As explained by Congressman Waxman, Medicaid is often the last resort:

> "AIDS has shown that Medicaid is shallow and inadequate. Many middle-class Americans are learning the hard way that, in most states, you can qualify only if you are completely disabled and have less than $1,500 to your name.
>
> AIDS has shown that we can produce medical miracles for the rich and plain neglect for the poor. AIDS drugs and treatments are priced for kings, while Medicaid is only for people who have been made paupers."

Even Medicaid coverage will not remove the problem of a PWA. In one documented instance, an HIV seropositive, young male without health insurance required relief from collection endeavours by a hospital for unpaid medical bills. His employment insurance was soon because of end, Medicaid did not fully cover his prescription costs, and he was barely able to pay his rent. The AIDS Law Project referred him to the local Consumer Bankruptcy Assistance Project.

7. Health Insurance Outside the United States

In most other countries, obtaining medical insurance is not as decisive to an HIV seropositive person because it is often obtained either at work or through a national health service. Within Australia, "Medicare" pays for HIV medical treatment. Health insurance is not an issue reasonable to HIV in Britain "because of the free availability of medical treatment of high quality under the National Health Service (NHS)." British law, however, has not been an obstacles to those employers who utilize pre-employment HIV testing, and a HIV seropositive employee may not have protection against removal within the first two years of employment.

Throughout Europe, the asymptomatic HIV seropositive employee has no duty to reveal and, generally, "when questioned has the right to remain silent or to lie." Sweden is an exception since the employer has both the right to test and to deny employment to those with HIV. The harshness of this policy is mitigated somewhat by the Swedish Social Security Scheme which will cover those HIV seropositive persons who are prevented from working. Should a worker become unable to work through HIV or any other illness, Belgian law has made provision to pay a guaranteed wage. In France, the person will be entitled to get social security. In Germany employers will provide payment followed by public health insurance.

Switzerland has no national health service. Medical care is given through private insurance plans which generally necessitate the insured to pay 10 per cent of all medical costs. "In the case of HIV and AIDS, this can amount to very high sums of money. For people without health insurance, the situation is obviously graver still." There is also discrimination, not only in insurance, but also in many pension funds which mandate that applicants not test HIV seropositive. Without joining a pension scheme, "it is practically not possible to get a job". Life insurance makes essential a HIV negative result, which is especially important in Switzerland since loans to professionals to establish a business practice "are often given only a conjunction with an insurance policy in favour of the lender in the amount of the loan."

In several European countries, health insurance is organized by an employer for employees and should an HIV seropositive person not be covered, then an employer might not want to employ an uncovered worker. French law prevents HIV exclusion and Belgian practice is to not exclude HIV-persons from group insurance. Within South Africa, insurers have expressed concern that in "several instances" an employer will offer work to an HIV seropositive person with a view to have the person "benefit from the company's group life and/or benefit scheme." This is because the group plan would not make essential evidence of HIV status" and also allows conversion to life insurance when the HIV seropositive worker leaves employment. Within the United States, testing is not regularly used in group health policies. In Uganda, insurers will not insure HIV "in the same way as if the illness were alcohol or drug related." Employees in Uganda are more worried about the employer-paid group insurance policy that provides a death payment for HIV or some other illness.

Canada has a National Health Service which makes available free medical care. Discrimination against HIV seropositive persons is prevented. As early as 1987, an employer in a collective bargaining agreement could not order an employee "to remain off work even where the employer is ready to maintain full pay and benefits" since such action could be "demeaning and corrosive to morale." Generally, HIV discrimination law is provincial and the matter is heard by a provincial administrative body such as a Board of Inquiry. There has been litigation when an employee was refused long-term disability benefits pursuant to the following clause: "If an employee has incurred medical expenses, or received care or treatment by a Physician during the 90-day period before the date his insurance becomes effective, no Income Benefit shall be payable for any disability resulting from the same or related cause until" the employee was not treated by a physician for 90 days or had been insured for 12 months. The Board of Inquiry decided that the above exclusionary clause did not offend the Ontario Human Rights Code partly because it was standard insurance practice for employers with less than 100 employees. The Code permitted distinctions that are reasonable and bona fide which would otherwise significantly increase an insurer's risk. But the court stressed the need to inform better all employees as to benefits and "to institute a review of all its contracts to make sure that the spirit of human rights legislation is observed, and particularly it is requested to review its P(re)E(xisting)C(onditions) clauses. It will file a report of its review with the Superintendent of Insurance within eighteen months. The OHRC in turn is asked to monitor the effectuation of this order."

Public health insurance will range from coverage of all workers in France, to two separate public funds in the Netherlands, to complicated German procedures. Not like the United States, worker's compensation or invalidity insurance schemes have nowhere "excluded HIV/AIDS sufferers." When there is hardship, it is "more as a result of administrative delays in receiving benefits than as a consequence of substantive limitations on the nature or extent of those benefits."

Life Insurance

1. United States of America

Not like medical insurance and HIV, which is a serious problem only in a few countries besides the US, gays and certain other groups everywhere have concerns over getting life insurance. Throughout much of the world, the issues are—(i) at what amount and under what conditions should mandatory HIV testing be required of applicants; and (ii) what questions may be asked of applicants which would protect the interest of the insurers, but not be unduly intrusive into an applicant's privacy. There is some concern that less expensive saliva tests might also be used by insurance companies, especially in developing countries.

Insurers must develop categories for risk of loss and one of the basic categories is health and often, unfortunately, lifestyles. Tied to lifestyles, some insurance companies also utilize factors such as an applicant's residence or occupation. Understandably, insurance companies are not interested to underwrite huge policies for HIV seropositive applicants and are not willing to cover persons with full blown AIDS. In order to test for HIV, companies have utilized blood tests which have been approved in all 50 states and the District of Columbia. It would be financially preventive, however, for insurers to require testing for every application, and therefore, several insurers require testing only for a policy of over $100,000. States occasionally have stringent requirements about informed consent, confidentiality, mandatory counselling, and disclosure of HIV tests.

AIDS exclusion clauses in life insurance policies are very rare. Life insurance policies are also unique in that state law generally set the time for an insurer to contest a misrepresentation upto two years. Understandably, insurers, when faced with an expensive payment, "have a strong financial incentive to allege misrepresentation" or failure to reveal the material facts. "Thus, in the case of a life insurance contract, the maxim 'fraud vitiates a contract' must be changed to 'fraud vitiates a contract, except for a life insurance contract which was issued more than two years ago."

Since an insurance agreement is in fact, an adhesion contract and as insurance companies are held to a good faith standard, courts will "resolve any uncertainty in favour of the insured." The following HIV issues in insurance contracts are illustrative of litigation results. In *Northern Life Insurance Co. v. Ippolito Real Estate Partnership*, a person with haemophilia took out six life insurance policies for business purposes. After Ippolito died of HIV, Northern Life sought, through a declaratory judgment, to annual the policies because the deceased had omitted material information on the amendment to the application. The deceased, after signing the first five policies, but prior to approval by the company, had experienced weight loss and sinusitis and did not reveal that he had twice seen a physician. The appellate court approved the trial court's decision for the deceased and arrived at a conclusion that as a matter of law there had been no material misrepresentation. The insurance company was given summary judgment on the sixth policy because Ippolio had verified he had not " suffered any....sickness or consulted or (had) been attended by a physician," when he earlier had been diagnosed with an HIV related illnesses. Thus, the court believed Ippolito wanted to deceive and his answers "contained misrepresentations material to Northern Life's risks." In *New England Mutual Life Insurance Company v. Johnson (executor)*, an insurance company attempted to annul a $50,000 policy because the insured misrepresented his relationship with his beneficiary lover, by only revealing him as a business partner. The judge criticized the company for having "searched through its files in an attempt to determine a way to escape its obligations" and gave decision that its actions were on a "bogus basis." The court further assessed the company with over $127,000 in attorney fees because if the deceased person's "illness was not one related with homosexuality, no attempt to annul the policy would have been made."

There is no obligation, generally, on the part of the insured to reveal his or her HIV status unless required by the insurer. In *Waxse v. Reserve Life Ins. Co.* the company was unsuccessful in attempting to annul the health policy because the insurer failed to reveal his HIV seropositive status. An opposite result was reached in *Sapp v. Paul Revere Life Insurance Co.*, Occasionally, an insurance company will litigate rather than pay a $10,000 policy. In *Hebert v. Magnolia Life Ins. Co.*, an HIV seropositive applicant, diagnosed with HIV in 1990, bought a $10,000 policy in 1991 and died in 1993. He answered "no" on an application question whether he had any medical examination in the last five years or whether he had any consultation/treatment which had been completed. The Court arrived at a decision that the applicant had made statements which were tended to deceive and which materially affected the insurer's risks. Both factors were necessary under Louisiana law for an insurer to escape responsibility.

British Isles

Other countries, of course, also deny to grant policies to HIV applicants and require blood tests if the policy is large and ask questions pertaining to HIV for smaller policies. In Britain, there was concern that individuals might be refused life insurance because they have had an HIV test or belonged to high-risk groups. Furthermore, it was "standard procedure" to test for HIV unmarried males who need life insurance with a view to obtain large mortgages. Unlike in the United States, mortgages in Great Britain often mandate life insurance.

In February 1987, a representative from an AIDS advocacy group informed the House of Commons Social Services Committee that individuals were refused life "insurance if they want to take out a joint mortgage with another man." Life insurance was also important for a self-employed person as security for an overdraft in business.

While there was no set amount of insurance that made essential a mandatory test, Midland Bank required tests for a male desiring £150,000 or a female desiring £250,000 policies, as well as all intravenous drug users and gays. Other firms generally tested for all policies over £40,000 for single males and £150,000 for everyone else. The general reaction of the insurance companies to HIV was to increase premiums up to 150 per cent for single males.

During the early 1990s there were not frequent attempts in Parliament to get the government to obtain assurances from life insurance companies to remove offensive/irrelevant questions on applications. One MP asked whether life insurance companies "will no longer ask questions of (applicants) that have the effect of putting people off taking the HIV test." The government responded that it was meeting with insurance representatives on this issue and conducting a study. The outcome of this study by the Association of British Insurers and the Department of Health had finally come to a conclusion that probably tens of thousands had put off taking an HIV test because of these questions. A government representative found this result to be "worrying".

By 1994, the Association of British Insurers (ABI) concluded that because HIV claims since 1987 (c. £50 million) were much lower than expected, it recommended that the question "Have you ever had an AIDS blood test?" be transferred with "Have you ever tested positive for HIV/AIDS or Hepatitis B or C or have you been tested/treated for other sexually transmitted diseases or are you deliberately awaiting the result of such a test?" It is still not certain as to whether the test question issue is resolved. By the end of 1994, only one-third of the 105 insurance companies had replaced the application wording. Applicants who are seronegative gay males still might have to pay higher premiums or accept an AIDS exclusion clause "in the early years of the policy."

Within the Republic of Ireland, insurance companies have "no immediate plans' to adopt the British example. The Irish Insurance Federation spokesperson said, however, that if the applicant had a negative HIV test, extra information would be sought only if the requested policy were "say over £100,000".

Africa

In Egypt, there is no need of HIV testing, although applicants must pass a certain number of medical examinations. An HIV seropositive person who does not reveal his or her condition will make the insurance contract a nullity. Sub-Saharan Africa has near about 2 per cent of the world's population, but 60 per cent of the world's HIV seropositive persons. Predictably, sub-Saharan Africans have difficulty in getting life insurance without testing.

In Zimbabwe, the government refused requests of insurance companies to test applicants for all policies over Z$50,000 (US$6,250) instead of the present limit of Z$100,000 (US$12,500). The Minister of Health of Zimbabwe declined to endorse the testing measure "since he is a strong supporter of the Geneva Convention banning (HIV) discrimination." The argument of the insurance company is that HIV accounts for 60 to 70 per cent of death claims during the first five years of the policy, and that one million of a ten and one-half million population is HIV seropositive. In 1993, 42 per cent (1,428) of all claims were pertaining to HIV, but between January and June 1994, only 111 of 2,888 tested applicants were HIV positive. At present, applicants, in order to avoid being tested, obtain endowment policies "which provide insurance coverage for up to 25 years of a person's life." It has been suggested that restrictions on HIV testing might "put an end to life assurance as a welfare option" in Zimbabwe as it did in Malawi.

In South Africa, HIV testing was set by the Life Office Association at R200,000. As HIV increased, insurers used AIDS exclusion clauses for those applicants unwilling to be tested. One South African company, Southern Life, has initiated a policy called "Exclusive Life Insurance", which makes essential all policy holders to be tested every five years. If the insured is HIV seropositive, the policy amount is subsided to 10 per cent unless the HIV "can be proved to be blood transfusion, rape, health procedures or other 'non-blameworthy' factors." At the work place, insurance companies, at the employer's request, busy in pre-employment testing for HIV since "job applicants are still not covered by any of the legislation implementing fair employment practices." Medical plans consisting of "employer operated schemes" have arbitrarily limited HIV claims. "Pension funds and provident funds have been curtailed to exclude" HIV.

Within South Africa, HIV has increased 10 times since 1990 to nearly 8 per cent of the black population. The mine workers, virtually all black, have been particularly hard hit by HIV. Consequently, the life insurance underwriter for the 350,000 National Union of Mine Workers wants to raise premiums by over one-third or curtail benefits for HIV. In Swaziland, the Swaziland Royal Insurance Corporation, as of 1 July, 1995, would mandate HIV screening for all life insurance policies over Rand 25,000. "Applicants have to prove that they do not have the virus with a view to qualify for a life policy on normal terms." In Uganda, HIV testing is utilized "for sums insured as low as $4,000."

Asia

According to the WHO, over one million Asians are HIV seropositive, with insurance issues being most debatable in Japan, Thailand, Singapore and Australia/New Zealand. Life insurers in Japan, are considering mandatory HIV tests for large life insurance policies. A physician group serving as advisors to life insurance companies had earlier arrived at a conclusion that life insurance applicants should be tested for HIV. This increase is also important as the industry is experiencing lower yields and also because policy-holders might be unwilling to pay increased premiums for higher HIV coverage. One major reservation to mandatory tests is the afraid of "how well applicant's privacy could be protected, no matter how strictly they guard test results," and whether HIV human rights might be violated by rejection. Should firms introduce questionnaires related HIV, which is considered as more controversial than testing, they would only have two years to set aside applications for false statements.

In Thailand, instead of emphasising more testing, the National AIDS Prevention and Control Administrative Committee has proposed to the Prime Minister that a regulation do not allow compulsory HIV testing by insurance companies. In addition to the usual arguments, viz., improper counselling, failure to keep results confidential, the Committee emphasised that many HIV seropositive persons "do not suffer from any serious infections, if they get the right medical treatment." The Committee instead urged that HIV seropositive persons be allowed to get insurance at a higher premium.

Presently, insurers can deny payment within one year of a policy in a group scheme if an insured intentionally failed to reveal his or her HIV status. Applicants in high-risk provinces must take HIV blood and saliva tests for any policy, and the remainder of the country must take a test for a policy over B75,000. Thai insurers have argued not successfully that no benefits be paid to an HIV seropositive person if he or she develops HIV within five years, or alternatively, have unsuccessfully tried to develop a sliding timescale for payments.

In Singapore, some particular occupations have been listed as "high-risk" groups which make essential mandatory tests for insurance. A Prudential Assurance spokesperson specifically listed male hairstylists, fashion designers and dancers [as tending] to be effeminate. We want to make sure they are not homosexuals." While Prudential denoted it might insure some groups if they tested seronegative, other insurers said they would not accept any risk group members as policy-holders. While testing is generally required only for policies of S$500,000 and above, it is mandatory for risk groups. Any misstatement related to a lifestyle would result in the contract being invalidated. Insurers have considered genetic testing not practicable.

Australia and New Zealand

The law of Australian insurance is federal, and state anti-discrimination agencies are prevented from dealing with insurance complaints. The Insurance Code of Practice now prevents an insurance company from basing its decision solely on an applicant's lifestyle. Nor may any prior negative tests be utilized, which should eliminate the fear of individuals voluntarily taking HIV tests. National Mutual, one of Australia's largest insurers, has also agreed to remove a clause that excluded HIV seropositive persons from getting payments in group life insurance. Previously, a person would be excluded from getting moneys if HIV were contracted within two years of the policy date.

This action by National Mutual was based on an independent study that the HIV spread in Australia "had not been as wide as insurers expected". The Trowbridge Report, an independent study commissioned by the federal government said that "there was no statistical proof to support exclusion clauses (by life insurance companies and superannuation funds) purely on the basis that applicants had the AIDS virus."

It is still not certain whether the Disability Act and Trowbridge Report would lessen fears by gay spokemen that it is "almost impossible" for gays to purchase life insurance. Australia has prepared, since 1988, a Code of Practice on Underwriting in Relation to AIDS, whose guidelines state that no decision will be based on sexual orientation or on a negative HIV result. In reality, "there is growing concern that there is a slightly less than zealous adherence to the guidelines and principles".

In New Zealand, life insurance claims for HIV did not suggest that HIV applicants were deliberately purchasing life insurance. In 1989, the industry followed a voluntary code for HIV guidelines concerning testing and counselling which asked certain special questions about sexual practices rather than lifestyle. The head of New Zealand's insurance industry stated "AIDS and HIV exclusions may also be used, especially in group life insurance, disability insurance, mortgage repayment insurance, and direct marketed policies, while non-guaranteed premium rates may become more common." The New Zealand Human Rights Act of 1993 allows discrimination insurance for HIV or gay status only if the discrimination is based on actuarial data, or if that is not available, the discrimination is based on either reputable actuarial opinion or medical data.

Europe

In the Netherlands, insurers as of 1993, pursuant to a Code of Conduct with the government, may not ask life insurance applicants whether they have had HIV tests, but only whether they have had an HIV seropositive result from such a test. Tests for life insurance may be provided for only for a policy over $f.200,000. If the policy is under that, the applicants are asked "Have you got AIDS?" and "Have HIV antibodies been found in your blood (are you seropositive)?" Legislation would have been enacted had not the above agreement been reached. In Belgium, any policy over BF5 million requires an HIV test.

In Denmark, the National Insurers Association consulted gay groups before issuing guidelines. Testing for HIV is required for policies over DKK 2M; for policies over DKK 1M, a certificate of health is required from the family physician. For cheaper policies, an applicant is asked about test information. Seronegativity is also required for an annual disability annuity of DKK 200,000. In Norway, all life insurance applicants "must confirm that they have not undergone a blood test which shows that they are HIV seropositive." Germany has not had mandatory testing, but insurers are starting to ask applicants to reveal HIV test results. Applicants seeking a DM250,000 policy must undergo a medical examination. The company may require an HIV test.

France conducts its insurance industry and the issue of HIV pursuant to an agreement between the Minister of Economics, the Minister of Health, and the insurance industry. The insurer may test for seropositivity. If the applicant gives his assent prior to the examination, the test is part of a full medical examination by a physician and the HIV results are given to a physician. The agreement also contains provisions for counselling and confidentiality. The Code of Conduct prohibits "questions pertaining to the intimate nature of private life, and, in particular, the sex life of the person applying for cover."

Testing is generally important only for policies over FF1 million. Yet, testing itself is not seen as controversial because "one in four men and women had taken the test." This ratio rises to just over one in two of all people between 25 to 34. A more serious problem is the requirement of a life insurance contract to insure real property loans. Until 1991, PWA were effectively precluded from such insurance. Pursuant to a 1991 agreement, HIV seropositive persons may get loans up to FF1 million for up to 10 years at a 4 to 6 per cent price increase.

In Sweden, life insurance companies may test and do test gays or those who have multiple partners. All applicants must inform a physician about their total sexual history. Should an applicant provide false information and later die from AIDS, the beneficiaries would get nothing. In Italy, applicants for policies over LIT 300 million are required to take an HIV test. An applicant for a lesser amount may be required to be tested if from the application "it seems to be important to seek.more information as to the risk."

Canada

Within Canada, the Canadian Life and Health Insurance Association utilized guidelines in 1987 that prohibited even indirect questions related to the applicants "sexual orientation" or on past seronegative test results. The Canadian Life and Health Insurance Association Incorporation (the Canadian trade association for about 100 companies) has taken a decision that applicants would be tested only for policies over C$100,000. Testing for smaller policies would occur only if there was a history of promiscuity, e.g., sexually transmitted diseases.

Other Matters

Policies Against Contracting HIV

Insurance companies across the world have formulated policies in case the insured contracts HIV. In Canada, an applicant can pay C$4 and get a $100,000 policy if the applicant becomes HIV seropositive during a trip. The insured must get two tests—one, 14 days after returning, which should be seronegative; and the other, 180 to 210 days after returning, which should be seropositive.

In Italy, an insurance policy has been given that will cover the applicant if he accidentally contracts HIV. The policy will be available to health care professionals, police personnel, and members of volunteer groups and later will be extended to dentists. In South Africa, SANA (the South African Nurses Association) has developed short-term insurance policies for nurses who may contract HIV through work. Applicants would not have to take a blood test or a medical examination and need only sign a "declaration of health."

In Great Britain, a "critical insurance policy, pays a lump sum for cancer, heart attacks, and strokes, but usually excludes HIV. Some companies will cover HIV if it is contracted through blood transfusion or from medical occupation". Australian insurers have given coverage for police, medical providers and others who contract HIV through employment. The insured would get $200,000 or twice one's annual salary, whichever is lower.

Within the United States, various insurers will give HIV insurance to health care workers who contract HIV in the course of employment. One insurer will give, through its HIV carrier protection plan, up to $250,000. The insured must take a test and report any workplace incident within 24 hours and then take a blood test within five days. A labour contract provision has given special disability insurance of $100,000 to a nurse who get HIV through employment. The American Medical Association also formulates a nationwide plan of a lump sum insurance amount of up to $500,000 to a physician who contracts HIV.

Death Futures

Some entities have offered to purchase life insurance policies of PWA through a Life Insurance Buyout. The purchaser becomes the irrevocable beneficiary, and the PWA gets remuneration that can be used for medicine, vacations or any other purpose. The purchaser will also continuously pay premiums until the death of the insured. The amount often depends upon how much time the HIV seropositive person has left. The buyout can extend from 30 per cent to 80 per cent. There are concerns whether the proceeds are taxable by the IRS or whether the payment would result in a loss of Supplemental Security Insurance/Medicaid benefits.

Two 26-year-old Americans have auctioned their policies in London. The first policy, paying $75,498 is hoped to sell for $60,000, and the insured has a life expectancy between 1.5 to 2 years. The second policy worth $100,000 should sell for $90,000 since the insured has only 13 months to survive. The purchaser must insure that the policy is unencumbered (i.e., not committed to mortgage repayment), that the insurance company has a proved history of stability, and that the insured is neither under any duress nor suffering from dearth of capacity.

A new business has formed to deal with these "death futures." Life Partners, Inc., for instance, "is one of the biggest of about 30 companies that invest in policies on their own or match buyers and sellers for fees or (3 to 5 per cent) commissions." In February 1995, Dignity Partners, Inc., which had purchased policies from HIV seropositive persons, "closed a $35 million deal" with Ironwood Capital Partners, Ltd.

For historical reasons, the British industry is "far less regulated in comparison of the United States." Within Great Britain, one might make effort to "surrender" a life insurance policy and one's success in obtaining moneys paid will increase if the policy has been in effect for over five years. An HIV seropositive person might get more money should he or she auction it or sell it to a company specializing in purchasing a policy from "people with life threatening conditions." An HIV seropositive person might be able to obtain the trustees of an occupational pension plan to pay immediately a lump sum on the term that he or she has less than 12 months to live. Parliamentary attempts to remove the requirement of "receiving a medical certificate stating he will unquestionably die within 12 months" have been unsuccessful.

Insurance of Coverage of Tort Actions of HIV

Insurance may cover an HIV seropositive person's negligent actions, but not those that are intentional. For instance, in *Christian v. Estate of Rock Hudson*, the jury concluded that Hudson's lover should be awarded $21.75 million as Hudson had not informed him of his HIV seropositive status while continuing intimacy. The amount was curtailed by the trial judge to $5.5 million.

One month after the jury award, Hudson's homeowners' insurance company filed a request for a declaration that it had no obligation to indemnify or defend Hudson's estate as the policy was not applicable to damage "which is expected or intended by the insured." The 9th Circuit, interpreting what the California Court would do, concluded that for Hudson to engage in unprotected sex for eight months after percepting he was HIV seropositive was an inherently harmful act which was exacerbated "by the seriousness and deadliness of AIDS." Since Hudson had deliberately misrepresented that he did not have HIV, the insurance company had no obligation to his estate under a homeowners' insurance policy. In Germany, an insurance policy will generally pay out if the insured is liable for infecting another, as long as the insured is not grossly negligent or intentional in acting to transmit HIV. Italian insurance companies also would accept liability.

Blood Transfusions

Blood transfusion responsibility and HIV is an issue that is beyond the scope of this section which is concerned only with the responsibility of the insurance coverage of a defendant. Nevertheless, some preliminary comments are necessary. In the United States, HIV seropositive blood transfusion recipients and persons with haemophilia have usually been unsuccessful either in litigation or in obtaining a settlement with blood product defendants or their insurance companies. There are many reasons for the plaintiffs' lack of success: unlike Canada, plaintiffs may sue neither in product responsibility nor implied warranty; plaintiffs' difficulty in proving negligence is exacerbated by utilization of a professional rather than an ordinary standard of care; there are also statute of limitation problems and often an inefficiency to discover a donor's recognition as well as the huge expenses of discovery. When plaintiffs do succeed at trial, the reward is often reversed on appeal or a new trial is mandated.

It appeared that a class settlement may have resolved the issue of allegations against manufacturers of blood products by HIV infected persons with haemophilia. In fact, a tentative settlement of $140-$160 million had been reached. Suddenly and unexpectedly, a federal judge granted partial class certification to the litigants. The chair of the committee representing the persons with haemophilia then denounced the offer as "absurdly low."

The court of appeals, however, reversed the class certification partly because it doubted that there was constitutional authority for one trial under "a law that is only an amalgam, or averaging of the non-identical laws of 51 jurisdictions." The impact of this reversal would make essential hundreds of separate cases and comprehensive costly discovery, subject to the laws of a number of jurisdictions. This is a terrible burden for attorneys operating on contingency fees and for clients who are responsible for court costs.

For insurance companies, such a settlement could have been a nightmare. Some of the defendants were "in litigation and negotiations" with insurers. One defendant, Baxter, sued in California, "seeking to force hundreds of liability insurers to defend and indemnify it against claims by (HIV) hemophiliacs." Insurers such as Zurich American emphasised it "provided no coverage for this sort of claim against Baxter. Therefore, we will not contribute to the reported settlement."

Insurance companies commonly pay the defendant's litigation costs and often all or part of settlement or unfavourable decisions. In the United States, however, only in rare instances they are directly involved in litigation, e.g., when a state law prohibits a charitable hospital from being sued which makes essential it being substituted by the insurance company, or when the widow of an HIV seropositive person, who contracted HIV from a blood transfusion before 1982, sued her homeowner's insurance policy which would pay the balance of the mortgage in case of accidental death.

It would seem that there must be a better approach than the adversarial system in blood bank litigation. One author has suggested the set up of a strict accountability "compensatory system similar to the National Vaccine Injury Compensation Programme. This would give swift, certain compensation to HIV transfusion victims while they are still alive." Insurance companies would benefit because an occasional "multimillion dollar judgment (has) started to trickle through their defenses."

In Germany, a Parliamentary AIDS Investigating Committee has come to a conclusion that about 60 per cent of Germany's over 2,300 HIV seropositive persons with haemophilia would not have become HIV seropositive between 1983 and 1987 had blood supply companies applied known screening procedures. The German Red Cross, for instance, utilized untested blood products through 1987 because "to acquire the required testing equipment was too expensive."

Compensation or indemnification of victims has not been as problematic in Germany because of a peculiarity of industry/ insurance payments. In 1978, about 130 German insurers and re-insurers, as well as pharmaceutical companies, created a "pharma-pool" to compensate injured parties in strict or product liability claims against pharmacy companies. By the end of 1994, the pool paid over DM120 million to over 1,250 HIV seropositive persons with haemophilia infected by blood products. The settlements ranged from DM20,000 to DM500,000. The insurance industry stressed that they are in no need of proof that a specific product caused HIV, "proof that most of the hemophiliacs would have had problem in supplying." The payment was made for loss of earnings and other material damages, but not pain and suffering since German law provides compensation only for proved negligence.

The German government, created, in 1994, developed a new fund (DM700 million) to compensate those HIV seropositive persons with haemophilia who have not received DM200,000 or more in settlement. Apart from the federal government, the states and drug industry have indicted a willingness to contribute. German insurers had denied to contribute partly because they claim to have already paid an average of DM60,000 per claimant. The government has threatened the companies with legislation that would force contributions, especially since the fund is grown to DM400 million and earns DM30 million p.a. in interest.

France, not like Germany, has an insurance industry that had been quasi-public. Furthermore, the actions of the French National Transfusion Centre to release feasibly HIV tainted blood for transfusion resulted in about 7,000 HIV infections, 1,200 of whom were persons with haemophilia. This has resulted in criminal prosecution, as well as serious questions of responsibility.

The French Insurance Companies Federation raised objection to a governmental proposal of compensation through a "special tax on damage insurance policies" which would raise approximately FF10 to FF14 billion. Ultimately, a compromise was made whereby insurance companies agreed to pay FF1.2 billion and the government became agree to replenish the fund after exhaustion. The trade body for the French insurance industry accepted the compromise "for the sake of national solidarity." Victims who accepted compensation, the amount of which was based according to circumstances, waived their right to further litigation. The state-owned UAP and Assurances Generales de France became agree to pay, respectively, FF109 million and FF68 million. Group AXA, a major private insurer, paid FF85 million. Perhaps this agreement was induced by the afraid of insurers that awards for HIV seropositive transfusion to about 400 plaintiffs averaged between FF1.5 million and 2.5 million.

In few countries, litigation has been a viable alternative for HIV seropositive persons with haemophilia. In the Netherlands, an individual became HIV seropositive when injected with properly not cleaned needle used on an AIDS patient. The insurer accepted liability and paid $86,000 as compensation and an additional $57,000 for pain and suffering. When the victim rejected the $57,000 for pain and suffering. When the victim rejected the $57,000 and demanded $400,000, the Supreme Court awarded him $170,000 for pain, "the highest amount awarded in the Netherlands."

In other countries it is not easy to sue a hospital for negligence related to HIV seropositive transfusions. In Romania, the parents/ guardians of children with HIV have started litigation against a government and medical system which "had benefited from a quasi-immunity under a half century of communism." They are suing for $162,000. "Equally novel is the attempt to cite individual doctors for malpractice. 'Professional liability is a reality when it is linked with a system of professional insurance, which does not exist yet in Romania'."

Within Australia, the vast majority of litigated cases have been lost by HIV seropositive persons with haemophilia largely because of the difficulty of proof. Fortunately for victims, almost all Australian states have settled claims. In one case, litigation costs totalled $15 million after an 87-day trial, with a payment of $87,000. In Victoria, federal state and insurance companies made a group settlement with 112 HIV seropositive persons who medically acquired HIV.

Great Britain and Canada have essentially settled all blood transfusion claims by creating a governmental fund. In Canada, unlike Great Britain, insurance companies have become agree to make substantial payments in the settlement with persons with haemophilia on the condition that the recipients sign a release or waiver of litigation. The insurance payments will profit mainly spouses and children of HIV seropositive persons with haemophilia and blood transfusion recipients. Perhaps one major cause behind the settlement is that the judiciary has twice ruled against class action litigation by Canadians infected with HIV through transfusion or plasma.

Conclusion

Insurance companies are, of course, in business to make a profit. All countries, however, impose a specially high standard by insurers. For insurers to simply deny to insure people with different lifestyles is not only unfair, but irrational. Related individuals with HIV, governmental subsidy of insurance for PWA would be ideal as many people who are asymptomatic have many long years ahead of them. In a number of countries, such a suggestion would be considered unrealistic. Certainly for society to do nothing means that HIV seropositive individuals are forced to depend totally on charity or on programmes such as Medicaid in the United States. By not offering HIV seropositive persons early medical care, society will pay much more through programmes such as Medicaid.

Fourteen

Role of NGOs

Acquired Immuno-deficiency Syndrome (AIDS) was first identified as a disease among homosexual males in USA in 1981. By the time the virus that causes AIDS – the human immuno-deficiency virus (HIV) – was isolated in 1983, the infection had spread across the globe. According to recent records, by mid-1996 HIV had infected a cumulative total of 28 million people, including 1.5 million children. Near about 5 million of these individuals are from Asia.

As the AIDS pandemic continues to spread throughout South-East Asia, a number of different organizations are becoming involved in the prevention and care of HIV/AIDS. Non-governmental organizations (NGOs) have a special part to play in this effort. Their community-based action can help a lot strengthen the national AIDS response. While maintaining their autonomy, specific interest and areas of work, NGOs and national AIDS programmes (NAPs) share common aims and objectives in AIDS prevention and control.

Experience however shows that while the number of NGOs engaged in AIDS-related issues has increased quite appreciably over the years, the technical and managerial capacity of many NGOs needs strengthening. Moreover, AIDS as a complex issue, it may be important for NGOs to have a deep knowledge of the issues, so that they could respond more effectively.

Role of NGOs in National Response to the AIDS

A number of different population groups such as commercial sex workers, those who indulge in unprotected sex and with multiple partners, injecting drug users (IDUs) and sexually transmitted disease (STD) patients, are at high risk of contracting HIV/AIDS. The sexual partners of these individuals are also especially vulnerable. These marginalized high risk groups are more accessible to NGOs than to government programmes. The role of NGOs is very important as:

- They are people-oriented, and are better acquainted with and more sensitive to the requirements and concerns of those affected by HIV/AIDS;
- The close interpersonal interaction which NGOs have with people in the communities they work in is extremely beneficial for implementing the behavioural interventions essential for HIV/AIDS prevention;
- NGOs often work in areas and regions which are not generally covered by government programmes;
- NGOs are not under the same political hurdles as government programmes are. They therefore have greater flexibility and the capacity to accommodate changing programmes and public needs and can innovate and implement new initiatives without major constraints;
- NGOs are more efficient and effective in the use of resources and can provide support directly to people and communities.

Above all, NGOs can play an important collaborative role in the planning, implementation and evaluation of the National AIDS Programme. Their activities widely reflect the national and regional priorities of the national programme which focuses on the modes of spread, the predominant risk groups involved and the rates of spread in various population groups and geographic areas.

This document aims to help NGOs to:

- become conversant with the strategies for HIV/AIDS prevention and control, as well as with the impact the epidemic could have if it continues its unabated spread;
- know the risk factors and understand priority interventions required for prevention of HIV transmission and the care of people with HIV/AIDS and their families;
- identify specific roles that they could play in the national response to the epidemic;
- suggest and develop mechanisms for collaboration, build alliances and promote information exchanges with other NGOs, National AIDS Programme Managers and international organizations.
- draft proposals for funding of specific projects.

Understanding the Regional Situations

Though most countries in the South-East Asia Region (SEAR) of the World Health Organization have so far reported comparatively small numbers of AIDS cases, the rate of spread since the late 1980s has been surprising. The virus is now spreading not only among people with high risk behaviour but also in the general population.

The total number of AIDS cases has gradually increased, particularly during the 1990s. By 1 January 1997, the SEAR countries had reported more than 49,000 AIDS cases to WHO. Given the long latency period of the virus, the problems of under-recognition and under-reporting in the countries, this figure can be completely misleading. By the year 2000, in conformity with estimates, there will be nearly 10 million HIV infections in the region and the number of full-blown AIDS cases may reach the two million mark.

India and Thailand currently account for more than 95 per cent of the cases reported from the region. Table 14.1 shows the number of cases as reported and the estimated number of HIV infections in various countries of South-East Asia.

TABLE 14.1
AIDS AND HIV INFECTIONS IN SEAR COUNTRIES AS ON 1 JANUARY, 1997

Country	*Reported AIDS Cases*	*Estimated HIV Infections*
Bangladesh	7	<20000
Bhutan	0	75
DPR Korea	0	<100
India	2996	2500000
Indonesia	110	95000
Maldives	3	60
Myanmar	1349	350000
Nepal	53	5000
Sri Lanka	68	6000
Thailand	44471	800000
Total	49057	>3750000

HIV Infections

The rates of spread of HIV in Asia vary geographically and by population subgroups. In certain parts of Thailand, India and Myanmar, HIV seroprevalence has approached the levels of 40 per cent to 60 per cent among commercial sex workers and injecting drug users. Also, other population groups of present STD patients, truck drivers and professional blood donors have shown rapid increases in HIV infections in most countries of the region. Even those SEAR countries which at present have low rates of prevalence of HIV are likely to present scenarios similar to those in Thailand and Myanmar, because risk behaviours such as injecting drug use (IDU), unprotected sex with a number of partners, along with high rates of untreated STDs—which encourage the spread of HIV-are widespread in the region. By 1995, HIV infection rates among pregnant women had increased to 2.5 per cent in Bombay, India; 8 per cent in Chiang Mai, and 3 per cent to 7 per cent in parts of Myanmar.

Epidemiological Factors

Certain important epidemiological aspects of the AIDS pandemic which have been noticed in Asia should be kept in view while planning any HIV/AIDS prevention activity. HIV infections do not uniformly affect all population. They disproportionately affect individuals with high risk behaviours and practices and their partners. The high risk behaviours and practices associated with HIV transmission are (see Table 14.2)

- Unprotected sexual relation with multiple partners, between males and females, and between two males;
- Sharing and re-use of inadequately sterilized needles and syringes by IDUs or within the health care settings, and transfusion of HIV infected blood or blood products;
- Besides, HIV is transmitted perinatally. From an infected mother to an infant or fetus, the transmission can take place in the post-partum as well as perinatal period.

HIV infections are introduced into different geographical areas and populations not at the same times. For example, in Bangkok, the infection which spread rapidly among the IDUs in 1988 later passed through to other high risk behaviour and subsequently to the general population. A similar pattern is being repeated in different parts of India and Myanmar and is also likely to occur in other South-East Asian countries. The latency period—that is, the time between becoming infected with HIV and the onset of AIDS—is unusually long, about eight to ten years. Once an individual develops AIDS, the survival time seems to be less than two years.

TABLE 14.2
HIV TRANSMITTED THROUGH DIFFERENT ROUTES

Route of transmission	*Percentage of infections*
Sexual intercourse	85-90
Blood Transfusion	3-5
Injecting drug use	3-5
Medical equipment and needles	0-1
Perinatal	2-5

Since sexual transmission responsible for around 85 to 90 per cent of HIV infections in Asia, it is important to concentrate efforts and resources of the prevention programme on promoting safe sexual behaviour among individuals with high risk behaviour and in the general population.

Existing evidence suggests that appropriately targeted interventions initiated early enough in the epidemic and sustained over time can cause delay the progress of the AIDS pandemic.

WHO Guidelines for National AIDS Programmes

In 1994, WHO developed guidelines for National AIDS Programmes (NAPs) in terms of the important role played by and support needs of NGOs. This document underlines WHO support to the process of capacity building in NGOs and community groups.

Besides providing technical and material support to NGOs, WHO has laid stress on the need to increase access to information by contacting various networks and interface organizations, by recognising intermediary organizations which can serve as support centres and be centres for providing technical assistance to other NGOs and community-based groups. National AIDS programmes should facilitate information exchange through setting up consortia, organising regular meetings and briefings, and by distributing pertinent documents and research findings.

NGO representation in planning and policy development is necessary. This can be achieved by including them in national committees, planning teams and in review and evaluation of programmes. Most importantly, we should try our utmost to increase access by NGOs to technical and financial support through training programmes, sharing of technical resources and liaison with the international donor agencies.

Support from National AIDS Programmes and other Sectors

NGOs with their limited resources can expand their activities through mutual collaboration, particularly through the National AIDS Programmes. In most SEAR countries, the National AIDS Programmes realize the need of NGO participation in the battle against AIDS. However, increasing effective working partnerships is sometimes disturbed owing to management and administrative problems.

To facilitate coordination activities, NGOs should seek out more opportunities to express their concerns to the National AIDS Programmes and other agencies. The problems arising out of differences in goals, interests and objectives of the different organizations can best be settled through frank discussions, both formally and informally, between all those involved.

The collaboration between NAPs and NGOs should work under the following broad areas of understanding.

National AIDS Programmes Should

(1) take liability for building a multisectoral response involving various partners, including NGOs, and accommodating divergent views and approaches;
(2) ensure that all those concerned with AIDS work are considered equal partners;
(3) accept that the different organizations involved may work with different mandates and styles, and attempt to minimize the politics involved while encouraging consensus in decision making;

(4) ensure that the process of collaboration should be opened and participatory, and build relationships among partners to form jointly-accepted goals and strategies; and
(5) supply technical and material support to and share resources with NGOs so that they can work effectively to support the overall national response to HIV/AIDS.

And NGOs Should

(1) participate actively in formulating and implementing common programme objectives and priorities to strengthen national efforts;
(2) accept and incorporate the national objectives and priorities into their work;
(3) maintain constant consultations and exchange information with the communities that they represent;
(4) support communities in ensuring important issues, plan and implement activities, and communicate these to the NAPs; and
(5) use resources as per national policies and strategies.

Mechanisms and Structures of Collaboration

The strategies of collaboration and coordination have to be country-specific, since goals and targets will be defined according to the needs of the country programmes and the institutional and human resources available. The modes of collaboration in the different countries will also depend on the varying structures of government and of NGOs. In general, the following mechanisms may be helpful in building and maintaining a multisectoral alliance.

National AIDS Committees

A national level committee under the leadership of a minister or a senior policy planner or a high level of authority may be an ideal structure or umbrella to draw multisectoral participation. If adequately flexible, it can help enhance the initiatives and activities of all partners involved.

Committees should have representation from all major sectors both private and public and will meet regularly and serve as a forum for free and frank discussion about programme policies and activities. Sub-committees or Working Groups may be formed to establish coordination between specific issues and activities. The representation of NGOs should reflect the extent of their involvement in the national programme.

It is potent that NGOs working in the programme areas as well as those with special technical capabilities are represented on the committee.

The responsibilities of National AIDS Committees include:

1. Setting overall policy framework and goals for the programme;
2. Participation of representatives from all sectors concerned in the country AIDS programme;
3. Acting as a democratic forum to sort out differences on policies and plans and to achieve a consensus, and
4. Resolving conflicts among political, public and technical authorities.

An NGO representation is also essential in the separate sub-committees as relevant.

NGO Co-ordinating Groups and Networking

Different mechanisms such as NGO networks, coordinating groups, and consortia are important for a collaborative process. The tasks of such groups may consist of:

1. Ensuring NGO representation and input into regional and national level committees and management teams;
2. Establishing coordination among members;
3. Supporting NGO participation in policy development and AIDS programme planning and implementation.;
4. Strengthening the administrative and technical capacities of the partner NGOs; and
5. Establishing exchange of information and sharing of experiences and resources among NGOs.

NGO Fora and Umbrella Organisations

NGOs working on HIV/AIDS or concerned activities may want to establish a representative forum to harmonize their activities with the government and private sector. The forum could consists of a group of people from selected NGOs. Representation could also possible through a nodal agency or umbrella organization. Such an organization can work as the NGO's representative to the government on management and administrative issues.

It is important that NGOs, NAPs and private and public sector organizations involved in the programme resolve important policy and operational conflicts in advance so that all activities in the country are according to national policies and strategies. An effective coordination among the NGOs, NAPs and other agencies can also help strengthening the technical, management and administrative skills of the smaller NGOs. NGOs often find bureaucratic procedures extremely burdened and are apprehensive of their involvement in projects needing improved technical and administrative resources. An NGO umbrella agency may be able to take on the accountability of helping NGOs with proposal writing, dealing with administrative matters and setting up monitoring systems. It may also provide programme support such as funding and financial management, and technical assistance in other areas.

The proposed terms of reference of the umbrella organization are given in Annexure 1.

Information Exchange

For NGOs wanting to get involved in AIDS activities, the first step is to find out about other NGOs working in the area, establish contact with them and know about their ongoing projects. NGO collaborative mechanisms such as fora, networks or umbrella organizations can facilitate informal and formal information exchange. Endeavours should be made to supplement the existing programmes in accordance with local needs and available resources. For example, there may be many NGOs working in the red-light areas and they may all be working chiefly to promote the use of condoms among the sex workers, ignoring other issues such as education of clients of sex workers, continuously condom supply, STD treatment, and so on, that may directly help sex workers deal with problems regarding AIDS.

NGOs which have been working in the sphere of AIDS and are familiar with the issues related to it can, through information exchange, help other NGOs which are not yet involved or not motivated to get involved in the AIDS programme. Organizational meetings also prove helpful for various NGOs to:

- identify common goals and areas of expertise;
- resolve differences and resolve work-related problems;
- find ways to interlink activities for the best use of their resources;
- decide who can do what best and how different NGOs can combine their resources.

Technical Resource Materials and Support

There are several foundations, NGOs and other private organizations working in the sphere of AIDS/HIV. Some of them with international links, make available funding for various projects. Organizations like the Asia Pacific Council of AIDS Service Organizations (APCASO), the Global Network of People Living with AIDS (GNP+), and the International HIV/AIDS Alliance are support groups and information sharing networks that can provide assistance and guidance to NGOs.

The addresses of these organizations are given below:

APCASO
Yayasan Citra Usadha Indonesia
Jalan Belimbing Gang Y No. 4
Denpasar, Bali 80231
Indonesia
Tel: (62-361) 222-620
Fax: (62-361) 229-487
E-mail: ycui@denpasar. wasantara.net.id
Contact Person: Dr Tuti Parwati Merati, Chair

APN+ (TheAsian Network of People Living with HIV/AIDS - the regional subgroup of GNP+)
62B Race Course Road
Singapore 218568
Coordinator: Paul Toh
Tel: 65-295-1153
Fax: 65-295-5567
E-mail: paultoh@pacific.neg.sg

International HIV/AIDS Alliance
Barratt House
341 Oxford Street
London W1R 3BH, U.K.
Tel: 44-171-491-2000
Fax: 44-171-491-2001
E-mail: 100302.3011@compuserve.com

WHO and UNAIDS regularly produce and update information on various aspects of HIV/AIDS policies and programmes. The Director of European Funders of HIV/AIDS Projects in Developing Countries is also a useful resource. It may be obtained by writing to UK NGO AIDS Consortium for the Third World, Fenner Brockway House, 37/39 Great Guildford Street, London SE1 OES, United Kingdom. Fax: 44-71-401-2124, Tel: 44-71-401-8231), E-mail: ukaidscon@gn.apc.org Price: Pounds 10.00 (Europe), Pounds 12.50 (Australia, Canada and USA), free to developing countries. The WHO South-East Asia Regional Office regularly products AIDS-related documents and publications many of these can be of use to NGOs in their work.

Resource Mobilisation and NGO Activities

Funding often depends completely on how well a project proposal has been written. However a number of NGOs do not have the expertise for writing good project proposals and this severely hinders their fund-raising capacity. Such limitations may prevent the involvement particularly of smaller NGOs in activities for which they may otherwise be best equipped.

Most national programmes and other bilateral and multilateral agencies have standard guidelines for funding AIDS-related projects. These guidelines should be distributed by NAPs to NGOs in the country. NGOs can seek guidelines either from the National AIDS Programme or funding agencies.

NGOs Take the Lead

Non-governmental organizations play an important role everywhere, but they are especially important in those countries where government action is constrained by strong cultural or religious traditions. Among the many examples:

- *The Syrian Women's Union* plays a sincere part in raising awareness about HIV/AIDS, conducting seminars for health personnel, running workshops on education and counselling, and helping design information materials. Members of the Medical Services Office of the Union, in collaboration with the Ministry of Health, have also visited prisons and social work schools to give out information on AIDS and how to prevent it.
- *The Egyptian AIDS Society*, established in Alexandria in mid-1992 and funded largely by local businessmen, has talked about AIDS on television and held information days in universities, secondary schools and family planning centres. It has also organized information workshops for medical professionals, social workers and police officers. The society aims to give social and financial support to people with HIV infection and AIDS and their families, and to provide counselling to those who need it.
- *The Pakistan AIDS Prevention Society* was formed in 1990 by a group of people, including teachers and trade-unionists, who saw the need for broad-based community action. Its work is public information and education. Major objectives are to dispel prejudice, stigma and discrimination in a country where ignorance and denial of AIDS are still widespread.
- In 1992, *the Arab Scouts Movement*, a pan-Arab organization, brought together members from all national scout organizations for a meeting that focussed, among other things, on AIDS. The meeting agreed that all national societies should provide their members with information on AIDS and how to protect oneself from the virus, so that they could spread the word among their families, friends and communities.
- In 1989, in Ljubljana, Slovenia, a group of drug users attending a psychotherapy programme threatened with closure, started *Stigma*, a self help organization to look after the interests of drug users and give them information about AIDS. Despite public resistance and an uncertain relationship with the authorities—including the health

services and police—*Stigma* has established drop-in information centres for drug users in three towns. Volunteer staff offer advice and counselling and the Ljubljana branch runs a needle-exchange programme. *Stigma* also operated telephone hotlines; publishes information materials and a newsletter; and takes advantage of any opportunity to campaign for the rights of drug users, and to promote safer drug injecting and sexual behaviour.

- *GAPA/RS* is an AIDS prevention programme for prisoners in the state of Rio Grande do Sul, Brazil. Its central activity has been the production of an eductional comic book that incorporates AIDS information in the story of a man in prison. Six prisoners in Porto Alegre were involved in creating the story line and characters, so the comic has an authentic and credible voice, and conveys a positive image of prisoners. The comic raises issues of injecting drug use and unsafe sexual behaviour, and messages are reinforced by the inclusion of puzzles and quizzes for the reader. A condom is given away with each comic. The programme, which is to be adopted in other states, includes a video version of the story for showing in prisons.

Part-VI

AIDS, Women and Human Rights

Fifteen

AIDS, Women and Human Rights

History of Human Rights

Some experts claim that human rights lay the very foundations of international law. The earliest records of legal dealings among peoples, traceable to relations among the city-states of classical Greece, emphasised the need to respect the rights that citizens enjoyed under Natural Law by virtue of their human status. The regard paid to the protection of diplomatic representatives of other city-states upon the outbreak of war reflected their entitlement to human rights. Anthropologists tracing the development of law, and its contribution to order, have interpreted law, including the laws of warfare, as a means of limiting violence and savagery and of preserving the respect that citizens owe to each other through the common bond of their human status.

The historic rules of humanitarian interference provided exceptions to the otherwise absolute claims of national sovereignty. The concept of sovereignty among nations governed the international legal order defined by Natural Law principles and endorsed by European religious authorities during the evolutionary phase of modern international law. The sovereign equality of members of the community of nations precluded one nation from interfering in the domestic affairs of other nations. If a state dealt inhumanely in its territory with the citizens of another state, the national state had legal rights of humanitarian interference. The historic laws of war among states, more ancient than the laws of peace, necessitated confinement of hostilities to combatant forces of hostile nations, and provided immunity from attack for their civilian populations on the basis of humanity.

The limitation of humanitarianism under the legal doctrine of sovereignty was that international law provided no supervision of a state's treatment of its own citizens. International law regulated the rights by which a state could claim that individuals and populations were its citizens, for example, on territorial acquisition and transfer between states, but when an individual's nationality was not legally questioned, that individual's subjection to the sovereign power of his or her nation-state within its territory was complete. Nations whose treatment of citizens fell short of the perceived standard of civilisation maintained by the historic European nation-states would have been considered not to be members of the community of nations whose practices furnished the content of international customary law, but recognised members were free from the scrutiny of others relating treatment within their territory of their own citizens.

Women's special requirements of international safety were recognised in the early decades of the present century through a series of international agreements. Their aim was not to liberate women within their homes, but to protect them in industry outside the home, and to protect them from sexual and other personal vulnerability that might destroy the integrity of family units. The International Convention Respecting Prohibition of Night Work for Women in Industrial Employment, of the year 1906, was the first international convention supported by the International Labour Office, protecting women in the workforce, which was reinforced by other conventions revealing humane protection of women such as the Convention relating to Employment of Women Before and After Childbirth of the year 1919. Similarly, the International Convention for the Suppression of Traffic in Women and Children, of the year 1921, was the first of a series of international conventions reflecting humane and moral concerns for protection of women and families. These treaties were open to adoption by states as an act of sovereign authority but were not mandatory, as is international customary law, on states that did not endorse them.

The conclusion of World War II marked a turning point in international tolerance of states' absolute sovereign authority over their own citizens, and over individuals who had become stateless by declarations of governments of territories which they had fled and who were, therefore, not amenable to protection under the laws of humanitarian interference. The conduct of Germany and of administrations in other countries cooperating in the German war effort regarding their Jewish and other citizens, gypsies and homosexuals, culminating in policies for their extermination, was considered a violation of any powers that could legitimately be claimed by even sovereign authorities. Such conduct amounted to punishable crimes against humanity committed by governmental and military leaders and those exercising powers derived from sovereignty.

To recognise the violation of humane and civilised conduct that had been evidenced recently the United Nations, which was created in the year 1945, drafted the Universal Declaration of Human Rights in the year 1948. The document was entitled a Declaration to confirm that it was not attempting to create new law but simply to declare the international law on human rights that existed before, and that had been violated in cases preceding the Declaration and inspiring its expression in concrete language in 1948. Being a declaration, the 1948 text was not itself legally binding. However, to provide direct legal force and definition to the spirit of the Declaration, a number of international conventions was implemented which has formed the modern international foundation for human rights law. These legal instruments have provided a set of human rights principles so widely accepted as to be understood on various grounds to have become international customary law which is legally binding on states without their express acceptance or confirmation. The modern international legal order demands the governments to respect international customary law in their international and domestic affairs as a attribute of their legitimacy as governments capable to be validated as such.

International Foundations of Human Rights Law

The modern international human rights law is established on international, regional and subject-specific conventions animated by the Universal Declaration of Human Rights. The general conventions are the International Covenant on Civil and Political Rights (the Political Covenant) and the International Covenant on Economic, Social and Cultural Rights (the Economic Covenant). The regional conventions are the European Convention on Human Rights, the American Convention on Human Rights and the African Charter on Human and Peoples' Rights. The leading specialized conventions are the International Convention on the Elimination of All Forms of Racial Discrimination (the Race Convention), the Convention on the Elimination of All Forms of Discrimination against Women (the Women's Convention) and the Convention on the Rights of the Child.

All these conventions have founded committees to monitor state consent with their provisions through mandatory, periodic state reports, and some committees receive complaints of violations that citizens make against states. The treaty committees may conduct investigations and present views on complaints of state violations. The committees can also offer help to states on the scope and content of obligations arising under the terms of each and every article of the conventions.

Leading provisions of different conventions applicable to HIV infection and the maintenance of health can be recognized by reference to named rights under their peculiar articles. It is necessary to observe the functional interdependence of individual rights with respect to the socio-economic and cultural dimensions of women's health status. The necessity of applying all human rights to improve women's status within societies and hence their negotiating ability within sexual relationships was underscored by the Platform for Action accepted by the Fourth World Conference on Women in Beijing in 1995, the Beijing Platform for Action). This Platform explained that :

> The human rights for women contain their right to control and decide freely and responsibly the matters connected to their sexual relationships, including sexual and reproductive health, free of coercion, discrimination and violence. Equal relationships between men and women in matters of sexual relations and reproduction, having complete respect for the integrity of the person need mutual respect, consent and shared responsibility for sexual relationship and its results.

Some of these rights may at first appear more distant from women's health can be shown in practice to be more proximate, or to be an important component of exercise of a right more clearly connected to health. For instance, the right to education is basis of literacy, without which individuals cannot learn various precautionary strategies for the maintenance of their health.

Many human rights, found in different international and regional human rights treaties, can be applied to women's health concerns. For instance, readers' literacy is of limited value if authors and publishers do not enjoy the right to provide information. Women's health is impressively aided by women's access to education and literacy and on the right to provide to others the information they have for example, on matters of safe and effective control of unwanted pregnancy and transmission of STDs.

The Committee on the Elimination of Discrimination against Women (CEDAW), the institution established by the women's Convention to volunteer compliance of States Parties with its terms, had paid special attention to how women's subordinate and dependent status in various communities denies and compromises their opportunities for self-defence against HIV infection. CEDAW has attracted attention towards the requirement to prevent discrimination against women in national AIDS tactics and has suggested that "programmes to combat AIDS should give special attention to the rights and requirements of women, and to the factors connecting to the reproductive act of women and their subordinate position in some societies that make them vulnerable to the infection of HIV."

The Obligation of Non-discrimination

Probably the most basic right in social existence, persons' right to non-discrimination on such basis as race and sex has now been so globally endorsed and recognized as a minimum condition of civilized behaviour as to have passed from the law grounded on acceptance of treaties to become international customary law, that binds all states without their clear agreement. States are not legally free to claim a general exemption from this obligation on the basis that they have not subscribed to a peculiar international convention. It is hardly demonstrable that the practice of states falls short of full observance of this obligation, and equally demonstrable which the incomplete nature of the international legal order sets states that violate this obligation from regular condemnation and sanction. The Race Convention has been broadly adopted by states, and the Women's Convention was brought into legal effect rapidly and now has over 140 states parties. Nevertheless, international entities, such as the Holy Sea and many Islamic States, which claim religious inspiration and moral authority for their behaviour, have declined to validate the Women's Convention, or have restricted their acceptance by such extensive reservations as to create doubts about if they are member states in law.

Sex and Gender Discrimination

The liability of women's to be excluded from similar rights with men, on the basis, for example, of religious principles that exclude women from having equal spiritual influence with men within religious hierarchies, and women's shut out from or subordinate representation within military groups that form governments or that are strongly effective on them, are illustrations of discrimination on the basis of both sex and gender. Sex discrimination against women as such and negative gender stereotyping that confines the social acts of women are both sources of women's health disadvantage, and their excessive vulnerability to HIV infection. Women's liability to suffer compromised health on the basis of gender is uncovered by the wide description of "health" provided by the Constitution of the World Health Organization (WHO), which has been accepted by all the states that are members of the WHO. "Health" is said to be "a state of complete physical, mental and social well-being and not merely the absence of disease or infirmity." UN member states accepted the programme of action at the 1994 International Conference on Population and Development held in Cairo, which was built on this explanation to define reproductive health as:

> "a state of complete physical, mental and social well-being and not merely the absence of disease or infirmity, in all matters concerning the reproductive system and to its functions. Reproductive health thus implies that people are able to have a satisfactory and safe sexual life and that they have the ability to reproduce and the freedom to decide when and how often to do so. In this last condition,

> there are the right of men and women to be acknowledged and to have access to safe and effective methods of family planning of their choice, along with other methods of their choice for regulation of fertility which are not against the law, and the right of access to suitable health-care services that will secure the women to go safely through pregnancy and childbirth and provide the couples with better chance of having a healthy child".

A large number of the disadvantages that fluctuates women's health arise from gender discrimination in their society, and from political, economic, spiritual and other sources of subordination that affect women's self-determination and self-esteem, giving rise to frustration and depression reflected in the absence of social and mental well-being.

The sex is a topic of biological classification but gender is a social frame applied by our societies through culture and social psychology. Gender concepts affect social institutions including the family, individual role expectations and aspirations, and, for example, the cultural senses of order, propriety and nature. For instance, authority is seen as male gendered, honestly exercised by male gendered institutions like governments, military administrations, religious, judicial and academic hierarchies and professional associations. Male gendered features are strength, decisiveness and willingness to oppose adversity and to struggle for ascendancy. Female gendered acts are subordinate and centre on service to others, especially in families, such as through housekeeping, child-care and nursing the infants disabled elderly and sick. Female gendered features are submission, indecisiveness and weakness.

Among the health care professions, nursing is female gendered. Nurses are considered historically the compliant handmaidens of doctors and constitute at most a subordinate profession. In many countries nurses still wear the modest convent garb of nuns, and are paid as meanly as others in lowly-esteemed services, such as domestic helpers and kitchen hands. Likewise, birth attendants and midwives are often considered secondary health care professionals to obstetricians, whose services, though delivered exclusively to women, are considered male gendered.

The acts which defy a prevailing social gender formation are frequently described as "unnatural", and explained as defying an order that is set without the influence of societies and cultures, for example by authoritative interpretation of divine will. By these rationalizations states claim that they have no responsibility of the discrimination they practice on the basis of gender. They may indicate toward the legislation that prohibits discrimination on the basis of sex, and disclaim accountability for the results that perpetuate the disadvantage which women suffer in practice. That is why the Women's Convention considered it necessary to reiterate the prohibition of discrimination on the basis of sex contained in the Universal Declaration and the Economic and the Political Covenants, observing that "despite these various instruments, extensive discrimination against women continues to exist". The Convention in Article 5(1) also provides that states should "take appropriate steps to modify the social and cultural patterns of behaviour to eliminate prejudices and customary and other practices based on the inferiority or superiority of either sex."

Gender Discrimination and HIV Infection

The health of women is prejudiced on the basis of their gender when in childhood, girl children are fed upon scarce food supplies only after boy children's appetites are completely satisfied. In many societies, girl children are regarded as a burden and detriment to the families, their births being at times a source of condemnation to their mothers. Health status is again compromised when girls become marriageable in early adolescence, at an age less than that for boys, and when after marriage women have no control over the timing of sexual intercourse, their husbands' sexual activity outside marriage, or husbands' use of safety measures to prevent from sexually transmitted diseases including HIV-infection. Women are frequently defenceless to the risk of HIV infection because of their subordinate and servile family and social status that the elimination of discrimination on the basis of both sex and gender should relieve. It is unauspicious that the population among which infection and AIDS are rising very rapidly comprised of women of reproductive age group.

The Beijing Platform for Action explained that

> "AIDS and other STDs, the transmission of which is sometimes a result of sexual violence, are having a desolating effect on women's health, especially the health of adolescent girls and young women. They often have no power to insist on safe and responsible sex practices and have little information and services for prevention and treatment. Women, representing the half of all adults newly infected with HIV and other sexually transmitted disease have highlighted that social vulnerability and the unbalanced relationships between women and men are barriers to safe sex, in their efforts to control the spread of sexually transmitted diseases. The results of AIDS reach beyond women's health to their act as mothers and caregivers and their participation in the economic support of the families. The social, developmental and health consequences of AIDS and other sexually transmitted diseases need to be seen in the light of gender perspective".

The gender discrimination can be seen even within otherwise enlightened health care systems. "Mandatory" HIV testing is generally taken to mean that testing is necessary only if individuals want to avail themselves of a particular right, service or opportunity. For example, donors of blood for transfusion will be subject to mandatory testing, but do not have to volunteer to donate. Oppression of women takes place when testing is mandatory for receipt of medical services that women cannot conscientiously forgo, especially existing services concerned with pregnancy, childbirth and care of the newborn. Mandatory testing becomes coercive and discriminatory when hospitals' regular practices that are gender-neutral on their face are applied to medical services which only women seek. Further, pregnancy and neonatal care arise not out of illness, but out of women's conscientious concern for themselves and for the children they bear. The practice of global precautions in delivery of these services decreased the requirement for HIV testing of women and their infants.

The gender and sex discriminations keep on to operate in present times to predispose women in many cultures to unduly high levels of HIV infection. A stereotype of women is that they are sexually humble and passive, and that only "loose" girls prepare themselves for sexual activity. The pervasive difficulty that young girls face in the quest for such birth control measures as condoms, which may draw communal attention to them, is provoked for adolescent girls, in that their prestige and value in marriage may be defamed if they compete for increasing the supplies of condoms against the males fixed to be their sexual partners. An obstetrician in Zimbabwe has noticed that "adolescents have very tough task to find condoms in the rural areas. Community-based distributors chiefly responsible for contraceptive pills and condoms in such areas do not cater for adolescents. A rural or small-town boy, let alone girl, could hardly obtain a condom without the whole community talking about it. This problem requires urgent attention because about 30 per cent of teenager pregnant girls are HIV positive."

The uneducated and illiterate adolescence women have few means of sustaining themselves outside their parents' homes before marriage. The gendered conditions of access to economic opportunities even for the literate deprive women of means to get into all but the most modest forms of industry. Women's service opportunities are limited, and then confined to service functions of a domestic character, generally paid at minimum wages where minimum rates are legislated and enforced. Accordingly, some young women are denied opportunities for self-sustaining services, except by prostitution. Even afforded the most dignified title of sex workers, they may acquire little, but remain exploitable and at high risk of HIV infection through inability to enforced condom use by their indiscriminate clientele.

The traditional gender discrimination often increases women's vulnerability to HIV infection. The women who are married to considerably older men, face early widowhood under legal regimes that exclude or minimize widows' rights of property inheritance. The widows become burdens to their husbands' families, but are unable to rejoin birth families that were relieved to give them in marriage. As their fathers' daughters, their inheritance, if any, will be secondary to that of their brothers. In societies where survival depends on land holding, subsistence agriculture and modest husbanding of cattle, women's inability in law and fact to acquire land denies them means to support themselves and their families in widowhood; their sons may be supported by their deceased husbands' families, but they remain responsible for the welfare of their daughters. Further, prostitution may be their only means to support themselves and their families. Enforcing the laws of sexual and gender equality in the areas like inheritance, land holding, education and training, similar employment opportunities, equal pay for equal work and, for example, bank loans and other forms of commercial credit, though not immediately concerned to considerations of infection and disease, would afford women opportunities in life that would decrease their vulnerability to HIV infection derived selling their bodies to which sex and gender discrimination may entrust them.

Some Other Internationally Protected Human Rights

(i) The Rights to Life and Survival

The degree to how far international human rights law must develop to contain the rate of HIV infection and to defend women's fundamental rights more effectively is the narrow meaning that international practice has provided to the right to life and survival. The right originates at the beginning of the Universal Declaration, the Political Covenant, the three regional human rights conventions, and, for example, the Children's Convention. The mysterious record of HIV infection and AIDS connects infection closely to premature death and denial of the right to life. Present experience reveals that the right has been applied, however, only to the issue of due process of law advancing a judicial sentence of capital punishment. Considerable scope, therefore, exists to widen this concept to create and enforce legal claims of AIDS patients to life-prolonging care, of HIV positive persons to treatment to postpone the onset of AIDS, and, for example, of those at high risk of HIV infection to preventive care and education. Interests growing under various conventions may be tied together in resistance of HIV infection. For example, women's ways to protect their health through provisions of the Women's Convention would protect their children, whose rights are mentioned in the Children's Convention.

(ii) The Right to Health Care

The right to health care is mentioned in the Economic Covenant, Article 12(1) of which recognizes "the right of everybody to the enjoyment of the highest attainable standard of physical and mental health". The Article again recognizes some steps to be taken for this purpose, and indicates many points of intersection between rights to health care and other rights that relate to health protection and promotion. The Article acknowledges that health care includes the avoidance of HIV infection, but also that those who are HIV positive enjoy rights to the highest health status they can get, including maintenance of a symptom-free condition, decrement of symptoms in the shortest possible period when they occur, and experience of maximum health after the onset of AIDS, including the postponement and maximum treatment of mental deterioration related to AIDS, like clinical depression and AIDS-related insanity.

The HIV infection affects the immune system. In the same way, pregnancy affects a woman's immune system, since the placental, embryonic and fetal tissues are genetically distinct and would be at risk of denial by the woman's normal immune reaction to foreign tissues. Thus, pregnancy can aggravate vulnerability to HIV infection and to opportunistic infections related to AIDS. The HIV infection during pregnancy can provoke the risk of maternal morbidity, and mortality. Danger to a woman's life from pregnancy gives an indication for medical termination of pregnancy. This is accommodated in even conservative abortion laws, which access the procedure when there is risk to life or danger to enduring health. Legislation may expressly permit abortion because of HIV infection, for instance in Guyana.

The right to health care is afforded considerable amplification in the Women's Convention. It is for each and every woman to decide whether she wants to have pregnancy knowing that she is HIV infected, and whether she wants to risk HIV infection through pregnancy, for example, by having the child of an HIV positive partner. The woman's right to health needs, however, that she can decide to reduce the chance of unwanted pregnancy through birth control means. Therefore, Women's Convention in Article 12 instructively provides that

> "States Parties should take all the suitable precautions to eliminate discrimination against women in the field of health care in order to guarantee, on a basis of equality of men and women, permission to health care services, including those of family planning."

The health care services affiliated to family planning contain information on the use of condoms, and access to them. The use of condom reduces unnecessary pregnancy and abortion, and is helpful in the reduction of sexually transmitted diseases, including AIDS. This is beneficial that condoms serve the goals both of family planning and of reducing the spread of HIV infection. The use of condom is justified on both of these grounds but societies and institutions that resist the use of condoms as an illicit or unnatural means of fertility control deny human rights of both birth control and protection of health. The states parties to international conventions that obey the right to health care compromise the integrity of their observance of human rights if they deny access to condoms.

The provisions in human rights laws on health care, including measures of family planning, raise the pervasive jurisprudential question of whether rights acknowledged in established human rights conventions are negative or positive rights, or impose obligations that consists of both negative and positive components. Negative rights are so called because they lay on only negative obligations on states, meaning obligations not to deny or obstruct peoples actions taken in pursuit of their rights. Peoples are to be legally free to take care of their own health and other interests as they see them, subject only to legal regulation relating the safety and virtue of the means they select to employ. When these measures involve medical treatment, for example, states can regulate the training and qualifications of practitioners named to provide such treatment.

Freedom of religion and conscience are individual rights, and contain freedom from enforcement of the religious and conscientious convictions of others, and of institutions and governments. States are not entitled to deny services of which people can avail themselves by invoking, for example, religious principles. People are free to offer, use or reject services on the grounds of their own religious, moral, social, political or other convictions. Those acting in conformity with their convictions are not to be obstructed by police or other state officials on the grounds of an asserted public morality or state religion. States are legally entitled to subscribe to a preferred moral vision and to a state religion, obviously, but not to impose such a religion by legal sanctions against nonconformity. There is a relationship between positive and negative duties in that, where states have laws that deny or obstruct negative rights, their acceptance of international human rights conventions may need that they take positive steps to amend or repeal such laws and modify these practices, but in general this will not change such rights into positive rights.

The meaning of a positive right is that its application is dependent on a state's acceptance of a positive duty to apply its resources in a affirmative way to make available services and instruments for the duty of providing an opportunity of which individuals may benefit themselves. For example, the right to health care need only be a negative right for those with the means to benefit themselves with the services and instruments, such as pharmaceutical products, that enhance their health status, but would have to be a positive right for states to be compelled to make provision for those who have no resources for self-determination of their health status, and who can achieve a state of sound health only through services and concerned instruments, including medicines that the state makes available.

In many cases, health services that individuals cannot manage for themselves are not provided by states, but are made available by international aid through international agencies or foreign government programmes, or by efforts of national non-governmental organisations. If national government has no obligation under international human rights conventions to manage for these health services, for example by reaching agreements with international or national suppliers, the right to health care would not offer more than a negative right. Although such health services would not have to be made available through efforts of government, an obligation would take over binding governments not to deny nationals access to such health services, and not to obstruct their delivery through, for example, provisions on import of means which are not related to the safety of the particular health services, or on entry of specialized health personnel. Thus, nations that are unable to manage for the means to contain the rate of HIV infection should accommodate international and national efforts for this purpose, and modify legislation that obstructs the effective delivery of such services. For example, legislation restricting the import of condoms or use by unmarried people on moral basis would obstruct AIDS preventive programmes.

(iii) The Right to Liberty and Security of the Person

The right to liberty and security of the person has its legal grounds in the Political Covenant rather than the Covenant that acknowledges social and cultural rights. It reveals that liberty and security were observed under the Universal Declaration primarily as political interests that are vulnerable to exclusion and limitation by the unlawful exercise of governmental power. In relation of HIV infection, rights to liberty and security may seems to be personal rather than political. However, governmental conduct may directly and indirectly influence the extent to which individuals may maintain their liberty and security against the possible risk of HIV infection, and against defective health care services when they are infected. The right to liberty and security closely crosses the right to health care when the policies of the government deny individuals the means to defend themselves against infection. For example, if government does not need HIV screening of blood donations that contribute to the national blood supply, patients who need blood will be denied security against HIV infection if they could not store their own blood in anticipation nor get donations in advance from family members and others they are familiar with to have minimum risk.

The denial of liberty and security by the government against HIV infection has more obvious political effects when governments fail to maintain security against sexual violence and abuse. Women's vulnerability to rape in the incidence of military turmoil is well documented, but they are also at risk in nations not in a general state of armed conflict when, for example, police and prison authorities abuse women prisoner after conviction. Men who commit rape, whether for political benefits of ethnic dominance or as an act of gender superiority, will not restrain themselves for fear of spreading STDs and will not use condoms unless they fear possible infection.

It becomes the duty of governments to enforce the restraints against sexual and other abuse on military, police, prison and refugee management personnel whose access to victims is dependent on governmental powers. The states will be in breach of obligations of similarity before the law under the Political Covenant if they fail to oppose and prevent such abuse, to investigate accusations of abuse by acceptance of women's complaints and evidence in relation of international standards of legal process, and to punish abuse heavily. For example, if the testimony of a woman is not given the same procedural weight as the testimony of a man and if a woman confirming sexual relations with a man meets undue obstacles in proving that she did not consent, and she therefore becomes liable to prosecution for fornication, her rights to equality before the law and to security of the person are violated. The violation of human rights is compounded when the convicted woman has also been infected, and is then abused and refused suitable care in delay.

In many institutions maintained by governments, such as prisons, mental hospitals and orphanages, and those in which there is no military or politically influenced action, residents or detainees who are supposed to be HIV positive suffer discrimination and are refused health and other services such as dental and sanitary care, considered to present caregivers with a risk of infection. Inversely of this, however, residents and detainees in these institutions may themselves be refused protection against infection. Homosexual rape of prisoners and mental health detainees is a common phenomenon. Again, consensual sexual activity is known to occur in single-sex institutions such as prisons. Institutional authorities frequently deny to make condoms available, and brand them as contraband when taken in from outside, on the basis that such sexual acts are violation of institutional rules. Drug taking is also familiar in many prisons, and because needles are scarce they tend to be shared, increasing the risk of transmission of HIV. Prison authorities have denied to implement or permit needle exchange programmes in prisons on the same basis as they denied to allow condom supplies. Such policies violate the rights of victims to security of the person. The moralistic answer, that there would be no risk if people in institutions refrained from sexual and drug taking activities, fails to identify sex as a natural part of life and the range of compulsive addictive habits.

A very familiar expression of the right to liberty is the right to foreign travel, whether for business purposes, employment or recreation. The international human rights movement has not significantly weakened the sovereignty that states may exercise over whether foreigners may enter their territory, except for obligations concerning refugees. An early universal reaction to HIV infection and AIDS was to presume that infection originated outside of countries, and that they could protect their citizens by broader controls on entrants, including requiring evidence that those proposing more than brief visits were HIV-negative. Regulations were inserted by many countries that violated international travel agreements made by WHO. A few countries proceeded further, in breach of the long standing provision of international law that countries cannot deny return of their own citizens, and required citizens who had spent some time abroad, such as students to present evidence of being HIV-negative. Such requirements are perhaps more acceptable if their task is to provide appropriate care on return rather than to prevent return but they might still hinder persons from return who would suffer stigmatization if they are HIV-positive.

There are evidences that a significant percentage of foreign visitors are sexually active abroad, including businessmen who are incidentally "entertained" and men who travel on cautiously promoted "sex junkets" to nations where sex workers are familiar with the entertainment industry. Compulsory HIV testing may be offensive, and useless when conducted on travellers' returning within the incubation period following the infection. Similarly, compulsory testing of immigrants may violate anti-discrimination laws. Nevertheless, human rights law do not preclude states from making health clearance a condition processes of visitors and immigrants. Restricting individuals who present a serious risk of infection to a country's population due to HIV infection may be different from restricting them due to other infections, or on the basis of the costs their care would impose on nationally funded health services. Blanket restrictions on entry may be less defensible, however, than case-by-case decisions taking reference of such factors as individuals' life style and family conditions.

(iv) The Right to Freedom from Torture or Ill-Treatment

The right to freedom from torture or ill-treatment is closely related to liberty and security of the person, and equally violates international human rights law when governments fail to exercise essential discipline on their military, police, prison and the like personnel. The Inter-American Commission on Human Rights defined the rape of a women by military personnel in Haiti as torture, which would be provoked were HIV infection to be transferred to victims. Torture tends to be understood as willful cruelty imposed in direct or indirect pursuit of a public or political purpose. The personal conduct of an HIV-positive person that recklessly or even deliberately risks the infection of another, for example through unprotected sexual intercourse, would not constitute torture. However, if states do not employ the means to investigate, prosecute, convict and punish such conduct, their tolerance of this ill-treatment would give rise to a violation of their obligation under the Political Covenant and, for example, relevant regional human rights agreement.

The nations must prepare themselves to deliver their international duties, and so be able to act diligently and in good faith to protect the human rights of the citizens against ill-treatment even when the violation is by a person not acting under the authority of the state. These persons are not directly bound by international human rights law, but must be responsible to preventive and punitive control by the laws of states, and to the competent enforcement of these laws. For example, persons who are found positive on HIV testing should be subject to counselling by public health personnel against the negligent spread of HIV infection.

As the torture arises from activities to enhance the purposes of states in military, political and strategic spheres, not only is the notion itself male gendered, but victims of torture, primarily military, political and strategic enemies of govenments in the search of power and authority, are also conceived of in male gendered terms. The image of the shackled and tormented victim of torture is necessarily male. Male torture victims really exist, and their victimization through sexual and other cruelty is documented, but less visible have been the countless female victims of ill-treatment through which state personnel have forwarded their purposes.

The women have to face multiple vulnerabilities to sexual and other types of torture. They are vulnerable to torture in their own right if they disregard the gendered expectations of their subordination and passivity and become bold leaders in protests against political, social and other injustice. They are at risk if militia want to assert ethnic dominance, the ethnic inferiority of the populations to which women belong, and that particular populations should be "cleansed" from the areas in which they have settled. Women are also vulnerable to torture for the instrumental purpose of threatening, punishing and mortifying their husbands, brothers, fathers and sons for their military, political and other activities. Women's victimization is provoked not only by risk of their suffering HIV infection but also when they are considered depressed within their own families and communities by even the unintentional loss of virginity, which is stigmatizing for women but not for men. Their rape is compounded by its results of rendering them unable to marriage in their own communities and unacceptable into any other that also practices gender discrimination in accepting only virgin brides.

The vulnerability of women to ill-treatment and torture in private sector employment can involve international human rights conventions against ill-treatment, and probably contribute to infection indirectly. In many work fields, women become vulnerable to sexual harassment including intercourse which they cannot resist because of their economic dependency on their employers. Beyond this, they may be forced to deal with others, such as through care giving, in unsafe manners that expose them to infection. Further, women who are or who may be HIV-positive may be compelled to hide infection and their health vulnerability, and perhaps forego essential treatment, lest they may fired off their employment. Enforcement of human rights laws against industrial and other ill-treatment would encourage such women to protect their health, integrity, and employment.

(v) The Right to Marry and Found a Family

The modern international human rights movement was triggered mainly by state policies of destruction of ethnic and racial groups, including laws against their intermarriage and on enforced sterilization. The human rights reaction is the emphasis on rights of marriage and family foundation included in all of the advancing international, regional and specialized human rights conventions. Limitations on rights of marriage are permitted only on narrow basis such as mental and physical immaturity, incest prevention and severe mental impairment. An unresolved jurisprudential matter is whether the human right to found a family is contingent on marriage, or if the right to found a family can be separated from marriage in a similar way that people unwilling to form families are free to marry.

Some of the jurisdictions have already reacted to HIV infection by ordering that an HIV test be made a condition of the grant of a licence to marry. Such laws are not only offensive to human rights laws of non-discrimination on the basis of disability, but may be ineffective if their purpose is to retard the marriage by infected persons. Of course, this would also offend the right of freedom to marry. In many societies, co-habitation and childbirth without marriage are a common thing and policies for containment of AIDS through control of marriage would be trifling. Such legislation is equally trifling to oppose homosexual spread of HIV, since same-sex partners are not permitted to marry.

Of course, denial of same-sex marriage may be fruitful, since the spread of HIV would be limited by encouraging and facilitating HIV-positive partners to stand with each other and not be sexually promiscuous. In many societies too, a legislative supposition that heterosexual intimacy does not take place before marriage is naive. The societies in which the supposition is justified, furthermore may be suspicion in their general respect for human rights, since they tend to be those in which virgin women's human rights of self-determination in social and association are very frequently violated in the enforcement of their virginity.

The vindication that laws mandating pre-marital testing for HIV are made only to ensure that prospective marriage partners are properly informed may be more defensible, but is patronizing in presuming that legislation has an important role in enforcing the obligations of prevention against HIV infection that partners in marriage owe to each other. The legislation would ravish human rights against discrimination against HIV-positive persons where it does not enforce equally to other sexually transmitted diseases. Where the sexes are equal, women do not need legally mandated information or protection against risks of sexually transmitted diseases contracted by husbands, and men do not need such legislative protection against their wives. Such legislation reveals that countries are in violation of their human rights obligations to gain similarity of the sexes.

Legislation of this type also reveals the risk of gender inequality if it reflects men's perceived requirements of protection. It proposes that women are both inherently deceivers of men, and sources of uncleanliness and venereal infection. The cultural formation of women as potential carriers of pathogens is historically profound, denigrating women as liable to be unclean, sexually promiscuous and inclined to prostitution. It is a barrier to women's rights of marriage if they are asked to demonstrate, for example, through evidence of chastity that they are able to be wives and mothers.

The right to found a family depends on the capacity for procreation and on the power of both mothers and children to survive pregnancy and childbirth. The capacity for procreation is generally a negative right, in that the responsibility of states is not to interfere with pregnancy or adoption. However, infertility may need medical treatment, and, where such services are present, medically assisted reproduction, to help infertile persons the opportunity to bear children. The duty of states to arrange for medical treatment, including reproductive technologies, is not defined as a positive right by international human rights law. However, where such treatments are provided by a state, and where a state notices its negative duty to permit such services to be available, the state is bound by the human rights law not to permit discrimination against people who are disabled because of AIDS.

Observance of the duty not to provide permission for discrimination that obstructs HIV-positive people's right to found families can introduce a conscientious dilemma. It has been observed that HIV infection aggravates the risks of pregnancy through further compromising biological immunity, and that pregnancy may be therapeutically contraindicated for a healthy woman whose partner is HIV-positive. Nevertheless, human rights laws indicate that counselling should be non-directive, and women should be allowed to exercise their right to found a family with informed autonomy. The information that their children on birth will be at risk of submit to HIV-infection, and that the women themselves may not long survive childbirth, are important things that women will take into account. They will not essentially be deterred, however, from initiating pregnancy, for example, where this risk does not overwhelm other risks they and their newborn babies would generally face. In any incident, the choice must be made by them and not by their counsellors.

The HIV-infected pregnant women have the same right to prenatal care, help in labour and postnatal care as a healthy women, and their children are entitled to the same care as those of healthy mothers. Different treatment is not essentially discriminatory, however, and care may appropriately be provided by personnel and facilities that are able to apply global precautions so as to minimize the risk of infection to helping personnel and other recipients of health care. Counselling should be offered to women in such cases as prenatal care, methods of delivery that may reduce the risk of HIV infection to a child, breast feeding, and management of a newborn infants. Counselling should be offered in addition to women's partners. If they are HIV positive they are factors to risks that women may face in having their children, and if women are HIV infected, their partners are equally involved in the risks of their pregnancy. Both partners have significant decisions to make in practice of their right to found a family.

(vi) The Right to Private and Family Life

The right to marry and found a family is an essential component of the right to private and family life, but the latter one goes considerably further. The right to private life reinforces duties of secrecy and privacy that arise in relations between health care givers and patients. Confidentiality is of special importance regarding AIDS because in various social environments these conditions are widely stigmatizing, and related to lifestyles that result in social condemnation, marginalization and alienation. Legislation orders reporting of HIV infection is consistent with human rights laws where public health authorities that receive reports are bound to respect the secrecy of their data, and to undertake public health protection without undue exposure of identities of reported people.

The right to private life may be compromised where public health legislation grants quarantine of infected persons. Since a withheld person will not stop to present a risk of infection, detention and separation may persist for some time. Public health authorities may not consider the public to be secure unless, for example, infected persons' undertakings of conduct, modification or lifestyle change are credible or can be reliably policed. Historic evidences exist of infected persons being kept in detention for over 26 years, and the experience might have been internationally replayable under the impact of the AIDS pandemic, subject to limitations and alternatives forced by international human rights law. Legislation may be dysfunctional and in transgression of human rights law, for example, when it blocks the wish of two HIV infected persons to establish a permanent household between themselves, and live a private life together that presents no risk to public health. The European Court of Human Rights has noticed violation of the right to private life, for example, in Irish legislation that criminalizes homosexual relations among consenting adults. Partner notification necessitates may also be dysfunctional if women are vulnerable to family violence and other types of spousal abuse.

The right of HIV-positive citizens to adopt children is generally contentious, but may be defended on the basis of the rights both of non-discrimination and of private and family life. The claim to the right may be opposed because of children's superior rights to safety and to placement where they would find a minimally interrupted upbringing. Children's rights may be consistently invoked in favour of their adoption by parents' same-sex partners, however, for example where the partners are concerned with their care and would continue to perform parental functions after the death of the real parent.

(vii) The Right to the Benefits of Scientific Progress

The Economic Covenant directs the human right to the benefits of scientific development, but the issue has a political aspect in that the Covenant anticipates scientific developments offering benefits to all persons without discrimination. Applied to HIV-positive persons, the right includes the negative factor that private initiatives to grow and apply evolving scientific knowledge for their benefit should not be damaged, and the positive factor that states should ensure that the new knowledge that comes from the initiatives they sponsor will be made available without discrimination on such basis as sex, race and physical or mental disability. The negative right relates tolerance, for example, private pharmaceutical companies and other research under regulations that are neither prohibitive nor unduly restrictive, and under situations of participants' free and informed consent that matches to international standards. It also includes permitting research, for example, to develop and test an HIV vaccine and to reinforce hindrance to infection and delay of the beginning of AIDS.

This remains difficult, however, to argue that states or international institutions have a positive legal duty, as opposed to a moral duty, to support AIDS research in priority to research into other infections, since states may have no legal obligation to support health research at all or by any particular method. Those whose situations are studied may timely enjoy benefits, but it is not discrimination against those whose inabilities are not recorded by state initiative that others are treated more favourably. Discrimination is refusal of an entitlement, but where there is no entitlement there is no discrimination when some gets benefits and others do not. States are free to pursue whatever health research strategies they find most suitable to their requirements. Further the science whose benefits must be provided is not limited to biomedical science but includes, for example, social science. Similarly, the science may direct preventative health care rather than curative treatment. Accordingly, states may release any positive obligations they have under the Economic Covenant by pursuing programmes of preventive community health care to prevent the spread of HIV rather than by sponsoring clinical research to help persons living with AIDS-related disorders.

The requirement of more deep research into HIV infection, its prevention, and in time, its cure is self-evident from increasing statistics of infection. An important challenge is development of gender-sensitive studies that direct women's special vulnerability to infection in the ordinary behaviour of their lives. Sufficient knowledge is present to achieve behavioural change that would considerably decrease the rates of infection, but the gendered working of many cultures and societies refuses women sexual and reproductive self-determination. Women who have no real alternatives in her life to early marriage to partners they do not need to be sexually abstinent outside marriage or to use condoms within marriage are refused means of self-protection against HIV and unwanted pregnancy. They have a proper claim to research to develop effective female-controlled means of resistance against STDs and unwanted pregnancy. A female condom has been developed, for example, but women may be unable to overcome partners' hostility for using it. The right to scientific development may not support the means to hold states to account for their insufficient research initiatives in this regard, but respect for human rights against sex and gender discrimination may condition more sensitivity to women's special requirements by both private and public supporters of biomedical research.

Governments consigned themselves through the Beijing Platform for Action to "sponsor and expedite action-oriented research on reachable methods, controlled by women to prevent AIDS and other sexually transmitted diseases, on strategies supporting women to protect themselves from sexually transmitted diseases including AIDS, and on means of care, aid and treatment of women, making sure their involvement in all respects of such research."

(viii) The Rights to Information and Education

Education, information and the power to acquire, process and apply knowledge properly are necessary tools for self-determination. Individuals must be capable of understanding particularly the means of transmission of HIV, and strategies to lessen the risk of infection, to themselves and others that they can apply effectively in the circumstances of their lives. It is commonly seen that knowledge is power and information and its proper use empower individuals to exercise autonomy and duties. Accordingly, rights to information and to the accomplishment of understanding of uses of information support most if not all of the human rights considered before in this lesson.

The European Court of Human Rights has reported a human rights violation when a government tried to limit information for fear that citizens would use it for purposes the government disapproved. The Court thereby enforced a limit on governmental means of censorship of information that citizens could use for self-determination because such censorship ravished individuals' human rights. The case related to reproductive self-determination and access to abortion services, but the Court's decision is applicable to information related to HIV infection and management of AIDS.

International experience shows how women may be refused the opportunity to protect their health, including against HIV infection, due to sex and gender discrimination in education. In many societies, the education of girl children is not considered as significant as the education of boy children; girls admitted in schools may more easily be kept away to help mothers in household work; and girls' education may be prematurely stopped by early marriage. Moreover, some schools expel girls who become pregnant while boys who cause pregnancy have no similar sanction.

The literacy levels among girls are generally lower than levels among boys, and states do not provide resources to encourage and facilitate families to admit their girl children in schools. A disincentive to families to invest in girls' education is the devaluation of women's education in their employment, and the concept that a woman's only proper destiny is care-giving in the home. Global recognition of the high percentage of women who are chiefs of households, and of women's valuable contributions to their families' economy, would lead to recognition of how important it is that women be informed and educated for the release of the functions even conservatively regarded to define women's function.

The conservative hindrance to the education of girls, and of other marginalized social under-classes, must not be underrated. Literacy permits individuals to develop sensitivities to their own situations, to gain awareness of the injustices and subordination to which they are subject, and to need that they and their perceptions be observed seriously, be respected, be treated equally with others and be effective in future developments. The principle that individuals can make their own destiny and defences, and escape regulates exercised, for example, by those who traditionally have defined natural and supernatural powers that governs individuals' destiny challenges traditional power within societies. Prevention of information has long been the instrument of politically and otherwise oppressive forces protective of their power. Only in recent years, for example, has the Roman Catholic Church discontinued its list of Prevented Books, which limited the literature that observant members of the Church could read in good conscience. Some Islamic authorities carry on to consider the abandonment of faith by reception of various ways of thinking, namely apostasy, as properly punishable by death. Conservative powers are willing to tolerate HIV infection and death, probably seen as the eternal ordained wage of sin, rather than tolerate the challenge to their traditional values represented, for example, by condom use to reduce the risk of sexually transmitted disease.

(ix) Associated Rights

Closely related to the rights to information and education are rights to communicate and apply the understandings which individuals have developed through informations and interpretation. The human rights to freedom of thought, conscience and religion, to political participation and to assembly and association, mentioned in the Political Covenant and, for example, the regional human rights conventions, both contribute to and depend on rights to information and education. Knowledge is power and power is used in political, social, spiritual and other related ways. Political power can achieve and secure rights to information and education, but democratic political power commonly depends on rights to assembly, association and collective action.

Development in the public health and health education in a community is commonly possible through collective and political initiatives, and initiatives can become effective through the use of historical, social and strategic understandings. Though these associated rights are of immense democratic favour in themselves, they can be of decisive importance in health protection and promotion, regarding hindrance to HIV infection and to other dangers to life, only when used interactively with each other. The indirect implication for health that each of these rights has separately becomes direct when they are used in association.

Domestic Application of International Human Rights Law

The international law was taught in post-medieval Western Europe, for instance by Gentili, the Professor who first taught the subject at Oxford University in the last phase of the 16th century, as The Law of Nature and Nations. As part of Natural Law, international law was an innate component of all laws, and all countries governed by law essentially included international law as a factor of their jurisprudence. Subsequent developments led to a distinction, however, in how domestic legal systems observed the international law. The Monist theory kept faith with history and observed the international law to be directly usable by domestic courts, although subject to domestic legislation that could direct courts differently. In contrast, the Dualist theory observed the international and domestic legal systems to be separate, the law of nations not being applicable to the domestic legal system.

Practically, few states applied either theory in its original form, and modern states define the domestic importance of international law according to historical and political influences. The modern constitutions of some nations, such as Germany, explicitly afford the principles of international law priority over national law where the two seems to be in conflict. Accordingly, international human rights law dominates within the domestic legal system over any contrary provisions within that system. Other nations have achieved the same effect with respect to human rights principles, but not essentially other provisions of international law. Countries in the English common law tradition do not provide domestic effect to international ties unless they have been provided the power of domestic law by explicit national legislation, but treat international customary law as essential part of domestic customary law. In yet others, provisions of constitutional law allow the state's ratification of certain international ties to be self-executing meaning that they become directly applicable within the domestic legal system, while other international ties do not have that effect but need explicit adoption by legislation. Where international law is not adopted into domestic law, however, domestic courts of all nations will normally try to avoid dissimilarities in their interpretation of domestic law so as not to put their nations in breach of their international duties if that result is avoidable.

The domestic laws of the states which are applied in ways that ravish international human rights law may be exposed and blamed by international human rights courts, when states are subject to their jurisdiction under human rights conventions. Condemnation is possible even relating matters that states claim to be of moral concern. For example, the European Court of Human Rights has criticised criminalization of homosexual relationships between consenting adults when the applicable national law was internally accepted as upholding moral values. As the international jurisprudence on human rights develops, such rights as those to non-discrimination on the basis, for example, of sex or disability are being identified to form part of international customary law, and therefore to be transformed into various national legal systems, and to be independent of states' legislative adoption of a peculiar convention.

This may be expected that international human rights law applicable to HIV infection and its prevention will develop to set international norms by which the humane character of states' domestic laws and practices will be assessed. Further, although individuals as such are not normally governed by international law, for example, concerning acts of domestic violence and those liable to transmission HIV infection, countries themselves are responsible under international law to take suitable preventive, remedial or punitive action when those subject to their jurisdiction violate doctrine of international human rights law. In case of some more extreme cases, citizens may face direct legal accountability under international human rights law for war crimes and crimes against humanity. Accordingly, international human rights law related to HIV infection will have sufficient potential for both international and domestic compulsion.

Under Strategic Objective C.3 of the Beijing Platform for Action, governments agreed to apply gender-sensitive initiatives that address sexually transmitted diseases, AIDS, and sexual and reproductive health matters that include re-examination and amending laws "that may help to women's susceptibility to HIV infection and other sexually transmitted diseases, including ordaining legislation against those socio-cultural practices that help to it, and implement legislation, policies and practices to defend women, adolescents and young girls from discrimination concerned to AIDS". Significant efforts are made in several areas, including Asia, to review laws and policies and enact new laws that enhance the protection and improvement of reproductive health, including the prevention and treatment of AIDS. The challenge is to ensure that such efforts are geared up and developed in a gender-sensitive way.

Part VII

AIDS and Ethics

Sixteen

AIDS and Ethics

AIDS, a very serious epidemic to strike advanced nations in more than a generation, has posed an extraordinary array of ethical challenges. Most of these challenges also confront the poorly developed nations. Among the matters that have drawn attention are: the duty of the state to take preventive measures against the spread of the disease; the obligation of physicians to care the needy; the limits and significance of medical confidentiality; the obligation to have informed consent previous to testing and starting treatment; the functions of counselling suffering individuals about their duties to partners and of helping the women who are infected as they are forced to make reproductive decisions; the contradiction between the cannons of research and the cannons of care; the limits of acceptable guarantee by insurance companies; the rights of people with costly medical conditions to emigrate; and, finally, the duties of the advanced industrial states toward poorly developed states.

Despite the special context of the epidemic during the past decade, what is important about the issues that have been pressed forward is that they all are not new. What is new is the frequency of the discussions, the broad participatory nature of the debate, the political forces called into action the needs they have cited, the solutions they have sought to fashion, and the degree to which efforts have been made to shape a global consensus on the ethics of prevention and care. More strikingly, AIDS has provided a chance to rethink of the traditions of public health in relation to human rights.

As a fatal illness spread in the context of the most essential relationships and as a public health threat, AIDS has compelled us to confront questions regarding the suitable role of the state in controlling morbidity and mortality. In doing so, it has required a reconsideration of the ethical limits on state power in the form of a grave social threat. As a disease of the social vulnerability, HIV infection and AIDS have forced us to face issues involving the role of the state in protecting the poor in moments of social stress. As a disease that has devastated large number of poors without appropriate health insurance, AIDS has required us once more to consider what justice demands, in terms of the protection of people against the costs associated with illness. So the roles of government in improving the public health, defending the poor and assuring good health care services have all been required by the AIDS.

The Ethics of Prevention and Protection

AIDS, an epidemic, is a blood-borne, sexually transmitted disease. It is transmitted by infected persons to the healthy persons during sexual intercourse (homosexual or heterosexual), through needle sharing by drug users and by pregnant women to their children. The infections were also transmitted through blood transfusions and to those dependant on clotting factor for haemophilia. This is no longer a problem in advanced industrial nations, although it lingers on as a challenge in poorly developed nations. Therefore, AIDS is pre-eminently a behaviourally transmitted disease. In the absence of a vaccine, transmission of HIV can only be prevented through modifications in behaviour. Those who are infected must use condoms during sexual intercourse, and those who are uninfected must do so to protect themselves against the infection. Intravenous drug users must not share needles. The risk of paediatric AIDS can be overcome completely only if infected women do not bear children.

It is such biological facts that provide the grounds for public health strategies made to prevent AIDS. It is these facts that raise questions about the moral responsibilities of those having to behave in ways that limit the prospect of spreading a fatal disease; and of the nation to make policies that will facilitate the radical modification of sexual and drug using habits.

Before discussion of these issues it is important to note a matter of overarching necessity in a discussion of the ethical issues posed by an epidemic like AIDS: the scope to which the ethical norms that should inform AIDS policies can be contemplated transnational; the extent to which such patterns are so culture-specific that they can only be use to judge policies and practices in given societies. While we cannot engage with the wide theoretical issues applied in this matter, it is important to identify some of the most fundamental questions posed by AIDS prevention measures: should cultural views that subdue women and restrain their freedoms to defend themselves in sexual relationships be tolerated in the name of cultural differences? Should cultural conservatism about homosexuality, drug use, prostitution, or sex education affect AIDS prevention programmes such as sharing of needles, explicit sex education, or condom availability? Should Western liberal views about the pre-eminence of individual freedom and autonomy regulates public health policies on testing and secrecy?

Such types of questions take on special importance in light of the fact that a central tenet of efforts to promote the adoption of behaviours that will limit the transmission of HIV is that they be culturally sensitive. Two arguments are typically formed on behalf of the centrality of cultural sensitivity. The first is pragmatic and instrumental; the second one is ethical. The pragmatic-instrumental claim affirms that AIDS prevention measures that are not culturally sensitive will be ineffective. They will meet to failure because they will not reach their intended audience, will not be understood by those who are reached, and will not be acquired by those who understand. They may, in fact, provoke immediate opposition.

Another claim on behalf of cultural sensitiveness, less often made explicitly but nevertheless of central significance, is ethical. The basic doctrine of ethics that individuals should be treated with respect and that their dignity should not be injured is by extension applied to cultures. Cultural sensitiveness is thus required of us by the ethics of pluralism. A failure to honour the cultural integrity of others is almost characterized as a duty of the values of the dominant and powerful on the subordinate and marginal. The insistence on cultural sensitiveness is premised on an egalitarian ethos, on the ethos that should inspire public policy in multicultural democratic societies. Both arguments have great values. Yet the claims on behalf of cultural sensitiveness may, in fact, be overstated. The demands of AIDS prevention may necessitate a confrontation with cultural patterns that sustain norms of behaviour which foster the transmission of AIDS.

In the list of bitterly fought issues raised in the context of AIDS prevention has been the question of whether literacy should stress the moral duties of those who are infected or the significance of self-protection for the uninfected. Of greater instant in the developed countries has been the political controversy excited by the centrality of educating gay men and drug users about how they should change their behaviours to defend themselves and others. Social conservatives opposed to homosexuality and all extramarital sex have objected to the "legitimization" of what they think to be immoral nature in the name of public health. Of course, efforts have been made to enforce restrictions on the language and content of messages designed to inform and shape AIDS-related behaviours. Likewise, those who view drug use as morally reprehensible have objected educational efforts designed to teach intravenous drug users about how they might continue to use drugs without having themselves at risk of a fatal infection. They have opposed the distribution of sterile injection instruments through needle exchange programmes and the lifting of prohibitions on the sale of injection instruments to drug users.

Such type of objections, in the name of morality, has paradoxically imposed restrictions on the state's first ethical responsibility related to the AIDS epidemic: to protect the vulnerable. This is no accident that those who have the burden of that failure was already socially vulnerable.

In developing countries the epidemiological pattern of HIV transmission is much different from that which exists in Western Europe and North America. Heterosexual nature is the dominant mode of HIV transmission. The central ethical challenges posed by this fact are the necessity of broad condom education for men and women and the provision of condoms at affordable prices. Frankness in sexual education has often met with conservative hindrance, paralleling in a way the experience in economically strong nations. As important, the pattern of HIV transmission obliges a confrontation with the subordinate status of women which refuses them the capacity to control their own sexual lives. Here we have underscored the most disturbing dimensions: as long as women are subordinate, they will not be successful to protect themselves against HIV; but to end that subordination will need far-reaching social modifications. Whether such modifications can occur at a pace that is compatible with the threat by HIV still remains an open question.

Historically, as countries confronted the challenge of the epidemic, they tried to rely on policies that were marked by an authoritarian perspective. Indeed, traditional public health service in Europe and North America centred on mandatory case search, reporting the cases to public health registries, contact tracing, necessary treatment, and at times quarantine and separation. The nature of the infections threats with which public health officials had to deal and dominating conceptions of the appropriate relationship between the individual and the nation dictated the shape of public health service. AIDS has provided the occasion for a challenge to the traditional approach to public health service.

In the United States and other nations bound by the liberal tradition, ethical considerations, pragmatic concerns, and extraordinary efforts on the matter of AIDS service organizations have helped to the adoption of public health strategies to control the spread of HIV that may be defined as voluntaristic—emphasizing mass education, counselling, and respect for privacy. Indeed, both in the United States and other countries what might be termed "HIV exceptionalism" has prevailed public health policy. A focus on voluntarism has also informed the policies put forward by the Global Programme on AIDS of the World Health Organization. That in turn has contributed to make policies all over the world. This general consensus has affected policies on discrimination, the protection of confidentiality, and the use of the compulsory powers of the nation to restrict those whose behaviours are thought to have a risk of HIV transmission.

Discrimination and Public Health

AIDS proved to be the first major infectious threat with which advanced industrial societies had to contend in almost a generation, and because the causative agent was not diagnosed until three years after the first case was reported, it is not astonishing that it provoked considerable social anxiety. How was it transmitted? Who posed a risk? Who was vulnerable? That AIDS was a disease of socially marginal, and not infrequently despised, persons only intensified the urge toward discrimination. Employers, landlords, school personnel, and even the employees of some health-care institutions witnessed a willingness to exclude those with the new disease. With the discovery of HIV, and the development of a test that could identify antibodies against the virus, the potential scope for discriminatory acts increased, despite the epidemiological evidence about how infection was transmitted.

In the United States, the Centres for Disease Control moved rapidly to contain the irrational impulse toward exclusion. Towards the end of 1985, guidelines to restrict the spread of HIV in schools and the workplace were issued. Early in 1986, broad guidelines for health care workers on preventing the spread of infection while encountered in invasive procedures were published. In each instance, the aim was to convey the information, to give protection, and to prevent panic. The message was clear: HIV could not be casually transmitted, and so there were no public health basis for exclusion of infected persons who otherwise were capable of performing their expected duties. There were thus no grounds for mandatory testing for HIV. In relation to the health-care setting, universal blood and body fluid precautions would defend workers not only from HIV, but also from the far more infectious hepatitis B. In the absence of any significant risk, there was no possible ethical basis for discrimination against individuals with HIV. Indeed, the absence of demonstrable risk and the irrational nature of discriminatory practices imposed on the government a positive ethical responsibility made on the principle of justice to protect those who are at risk from discriminatory actions.

The condition in health care has not been so clear. The unresolved query to the appropriate response to HIV-positive clinicians has continued to fester, even in actions that have by and large sought to protect the rights of individuals with HIV. Debate on this matter has been called by the single, still unexplained case of a Florida dentist to whom the only cases of HIV infection in patients linked to a clinician have been identified. Some people have argued that although professionals have a moral responsibility to assume some risks—particularly those that are quite small—in caring for their patients, patients do not have an equivalent responsibility to expose themselves to even small risks when being cared for. Dismissing as irrational those who would refuse all infected health-care workers, whatever their roles, the right to engage in clinical work, many have asserted that doctors whose invasive work can make their patients at some risk ought not to engage in those procedures. But the logic of this perspective leads to bothering conclusions. If those who know themselves to be HIV-positive have professional responsibilities not to place their patients at risk, are there correlative institutional obligations to identify the infected, to exclude them from certain actions? Are they obligated to screen health-care workers, and if so, at what rate? Might concern about protecting patients provide the grounds for mandatory screening and surveillance after so much effort to anticipate such programmes? And if screening were to be acquired what would be the effect on an anxious social climate?

In thinking deep about these matters it would be useful to underscore the possible tension between the ethics of acknowledged consent and the ethics of protecting the vulnerable from discrimination. The ethics of informed consent has increasingly been formed by a commitment to the view that patients should be able to determine, for themselves, the level of risk, which is acceptable in relation to medical practice. Such a view denies the "objective" standard of the reasonable person or the doctor in determining which risks should be disclosed to a patient for his or her consideration. The ethics of anti-discrimination practice and policy is profoundly different. It refuses subjectivity; views it as the fount of irrationality. From that view, personal views about risk cannot override the rights of those with peculiar disabilities to work. A refusal, for example, to hire a person with limited hearing loss due to a belief that such an individual would represent some remote theoretical risk would never be countenanced under dominating conceptions of the rights of those with disabilities. Thus, the understanding of the disaster posed by the HIV-infected doctor will very much depend on whether it is defined necessarily as one that implicates the ethics of acknowledged consent of the ethics of disability rights.

Confidentiality and its Limits

There is, perhaps, no ethical matter involving AIDS that has got more attention than that of confidentiality. That gay men and those who have spoken on their behalf have placed such great pressure on confidentiality should come as no surprise. The history of oppression and the existence of anti-sodomy laws have made the protection of privacy a critical characteristic of the struggle for social existence. But the call for the protection of confidentiality has come as well from those vested with the duty for public health, including the World Health Organization, the Council of Europe, and the US Centres for Disease Control and Prevention. For them the protection of confidentiality was specific to the strategy to encourage mass behavioural change and to the task of encouraging people to go for testing and counselling.

The legal safeguards that countries have adopted, reflecting a degree of ethical considerations, however, are highly variable. An international survey of AIDS legislation undertaken for the World Health Organization in1991 revealed that 33 countries had peculiar confidentiality provisions relating to AIDS. Indeed, countries may have quite different cultural ideas of privacy. In the North and West, privacy is defined as the right of an individual to restrict access by others to some aspect of the person. Accordingly, the contemporary cultural expectation, reflecting significant changes over the past several decades, is that medical information concerning the person is kept secret and cannot be disclosed even to family members without the person's permission. In some parts of Africa and the Far East, however, privacy is understood in some other way. In many societies, issues of disease and death are seldom individual concerns but affairs of the family or even the entire society. In many traditional societies, too, issues of health and medicine—even death itself—become public. Thus, secrecy as a one-to-one exchange between clinician and patient-hardly exists. Here, in a stark way, the tension between cultural peculiarism and the claims of ethical globalization are made clear.

On the other hand, even in the developed countries of the northern and western hemispheres, the principle of confidentiality has required changes in light of pressing public health necessities. The doctrine of confidentiality is never complete and has always been subject to limits. In many countries, a central duty of public health officials has been to record the names in special registries of those with certain diseases. In part, such reporting of diseases has been deemed important for purposes of epidemiological surveillance. On other occasions, reporting has been thought of as necessary to adequate follow-up to ensure that persons with communicable conditions are appropriately treated. Finally, such reporting has been central to contract tracing.

Each of such public health activities has been used as a justification for requiring the reporting of the names of persons with AIDS and HIV infection. Provided the threat posed by the epidemic such nominal reporting of AIDS cases has generally not been subject to ethical challenges. In some countries, however, efforts have been made to achieve target of reporting without the use of names, thus showing the extraordinary sensitivity of confidentiality in the AIDS epidemic. More common has been the disputation over the reporting of persons with HIV, without the manifestations of AIDS. In some countries, only the latter is reportable.

In cases, where reporting by name does occur, the ethics of secrecy dictate that the identity of those with AIDS be shielded from unauthorised disclosure. The reporting by names is justified only on public grounds, and thus no disclosure to those who may have other reasons to want to have the identity of persons with AIDS is ethically justifiable. Those who are responsible for public health registries have a peculiar obligation to defend the integrity of the lists developed by reporting needs.

But what of the function of confidentiality in the clinical setting? What are the moral duties of a physician when an HIV-infected patient denies to inform identifiable, unsuspecting past or current partners about the risks of infection. In the United States a central legal principle emerged out of the widely discussed *Tarasoff* case, which held that under certain circumstances a clinician has an affirmative responsibility to protect unsuspecting targets of his patient's violent intentions. That case need not detain us here. What is peculiar is the underlying ethical doctrine that confidentiality, while critical, is not the only ethical value. Indeed, when vulnerable unsuspecting individuals are placed at risk, it may be obligatory to breach confidentiality.

In relation to HIV, concern has focussed on two very different situations: the possibility that an individual unknowingly infected by a previous partner might serve as unwitting agent of transmission to yet others or might lose the chance to commence early therapeutic intervention; in the case of an individual who has not expressed his or her infected status to a current partner, the focus has been on the probability of preventing the spread of HIV. As these matters were considered, it became clear that the process of warning past sexual partners did not need the identification of the source of potential infection. No public health goal would be served by breaching the cloak of anonymity of the index case. Where an infected individual denied to warn a current partner, the condition posed graver difficulties. It was not possible to give any effective protective warning without recognizing the source of risk.

Informing the dispute concerning how it might be best to proceed has been a deep concern about the results that could well follow were it to be widely believed that doctors would routinely breach confidentiality when presented with a patient who denied to warn past or current partners about the risk of HIV infection. Would the consequences be a reduction in clinical candour? Would patients be discouraged from knowing their HIV status? Would they be less accessible to the efforts of clinicians to convince them of the significance of warning those who might have been at risk? In sum, would breaching confidentiality to warn unsuspecting persons result in a net loss from point of view of public health?

Starting in the latter phase of 1987, a number of efforts were made in the United States to resolve the issues concerned with the warning of unsuspecting third parties. Towards the end of 1987, the American Medical Association issued a broad set of statements on the ethical issues posed by the AIDS epidemic. In that document the AMA asserted the issue of warning in a forthright manner. Doctors were to try to convince patients of their obligation to warn the unsuspecting. If they failed in that job, they were to seek the intervention of public health personnel. Only if public health officials denied or were unwilling to take on the duty of warning was it the obligation of the doctor to act directly.

In mid-1988 when the Presidential Commission on the AIDS

Epidemic addressed this issue, it too endorsed the notion that doctors should have the right to breach confidentiality in order to warn the unsuspecting, despite the centrality of confidentiality in order to warn the unsuspecting, despite the centrality of confidentiality to its complete strategy. Reflecting, however, a commitment to professional autonomy, the Commission held that the decision about whether to breach confidentiality was to remain with the doctor and was not to be imposed as an issue of law. That too was the stance of a broad spectrum of public health officials, along with the Association of State and Territorial Health Officials, who chose to speak of a "privilege to disclose" rather than the responsibility to warn. The lingering ethical query is whether such a strategy meets the moral challenge clinicians face when confronted with patients who may risk the lives of their partners. This issue has been the source of enduring contradiction in nations such as Sweden, Denmark and The Netherlands.

Coercive Controls

An important question of how to respond to persons whose behaviour presents a threat to unknown partners has inevitably provoked discussion of the public health tradition of enforcing restrictions on liberty in the name of communal welfare. The spectre of mass quarantine has haunted all such discussion. Only Cuba has sought to quarantine all individuals with AIDS. In other countries the focus has been on the more limited case of individuals whose behaviours have places others at risk of HIV infection. Even such limited efforts have caused concern because of fears that they would give rise to egregious intrusions upon privacy and insidiously enforce deprivations of freedom.

In the US, fierce opposition has surfaced to all efforts to bring AIDS within the reach of state quarantine statutes. Moreover, more than a dozen states had done the same between 1987 and 1990, typically using the occasion to modify their disease control laws to reveal contemporary constitutional standards which detail procedural guarantees, and to require that restrictions on freedom shows the "least restrictive alternative" available to get a "compelling state interest".

Despite the intensity of the debate that has surrounded this issue, the only empirical study of the use of power of separation in the United States has found that state health departments have almost never used the authority provided by statute. During 1981-90 only 10 cases were registered, and in virtually each case the duration of confinement has been very short. Far more common has been the utilization of public health authority to warn individuals that their behaviour posed a risk. Such types of warnings have often been accompanied by "cease and desist orders". Public health efforts to separate the small numbers of individuals suspected to pose a behavioural threat to an "unsuspecting" partner have occurred in other nations typically reflecting on prostitutes.

The enforcement of statutes criminalizing behaviours related to the transmission of HIV or the application of general criminal law to such cases has equalized the political receptivity to laws extending the authority of public health officials to control the persons whose behaviour posed the risk of HIV transmission.

What are the ethical grounds of such statutes? Criminal law helps to express a society's profound abhorrence of peculiar behaviours. In doing so, the law threatens to punish the persons who violate certain social laws. It may also help as a deterrent. Some acts are globally the subject of criminal law. Other acts may be crimes only in certain societies. The enactment of criminal statutes that restrict the wilful and knowing infection with HIV of an unsuspecting sexual partner would fall within the morally acceptable use of criminal law. But the enforcement of such statutes has often served ends that raise profound ethical questions. To seek to punish activities that cannot possibly result in the spread of AIDS, serves only to underscore the penchant for repressive means in the face of complex social troubles.

Whatever the allure of such means and of the rediscovery of traditional public health approaches in the effort to prevent the spread of AIDS, it remains clear that the future results of the AIDS epidemic will be determined by the formation of a social and institutional milieu within which radical voluntary modifications in behaviour can occur and be sustained. Educational campaigns and counselling programmes most efficiently undertaken by groups related to the populations at risk, not repressive means, remain the centre-piece of such preventive effort.

The Ethics of Research

The AIDS epidemic has provided the situations for the emergence of a wide and potent political movement that has sought to reshape radically the conditions under which research has been undertaken in the United States. The implications for research in other countries with important pharmaceutical efforts are very distinct. The role of the randomized clinical trial, the significance of placebo controls, the centrality of academic research institutions, the dominance of scientists over subjects, the sharp difference between research and therapy, and the protectionist ethos that has informed research ethics since the end of the World War II have all been brought into query.

Although scholars related to the methodological requirements of sound research and ethicists committed to the protection of research subjects have played a significant role in the ensuring discussions, both as defenders of received intellect and as critics, the debate has been driven by the articulate demands of those threatened by AIDS. Most prominent have been the groups like the People With AIDS Coalition and ACT-UP, institutions made up primarily of white, gay people. But advocates of women's, children's and prisoners' rights have also made their demands heard. What has been so stunning and disconcerting to some, and exciting to others, has been the balance of challenge and response. Rather than the exchange of academic arguments, we have been witness to the mobilization of disruptive and effective political protest.

The threat of death has hovered over the process. "The shortage of proven therapeutic alternatives for AIDS and the belief that trials are, in and themselves, beneficial have led to the claim that people have a right to be research subjects. This is the exact opposite of the tradition starting with Nuremberg that people have the right *not* to be research subjects." It is this striking reversal that has led to a rejection of the model of research conducted at remote academic centres, with restrictive (protective) standards of access, and strict compliance to the 'gold standard' of the randomised clinical trial. Blurring the distinction between research and treatment"—A Drug Trial is Health Care Too"—those insistent upon radical reform have sought to open wide the points of entry to new "therapeutic" agents both within and outside of clinical trails; have demanded that the paternalistic ethical warrant for the protection of the vulnerable from research be substituted by an ethical regime informed by respect for the autonomous choice of potential subjects who could weigh, for themselves, the potential risks and benefits of new experimental treatments for HIV infection. Thus, demands have been made that women be called for trials in greater numbers; that prisoners and drug users be granted access; that children be included in trials at a much earlier point than had been considered agreeable. Moreover, the revisionists have demanded a basic reconceptualisation of the relationship between researchers and subjects. In place of protocols enforced from above, they have proposed a more egalitarian and democratic model in which negotiation would substitute the scientific authority.

The revamption of the ethics of research that has started under the effect of AIDS has implications that go far beyond the epidemic of HIV disease since the emerging new conceptions and standards could govern the conduct of the entire research effort. Protagonists, who have been locked in often acrimonious debate, foretell very different outcomes of the changing social standards of research. Proponents of the new ethos hold out the prospect of a revised regime that is both respectful of individual rights and the requirements of good science. Critics, on the other hand, have opined that the blurring of the distinction between research and treatment can only harm the desperate.

Another set of issues is raised by the question of research in less developed countries, particularly international collaborative research started by investigators in the advanced industrial nations. A body of scholarship has come out in relation to the ethics of international collaborative research. The Council of International Organizations of Medial Sciences has issued ethical guidelines for both biomedical and epidemiological research that are highly impressive. These guidelines necessitate ethical review of research proposals both in the country of origin and in the host country. They necessitate consent of the research subject, a favourable benefit-to-burden ratio, confidentiality, and a compensation for the subjects who are harmed during the research.

Probably the most important and controversial issue in

international collaborative research is the need to have infrastructure in the host country and to make the fruits of the research available to people in that community or similarly located populations. The central ethical question is—to what extent does the principle of distributive justice necessitate that therapeutic interventions emerged in the course of such research be made available to subjects in their communities?

This issue is relevant especially to the conduct of vaccine trials. For epidemiological reasons, it has been suggested that countries in Asia and Africa represent ideal settings for investigation into possible preventive vaccines. Large numbers of victims, and the tragically high incidence of infection, make countries in Asia and Africa ideal for the determination of vaccine efficacy. But no vaccine trial would be ethical—assuming that issues of consent could be resolved—if there was no confirmation that a successful vaccine would be provided by international agreement, despite the potential cost. Agreements like this must precede the conduct of vaccine trials.

The Ethics Concerning Care

For about four decades, health care workers in America, as well as in other advanced industrial societies, were largely shielded from what had been the regular experience of those who had in earlier times worked with the sick—the acquisition of their patients' infections and sometimes lethal diseases. Though never as total as many had come to believe, this invincibility was psychologically demolished by the intrusion of AIDS, beginning in 1981. AIDS forced physicians and health care workers to consider the fact that theirs was in fact a 'dangerous trade'.

In the early history of this epidemic, anecdotal reports began to surface about hospital aides leaving food trays at the doors the infected persons, and of nurses, physicians, and dentists refusing to treat patients with AIDS. The Centres for Disease Control confronted such behaviour by publishing in late 1985 and 1986 a series of reports in *Morbidity and Mortality Weekly Report* that sought to provide guidance for sound infection control practice and a rational social policy.

Faced with the challenge posed by the threat of patient

abandonment, those committed to stanching the emerging trend turned to history in the expectation that a clear lesson on responsibility of physicians would emerge. Physicians had, after all, been called to respond when epidemics were more frequent, when morbidity was awesome. For those who had hoped to discover a clear message from the chronicles of the past, the turn of history proved a disappointment. Although some physicians had stayed to care for their patients, many had fled. Sometimes, they did so in order that they might attend to their fleeing patrons, sometimes to protect themselves. Perhaps most significant as a reflection of the extent to which many physicians refused to be with those afflicted in earlier plagues was the need to make arrangements for the care of the patient through the special institution of the 'plague doctor'. Appointed by local merchants and the political elites, these physicians took up where others had failed.

If history presented no clear guidance, what of the codes of ethics that have expressed the ambitions of the guilds and associations of medical practitioners? Surprisingly, such codes had been silent on the duty of physicians to treat during the epidemics. In the United States of America, the AMA code of 1847 was unique in its forthright assertion of such a responsibility, "And when pestilence prevails, it is their duty to face the danger and to continue their labours for the alleviation of suffering, even at the jeopardy of their own lives." This provision remained in the code until 1957, when a revised statement eliminated the stipulation that must certainly have been an anachronism. Ultimately, the era of epidemics had come to an end in the advanced industrial countries.

Remaining in the code was a provision—first incorporated into the AMA's statement of professional responsibility of 1912, which in the absence of a strong assertion of a duty to care was to be a point of great confusion when AIDS faced American medicine. "A physician shall, in the provision of appropriate patient care, except in emergencies, be free to choose whom to serve." Amending the blunt articulation of an unencumbered professional freedom, the AMA's Judicial Council has stated that refusals to treat on the basis of race, religion, or creed were unethical. In November 1987, the Council ruled that "A physician may not ethically refuse to treat a patient whose condition is within the physician's current realm of competence solely because the patient is seropositive." In doing so the AMA joined the American Nurses Association, which had, a year earlier, denounced discrimination against the AIDS patients.

Philosophers attempting to struggle with this issue, stressed the importance of a 'social' responsibility to guarantee each HIV-infected individual access to health care; the responsibility of the health care *professions* as collective entities to provide appropriate care to the needy, rather than the responsibility of each individual health care worker to treat. In brief, some argued, if somewhat reluctantly, that as along as the needs of the HIV infected were met, there might be no strong ethical grounds for insisting that each health care worker share in the responsibility.

Others have asked for a more universal obligation. Thus, did physician-philosopher Edmund Pellegrino opine, "to refuse to care for AIDS patients, even if the danger were greater than it is, is to abnegate what is essential to being a physician."

For those who have stressed a universal obligation to treat, it is clear that the relatively low risk of infection has been central. Had the risks of HIV transmission been very much greater, it would have required an ethics of heroism to insist that each health care workers bear the responsibility of assuring adequate and proper health care to the infected. Given the level of risk entailed in the face of HIV infection, even among surgeons and obstetricians, those who stress the obligation to treat opine that it was not heroism but more straightforward duty that is inherent.

The point of access to care is not, however, primarily raised by the spectre of physician abandonment. Rather, it rests on the problem of access to care on the part of the poor.

In the United States of America, which unlike other economically advanced nations does not guarantee access to care on the part of its citizens, the striking contrast between important clinical advances in the care of the AIDS patients, and the social organization of American medicine led the National Commission on Acquired Immune Deficiency Syndrome to warn, in a December 1989 report to the President, that medical milestones would "mean little unless the health care system can incorporate them and make them accessible to people in need." The presence of a medically disenfranchised class meant that for many, access to care was almost solely through the "emergency room door of one of the few hospitals in the country that treats people with HIV infection and AIDS".

The point of how to assure access to care and, more importantly, the question of what degree of care to provide in nations that are poor and that can provide only rudimentary health care services presents very difficult ethical questions. No simple answers are possible in situations where so many pressing health care needs go unfulfilled. A basic ethical principle would necessitate that the infected persons should not be discriminated against because of that fact; that they receive no less than other gravely ill persons. Ultimately, the choices made within conditions of severe constraints make clear how the resolution of pressing human needs in the less developed nations will require support and help from economically advanced countries.

AIDS and the World

AIDS concerns unfortunately, the most advanced technological societies, like the United States of America, with the poorest nations of Africa, Asia and Latin America. The vast proportion of AIDS in the world exists outside North America and Western Europe. In the next decade, the already stark contrast will become even sharper. In the face of the social catastrophe now making itself felt, it will be critical to face the question of what the rich nations of the world owe the poor as the latter faces the issues of prevention and treatment. The social, economic and political realities of general assistance to the Third World cannot be ignored as we face the AIDS pandemics. The basic fact is that advanced industrial world does very meagre to meet the needs of the Third World, in terms of food, health care or other basic needs.

This is all too easy to imagine the development of expensive therapeutic agents that will be reserved for those who fall ill as a result of HIV infection in the advanced industrial societies but which will not be available the ones similarly placed in Third World nations. The use of AZT during pregnancy poses a paradigm challenge. Here is a therapy that could radically reduce HIV transmission. It is in the less-developed world that paediatric AIDS poses such a significant problem, yet the cost of AZT places it out of reach of the needy. As noted above, if and when a vaccine were to be developed, will it be made available to those most in need? And who would pay the cost of production and distribution for those countries which are too poor to bear the cost?

AIDS, due to its dramatic features, underscores the limitations of our capacity to conceive of and act upon notions of shared responsibility across national boundaries. At stake, of course, is the issue of justice and the global distribution of resources.

Conclusion

For recognising the extent to which efforts to control AIDS will call forth sharp ethical and social disputes is not, however, the end of the analysis. It is, in fact, just the beginning. Which values—with what impact on the lives of men, women and children, with what implications for democratic social life, with what likely aftermath for the further spread of HIV infection—should lead us? This is the critical ethical question raised by the AIDS pandemic.

Seventeen

HIV Screening: The Ethical Issues

The test developed to detect antibody to the AIDS virus—and first used on a large scale in blood banking—was mired in controversy. Uncertainty about the significance of the test's outcome and about its quality and accuracy provided the technical substrate of disputes that inevitably took on a political and ethical character, since issues of privacy, communal health, social and economic discrimination, coercion and liberty were always involved. How would the test be carried out outside the context of blood banking? Would groups at increased risk for AIDS be encouraged to adopt the test? How forceful would such encouragement be? How would those who agreed to be tested be counselled about the test's significance for themselves and others? Would and could the results be kept confidential? Would the initially voluntary testing be a prelude to compulsory screening? What would be the consequence of testing for the right to work? To go to school? To obtain insurance? To bear children? To remain free? Each of these questions would force a confrontation over the fundamental matter of the relationship between the defence of privacy and the protection of the public health; over the roles of voluntarism and force in the social response to the threat of AIDS.

Out of the debate that swang around about the antibody test there emerged a broad voluntarist consensus. Barring clearly circumscribed circumstances, testing was to be done under conditions of voluntary, informed consent, and the results were to be protected by strict confidentiality safeguards. In the United States, to underscore the value of protecting the privacy of tested individuals the option of anonymity was made broadly available. This consensus was backed by gay leaders, civil libertarians, bioethicists, public health officials and by professional organizations representing clinicians. But as broad as the consensus was, it was also fragile based as it was on diverse interests and commitments.

In this chapter five broad issues are being addressed: screening and behvioural change, screening for clinical purposes, screening for safety, screening in blinded seroprevalence studies, and changing technologies in screening.

Screening and Behavioural Change

Even before the screening of the blood supply had started in mid-1985 it was explicit that the new antibody test would be enlisted in the effort to achieve the overriding public health goal of mass behavioural change. What was the matter of wider controversy and what has remained a matter of controversy was how much of a role. For public health officials who faced the fearful challenge of affecting the most intimate behaviours and for whom the legacy of other health promotion campaigns gave little cause for optimism, the test seemed a technology that could encourage the desired changes. Those who tested positive could be counselled about the urgency of behavioural changes to the prevention of the spread of HIV. Those who tested negative could be counselled on the importance of self-protection. Opponents of too great a reliance on testing—often representatives of the gay community and of civil liberties groups—were afraid of the social consequences of being recognised as infected with HIV. It was mass education and individual couselling they argued, that were crucial. From this perspective testing with all of its technical uncertainties was too costly and too dangerous.

Over the past many years the bitter edge has all but vanished from the dispute. Public health officials have identified that an extraordinary change has taken place in the behaviour of gay men, for instance, a change that could in no way be directly related to the availability of testing. Representatives of those most at risk have come to recognize that for specific mass campaigns of education have been not sufficient to motivate behavioural change, that the more direct and targeted efforts concerned with test-linked counselling are necessary. What remains a matter of controversy is how aggressively to press for testing among those groups where the degree of behavioural change thus far attained gives reason for concern, even alarm—intravenous drug users and their sexual partners for example. In a number of developing countries, where patterns of transmission powerfully affect the heterosexual population testing of women, particularly sex workers, has resulted in sharp controversy.

Contributing to the always fragile consensus on testing for behavioural change has been a credit on the part of public health officials of the need to win the confidence of those most at risk for HIV infection. The fears that the confidentiality of test results would be breached, thus exposing the infected to stigma and discrimination, public health officials have often responded by embracing the cause of confidentiality and legislation to protect the social and economic rights of individuals with HIV infection. What ethics required following the duty to respect the dignity of each individual, the public health postulated as well. Absent careful assurances of confidentiality and protections against irrational discrimination, it would not be possible to encourage those at risk to come forward for testing.

Screening for Clinical Purposes

Early in the history of the epidemic, when medicine was all but ineffective before the opportunistic diseases that afflicted those with HIV infection, the question with which some patients and several of their advocates confronted those who suggested antibody testing was, "Of what advantage will a positive finding be for *me*?" Furthermore, this was not a test like any other typically employed by clinicians and typically covered by the broad general consent implied in an agreement to be treated.

Rather, it was argued, the antibody test was for social and psychological causes more like those invasive procedures for which special consent was required. Faced with such challenges, and the undeniable fact of social stigma related to HIV infection, physicians, their professional associations and public health officials agreed that an exact standard of consent for HIV testing was proper: specific informed consent was to be sought from patients or their surrogates. To a number of clinicians, however, such requirements represented an unacceptable intrusion into the therapeutic relationship, an obstacle designed to disrupt sound diagnostic work.

The early history of HIV testing in developed countries may still apply in the developing world, where effective treatment is still beyond the reach of much of the population. What purpose, critics may ask, is served by requiring poor people to be tested when there is little personal benefit that may accrue?

Now that there have been some significant advances in the capacity of medicine to control the life-threatening illnesses faced by HIV-infected individuals in the North and West, given the aspirations of physicians and researchers for the prophylactic use of therapeutic agents like Zidovudine may slow the progression of HIV disease, that other medications may prevent pneumocystis pneumonia, and given the range of clinical trials for which the infected may be eligible, the picture for patients is very different from that which had prevailed just a short time ago. Under such circumstances it is feasible to answer the question, "Of what advantage will a positive finding be for me?" rather differently than in 1985. It is possible to respond, "Though we are nowhere close to a cure for HIV infection, there are several interventions that may extend your life if we move aggressively." Under such circumstances pressure has begun to mount on the part of clinicians to loosen the requirements for particular informed consent before testing occurs. In brief, clinicians have begun to assert that the time has come to return AIDS to the "medical mainstream".

Although it is feasible to appreciate the impatience expressed in this perspective, it is potent at this juncture to resist the pressure for routine unconsented testing. In the first place, as much as the clinical picture has begun to change, there is no definitive therapeutic course for HIV-infected but otherwise asymptomatic individuals. At the same time the feasibility of stigma and of discrimination remains an ever present threat to the social well being of the infected. Given these conditions the arguments for particular informed consent remain as pertinent as they ever were. But even were the clinical picture to improve dramatically the moral grounds for emphasising on informed consent before HIV testing would not change. It is an established principle of medical ethics that competent adults have the right to decide whether or not to undergo treatment, whether or not to discontinue treatment already begun. Certainly, the principle that limits the paternalistic authority of the physicians under therapics in the interest of the patient extends to the authority to order those tests that would serve as the basis for commencing treatment.

But if respect for the autonomy of the patient requires that physicians exercise restraint, the physician's ethical liability to take appropriate care and the principle of beneficence, now require that physicians properly offer HIV antibody testing in those situations *where therapies are available and accessible* to patients at risk, either geographically or socially. Only by properly offering such tests can patients be given the opportunity to learn whether or not they are infected. Only then can they exercise their right to choose whether or not to initiate therapy or enter available clinical trials. In urging patients to undergo testing physicians must explicitly define the risks related to being identified as infected and the benefits that *may* be associated with treatment. An effort to persuade a patient by exaggerating current therapeutic possibilities or the benefits that might follow from participating in clinical trials entails a deception that deprives the individual of the right to make a fully informed decision in the face of a very difficult situation.

More complex still is the question of whether the existing situation justifies the routine or essential screening of infants born to mothers at increased risk for HIV infection. In more developed countries pediatricians have for some time now opined that the early identification of infected newborns provides an opportunity to begin aggressive intervention, containing the prophylactic administration of drugs to prevent pneumocystis pneumonia. Others have been more sceptical of what can be done. They have argued that the long-term advantage to infected children of early clinical intervention is by no means clear. What the test does is to recognise the existence of an infected mother. Certainly, before such recognition is permitted to occur without consent it should be important to demonstrate more than a theoretical benefit to the infant.

This debate takes place against a background of widely accepted mandatory or routine testing of newborns to allow the recognition of those in need of special treatment. Screening in these instances is held to represent a legitimate exercise of the states power to protect the vulnerable. Screening for PKU is paradigmatic. Early recognition is critical so that a special dietary regime can be started. The failure to undertake such a therapeutic intervention can be destructive for the child. A definitive diagnostic test, a definitive therapeutic intervention, an essential to act quickly—these are the conditions that provide the empirical and moral grounds for the routine screening of newborns without first seeking parental consent.

None of these conditions prevail in the case of HIV. There is, therefore, no basis for mandatory newborn screening. That the current test is, in fact, a test of the mother makes the argument against unconsented testing all the more compelling. Were a therapy for such new born available the clinical foundation would exist for making a claim on behalf of the vulnerable child. Such a claim might well be sufficient to establish the grounds for testing without prior parental consent.

In spite of the enormous attention devoted to the question of newborn testing in the late 1980's and early 1990's, that issue will, in all likelihood, be superseded by pressure to recognise HIV-infected pregnant women. That pressure will stem from a proper research finding in early 1994 that showed a sharp reduction in HIV transmission from infected pregnant women to their foetuses when AZT was administered during pregnancy and delivery and to the newborn for six weeks after birth. Following this finding, obstetricians and pediatricians proceeded to assert that the regime surrounding testing should be liberalized so that all infected women could be identified and offered treatment. Some have called for mandatory testing during pregnancy, using as a model testing for syphilis and hepatitis B. While avoiding mandatory treatment as ethically unacceptable and practically not possible, advocates of mandatory screening have asserted that women who learn of their HIV infection will be more likely to accept voluntary treatment. More common, several physicians have asserted that the stringent requirements of informed consent with pretest counselling should be replaced with a strong recommendation to undergo testing with an informed right of refusal. Such proposals clearly seek to shift the burden of decision—making to those women who would reject HIV testing. The foundation for such a shift, it is argued, is the advantage for the foetus which might have been infected had its mother not been identified and offered AZT treatment. Here, as in the situation of mandatory screening, there is an assumption that while women might not be interested to undergo testing, they will, once they know they are infected, undertake therapies designed to protect the children they will bear.

In spite of such proposals, the posture of the United States Public Health Service has been steadfastly voluntarist. The outcome of ongoing consultations among broad constituencies, this rejection of mandatory testing or near-mandatory testing has been premised on the assumption that when completely informed of the advantages of AZT treatment in the period of pregnancy, the vast majority of women at risk will accept voluntary HIV testing. Non-coercive testing would, it is asserted, provide the context of a therapeutic alliance conducive to the beginning of treatment with AZT during pregnancy.

Much will rely on whether the assumptions of the Public Health Service prove correct. If most infected women are recognised, and if the rate of vertical HIV transmission declines dramatically, it is less likely that mandatory measures will be followed. If, however, that does not turn out to be the case, the voluntarist approach will be not easy to sustain.

Screening for Safety

Because AIDS represented the first major infectious disease with which advanced industrial societies had to contend in almost a generation, and because the causative agent was not recognised until three years after the first case reports, it is not surprising that it provoked considerable social concern. How was it spread? Who posed the risk? Who was endangered? That it was socially marginal and not infrequently despised individuals who seemed to be epidemiologically at increased risk only intensified the urge towards discrimination. Employers, landlords, schools and even some health care institutions evidenced a willingness to exclude those with the new disease. With the discovery of HIV, and the development of a test that could identify antibody to the virus, the potential scope for discriminatory activity increased in spite of the epidemiological evidence about how infection was spread.

The World Health Organization, Council of Europe, and international AIDS organizations have largely opposed exclusion of persons with HIV infection in the workplace, schools, and other public places. Anti-discrimination provisions have been among the earliest and the most consistent pronouncements of the Global Programme on AIDS.

In the United States, the Centres for Disease Control moved swiftly to contain the irrational impulse towards exclusion. At the end of 1985 guidelines to stop the spread of HIV infection in schools and the workplace were issued. Early in 1986 detailed guidelines on stopping the spread of infection when health care workers were engaged in invasive procedures were published. In each example the aim was to give information, to provide protection, to prevent panic. The message was clear: HIV could not be casually transmitted and so there were no grounds for exclusion from school and workplace of infected individuals who were otherwise capable of performing their expected functions. In the perspective of the health care setting, universal blood and body fluid precautions would protect workers not only from HIV but from the far more infectious hepatitis B. Screening would only give illusory protections.

Although there are still shameful occurrences of efforts to exclude or isolate school children with AIDS or HIV infection, and although cases of discrimination by employers continue to exist, they are almost widely deplored as irrational, unscientific and ethically retrograde.

The situation in health care has not been so explicit. The comparatively few cases of transmission that have occurred as a result of needle sticks, and the even smaller number of transmissions linked to blood splashes, have provoked distress among health care workers, particularly among surgeons, obstetricians, nurses and emergency room personnel. Persons whose work continuously brings them into contact with their patients' blood have felt vulnerable. On rare occasions they have asserted the right to refuse to care for the infected. Far more frequently, such clinicians have openly challenged the adequacy of the recommendations for universal blood and body fluid precautions. Instead, they have postulated the right to know whether or not their patients are infected, and the right to screen on a routine or mandatory basis for HIV infection. The level of vigilance demanded by the threat of a lethal infection could not, they have argued, be maintained at all times. The conflict between public health officials who have declared that universal precautions are sufficient, and clinicians who have asserted that they are not, has not abated; really, it has intensified. A deep fissure has thus emerged, rupturing the broad alliance which had existed within the medical profession.

In several less developed countries, there is not sufficient sterilization of instruments and lack of gloves and equipment important for effective infection control. Health care workers claim the right to protect themselves and their patients, urging that infection control equipment must be a priority.

Paralleling this debate has been the unresolved question of the substantial measures to protect patients from HIV-infected clinicians. Debate on this matter has been driven by the single, still unexplained case of a Florida dentist to whom the only cases of HIV infection in patients linked to a clinician have been traced. Some are of the view that although professionals have a moral duty to assume some risks—particularly those that are quite small—in caring for their patients, patients do not have an equivalent duty to expose themselves to even small risks when being cared for. Dismissing as irrational those who would refuse all infected health care workers, whatever their functions, the right to engage in clinical work, many have asserted that physicians whose invasive work can place their patients at some risk ought not to engage in those procedures. But if those who know themselves to be infected with HIV have such professional duties, are there correlative institutional obligations to recognise the infected, to exclude them from certain functions? Are they obligated to screen health care workers and, if so, at what frequency? Might concern about protecting patients give the basis for mandatory screening and surveillance after so much endeavour to forestall such programmes? And if screening and surveillance were to be adopted, what would be the impact on a concerned social climate?

Seroprevalence Studies

When the Centres for Disease Control announced that it would initiate to undertake blinded seroprevalence studies in order to track the course of HIV infection in the United States, the media assumed that the stage had been set for a bitter conflict between public health officials and the proponents of civil liberties, gay rights, and medical ethics. In fact, no such conflict occurred.

Those who had proposed the studies made the following arguments: Samples drawn from gay men at testing sites, from blood donors, and recruits to the armed forces did not give a wider base for determining the spread of infection in the general population. Nor did such samples provide a very good base for determining the level of infection among those most at risk. Selection bias was necessary. Only with blood drawn for other objectives in hospitals and clinics would it be possible to develop accurate epidemiological data—data critical to an understanding of the course of HIV infection, to the evaluation of preventive interventions, to the planning for needed health care and social services. But would such efforts represent a violation of the moral rules of voluntariness, and would they represent an unacceptable intrusion upon privacy?

From the perspective of those worried about the protection of individual rights and for whom the threats of stigmatization and discrimination in the face of the AIDS epidemic were of deep concern, these were critical questions. Neither voluntariness nor privacy appeared threatened by the proposed seroprevalence studies. The blood being subject to analysis had been drawn for other purposes presumably with consent. Because the samples were to be stripped of identifiers, because the findings produced could not be linked to specific persons, and because the data produced could not only be statistical, no threats to privacy were posed.

Ironically, what *few* objections were raised to blinded seroprevalence studies came not from those worried about individual rights but from some public health officials and clinicians. It was briefly the features of blinded seroprevalence studies that recommended them to those worried about privacy that such opponents found most disturbing. Stripping samples of identifiers made it not possible to relate results and persons, made it impossible to inform the infected about their own serological status, about the hazard they might inadvertently pose for others. These purposes were not significant. Yet to public health officials and those who studied the moral issues posed by the AIDS epidemic the overall benefits of blinded seroprevalence studies seemed, on balance, to provide a warrant for them.

It is noteworthy, the rather unhampered conduct of such studies in the United States was not repeated in Europe. In Great Britain a forceful attack on the ethics of such surveillance by those who saw such studies as entailing an unacceptable invasion of privacy was joined by public health concerns about the conduct of investigators that would not allow investigators to inform the infected. Finally, some in the Ministry of Health believed that the quality of the data produced by studies would in fact be poor. It was only at the end of 1988 after a protracted discussion that a decision at the highest levels allowed Great Britain to pursue a research course first allowed by the United States and strongly supported by the WHO Global Programme on AIDS.

Strikingly, as the epidemiological advantages of blinded seroprevalence studies have become ever clearer, controversy has surfaced in the nation where the broad scale application of the approach faced virtually no resistance. In 1995 in the United States, a broadly based political challenge to blinded seroprevalence studies involving newborns was undertaken. How, it was argued, could one justify the failure to inform a mother that her child was effectively infected with HIV? Did not the prospect of early therapeutic intervention render such endeavours ethically unacceptable? Was this not but a latter-day version of the infamous Tuskegee syphilis experiment in which poor African-American men were refused the knowledge that they had syphilis following the desire to trace the natural history of the disease? (Begun at a time when there was little that could be done for individuals and syphilis, the experiment continued through the 1960's, two decades after discovering that penicillin could cure syphilis). Could the justification of blinded seroprevalence at a time of therapeutic impotence be carried over to a period marked by a commitment to early intervention?

So forceful was this challenge that the CDC was compelled to suspend its funding for such endeavours. At a deeper level the challenge does raise an important ethical question about the point at which the ethical justification for blinded seroprevalence may need to be resisted as the therapeutic picture changes.

Changing Testing Technologies

A striking departure from the conventional approach to HIV testing has been proposed in some developed countries, one that would permit individuals to acquire a blood sample in the privacy of their homes, send it to a laboratory where it would be analyzed, and then receive the results by telephone after entering a unique code number. Those who were negative would get this information by a recorded statement that would contain information about the importance of safer sex. Those who tested positive would get the results from a telephone counsellor. The proposed sale of over-the-counter HIV test kits would drastically change the role of health professionals at critical junctures in the testing process.

The proposed test kits, which have been under review by the Food and Drug Administration, gave rise to a number of questions: Would they be used by people at risk for HIV infection who thus far have not been tested? Would those tested suffer because they would not get face-to-face counselling? How would such testing affect public health practices?

When first proposed in 1987 home-access HIV testing met with virtually unanimous opposition. The American Medicine Association, the Centres for Disease Control and Prevention (CDC), and the gay community all opposed the idea as threatening the foundations of America's formal HIV-testing policy, predicated on the importance of pre and post-test counselling. With so forceful a public reaction, it is not surprising that in 1989 the Food and Drug Administration prevented marketing of the test, expressing scepticism about "whether a lay person can reliably and safely perform the test and interpret the results without advantage of medical advice and professional counselling.

The reconsideration of home testing has been made feasible by a profound shift in the political climate and by refinements in the ability to offer counselling by telephone. No longer is there a solid wall of opposition from the people engaged in public health, medicine, gay activism, and service to patients with AIDS. Support—some cautions, some enthusiastic—has come from those who in the past viewed home-access testing as anathema.

The controversy over the home-access HIV test raises some public policy issues unique to AIDS and other issues that touch on matters with even broader implications—the role home diagnostic techniques should have in the evolving practice of medicine and the extent to which federal regulatory bodies should protect people from technically accurate devices that may produce psychologically burdensome results.

The challenges threw by such home access testing are limited in terms of the worldwide HIV epidemic, because of the quite conspicuous extent to which home telephones are a rarity in parts of Africa and Asia where the epidemic is raging. But the challenge does open up a vital question about the extent to which individuals should be permitted to discover their HIV status without the guidance of medical professionals at every important juncture of the process.

The home access test challenges the traditional model in a confined way. But future technologies may allow for home testing in a way that throws a much more fundamental challenge. The future holds out the feasibility of a true home test—like the pregnancy test—that would allow an individual to discover in the privacy of his or her home, without a laboratory, without a telephone counsellor, his or her HIV status. Such tests would, in principle, be more widely accessible. Such home HIV tests will put vital ethical and policy questions that have yet to be addressed—issues of the extent to which individuals should have the right to initiate such self-diagnosis; the extent to which the harm that might befall such individuals as a result of such self-diagnosis provides the warrant for limiting access to such tests for both reasons of paternalism and the common good.

Conclusions

The HIV test, a simple technological measures, has been the subject of ongoing debate because what it reveals has such profound significance for both individuals and the communities within which they live. The issues highlighted by the HIV test may change as the therapeutic context changes, and as the technologies of testing themselves undergo transformation. But what cannot change is the inevitability of careful analysis of the ethical and social implications of policies designed to guide the use of the test. By the very nature, such policies compel us to think our matters of privacy, dignity and social welfare. As such they compel us to face the most important questions of ethics and human rights presented by the AIDS.

References

1. Bayer, R. *Private Acts, Social Consequences: AIDS and the Politics of Public Health*. New York: The Free Press, 1989.
2. American Association of Physicians for Human Rights (November 12, 1985). Mimeo.
3. Northern California Branch, American Civil Liberties Union: AIDS and Civil Liberties. San Francisco. Northern California Branch, ACLU, March 1986.
4. Bayer R. Levine C., Wolf S.M.: HIV antibody screening: an ethical framework for evaluating proposed programs. *Journal of American Medical Association 1986*, 256:1768-74.
5. Association of State Territorial Health Officials: ASTHO Guide to Public Health Practice: HTLV III Antibody Testing and Community Approaches. Washington DC: Public Health Foundation, 1985.
6. American Medical Association: *Report of the Council on Ethical and Judicial Affairs: Ethical Issues Involved in the Growing AIDS Crisis*, Chicago, 1987.
7. Coates, T.J., et al: AIDS Antibody Testing: Will It Stop the AIDS Epidemic? Will It Help People Infected With HIV? *American Psychologist*, 1988, 43:859-64.
8. Centres for Disease Control: *Recommended Additional Guidelines for HIV Antibody Counselling and Testing in the Prevention of HIV Infection and AIDS* (April 30, 1987). Mimeo.
9. Surgeon General's *Report on Acquired Immune Deficiency Syndrome*, Washington, DC. 1986.
10. Institute of Medicine and the National Academy of Sciences: *Confronting* AIDS. Washington, DC: National Academy Press, 1986.
11. *Report of the PresidentialCommission on the Human Immunodeficiency Virus Epidemic*. Washington, DC: 1988.
12. Levine C. and Bayer R.: "The Ethics of Screening for Early Invention in HIV Disease," *American Journal of Public Health* (December 1989), Vol. 79, No.12, pp. 1961-67.
13. Bayer R.,: "Womens Rights, Babies' Interests: Ethics, Politics, and Science in the Debate of Newborn HIV Screening," in *HIV Infection in Women*, H. Minkoff, J. DeHovitz, and A. Duerr, eds., (New York: Raven Press, 1995), pp. 293-307.

14. Bayer R.: "Ethical Challenges Posed by Zidovudine Treatment to Reduce Vertical Transmission of HIV" (Editorial), *The New England Journal of Medicine* (1994) Vol. 331, No. 18: 1223-25.
15. Hoffman C. and Munson R.,: "Ethical Issues in the use of Zidovudine to Reduce Vertical Transmission of HIV", (letter to the Editor), *The New England Journal of Medicine* (1995), Vol. 332, No. 13:891.
16. Minkoff H. and Willoughby A.,: "Pediatric HIV Disease, Zidovudine in Pregnancy, and Unblinding Heelstick Surveys: Reframing the Debate on Prenatal HIV Testing, *Journal of the American Medical Association*, October 11, 1995, Vol. 274, No. 14:1165-68.
17. Recommendations of the US Public Health Service Task Force on the use of Zidovudine to reduce perinatal transmission of human immunodeficiency virus. *MMWR* 1994:43 (RR-11): 1-20.
18. World Health Organization, Consensus Statement from the Consultation of AIDS in the Workplace, Geneva, 27-29 June, 1988, WHO/GPA/INF/ 88.7.
19. World Health Assembly, (40th), Global Strategy for the Prevention and Control of AIDS, 15 May 1987. WHA, 40/26. World Health Assembly, (41st), Avoidance of Discrimination of Relation to HIV-Infected People. WHA, 41/24, May 13, 1988.
20. Centres for Disease Control: Recommendations for preventing transmission of infection with human T-lymphotropic virus type III/lymphadenopathy-associated virus in the workplace. *MMWR* 1984, 34:681-86, 691-95.
21. Centres for Disease Control: Recommendations for preventing transmission of infection with human T-lymphotropic virus type III/lymphadenopathy-associated virus during invasive procedures. *MMWR* 1986, 35:221-23.
22. Centres for Disease Control: Update: Acquired immunodeficiency syndrome and human immunodeficiency virus infection among health-care workers. *MMWR* 1988, 37: 229-39.
23. *New York Times*, November 9, 1987.
24. Gostin L.,: "HIV-infection physicians and the practice of seriously invasive procedures", *The Hastings Center Report* 19:1:32-39 (1989).
25. Bayer R.,: "The ethics of blinded seroprevalence testing," *American Journal of Public Health* (1993), Vol. 83, No. 4.
26. Bayer R., Lumey LH and Wan L.,: "The American, British and Dutch responses to unlinked anonymous HIV seroprevalence studies: an international comparison," *AIDS* (UK) (April 1990). Reprinted in *Law, Medicine & Health Care*, (Fall-Winter, 1991) Vol. 19, No. 3-4.
27. Bayer R., Stryker J. and Smith M.,: "Testing for HIV infection at Home," (Sounding Board) *The New England Journal of Medicine* (1995) 332:1296-99.
28. Banned at home: Food and Drug Administration ruling on AIDS test. *Time*. April 18, 1989.

Index

ENCYCLOPAEDIA OF AIDS

ENCYCLOPAEDIA
OF
AIDS

(In 7 Volumes)

(Volume 2)

Editor

Dr. G.C. Satpathy

PUBLICATIONS

KALPAZ PUBLICATIONS

DELHI - 110052

ENCYCLOPAEDIA OF AIDS
(*Health, Reference*)

Rs. 7000 (Set)
Rs. 1000 (each volume)

ISBN: 81-7835-112-9 (Set)
ISBN: 81-7835-133-1 (Vol. 2)

Published in 2003 in India by
Kalpaz Publications
C-30, Satyawati Nagar
Delhi-110052
e-mail: kalpaz@hotmail.com

Laser Typeset at: Alphabet, Delhi
Printed at: Mehra Offset Press, Delhi

Contents

Preface

The later half of the twentieth century will be remembered in the history of medicine for two remarkable events, one good, that is the eradication of smallpox, and the other one bad, when the world was alerted to the first case AIDS in 1981, now running in a pandemic proportion. In a little over two decades it is estimated that over 36 million people are now infected with HIV/AIDS with 5.3 million being infected every year. India alone has about 4 million HIV/AIDS patients, the second highest number among all nations. Now it is well perceived as a serious threat to humanity, and the control of this epidemic lies not only in the hands of physicians alone but the entire society must involve to the task. No cure or vaccine is yet in sight. So the only mode of controlling it is prevention. The key to prevention lies in information, education and communication.

Twenty years of observation and study of the syndrome has generated profound interest among all branches of medicine, social activists, research workers, public health issues, health and sex education strategies, with innumerable clinical and pharmacological research being conducted on it all over the world. It is not possible to compile the whole saga of AIDS, which is unique in many ways and not yet fully understood. We have tried to accumulate as much information as possible in this seven-volume encyclopaedia, probably the first such attempt made ever. Since the process of acquiring information is never-ending, we hope to provide more and more information in future.

It has been a herculean task to compile the huge materials systematically, besides being an unique experience. In spite of the best efforts for accuracy and perfection, there may be shortcomings, which may be excused. It will be a success story for us if by this work the society to which the work is dedicated is benefited at large. The study does not end here. It shall be a continuous series in future with comprehensive details having a deep bearing on the subject.

Guwahati-23
Rathyatra-2002

Dr. G.C. Satpathy
MD, IPM

Acknowledgements

During the course of this research work, I happened to visit several academic fora which willingly afforded their support and facilitated my work. These are the Ministry of Health, Govt. of India, World Health Organisation, health departments of the States and academic institutions of higher learning. I have used the material from published works including scholarly journals and magazines to fill up the gaps in these volumes.

I have also taken academic support from several sources, which include universities, institutes, centres for higher learning, Acts passed in this direction, Statistical Year Book (UNESCO), voluntary organisations, legal luminaries, social activists, prison management, legal issues of AIDS, Legislation Enquiry Commission on HIV Law, Sri Lanka, Prevention of Brothels Act, Myanmar, Laws of HIV/AIDS in Pakistan, Documents in sub-Saharan, Africa, European Council Recommendations, UNESCO Courier, Philippines Overseas Employment Agency, Foreign Exchange Regulations Deptt., Central Bank of the Philippines, National Advisory Committee on AIDS in Singapore, Vietnamese National AIDS Committee, National Blood Transfusion Centre in Cambodia, Infectious Diseases Act, Thailand, AIDS Prevention Act in Korea, Labour Protection Law, Thailand, Social Security Act, Thailand, Homosexual Law Reform Act, 1986, Universities of Nairobi, Manitola (in Canada) and Washington, Institute of Systemic Therapy, Harare, Zimbabwe, The AIDS Service Organisation, Kampala, Uganda, Health Economics and HIV/ AIDS Research Division, University of Natal, Durban, School of

Public Health, University of Natal, South Africa Institute for Medical Research, Johannesburg, Centre for African Family Studies, Nairobi, Kenya, Malwai Institute of Management, Malwai.

I feel much grateful to these institutions and learned authors whose writings have proved useful in the texts of these seven volumes.

The publisher and myself feel much beholden to the panel of highly qualified and experienced advisers who are distinguished in their respective fields, for their valuable and timely guidelines, contributions and encouragement in making this work an epoch-making one.

I am grateful to several other research institutes and NGOs etc., scholars whose writings have been used in these volumes.

I am extremely grateful to my wife, son Anurag and daughter Anamika for their consistent encouragement to me during this stupendous research work.

Dr. G.C. Satpathy

Our Distinguished Panel of Advisers

1. Dr. A.K. Das, MD, MNAMS, Ph.D., FICA	Dean and Director-Prof. Dept. of Medicine, JIMPER, Pondicherry
2. Mr. D.K. Arya IPS (Retd.)	Former Director General, BSF
3. Dr. K.V. Dakhina Murty MD, DM, DNB, FISN	Prof. & Head, Deptt. of Nephrology, Nizam's Instt. of Medical Sciences, Panjagutta, Hyderabad
4. Maj. Gen. K.K. Ganguly	VSM (Retd.)
5. Col. M.K. Bhandari MD, FICA	Asso. Prof. of Medicine, Armed Forces Medical College, Pune
6. Dr. M.C. Dash	Vice Chancellor, Sambalpur University, P.O.: Jyoti Vihar, Orissa
7. Dr. N.C. Borah MD, DM	C.M.D. GNRC Hospitals Ltd. Dispur, Guwahati
8. Dr. P.C. Bhattacharya MD	Sr. Consultant, downtown hospital Dispur, Guwahati
9. Dr. S.B. Gupta MD	Physician and Cardiologist Central Railway Hospital, Mumbai

Introduction

As far as HIV/AIDS is concerned, spreading through out the world more than 114 countries. There are many causes of spreading this monstrous disease. Injecting drug, homosexual activities, bisexual or heterosexual activities and inadequate education among the people are believed to havc been the main causes of reaching out this disease to the more wider areas of the world.

The impact of HIV/AIDS on economy, production and the national income expected to be larger extent possible in future if it would not have taken proper action in the near future. Not only the actions but disseminating, processing and compiling information of HIV/AIDS could prevent it to a great extent.

It has been Proved that it affects the younger people at the age of 15 to 25 years. It will have many consequences on health production and growth and income of the country. On the one hand it reduces the income and wealth production in the economy and on the other there are many macro economic consequences in case the disease become uncontrollable.

As far as the third world economy is concerned they are facing acute unemployment, under employment and foreign exchange imbalances which are the hurdles in the way of their development path. Those countries are mainly depending the overseas contract workers OCW's for Foreign exchange. If the HIV/AIDS had affected the OCW's, it would have been increased the cost significantly and reduce the employment opportunities abroad. It will reduce or dry up the foreign remittance from the OCW's from the abroad. This is the macro economic side of the story.

Micro economic side will also have significant impact on the economy. It could impose costs at the micro level in the form of medical care costs and the external costs imposed by HIV/AIDS positive individuals who infected others. These consist of men and women employed overseas belong to the most productive age group and embody substantial amount of human capital.

The following are the examination of Philippines, Malaysia, Latin America and Africa areas.

In Philippines, because of domestic unemployment problems they are facing, Overseas work becoming increasing in mitigating unemployment. From the OCW's Filipino is getting 8 per cent of foreign exchange. In so far as in Philippines of the 335 persons found as sero-positive, 39 had been employed and contracted the HIV overseas. It is important to note that HIV/AIDS epidemic has created macro economic and micro economic problems on the OCW's in the country and in the long run it may reduce the inflow of foreign remittance.

In Malaysia, spread of the AIDS epidemic cannot be treated or considered as a major issue. By International Standards Malaysia has a low sero-prevalence rate and the consequence of AIDS on its economic and industrial programmes have been very less. Anyhow, the characteristics of the disease in Malaysia and the countries geographical location suggests that the consequences could be high in near future unless the government implement prevention measures.

Latin America and the Caribbean islands is getting increasingly susceptible to HIV/AIDS infection. A WHO estimate puts the number of adults infected with the killer disease at 1.5 million. Urban homosexual and bisexual men, injecting drug users of commercially supplied blood and blood products are identified as the high risk groups and they were the ones who initially spread the disease.

Sub-Saharan Africa, the most poor and Strife-torn part of the world, the monstrous epidemic spread of HIV/AIDS began 15 years ago. There are 9 million people found to the HIV/AIDS infected, experts are of the opinion that it is the half of the total AIDS infected people.

According to the WHO estimates in 1994 over 2 million men, women and children believed to be ill with AIDS. By the same estimates, it has been increased cumulative total of 5 million AIDS patients by the end of the year 2000.

Editor

One

Sri Lanka: Mechanisms for Consultation

Introduction

Legislation is an endeavour of the executive. Being an instrument of social policy its success depends on the acceptance of the people who will be affected by it.

Legislation

The administration is the source of most legislations. Administrators in the course of furthering government policy or what has been termed as the momentum of administration find gaps in the legislative framework or entire areas that are not regulated by legislation. They then take measures to engulf what they perceive to be gaps in the law or to bring in new legislation to regulate the unregulated areas. In doing so, they consult the people who will or who are likely to be affected by the legislation. When interest groups are well-organized they themselves may provide the impetus for legislative change. In such cases, it is always prudent for the policy-maker to consult other groups before deciding on the policy or legislation. These consultations between policy-makers and interest groups take place at an informal level and, generally, on an *ad hoc* basis if and when the need for consultation arises.

White Papers

A different mechanism for consultation is the use of white papers. A white paper provides of a broad outline of the proposed government policy and sometimes has attached to it a draft bill giving effect to this policy. This is useful when the government is not committed to a policy in dealing with a certain social issue or in cases where it is not certain how it should address itself to the problem. The purpose of white paper is to elicit a response from the public as to how the government should act in addressing itself to the problem. It is a very effective mechanism for consultation of. Firstly, it enables the broadest possible consultation. Consultation is not confined to the stronger and better organized interest groups as any member of the public can make representations for or against the policy outlined. Secondly, it clarifies the issues which underline the proposed policy. As often is the case, things may not be as simple or clear-cut as they appear to be at first glance. A social issue has to be seen from different sides. To take an example, a policy that addresses the problems of drugs or HIV purely as a law and order problem will be less effective than a policy that takes account of the several social factors which give rise to such issues.

The use of white papers should be encouraged. But, in situations which require quick policy or legislative responses this mechanism may not always be feasible option.

Enquiry Commission

The other important mechanism for enabling the participation of the public in the formulation of policy is the commission of inquiry. In Sri Lanka, there are three types of commissions—a departmental commission, a commission of inquiry under the Commissions of Inquiry Act, and a special presidential commission of inquiry under the Special Presidential Commissions of Inquiry Act.

(A) There are a few departmental committees in the Ministry of Health, including one on mental health comprising officers of the ministry, academics and representatives of NGOs. The departmental committees have three advantages over the formal commissions of inquiry: their proceedings are more informal and participation in them is less inhibited; they are not difficult to set up, and unlike commissions of inquiry, the membership can be expanded from time to time to accommodate interests which have inadequately or not been represented.

(B) The presidential commissions of inquiry have to be presided over by sitting judges. They may not be an appropriate vehicle for the consultative process. Apart from the difficulty in getting them to serve on these commissions, judges may not be the best equipped to do it. They may have the expertise to ascertain the facts, but recommending policies based on an analysis of facts may require a multidisciplinary approach.

(C) Commissions of inquiry appointed under the Commissions of Inquiry Act have no such decents. Compared to a departmental committee, a commission of inquiry has greater visibility, by reason of the fact that the members are appointed by the President, and a vast panoply of powers- to summon witnesses, to visit persons to give evidence on oath, to produce documents, etc. Thus it has all the powers required to investigate a problem with great thoroughness. These powers also enable a commission of inquiry to have a wider reach. While commissions of inquiry call for representations from the public through advertisements in newspapers and the like, they have been explained as providing a unique channel through which private individuals and interest groups can take part directly in the making of public policy. On the other hand, the formal procedures of a commission of inquiry may deter affected parties from making representations before it.

Commissions on HIV Law

The statue which institutes the Law Commission, it enjoins to bring the law under review, both procedural and substantive, with a view to its systematic development reform. In formulating proposals for reform, the commission endeavours to consult as broad a range of interests as possible and, certainly, the ministries concerned. The proposals for reform made are subject to ratification by the Minister of Justice.

Reforms in HIV Law

Governments should undertake broadest possible consultation before embarking on law reform in sensitive areas like HIV. The hastily taken legislative initiatives may contain conceptual flaws and its mechanics of implementation may aggravate the problems posed by the HIV epidemic.

HIV/AIDS Laws in Sri Lanka

AIDS—a catastrophe of major proportions, with an estimate of 10 million infections in the world—has posed a serious menace to humanity. With the magnitude alarmingly rising, the disease requires the development of legislation within the legitimate rights of the patient. To face this challenge, there are many legal and ethical issues to be resolved.

With more than 10 million infections in the world today AIDS is taking the form of a catastrophe. It is need of the hour to develop legislations, far providing succour to the patients.

There are not any specific laws in Sri Lanka relating to AIDS. So we have to take into consideration the rubric of the prevailing laws, of which the relevant are:

1. *Contagious Diseases Ordinance No. 8 of 1866*—which suggests that every case of smallpox, cholera or other disease which may from time to time be named by the Minister should give information to a police officer or *grama seva niladhari*. Even if no regulation has been made under this ordinance to cover AIDS specifically, the executive has still to make use of the broad statement ("other disease") in the section of the law to the benefit of finding a solution AIDS-related issues.
2. *Quarantine and Prevention of Diseases Ordinance No. 3 of 1897*—is the most relevant in this context. The Quarantine and Prevention of Diseases Ordinance in Sri Lanka governs the rights and obligations of the health authority in respect of identification and control of contagious diseases. Through this Ordinance, the Minister of Health has been empowered to issue regulations specifying a disease as contagious.. The Ordinance establishes the prevention and spread of disease in and outside Sri Lanka. The Ordinance needs a physician who is reporting a case of HIV infection to identify the individual who is the subject of the report, by name, race, sex, age and place of residence and the nature of the disease shall report the concerned authorities

within 12 hours. It also empowers the authority to take the infected person or person suspected of being infected to some public hospital or other place for such period as the proper authority shall suggest.

There is no section in the Ordinance to keep the confidentiality of personally identifying information pertaining to cases of certain specified diseases, such as HIV/AIDS.

Voluntary Diagnosis

Consent to Treatment

The law of consent to medical treatment raises many unresolved questions like whether a physician must obtain a patient's specific informed consent before an HIV-related test can be legally administered or whether a physician could rely upon a patient's implied or tacit consent to perform an HIV-related test. Discussions with some physicians in Sri Lanka revealed that HIV anti-body tests are being done without obtaining specific informed consent.

Testing of People at High Risk

It is suggested that many of the problems related to universal compulsory HIV testing could be avoided if compulsory testing were confined solely to individuals, with a relatively high incidence of infection, such as men who are gay, bisexual, injecting drug users, haemophiliacs and their sexual partners. Some of the laws which have a bearing on high risk behaviours are the Vagrants Ordinance No. 4 to 1841 where indecent behaviour of persons in public is declared guilty of an offence liable for prosecution, and the Brothel's Ordinance No. 5 of 1880 deeming brothels as illegal and any person who helps in the management of one shall be guilty of an offence.

The penal Code No. 2 of 1883 is of vital importance wherein whoever maliciously, unlawfully or negligently does any act which is likely to spread the infection of any disease dangerous to life shall be punished. These are cognizable offences, in which a police officer could book without a warrant and implement an investigation according to the Criminal

Procedure Code No. 15 of 1979. The Children and Young Persons Ordinance No. 48 of 1939 resolves to safeguard young persons from being exploited for immoral or indecent purposes. Moreover, necessary legislation is to be implemented to strictly forbid prostitution, homosexuality, paedophilia, child abuse and sexual exploitation of children, as these have great potential to spread the HIV.

Testing of Foreigners

The Immigrants and Emigrants Act No. 20 of 1948 empowers the authorities to deny *prima facie* the entry of persons to the country for medical reasons. This could include a person with HIV being refused entry into the country.

Applicants for Insurance

HIV-related tests could be done on applicants for individual policies, but it is not a requirement. Anyhow, even if an HIV test were not done and if the application is aware that his is HIV-positive, it is his duty to uncover every, fact within his knowledge that is material to the insurance, failing which will make the contract voidable by the insurer.

Donors of Blood Products or Bodily Tissues

The compulsory HIV anti-body testing of donors of blood, organs, tissue, ova, semen or other human body parts and fluids, has been universally sanctioned by public health officials as an urgent and effective means of preventing the spread of HIV infection. With the development of the HIV anti-body test, the normal practice in Sri Lanka is to test all blood donors. The current methodization and practice in the area of human tissue donation is vague. The transplantation of Human Tissues Act No. 48 of 1987 deals with the donation of human tissue for transplantation purpose. In the wake of the AIDS epidemic, several countries have improved their legislation in connection with transplants and transfusions to make HIV screening compulsory before any transplant and transfusion. It is desirable to improve the transplantation of Human Tissues Act by introducing a similar requirement.

AIDS Related Fundamental Rights

The Constitution of 1987 of Sri Lanka has given over an entire chapter on "Fundamental Rights". It enumerates many rights, the violation of which is justifiable in a court of law. For example, according to Article 14(g), (h) and (i) of the Constitution, every citizen is enabled to the freedom to engage by himself or in association with others in any lawful occupation, profession, trade, business or enterprise, the freedom of movement and of choosing his residence within Sri Lanka and the freedom to come back to one's own country, which means even an HIV-positive citizen has all the above rights. But, according to Article 15(7), these rights shall be subject to such bounds as may be prescribed by law in the interest of national security, public order and the protection of public health or morality. So, an HIV-positive citizen has all the above rights but they could be restricted principally for the protection of public health, and thus other rules, regulations and laws that enable identification of AIDS patients and thereby check the spread of the disease should not in any way be considered as a violation of anyone's fundamental rights. However, the Article 11 of the Constitution confers upon any individual (even an AIDS patient) a fundamental right that is non-derogable.

Two

Economic Fallout of AIDS in South-East Asia

Introduction

As far as the AIDS in South-East Asia is concerned, the main reasons are poverty in the area. The other section of the people who are most affected are ethnic minority and women. They are bearing brunt of it. The area consist of the poorest people live and it is predicted the most vulnerable to the most monstrous disease like AIDS. The costs, direct and indirect will destruct their economy in the near future.

Efforts to contain HIV virus notwithstanding, the epidemic imposes major economic costs on the countries and subregions of Southeast Asia where prevalence rates are high. The economic costs are mainly the direct costs of care, particularly in hospital settings. The epidemic is spread in a nonrandom pattern and the poor are more at risk than those who are economically well off. In Southeast Asia the two subgroups of the poor who are most at risk are ethnic/tribal groups and women.

One must also assess existing and possible health policy responses to the epidemic in light of the epidemic's differential consequences on different sub-population groups. It suggests the urgency for responses that are more consistent with geographical, cultural, political, and economic realities. In particular, policymakers need to examine the present importance on individual volition as the cause of the epidemic and changes in individual behaviour as the key to preventing its spread.

Even though the ultimate longer-term dimensions of the HIV/AIDS epidemic cannot yet be forecast with any degree of confidence, a plausible range of estimates. For the year 2000, by the World Health Organization's current suggest a cumulative total of about 30 to 40 million HIV infections in men, women, and children, of which more than 90 per cent will be in the developing countries. The projected cumulative total of adult AIDS cases is close to 10 million, of which again almost 90 per cent will be in the developing countries. South and Southeast Asia may have greater numerical increments in HIV infections because of the very large populations involved.

The Question of Costs

Though the HIV/AIDS epidemic is not yet alarmingly widespread in Southeast Asia except in Thailand, the economic costs for society are fairly large. Moreover, the inherent inertia as well as the existence of those factors and conditions favourable for the spread of the epidemic suggest that the scale of the epidemic is likely to grow.

The likely economic impacts of the epidemic has both direct costs as well as indirect costs. There are intergenerational and long-run costs and equity and distributional impacts as well.

Direct costs consists of all costs associated with the prevention, diagnosis, and treatment of the epidemic and related diseases, including expenditures on hospital care, the services of medical practitioners and other health personnel, drugs, medical equipment, and long-term care, as well as incidental costs such as transport costs. Also included in this category are control and prevention measures, including blood screening, health education, and the distribution of disposable syringes and condoms.

The calculation of indirect costs include lost output and income due to illness and premature death and lost productivity due to disability. Even though indirect costs are likely to be the largest component of total costs due to the epidemic they have received less attention than direct costs. A recent study of Thailand concluded that the sum of direct costs and losses resulting from declined productivity amounts to an estimated US$7.3-8.7 billion, with each death equivalent to a loss of US$22,000. Moreover, this figure did not include costs due to worker absenteeism, retraining, reduced direct foreign investment, and lower household savings. Health care costs per AIDS patient are calculated to be US$658-1,016 per year, which is about ten times the amount Thai households currently spend on health care.

Studies of the epidemic's consequences on equity and distributional issues are even less common than studies of indirect costs. Researchers have now realized that the epidemic spreads in a nonrandom fashion. The lack of randomness is owing to the heterogeneity of the underlying population base, which is endowed with differing abilities to handle risk and is also subject to different levels of risk. Equity, at least in terms of who is affected by the epidemic and who is most at risk, is an important issue as well as it is likely to have a major consequences on the course of the epidemic over time, and consequently on the total costs incurred. An understanding of the epidemic's differential consequence on different population groups may permit the design of more accurately targeted, cost-effective preventive measures while the epidemic is still in its early stages.

In identifying the epidemic's differential consequence one can break down population groups by a variety of classifications, for example, age, gender, racial background, or ethnic characteristics. Usually, populations are grouped by perceived behavioural patterns and discussions are in terms of high or low risk groups. However, populations can be classified by economic category. More precisely, equity issues using the conventional economic concept of poverty can be analyzed. The evidence proved that the AIDS epidemic could affect those groups that are least well off and are least able to resist its effects. This is due to poor people's lower information and knowledge base, the greater prevalence of drug abuse that entails use of needles and syringes among low-income groups, and their limited access to higher quality goods and services. The greater consequence on these groups, many of which are on the fringes of survival, will come through reduced labour remittances, reduced availability of labour and ultimately less food security and income. Thus, the poverty of some social groups will intensify as a result of the epidemic.

Implications of Poverty on HIV in South Asia

Conceptual and data problems in calculating poverty in Southeast Asia abound. At the most fundamental level, the Indochina countries and Myanmar have not collected data on poverty indicators and studies are rare, which is somewhat surprising considering their historical concern with broad-based social development. Even where indicators of relative or absolute deprivation exist, cross-country comparability may be limited. Nonetheless, the data in table 1 provide a rough indicator of the depth of poverty in Southeast Asian countries. In all cases, significant shares of the total population live below the poverty line, and in the case of the Philippines, the majority of the population were officially considered as poor. Furthermore, in all the countries the share of the population below the poverty line was more severe in rural than in urban areas.

Even in a country that has developed rapidly during the past twenty years and is regarded as a successful development case study, widespread poverty remains a major problem. The extent of poverty is also not evenly distributed. The majority of the poor were farmers or labourers, and that the vast majority lived in villages.

TABLE 1
SELECTED SOCIAL INDICATORS IN SOME ASIAN DEVELOPING COUNTRIES

Country	*Adult literacy rate, 1990 (percent)*			*Female literacy index, 1990 (north = 100)*	*Fertility rate 1990*
	Total	*Male*	*Female*		
India	48	62	34	35	4.2
Indonesia	77	84	68	72	3.3
Lao PDR	44[a]	—	—	—	6.7
Malaysia	78	87	70	74	3.8
Myanmar	81	89	72	76	3.9
Philippines	90	90	90	94	4.1
Thailand	93	96	90	95	2.4
Viet Nam	88	92	84	88	3.9

— = Not available

a. Data refer to 1989 overall literacy rate.

Source: UNDP (1992)

Profiles of the poor show that even though they had large families, there were very few income earners and the heads of house-hold had low educational levels. The poor depended much on income in kind and lacked basic amenities such as piped water and proper sanitation. Therefore, an accurate generalization of poverty in Southeast Asia would be that many of the poor live in rural areas and most of the rural populace are poor. While regional differentials in the incidence of poverty may not be as pronounced elsewhere in Southeast Asia, they still exist. A recent study of rural poverty in Asia (Asian Development Bank 1992) identified the following characteristics of rural poverty as important:

- Limited access to land and irrigation facilities;
- Slow adoption of modern agricultural techniques due to barriers that limit access to technology, information, and credit;
- Large family size and relatively low numbers of income earners;
- Fewer human capital resources, especially among women;
- Concentration in backward areas;
- Concentration among minority and ethnic groups.

Other characteristics of poverty would include the limited linkage with a market economy and limited access to public goods such as basic health services. The limited access is due to physical remoteness and unclear political and economic rights.

In the context of the HIV/AIDS epidemic in Southeast Asia the two most important features of poverty are gender and ethnicity. In other words, within the sub population group broadly referred to as poor, women and ethnic minorities are perhaps to be at risk and the least likely to be able to withstand the epidemic's effects.

Ethnic Diversity

The countries of mainland Southeast Asia are distinguished by marked ethnic and cultural diversity. Lao PDR, Myanmar, Thailand, and Vietnam each have one or more large river valleys, a perimeter of high mountains, and at least one plateau (Bowles 1977). In all the countries, major distinctions exist between the more powerful and numerous groups who live in the lowlands and the different ethnic groups who live in the mountains. The latter group are only tenuously associated with the lowland population because of differences in language, culture, and religion. The village is very much the center of economic, political, and social activity and smallholding agriculture is pervasive. Integration into the mainstream has also been prevented by limited political representation. Thus, in combination with other factors has conferred few economic benefits on the ethnic minorities. Although governments have tried to include these groups in national development programs, progress has been thwarted by limited acceptance of lowland values.

In addition to the many ethnic groups distinct to each of the Southeast Asian countries, most of the ethnic groups live in areas straddling modern borders. Prominent among these are the Lahu and Akha, who are found in Myanmar, Lao PDR, and parts of Yunnan China. The Lahu live in all these areas and in parts of Vietnam. The Lisu are found in Yunnan, Myanmar, and Thailand. In the western part of the region, the Kachin live in Myanmar, Yunnan, and Assam, India, while the Nagas and Hkamti Shan live in both Myanmar and Assam. The Wa live only in Myanmar or Yunnan.

Ethnic diversity and the large numbers of ethnic groups who straddle political borders are of more than anthropological interest in a study of the HIV and AIDS in Southeast Asia. The main reason is that opium cultivation and its use as a narcotic are widespread among these ethnic groups. This is not to say that all ethnic minorities are straddle political borders cultivate and use opium. Indeed, the borders of Myanmar, Lao PDR, and Thailand constitute the Golden Triangle, which produces at least 500 tons of opium annually, which is later refined into heroin and smuggled by various routes to its final destinations.

Opium cultivation and use have been a way of life in this area for generations. Recent developments, however, turned in drug abuse from opium smoking to intravenous heroin injection. The practice of sharing needles and syringes, combined with the frequency of injection, predominantly magnify the probability of contracting the HIV.

A major reason for concern with equity issues in general and ethnicity in particular in a discussion of the HIV epidemic is that should an epidemic driven by intravenous drug use take hold, the extent of structural poverty among ethnic minorities is such that few existing preventive measures are likely to be effective. Mountainous terrain, large expanses, and low population densities make the dissemination of information, whether on agricultural extension and income enhancement or AIDS prevention, very much difficult. Cultural, ethnic, and linguistic factors hinder greater participation in market exchanges and increased economic welfare. Ethnic groups and subgroups can each have their own language or dialect, customary law, and political, economic, and social arrangements that extremely different from those of neighbouring groups. The most important contributory factor to extensive structural poverty is perhaps the limited human capital endowment of many ethnic groups. The low levels of endowment, especially of female education, not only prevent access to remunerative occupations, but limit the ability to respond to traditional measures designed to prevent the spread of the HIV epidemic.

Gender Issues in South Asia

The major group of poor who are severely affected by the AIDS epidemic in Southeast Asia is women. The AIDS epidemic has virtually become a women's disease. As the epidemic spreads to more areas and progresses from being a disease of a few subgroups to that of the larger population, more and more women become infected. Moreover, there are strong reasons to believe that the epidemic affects women, especially poor women, more than men. Generally, women use health facilities more than men due to the biological division of labour, whereby women must deal with pregnancy, childbirth, and contraception. Women also have greater responsibilities in raising children and in health matters. However, in fulfilling these tasks, women always face significant problems, such as a lack of information and facilities limited financial resources to pay for the use of health facilities, or difficulties in using these facilities due to competing demands on their time. Thus, poverty directly prevents women from addressing their health care needs adequately.

In the context of the HIV epidemic, women are more vulnerable to infection because of epidemiological, sociological, and economic reasons. Epidemiologically, it is that the virus is more easily transmitted from men to women than the other way round is well established. Socially, women lack control over their own sexual lives or those of their husbands outside the marriage. Extramarital relations, as well as intravenous drug abuse or bisexual behaviour, are possible routes for the entry of the HIV into the marital union. Limited literacy, mobility, and access to information; and cultural and moral attitudes toward sexuality prevent women to insist for protected sex. They are not be able to discuss sexual matters in public, or even with their husbands. Social and sexual passivity make insistence on the use of condoms as protection against HIV infection difficult.

In Southeast Asia, absolute and relative poverty are the main reasons why women face a greater risk of infection by the HIV. Sex differentials in income are caused by a combination of customary sexual division of labour. Biological factors, limited demand for labour, and economic institutions that induce labour market stratification. Social and geographical movement induced by the disintegration of traditional economic systems make worse the vulnerability to HIV infection. Absolute poverty, in turn, control choice in areas that are basic to health, such as adequate food, housing, sanitation, and clean water; availability of adequate health care on demand; and the ability to plan into the future. Biased intra-household allocations of wealth also limit women's range of choices on matters relating to health and sexuality.

In extreme cases, lack of alternative work opportunities women may be induced to turn to prostitution. In Southeast Asia, prostitution is a major reason by which impoverished young women become infected and vector through which the epidemic is spread to the general population.

Though, estimating the number of individuals who are involved in behaviour that is illegal or of a private personal nature is extremely difficult, in Southeast Asia, Thailand probably has the largest number of prostitutes. In Southeast Asia, prostitution as an industry is not bigger, although in certain urban areas that are transportation nodes or are close to military bases it can be a major service industry.

A relatively new character of prostitution in Southeast Asia is that the supply source of potential entrants into prostitution is not limited to the rural hinterland of an individual country. Movement across borders is enthused by large cross-border real income differentials that in some cases are magnified by exchange rate distortions. An important determinant of the poverty of those groups who enter prostitution is their limited human capital assets, especially their low education levels. Several factors on the demand side contribute to the size of the prostitute population. The lack or impossibility of usual marital sexual relations due to seasonal or cyclical unemployment increases the demand for paid sexual services. External forces play a significant role on the demand side in increasing the number of prostitutes. In a number of Southeast Asian countries tourism, a major source of foreign exchange also play an important role in fuelling the demand for prostitutes, at least in the largest urban areas, is therefore much larger than in the immediate economic hinterland.

While some assert that prostitutes and prostitution did not necessarily spread the epidemic, this is more likely to apply to industrial countries where prostitutes have adopted relatively safe sexual practices, particularly the use of condoms. The situation in Southeast Asia is totally different and prostitutes have been an effective medium through which the epidemic has spread across the region and between various subpopulation groups. The rapid spread of the epidemic in Thailand is unlikely to have happened without the large number of prostitutes who transmitted the disease. In this region the use of safe sexual practices is reduced by ignorance of the effects of the virus, which in turn results from both the lack of relevant information and inaccessibility to existing information. Condom use is also curtailed by customer ignorance and the highly elastic labour supply of potential prostitutes, which reduces their bargaining power with brothel owners and customers. General ignorance about the disease is a factor in the low reported rate of condom use among prostitutes.

Furthermore, the frequency of condom use did not change substantially after the prostitutes were informed they were HIV-positive.

Two further distributional subissues related to the problem of poverty induced participation in prostitution. First, the HIV epidemic will increase existing social divisions and discrimination against prostitutes. Female prostitutes may be viewed solely as vectors of the HIV and not as possible recipients. Second, among prostitutes the lowest earning women have the highest probability of being infected. A recent survey of Chiang Mai brothels formed that those who charged B 30-50 per session had a prevalence level of 72 per cent, those who charged B 50-100 per session had a 30 per cent prevalence level, while those who charged over B 100 per encounter had a prevalence rate of only 16 per cent. Another survey revealed that the median infection rate for low-paid brothel prostitutes was 15.2 per cent and that for high-paid prostitutes it was only 4.8 per cent. The lower prevalence rate for higher-paid prostitutes was because they had fewer customers, and possibly also because some could insist on the use of condoms. However, lower-priced prostitutes, many of whom can not speak standard Thai, probably could not insist on relatively safe sexual practices.

The Preventive Strategy

The HIV epidemic is well common in some countries of Southeast Asia and its spread has been facilitated by the existence in a single region of all the known factors that are propitious for the increase of the epidemic. The combined presence and extent of a commercial sex industry, entrenched rural poverty, massive intravenous drug abuse, limited national health budgets, and marital heterosexual transmission is probably globally unique.

Given that the epidemic is at an early stage in most countries, and the limited number of preventive actions taken so far, the total economic cost to most Southeast Asian societies will rise. Moreover, the costs of the epidemic will fall disproportionately on the poor, especially prostitutes and ethnic groups. In other cases where the husband is the one who is infected, wives and widows will have to confront the household's reduced labour power and the possible removal of a critical source of old-age support. Rural economies that are dependent on non-mechanical sources of power for production and output are more likely to feel the decline in labour power. Insecure property rights, especially to land, make the situation even more severe. The epidemic's consequence is likely to be less in areas that can easily obtain more labour without paying higher wages or can raise the productivity of the remaining labour by using high-yielding crops and mechanization. The total consequence of the epidemic on any rural-based population depend heavily on the nature of the agricultural economy and the capacity to respond to changes in the macroeconomic environment.

The extent of the consequence will depend on the epidemic's prevalence and associated morbidity and mortality, the structure of the farm sector, the labour intensity of the farming systems, and the availability of support structures such as extension, credit, research, and development. Neither of these conditions is likely to hold in areas where ethnic groups primarily live. The economic circumstances of the poor are, therefore, worse once the epidemic becomes more widespread even if the economy as a whole is resilient and able to adapt to the changing conditions.

The epidemic's extent and the large costs incurred, which are related to its epidemiological and economic characteristics viz. lethality; communicability; difficulty to identify; long gestation period; concentration on the young, economically productive age groups, have led to a broad consensus among international development institutions of the need for proactive preventive policies before the epidemic spreads further. There is widespread acceptance that the disease irrespective of social or cultural boundaries and acknowledge that both domestic residents as well as foreigners can have the virus. For developing countries, their lack of financial, technical, and institutional capabilities for treatment and care mean that preventive strategies are the policy of choice as well as of necessity.

Actual interventions by governments to contain the HIV epidemic will be determined by the epidemic's stage and the predominant routes of transmission. In low-income countries, such as Myanmar and Lao PDR, where is public health facilities are limited, a cost-effective campaign should focus on the direct provision of health inputs and services. Particular attention is needed in establishing and maintaining a safe blood supply and reducing the probability of infection through contaminated syringes and needles in health settings. An integral part of such a program would also include establishment of more drug rehabilitation centers and providing addicts with legal and financial impetus to avail themselves of these facilities.

Countries such as Thailand, which are more developed economically, may use a different approach. In these countries basic health facilities are largely in place and the probability of infection through contaminated blood or infected needles and syringes, in medical settings at least, is low. A cost-effective strategy would be to allocate more resources to the dissemination of information, education, and communication (IEC) to prevent infection by promoting greater awareness of the epidemic and corresponding changes in individual behaviour. There is, however, a caution. In the absence of an effective vaccine or cure for HIV infection, education on how HIV is transmitted and how exposure to it can be reduced or eliminated is the most important way to limit its spread. The elevation of IEC activities to the central position of a preventive strategy is based on the implicit assumption that individual volition is the major contributing factor to the spread of the epidemic. It is assumed that all individuals are in a position to change their behaviour in response to a health threat with a minimal amount of cost and delay. This view may be much too simplistic and takes no account of the structural causes of poverty and their impact. The assumption also reduces the role of peer and communal pressure in promoting high risk behaviour. Moreover, disseminating information is expensive. In short, the technical problems involved in giving effective IEC cannot be minimized. Health messages that stress that behaviour change in the face of the HIV epidemic is desirable and possible will need to take into account the social norms and cultures of those to whom the messages are directed.

It can be concluded that given the epidemic's high costs, the need for preventive policies is commonly accepted. Responses to the epidemic would, however, differ from country to country depending on the extent to which the epidemic is widespread and the availability of basic public health facilities. While the provision of IEC need to be an important component of preventive measures, policymakers must recognize that cost-effective IEC must be well designed, targeted, and take into account major differences in socio-economic and cultural characteristics within the total population. A combination of these policies with those that address structural problems, such as rural poverty, rising regional income inequality, and limited national health budgets, are likely to hold the greatest promise for reducing the threat of the HIV/AIDS epidemic in Southeast Asia.

The South-East Asia Region

First reported in 1984 in Thailand, the South-East Asian region witnessed the rapid spread of HIV during the late 1980s. Besides people with high-risk behaviour, HIV infection rates have now begun to increase in the general population as well. Heterosexual intercourse is the major route of transmission in the region. At the beginning of a new millenium, the HIV epidemic continues to grow, invisibly and the number of people diagnosed with AIDS is increasingly rapidly. In the South-East Asia region it is estimated that 5 million people have been infected with HIV since the beginning of the pandemic. HIV is spreading fast and requires effective responses from all countries. As of 1 October, 2000, 152,939 AIDS cases have been reported in the South-East Asia region; more than 95% of which were reported from just three countries namely Thailand, India and Myanmar. Women and children are becoming increasingly affected by HIV; nearly 5% of AIDS cases reported were among children.

The South-East Asia Reason

TABLE 2
SUPPLY OF CONDOMS

	Condoms distributed (thousands)[a] *1991*	*Condom social marketing programme in 1992*[b]
Bangladesh	—	Yes
Bhutan	—	No
India	1,100,000	Yes
Indonesia	25	Yes
Maldives	0	No
Myanmar	29	No
Nepal	20	Yes
Sri Lanka	80	Yes
Thailand	31,950	Yes

(a) Compiled from answers by countries to the GPA questionnaire. The stated number of condoms distributed does not always include those sold by the private sector.

(b) Compiled from answers by countries to the GPA questionnaire and other information available to GPA.

TABLE 3
COUNTRY INFORMATION

	Total Popula-Lation (thousand)[a]	Popu-lation 0-14 Yrs. (%)[a]	Popula-tion 15-49 Yrs. (%)[a]	Popula-tion >50 yrs (%)[a]	Annual growth rate (%)[b]	Urban popula-tion (thou-sands)[b]	Infant morta-lity rate[b,c]	Life expec-tancy men[b]	Life expec-tancy women[d]	Gross national product per capita (US$)[d]	Male literacy rate in 1990[e]	Female literacy rate in 1990[e]
Bangladesh	122,210	41	49	10	2.4	22,288	106	53	53	210	47	22
Bhutan	1,650	41	48	12	2.3	98	127	48	49	190	-	-
India	896,567	35	50	14	1.9	235,509	87	60	61	350	62	34
Indonesia	194,617	34	52	14	1.8	60,229	64	61	65	570	84	68
Maldives	234	44	45	11	3.0	74	53	65	62	-	-	-
Myanmar	44,613	38	50	13	2.1	11,421	80	56	60	-	89	72
Nepal	21,086	43	46	11	2.4	2,633	98	54	53	170	38	13
Srilanka	17,894	31	53	16	1.3	3,930	24	70	74	470	93	84
Thailand	56,868	30	56	13	1.2	13,661	26	67	72	1420	96	90

(a) Estimate for 1993. Source: UN Population Division 1992.
(b) WHO estimate for 1993 based on data from UN Population Division 1992.
(c) Per 1000 live births
(d) Data for 1990. Source: World Bank (STARS) (April, 1992).
(e) *Source:* Statistical Yearbook (UNESCO, 1991).

TABLE 4

AIDS INFORMATION, EDUCATION AND COMMUNICATION (IEC)[a]

	AIDS & STD education included in school curricula (since)	*Frequency of AIDS messages on:*				*Free air time given to AIDS messages*			*Promotion of condoms*	
		radio		*television*						
		more often than weekly	*less often than weekly*	*more often than weekly*	*less often than weekly*	*yes*	*partly*	*no*	*through mass media*	*to vulnerable groups*
Bangladesh	no		x		x		x		yes	no
Bhutan	no		x			x			no	yes
India	no				x		x		yes	yes
Indonesia	no		x		x			x	yes	yes
Maldives	no	x			x	x			no	no
Myanmar	no		x	x		x			no	yes
Nepal	no	x		x				x	yes	no
Sri Lanka	1986[b]	x		x				x	no	yes
Thailand	1989	x		x		x			yes	yes

(a) compiled from answers by countries to the GPA questionnaire.

(b) STD only.

TABLE 5
HIV ANTIBODY TESTING[a]

	Laboratory testing facilities at		
	Central level	*provincial level*	*district level*
Bangladesh	x	x	x
Bhutan	x	x	
India	x	x	
Indonesia	x	x	
Maldives	x		
Myanmar	x	x	
Nepal	x	x	
Sri Lanka	x	x	
Thailand	x	x	x

(a) Compiled from answers by countries to the GPA questionnaire.

References

Asian Development Bank, 1992. "The Economic Impact of AIDS in Asia." *Asian Development Outlook* 1992. Manila.

Asiaweek, 1991. "Sitting on a Volcano." 19 July.

Bowles, Gordon T. 1977. *The People of Asia*. New York; C. Scribner's Sons.

Bunge, Frederica M., ed. 1981. *Thailand; A country Study*. Washington, D.C: The American University.

Heh, Toh Mun and Linda Low. 1990. "Economic Impact of Tourism in Singapore." *Annals of Tourism Research* 17:246-69.

Heyzer, Noeleen. 1986. "Working Women in South-East Asia." In Development, Subordination and Emancipation. Philadelphia: Open University Press.

Indochina Chronology. 1991. 10(4):8,16.

Krongkaew, Medhi, Pranee Tinakorn, and Suphat Supachalasai. 1991.
"Priority Issues and Policy Measures to Alleviate Rural Poverty: The Case of Thailand." Manila: Asian Development Bank. Processed.

Lebar, Frank M., Gerald C. Hickey, and John K. Musgrave. 1964. *Ethnic Groups of Mainland Southeast Asia*. New Haven, Connecticut: Human Relations Area Files Press.

Lewis, Gwyneth, Joel Finlay, and Roy Widdus. 1991. "AIDS Programmes in Transition." *World Health Forum* 12:297-306.

Manaloto, C. R., C. G. Hayes, L. P. Padre, G. Espinosa, A. Andrada, P. Mejia, D. Cano, and V. Basaca-Sevilla. 1990. "Sexual Behavior of Filipino Female Prostitutes After Diagnosis of HIV Infection." *Southeast Asian Journal for Tropical Medicine and Public Health* 21(2):301-5.

Mathews, Paul W. 1987. "Some Preliminary Observations of Male Prostitution in Manila." *Philippine Sociological Review* July/December:55-74.

Moselina, Leopoldo M. 1979. "Olongapo's Rest and Recreation Industry: A Sociological Analysis of Institutionalized Prostitution—With Implications for a Grassroots-Oriented Sociology." *Philippine Sociological Review* 27:176-88.

Muecke, Marjorie A. 1990. "The AIDS Prevention Dilemma in Thailand". *Asian and Pacific Population Forum* 4(4):1-28

Over, M., and M. Piot. Forthcoming. "HIV Infection and Sexually Transmitted Diseases." In D. T. Jamison and W. N. Mosley, eds., *Disease Control Priorities in Developing Countries*. New York: Oxford University Press for the World Bank.

Piot, Peter, and Marie Laga. 1988. "Prostitutes: A High Risk Group for HIV Infection?" *Sozial-und Pravantivmedicin (Medecine Sociale et Preventiv)* 33:331-39.

Smith, Martin. 1991. *Burma: Insurgency and the Politics of Ethnicity* London and New Jersey: Zed Books.

Smyke, Patricia. 1991. Women and Health. London and New Jersey: Zed Books.

Swaddiwudhipong, W., C. Chaovakiratipong, S. Siri, and P. Lerdlukanavonge. 1990. "Sociodemographic Characteristics and Incidence of Gonorrhoea in Prostitutes Working near the Thai-Burmese Border." *Southeast Asian Journal for Tropical Medicine and Public Health* 21(1): 45-52.

Tan, M., de Leon, B. Stoltzfus, and C. O'Donnell. 1989. "AIDS as a Political Issue: Working with the Sexually prostituted in the Philippines." *Community development Journal* 24(3): 186-93.

Tilman, Robert, ed. 1969. "Man, State, and Society." In *Contemporary Southeast Asia*. New York: Praeger.

UNDP (United Nations Development Programme). 1992. *Human Development Report*. New York: Oxford University Press.

Widdus, Roy, Andre Meheus, and Roger Short. 1989. "The Management of Risk in Sexually Transmitted Diseases." Daedalus (spring): 177-91.

WHO (World Health Organization). 1988. "Report: Regional Workshop on Safe Blood and Blood Products." Regional Office for the Western Pacific, Manila, Philippines, September 26-30.

———, 1992. *Current and Future Dimensions of the HIV/AIDS Pandemic-A Capsule Summary*. Geneva

Three

Legal Aspects of AIDS in Mongolia

Introduction

Prevention and Control of pandemic of AIDS is a priority for Mongolia. In order to prevent the HIV, the national AIDS programme was established.

The Programme attempted to achieve those objectives in 1991-1992 by :

- strengthening the National AIDS Reference Centre developing;
- development of HIV surveillance, including serosurveys of high-risk and sentinel population groups;
- training of health-care workers;
- conducting education activities, promoting condom use and safe sex, complemented by mass media campaigns and NGO involvement;
- mobilising additional resources; and
- refining existing AIDS legislation.

The National AIDS Programme is being implemented at the same time when the country is undergoing overall reforms and the view of Mongolia as being a low-risk country for AIDS must be revised. At present both external and internal factors are increasing the risk for the transmission and the wide-spread infection in the people of Mongolia. For example :

- Increased detection of AIDS cases in almost every country is alarming.
- Mongolia's contacts with the outside world are also increasing.

The number of international flights, trains, and local border communications, particularly with China and other Asian countries, has risen as well. Sexually transmitted diseases (STDs) in Mongolia during last few years show a tendency to increase.

Moderate increases in other STDs, such as syphilis, trichomoniasis, and chlamidia, have been observed. These trends may be explained by changes in Mongolian life styles, migration processes, the low cultural and educational level of the population, social unrest (i.e., unemployment, alcoholism, etc.) and obsolete facilities for the control and prevention of STDs. So far, Mongolia is considered as one of the few countries in the world to remain AIDS-free. The first case of HIV infection in Mongolia was reported in Ulaanbaatar in August 1992. This case triggered strong and political commitment from the Government. As a sign of its decision, the Government issued decree No. 18 which renewed the National AIDS Committee headed by the Vice-Prime Minister.

The new National AIDS Committee called its first meeting in September 1992 and approved the new version of the National AIDS programme, the plan of action for implementing the programme, and some other important documents. As a follow up to the Government decree No. 18, the Health Minister issued decree No. 128, which created the Technical Advisory Board, which has 17 members under the chairmanship of the Deputy Health Minister.

The newly-approved action plan for implementing the National AIDS Programme strengthens the capability of the National AIDS Reference Centre, develops an AIDS laboratory network based on existing districts (*aimak*) and cities, establishes STD/blood bank serological laboratories, and makes AIDS patient wards in the Central Infectious Disease Hospital. The plan also demands many educational measures. It also suggests the need for the including of AIDS/STD in the school curricular and incorporates AIDS into the teaching curricula of graduate and post-graduate training for medical students, doctors and health personnel. The plan suggests to use education activities to encourage condom use in sexual behaviour, as well as improving the commitment of the community and NGOs to anti-AIDS activities. The activities planned in the MTP were successfully implemented in 1991-1992 except for the KABP study which was not processed or analysed owing to the lack of computers and trained personnel in the National AIDS Reference Centre. WHO back up is crucial to the success of the National AIDS Programme.

To date more than 90,000 serum samples, mainly from blood donors, pregnant women and other high-risk and sentinel population groups, had undergone test for HIV. Only one test has been positive.

The draft law on AIDS was prepared jointly by the Ministry of Health and the Ministry of Justice and submitted to a working group of the Parliament, it includes regulations for preventing the spread of HIV/AIDS, the draft law emphasised the need to discourage discrimination against HIV/AIDS victims, their family members and relatives according to World Health Organisation resolutions (41.24 and 45.35). This draft law consists of many articles which regulate social relations as they affect state policies on the prevention, detection, and verification of AIDS and the treatment and counselling of HIV/AIDS patients on HIV/AIDS.

The draft suggests increases the responsibility of medical personnel and establishments to halt spread of HIV. The draft also draws attention to the personal responsibility of HIV-positive people to prevent the transmission of HIV. While it encourages voluntary screening tests, it also envisages coercive measures in case people with HIV or those suspected of having HIV fail to act responsibility. Finally, the draft law stresses the need for avoiding discrimination against HIV-infected people while preserving their anonymity and right to confidentiality.

Four

Prejudices against the HIV/AIDS Infected Patients in Hong Kong

Introduction

The first case of AIDS was reported in the mid 1980's in Hong Kong. The government is assuming a straightline increase at the rate of 25 per cent per annum. The target segments are the socially-and economically active people in the young and middle age groups.

Discrimination Faced by People with HIV/AIDS

Belief Discrimination with HIV/AIDS in Hong Kong

People with HIV/AIDS have been subjected to serious, irrational discrimination in Hong Kong and as well as. People with AIDS but HIV positive people who have not yet developed AIDS are often ill-treated. Following are the major areas in which people with HIV/AIDS in Hong Kong are discriminated against:

Hospital Services

Majority of doctors in the hospitals are reluctant to treat HIV/AIDS patients. Home help service agencies are reluctant to render their services to PWHIV/AIDS, even when the service needed is only meal delivery or accompanying the patient to the clinic or hospital. It has also been reported that some drug rehabilitation service agencies would conduct HIV antibody tests screen out those potential clients who are HIV positive.

Schools

Reportedly, HIV positive school children were in some cases required or requested by the school authorities to discontinue education in the school. While in the last reported incident the

Director of Education declared that schools which reject HIV positive students would face sanctions, the findings of a subsequent survey showed that 37 per cent of the secondary school principals and 41 per cent of the teachers decided that infected children should be kept in special schools. A small percentage of the principals and teachers remarked that infected children should not continue their studies at school.

Employment

The people with HIV/AIDS want to keep their HIV status out of fear of loss of opportunity to work. There have been incidents of PWHIV/AIDS being dismissed from employment or requested to leave partnerships.

Housing

Housing is another major concern of PWHIV/AIDS if their HIV status becomes known to others. A landlord who suspects his tenant of having AIDS requests the latter to move out. Even after their death the people with HIV/AIDS are discriminated against. The funeral barlours refuse to provide services to the victims of AIDS.

The government is considering a bill to deal with such discrimination.

Legislation on HIV/AIDS in Hong Kong

The Hong Kong AIDS Foundation has strongly emphasized that HIV/AIDS aspects should be covered by the Equal Opportunities Bill, and the establishment of an Equal Opportunities Commission which should be charged with the responsibility to adjudicate complaints of discrimination, but also take positive steps to promote the elimination of discrimination in the community.

The Hong Kong Government has expressed its desire to enact disability discrimination legislation in 1994-1995 and has set into motion the consultative procedure. At these consultations, the Hong Kong AIDS Foundation and other AIDS related organizations have raised the following points concerning HIV/AIDS:

1. Confidentiality of the complainants.
2. Blood screening – it should be regarded as discriminatory despite that it my be required for all employees or applicants.
3. Difficulty in proving discriminatory dismissal.
4. Prisoners' rights - their rights to lodge a complaint and the power of the proposed Equal Opportunities Commission to investigate complaints relating to correctional institutions.
5. Funeral services, where discrimination is against the deceased.
6. Discrimination based on suspected disability.

Five

The Impact of AIDS on the Economy of Malaysia

Introduction

The spread of the AIDS epidemic cannot be considered as a mere health issue. It would affect social and economic development by reducing the supply of skilled workers and the level of savings. By international standards Malaysia has a low sero-prevalence rate, and the impact of AIDS on its economic and industrial programs has been very less so far. Anyhow, the features of the disease in Malaysia and the country's geographical location suggest that the impact could be severe in the future unless the government introduces prevention measures as soon as possible.

In developing countries, particularly in Africa, the AIDS epidemic can any more be considered as only a health issue. AIDS can hinder the social and economic development of these countries by cutting down supply of skilled workers, and in the extreme case, by reducing the actual labor force. It can also have an adverse effect by reduce lessening the level of domestic savings as both the private and public sectors use more funds to cope with the impact of the disease. Foreign savings in the form of direct foreign investment may also come down. A main determinant of the level of foreign savings is the host country's economic performance, which is likely to deteriorate as skilled workers are not available and the drop in investment following the fall in domestic savings.

This study analyses the economic impact of AIDS on Malaysia. It gives importance to the industrial sector as it has played, and will continue to play, a significant role in Malaysia's economic development, and because the shortage of skilled workers has constrained its growth, especially in labor-intensive industries.

Growth of Economy and Industries in Malaysia

By international standards, Malaysia's economic growth was sudden and sustained. For instance, at the time of the Fifth Malaysia Plan, 1986-1990, the real per capita gross domestic product (GDP) grew at 4.2 per cent per year. A decrease in poverty rate from 20.7 per cent to 17.1 per cent and a growth rate in the income of the bottom 40 percent of households that was better than the that of the other groups accompanied this rapid growth in output. Malaysia could perform so by adopting a market-friendly and internationally competitive approach to development (World Bank 1991). Industrial sector had a major role, as illustrated during the period of the Fifth Malaysia Plan, 1986-1990. The industrial real value added grew at 13.7 per cent per year, more than the double of the target of 6.4 per cent (Malaysian Government 1991a, p. 20). This sudden increase resulted in the industrial sector contributing nearly half of the increase in GDP in that period. It also raised the sector's share in the GDP from 19.7 per cent in 1985 to 27.0 per cent in 1990. In the process Malaysia's economic growth reached its zenith in 1987 the industrial sector's share in the GDP for the first time went ahead of the agricultural sector, for long the mainstay of Malaysia's economy. The gap has increased consistently since then. The sudden industrial growth also affected employment. Employment in the sector grew at a rapid 8.6 per cent per year during 1986-90, and consequently accounted for 44 per cent of the new job opportunities. This increased the share of manufacturing in the country's employment from 15.2 to 19.5 per cent. The sudden increase in manufacturing has been accelerated by production for exports. Manufacturing exports grew at 31.0 per cent per year during the plan period, and in the process rapidly increased their share in the country's total merchandise exports, from 32.8 to 60.4 per cent. The labor-intensive electrical and electronics industry was major contributor (56.2 per cent) to manufacturing exports during 1986-1990. A long way behind was another labor-intensive industry, textiles, clothing and footwear, at 9.7 per cent, but this share was more than double that of the third most important industry, transport and transport equipment, at 4.7 per cent. Manufacturing industry is much more diversified than ever and it is very dependent on a small number of labor-intensive industries for its exports.

The rapid growth of Malaysia's economy led to labor shortages in the commercial agricultural, construction, and industrial sectors. Almost 300,000 illegal and legal migrant workers from Indonesia met the shortages of agricultural and construction workers in Peninsular Malaysia and some 500,000 illegal migrant workers from the southern part of the Philippines met the shortages in the east Malaysian state of Sabah.

The industrial sector suffered from a grave shortage of experienced technicians and production workers, particularly in the labor-intensive and rapidly growing industries such as electrical and electronic products, textiles and clothing, and wood and cork products. The shortage forced a severe constraint on the expansion of these industries.

This labor shortage and the contracted profitability in labor-intensive and low-technology industries as wage rates raised with rises in the standard of living have reflected in the government's move to encourage the expansion of capital-intensive and technologically sophisticated industries during the period of the Sixth Malaysia Plan, 1991-1995. Thus, the government would introduce steps to accelerate industrial restructuring, technological upgrading, human resource development, and industrial linkages that would affect industrial production and remove some of the constraints on growth imposed by the labor shortage.

AIDS and Economic Growth

The programme to stimulate economic growth and to upgrade the industrial sector, or to maintain the existing level of economic growth, could be detrimental if the country experienced a high incidence of AIDS. As pointed out that, AIDS can adversely affect social and economic development by reducing the quantity and quality of the labour force and by reducing savings. The reduction in the size of the labour force is an outrageous case, but it may happen as the disease could increase the infant mortality rate, as is happening in certain African countries, and reverse the decline in the adult mortality rate. If this happened, then Malaysia would become even more dependent on migrant workers, which would develop additional problems. The incidence of sexually transmitted diseases among male migrant workers is very high, and these diseases facilitate the transmission of the HIV during sexual relations. If the supply of labour is a constraint on industrial growth, then the consequence of AIDS will be direct and negative.

The consequence on the labour force is a decline in its quality. Most studies have shown that educational attainment is positively linked to economic growth, and it suggested that this link is more than a statistical one. The situation in Malaysia is not different. The country also require skilled and experienced workers in its industrial program. If this shortage were allowed to continue, it would create a severe constraint on the country's future industrial growth. Given the characteristics of AIDS, it can strengthens the problem by declining the overall level of skills of the industrial labour force and by changing its mix of skills adversely. First, it is disastrous, with the average survival time after its onset being less than a year in developing countries. Second, it affects commonly adults in their prime sexual and productive ages, thus it generates the maximum potential spread effect on the population and the maximum potential economic consequence on production. Third, the treatment of HIV-positive and AIDS patients has very high opportunity cost: not only would patients with curable diseases leave out on treatment, but other major activities such as educational spending will also lose out. Families with an AIDS victim would also be compelled to spend less on education.

These characteristics of AIDS would combine to produce two major adverse effects: reduction of most expensively trained group of workers in their most productive period, and declining the group of workers most needed for economic and industrial growth. It would create a negative effect on national output growth. This could be forced the country to turn to foreign labour, which could aggravate the situation. The incidence of sexually transmitted diseases is quiet high among transient male workers as these tend to seek comfort from prostitutes. It would again increases their chances of being infected by the HIV. If these migrant workers marry into the local population again the chance of spreading the virus to local women and their ensuing children. Unlike the situation in the industrial countries, in Africa and Asia AIDS has spread among men and women in nearly equal proportions, and is not limited largely to the homosexual community.

AIDS can also hinder a country's economic growth by declining the level of domestic and foreign savings available to it. Domestic savings are what was to be left out of income after deducting current expenditure. With the spread of the HIV and AIDS, current expenditure would rise in all sectors of the economy. Households may incur additional expenditures on health. The business sector would need to spend more as labour costs increase with, first, decreases in labour productivity, and second, increases in labour turnover, leading to additional training costs. It may have also to increase its expenditure on health and social programmes. The government sector is defied with the same costs, with perhaps the additional problems of having to look after raising numbers of orphans and sections of the population pushed below the poverty line on account of the disease.

All these expenditures are compelled on society by the spread of the epidemic and will, reduce the level of domestic savings for a given income. The net effect would be a lowering of investment, and hence of the rate of economic growth. In the process, foreign savings in the form of direct foreign investment would also be adversely affected. Empirical studies have suggested that the level of foreign investment is decided more by the host country's proven economic track record than the number and level of fiscal incentives it provides. This economic performance would decline after the AIDS epidemic has worked its destructive way through the nation's supply of skilled labour and domestic savings.

AIDS's Adverse Consequences on Malaysia's Industrialization and Society

The adverse consequences of AIDS on Malaysian industrialization through its effects on the quantity and quality of the industrial labour force. To have a picture of the cost of HIV infection and AIDS on other sectors of the economy, it needs some estimates of the direct and indirect costs on Malaysian society as a whole.

The publicly available data on AIDS in Malaysia did not suggest that it has had an adverse impact on the country's industrial programme. Ministry of Health official data pointed out that by the end of February 1992 the country had only 46 cases of AIDS, of whom 33 had died, and 2,900 HIV-infected persons (table 2). Reliable sources within the ministry suggested that the number of AIDS cases reported constitute about 80 per cent of the total number of cases, which would put the total number at around 58, and that the actual number of HIV-positive cases would be around 5,800, double the number officially reported. Even these unofficial figures, the impact of the HIV and AIDS on Malaysia's industrial growth to date would have been minimal. The numbers are simply not big enough to have aggravated the shortage of skilled workers, particularly as the available evidence proved that the cases have not been concentrated among the more highly skilled members of the labour force. Data from the Ministry of Health suggested that the largest group (17 per cent) comes from the ranks of the unemployed. This group does not consist of highly skilled, experienced, and expensively trained members of the labour force as the market for these has been very tight in recent years. This conclusion is supported by the fact that the five next most affected groups he, fishermen at 12.0 per cent, labourers at 7.0 per cent, workers doing odd jobs at 7.0 per cent, estate workers at 4.5 per cent, and truck and bus drivers at 4.5 per cent all draw workers from the lower end of the occupational and skill structure.

Many experts of the opinion that the number of injecting drug users among the Indonesian migrant population in Peninsular Malaysia is much less than that for the local population, and that HIV infection and AIDS are not a problem among them.

As in the case of Indonesian workers who are employed mainly in the estate, timber, and mining sectors and as maids. In 1989 they accounted for less than 2 per cent of the work force in the manufacturing sector, so that even if the prevalence of AIDS among the Indonesian migrant workers were higher, the consequence on industrial growth would have been insignificant.

The east Malaysian state of Sabah has large numbers of illegal migrants from the Philippines, but official figures suggested that cases of AIDS and HIV infection have not been reported in Sabah. This means that HIV infection and AIDS are not a problem among the migrant labour force.

Thus, both the absolute number of AIDS and HIV-infected cases and their distribution by occupation and skill suggested that the progress of Malaysian industrialization has not been directly affected by the disease so far.

TABLE 1
MALAYSIA: AIDS CASES AND DEATHS AND HIV-INFECTED PERSONS, 1985-1992

Year	*AIDS cases*	*AIDS deaths*	*HIV-infected persons*
1985	0	0	0
1986	1	0	3
1987	1	2[a]	4
1988	4	3	19
1989	6	3	177
1990	12	8	650
1991	14	14	1,672
1992[b]	8	3	375
Total	46	33	2,900
Male	40	28	2,804
Female	6	5	96

(a) Resulting from previous year
(b) Up to February 29.
Source: Ministry of Health, as reported in *Berita Harian*, April 16, 1992.

The costs imposed on Malaysian society in general have not been high. These costs comprise mainly of the direct costs of treatment and the indirect costs arising from the loss of productivity and income. Unofficial sources within the Ministry of Health pointed out that the annual direct costs of treatment in Malaysia (drugs, length of hospitalization, and the number of hospitalizations required per year for each AIDS patient) are around US$2,000 per patient. If this figure is true, this needs a direct total annual cost of around US$0.09 million for the forty-six official cases of AIDS for Malaysia, or almost US$0.12 million using the higher number of fifty-eight.

The epidemic's direct costs included the cost of control and prevention measures. The Ministry of Health runs the National AIDS Committee, whose programmes include routine testing of blood products before transfusion; testing for people infected with the HIV in forty-seven government laboratories; and giving educational materials, counseling services, and training programmes to all the people. The Ministry of Education has started HIV and AIDS education at the secondary school level under health education and chart out methods to trained teachers to deal with the matter. The Ministry of Social Welfare runs educational programmes on the epidemic.

The indirect costs of AIDS comprise the loss of output and income owing to illness and premature death and the loss of productivity from disability. The average survival time after the onset of AIDS is one year. If the person is unable to work during one year and upon death foregoes twenty-five years of output and income estimating, income lost with a social discount rate of 5 per cent and a per capita income of US$2,528 would create a future income foregone of US$38,300. For the thirty-three AIDS deaths in Malaysia, this would have meant a loss of future income of around US$1.26 million. A period of twenty-five years is used for the calculation because the retirement age is fifty-five and most AIDS deaths happen in the twenty-six to thirty age group.

It should be added the decline in productivity and output of those not infected with the HIV, but who are looking after those who are. The upper bound cost of this would be US$0.06 million, on the basis that one AIDS patient needs one non-HIV-infected person to care for him or her and the income lost per helper is US$1,264. The income lost is assumed to be half of the per capita income of US$2,528, as some of the helpers are housewives with a lower opportunity cost.

As from the table, adding all the direct and indirect costs of having 46 (58) AIDS cases, 33 AIDS deaths, and 2,900 (5,800) HIV-infected cases gives a total of US$10.4 million to US$11.0 million. This comprised between 15 and 16 per cent of the average annual health expenditure under the Fifth Malaysia Plan. These figures are relatively important, but when assessed in terms of their consequences on the manufacturing sector they did not amount to much, being less than one-fifth of 1 per cent of the value of net manufacturing output for 1989.

TABLE 2
MALAYSIA: ESTIMATED DIRECT AND INDIRECT COSTS OF AIDS AND HIV INFECTION AS OF FEBRUARY 29,1992

(US$)

Cost item	*Cost*
Direct	
AIDS treatment at US$2,000 per case	
46 AIDS cases	92,000
58 AIDS cases	116,000
Control and prevention measures at US$0.5 per Capita for a population of 18.4 million	9,200,000
Indirect	
Loss of income from 1 year of AIDS and 25 years After death for 33 AIDS deaths	
Discount rate of 2.5%	1,623,039
Discount rate of 5.0%	1,263,207
Discount rate of 7.5%	1,020,063
Decline in productivity from looking after AIDS Patients at US$1,264 per helper	
46 AIDS cases	60,672
58 AIDS cases	73,312
Total (direct and indirect)	
Low estimates	
Discount rate of 2.5%	10,975,711
Discount rate of 5.0%	10,615,879
Discount rate of 7.5%	10,372,735
High estimates	
Discount rate of 2.5%	11,012,351
Discount rate of 5.0%	10,652,519
Discount rate of 7.5%	10,409,375

A number of factors lead to this conclusion. First, even though the time period is short, the rate of increase in the number of AIDS and HIV-infected cases were increasing since 1989. This reflects only in part the improved surveillance programme to screen injecting drug users in government correctional institutions and medical centers and the likelihood that many of the cases left out unreported in earlier years. Secondly, while most of the AIDS cases are due to homosexual and bi-sexual contacts, most of the AIDS carriers (82.0 per cent) are injecting drug users. These are mainly heterosexual, and some of them are married. Thus, the AIDS issue will not be largely a homosexual one in Malaysia, and its reach will extend across the entire population. Through sexual activities, the injecting drug users can pass the HIV to their partners, and consequently to their children. Another channel of transmission is the use of contaminated needles. The problem is especially serious because of Malaysia's increasing drug problem and the observed increase in the incidence of HIV infections among intravenous drug users, from 0.14 percent in 1988 to 6.9 per cent in 1991.

Third, a large number of Malaysian men, found by the Ministry of Health at more than 100,000 per year, visit brothels in southern Thailand. The risk of contracting the HIV is high as the prevalence rate among Thai brothel prostitutes has increased dramatically.

TABLE 3
MALAYSIA: AIDS CASES AND DEATHS AND HIV-INFECTED PERSONS BY TYPE OF EXPOSURE AS OF FEBRUARY 29, 1992

Type of exposure	*AIDS cases*		*AIDS deaths*		*HIV-infected persons*	
	No.	*%*	*No.*	*%*	*No.*	*%*
Bisexual activities	12	26.0	8	24.2	8	0.3
Blood transfusion	5	10.9	4	12.1	10	0.3
Heterosexual Intercourse	5	10.9	2	6.0	58	2.0
Homosexual activities	6	13.0	5	15.1	22	0.7
Intravenous drug use	14	30.4	8	24.2	2,377	82.0
Perinatal	1	2.2	1	3.0	4	0.1
Prostitution	2	4.3	2	6.0	51	1.7
Tissue transplantation	1	2.2	0	0	3	0.1
Unknown	1	2.2	1	3.0	367	12.6
Total	46	100.0	33	100.0	2,900	100.0

Source: Ministry of Health, as reported in *Berita Harian*, April 16, 1992.

TABLE 4
MALAYSIA: ESTIMATED DIRECT AND INDIRECT COSTS OF AIDS AND HIV INFECTION BY THE YEAR 2000

(1991 US$ millions)

Cost item	*Cost*
Direct	
AIDS treatment at US$2,000 per case	
1,450 AIDS cases	2.90
2,900 AIDS cases	5.80
Control and prevention measures at US$0.50 per capita for a population of 22.66 million	11.33
Indirect	
Loss of income from 1 year of AIDS and 25 years after death for 1,450 AIDS death at:[a]	
Discount rate of 2.5%	131.90
Discount rate of 5.0%	102.70
Discount rate of 7.5%	82.90
Loss of income from 1 year of AIDS and 25 years after death for 2,900 AIDS deaths at:[a]	
Discount rate of 2.5%	263.80
Discount rate of 5.0%	205.40
Discount rate of 7.5%	165.80
Decline in productivity from looking after AIDS patients at US$2,324 per helper:[b]	
1,450 AIDS cases	3.37
2,900 AIDS cases	6.74
Total	
Low estimates	
Discount rate of 2.5%	149.50
Discount rate of 5.0%	120.30
Discount rate of 7.5%	100.50
High estimates	
Discount rate of 2.5%	287.70
Discount rate of 5.0%	229.30
Discount rate of 7.5%	189.70

(a) Calculated on the basis that the 1991 per capita income of US$2,528 is forecasted grow in real terms at 7 per cent per year to the year 2000 (Malaysian Government 1991b, p.69).

(b) Calculated on the basis that the income forgone is half the per capita income of US$4,648 in the year 2000, as some of the helpers are housewives.

Fourth, the calculated incidence rate of HIV infection among female prostitutes in Malaysia has increased from 0.3 per cent in 1989 to 1.3 per cent in 1991. The virus can be passed on to the male clients and from them to their girlfriends or wives and the children born. The rate of infection may increase further as it is difficult to police the inflow of prostitutes from Thailand. Of known HIV-infected cases among prostitutes in Malaysia, 82 per cent were foreigners, mainly from Thailand.

The above four factors can combine to create a marked increase in the number of HIV infections and AIDS cases in Malaysia in the near future. Any one can argue that the picture presented of the current situation may be somewhat optimistic because so little is known, particularly about the large migrant population, where the conclusions on their low incidence of HIV infection depend on rather indirect evidence.

Six

Legislation on AIDS in Myanmar

Introduction

Combating AIDS has been given top priority by the Government of Myanmar. A multi sectoral approach has been adopted. Participation of non-government organizations in AIDS control activities is being encouraged together with preventive steps regarding communicable diseases including AIDS, have been undertaken by the Ministry of Health, as reflected in newly-enacted the Prevention and Control of Communicable Diseases Law.

Eventhough there is no legislation which deals specifically with HIV/AIDS, certain provision concerning prevention of AIDS are contained in various laws.

AIDS Laws in Myanmar

Law for the Prevention and Control of communicable Diseases enacted in March 1995, the law establishes an administrative mechanism in order to prevent the outbreak of communicable diseases. It identifies functions and duties of the health officers as well as those of the public for environmental sanitation. Communicable diseases which require to be reported are also to be identified. The law prescribes measures to be taken in respect of an outbreak of a principal epidemic disease and identifies quarantine periods; specifies offences and penalties. It establishes the power to make rules (regulations) and procedures as well as to issue orders and directives. Under this Law, AIDS is classified as a "principal epidemic disease". Section 4 provides that when a Principal Epidemic Disease or a Notifiable Disease occurs:

(a) immunization and other necessary measures shall be undertaken by the Department of Health, in order to control the spread thereof;

(b) the public shall abide by the measures undertaken by the Department of Health under sub-section (a).

Section 5 puts forth the duties to be performed by the health officer when a principal epidemic disease or an identifiable disease occurs in an area to which he is assigned. Section 9 says that the head of the household or any member of the household shall report as soon as to the nearest health department or hospital principal epidemic disease cases. Section 10 deals with traditional medicine practitioners, health assistants and doctors and provides for reportage to the nearest health department or hospital if a case of principal epidemic disease or a notifiable disease is found. Section 11 prescribes the steps to be undertaken by the health officer in order to check the spread of a principal epidemic disease. Section 13 suggests that the health officer shall report the source of the principal spreading disease to the relevant Department of Health. Section 14 empowers an organization or an officer authorized by the Ministry of Health to issue an order prohibiting or restricting based on matters mentioned in that section. Sections 15 to 18 provide penalties regarding the failures to comply with or violations of the provisions of the Law. Section 20 provides that prevention, control of the spread, and necessary investigations in respect of AIDS shall be done in accordance with the orders and directives issued particularly by the Ministry of Health.

Prevention Laws on Using Syringe

The law prescribes that, no person may make, sell, possess or use any hypodermic syringe, or any other apparatus suitable for injecting any intoxicating drug, except under and according to the conditions of a license granted under the Act. This prohibition, anyhow, does not apply to medical practitioners, veterinary practitioners or persons who possess or use any syringe or apparatus on the prescription of a medical practitioner. Section 33 provides that whoever, in contravention of Section 13 makes, sells, possesses or uses any hypodermic syringes, or any other apparatus suitable for injecting any intoxicating drug, shall be punished with imprisonment for a term which may extend to six months, or with fine which may extend to one thousand kyats, or with both.

Thus, apart from the three kinds of persons, no person has any right to make or sell or possess or use any hypodermic syringes or any other apparatus used for injecting any intoxicating drug.

Disposable needles, however, are now available in the market openly. The Ministry of health has issued a directive to the effect that proper sterilization of syringes, needles, surgical equipment, and other skin piercing equipment (boiled for at least twenty minutes) be undertaken in every health care centre throughout the country.

The Prevention of Brothels Act

Enacted in 1949 and was amended in 1956, the act makes prostitution a punishable offence. Section 3 of the Act provides that any person who, in any public place or within sight of such public place by words, gestures, wilful and indecent exposure of her person or otherwise attracting for prostitution; or solicits or molests any person for the purpose of prostitution shall be punished with strict imprisonment for a term which may extend to one year or with fine or with both.

Section 5 sub-section (1) suggests that any person who knowingly lives, wholly or in part, on the earnings of prostitution shall be punished with imprisonment which may extend to three years.

Sub-section (2) provides that where a person is found to be living with, or to be in the company of a wroth, or is proved to have exercised control, direction or influence over the movements of a sex worker in such a way as to prove that he is helping, abetting or compelling her prostitution with any other person, it shall be presumed, until the contrary is proved, that he is intentionally living on the earnings of prostitution. Procurement as well as management of brothels are also offences under this Act.

Section 377 of the Penal Code penalizes unnatural offences and is would punish the offence of sodomy, buggery and bestiality. The offence means in having carnal knowledge against the order of nature by a man with a man, or in the same unnatural manner with a woman, or by a man or woman in any way with an animal.

Narcotic Drugs and Psychotropic Substances law, enacted in

1993, reabling the Narcotic and Dangerous Drugs law, 1974 was drafted to be in conformity with the United Nations Convention against Illicit Traffic in Narcotic Drugs and Psychotropic Substances. It has 31 sections. Section 9 of the Law provides for the registration of drug users at a medical centre recognized by the Government aiming at medical treatment.

Registered drug users undergoing medical treatment are requested to act in accordance with the directives issued by the Ministry of Health.

Under Section 15 of the law the failure to register at the place prescribed by the Ministry of Health or at a medical centre recognized by the Government for this purpose or to comply with the directives issued by the Ministry of Health for medical treatment is an offence liable to imprisonment for a term which may extend from a minimum of 3 years to a maximum of 5 years.

Section 10 provides for the deregistration of drug users. Section 11 prescribed the measures to be carried out by the Ministry of Social Welfare, Relief and Resettlement keeping in mind the rehabilitation and after-care of drug users.

Besides these laws, there is a practice to screen the blood for possible viruses at various blood donation centres. There is, however, no specific law for blood transfusion.

Seven

Law Reforms on HIV/AIDS in Maldives

The spread of HIV is very limited in the Island country of Maldives with a predominantly Muslim population. The first HIV case in Maldives was reported in 1991 and since then four more such cases have been reported.

The Constitution and the laws of Maldives are based on the principles of Islamic law, which guarantees fundamental rights and freedoms of the individual and also stresses on the rights of the public and society at large. There are adequate laws to control drug use, extra-marital sex etc. Such acts are illegal under Maldivian laws. Moreover, the Muslim population is very conscious of their religious duties and family values mainly because of the small size of the communities in which they live.

At present there is no HIV or AIDS related special legislation in the Maldives. The response of the Government to the HIV/AIDS problem has been very encouraging. It established a National AIDS Council which has a strong legal basis under Maldivian laws. This Council has formulated and implemented action programmes for the prevention of the spread of HIV and for the protection of the HIV/AIDS infected persons. There are some administrative arrangements as well to provide protection for the infected persons and to lessen possible discrimination.

There is no need for the compulsory testing or screening of any population sub-group. No particular group of the population is prevented from donating blood, though earlier, there was a strong move by health managers and experts to make testing mandatory for certain target groups, like seamen and those working in the tourist resorts.

Confidentiality of information related to persons infected with HIV has been preserved through administrative arrangements. But as the islands are very tiny, and thickly populated, it could be very difficult to preserve the identity of infected persons.

Maldivian law does not prosecute a person merely because one has contracted HIV. So, it is not likely for HIV infected persons to become reluctant to identify themselves or to go voluntary testing. A person might be prosecuted only if there is evidence to show involvement in any illegal act or such person has been engaging in 'immoral conduct.' Under the criminal laws it is an offence to knowingly or deliberately or recklessly spread HIV.

Administrative measures require that there should not be any discrimination of AIDS patients regarding employment. But this administrative order is only applicable to the civil service and government owned companies, and not to private sector employment. Similarly, there is no rule or regulation enrolling in a school a child who is infected with HIV/AIDS. But the right to education of such children is well protected.

Eight

Reasons behind Rapid Spread of HIV/ AIDS in Southeast Asia

World Health Organization believes that if effective HIV prevention programmes are not put in place, Asia will overtake Africa soon in terms of the number of new AIDS patients per year. HIV transmission rates in some population groups in south and south-east Asia today are as high as they were 10 years ago in sub-Saharan Africa. Fortunately, HIV rates in the general population are still comparatively low even in the worst-affected countries of this region. Asia thus has a chance to avert catastrophe.

WHO estimates that more than two million adults have been infected till date. Most infections thus far are thought to have been in India, Thailand and Myanmar, but the virus is spreading quickly among vulnerable groups elsewhere. The predominant modes of transmission are unprotected heterosexual intercourse and needle-sharing.

Homo-sexual transmission is also thought to play some role in the region, although this form of sexuality is often hidden.

In India, an indication of the population's vulnerability to HIV can be found in the millions of STDs occurring each year. In addition to being a "marker" for behavioural vulnerability to HIV infection, untreated STDs facilitate HIV transmission. Infection rates of up to 25 per cent were reported in 1992 from surveys among prostitutes in Mumbai.

Surveys among STD patients in Myanmar have found a steep rise in the prevalence of HIV infection. Given the fact that condom use is low, HIV can spread in this tiny country as a wildfire. Add to it the fact that, it is only a matter of time before people outside these particularly vulnerable groups are drawn into the circle of infection. Among pregnant Thai women attending antenatal clinics, for example, HIV prevalence has reached 4 per cent in at least five provinces.

The AIDS epidemic in south and south-east Asia gained an early foothold among injecting drug users in the region, and they remain hard-hit today. People who inject drugs are by no means a homogeneous group. Mostly, drug use tends to be associated with poverty and crime, as it is in industrialized countries. However, this kind of drug use is also comparable to alcohol use in some cases, especially among older people.

In recent years, however, the region's drug scene has begun to change. While older people have tended to smoke opium, younger people begin their drug use smoking heroin, a derivative of opium and eventually start injecting the drug in order to increase its effect. The tragedy, as it unfolds, has now attracted a lot of condemnation from societies. It has become even more pronounced since the emergence of AIDS. Drug users are summarily imprisoned, or confined in "rehabilitation centres" resembling prison camps, or even attacked and beaten to death in the streets. Even milder forms of stigmatization are hampering efforts to bring the HIV epidemic under control. Health authorities face a tough time in following up on drug users who are HIV-positive because visiting their homes can bring shame on their families and ostracism by friends and neighbours. The virus has spread rapidly in the area known as the Golden Triangle, where the territories of the Lao People's Democratic Republic, Myanmar and Thailand meet, and where most of the world's opium and heroin are produced.

In Myanmar, there has been an alarming rise in infection rates fuelled by poverty and by strict action against drug-taking. High prices of needles and syringes prompt many people to share these. The sharing of injection equipment is also encouraged by the fact that possession of needles and syringes—by anyone other than a health professional or a diabetic—is used by police as evidence of drug-taking, strictly punishable by law. Needle-sharing is practised, too, out of camaraderie. India, on the other hand, has been drawn into the drugs and AIDS vortex of the Golden Triangle and it gives a clear example of the dynamics of the epidemic among drug users. Heroin use became established among the people of the north-eastern State of Manipur, which borders Myanmar, in mid 80s and the practice of injecting the drug was soon widespread among users. Initially middle-class, well educated youngsters, Manipur's drug users are found in all strata of society, as they tend to be elsewhere in India, for example, in Nagaland, bordering Manipur to the north. In Thailand, where infection rates among injecting drug users are rising steeply, heroin use is implicated in the spread of HIV not only directly through the sharing of needles, but also indirectly through complex links with sex work. With a flourishing sex induces in cities attracting a lot of village women, the problem becomes more complicated. In some cases, families agree to allow their daughters to work off loans (debt bondage), and in some cases they "sell" their daughters outright.

People living in Shan State, Myanmar (formerly Burma), were familiar with AIDS several years before it was recognized by their government. It was known as "dangerous disease coming from outside".

In some cases, the recruits are imprisoned by the brothel-owners during their initiation into the business. Such stories are seldom told in the villages, however, for the young women who come back home dressed in modern clothes and make-up are too proud to relate the price they have had to pay for the modern life style and for the survival of their families.

Extremely high rates of HIV infection have been reported among illiterate women, who for a paltry sum work as prostitutes in local brothels and who get little information on AIDS/HIV. Contaminated blood transfusions contribute no less to the rapid spread to epidemic in parts of south and south-east Asia. In India, the trading of blood for transfusion and the preparation of blood products is big business and subject to very little control. Infection rates among donors are higher among professional donors than among voluntary donors. Though the Ministry of Health and the Indian Council of Medical Research have an official policy not to use blood procured from the open market (i.e., from paid blood donors) in government health services, blood screening facilities are in general available only in major cities.

The problems of India, Myanmar and Thailand could easily be repeated in other countries of the region—especially Bangladesh, Indonesia, Malaysia, Nepal and Sri Lanka, where illicit drug injection, high STD rates, male patronage of female and male prostitutes and/or low rates of contraceptives usage in both casual and long-term relationships are common. Countries such as Cambodia, the Lao People's Democratic Republic and Vietnam are also especially vulnerable to HIV infection as their people go through profound social and economic changes.

Nine

Laws on HIV/AIDS in Pakistan

All the factors that predispose a country to the growing spread of HIV/AIDS like the influx of migrants, unregulated blood transfusion system, prevalence of prostitution, and homosexuality, travel to and from the country-are present in Pakistan. Though the Constitution provides a certain degree of protection with regard to personal rights and liberties, there is no specific legislation which covers the area of HIV/AIDS. There are laws like the Infectious Diseases Act, that indirectly provide for restrictive approaches in law. Among the administrative regulations in place are those covering quarantine and isolation (though not HIV specific); and travellers entering the country for a period exceeding six months.

New legislation covering blood transfusion and selected policies are being worked out, the main features being the mandatory testing of all donated blood and the elimination of professional donors. A notification law exists in terms of which HIV/AIDS has been specially declared as a notifiable disease by the government.

Pakistan is affected by the laws in other countries. About 700 Pakistani HIV patients have been deported during the past two years from Middle East countries.

Pakistan has enacted certain laws that are general in nature. However, they cover many issues related to HIV.

Prohibition of Prostitution Law, Child Abuse Law, Hadood Ordinance, Law relating to Medical Termination of Pregnancy and Narcotics and Drugs Act, all have their specific role in combating HIV/AIDS in the country. Unfortunately, HIV/AIDS campaigns on the electronic media were not allowed earlier. Following the recent changes in policy, the electronic media has begun to carry low profile AIDS prevention messages, with no direct mention of condoms and sex.

Pakistan need to create legal/ethical committees at the national and provincial programme levels, and also integrate HIV counselling into legislation, more particularly workplace laws.

Serious efforts need to be made to integrate HIV concerns into its legislative and quasi-legislative systems. Donor agencies, like the WHO, which are the main financial partners in the National Programme, and are in the regular process of consultation with the National AIDS Committee, can play a leading role in formulating the programme for law review.

Ten

The Asian Experience

Introduction

For over a centrury, Asia has experienced drug-use problems in the form of large-scale epidemics that have caused social disintegration, civil unrest, and serious public health problems. They have enormous direct and indirect economic costs; and had impeded social and economic development. The multibillion dollar drug trade has caused wars and abetted them financially. It continues to be a financial resource used by militant organisations for purchasing arms. Despite strenuous measures to reduce drug-use problems, drug use is not under control. Though, the production of opiates has been reduced significantly in a number of areas, trafficking and consumption, however, remain issues of serious concern. Over the past several years, an increasing trend from opium to heroin use has been observed in many countries. Codeine and other narcotic and psychotropic substances are also being used at a significant level.

Produced in clandestine laboratories or produced legally by large pharmaceutical industries, these drugs reach the illegal markets.

Smoking or injecting has increased, together with an epidemic use of amphetamine-type stimulant (ATS), particularly of methamphetamine. Virtually all countries in South-East Asia are now affected. ATS use is generally higher among young adult males and among special occupational groups such as truck drivers, fishermen, and construction workers. Commercial sex workers have also been identified as a high-risk group related to ATS. Because all these groups have a high degree of mobility, they are hard to reach through traditional prevention and treatment services. In addition to the use of narcotics and psychotropic substances many Asian countries have identified inhalant use as a significant drug issue in their cities. Street children living in harsh conditions are the most affected group. The use of cannabis in its various preparations also continues to be widespread in most countries of the region.

The Vulnerable Users

The majority of drug users in Asia who are mostly poor and socially stigmatized pose the greatest challenge in Asia. They are prone to health hazards with little protection. Blood borne diseases such as hepatitis and HIV infection, abscesses and serious wounds from inadequate injecting equipment, and death from overdose are common. With HIV/AIDS epidemic has now become a major public health concern. Drug use has an intricate relationship with HIV/AIDS: HIV is transmitted through the sharing of contaminated needles and syringes and other equipment employed by drug users. In addition, alcohol and stimulant abuse often lower resistance to high-risk behaviour such as unprotected sexual intercourse. For want of a developed health infrastructure, drug users have fallen pray to the deadly diseases.

TABLE 1
DRUG USE IN SELECTED COUNTRIES OF ASIA (ESTIMATES)

Country	*Drug users (000s)*	*Opiate users (000s)*	*% injectors*	*% drug users Among HIV+*	*% HIV+among drug users*
Bangladesh	500-1000	N/E	10-17	N/E	2.5
China	540	majority	66	69.4	40.5
India	2250	500	25-90	N/E	1.3-68.4
Malaysia	300	200	50	77.0	10-27
Myanmar	300	majority	30	20-30	65.5-72.5
Nepal	30-50	majority	74.8	12.6	49.7
Pakistan	3000	1500	1.8-29	N/E	0.4-1.8
Sri Lanka	240	40	7.5	N/E	N/E
Thailand	1270	219	60	5.25	30-40
Vietnam	185	majority	no data	65.5	13.5-64.0

N/E = no estimates

Source: Regional Task Force on Drug Use and HIV Vulnerability, Drug Use and HIV Vulnerability Policy Research Study.

Strongly held beliefs about drugs and their adverse effects on the society, national experiences with drug use in the past. The extent and seriousness of past and present drug problems, and the interpretation of international conventions all have an impact on the development of policies and legal instruments directed at drug use. In a number of Asian countries, as elsewhere in the world the law prescribes severe punishments for all drug-related offences. The level of penalties and the stringency with which they are applied locally affect the feasibility of preventive interventions for drug users. Indeed, these penalities may actually preclude providing drug users with information.

Drug-use practices contribute significantly to the vulnerability of drug users. Many drug users in the region use narcotics such as opium and heroin, and a significant percentage inject. More often than not, injecting takes place in more public locations. Public injectors have little or no information about HIV infection mostly. The sharing of needles, syringes, and other drug-use equipment is common. The sexual practices of drug users is another important area that contributes to their vulnerability to HIV infection. Drug users condom use is often very low. Unprotected sex is often perceived to be less risky than sharing needles and syringes. They and their partners often act as a bridge to transmit HIV to other populations such as commercial sex workers, clients of commercial sex workers, and then to the general population.

With the onset of HIV/AIDS in 1980s in Asia, drug users were the first to be infected in most of the countries like China, Myanmar, Nepal, Thailand and Vietnam. The epidemic then spread from drug-using populations to other groups, and from there to the general population. Treatment and rehabilitation centres are often not readily available to drug users. In many countries, services provide detoxification only. In many regions of Asia, outpatient and substitution treatment as well as aftercare services are virtually absent. Professionals have limited knowledge about drug treatment and HIV/AIDS prevention.

The Action Plan

United Nations subcommittee of the Administrative Committee on Coordination, has spelt out a comprehensive policy response to drug use and HIV/AIDS in a position paper in September 2000. The principles of the policy include protection of human rights critical for the successful prevention of HIV/AIDS. The paper says that HIV prevention should start as early as possible and comprehensive coverage of the entire targeted population is essential. Recognizing the fact that the drug-abuse problems cannot be solved simply by criminal justice initiatives, it is said that to halt the epidemic requires a three-part strategy—preventing drug abuse; facilitating entry into drug-abuse treatment; and establishing effective outreach to engage drug abusers in HIV-prevention strategies that protect them, and their partners and families, from exposure to HIV (i.e., promoting the acceptance of substance abuse treatment and medical care).

The Asian Strategy

At the Government level, HIV/AIDS issues are usually addressed by the Ministry of Health. Earlier, there was little communication and less cooperation between these government entities. Because of this, the process of developing and reviewing drug and HIV policies in Asian countries is difficult. In many countries, drug-control legislation was made prior to the onset of the HIV/AIDS epidemics, and it is usually based on the United Nations Drug Control Conventions most of the ratified by most countries of Asia. In Asian countries, drug policies are not supportive of effective HIV prevention among drug users. Drug problems are not generally accorded high funding priority. There are few government programmes in the region that directly address problems presented by the interface between drug use and HIV/AIDS. Governmental measures to check the spread of HIV among drug users and their sexual partners, are often localized, short term, under-funded, and insufficient in scope. Adherence to traditional values is in tense many of the countries, making debate on HIV/AIDS prevention and sexual behaviour sensitive. Drug treatment almost invariably focuses on detoxification treatment. Drug-treatment personnel are often non-specialists in the drug field.

Role of NGOs

A great number of Non-Governmental Organizations (NGOs) are engaged in fighting the drug menace. The International Federation of Non-Governmental Organizations against Drug and Substance Abuse, established in 1981 and based in Kuala Lumpur, currently has 54 members. Forum, another federation of non-governmental organizations, currently has approximately 15 members. Though at the apex level, NGOs are better informed and equipped to deal with the problems, at the micro levels, there seem to be not much information of the strategies and policy to meet the problem. Another feature of Asian NGOs working in the field of drug use is that they rarely include drug users themselves. In most of the cases, these organizations work for drug users—or even against drug users—but not with drug users. Some organizations that are closely affiliated with law-enforcement agencies understand their mission as a "war against drugs". Interventions developed by such organizations often embark on a fear approach, reinforcing stereotypes of drug users. They sometimes practise wild and degrading treatment approaches such as "cold turkey", a method of withdrawal without any supporting medication, or "haircuts," which entails humiliating a drug user in public if he or she has not adhered to the rules of the treatment facility. These organizations naturally experience problems in reaching out to drug users, identifying their needs, and developing feasible low-threshold programmes—encouraging drug users to seek help.

In the field of HIV/AIDS, a great number of national and international organizations, addressing the needs of people living with HIV/AIDS, are now involving them in the daily operations of the organization. In fact, since the launching of what is called the Greater Involvement of People Living with HIV/AIDS (GIPA) at the Paris AIDS Summit on 1 December 1994, it has become standard for non-governmental organizations to include people with HIV/AIDS. Interestingly, in case of drug use and HIV/AIDS there is a similarity in policies between governmental and non-governmental organizations. NGOs working in the drug field state that HIV/AIDS is a health issue that should be dealt with by those institutions specializing in health issues. As a consequence, few NGOs work with both drug use and HIV/AIDS. It should also be noted that drug NGOs have relatively little experience in working with HIV/AIDS, and HIV/AIDS NGOs generally lack adequate knowledge about drug issues. The prime reasons for such a trend include: isolation and marginalization; resource shortages; lack of institutional capacity and skills relating to programme design, implementation, and evaluation; lack of information, such as documentation or research on effective models and interventions, and few suitable mechanisms for sharing information and slow or non-existent governmental responses, and little support for non-governmental responses.

Other Organizations

Until September 2000, the United Nations International Drug Control Programme (UNDCP) together with the International Narcotics Control Board (INCB) advocated an abstinence-only policy to lesser drug use, believing this would lead to a reduction in the incidence of HIV infection among drug users. Both UNDCP and INCB insisted on adherence to international drug-control conventions, that exclude the use of narcotics for other than medical or scientific purposes. The Chief sponsor or partner organizations of UNDCP and INCB were usually powerful national drug-control agencies. The World Health Organization as well as UNAIDS, which began its operations in January 1996, promoted various pragmatic risk-reduction strategies, including information campaigns, peer outreach, drug-substitution therapy, and needle- and syringe-exchange programmes. In June 1998, the United Nations General Assembly adopted the Declaration on Demand Reduction, which called for addressing the adverse health consequences of drug use; and in April 1999, UNDCP became a cosponsor of UNAIDS. A similar split can be observed in regional intergovernmental organizations such as the Association of South-East Asian Nations (ASEAN) and the South Asian Association of Regional Cooperation (SAARC). It was not until September 2000 that United Nations bodies and entities agreed on a common and system-wide position with regard to drug use and HIV/AIDS.

The Holistic Outlook

Since the early 1990s, some programmes began operating in different Asian countries to address both drug use and HIV/AIDS. One of the first of these was the Lifesaving and Lifegiving Society (LALS), an outreach needle-exchange programme in Kathmandu. The LALS carefully observed the effects on the growing epidemic of HIV/AIDS among drug users in this country. During the same time, similar programmes began operating in other Asian countries; these included: Sharan (New Delhi, India); Ikhlas (Kuala Lumpur, Malaysia); the SHALOM Project (Manipur, India); Save the Children Fund (Ho Chi Minh City, Vietnam); AIDS Surveillance and Education (ASEP) (Cebu City, Philippines) and HIV/AIDS Prevention and Care Project for the Hilltribes of Northern Thailand (HAHP).

Funds were collected through fundraising activities in the local communities or were provided by foreign donors. Programmes whose prime focus was rehabilitation also began to expand their activities to include prevention of HIV infection by means of information, communication, and education campaigns, peer outreach, needle and syringe-exchange programmes, and drug-substitution programmes. By 1996, the number of programmes addressing drug use and HIV/AIDS had slowly increased. Although these programmes were small, they were influential and demonstrated that it was possible to lessen the risk of HIV transmission among drug users.

Eleven

HIV/AIDS in Caribbean and Latin America

Introduction

Latin America, the Caribbean islands is getting increasingly susceptible to HIV infection. A WHO estimate puts the number of adults infected with the killer disease at 105 million. Urban homosexual and bisexual men, injecting drug users and users of commercially supplied blood and blood products are identified as the high risk groups and they were the ones who initially spread the disease.

Thus far, there have been about a quarter of a million AIDS cases in adults and children in this region. Brazil, whose population is around 150 million comes out as the fourth largest country in the world and has the highest number of reported AIDS cases in the Americas, after the USA—40000. As of December 1992, Colombia and Venezuela together had reported over 5000 cumulative AIDS cases, and Argentina over 2000 cases. The ratio of infected people to per 100,000 population was 5.6 in 1991 in Brazil, but far higher rates were observed in some Caribbean islands where the population is much smaller.

In Brazil—only 7.5 per cent of reported AIDS cases were caused by heterosexual transmission in 1987 but the figure went up to 23 per cent by 1992. Primarily for this reason, women are increasingly affected: the male/female ratio was 28 to 1 in 1985 and only 5 to 1 in 1992. Studies among pregnant women attending antenatal clinics in Sao Paulo state between 1987 and 1990 found that seroprevalence increased consistently during the period, from 0.2 per cent to 1.3 per cent.

The situation in Central America is also causing grave concern. In 1991, 0.6 per cent of male police employees in

Guatemala City were found to be infected. Meanwhile, in San Pedro Sula, Honduras, studies among pregnant women conducted in 1991 brought to light infection rates of 3.6 per cent. In a nearby commune close to the Guatemalan border, a 1992 HIV prevalence study of sex workers, whose clients are mostly truck drivers, found around one-third to be infected. This reveals the fact that people doing certain jobs are particularly vulnerable to the infection. Around 10 per cent of STD clinic attenders in Honduras were also infected with HIV, reflecting the close epidemiological link between HIV infection and the conventional STDs.

In many parts of Latin America, as elsewhere in the world, men are by tradition permitted to seek sex prior to and outside of marriage, while women are expected to remain virgins before marriage and monogamous thereafter. A study in Mexico observes that it is socially acceptable for men to have sex with a homosexual partner provided they take the active, insertive role in anal intercourse—a role regarded as "macho", i.e. super-masculine. The same sex partner who in "passive" may be a boy who sells sex occasionally for the price of a new shirt or pair of shoes. In Peru, where more than half a million children under the age of 14 live in families struggling below the poverty line, this form of occasional prostitution is known as *fleteo*. Or the relationship can take the form of sex barter whereby, as has been observed in Mexico, apprentices in the construction trade may be afforded some degree of protection (e.g. job stability) in exchange for sex, rather than money.

In some parts of Latin Amercia, HIV transmission through needle-sharing during drug abuse is causing special alarm. In Brazil, the proportion of reported AIDS patients who injected drugs rose dramatically between 1986 and 1991. One of the worst affected cities is Santos, the port city of Sao Paulo, which bustles with shipping traffic, trade and tourism. The injecting of cocaine—especially dangerous because it may involve 5-6 injections a day to be high for a longer time—is said to be reaching epidemic proportions, and serosurveys in Santos have found rates of HIV infection of 50-60 per cent among users. This reinforces the fear that certain development patterns can cause "high risk areas".

Since the mid to late 1980s heterosexual transmission has increased steadily, principally between bisexual men and their female sex partners, between male and female drug injectors and their sex partners, between female sex workers and their male clients, and between the latter and their regular partners. In the Caribbean, which has some of the highest per capita AIDS rates in the world, heterosexual intercourse is the main mode of HIV transmission. Alarmingly, AIDS is occurring in ever-younger people. The Caribbean Epidemiology Centre reports that young people in the age group 15 and 29 now account for more than 50 per cent of all AIDS cases—up from 30 per cent in 1986. Teenagers are thus fast becoming victims.

Elsewhere, too, young people are at risk. In a survey in Rio de Janeiro, some 44 per cent of men aged 15-49 reported engaging in sexual intercourse outside a regular partnership. But among young men aged 15-19, the proportion of this kind of sexual behaviour among youngsters was around 60 per cent. Rates as high as this were not seen among similar samples of male teenagers surveyed in other parts of the world.

An important early factor in the spread of HIV in some areas of South America was the large number of men whose primary relationships were with women but who also had sex with other men. For example, a study of women diagnosed with AIDS in Mexico up to December 1990 showed that, of those for whom information was available about their sex partner, 46 per cent had a bisexual partner. Considering the fact that the sexual preferences of many men are not known, this figure is quite alarming.

While sexual exposure to bisexual men and to male or female drug users accounted for a significant proportion of HIV infections among heterosexuals early in the epidemic, today their overwhelming risk factor is associated with exposure to another heterosexual. This is especially true where heterosexual transmission is spurred by a high prevalence of STDs and other genital tract infections, due to inadequate access to preventive methods early detection and treatment, and by poverty and social misery which favour unprotected sex with many partners, frequently as part of a strategy of survival through sex work. If AIDS prevention is to be successful, strategies must be found for confronting or circumventing these conditions, for they exist to varying degrees in practically every country of the region. Moreover, political stability and people's participation in the preventive programmes and drives is also essential.

Twelve

HIV/AIDS in Pacific and the East Asia

HIV started spreading in East Asia and Pacific the mid-eighties. The immense diversity cultures, political systems and socio-economic environment acted as a breeding ground for the rapid increase in the various forms and patterns of HIV infection.

In 1994, WHO estimated that the region in total had more than 25,000 infections in adults. Japan estimated that the cumulative total in that country was around 11,000 at the end of 1992, a 3,000 increase within one year.

Less than 1000 AIDS cases have been found from the region. Japan has reported the highest number: a total of 566 till April 1993. But other smaller islands—notably French Polynesia, New Caledonia and Guam—have a higher rate of AIDS cases per 100,000 population.

In Japan, most cases thus far have been in men with haemophilia found to have received contaminated factor VIII, and HIV infections have been reported in people with haemophilia in Hong Kong and China (Province of Taiwan) as well. These commercial products were always prepared from what is known as "source plasma" extracted from paid donors, without the availability of HIV testing and viral inactivation procedures. Transmission through blood transfusions has been less, as HIV testing of blood transfusion was started at the same time as in most developed countries. By 1990 the rate of heterosexual infections in Japan began to rise amazingly, marking the beginning of a new trend in the pattern of HIV transmission in that country. As in the case of Filippino, in 1990 under half of all reported HIV infections and AIDS cases in Japan were in women, by 1992 women outnumbered men by about three to two.

AIDS in Hong Kong has mainly affected homosexual and

bisexual men. In French Polynesia also, more than half of all cases have been in men who have sex with men, at the same time more than 20 per cent have been linked to heterosexual transmission. In Papua New Guinea, more than half of all HIV infections have been transmitted heterosexually.

Very little cases of AIDS have been reported from the vast territory and population of China, though serological surveys shown that HIV has taken root among injecting drug users in the south-western province of Yunnan, which has a border with Myanmar in the Golden Triangle area. The total number of people involved in injecting drug use, which is illegal, highly stigmatized and therefore hidden, are unknown. But infection rates of 10-35 per cent among drug injectors were found in 1990. Most affected are minority groups living in the mountains close to the China/Myanmar border, where people cross freely for personal visits or to trade with neighbouring villages. Drug use in this area is mainly a male habit.

A wide range of demographic and economic features could affect the dynamics of the HIV/AIDS epidemic in this region: its vast population size, its population density far greater than that in Africa or Latin America, and its expanding urban economies leading to huge population shifts from rural to urban areas, encouraged by hopes of greater economic opportunities. On the positive side, half a century of investment in education has improved Asia's literacy rate and hence easy to reach with information on AIDS; many rural people have access to television and other media; and family planning programmes have been established for nearly 30 years, giving a good infrastructure for condom distribution and STD care. Where condoms are already become a popular family planning method, the challenge is to induce men to see them as effective tools for disease prevention and to use them above all for casual sex—the behaviour through which HIV is spreading so rapidly.

Thirteen

HIV/AIDS in Sub-Saharan African Area

Sub-Saharan Africa, the most poor and strife-torn part of the world, the epidemic spread of AIDS began 15 years ago. There are 9 million people found to be AIDS infected, experts are of the opinion that it is half of the total AIDS infected people. According to the WHO estimates in 1994 over 2 million men, women and children believed to be ill with AIDS. By the same estimates, it has been increased cumulative total of 5 million AIDS by the year 2000.

The vast majority of HIV-infected adults in sub-Saharan Africa are found to have acquired the virus through heterosexual intercourse; and infected women overrun men by 6 to 5. One reason is that the frequent presence of other STDs, which facilitate HIV transmission. Mostly because of a lack of effective STD care women in the developing world are found to have gonorrhea rates 10-15 times higher and syphilis rates 10-100 times higher, than women in industrialized countries.

Not less than 5 million women of childbearing age have been infected and WHO calculated that as many as 1 million children are infected prior to or during birth, or through breast-feeding. This number is expected to swell considerably by the starting of the century. Most such children have brief lives, many never know what it is to feel healthy, and some are given up by mothers who, ill themselves, are unable to cope with the burden of a dying child.

In this region, transmission through the transfusion of HIV-infected blood perhaps accounts for less than 10 per cent of all HIV infections. Practices such as ritual scarification and the use of ineffective sterilized skin-piercing instruments are believed to account for a relatively small proportion of infections.

In almost all areas of sub-Saharan Africa, transmission of HIV through infected blood and blood products is being curtailed as appropriate screening of donated blood is introduced. Other criterias being taken to protect the blood supply include recruiting donors from among low-risk population groups, on a free and unpaid basis so as to discourage unsuitable donors, enthused only by money, from coming forward. Countries are also being encouraged to change their guidelines on transfusion to make sure that the procedure is only carried out when absolutely necessary and that saline solutions are used as blood substitutes whenever possible.

The injecting of drugs for non-medical purposes has usually been rarity in sub-Saharan Africa. However, there are some signs that the practice may be catching on, particularly in port areas and among educated and rich city-dwellers.

The area hardest hit by the AIDS is central and east Africa which accounts for one-sixth of the region's population. In several towns and cities, a quarter or even one-third of all men and women aged 15-49 are believed to be HIV-positive.

In 1990, the infection rate was more higher in urban than in rural areas. But the differential has since declined, and very high infection rates have been recorded in some rural areas—notably in those where good roads or navigable rivers promote movement to and from towns and cities.

The HIV/AIDS epidemic is well established in west and southern Africa as well, and was travelled the trade routes with truckers and migrant workers who form liaisons away from home or have casual sex partners. In Zimbabwe only more than 6,00,000 people have been infected with HIV.

In the major urban areas of Botswana, studies proved that almost 18 per cent of people aged 15-49 are infected with HIV. And in South Africa nationwide sentinel surveillance among antenatal clinic attenders pointed out that the number of HIV-infected people doubled between 1990 and 1991. Sentinel surveillance data from Nigeria in early 1992 revealed that extensive HIV spread in the country, with rates of 15-20 per cent in certain groups of female prostitutes. In Abidjan, Cote d'Ivoire, where AIDS is becoming one of the major cause of death among adults,

HIV prevalence in the general population is believed to be 10-12 per cent.

> "An environment of death"
>
> "This is an environment of death," says Protase Karani, who heads a Tanzanian home-based care team in Kagera Region on the shores of Lake Victoria. "So many people in the villages round here have died that those in the sexually active age group are frightened and unsure. Nobody is prepared to do anything very permanent."
>
> When a man sees his wife die of AIDS and his son or daughter returns from the city also sick, why should he invest in the future? Asks Karani. Why should he spend money on coffee trees that will take several years to mature or plough more land than necessary to feed his family this year? "Today many people are spending whatever money they have on drink because they say: 'What is the point? I shall die soon too.' That's what I mean by an environment of death."
>
> In Kasheni a Tanzanian village bordering Lake Victoria, village chairman Gerald Ndyekobola turns the yellowed pages of a well-worn personal file in which he keeps photographs of villagers who have died. Among the portraits and snapshots of family groups is a photo of eleven fit and smiling young men who made up the local football team. More than half the figures are now marked with an ink cross indicating that they have become casualties of the epidemic.
>
> Ndyekobola recalls a market in nearby Rukunyo, where Tanzanian and Ugandan traders did brisk business in second-hand clothing sisal, bicycle tyres and other goods. Then people began to fall ill. When it was discovered that the sickness was AIDS, traders drifted away the market died, and the surrounding bars and hotels gradually closed their doors.

The spreading of HIV in sub-Saharan Africa has been increased by mass population movement due to war poverty, drought and poor development decisions. "The fact that HIV thrives on social unrest and poverty is clearly illustrated by the situation in this country," said Professor Nicky Padayachee, an epidemiologist in Johannesburg. Several years of clashes between rival political groups in the townships and rural villages of the troubled KwaZulu-natal province have generated a kind of fatalism, which is reflected in an reluctant to take precautions against infection on the grounds that it is no more good. Family life and education have been broken as people fled their homes and the violence. According to one survey among 5000 people in the north of the province found that HIV seroprevalence—1.2 per cent at the end of 1990—doubled in the next six months. It would be amazing if similarly rapid HIV spread were not occurring in war-ravaged populations across the continent, from Liberia to Zaire, Angola to Mozambique, in some cases through rape by soldiers.

Some experts believed that homosexual intercourse played major role in HIV transmission in Africa, although homosexuality is so heavily denounced in this part of the world that little is known about its extent or associated behaviours. It is clear, however, that the route in Africa is heterosexual intercourse.

One reason for optimism is that the rural areas of sub-Saharan Africa are less affected by HIV/AIDS than the cities and towns although the differential appears to be declining. But even in cities where HIV prevalence is high is not less than 20 per cent—but it is important to bear in mind that 80 per cent of the adult population is *not* infected. These people can avoid infection if the right information and services get to them properly. Another reason for optimism is that in many countries close to half the population is under 15 years old and in many cases not yet sexually active. If effective AIDS education campaigns are implemented for youngsters there are ground for hope that the next generation will be saved from the disastrous disease.

TABLE 1
SUMMARY OF DOCUMENTED EXAMPLES OF COLLABORATION IN SUB-SAHARAN AFRICA (1987-1999)

Country	*Project/ institution*	*Initiated/ supported by*	*Objectives*	*Methods*	*Achievements/findings*
Botswana	Seminars for traditional healers on AIDS, 1993	Ministry of Health	- Sensitization of traditional healers to AIDS - To coordinate activities of traditional healers with district health teams	No information	Seminars held sporadically with traditional healers on various diseases including Aids
	Botswana Dingaka AIDS Awareness and Training Programme, 1991-1993	CIDA, WHO, Ministry of Health	- Providing a forum for exchange of information and experiences between traditional healers and biomedical health practitioners - Promoting cooperation and collaboration for health services - Creating awareness on AIDS among traditional healers - Training core trainers who will, in turn, pass on the information to other traditional healers in selected pilot areas	- 2-week TOT held with 12 traditional healers on AIDS from 6 districts of Botswana - Independent evaluation interviewed 32 traditional healers, 19 nurses and 20 medical doctors	- Trained traditional healers trained, on average, 45 other traditional healers per district in 2 years - 72 per cent of traditional healers said they had changed something in their practice in relation to AIDS training - 80 per cent said they recommend condoms - Educational video produced - Flip chart addressing practices of traditional healers produced

(Contd.)

(Contd.)

Country	*Project/ institution*	*Initiated/ supported by*	*Objectives*	*Methods*	*Achievements/findings*
Cameroon	KABP survey of traditional healers, 1990	NACP Natio-nal traditional medicine programme	- To sensitize and introduce traditional healers to HIV/AIDS control.	- National seminar on traditional medicine and AIDS to be conducted	No information
Central African Republic	Action to Define, Broaden, and Strengthen the Role of Traditional Practitioners (ADERT), 1995	Ministry of Health, University of Bangui, World, AIDS Foundation, CDC, CIDA, University of Washington, USA	- To identify and reinforce aspects of traditional medicine believed to promote public health, while discouraging those that have negative health impacts - To enable traditional healers to deliver preventive messages, support persons living with HIV/AIDS and modify their own risk practices	- Focus groups to identify training topics and methods - Working group of traditional healers and Ministry of Health staff to develop curriculum. - 103 traditional healers at 4 locations (urban and rural) completed 6-day training - 96 traditional healers completed pre-and post-KABP questionnaires	Traditional healers' knowledge improved, except with regard to their own risk practices. Repetitive rather than single training model suggested.
Ghana	Unit for traditional medicine established in Ministry of Health, 1990	WHO, Ministry of Health	- To involve traditional healers in primary health care.	- Establishing a dialogue with traditional healers	Recommendations for involving traditional healers in management and treatment of AIDS
	Training manual for traditional healers	Save the Children	- To produce a document to systematically train traditional healers in AIDS prevention and care	- Production of training manual	No information

Country	*Project/ institution*	*Initiated/ supported by*	*Objectives*	*Methods*	*Achievements/findings*
Guinea	Ministry of Health, traditional medicine unit. Integration of traditional healers into health activities, 1985.	Ministry of Health	- To identify the factors within traditional medicine that can increase the effectiveness of the fight against AIDS in Guinea - To increase traditional healers' knowledge of modes of HIV transmission and prevention, clinical manifestations, care and support.	- Survey of STDs known to traditional healers - Research on traditional treatments for fertility, AIDS, STDs - Baseline survey of traditional healers' knowledge of AIDS - 2 workshops organized for traditional healers - Each district has a physician in charge of traditional medicine	Traditional healers are registered with Ministry of Health. Research on 898 traditional healers since the beginning of the programme found that increasing numbers of traditional healers refer to health centres (using referral forms), hospitals and other traditional healers for diagnosis and treatment. Biomedical health providers also refer back. Traditional healers keep records on numbers of cases and treatment.
Liberia	Anthropological Research on STDs, 1988	SOMARCH/ USAID Johns Hopkins University, USA	- To learn how to promote condoms to limit the spread of HIV	- Focus group discussions with 53 participants - Conducted interviews with 103 traditional healers	- Traditional healers advise against prostitutes. - Traditional healers should be taught STD diagnosis and referral because people believe in traditional medicine for STDs.

(Contd.)

(Contd.)

Country	*Project/ institution*	*Initiated/ supported by*	*Objectives*	*Methods*	*Achievements/findings*
Malawi	Training on AIDS for traditional healers, 1992	International Eye Foundation, Malawi International Centre for Eye Health, UK	- To better understand the practices and roles of healers in their communities - To promote greater communication between traditional healers and the formal health care sector - To educate traditional healers about HIV/AIDS and STD transmission and prevention - To encourage community-based HIV/AIDS prevention and care by traditional healers.	- Series of orientations and focus group discussion were held with traditional healers - An eye care programme formed the initial base of contact and collaboration between project staff and traditional healers - Baseline and follow-up (6 months post-training) were conducted with 89 traditional healers - One-day training sessions were held in 14 sites in one district (334 traditional healers)	- Increase in community education, condom distribution, and patient counselling activities 6 months post training.
Mozambique	Anthropological research and training on AIDS and STDs for traditional healers, 1991-1994	Ministry of Health, Swiss Cooperation	- To improve intersectoral cooperation in the prevention and treatment of STDs - To identify and reinforce aspects of traditional medicine believed to promote public health, while discouraging those believed to have negative health impacts	- Conducted interviews with 51 traditional healers specializing in STDs to develop training strategy - 5 Focus group discussions were held, with 7 traditional healers per group - 2 one-week workshops in 2 provinces	- Developed culturally appropriate strategy for the NACP involving traditional healers for STDs. - 30 traditional healers participated in workshop on STDs in 1991. In 1994, follow-up with 21 traditional healers; 8 clients were interviewed and showed increased knowledge on HIV transmission, condom use and promotion.

Country	Project/ institution	Initiated/ supported by	Objectives	Methods	Achievements/findings
Namibia	Anthropological research on traditional medicine, 1995	PhD thesis fieldwork	- To analyse traditional healers' patients' health-seeking behaviour for illness in general	- Quantitative and qualitative methods	No information
Rwanda	AIDS research project (Project San Francisco), 1990	University of California, San Francisco, USA; Ministry of Health	- To analyse health-seeking behaviour of women patients with regard to AIDS and traditional medicine - To analyse knowledge, attitudes, practices surrounding AIDS and STDs	- Quantitative and qualitative methods including questionnaires, and in-depth interviews among 40 women involved in a prospective cohort study - 25 traditional healers interviewed on KABP on AIDS	- Majority of women used both bio-medical and traditional systems and believed in greater effective-ness of traditional medicine for certain AIDS symptoms. - All traditional healers had heard of AIDS, knew modes of transmission, signs and symptoms and that there was no treatment or vaccine.
Senegal	Promotion of Traditional Medicine (PROMETRA), 1981	Centre for Expe-rimentation of Traditional Medicine, Senegal Tulane School of Public Health, USA Morehouse School of Medicine, USA	- To promote traditional medicine	- 383 healers organized into an association called PROMETRA - Conducted training on diarrhoea and family planning, but not yet on AIDS - Needs assessment conducted prior to training.	- 87 per cent of interviewed patients were satisfied with traditional healers' services. - 67 per cent physicians inter-viewed stated they referred patients to traditional healers.

(Contd.)

(Contd.)

Country	*Project/ institution*	*Initiated/ supported by*	*Objectives*	*Methods*	*Achievements/findings*
Sierra Leone	Counselling training for traditional healers, 1992	National STD/ AIDS Control Programme	- To train traditional healers in HIV/AIDS counselling	1-day training held with 150 traditional healers.	- 150 traditional healers trained in HIV/AIDS counselling - 80 per cent of people with HIV/AIDS prefer traditional medicine treatment.
South Africa	Training of trainers for healers, 1992	AIDSCAP, USA AIDSCOM, USA Ministry of Health, South Africa	- The initial goal was to determine the level of interest, knowledge, and skills of traditional healers in HIV prevention and whether they could serve as effective agents of behaviour change. - The ultimate goal was to engage traditional healers in combating HIV/AIDS in South Africa through training other healers and incorporating HIV/AIDS prevention into their practices.	- 1-year feasibility study - Preliminary 5-day workshop (Nov. 1992) 28 traditional healers 3 follow-up workshops (July 1993, Nov. 1993, July 1994)	- 630 traditional healers trained by 28 trained traditional healers on basic AIDS facts. - 7-month follow-up:> 80 per cent retained correct STD/AIDS information and practised counselling
	Pilot survey of traditional healers, 1992	Centre for Natural and Traditional Medicine, Washington, DC, USA	- To assess traditional healers' potential for AIDS prevention and care	No information	- Survey found traditional healers had high knowledge about AIDS, were treating symptoms of AIDS; and concluded that, "traditional healers are a force that cannot be ignored in the fight against HIV/AIDS".

Country	*Project/ institution*	*Initiated/ supported by*	*Objectives*	*Methods*	*Achievements/findings*
	Training programme for traditional healers in KwaZulu-Natal, 1994	AIDS Foundation of South Africa, National Traditional Healers' Association of South Africa	- To increase AIDS prevention, education and management in KwaZulu-Natal by providing training and resources to traditional healers - To help trained traditional healers become accepted by the biomedical system in KwaZulu-Natal	- Project emphasized strengthening resources in disadvantaged communities.	- Traditional healers could identify signs and symptoms of AIDS after training. - Traditional healers identified need for rural AIDS hospices and trained homecare personnel to care for persons living with HIV/AIDS. - 75 per cent traditional healers believed they could cure AIDS before training, none after
	Training of traditional healers in HIV prevention and collaboration, 1998	Government of South Africa	- To train traditional healers in every province of South Africa on AIDS prevention - To build collaboration between traditional and biomedical health systems	- 3-day workshop for traditional healers in every province of South Africa, using participatory methods	- Prevention training was successful, but collaboration was not. Recommends using traditional healers to train traditional healers because traditional healers respect their fellow-members.

(Contd.)

(Contd.)

Country	*Project/ institution*	*Initiated/ supported by*	*Objectives*	*Methods*	*Achievements/findings*
Uganda	Traditional and Modern Health Practitioners Together against AIDS (THETA), 1992	Doctors without Borders, The AIDS Support Organization, NACP, Ministry of Health, Uganda AIDS Commission, Rockefeller Foundation	- To provide training for traditional healers in community counselling and HIV/AIDS education, basic clinical diagnosis and patient management - To provide a resource centre for information sharing on traditional medicine and AIDS - To advocate for traditional medicine among health professionals and other scientists in order to build a true collaboration	- Community mobilization, traditional healers training in AIDS education and counselling in 7 districts in Uganda, with 40 traditional healers per district since 1993 - Traditional healers' training in patient management with 30 traditional healers in Kampala in 1 year - Resource centre collects and disseminates information on traditional medicine and AIDS - Promoting collaboration between traditional medicine and biomedicine	- Increased couselling and AIDS education by trained traditional healers and increased knowledge and condom use among clients of trained traditional healers - Over 120 traditional healers trained and more than 96,000 persons benefited in 2 years - Collected a wide variety of materials on traditional medicine and AIDS - Produced 2 videos in Uganda and English for educational and informational use
	Community based home care, 1993	CONCERN, Ireland Ministry of Health, Uganda	- To train volunteers to provide care and support to the sick using a primary care herbal kit developed by the project - To disseminate information on herbs and disease	- Workshops centred on skills and confidence-building in giving out herbal medicine	- Traditional healers trained 68 volunteers involved in home care and distributing herbs for common AIDS-related symptoms

Country	*Project/ institution*	*Initiated/ supported by*	*Objectives*	*Methods*	*Achievements/findings*
United Republic of Tanzania	Tanga AIDS Working Group (TAWG), 1990	Initiated by a physician and traditional healers. Family Health International, Shaman Pharmaceutical Company, Evangelische Zentralstelle fur Entwicklu-ngshilfe, GTZ	- Raise HIV/AIDS/STD awareness among traditional practitioners in 3 districts to safeguard both practitioners and clients from being infected during practices - Train traditional healers as community based HIV/AIDS/STD educators and home-care providers for persons living with HIV/AIDS and their families - Promotion of community-based condom distribution	- Series of sensitization meetings between local govt., district PHC committees, village health committees, communities and traditional healers - 2 types of participatory approaches - ZOPP and LEPSA - were used to identify and train key people at the grassroots level - TAWG trained 120 traditional healers in 3 districts in 1994 - Health personnel at each health facility were trained to support the programme	- 160 traditional healers have been trained in HIV/AIDS and health information. - Healers are involved in collaborative clinical work, AIDS education, counselling, home visits and village theatre groups. - Training manual produced
Zaire	Workshops with traditional healers, 1989	CONNAISSIDA, Zaire Traditional Healers' Association	No information.	- Action research using 2 experimental risk-reduction workshops with women in low-income area.	- Demonstrated traditional healers' pragmatism and the role they can play in promoting behaviour change for safer sex practices.

(Contd.)

(Contd.)

Country	*Project/ institution*	*Initiated/ supported by*	*Objectives*	*Methods*	*Achievements/findings*
Zambia	AIDS workshop, 1987	Traditional Practitioners' Association of Zambia, Ministry of Health	- To exchange ideas and experiences on AIDS and gain traditional healers' support in fighting its spread.	- Dialogue between the Ministry of Health Education Unit and the secretariat of the Traditional Practitioners' Assn. of Zambia - Workshop held with 40 traditional healers	- 40 traditional healers attended - Knowledge increased, misconceptions still strong
	AIDS research, training and follow-up 1994-1996	Ministry of Health, USAID, Morehouse University School of Medicine, USA	- To educate traditional healers about HIV/AIDS and STD transmission, prevention and care - To enable traditional healers to educate their patients about these issues and motivate them to avoid high risk behaviour	- 25-40 prominent traditional healers selected to participate in 3-day workshops on AIDS between June 94 and Nov. 95. - Trained traditional healers attended monthly or alternate month follow-up meetings led by health centre staff	- 2000 traditional healers trained on AIDS facts and 120 traditional healers trained in community education. - Knowledge increased, traditional healers started selling condoms through a social marketing programme.
Zimbabwe	AIDS workshops, 1988	Zimbabwe National Traditional Healers Association (ZINATHA), Ministry of Health	No information	No information	- Workshops organized to train traditional healers in AIDS and counselling. - Pamphlet in local language designed for traditional healers and AIDS

Abbreviations:

AMREF	African Medical Research Foundation
BHP	Biomedical Health Practitioners
CDC	Centres for Disease Control and Prevention
CDD	Control of Diarrhoeal Diseases
CIDA	Canadian International Development Agency
KABP	Knowledge, Attitudes, Beliefs and Practices
MOH	Ministry of Health
NACP	National AIDS Control Programme
PHC	Primary Health Care
SOMARC	Condom Social Marketing Programme
TH	Traditional Healers
TM	Traditional Medicine
TOT	Training of Trainers
WHO	World Health Organization

TABLE 2
COUNTRY INFORMATION

	Total Population (Thousands)[a]	Population 0-14 years (%)[a]	Population 15-49 Years (%)[a]	Population >50 years (%)[a]	Annual growth rate (%)[b]	Urban population (thousands)[b]	Infant mortality rate[b, c]	Life expectancy men[b]	Life expectancy women[b]	Gross National product per capita (US$)[d]	Male literacy rate in 1990[e]	Female literacy rate in 1990[e]
(1)	(2)	(3)	(4)	(5)	(6)	(7)	(8)	(9)	(10)	(11)	(12)	(13)
Algeria	27070	42	47	10	2.7	14657	60	65	68	2060	70	46
Angola	10276	47	43	10	3.7	3145	123	45	48	-	56	29
Benin	5075	47	43	9	3.1	2044	87	45	48	360	32	16
Botswana	1352	45	45	9	2.9	383	59	58	64	2040	84	65
Burkina Faso	9788	45	45	11	2.8	1727	117	47	50	330	28	9
Burundi	5995	46	45	9	2.9	345	105	46	50	210	61	40
Cameroon	12547	44	45	11	2.8	5392	62	55	58	960	67	43
Cape Verde	395	44	46	11	2.9	121	39	67	69	-	-	-
Central African Republic	3258	45	44	12	2.6	1597	104	45	49	390	52	25
Chad	6010	43	45	11	2.7	2092	121	46	49	190	42	18
Comoros	607	49	43	8	3.7	179	88	56	57	-	-	-
Congo	2441	46	44	10	3.0	1030	82	49	54	1010	70	44
Cote d'Ivoire	13397	49	42	9	3.7	5657	90	50	53	750	67	40
Equatorial Guinea	379	43	45	12	2.5	113	116	47	50	-	-	-
Ethiopia	54628	46	44	10	3.0	7058	121	46	49	120	-	-
Gabon	1279	34	49	17	3.3	617	93	52	55	3330	74	49
Gambia	932	44	45	11	2.6	226	131	44	47	-	39	16
Ghana	16446	45	45	9	3.0	5811	80	54	58	390	70	51

(1)	(2)	(3)	(4)	(5)	(6)	(7)	(8)	(9)	(10)	(11)	(12)	(13)
Guinea-Bissau	1028	41	46	13	2.1	218	139	42	45	-	50	24
Kenya	26090	48	44	8	3.3	6766	65	57	61	370	80	59
Lesotho	1882	41	46	12	2.5	405	78	58	63	530	-	-
Madagascar	13259	46	45	10	3.3	3412	109	54	57	230	88	73
Malawi	10694	49	42	9	3.2	1356	141	44	45	200	-	-
Mauritius	1109	28	57	15	1.0	450	21	67	74	2250	-	-
Mozambique	15322	45	45	11	2.9	4796	145	45	49	80	45	21
Namibia	1584	45	45	11	3.2	469	69	58	60	-	-	-
Niger	8529	48	43	9	3.3	1838	123	45	48	310	40	17
Nigeria	119328	47	44	9	3.1	44802	95	51	55	290	62	40
Rwanda	7789	50	42	8	3.4	457	110	45	48	310	64	37
Senegal	7948	45	45	10	2.7	3279	79	49	51	710	52	25
Sierra Leone	4494	45	45	11	2.6	1552	142	42	45	240	31	11
Swaziland	814	43	47	10	2.7	237	72	57	60	-	-	-
Togo	3885	46	44	10	3.2	1160	84	53	57	410	56	31
Uganda	19246	49	44	8	3.0	2300	103	41	43	220	62	35
United Republic of Tanzania	28783	48	44	9	3.3	6573	101	49	52	110	-	-
Zaire	41166	48	43	9	3.2	11789	92	50	53	220	84	61
Zambia	8885	48	44	8	2.8	3778	84	43	45	420	81	65
Zimbabwe	10898	45	47	9	2.9	3332	59	54	57	640	74	60

a. Estimate for 1993. Source: UN Population Division 1992.
b. WHO estimate for 1993 based on data from UN Population Division 1992.
c. Per 1000 live births
d. Data for 1990. Source: World Bank (STARS) (April 1992)
e. Source: Statistical Yearbook (UNESCO, 1991).

TABLE 3
REPORTING OF HIV AND AIDS

	HIV Infection first Reported[a]	*No. of AIDS cases reported* 1991[b]	1992[b]	*Cumulative no. of AIDS cases reported by 1st July 1993*[b]
Algeria	1985	32	40	138
Angola	1985	130	187	608
Benin	1985	113	218	465
Botswana	1985	-	189	439
Burkina Faso	1986	-	0	1307
Burundi	1983	1565	1583	7131
Cameroon	1985	510	1347	2174
Cape Verde	1986	13	13	65
Central African Republic	1984	840	416	3730
Chad	-	94	363	899
Comoros	1988	1	0	3
Congo	1986	1077	1785	5267
Cote d'Ivoire	1985	3894	3863	14655
Equatorial Guinea	1988	2	12	31
Ethiopia	1984	924	3230	4861
Gabon	1986	98	177	392
Gambia	1986	56	56	240
Ghana	1986	903	2699	10285
Guinea-Bissau	1989	30	116	288
Kenya	1980[c]	9202	6762	31185
Lesotho	1986	28	131	219
Madagascar	1987	0	0	4
Malawi	1985	-	4655	26955
Mauritius	1987	-	6	16
Mozambique	1986	178	322	737
Namibia	1986	-	0	311
Niger	1987	212	290	795
Nigeria	1986	57	225	552
Rwanda	1983	-	2908	9486
Senegal	1986	125	323	911
Seychelles	1987	0	1	1
Sierra Leone	1987	52	32	95
Swaziland	1986	92	156	248
Togo	1987	628	675	1953
Uganda	1983	8706	4421	34611
United Republic of Tanzania	1983	12059	4579	38719
Zaire	1986	3120	1181	21008
Zambia	1985	1646	1276	7124
Zimbabwe	1985	4557	3472	14023

a. Compiled from answers by countries to the GPA questionnaire.
b. Based on other information reported to WHO/GPA by countries.
c. HIV statistics.
d. Sex not identified in 157 cases.

TABLE 4
THE NATIONAL AIDS COMMITTEE (NAC) AND THE NATIONAL AIDS PROGRAMME (NAP)A

	National AIDS Committee			
	Year Established	*Chairman's position*	*NGOs repre-sented (since)*	*full-time NAP manager (since)*
Algeria	1989	Medical Professor	No	No
Angola	-	Vice Minister of Health	—	1991
Benin	1987	Minister of Health	Yes	1989
Botswana	1988	Permanent Secretary Ministry of Health	Yes	1992
Burkina Faso	1986	Minister of Health	1989	1989
Burundi	1988	Minister of Health	Yes	1989
Cameroon	1985	Inspector General of Health	1985	1988
Cape Verde	1987	Medical Doctor	Yes	1988
Central African Republic	1986	Minister of Public Health and Social Affairs	1992	1987
Chad	1988	Minister of Public Health and Social Welfare	Yes	1991
Comoros	1988	—	No	1990
Congo	1987	Minister of Health and Social Affairs	1990	1987
Cote d'Ivoire	1987	Minister of Health and Social Welfare	1991	1989
Equatorial Guinea	1988	Minister of Health	Yes	1988
Ethiopia	1986[b]	Director of Armed Forces General Hospital	1989	1987
Gabon	1987	Minister of Health and Population	1990	1990
Gambia	1987	Director of Health Services	1987	1987
Ghana	1990	Medical Doctor, Private Practitioner	1990	1987
Guinea-Bissau	1987	President of the Republic	1992	1992
Kenya	1985	Head of Microbiology Department, University of Nairobi	Yes	1988
Lesotho	1985	Director of Laboratory Services	1985	1988
Madagascar	1990	Minister of Health	—	1988
Malawi	—	—	Yes	1989
Mauritius	1987	Chief Medical Officer	1987	1991
Mozambique	1988	Deputy National Director of Health	1990	—
Namibia	—	—	1991	1991
Niger	1987	Minister of Public Health	No	1990
Nigeria	1988	Minister of Health and Social Services	1988	1988
Rwanda	1987	Prime Minister	Yes	1989
Senegal	1986	Public Health Director	1986	1987
Seychelles	1987	Principal Secretary	No	—
Sierra Leone	1986	Chief Medical Officer	1987	1986
Swaziland	1987	Minister of Health	1987	1990
Togo	1987	Minister of Health	1990	1992
Uganda	1987	Minister of Health	1987	1987
United Republic of Tanzania	1989	Principal Secretary, Prime Minister's Office	No	1988
Zaire	1985	Minister of Public Health	1990	1988
Zambia	1989[c]	Deputy Director of Medical Services	1990	1990
Zimbabwe	1990	—	1990	1988

a. compiled from answers by countries to the GPA questionnaire, updated where possible by other information available GPA in mid-1993.

b. A Technical Advisory committee.

c. A National AIDS Committee was established but it was disbanded in 1990 and not reconstituted since. There is management committee.

Fourteen

HIV Laws in Europe

Introduction

In Europe HIV/AIDS legislation has been made to compiling processing and disseminating information on all aspects of health problems on HIV/AIDS. It is mainly to prevent this monstrous disease from Europe.

Historical Perspectives

In keeping with its traditional function of arranging, processing, and disseminating information on all directions of health legislation, WHO's Health Legislation Unit in Geneva has been cautiously monitoring all significant regional, national, and subnational developments in the field of HIV/AIDS legislation in Europe. Following passeges describes the major legislative and regulatory developments that have come about during the period 1983-1995. As one reviews the complex legislative scene in late 1995, it is helpful to bear in mind that legislative activity on HIV/AIDS in Europe commenced in the spring of 1983. It was on 8 March 1983 that regulations were taken in Sweden by the National Board of Health and Welfare which stated it to be a matter of urgency "to survey suspected and confirmed cases [of AIDS] in order to provide the information needed to determine whether preventive measures are required."

It is important to note that France appears to have been the first jurisdiction to draw attention to what was then described as "the possible transmission of AIDS through blood transfusions." The circular was issued by the Directorate-General of Health on 20 June 1983; three days later, on 23 June, the Committee of Ministers of the Council of Europe issued a recommendation (R [83] 8) on the blood safety issue. Governments of the Member

States of the Council of Europe were suggested to, *inter alia*, provide all blood donors with information on AIDS, so that "those in risk groups will refrain from donating." It is important that on 20 January 1984, the European Parliament adopted a resolution on "an emergency Community programme of research into and measures to combat AIDS disease"; this included a call on what was then known as the Commission of the European Communities presently European Commission) to change the Council of Europe's non-binding recommendations on blood safety into "binding Community law".

Another major event in this sphere in 1983 was the adoption on 3 November, by the Parliamentary Assembly of the Council of Europe, of Resolution 812 (1983) on AIDS. While the term "human rights" did not actually appear in the text of the Resolution, one of the preambular paragraphs reaffirms the Assembly's "unshakeable attachment to the principle that each individual is entitled to have his privacy respected and to self-determination in sexual matters." The Assembly changed the Recommendation and Resolution, both adopted in 1981, that addressed the issue of discrimination against homosexuals, and expressed its concern at the "inaccuracy in the information circulated on AIDS by some of the media, whose sole concern is sensational news." It pointed out that "campaigns of this kind establish a link between AIDS and homosexuality, so spreading anti-homosexual reactions." In which it appears to have received relatively little attention at the time, was certainly the precursor to many subsequent developments, culminating in the Declaration adopted by the Paris AIDS Summit on 1 December 1994.

In 16 March 1983, the Federal Ministry for Health and Environment Protection of Austria delivered a Decree containing a series of preparatory recommendations addressed to health and laboratory personnel according to the provisions were introduced in Greece by a Circular of 14 July 1983.

WHO has been guiding the literature on the legal/ethical aspects of the epidemic and, rather surprisingly perhaps, only one book devoted to these issues was published in Europe during the period 1983-1986.

There have, certainly, been many other milestones in the

development of HIV/AIDS legislation. Thus, it appears that Austria was the first Europe country made (on 16 May 1986) a fairly comprehensive statute on AIDS. Known as the AIDS Law which include provisions on the following aspects:

- Notification of AIDS cases and deaths from AIDS
- Preservation of confidentiality
- Prevention on AIDS-infected persons engaging in prostitution
- Testing of prostitutes
- Counselling of seropositive persons
- Approval of diagnostic kits
- Encouraging of epidemiological studies on AIDS
- Preparation of a plan of information proliferation
- Funding of institutions and associations concerned with counselling and care in the AIDS context.

Provisions on different aspects of AIDS research also appeared at an early stage. Thus, by 15 October 1983, a Notice was issued in Germany aimed at the promotion of research and development projects concerning AIDS. In Slovakia, a reference laboratory for AIDS was started by a Directive dated 17 January 1984; its aim included research on AIDS and the coordination of testing for infection.

One of the first European countries to start mandatory screening was Austria, as mentioned above. More all-inclusive provisions that could be described as "coercive" appeared in the German Land of Bavaria in May-June 1987. The first provisions in Europe concerning HIV in the immigration context had been introduced by a Notice of 19 May 1987 of the Bavarian Ministry of the Interior and indeed the same Ministry after that issued provisions requiring applicants for posts in the Civil Service and the judiciary in Bavaria to be tested for HIV infection. The year later, the Ministry of Health of what was then the USSR issued regulations requiring the following to be tested:

- Blood and tissue donors.
- Nationals returning from assignments abroad of more than one month's duration.
- Aliens intending to stay in the country for more than three months.

- Persons including to "high-risk" groups, i.e., recipients of multiple blood transfusions, drug-dependent persons, homosexuals, and prostitutes.
- Contacts of AIDS patients or carriers of the virus identified in epidemiological investigations.

A number of European countries started what are known as "alternative testing sites" at a relatively early stage, mainly in response to particular provisions contained in a Council of Europe Recommendation (R[85]12) of 13 September 1985. There have been a trend towards the introduction of mandatory testing programmes was to some extent pre-empted by a series of international recommendations, developed both by WHO and by other European institutions. Thus, an European Community test dated 15 May 1987, formulated the basis of community policy on various aspects of AIDS. One of the preambular paragraphs emphasized "the inefficacy, in terms of prevention, of recourse to any policy for systematic, obligatory screening, particularly during health controls at frontiers."

Few countries were as early as Norway in developing an comprehensive programme for the control of AIDS. Thus, a Circular dated 2 July 1985 issued by the Director-General of Health Services addressed the following aspects, *inter alia*:

- Aims and basic principles.
- Epidemiological surveillance.
- Measures should be adopted to prevent the spread of infection.
- Moral issues.

By 1987, France and Belgium introduced legislation waiving certain restrictions on the advertising of condoms and provisions designed to facilitate access to clean syringes and needles. In the same year, France issued mandatory standards for condoms.

Norway was one of the countries that first addressed the problem of transmission of AIDS in the dental context (a Circular of 7 February 1986 concluded that there was no risk of transfusion of the disease from one dental patient to another in the dental care provided under normal conditions of hygiene); Specially integrated programme for the control of HIV infection in dental services, and in laboratories, were started in December 1986.

As regards institutional mechanisms, a National Commission for the Coordination and Monitoring of Programmes for the Prevention of AIDS was started in Spain in June 1987, by a Decision of the Council of Ministers. A National AIDS Control Commission was started in Italy by a Ministerial Decree issued in January 1987. The first provisions concerning the prescribing of zidovudine (formerly known as AZT) appeared in Austria, the Netherlands and Span of 1987.

One of the European countries to identify infection by what was then known as HTLV-III as a sexually transmitted disease was Iceland (by a Law dated 7 April 1986).

By 1987, Denmark was also established compensation mechanisms for persons with haemophilia and blood transfusion recipients infected with HIV as a result of treatment in Hospitals.

In 1988, United Kingdom was also enacted legislation concerning access to HIV-testing kits.

Particularly all inclusive legislation has been made in Sweden on diverse forms of potential HIV transmission in the hospital/laboratory context; as an example, detailed provisions were issued in April 1987 designed to prevent the transfusion of HIV through infected wastes.

Features of HIV/AIDS Legislation Europe

It must be recognized that the legislative responses to HIV/AIDS from country to country have appeared major differences, both quantitatively and qualitatively. The reasons are many; one self-evident reason is the fact that measures that need legislative (or regulatory) intervention in one country may be adopted elsewhere without resorting to primary or secondary/subsidiary legislation. This is true for the 15 Member States of the Brussels-based European Union as it is for the 34 Member States of the Strasbourg-based Council of Europe. Perhaps the best example of this point is the fact that, at least one country that is a Member State of both institutions, namely Ireland, has so far not made legislation of any nature on HIV/AIDS. Legislative intervention in the Netherlands were limited to three Decrees, all issued in 1987.

The reason why some countries have tended to make a

substantial amount of "hard law", i.e., statute law and implementing regulations or the equivalent and others have choosen to rely on "soft law", i.e., guidelines, circulars or the equivalent are grounded in the legal, administrative, social and political customs and contexts.

The following paragraphs will give you some idea of legislative provisions in European countries. It is not thorough examination of all the laws made by the countries nor the backdrop such legislations.

Albania: There are particular provisions on AIDS in Law No. 7761 of 19 October 1993 on the control of communicable diseases. Thus, provision is adopted for the establishment of a national commission to address issues in the prevention and control of AIDS. Provisions on blood safety need all blood donors to be tested for HIV infection on each occasion when they donate blood. A Resolution of the Council of Ministers, dated 13 March 1995, gives for the free supply of medicaments to persons suffering from AIDS and undergoing treatment on an out patient basis.

Andorra: An interministerial Commission on the AIDS Prevention and Control Programme was started by a Decree of 23 June 1994; its remit focuses mainly on activities in the field of health education and prevention.

Austria: An Ordinance of 1994 concerned in detail with quality control and quality assurance within the conditions of the diagnosis of HIV infection and on the modalities for doing HIV tests; Previous Ordinance of the same year addressed the issue of evidence of the presence of HIV infection and indicator diseases for AIDS. On the subject of notification, a 1993 Decree shown that seropositivity, alone, is not subject to notification.

Belgium: There have been many noteworthy items of legislation in these years. For example, provisions need testing for HIV-1 and HIV-2 are included in the Law of 5 July 1994 on blood and blood derivatives.

Bulgaria: The conditions and laws governing testing for HIV infection were started by an Order issued by the Minister of Health on 2 April 1992. Provisions on mandatory testing covered:

1. All blood units obtained from donations.
2. Tissue and organ donors.

3. Sperm donors.
4. Milk donors
5. Children born from HIV-infected mothers
6. All the foreign nationals spending more than one month in Bulgaria for purposes of study or for professional reasons, and immigrants, irrespective of the length of their stay.

As well as the provisions on voluntary testing (under conditions of strict confidentiality). Health personnel giving care to pregnant women are needed to inform them of the risks incurred by the offspring of HIV-infected mothers and to ask them to undergo testing and particularly, to have blood withdrawn for the purpose. An order issued two months later, i.e., July 1992, started requirements for the testing of blood products for HIV-1 and HIV-2.

Croatia: A Law made in September 1992 on the control of communicable diseases includes provisions requiring (a) the notification/reporting of cases of AIDS and also cases of seropositivity for HIV and (b) all health institutions to test blood, organ, and semen donors for HIV infection.

Denmark: the provisions for notifying (a) AIDS cases and (b) seropositivity for HIV were defined by an Order of December 1993. In April 1993, a Law was made providing for the payment of compensation to HIV-positive minors, persons contaminated as a result of blood transfusions, etc. Two items of subsidiary legislation (a Circular and Guidelines) were introduced in September 1994; these formulated the detailed modalities for the testing of donated blood for HIV-1 and HIV-2.

Estonia: Two items of HIV/AIDS legislation have already been reported to WHO. The first is the Penal Code of May 1992, which includes a Section (119-2) entitled "Infection by the AIDS virus." The other is a Decree, ordered in May 1992, which started AIDS Prevention Programme in the Republic.

France: There is probably no country in Europe that has observed as much legislative activity relating to HIV/AIDS as France. Only a small selection—not necessarily representative—is cited below:

- International coordination of AIDS control was addressed in a May 1994 Decree.

- Measures to avoid any risk of HIV-1 or HIV-2 infection are included in a Decree of February 1992. (amended in May 1994) framed to prevent the transmission of infectious diseases in the use of human organs, tissues and cells.
- A Circular issued in August 1994 concerned with the establishments of an experimental programme for "therapeutic accommodation" for persons suffering from AIDS.
- AIDS control is stated to be an important requirement of public health—with absolute priority being given to prevention—in another Circular issued in August 1994.
- A whole series of legislative texts have addressed the issue of transfusion safety, including the institutional, organizational and administrative aspects.

Germany: There has been few Federal legislation on HIV/AIDS, and legislation at the Land level other than in Bavaria has also been limited. The October 1983 Notice referred to above was cited by only two instruments, viz. 1985 Guidelines of the Federal Health Office on the detection of anti-LAV/HTLV-III antibodies in blood, and a Laboratory Notification Ordinance of December 1987 giving for the anonymous reporting of positive confirmatory tests to the Central AIDS Infection Registry of the above-mentioned Office.

A significant development was the promulgation, on 24 July 1995, of a law on humanitarian help for persons who have become HIV infected through blood products. This created a foundation known as the "Humanitarian Assiatance for Persons who have become HIV-infected as a result of Blood products". The provision of the foundation is DM 250 million.

Italy: Only a small number of the many major items of HIV/AIDS legislation made recently. They include Decrees of September 1991 and October 1992 of the President of the Republic, which address the issue of the establishing of services for the domiciliary treatment of persons affected by AIDS and associated pathological conditions; a Law made in February 1992 which stipulates compensation programme for persons who have become HIV infected as a result of the administration of blood or blood products; a series of legal instruments ordered in 1992 and 1993 on HIV/AIDS in prisons; a December 1992 Decree demanding all donated blood and plasma units to be tested for HIV-2; and an April 1994 Decree of the President of the Republic adopting the "AIDS Project-Objective for 1994-1996" which places stressed on prevention, care training, coordination and research.

Russian Federation: A Federal Law on the Prevention of HIV infection was made on 30 March 1995. Specific detailed provision on "Guarantees by the State" are contained in Section 4. Thus, the following are guaranteed:

- Regular dissemination of information to the population, mainly through the mass media, on available means for the prevention of HIV infection.
- Epidemiological surveillance on the spread of HIV infection in the territory of the Russian Federation.
- Development of means for the prophylaxis, diagnosis and treatment of HIV infection; and the monitoring of the safety of medical preparations, biological fluids and tissues used for diagnostic, therapeutic and scientific purposes.
- Availability of medical testing for the tracking down of HIV infection including anonymous testing, followed by counselling before and after testing, and the assurance of the safety of such medical testing both for persons being tested and for persons performing the test.
- Free provision of all types of qualified and specialist medical care to HIV-infected persons who are citizens of the Russian Federation; the free supply of medicaments to such persons within the groundwork for out-patient or in-patient care; and free transport for such persons to and from the place of treatment within the limits of the Russian Federation.
- Development of scientific research on the issues of HIV infection.
- The inclusion, in the teaching programmes of education institutions, of thematic issues as part of moral and sexual education.
- Social and housing facilities to HIV-infected persons who are citizens of the Russian Federation; and provisions for such persons to get training, professional retraining, and work adjustments.

- Training of specialists for performing measures for controlling the spread of HIV infection.
- Development of international cooperation and day to day exchange of information within the framework of international programmes for controlling the spread of HIV infection.

A Chapter in the Law devoted to "Medical care for HIV infected persons" includes general procedures on testing, followed by particular provisions on voluntary testing, mandatory testing, restrictions for the entry of aliens, the consequences of tracking down of HIV infection, the right to a second medical test, certain rights of HIV-infected persons and the development of a programme for the controlling, diagnosis and treatment of HIV infection. Another Chapter concerned "Social protection of HIV-infected persons and members of their families", while the penultimate Chapter described the "Social protection of persons exposed to a risk of HIV infection in the performance of their professional duties."

Spain: A Crown Decree of April 1993 prescribed that the National Commission for the Coordination and Monitoring of AIDS Prevention Programmes fulfilled as the agency responsible for coordinating the programmes for HIV/AIDS prevention and control undertaken by the Public Administrations. A Crown Decree-Law enacted in May 1993 established a programme of social assistance to persons infected by HIV as a consequence of provisions carried out within the public health system including HIV-infected persons with haemophilia and blood-transfusion recipients who were treated before mandatory testing for HIV infection was instituted. A special commission—Commission on Assiatance to Persons affected by HIV—was started by a July 1993 Order.

Switzerland: Two fairly recent items of Federal legislation are important. The first, an Ordinance of February 1993, demanded the authorization of the Federal Office of Public Health for the marketing of *in vitro* diagnostic kits, including those aimed for the diagnosis of HIV infection. The second, the Ordinance on HIV studies of June 1993, started stated standards and criteria for carrying out epidemiological studies on HIV.

Ukraine: An extensive Law on the Prevention of AIDS and the Social Protection of the Population was made in December 1991. It establishes compulsory testing for *inter alia*, persons involved in prostitution, and self-injecting drug-dependent persons as well as aliens under certain conditions. There are provisions desired to safeguard confidentiality. Successive Chapters deal with: (a) the obligations of HIV-infected persons and all persons subject to "medical testing" for AIDS; (b) social protection of HIV-infected persons, persons suffering from AIDS, and members of their families; (c) social protection of members of the "medical professions" at risk of being infected with HIV; and (d) liability for violating the legislation on the control of AIDS.

European Council: Two recent Recommendations issued by the Committee of Ministers should be mentioned. One of these, Recommendation R (93) 6 of 18 October 1993, addresses "prison and criminological aspects of the control of transmissible diseases including AIDS and related health problems in prison [sic]." Details of the principles and policies continued in the prison and criminological contexts are formulated in a lengthy appendix. The other, Recommendation R (94) 10 of 10 October 1994, addresses the problem of "early pharmacological intervention against HIV infection." One of the criteria for such intervention is stated to be "full protection of a person's privacy, as well as full respect for a person's free choice."

Assessment

Writing a decade ago, a well-known former US Assistant Secretary for Health, Edward Brandt, in 1985, referred to the need for the scientific community to "study this[AIDS] epidemic and the total societal response to it." Legislation is surely one of these responses and this chapter has sought to illustrated how the European countries and intergovernmental institutions have addressed the complex and interrelated problems that have arisen over the years. The international context has been, and continues to be, at critical juncture and the various measures and instruments adopted by WHO and by other institutions, within the United Nations system, have influenced the current, and constantly evolving, configuration of HIV/AIDS legislation in Europe.

In the coming years, the human rights and social dimensions of AIDS would play a major role in the legislative responses to AIDS by European jurisdictions. It is obvious that WHO and the various United Nations bodies that have considered AIDS and AIDS-related problems, have been placing increasing stress on these dimensions. It is important that resolution 1995/44, adopted on 3 March 1995 by the Commission on Human Rights, included a call upon all states.

"...to take all the necessary steps, including appropriate and speedy redressal of procedures and the introduction of protective legislation and appropriate education to combat discrimination, prejudice and stigma, to ensure the full enjoyment of civil, political economic, social and cultural rights by people living with HIV/AIDS, their families and associates and people presumed to be at risk of infection, with particular attention to women, children and vulnerable groups, and to address such concerns within their activities in the context of the United Nations Year for Tolerance, 1995."

More importantly, the Commission called upon all States to:

"...ensure, where necessary, that their laws, policies and practices, including those introduced in the context of HIV/AIDS, respect human rights standard, including the right to privacy and integrity of people living with HIV/AIDS, prohibit HIV/AIDS-related discrimination and do not have the effect of inhibiting programmes for the prevention of HIV/AIDS and for the care of persons infected with HIV/AIDS."

In an address to the Forty-seventh Session of the Sub-Commission on Prevention of Discrimination and Protection of Minorities of the Commission on Human rights in Geneva in 1995, Peter Piot, Executive Director of the Joint United Nations Programme on HIV/AIDS, stated that :

"A key part of the multisectoral response is the human rights response. UNAIDS will be a strong advocate for the respect of human rights in the context of HIV/AIDS and will incorporate human rights concerns in all its activities. Furthermore, we intend to develop a partnership between the public health community and the human rights community and to help ensure that human rights concerns are part of the national response to HIV/AIDS in every country."

He went on to add that :

"...the epidemic has forced us to reconsider what 'public health' means in the context of transmissible diseases and what it means as a valid limitation on human rights. Many of the drastic measures that have historically been directed against sick people in the name of public health are clearly *not* appropriate or useful in the context of HIV/AIDS. Only now are these measures being challenged on the basis of human rights. Thus, there is a need to clarify the meaning of the public health limitation on human rights and to subject it to the human rights scrutiny it deserves."

Before many years ago, the Lancet published an editorial that contained the following affirmation: "Public-health legislation and related measures have probably done more than all the advances of scientific medicine to promote the well-being of the community in Britain and in most other countries."[10]

To what extent has legislation on HIV/AIDS in Europe helped to stem and contain the spread of HIV/AIDS since 1983? The time is probably, not yet ripe to give an authoritative response to this crucial question. What is obvious is that many, in Europe and elsewhere, will have much to contribute in the years to come in delivery what role legislation has played, in protecting the blood supply and in combating discrimination. It is obvious that at least in some countries, the political dilemmas described by Rita Sussmuth, a former Minister of Health of the Federal Republic of Germany (1986-1988) and President of Bundestag, are still on the agenda. In a special issue of the UNESCO Courier (June 1995) devoted to AIDS, Sussmuth raised the following question: Can the epidemic be contained more effectively by coercion or by a liberal policy based on education and individual responsibility?

It is important that there is an international consensus, indeed a powerful consensus, that the second of these alternatives is the optimal one at this point of time and for the foreseeable future. In other words, most would be in agreement with the affirmation by Porter that "History says no to the policeman's response to AIDS."[11]

References

1. W Eberback. Rechtsprobleme der HTLV-III-Infektion (AIDS). Berlin (West): Springer-Verlag 1986.
2. Many of the important items of legislation on the control of HIV/AIDS referred to in this article have been reported in the WHO quarterly journal, the *International Digest of Health Legislation*. The reader is also referred to *Legislative Responses to AIDS*. Dordrecht and Boston: Martinus Nijhoff, 1989. Furthermore, reference should be made to the regularly updated listing, produced by WHO, entitled "Tabular information on legal instruments dealing with HIV infection and AIDS" (the current version of this document, WHO/GPS/HLE/94.1 was produced in July 1994).
3. Cattrorini P *et al. Comparison and Analysis of European Legislation on AIDS from the Ethical and Legal Standpoint* Milan: International Research Centre on Ethical, Legal and Forensic-Medical Questions Related to AIDS and Scientific Institute H. San Raffaele. In preparation.
4. Kirp DL, Bayer R., eds. *AIDS in the Industrialized Democracies: Passions, Politics, and Policies*. New Brunswick, NJ: Rutgers University Press, 1992.
5. Swiss Institute of Comparative Law, *Comparative Study on Discrimination Against Persons with HIV or AIDS*. Strasbourg: Council of Europe, 1993.
6. Foyer J, Khaiat L, eds. Droit *et Sida: Cmparaison Internationale*. Paris: CNRS Editions, 1994.
7. Manuel C., San Marco J-L, eds. *Sida: Les Enjeux Ethiques*. Paris: Doin Editeurs, 1994.
8. Feuillet-le Mintier B ed. *Le SIDA: Aspects Juridiques*. Paris: Economica, 1995.
9. Brandt EN. Implications of the Acquired Immunodeficiency Syndrome for health policy. *Annals of Internal Medicine* 1985; 103:771-3.
10. Anonymous. [Editorial] *The Lancet* 1978; 2:354-5
11. Porter R. *British Medical Journal* 1986; 293:1589-90.

Fifteen

Economic Impacts of the HIV/AIDS on Overseas Contract Workers in Philippines

Introduction

In mitigating the domestic unemployment problems, overseas work has been playing a major role on Filipino work force. From the OCW's Filipino is getting 8 per cent of Foreign Exchange. It is important that HIV/AIDS epidemic has created macro economic and macro eonomic problems on the OCW's in Philippines and in the long run it may reduce the inflow of foreign remittance.

Filipino overseas contract workers (OCW's) are very much significant to the Philippine economy. The men and women employed overseas belong to the most productive age group stands for substantial amounts of human capital. Their deployment overseas represents an effective methods against widespread unemployment and underemployment in the Philippines. Moreover, for an economy strapped by huge balance of payments deficits, their remittances are an important source of foreign exchange reserves.

Though, the burden that goes with being able to perform their economic role weighs heavily upon the OCW's: while seeking jobs abroad, they are always exploited by unscrupulous recruiters; abroad, they are subject to victimize by employers; and their dislocation into disparate cultural environments subjects them to physical and emotional stress. The Philippine Department of Health has recognized that one of the most serious risks OCWs face was the HIV and AIDS. In the Philippines, of the 335 persons found as sero-positive, 39 had been employed, and contracted the HIV, overseas.

HIV infection and AIDS among OCWs inflicted three types of costs on the Philippine economy: (a) the costs representing the resources used to provide medical care and the income fallen down as workers fall ill and die of AIDS; (b) the external costs imposed by those infected with the HIV and AIDS who knowingly or unknowingly disseminate the virus to others; and (c) the inefficiencies enforced by HIV infection and AIDS on the labour market as workers find working abroad less desirable and as overseas employers remodelled their recruitment efforts to less risky pools of labour. The first set of costs is common to all incurable diseases, while the second set is a feature of communicable diseases. The third type of costs is lone to the AIDS epidemic and the OCW sector of the Philippine labour market. It is very much important because such costs are expressed in terms of reduced foreign exchange inflows.

HIV/AIDS among Filipino OCWs

As per official records in 1991 as many as 476,693 Filipinos were deployed as overseas contract workers. But, media reports suggest that the actual numbers are double than the official figures if one includes those who leave without going through official channels. Filipino OCWs represent 2 to 5 per cent of their working age population. Over the years the number of OCWs has been increasing, especially as new markets have opened up. As per the Table 1 over half are in the Middle East, a market that opened up in the 1970s, about a third are in Asian countries, a market that only opened up in the 1980s.

According to the National Statistics Office data (table 2) that men OCWs outnumbered women OCWs 1.5 to 1. Among men, the thirty to thirty-nine age group has the highest stint among workers (38 per cent), followed by the twenty to twenty-nine age group (26 per cent). The revert process have taken place among women OCWs where 47 per cent fall in the Twenty to twenty-nine age group and 33 per cent are in the thirty to thirty-nine age group. From both men and women, over 70 per cent of OCWs belong to the twenty to thirty-nine age group, which constitute the most economically productive age group.

Not only are OCWs of prime age, they also contained considerable amounts of human capital. As per the available data the level of education among OCWs reveals that 61 per cent graduated from high school, while about 55 per cent had some college-level training.

TABLE 1

NUMBER OF FILIPINO OCWs BY REGION, 1984-1991

Region	*1984*	*1985*	*1986*	*1987*	*1988*	*1989*	*1990*	*1991*
Africa	1,843	1,977	1,847	1,856	1,958	1,741	1,273	1,964
Americas	2,515	3,744	4,035	5,614	7,902	9,962	9,557	13,373
Asia	38,817	52,838	72,536	90,434	92,648	86,196	90,768	132,592
Europe	3,683	4,067	3,693	5,643	7,614	7,830	6,853	13,156
Middle East	250,210	253,867	236,434	272,038	267,035	241,081	218,110	302,825
Oceania	913	953	1,080	1,271	1,397	1,247	942	1,374
Trust Territories[a]	2,397	3,048	3,892	5,373	6,563	7,289	7,380	11,409
Total	300,378	320,494	323,517	382,229	385,117	355,346	334,883	476,693

a. The Trust Territories of the Pacific Islands consist of more than 2,000 islands administered by the United States under a United Nations strategic-area trusteeship.

Source: Philippine Overseas Employment Agency data.

TABLE 2

OCWs BY AGE AND GENDER, OCTOBER 1991

(in thousands)

Age group	*Both sexes*	*Men*	*Women*
15-19	17.4	1.4	16.1
20-24	102.0	36.5	65.5
25-29	147.5	77.0	70.5
30-34	143.4	86.1	57.2
35-39	115.2	77.9	37.3
40-44	92.3	69.5	22.9
45 and over	103.3	81.7	21.6
Total	721.1	430.1	291.1

Note: The total number of OCWs is higher than that shown in table 1 as the figures above include both legal and illegal workers.

Source: Highlights of the October 1991 *Survey on Overseas Workers.*

Overseas employment is not only an important outlet for unemployment and underemployment pressures, it is also an important source of foreign exchange for an economy facing chronic balance of payments problems. Dollar remittances have been increasing steadily despite falling wages abroad. Filipino workers in North America account for the biggest share of remittances, followed by those from the Middle East and Europe. The share of remittances in total dollar inflow to the Philippines increased from 3 per cent in 1984 to close to 8 per cent in 1991.

The first case of HIV in the Philippines was found in 1984, and by June 1992, 335 cases had been reported. According to the latest reports by the Philippine Department of Health indicated that as many as 4,000 to 7,000 Filipinos may be infected.

TABLE 3
OCWs' REMITTANCES BY REGION AND TYPE OF WORKER, 1989-1991

(US$ thousands)

Region	*1989*	*1990*	*1991*
Asia	74,918	75,321	86,487
Sea-based	22,316	19,112	36,062
Land-based	52,602	56,209	50,425
Africa	33	25	18
Sea-based	2	0	0
Land-based	31	25	18
Americas	474,532	799,823	1,162,480
Sea-based	131,072	210,798	276,466
Land-based	343,460	589,025	886,014
Europe	48,310	92,677	109,483
Sea-based	14,351	39,225	57,223
Land-based	33,959	53,452	52,260
Middle East	129,362	105,362	101,977
Sea-based	1,672	997	739
Land based	127,690	104,365	101,238
Oceania	24,544	19,673	5,144
Sea-based	79	603	78
Land-based	24,465	19,070	5,066
Others[b]	221,367	88,194	34,702
Sea-based	48,323	16,938	4,658
Land based	173,044	71,256	30,044
Total	973,066	1,181,075	1,500,291

Source: Foreign Exchange Regulations Department, Central Bank of the Philippines.

Based on reported HIV and AIDS cases, sexual relations are the main way of transmission in the Philippines in which 50 per cent heterosexual, 13 per cent homosexual, and 5 per cent bisexuals. Unlike in Thailand, less than 1 per cent of reported cases in the Philippines contracted the virus through intravenous drug use. Some 33 per cent of patients believed that they had contracted the virus abroad, 46 per cent believed that they were infected in the Philippines.

As per the 335 reported cases, 166 are men and 169 are women. While the number of cases among men showed a steadly upward trend, the trend among women is erratic (table 4). This observation may be due to underreporting by women owing to the greater social stigma borne by female patients.

The average age of sero-positive individuals in the Philippines is almost thirty, twenty-seven for women and thirty-two for men. Of the reported cases, over 70 per cent are in the twenty to thirty-nine age group (table 5).

A major portion of those persons reported as being HIV-positive or diagnosed as having AIDS are relatively skilled. Among 59 per cent are professionals, managers, and sales, service, and production workers (table 6).

TABLE 4
NUMBER OF HIV/AIDS CASES BY GENDER, 1984-1992

Date diagnosed	*Men*	*Women*	*Total*
1984	2	0	2
1985	3	7	10
1986	4	25	29
1987	12	26	38
1988	16	18	34
1989	20	19	39
1990	29	38	67
1991	54	25	79
1992[a]	26		37
Total	166	169	335

a. January-June
Source: Field Epidemiology Training Program, Department of Health.

TABLE 5
NUMBER OF HIV/AIDS CASES BY AGE, 1984-1992

Age group	*1984*	*1985*	*1986*	*1987*	*1988*	*1989*	*1990*	*1991*	*1992*
Under 15	0	0	0	0	1	0	1	0	0
15-19	0	0	1	2	2	1	1	6	0
20-24	0	3	14	12	5	7	18	16	7
25-29	0	2	6	9	7	11	16	17	6
30-34	1	1	2	2	5	8	11	12	5
35-39	0	2	2	4	2	6	1	10	4
40-44	0	2	1	2	1	3	5	1	2
45 and over	0	0	3	7	11	3	14	17	13
Total	1	10	29	38	34	39	67	79	37

a. January-June.
Source: Field Epidemiology Training Program, Department of Health.

TABLE 6
NUMBER OF HIV/AIDS CASES BY MAJOR OCCUPATIONAL CATEGORY, 1984-1992

Major Occupational Category	*1984*	*1985*	*1986*	*1987*	*1988*	*1989*	*1990*	*1991*	*1992*[a]
Professional, technical, and related workers	1	0	1	1	5	4	8	6	4
Entertainers	0	8	26	22	0	3	6	7	0
Managers, executives, and administrative workers	1	0	0	1	9	0	0	0	0
Clerical workers	0	0	0	1	0	1	1	2	0
Sales workers	0	0	0	0	0	0	0	0	0
Service workers	0	0	1	2	4	3	12	9	7
Farmers, loggers, and related workers	0	0	0	0	0	0	0	0	0
Production and process workers	0	0	0	3	0	2	8	2	0

Note: Figures do not add up to total HIV/AIDS cases (335) because some HIV-positive individuals (housewives, retirees, children, and so on) were not employed at the time of diagnosis, while the rest did not record their occupations in the AIDS registry.

a. January-June.
Source: Field Epidemiology Training Program, Department of Health.

An astonishing pattern that emerged from the profile of Filipino OCWs and sero-positive individuals is that both are in their prime economically productive and sexually active age and both possess skills that permitted mobility between the domestic and international labour markets.

In 1984, two persons were found as having HIV, one of them an OCW. As of June 1992, 39 (or 12 per cent) of the 335 reported HIV-positive persons clasified that they had been working abroad and believed they had contracted the disease there. According to a report by the Research Institute of Tropical Medicine of the Philippine Department of Health on a study of blood samples ranked OCWs are more affected HIV-positive than prostitutes.

Filipinos working abroad are at risk of contracting the HIV for different reasons. First, many of them work in occupations considered high risk wherever they are employed, for example, entertainers and service workers, some of whom probably work as prostitutes. Second, those with doubtfully authenticated travel papers and work permits have subjected to various forms of sexual abuse and exploitation. A number of female workers are reported to have increase succumbed to sexual exploitation for job security or to increase their salaries, which fall short of what they actually contracted for. Third, workers abroad, especially sea-based workers, may be prone to engaging in high risk sexual activities by hiring prostitutes, having homosexual relations, or having multiple partners because of being separated from their families for long periods and being exposed to different cultural environments.

Impacts of HIV/AIDS on Economy

The family or household is the best place to begin examining the economic consequences of a disastrous illness such as AIDS. The typology of economic effects serves as an excellent framework for assessing the cost of HIV infection and AIDS for two major reasons: (a) it is based on the timing of economic effects; and (b) it explicitly taken into account the cost of household coping mechanisms, if it is avoided would underestimate the economic impact of the disease.

According to the table 7, costs are already incurred before infection. The direct costs including the cost of avoidance and preventive measures, and the indirect costs which included those associated with changes in occupational choice, which in the case of OCWs is whether to seek employment at home or abroad.

TABLE 7
A TYPOLOGY OF ECONOMIC CONSEQUENCES OF HIV/AIDS

	Timing of impact			
Type of Impact	*Before infection*	*Period of latency*	*During illness*	*Death and after*
Direct	Cost of avoidance and preventive measures	Cost of testing and out-patient care	Cost of in-patient care	Funeral costs
Indirect	Occupational choice	Reduced productivity of ill member	Reduced productivity of ill member	Reallocation of labour and other productive assets
	Precautionary savings	Changes in consumption and investment	Changes in consumption and investment	Changes in consumption and investment
	Insurance	Reallocation of labour for health maintenance	Reallocation of labour for health maintenance	Poor health of surviving family members, e.g., perinantal transmission
		Cost to others infected by the afflicted individual	Distility of infected individual to other family members	
		Distility of infected individual to other family members		

Source: Over and others (1991).

Once people are infected with the HIV and enter the period of latency, they should incur a number of costs. Direct costs included expenses on testing and out-patient care. The indirect costs included reduced productivity of the infected household member, transform consumption and investment patterns in anticipation of future medical expenditures, reallocation of family labour supply to maintain the sick person and to compensate for the lost income and the psychological costs to the infected individual and to other family members.

The major cost that could materialize during the period of latency, particularly if individuals are unaware that they are infected, is the external cost to others to whom the infection is transmitted. Upon returning home, these OCWs are giving the disease through sexual relations with their spouses or partners. Certainly, HIV infection and AIDS will spread much faster than if the OCW took this social cost into account.

At the time of illness, in-patient care is the main item of direct cost. Indirect costs will include reduced productivity or complete loss of the sick family member's income and the cost of labour supply adjustments by other household members, not only to maintain the sick person, but to compensate for the lost income. Such losses are expressed in terms of incomes foregone because of reduced human capital investment as family members left school to join the labour market.

After the death of the AIDS patient, the direct costs include funeral expenses, legal fees, and other related expenditures. Indirect costs include those associated with more permanent reallocation of labour and other productive assets, transform consumption and investment patterns, and possibly poorer well-being of surviving family members as the level of household income is reduced in absolute terms.

Sixteen

HIV/AIDS in North Africa, the Horn of Africa and the Eastern Mediterranean Area

North Africa and the eastern Mediterranean area gave us a two different epidemiological pictures. In the Horn of Africa as well as Southern Sudan, like sub-Saharan Africa pattern of HIV transmission is high in some communities. So far as the other parts of the region is concerned, lack of information is available, the magnitude of the transmission of HIV has not been well documented.

Worst affected are the huge territories of Ethiopia and Sudan parts of the Maghreb, and Djibouti. The first International Arab Conference in March 1988 on AIDS held in Egypt come to the conclusion by many countries in the region that risk factors seen elsewhere in the world—social instability and poverty, commercial sex, drug injecting and homosexual behaviour between men—existed in their populations and that the mobility of people in a region where so many migrants in search of work or education denotes that no country can be isolated from the threat.

Till mid-1993, less than 1400 AIDS cases had been reported to WHO, with only one country reporting no cases. There are considerable under-recognition and under-reporting in many countries, otherwise the actual number of cases is considered to be much higher. From statistics, it has been drawn that 75% are in males and 25 per cent in females, the majority due to sexual transmission.

A booming sex industry has established itself in and around the busy Red Sea port of Djibouti, as women fleeing crippling poverty and war in neighbouring countries found a chance to make a living. According to Djibouti's national AIDS programme in January 1993, the clients of street prostitutes serve to be local men, while the bar girls cater for foreign sailors and military men and the local elite. As per the analysis, HIV infection rates of 51 per cent have been found among street prostitutes, 22 per cent among bar girls, and 12 per cent among men attending STD clinics.

In southern Sudan, where civil war torn apart much of the population, the HIV/AIDS problem continues to grow. The number of AIDS cases reported in 1991 was 40 per cent higher than the 1990's. Heterosexual intercourse was reported in 1991 as being the main cause of transmission behind 94 per cent of cases. In southern Sudan relationships between the sexes are traditionally less confined than in the Muslim north, but even in some northern population groups premarital sex is considered as a means of testing the fertility of girls and increasing the population.

In the northern city of Khartoum, the Sudanese capital where all donated blood is tested the proportion of HIV/infected samples increased tenfold between 1987 and late 1992.

Though efforts are being made to guarantee safe blood supplies in major hospitals throughout Sudan, severe shortages of facilities, equipment and materials mean that only about 30 per cent of donated blood is tested for HIV. Tests conducted before 1990 on 33 recipients of blood established that 16 had contracted the virus. Varying levels of transmission through contaminated blood have been also been reported in Algeria, Egypt, Libyan Arab Jamahirya, Islamic Republic of Iran, and Tunisia.

Ethiopia, which has a long border and many social problems with Sudan, is probably open about its epidemic. "We have here the same preconditions for a rapid spread of AIDS as existed in Uganda: civil war, the displacement of people, a deteriorating economy," says Dr Mekonnen Bishaw, head of social science at Addis Ababa University. "All the conditions exist for an explosion of HIV infection and it's very worrying."

Till end of 1991, Ethiopia had reported 1631 cases of AIDS. But serosurveys in urban centres have established extremely high levels of HIV infection in certain population groups, and by 1993 the Ministry of Health was using a working estimate of close to half a million infections.

The much-affected population groups in Ethiopia, which has a population of around 50 million, are female prostitutes and their clients. At least 2,00,000 women are found to survive through prostitution, most of them from northern rural areas where poverty, war, drought and famine have driven them away from the land. The majority are little educated and unskilled, but even educated women are employed in bars and brothels as the economy deteriorates.

Members of the armed forces accounted for 17 per cent of the AIDS cases reported in Ethiopia until 1991, twice the proportion accounted for by female prostitutes. The national AIDS programme felt that infection rates will rise sharply in rural areas—where the majority of Ethiopia's population lives—as soldiers from what was Africa's biggest army return home, after the long civil war, to become farmers.

Among long distance lorry drivers, HIV infection rates were reached 15-20 per cent as long ago as 1990. Most drivers travel the main road between Addis Ababa and the port city of Assab, presently in Eritrea. Cases of AIDS and HIV infection are growing together all along this route in towns full of hotels and bars supplying for a highly mobile population of merchants, businessmen and other travellers.

The administration of injections by unqualified health practitioners are contributing to HIV transmission. Ethiopian people, especially rural people, using injections to be more effective than tablets, says Dr Hailu Negassa of the Department of AIDS Control. Many community health agents or traditional birth attendants—or even just cleaners at hospitals who have accessed to supplies of needles and syringes—have set up private clinics to exploit this belief. "These people are accepted by their communities and we think it is a problem," says Negassa.

Injecting drug use plays major role in the spread of HIV in the Maghreb countries of North Africa, which have strong historic and economic links with Europe. In Tunisia, needle-sharing accounted for around three-quarters of AIDS cases in 1992, most of which have reportedly occurred among Tunisians who visited Europe for work or study. Very much information is not available on AIDS in Mauritania, but there are thought to be many drug users at high risk of infection. An HIV prevalence of about 14 per cent was found among injecting drug users known to police authorities in one gulf state in 1989.

The abundance of men among injecting drug users helps

explain why, among the region's AIDS cases, men outnumber women. Open sex between men is another factor. However, in parts of the world where homosexual and bisexual behaviour is condemned, it is important to get information about this transmission route in a useful way.

Of the approximately 1500 HIV infections among resident and immigrant expatriates found over the past seven years in one Gulf State, one-third were found to have occurred during 1992 alone, showing the rapid evolution of the epidemic in the region.

Although some countries of the region affirmed that AIDS would never be a major problem for them because the cultural and moral values of their societies are no longer conducive to the spread of HIV many countries demonstrate great willingness and determination to confront the epidemic. A positive sign is that religious leaders have more aware in response to AIDS, and many advocate a compassionate attitude towards people with the disease. It is also promoting that where religious and cultural sensibilities limit frank discussion about sexuality and make it difficult for officials to promote condoms, independent, non-governmental groups have sprung up to take action.

Sex Work and Begging

Berhane, a fragile woman in her mid-twenties, works in a bar in Nazareth, Ethiopia, serving "tej"—a thick yellow alcoholic drink made from honey. She was married at the age of nine. After her children died at the ages of four and two, she fled rural poverty and an abusive husband for the city, where work as a barmaid was all she could find. As the bar owner gives only board and lodging in return for her work, cash has to be earned through prostitution. "This life is not much better than what I ran away from, but what can I do?" she says. "At least it's better than begging."

Almaz also chose sex work as the only alternative to begging. Moving from the north to live with relatives in Addis Ababa on the death of her parents, she had to drop out of school when her aunt there died. She works at the lower end of the sex industry in a "red light"—a tiny rented room which is also her home. All along the narrow alleyway, doors open on similar dingy rooms. Outside, young women in colourful dresses chat, comb their hair, lean against the door-jambs and wait for clients.

Seventeen

Review/Reform of HIV/AIDS Law in Malaysia

Introduction

Government policies on issues related to HIV and AIDS can enhance or hinder AIDS control and care activities. For example, insufficient educational and economic opportunities may cause increase in the number of those who provide sexual services for money. Lack of confidentiality may generate barriers for those who intends to start preventive measures or seek early diagnosis and treatment of AIDS and other STDs.

Legislation Process

HIV infection, a disease attached with certain behaviours, has a major socio-cultural impact on the affected community. The development of effective responses to the epidemic need policies and measures which generate an environment that enables, encourages and sustains voluntary behaviour change, care and support of those affected. This can be achieved by empowering individuals and communities to protect themselves against HIV and ensuring that people living with HIV remain integrated within society, are free from discrimination, and are participating during the process of policy formulation.

In fact, the key objectives of preventing the spread of disease as well as limiting the impact of HIV infection on individuals, groups and societies cannot be achieved without the active support, cooperation and involvement of many agencies and organizations both in the public and private sectors. This includes people affected by the epidemic, the communities, and the legal, health and other professions. To strengthen the process of consultation, cooperation and collaboration, both formal and informal consultative structures need to be established. Informal consultative activities such as seminars, workshops and conferences can facilitate the formulation of more enhanced policies tied together with the viewpoints of all affected parties. Such policies stand for result oriented implementation and are less likely to meet with resistance. The recommendations of these informal consultative activities are generally discussed in formal national level committees for further action. A top level formal consultative structure can make a significant contribution to the efficacy of an AIDS control and prevention programme. This could overcome barriers among members by enhancing mutual understanding. This can be achieved because deliberations and consultations take place during discussions of some particular issues or policies. Multisectoral national committees can also create synergy, which is sometimes available only through sharing or joint working, for example, reducing service gaps. Through outreach services, the NGOs complement governmental efforts in preventing HIV/AIDS because they have strong tie-ups with individuals and groups in the communities, particularly those at high risk. These committees can act as coordinating bodies to avoid unnecessary duplication, maximizing the contribution of each agency and ensuring optimum use of skills and resources.

Administrative Reforms on AIDS

The government is responsible for announcing the national policies that can develop the framework within which intervention activities for HIV/AIDS take place. However, multisectoral involvement, cooperation and consultation are essential for the development of policies which reflect the needs and interests of various communities and individuals. Before contemplating the setting up of new and autonomous administrative structures, the government should take into account the strengthening present structures.

As far as the Malaysia is concerned, it was decided that the prevention and control of AIDS should be correlated into the existing medical and health services handed over through various outlets, i.e., through all government hospitals and health centres. Recognizing that a top level multisectoral national committee is generally the most effective way to achieve multisectoral involvement, cooperation and consultation, a committee chaired by the Director of Health was constituted in the Ministry of Health in April 1985. Later, the committee was renamed as 'The AIDS Task Force'. The Task Force has empowered to formulate the policies and to coordinate the AIDS prevention and control programme. A total of 28 members stands for various organizations – including Ministry of Education, Ministry of Information, Ministry of Youth and Sports, Prime Minister's Department, armed forces, Religious Department, universities, various medical bodies, the health sector, as well as non-government organizations-are on the committee. Serving the Task Force are several standing and *ad hoc* committees. For each state, a state coordinating committee on AIDS has been formed and made responsible for the implementation and coordination of AIDS prevention and control activities.

In 1992 a ministerial level committee on AIDS, chaired by the Minister of Health, was established by the Cabinet. Its members include the Ministers of Information, Education, National Unity and Social Development, Justice and Law, Culture, Art and Tourism, Youth and Sports, Home Affairs as well as staff attached with Prime Minister's Department. The role of this committee is to advise the Cabinet on all matters relating to the prevention, control and management of HIV/AIDS in the country, and also to facilitate inter-ministerial coordination in this area.

In September 1993, the Health Division was restructured and a Section on AIDS/STD was officially established within the Disease Control Division. As a result the AIDS Task Force was reconstituted into two main committees, i.e., the National Technical Committee and the National Coordinating Committee on AIDS. One of the functions of the AIDS Section is to assist as a secretariat to the ministerial level Committee, National Technical Committee, National Coordinating committee, and several national level subcommittees. The staff of the AIDS Section consisting of five public health doctors, two health education officers, and two assisting personnel.

The National Technical Committee, chaired by the Director-General of Health, is responsible for the formulation, controlling and evaluation of policies and the review and approval of recommendations made by various subcommittees on technical matters pertaining to the prevention, control and management of HIV/AIDS. The members include chairmen of various subcommittees, representatives of various technical programmes, directors of the Ministry of Health, universities, and representative of various professional bodies.

The National Coordinating Committee chaired by the Secretary-General of Health consisting of the secretaries-general of various ministeries including those of Information, Education, National Unity and Social Development, Justice and law, Culture, Art and Tourism, Youth and Sports, Home Affairs and the Prime Minister's Department, as well as the Deputy Secretary-General of Health, both finance and services, and the Legal Advisor to the Ministry of Health. This committee gives a platform for intersectoral consultations and discussions on social, cultural, religious, legal and other related issues. This committee also appoints working groups to review specific problems evaluate and approve the recommendations of various sub-committees.

Coordination with NGOs

The Ministry of Health in its effort to strengthen collaboration and consultation with NGOs working with HIV/AIDS problems responded to their call to help in the formation of the Malaysian AIDS Council (MAC), which was registered with the Registrar of Societies in July 1992. The Malaysian AIDS Council is an umbrella organization which collaborates AIDS-related NGOs. The Council's educational, preventive and care activities complement, supplement and assist the government's efforts. Among the coordinated projects and AIDS- related activities of its affiliates are submission of project proposals to the Ministry of Health for financial help and managing approved funds channelled through the council. The main important function is their participation in the national level committees and subcommittees representing the organizations, groups and individuals whose interests need to be taken into account.

Its affiliates are both AIDS specific NGOs and non-AIDS specific NGOs that have incorporated the AIDS agenda into their existing project structures. The Malaysian AIDS Council has a membership of 22 NGOs consisting various community based groups, health and legal professional associations, religious organizations, organizations addressing the needs of women and children, and social marketing affiliates, which are helped in various AIDS prevention and care efforts.

Eighteen

Threat of AIDS and its Prevention in Singapore

HIV/AIDS in Singapore

By 31 December 1994, 308 Singaporeans were reported to be HIV infected. Among them, 44 were AIDS cases 180 were asymptomatic carriers, and 84 have died. The number of reported cases of patients has raised since the first HIV infected Singaporean was found-from 2 cases in 1985 to 17 cases in 1990 and 86 cases in 1994.

Different ways of HIV Infection Among Singaporeans

Out of 308 HIV infected Singaporeans 295 (95.8 per cent) contracted the venereal disease, 7 (2.3 per cent) by intravenous drug use, 4 (1.3 per cent) through renal transplant overseas, 1 (0.3 per cent) through blood transfusion overseas and 1 (0.3 per cent) through the prenatal route. Since 1991, heterosexual contact has become the most common channel of HIV transmission among Singaporeans. In 1994, it accounted for more than 72 per cent cases of HIV transmission. Most people have contracted the infection through casual sex with prostitutes in Singapore and overseas.

The AIDS Patients in Singaporeans

Out of the 308 Singaporeans who have been detected to be HIV positive, 281 (91.2 per cent) were males and 27 (8.8 per cent) were females. At the time of diagnosis, 78 per cent were between the ages of 20 and 39 years. Moreover they were mostly single (71 per cent). Only 21 per cent were married, while the rest were either widowed or divorced.

National AIDS Prevention Programme in Singapore

The control and prevention of AIDS comes under the purview of the Ministry of Health with the active involvement of other

Government Agencies and community groups fighting against AIDS in Singapore. The National AIDS Control Programme came into force effect 1985.

The programme addresses issues dealing with:

- Education for all
- Legislation
- Protection of the national blood supply through routine checking of blood and blood products
- Take care of the infected
- Counselling those with high risk of infection
- Monitoring the disease
- Conducting Training to the personnel
- Conducting research and studies.

Two Committees were introduced to help the programme: the National Advisory Committee on AIDS, which gives community feedback on the AIDS education programme, and the AIDS Task Force, which advises the Ministry of Health on medical and scientific issues in connection with AIDS.

Legislation Process

While efforts were continuously being made to educate the public on HIV infection/AIDS, certain legal steps have also been taken to control the disease in the interest of both the infected as well as the general public. HIV infection and AIDS were made detectable diseases under the Infectious Diseases Act in 1985. To get more effective control of AIDS in Singapore, the Infectious Diseases Act was amended in 1992 and included the following provisions:

- The Director of Medical Services has the right to enjoin any person who has been diagnosed as having AIDS or being infected with HIV to go through counselling or to comply with the security measures.
- It is an offence for any person who intentionally commit any act which is likely to transmit the disease to another person, e.g., sexual intercourse with another person or donating blood at any blood bank in Singapore.

Moreover, the Infectious Diseases (Amendment) Act also keeps secretly the identity of a HIV infected person, so as to prevent discrimination against such person and encourage those who are at danger of infection to join with counselling and HIV testing.

Screening of the National Blood Supply

Strict and effective measures are being undertaken to safeguard the National Blood Supply from HIV infection and other blood-borne diseases. These measures include:

- Testing of blood and blood products for HIV, syphilis and Hepatitis B and C.
- Strict donor selection at the pre-donation stage is executed using a specially featured questionnaire. All potential donors are interviewed and have to follow a detailed questionnaire on past and present risk activities in connection with HIV infection. Persons at risk of such diseases are to exempt themselves from giving blood. The potential donor is then counselled by a doctor, after which he signs a declaration stating that he has not made a wrong statement. Offenders with wrong declarations may face prosecution. This is to prevent anyone indulging in high-risk behaviour from donating blood that may be infected. Singapore also has infrastructures for autologous blood donation to permit persons to store their own blood for elective operation. This measure has abolished the risk of a patient contracting blood borne diseases, such as AIDS, from other people's blood.

Managing the Infected

Individuals who perceive themselves to be at risk of infection are motivated to go through HIV test. Cases are managed at the Communicable Disease Centre by doctors and other staff who are expertised to handle such cases. Patients are counselled to ensure compliance with treatment, care and follow-up measures. All patients with AIDS/HIV infection are counselled regularly. Infected persons and their sex partners are counselled and screening is carried out for those who have been exposed to the infection. Person-to-person counselling is provided for those with dangerous behaviour. An AIDS Telephone Helpline was started in 1987 to made available personal counselling to the public. Recorded information on AIDS in the four major languages is also given.

Controlling the Situation

Surveillance of the AIDS situation in Singapore is based on the collated results of:

- Voluntary confidential blood diagnosis
- Screening of prostitutes.
- Unlinked sentinel surveillance of selected groups in the population at a higher risk of the infection, such as patients with venereal diseases, Hepatitis B and tuberculosis, and pregnant women.

Training Programme

The Ministry of Health works closely with other related ministries, community groups and international agencies in the training of personnel for the effective control of AIDS. All medical and paramedical personnel have been issued with 'Guidelines for Preventing Transmission of Blood-borne Infection in a Health Care Setting'. They are continuously reminded of the importance of effective infection control procedures based on global precautions.

Workshops have been held for prison and drug rehabilitation officers to give them awareness on AIDS, how to deal with infected inmates, and how to counsel those participating in high-risk activities. Teachers have been trained to organize educational programmes on AIDS/HIV infection for students in their schools and institutions.

Community Participation

A voluntary organization, Action for AIDS, Singapore, was started in 1988. Its operations complement the government's efforts in controlling AIDS. Its objectives are to organize educational activities in connection with AIDS and HIV infection; support welfare activities to avoid discrimination against patients and families; and promote research in areas related to HIV infection and AIDS.

Nineteen

Control of AIDS in Vietnam

Introduction

Since the first case of AIDS reported in 1990 in Vietnam the number of AIDS patients has drastically increased as of 30th March 1995, there were over 2,000 HIV positive cases, 131 AIDS cases and 54 deaths. Eventhough the attack reached into the South-East Asian country comparatively late, it is spreading very rapidly. If Vietnam does not implement timely and effective steps to stop its spread, it will have to shoulder a heavy social-economic burden.

The reason behind the HIV/AIDS infection in Vietnam is due to high rate of transmission through intravenous drug use tentatively (72.2 per cent). Transmission through illegal sexual relations accounts for only 4.4 per cent of the cases. Males have been disproportionately infected (86.1 per cent). The first measure taken by the Vietnam Government was to form Vietnamese National AIDS Committee (NAC) for the prevention and control of HIV/AIDS. The Minister for Health is its president. The NAC is changed with coordinating state bodies, social organizations and the public in preventive activities. A strategic policy on prevention and control of HIV/AIDS has been formulated by the Vietnam Government, incorporating short-term and long term plans which have been evolved out of the general policies of the international community. An important point stressed by the National Programme on prevention and control of HIV/AIDS is that HIV/AIDS is not merely a medical issue. To prevent the danger of the spread of HIV/AIDS, it is necessary to ensure the association with the social organizations, state bodies and community groups.

Legal Publications Connected to the Prevention and Control of HIV/AIDS

On 2nd December 1989, the Chairman of the Council of Ministers, in anticipation of the threat of HIV infection, issued instruction No. 339/CT, for the prevention and control of HIV/AIDS. In this document, he entrusted ministries, branches and provinces the responsibility of teaching the public about the effective measures necessary to prevent the disease.

The document also concentrates as the close observation of groups at high risk, such as prostitutes and intravenous drug adicts. Decree No. 16/CP, issued by the Vietnam Government on 18th December 1992, confirm the principle of non-discrimination towards HIV/AIDS patients. It also encouraged Vietnamese and expatriates to undergo HIV testing.

The Decree recognized the principle of right to confidentiality with regard to name, age and address and of the result of tests, if requested. Moreover, health institutions were responsible for testing for HIV blood and semen donors and donors of tissues or other organs.

Another important issue was the rights and obligations of persons infected with HIV/AIDS. The Decree provided that it is strictly forbidden for anyone who had HIV/AIDS infection to deliberately transmit the infection to others. They were responsible for protecting the community.

The Decree sets out the responsibilities of doctors and health staff. It also gives state incentives for them.

Legal Publications Indirectly Dealing with the Prevention and Control of HIV/AIDS

- Law on the protection of people's health provides for the compulsory treatment of infectious disease like AIDS which are transmitted through unsafe sex, drug use.
- Ordinance on immigration, residence and travel by expatriates in Vietnam provides the conditions for issuing visas, consistent with the prevention and control of diseases and the safety of the community.
- Ordinance on marriages between Vietnamese citizens and expatriates, issued by the Standing committee of the

National Assembly, provides the conditions, subject to which marriages can take place.

- Penal Code makes the violation of the rules of confidentiality in HIV testing an offence.

The Constitution includes a provision in Article 61 dealing with social evils such as prostitution and intravenous drug use. Their regulation could play a vital role in the prevention and control of HIV/AIDS. Resolution No. 05/CP deals with the control of prostitution and resolution 06/CP with the prevention, control and supervision of drug use.

The Vietnam Government has taken steps to abolish prostitution in any form, especially in cities and tourist and industrial centres. It has also introduced public awareness campaigns on the harmful impacts of prostitution, especially the transmission of HIV. The Government has given the changes to the ministries and its branches responsible for the prevention and control of drug abuse and prostitution the special task of controlling the spread of HIV.

Decree No. 53/CP announced by the Government provides for the stringent punishment to be taken against state employees especially directors of hotels and owners of restaurants, involved in prostitution and drug related crimes – e.g. they can be dismissed.

Legal Publications Relating to Professional Rules in Medical Settings

The Ministry of Health has announced regulations on blood transfusion and on treatment of HIV/AIDS infection. Health experts are responsible for consulting with HIV/AIDS infected people so as to enable them to understand their disease; for encouraging them to seek treatment and actively participate in communication strategies on the prevention and control of HIV/AIDS; and instructing the patients' families to take care of them and avoid discrimination.

Assessment

The Vietnam Government has taken various steps, including legal measures, for the prevention and control of HIV/AIDS.

While the legal publications released by the Government and its branches so far have, by and large, specially addressed the prevention and control of HIV/AIDS, these texts are not very effective or systematic. Vietnam badly needed laws promulgated by a legislative body, which address basic matters in the prevention and control of HIV/AIDS.

A draft Ordinance with advanced provisions to prevent and Control of HIV/AIDS infection is aimed at meeting these requirements. Its formulation has highlighted several difficulties, especially in balancing the rights of the individual against public interest in matters related to the prevention and control of HIV/AIDS. For example, concrete provisions were needed not only to satisfy the requirements of non-discrimination of the infected, but also to ensure the safety of the public.

Twenty

AIDS in Indonesia

Introduction

Indonesia is a country where the government had set up a National AIDS Commissions even before the first report of HIV infection came out. At present reports of AIDS patients, from 17 out of 27 provinces have become a threat to the country. Still the preventive programmes are in full swing. Widespread Commercial activity, like awareness of the seriousness of the disease and premarital and extra-marital affairs make the work of the Commission a challenge.

Report of AIDS from Indonesia

Indonesia's first report of AIDS infection came out in 1987. By February 1995, 69 cases of AIDS out of 282 HIV positive people had been identified. But according to WHO, there were 50,000-60,000 cases—this suggests that the increase has been far more dramatic. HIV epidemic in Indonesia seemed to be spread like in other Asian countries, i.e., appearing first in the homosexual community, and later in people in situations of risks, such as prostitutes, their clients and drug users. Incidentally, spread throughout the population, infecting both men and women. Most of the infected people (96 per cent) belong to the group of 15-49 years. Sexual transmission is the primary mode of infection. Eighty per cent of the cases seemed to be infected through this mode (55 per cent heterosexually and 25 per cent through homosexual and bisexual contact). Though the total number of reported HIV/ AIDS cases was regarded as very less, the reports have come out from 17 out of 27 provinces in Indonesia and which include all the socio-economic strata. Certain factors that lead to the sudden spread of HIV infection are present in Indonesia i.e., a widespread commercial sex industry, high rates of sexually transmitted diseases (STDs), low awareness of STD and HIV infection prevention, high labour migration, and the prevalence of premarital and extra-marital sexual activities.

Attempts to Control AIDS in Indonesia

In 1986, before the first report of AIDS case came out from Indonesia, the Indonesian Government formed the National AIDS Commission. It was reorganized into the AIDS Prevention and Control Commission in 1994 through a Presidential Decree. Coordinating Minister for People's Welfare, was the head of the Commission which included several ministers and other heads of government institutions. A National AIDS Strategy was put into practice in June 1994. It gives instructions on the framework and guidelines for all preventive and control activities.

The strategy states that the government should lead and guide the efforts and help create a supportive environment. Certain principles of the strategy, among others, are that all approaches should consider the religious and cultural values found in Indonesia; all activities should first of all aim to strengthen the resilience and welfare of the family and the traditional social back up systems rooted in the community; and that there should be no discrimination in helping the people living with HIV infection, whose dignity and self-respect should not be affected.

In February 1995 the strategy took an important step for the promotion of the concept of AIDS Conscious Prosperous Family. The government remarked that the HIV epidemic awareness campaign should begin with the family since it is the first and foremost institution which moulds people's attitudes and behaviours, including those pertaining to sexual matters. According to the Minister of Population, the number of AIDS conscious families to date is only 1,000-2,000, out of 40 million families (Kompas, 7 February 1995). Various programmes were put forth to increase this number.

Laws Relating to the HIV Epidemic in Indonesia

As the HIV epidemic in Indonesia was something there were only a few laws and regulations that directly deal with it. In 1987, when the first report of AIDS case came out, several ministries, and the President himself, have enacted various law and regulations relating to the HIV epidemic.

The Minister of Health (MOH) enacted Decree no. 484/1987 to form a National AIDS Committee in 1987. This Committee was limited to representatives from various sectors in the Ministry of Health. In 1988 the MOH designated HIV/AIDS as a notifiable infections disease and formed guidelines for the reporting of AIDS and HIV positive cases. In 1989 the MOH enacted a new Decree – no. 301/1989 – to reorganize the National AIDS Committee. The Director-General of Communicable Disease Control and Environmental Health of the MOH issued circular No. 5 of 3 January 1991 which put forth some guidelines to be followed by port health authorities, indicating that HIV/AIDS infection should not interfere with international/tourist travel.

The Director-General – in his capacity as Chairman of the National AIDS Committee-also issued Decree no. 61/1991 clearly stated on the appointment, within the National AIDS Committee, of technical advisory groups dealing with health education, case management, observation, laboratories and blood banks, and research in the same year. Between 1990 and 1992, some newly-enacted laws, e.g., Health Law and Immigration Law, had already covered the issue of HIV/AIDS. The Minister of Health put forth technical guidelines on the care of AIDS patient in the same year. In 1993-94, the President of the Republic of Indonesia issued a Presidential Decree on the National AIDS Prevention and Control Commission. The status of this Commission has been upgraded from ministerial level to the national level.

The Coordinating Minister for People's Welfare, in his capacity as the Chairman of the Indonesian National AIDS Commission, released the Indonesian National AIDS Strategy in July 1994. The strategy includes basic principles, programme areas, roles and responsibilities of the government and the community, international cooperation and financing. Another measure taken to control to the HIV epidemic is the Decree of the Coordinating Minister for People's Welfare/Chairman of the National AIDS Commission, No. 05, 22 February 1995, on the National HIV/AIDS Prevention and Control Programme for the Sixth Five year

Development Plan. The programme for 1995-99 included issues relating to information, education and communication, prevention measures, HIV testing and counselling, treatment, care and other health services, research and development, monitoring and evaluation, training, international cooperation, institutionalization, and laws and regulations. The section on each issue includes targets, strategies, activities, output indicators and coverage in units per year. Besides, these law and regulations that are directly related to the HIV epidemic, there are others which are indirectly related, e.g., the law on infectious disease control. Since it was enacted in 1984, HIV infection is not mentioned. Since the law, needed to be amended taking into considerations that the HIV epidemic is a new and spreading social issue that can, among other things, pose a threat to human rights. The legislative steps should include all the issues arising out of the prevention and services efforts, as well as ensure protection for the community.

The objectives of the Prevention Component of the National HIV/AIDS Prevention and Control Programme for the Sixth Five year Development Plan are: (a) to provide possible help and information for preventing the spread of HIV infection; (b) render help in preventing and controlling STDs; (c) to perform screening procedures to prevent HIV infection through blood and blood products; and (d) to provide medical services that implement universal precautions.

Legislation should be implemented to deal with particular issues such as the provision of STD diagnostic and treatment facilities; standard procedures for applying HIV prevention measures including universal precautions; the procedures for blood and blood products screening; and providing health services to AIDS patients. The services component of the National HIV Programme aims of (a) to provide facilities and continuing humane and non-discriminative treatment and care; (b) to ensure individual health and safety for those who help AIDS patients in health facilities; (c) to develop skills and commitment at the family and community level, in taking care of AIDS patients and (d) to make and develop laws and legislation connected to the standards of care and case management, which should be ethical, technically accurate, non-discriminatory and humane. Rules and regulations which may back these objectives include regulations on hospital standards of care for HIV/AIDS patients, non-discrimination in labour and education sectors, and on insurance system for AIDS patients.

To conclude, the upcoming reforms and new legislative texts should back the three approaches in the National AIDS Strategy: (a) religious and cultural approach, (b) family function approach, and (c) public health approaches, which acknowledge public interest as well as individual rights. All laws and regulations should ensure safety for the entire community having HIV/AIDS patients, the health providers, as well as the general community. However difficult it may be, efforts should be taken to balance public interest and individual rights. Ultimately, information on legal matters relating to HIV/AIDS should be made available among all levels of the government and its various sectors, and the general community all over the country. The role of the press is vital, as is of the law enforcement officers who should also be well-informed and skilled in facing legal cases relating to HIV/AIDS.

These measures should also include different issues arising from the implementation of the National of the National HIV Epidemic Prevention and Control Programme e.g. blood and blood products screening, blood testing help to AIDS infected babies and counselling.

Twenty One

AIDS in Cambodia

Introduction

Cambodia is a country having enough possibilities of intermingling of different people specially, because of its geographical factors. HIV infections was first detected among the blood donors in the country, and later among the sex workers. In 1994, 401 donors were reportedly found to HIV positive. A comprehensive plan has been done to prevent and control the menace in the country. Still some social taboos make the programmes unreachable to the mass.

Reports of AIDS from Cambodia

By January 1995, in the Cambodia more than 1,000 people have been reported as HIV infected. The first cases of AIDS in Cambodia were diagnosed in 1994. HIV infections were first reported among volunteer blood donors, when three donors tested positive for antibodies to HIV in Cambodia in 1991. Since then, each year the number has escalated in the numbers infected in this group. In 1994 alone, 401 donors were found to be HIV positive. This sudden increase in infected cases is also vivid among other groups such as sex workers.

Based on the available data it is estimated that at least 6,000 people in Cambodia may be HIV seropositive. Anyhow, this is considered to be a conservative estimate.

Major Factors

Cambodia is a country having huge shifts in populations, porous borders, socio-economic disruption and limited public services. These factors led to our increase in the sexually transmitted diseases which are seen as an indicator of HIV transmission.

According to Dr. Michael Merson, Executive Director of the Global Programme on AIDS, a comparison of HIV trends among blood donors makes it clear that Phnom Penh may experience an even larger epidemic than Chiang Mai, the worst-affected city in Thailand.

According to the available data the risk behaviour can be characterized as primarily sexual. As a result of economic liberalization, the influx of foreign businessmen, expanding tourism, increase in the number of relief and development personnel and United Nations Peace-Keeping Force (UNTAC), the sex trade has increased rapidly since 1991. In one commercial sex area only in Phnom Penh, it is estimated that there are about 1,000-2,000 workers. There are many other such easily identifiable smaller areas in Phnom Penh, besides certain locations such as bars, dance halls and massage parlours. Moreover there are many 'indirect' sex workers such as hotel workers, beer and cigarette promotion staff and peddlers also indulge in prostitution. Outside Phnom Penh the pattern is repeated with commercial sex work increasing in economic centres, most notably in the western provinces and in the ports of Sihanoukville and Koh Kong.

The United Nations International Drug Control Programme and the WHO Programme on Substance Abuse have got no ample evidence of a serious drug problem in Cambodia, they fear the capability for such a problem given the proximity of Cambodia to opium producing countries and development trends that could increase drug abuse in the years ahead (urban migration and a limited urban infrastructure and job market to absorb increases in the population).

Injections, as a mode of treatment of illness in Cambodia should be noted as a potentially major route for the transmission of HIV. Injections for treatment exceeds the availability of sterile needles and syringes making re-use without sterilization between patients. Also lack of barrier protection places could make a health personnel infected.

The National Blood Transfusion Centre started screening volunteer blood donors for antibodies to HIV in 1991. Provincial transfusion centres now work in nine provinces, but unscreened blood is still in used in certain parts of the country.

Measures Taken for AIDS Prevention and Control in Cambodia

Main Objectives

1. To lessen HIV transmission
2. To reduce the morbidity and mortality related to HIV infection

The National Plan stands for a nationwide effort to prevent and control HIV/AIDS. It addresses programme strategies and specific target areas of implementation for reducing HIV transmission and associated morbidity and mortality. Recommended by the World Health Organization's Global programme on AIDS to all countries with national AIDS programmes, the strategies have been adopted to the special needs of Cambodia. The Plan, which comes at an appropriate time, can be used to mobilize the large number of intergovernmental organizations working in Cambodia. There is good potential for a far-reaching and well-coordinated control programme.

The Plan aims at the following assessed needs for the period 1993-1998:

1. Prevention of sexual transmission.
2. Prevention of transmission through blood.
3. Prevention of perinatal transmission.
4. Surveillance for HIV/AIDS and STDs.
5. Socio-economic impact studies and research.
6. The care and management of HIV infected individuals.

Obstacles in Programme Implementation

As the primary mode of HIV transmission is sexual for prevention and control efforts issues concerning sex be addressed. Cultural and social taboos, however, inhibit open discussion on sexual matters among the population.

In Cambodia, these social taboos can affect the implementation of programme strategies critical to HIV transmission prevention and control such as encouraging the use of condoms, education campaigns for the general public and specific target groups, including commercial sex workers, and the care and management of venereal diseases.

Laws to Safeguard AIDS

As there exists no law or bill yet to safeguard the rights of AIDS patients, health education materials have been used to erase the fears, prejudices and misunderstandings among the general public. The message of compassion for the infected and of the sense of responsibility of the non-infected have been often stressed on TV, radio and other media. A STD clinic in the centre of a red-light area gives free STD care and health education information to commercial sex workers (CSWs)-this project was meant to send a signal to the public that CSWs should not be marginalized. Besides, the training at central and provincial level for health care workers is made to make them aware of the fact that mandatory testing before the provision of medical services is not useful; health care workers should, instead, follow the universal precautionary guidelines to keep away from HIV infection. National blood transfusion centres, while searching for blood donors, observe strict confidentiality regarding the identity of individuals found to be HIV positive and arrange for their counselling at the National STD Centre. Thus, besides legal measures, health education can play vital role in safeguarding the rights of HIV infected people and in preventing the spread of infection to the non-infected.

Furthermore, since 1993 the Kingdom of Cambodia has adopted a new Constitution which gives importance to human rights as defined in the Universal Declaration of Human Rights, and the conventions on human rights and the rights of women and children. Anyhow, future laws related to HIV to be adopted by the national bodies cannot be in contravention of the national constitution which is the greatest law of the land.

Twenty Two

Ethical Legal Aspects of HIV/AIDS in Thailand

Introduction

Thai Society was subjected to increasing dilemmas due to the advent of HIV/AIDS. As a corollary to an estimated half a million (out of 60 million) of the populace having HIV/AIDS infections, have generated controversies not only of the epidemiological nature but also the socio-economical, political-legal consequences. Problems created by poverty, discrimination, budgetary tug-of-war, and the presence of draconian practice make it explicit that HIV/AIDS is not simply a medical disease. It is also a socio-economic and political disease. From the angle of law, HIV/AIDS is unmarking loopholes and pitfalls as never before. In a word, HIV/AIDS is equally a "legal" disease.

The law stands for and its interrelationship with ethics pose many challenges to the dimension of HIV/AIDS. On another front, existing laws seem to be remedial by nature. More often than not, they address grievances after the event, rather than provide for preventive action. Sanctions against different acts abound in the legislation available, but they fail to tackle the root causes of the problem. While many laws seek to proscribe and punish, there is a paucity of laws and related measures that seek to help, protect, and check.

Laws Concerning Public Health

The Infectious Diseases Act 1980, provides for broad discretion on the part of the medical authorities to implement steps, even those verging on the draconian. By section 8, the authorities are empowered to order infected persons to appear for examination, to detain them, and to order ways of protection, such as orders to desist from action which may lead to the spread of the disease (including sexual intercourse). Non-compliance may lead to fines. Under Section 10, the Minister of Public Health or provincial governors may cause infected persons to quit their job. Violations of these orders may lead to fines and/or imprisonment.

Thailand Case

Succeeding legislation, under the umbrella of the 1970 Act dealt with the question of reporting and notification. By ministerial announcements of 1985 and 1986, AIDS was mentioned as one of the "the diseases requiring notification," indicating that householders, doctors in charge of hospitals, or the equivalent had to report news on infected persons to the health authorities within twenty four hours of discovering the illness or suspicion of illness. Fines could be imposed on those who do not report such cases. This obligation overrode the general confidentiality principle related to doctors and patients discussed below.

It is clear from this Act and subordinate legislation that at the time when AIDS was numbered as one of "the diseases requiring notification," the public health authorities had broad powers to subject those with AIDS to their discretion, including coercion and draconian measures. Later on in 1991 AIDS was detected from the list of diseases requiring notification. These were in conflict with international human rights standards espoused by the World Health Organization, which advocate voluntariness and humane steps with safeguards against discrimination.

As regards surveillance, the AIDS/ARC (AIDS related complex) voluntary reporting system and the Biennual Sentinel Seroprevalence Surveillance system are the two major source of information but it is difficult to establish the exact national statistics in regard to those with HIV/AIDS.

The National Plan for the Prevention of AIDS lays down guidelines on the type of testing permitted but the realities are still a far cry from that which is advocated by the National Plan. Reports of compulsory or hidden testing without informed consent continue to appear. On another front, access to counselling is not always guaranteed, and the quality of counselling is not always good.

Under the relationship between doctors and patients, by reason of national medical ethics, doctors are obliged to care for their patients. However, in practice, there are instances where doctors and hospitals shun those with HIV/AIDS. A related problem is that there is no general social welfare legislation or provision to provide free medical care to the needy. En passant it may be added that even if the poor victims had some access to medical facilities, they tend to suffer from a lower quality of medical treatment. The issue of vaccine trials has led to heated debate in Thai society. In 1992 a National Plan for HIV/AIDS Vaccine Development and Evaluation was adopted with national guidelines for reviewing HIV/AIDS vaccine studies in Thailand. It recognized the role of various national institutions in considering whether to approve the trials of specific vaccines in the country.

The dispute is dependent upon resolution through various governmental committees concerning the green light for the vaccines to be tested. The National AIDS Committee is, in theory, the primary entity for guiding the process but it has not met since 1991.

Discrimination

There is not any general law providing redressal against discrimination in the Thai constitution.

Thailand has witnessed crores of coup d' tat and there were many constitution drafted. The constitution does not confer direct rights upon citizens to challenge the administrative actions in court.

Regarding the discriminations concerning treatment, accommodation, education and access to services and facilities, there are generally no legal provisions to help the victims on the immigration front, the foreigners with HIV/AIDS are denied entry. Also, there is no substantive law on privacy. Accept in matters of confidentiality on the part of medical personnel and other authorities in caring for those with HIV/AIDS is proffered by section 323 of the Criminal Code. The main exception is the presence of the labour legislation, such as Revolutionary Decree No. 103 of 1972, which has provisions against discrimination in employment, and a special labour court to provide redress. However, no case concerning discrimination by reasons of HIV/AIDS has yet come to court, even though it is common knowledge that several employers have been dismissing those with HIV/AIDS from employment. One can surmise that an essential reason for this is the fear of exposure of one's identity if one takes action in court.

In the National Plan for the Prevention of AIDS, there is a specific section on human rights and social assistance which calls for measures against discrimination and to protect confidentiality. However, these aspirations are not reflected in the current law and practice in terms of effective redress. Here, it should be noted that the Thai legal approach is based upon a dualistic system; international law is not automatically part and parcel of Thai law. In order for international law to be invoked in Thailand, it is necessary to transform such law into local law through parliamentary legislation or the equivalent.

Gender Issues

In a recent study it came to the fore that women are more vulnerable to AIDS/HIV. This is due to a variety of reasons. A cross-over link of the disease into the family system. Prevalence large numbers of female sex workers, due to ingrained socio-cultural impediments, women's role in sexual negotiation including resistence to use condoms.

Notwithstanding, many legislative improvements concerning the status of women in Thailand, there remains much discrimination in practice. Women are also victims of the pressures of triple burden—domestic work, child rearing, and service-related work, all part and parcel of socio-economic needs. In the National Plan for the prevention of AIDS their is provision of assistance and care for all those with HIV/AIDS and their families, in reality the answers are not yet forthcoming, especially in the case of women.

Right to Information

As there is not any specific law guaranteeing access to official information, the doctors are not under compulsion to divulge the relevant information much to the chagrin of the patients. Yet instances of complaints by patients against doctors are rare in this country, as there is much reverence towards them.

On the fronts of broadcasting, censorship, pornography and advertising, there is a myriad of laws. The press in Thailand is in the hands of the private sector; it is the freest of the mass media in Asia. There has been a variety of educational programmes on television, radio and the press on the prevention and control of AIDS. These have included advertisements, films, plays and publicity spots to raise public awareness of HIV/AIDS and promote precautions, such as the use of condoms. But culturally there has been a reticence towards sex education at schools.

Whereas a range of campaigns is carried out by non-governmental organizations, bolstered by various mass media programmes.

Incarceration and Related Institutions

Till the recent past, prisoners were tested for HIV/AIDS without their consent and were segregated if they tested HIV-positive. However, the more liberal policy of the Public Health Ministry and the National Plan for the Prevention of AIDS has now influenced the prison system to take a more humanitarian approach. In theory, there is now no mandatory testing and segregation. There is part of the invisibility factor surrounding prisons, which requires greater openness of monitoring, precisely because the prison system is also an environment where needles are shared between those who inject drugs and unprotected sex is a corollary of the environment—all of which lend themselves to the risk of contracting HIV. Condoms are not generally available in prisons, but prisoners are given three condoms upon discharge from these institutions. Needles and other implements affiliated with drug injection are prohibited. Although some education and counselling on AIDS is available in prison, it tends to be ad hoc. The current situation remains vague. Ideally, it would be best if prison authorities could follow the National Plan for the Prevention of AIDS strictly for the purpose of implementation.

Wage and Employment

Despite the National Plan for the Prevention of AIDS which rejects compulsory testing of potential and actual employees, transgressions are always there. Rejections of potential employees on the basis of HIV/AIDS and dismissals of actual employees due to HIV/AIDS are common. There are a number of laws on employment with implications for HIV/AIDS. These range from the provisions on the Civil Code on employment contracts to specific laws on labour protection and labour relations. The most pertinent is probably Revolutionary Decree No. 103 of 1972 which stipulates the rights of employees in regard to unfair dismissal, remuneration and safe working conditions. However, even though employees dismissed by reason of HIV/AIDS could sue the employer under such labour protection law, this has not taken place for the reason already noted, namely fear of exposure of identity.

There was a provident fund for employees, and disability support was given only for harm incurred in the course of employment. In 1990 a new law was enacted to provide extensive social security to workers and their families through the establishment of a social security fund to cover injuries and diseases suffered by workers even if they are not related to the work. Although there is some HIV/AIDS education in the workplace, the expectations of the National Plan for the Prevention of AIDS which call for extensive education have yet to be realised.

Criminal Law

The criminal law is relevant to those who transmit HIV to other persons. The provisions of the dangerous Drugs Acts 1979 could also be used to detain those with HIV/AIDS where they are related to drug addiction was broadened in 1991 with a new law on the rehabilitation of drug addicts.

There are variety of pertinent laws on immoral trafficking. On the issue of sex workers, there is a variety of pertinent laws. The Criminal Code like the which prohibits sexual intercourse with those under fifteen years, even if they consent. The other two laws are relevant: the Prostitution Suppression Act 1960 and the Entertainment Places Act 1966.

Notwithstanding this legislation, prostitution is rampant in Thailand, indicating poor implementation of the law. When the Act is enforced, it tends to be the prostitutes themselves rather then the procurers who are punished. The law also fails to take into account the root causes of the prostitution, thereby being confined to a remedial approach. If there are no real incentives for prostitutes to change their profession, particularly through alternative livelihoods, medical risks may be only a step away, and the legal framework may aggravate the situation. Current proposals to reform this law include a ban on exploiting minor children for carnal pleasures. The 1966 Act also covers entertainment places such a massage parlours and bars which could be haunts for prostitution.

The prostitution trade in the country affects both men and women, although the figures are larger among women. A worrying trend also is the sale and trafficking of children into prostitution. Recent instances point to an underground trade of children and women trafficked for prostitution between China, Laos, Burma, Cambodia, Vietnam and Thailand. Many are then infected with HIV. It is worth mentioning that homosexuality is not illegal in Thailand. Although this group was initially the most affected group at the start of the epidemic in Thailand, this is no longer the case. By contrast, recent trends highlight the problem of prostitution as the factor most closely linked with the rapid spread of this pandemic.

Legal Process

Contrary to the Thai legal process adherence to the maxim "ignorance of the law is no excuse," it is peculiar that an obligation upon the state to disseminate the law to the people is lacking. Thus, many people simply do not know the law. It is a fact that 70 per cent of the population are rural based with few means of access to the legal structure which is situated in towns. The people are not litigious in the sense of the developed world—disputes tend to be settled at the local level rather by means of formal courts of law. Limited legal aid and assistance, provided by both governmental and non-governmental sectors, are available under the formal system. However, there is a need to ensure that the informal system also abides by the national law and procedure. Too much discretion on the part of the informal system may lead to a conflict between the informal system and the formal structure based upon legislation and the judiciary.

Conclusion

In a nutshell, it may be surmised that, like other countries, Thailand has a myriad of laws relevant to HIV/AIDS. In several instances, they are remedial rather than preventive. At times, they are reactive, indeed reactionary, rather than proactive and humane. Legislative aspirations are plagued by poor law enforcement.

The current beacon light for better performance towards those with HIV/AIDS is the National Plan for the Prevention of AIDS with its multi-pronged strategies of public relations and education, rehabilitation and medical help, protection of human rights and social assistance, and research and evaluation. However, the Plan suffers from the fact that it pretends to be persuasive rather than binding. It is also threatened by lack of continuity when there is a change of government. A key challenge will be how to ensure that the Plan itself is able to transcend such change and avoid the internecine skirmishes between some bureaucrats who view AIDS-related budgets and programmes as another source of power.

The law alone will never suffice, unless it encompasses and bolsters an inter-disciplinary and cross-sectoral perspective. It has to be posited in the framework of both preventive and remedial strategies. It should move away from the reactive to become proactive. It should shun inhumane action but espouse humane principles and practices. Keeping in mind the points delineated in the course of the discussion one can move away from a purely legalistic and juridical approach to law to adopt a more comprehensive and people centered vision of desired laws policies and practices in the process of making a formidable alliance.

Twenty Three

The Economic Fallout of AIDS on Korean Republic

Introduction

The wide ranging HIV infection has a far reaching impact on Society as a whole AIDS is different from other diseases due to several reasons:

(a) It is 100 per cent preventable if proper measures are taken
(b) Direct medical expenditure on AIDS is less due to unavailability of medicines.
(c) The latency period between initial infection and diagnosis of AIDS is around ten years.
(d) The disease can easily be transmitted to others from the people who are unaware that they are infected.
(e) The incidence of this disease is higher among the most productive population of an economy.

Thus the social costs of AIDS from disability to premature death could be extensive.

Prelude

AIDS has a number of economic fallouts in an economy. In the case of AIDS, indirect costs such as opportunity costs and production impacts make up a large share of total costs. The economic fallouts of AIDS would be especially significant in the Republic of Korea provided the country's low unemployment rate of 2 per cent. Tight labour markets imply that AIDS would affect the labour supply, and consequently the economic growth. AIDS mortality will induce more foreign labour to move to Korea, perhaps bringing more HIV-infected persons into the country.

Korea has paid little attention to the economic consequences of AIDS. The socio-economic impact of AIDS, and its economic impact has not been undertaken for studies primarily due to the levity on the part of government as well as the citizenry. In addition, the prevalence rate of HIV, even among high risk groups, is very low. As of the end of March, 1992, the health authorities reported 185 AIDS and HIV cases.

Comparatively small number of reported AIDS and HIV cases than other developed and neighbouring countries does not signifies that Korea is safe from or immune to the endemic, or that it can ignore the economic impact of AIDS. Rather, the reported statistics suggest only that Korea is in the early stage of the AIDS epidemic and it needs in-depth research on the economic fallout of AIDS. Such studies would proffer policy discussions on what the government could do, who should be involved, and which would be the most appropriate and cost-effective strategies.

Objectives of the Study

This study focussing on the epidemic's economic impacts, has four main objectives. First, it estimates the number of HIV sero-positive subjects for different risk groups of Korea's population. Identifying these cases, this study aims to inform the public about the risk of infection by these unidentified HIV-positive cases. Second, the study calculates the direct and indirect economic costs of AIDS and HIV infection based on a human capital approach. Third, based on the above estimation, the study aims to deliver a message to the health authorities that if they are to prevent a socio-economic catastrophe caused by the spread of AIDS, now is the time for Korea to act accordingly. Fourth, the study also tries to convey the same message to the public, that an increase in awareness and a change in sexual behaviour are must.

Literature Review

Researchers have carried out a number of studies on the economic impacts of AIDS in other countries. Economists appear to be the "third wave" to consider the implications of AIDS, after initial involvement by epidemiologists and clinicians, followed by social and behavioural studies. However, most of these studies are by scholars in occidental countries. AIDS and HIV infection are at the outset of affecting the health care systems and economies of the developing countries, including Korea. A carefully designed economic analysis is required for the countries currently marginally affected.

How the Number of HIV-Positive Cases estimated?

Reports of HIV infection varies considerably from country to country. The interaction between demographic, behavioural, and political factors determines the features of HIV epidemic (over and Piot 1991). Determining the causes of the proliferation of the HIV may give vital information for those involved in holding preventive strategies and programmes.

The Different Stages of AIDS Infection in Korea

Perceiving the spread of HIV-positive cases in Korea over time, one finds that AIDS has spread through the following stages. The first stage is when AIDS is imported by foreigners. Another vital source of transmission during this import stage is through blood transfusions and blood products.

The second stage (the first stage of domestic transmission) is when transmission occurs among homosexual and bisexual men and intravenous drug users. Once the virus has been introduced, it soon spreads through people who practise non-heterosexual behaviour. The third stage is when transmission takes place through heterosexual contact. Heterosexual transmission results in enveloping HIV infection rates among groups who are typically not under high risk groups, such as housewives. The result is an increase of infection among women, and subsequently their children. Recent statistics show that Korea has just reached this stage. In extreme cases this leads to a situation where the epidemic takes the shape of a catastrophic and results in serious social and economic problems. Some African countries have at present reached this point.

As Korea has only just begun to enter the third stage of transmission, and given the relatively lesser cases arising from the first and second stages compared to Western or other Asian countries, if preventive measures are adopted in time, AIDS may not pose serious threat to Korea's society or economy.

HIV Infection in Korea

Since the first detection of AIDS in the early 1980s, researchers have paid much attention to its prevalence rate and the number of cases expected in the future. Yet despite the number of studies carried out to date, no study has produced numbers and quantitative methods that are welcomed by all. A universally accepted way to estimate the number of HIV infections is virtually nonexistent, due mainly to the disease's unique nature, differences in transmission routes, and differences in the distribution of infected groups. Special cultural practices enhance the transmission of the HIV in particular areas once the virus is introduced.

Korea is different from other countries in many respects. It has a different distribution of the at risk population, a different degree of exposure to risky behaviour, and even various patterns of sexual behaviour. Thus, the same estimation techniques used in for other countries cannot be used in Korea, and Korea specific approach is desirable.

CHART 1
KOREA: ROUTES OF HIV TRANSMISSION

Domestic transmission	- Population at large - Homosexual and bisexual males - Hemophiliacs - Prostitutes
Foreign import	Sailors and Korean workers returning from abroad Foreigners legally or illegally staying in Korea

In Korea, Homosexuals are not subjected to compulsory HIV testing. They are declared as HIV-positive only when they submit to voluntary testing or donate blood. Thus, the number of cases reported to the health authorities does not adequately reflect the actual number of HIV-positive homosexuals.

Hemophiliacs

Most HIV contagion among hemophiliacs occurred before 1985, when thermal dis-infection of blood products was introduced. The National Institute of Health of Korea estimates that as of March 1992, Korea had about 1,500 hemophiliacs. The sero-prevalence rate of hemophiliacs is estimated at 2 per cent, resulting in an estimate of thirty HIV-infected hemophiliacs, substantially lower the Japan (40 per cent).

Prostitutes

As prostitutes are subject to mandatory HIV testing, the 25 reported cases out of the 1,305,428 people tested by the end of 1991 are probably close to the actual number of HIV infections in this group. But their are few caveats such as few cases gone undetected in the case of high profile prostitution in Star Hotels.

The Population as a Whole

The number of HIV contagion through heterosexual contact has increased, specially among women (table 1). The focus of the HIV and AIDS epidemic has shifted form an early concentration among homosexual men to the heterosexual population.

CHART 2
KOREA: SERO-POSITIVE RATES BY EPIDEMIOLOGICAL GROUP AS OF DECEMBER 1991

Epidemiological Group	*Number of people tested (A)*	*Number of positives (B)*	*B/A (%)*
Sailors	182466	78	0.0427
Prostitutes	411425	11	0.0026
Entertainers	1894503	14	0.0007
Blood donors	4733921	27	0.0005
Total	7222315	130	0.0018

Source: National Institute of Health internal report (1992).

The chance of infection for a Korean not in the traditionally at risk groups is not available. Anyhow, the sero-positive rate of blood donors (0.0005 per cent) can be used as a proxy for such a probability. Table 2 indicates the sero-prevalence rates among various epidemiological groups. So an adjustment that takes account of the difference in sex ratio between blood donors (9 men: 1woman) and the average population (5:5) is required. Taking the sample of 185 Korean individuals in representative of the population of HIV-positive individuals, the blood donor seroprevalence rate is adjusted through the following equation:

$$Y = X \frac{\sum_{i=1}^{2} A_i C_i}{\sum_{i=2}^{2} A_i B_i} \quad i = 1, 2$$

where

Y = sero-prevalence rate after sex ratio adjustment

X = sero-prevalence rate among blood donors (male and female together=0.000005 or 0.0005 per cent, table 2)

1 = male, 2 = female

A = proportion of 185 confirmed HIV-positive blood cases. A_1 can be shown to be the probability that a person is male conditional on testing positive for the HIV. Similarly, A_2 should be considered to mean the probability that a person is a female conditional on testing positive for the HIV.

B = distribution of blood donors: $B_1 = 0.898$, $B_2 = 0.102$

C = population distribution: $C_1 = 0.50$, $C_2 = 0.50$

A new sero-prevalence rate adjusted to the sex ratio of the total population (Y) is 0.000314 per cent. This is multiplied by 40 million (the total population of Korea) to reach at the number of estimated HIV-positive cases among the majority of population, that is, 126 persons. Most of them are infected through heterosexual contact.

Sailors and Returning Expatriates

Sailors are subject to compulsory HIV testing at the port of arrival on their return from overseas. By the end of 1991, a total of 182,466 sailors had been tested and 78 of them had tested positive, indicating a sero-prevalence rate of 0.427 per cent. It shows the highest rate among all the epidemiological groups in Korea.

Every year many a Korean returns from working or studying overseas, they are not subject to compulsory HIV testing, establishing the number of HIV-positive cases among this group is not so easy. The number of HIV-positive cases among expatriates Koreans is estimated using data on the total number of Koreans returning from epidemic areas.

Foreigners in Korea

A lot of foreigners are working in Korea due to the high wages in Korean labour market. Twelve foreigners were found as HIV-positive by the health authorities from 1985 to March 1992, and were compulsorily deported to their native country. As only foreign entertainers who wanted to stay for longer than ninety-one days are subject to compulsory HIV testing, the twelve reported cases are probably just the tip of the iceberg.

Total Estimated Sero-positive Cases

Table 3 presents the estimated numbers of HIV sero-positive individuals among different groups. By March 1992, 185 AIDS and HIV cases had been officially detected by the health authorities. Any how, based on very conservative estimates, this study shows that Korea had minimum of 494 HIV-positive individuals by the end of 1991.

CHART 3

KOREA: ESTIMATED NUMBER OF SERO-POSITIVE INDIVIDUALS, 1991

Groups	*Number*
Homosexual and bisexual men	144
Hemophiliacs	30
Prostitutes	25
Population at large	126
Sailors	78
Koreans returning from abroad	70
Foreigners in Korea	21
Total	**494**

The estimation aims at informing the public that many more people are HIV-positive than officially reported. In most of these cases, the patients are probably unaware that they are infected and continue to have sex without necessarily taking the proper precautions. It is this point juncture that intervention is appropriate to encourage people to take precautions, especially during sexual contact with a new partner.

AIDS Treatment and its Cost

The expense on AIDS refer to both direct and indirect costs. Direct costs consist mostly of health care expenditures arising from drug consumption, out-patient visits, in-hospital treatments, and public expenditures for AZT and HIV testing. Indirect costs mean the value of foregone production due to disability and premature death. In estimating indirect costs this study made no effort to estimate the monetary value of social support services and public health information given by volunteers or nonprofit organizations. The study also did not consider psychological costs and intergenerational effects owing to AIDS calculating indirect costs due to the problem of obtaining data on such costs.

This study computes lifetime economic costs for representative AIDS patients, a thirty-year-old man and a thirty-year-old woman.

Direct Medical Expenditure

Hospital Costs. After the onset of HIV-related illness, a patient's life span can range from a few months to two years. Patients in the industrial countries average one to two years, while those in the developing countries usually live for about six months (WHO/GPA 1991). This is the period when a patient needs intensive hospital care.

Indirect Costs

The indirect economic costs of AIDS and HIV are calculated based on the human capital approach, which is used to make the proper allowances for losses arising from disability and/or death. The study assumes that average wages and labour force participation rates of persons with AIDS are the same as those for the general population.

A precise expression for the loss to the economy calculated on this method would be:

$$L = \sum_{t=a}^{n} Y_t P_t^a (1+r)^{-1(t-a)}$$

Where

Y_t = expected gross earnings of the person during the tth year

P_t = probability in the ath year of the person being alive during the tth year

R = the social rate of discount expected to apply during the tth year.

CHART 4
KOREA: ECONOMIC COSTS OF THE PREMATURE DEATH OF AIDS PATIENTS

(won and US$)

Discount rate (%)	*30-year-old man*	*30-year-old woman*
3.0	W 177,505,924 ($227,572)	W 89,076,333 ($114,200)
1.5	W 226,427,956 ($290,292)	W 111,205,381 ($142,571)

Note: Exchange rate used is US$1 = W 780.

Total Expense

Chart 4 sums up the economic costs incurred by a thirty-year-old male AIDS patient. The indirect costs of premature death are the present value of future earnings using a 3 per cent discount rate. The chart shows that the indirect social cost (US$241,794) is about fifty-seven times as much as the direct health care cost (US$4,225). The largest component of the cost of the AIDS epidemic is due to work time lost and future earnings foregone rather than to direct medical care expenditure. The result of this analysis is according to earlier studies by Fox and Thomas (1987), Hardy and others (1986), and Scitovsky and Rice (1987).

Direct costs are comparatively less partly because the medical technology for treating AIDS is currently scarce, specifically in the developing countries. Another reason for the high indirect costs, particularly the high mortality costs, is that most of the infected are in their most productive years. Eventhough, the direct medical care costs of AIDS are not negligible, they are far surpassed by the indirect expenses due to premature death.

CHART 5
KOREA: THE ECONOMIC COSTS OF AIDS: THE CASE OF A THIRTY-YEAR-OLD MAN

(won and US$)

Type of cost	*Cost*	*Estimated amount*
Direct medical Costs	Out-patient costs: immune tests and AZT prescription	W 1,728,000 ($2,215)
	Hospital costs	W 1,567,512 ($2,010)
	Sub-total	W 3,295,512 ($4,225)
Indirect costs	Disability loss	W 11,093,394 ($14,222)
	Premature death	W 177,505,924 ($227,572)
	Sub-total	W 188,599,318 ($241,794)
Total		W 191,894,830 ($246,019)

This indicates that from the social point of view, the economic costs of the AIDS epidemic are not health expenses but the loss of productive labour.

Synopsis

This study is focused on the economic fallout of the pandemic. Two points are worth mentioning. First, the health authorities' official statistics cite 1£5 AIDS and HIV cases in Korea, but this study estimates that a more likely figure is around 494 cases. The number itself is not high compared to other countries, including Japan, but what is significant is that many cases of undetected HIV exist. Most of these people are unaware that they are infected, and there is a chance to spread the disease. Second, the indirect social costs of AIDS are much more than the costs of direct health care.

Despite Korea's present low prevalence of the HIV and AIDS, it is not immune to the epidemic. The government should take steps now to protect the well-being of the existing population and future generations.

Research on the economic impacts of AIDS in Korea is needed, for example, on medical care costs, on the impact of AIDS on the shipping industry and on the labour supply, and the distribution of AIDS expenses.

References

Barnett, T., and P. Blaikie. 1992. AIDS in *Africa: Its Present and Future Impact*. London: Bellhaven.

Bennett, C., M. Cvitanic, and A. Pascal. 1991. "The Costs of AIDS in Los Angeles." *Journal of Acquired Immune Deficiency Syndromes* 4:197-203.

Bloom, D., and G. Carliner. 1988. 'The Economic Impacts of AIDS in the United States." *Science* 239:604-10.

Cho, Y. 1991. "Life after HIV Infection." *Korean Journal of Epidemiology* 13(1).

Choo, S., and D. Chang. 1990. *Report on HIV High Risk Group Population*. Seoul: Korea Institute of Health and Social Affairs.

Dunlop, D. 1987. *The Economic Impacts of the Disease AIDS: An Analysis of the Costs of the Disease and a Proposed Study Strategy in Poor Countries*. Boston, Massachusetts: Abt Associates.

Fox, D., and E. Thomas. 1987. "AIDS Cost Analysis and Social Policy." *Law Medicine and Health Care* 15.185-211.

Gillespie, S. 1989. "Potential Impact of AIDS on Farming Systems: a Case Study from Rwanda." *Land Use Policy* 6:301-12.

Hardy, A., K. Rauch, D. Echenberg, W. Morgan, and J. Curran. 1986. "The Economic Impact of the First 10,000 Cases of AIDS in the U.S." *Journal of the American Medical Association* 255(2).

Hellinger, F. J. 1991. "Forecasting the Medical Care Costs of the HIV Epidemic." *Inquiry* 28:213-25.

Hunter, S. S. 1990. "Orphans as a Window on the AIDS Epidemic in Sub-Saharan Africa: Initial Results and implications of a study in Uganda." *Social Science and Medicine* 31(6):681-90.

Kumio, I. 1988. "Report on One AIDS Risk Group." MPH thesis, School of Public Health, Yonsei University, Korea.

Norse, D. 1991. "Socio-Economic Impact of AIDS on Food Production in East Africa." Paper prepared for the VIIth International Conference on AIDS, Florence, Italy, June.

Ohi, G., I. Kai, H. Terao, Y. Kobayashi, W. Hirano, T. Hasegawa, K. Soda, and K. Fukutomi. 1988. "Cost-Benefit Aspect of AIDS Preventive Programmes: Its Limitation in Policy Making." In A. Fleming and others, eds., *The Global Impact of AIDS*. New York: Alan R. Liss.

Over, M., and P. Piot. 1991. HIV Infection and Sexually Transmitted Diseases. HSPR-26. Washington, D.C.: World Bank, Population and Health Resources Division.

Preble, E. A. 1990. "Impact of HIV/AIDS on African Children." *Social Science and Medicine* 31 (6):671-680.

Scitovsky, A., and D. Rice. 1987. "Estimates of Direct and Indirect Costs of AIDS in the U.S." *Public Health Reports* 102(1).

Soda, K. 1991. "Epidemiology and Control of HIV/AIDS in Japan." In *Current and Future Dimensions of the HIV/AIDS Pandemic: A Capsule Summary*. Geneva: Global Programme on AIDS World Health Organization.

WHO/GPA (World Health Organization/Global Programme on AIDS). 1991. *Current and Future Dimensions of the HIV/AIDS Pandemic*. Geneva.

World Bank. 1990. *Uganda: Economic Impact of AIDS-Study Outline*. Washington, D.C.: Eastern Africa Department, Human Resources Division.

Twenty Four

AIDS Prevention Act: Its Status in Korea

Background

The AIDS Prevention Act (HIV Law hereinafter) was first promulgated on 28 November 1987, supplemented by the AIDS Prevention Decree (Presidential Decree) of 18 June 1988 and by the AIDS Prevention Enforcement Regulations of 6 November 1990. The HIV Law, as amended consists of 28 Articles in 6 Chapters.

Though, the Korean constitution upholds the dignity and rights of everyone but it is not possible to respect everyone's human rights. Some articles of the Korean HIV Law stipulate segregation, compulsory detention and restriction of employment of the infected even though there are no specific measures for prevention and treatment.

The following aspects of the HIV Law need to be highlighted:

Not Proper Emphasis on Educating the People

The HIV Law does not contain any article which stipulates mandatory duties for the state and the local governments with regard to educating like people.

For example, Article 3 of the Korean HIV Law merely states that:

(1) The State and the local governments shall work out and execute counter measures to combat AIDS and to protect and control the people infected with HIV (hereinafter referred to as "infected") and shall pass the detailed information to those who are positive. (2) Citizens shall pay attention to prevention with adequate knowledge about AIDS, and cooperate actively in steps taken by the State or the local governments under this Act.

Due to the vital importance of educational activities, this type of article should stipulate specific items to be undertaken. Such as formal (school) education and non-formal (social) education can be stipulated, along with, community awareness by appropriate regulations.

Empowering the Anti-AIDS Committee

Under article 4 of the Korean HIV Law an Anti-AIDS Committee shall be established to decide on important matters concerning the prevention of AIDS and protection, control, etc. It is important to give more status to this Committee by placing it directly under the office of Prime Minister.

Needed Reforms in the Medical Diagnosis and Control System

The importance of consent and confidentiality of the person who receives medical examination for HIV test cannot be over emphasized. In this regard, the Korean HIV Law appears to be rather vague.

HIV Test on Foreigners

The Article regarding the regulation of testing of foreigners is unclear and impractical. Article 8 of the Korean HIV Law states that:

> "Foreigners entering the Republic of Korea from foreign countries, and who wish to stay for more than 91 days, must present to the Minister of Health and Social Affairs a written confirmation of the negative antibody test result issued within one month before entering the country. If it is impossible to present such document, the person must undergo medical examination at an institution designated by the Minister of Health and Social Affairs within seventy two hours after entering the country".

Though testing is prescribed by this Article, there is neither the way for informing foreigners nor a penal provision to meet instances of contravention. This Article is a glaring example of the impracticability of some provisions of the Korean HIV Law.

International trends show that women are equally vulnerable to HIV/AIDS and an increasingly juvenile population is exposed to this epidemic every year. Consequently, the formulation of special articles in the HIV Law to deal with these issues should be seriously considered. Efforts should be made to raise the status of women through legislation.

Legal Provision Needed to Support the NGO's

Without the active support of NGO's the AIDS Programme cannot be carried out. Despite this ground reality there is not any provision in Korean HIV law to extend financial and administrative support to NGO's .

Conclusion

The AIDS programme in Korea is in the primitive stage of development, it is quiet evident that there are many sectors which requires reform.

Twenty Five

Economic Consequences of AIDS on Transport Sector of Thailand

Introduction

The phenomenal rise of AIDS and its consequent economic fallouts has severely damaged not only national economy and household but its bearing is also on the sectors, prone to AIDS such as transport and tourism. Here it would be worth mentioning that the final AIDS related costs are burdened on customers through price rise. To halt this scourge it is desirable to disseminate information and specifically develop prevention activities.

Significant strides has been made in the fight against AIDS since it was first recognized in 1981. As per WHO researchers have developed some 150 experimental drugs and vaccines and that at least 13 vaccines made either to prevent infection or to prevent those who are infected from developing full-blown AIDS are now being tested worldwide. It is very difficult to predict when a vaccine for general public use might become available. Until then, the only response to the epidemic is prevention.

Asian countries face a major challenge due to the rapid spread. Most have already made or plan to make major prevention efforts, for example, in 1991 Thailand spent almost US$107 million on prevention and with the financial assistance of the World Bank.

The Chapter aims at highlighting the effect of the AIDS epidemic on business activity and to develop a methodology to assess the economic impact of AIDS on a specific sector. An application in the transport sector has been used to illustrate the methodology by assessing the economic impact of AIDS on the trucking industry in Thailand. Which has probably the lowest concentration of treatment facilities.

Developing the Methodology to Assess the Economic Consequences of AIDS at the Sectoral Level

The scourge of AIDS can affect business enterprises via a number of channels: directly when members of the labour force become ill, and, to a lower extent, indirectly because of demand reduction due to declined household incomes or reallocation of income to health expenses. This chapter will therefore address the consequence on enterprises' labour forces and will be more of a financial than an economic study as it will focus on the additional financial costs enterprises will have to bear because of AIDS.

To assess the impact of the HIV and AIDS on a sector's enterprises through their labour force three pertinent questions must be answered:

(a) How many workers will be infected?

(b) How much will AIDS cost the enterprises directly and indirectly?

(c) Who will finally bear these additional costs?

The number of workers infected in a sector will depend on the level of sero-prevalence among the workers, which will vary with their occupation. Assessing the costs of infection to enterprises needs an analysis of all relevant costs and how they will be shared between the government, households, and enterprises. The primary costs are those for medical care, employee sick leave, and employee replacement. The proportion of medical care and sick leave costs enterprises must bear will depend on the existence of a social security system and/or on social customs in the sector. Sick leave and replacement costs will vary widely with occupation and labour market conditions. Given the direct costs per employee living with AIDS, the indirect costs per employee (infected or not), and the total number of employees in each occupation each year, one can estimate the total cost of AIDS that a sector's enterprises must bear.

Depending on the conditions of market in the transport sector, transport enterprises will be able to transform all or some of the cost to their customers, that is, other sectors of the economy. If they have to bear all the costs themselves, the impact for private companies and state-owned enterprises will be very different. The effects for all enterprises may vary from a declined profit margin to a complete cessation of activity, depending on the enterprise's size and financial health. In the case of state enterprises the cost could be changed to the government. Depending on government policy, the final cost will be borne indirectly by private enterprises, and/or by other sectors of the economy and/or by taxpayers.

The methodology used in this chapter can be used to an entire sector, to a subsector, or to an individual enterprise. In this last case one must be careful to take the enterprise's size into account. For a large enterprise one can predict that HIV prevalence is the same as for the sector as a whole, but for very small enterprises this assumption may not be valid.

The Existence of HIV Infection in a Sector

Some jobs carry a higher risk of HIV infection than others. Thus, the first step is to identify these jobs. The workers whose jobs take them away from their families for long periods of time or where behavioural norms include intravenous drug use, sexual relations with prostitutes, or multiple sex partners make a higher proportion of these workers as being in high risk occupations (HROs).

The existence of HIV infection among workers in high risk occupations. There are two main ways of calculating the prevalence of HIV infection among high risk occupation workers in a given country. The first is from sociological studies of the specific HRO workers and national data on HIV infection and AIDS. The second is by carrying out sero-prevalence surveys of HRO workers.

Using Available Studies and Data. To study the risk of HIV infection HRO workers face, data are required on their lifestyle, behaviour, job environment, and whether they are in any way related to high risk groups.

The first step is a qualitative research study using observations, small group conversations, questionnaires, and interviews with a limited sample of workers. Although some may criticize such an approach as not representing an entire HRO, it will, at low cost, give a rough calculations of the risk HRO workers face. If the limited qualitative study suggests an HIV existence rate noticeably higher than among the general population, the next step should be a more quantitative study of a national sample of HRO workers to determine the findings and justify a sero-prevalence survey.

Given information about the behaviour patterns of HRO workers, their connections with high risk groups, and data on HIV prevalence rates among the general population, one can calculated a rough estimate of the HIV prevalence rate among the HRO workers under consideration.

Using Sero-Prevalence Surveys. A survey based on HIV tests would probably give the most acceptable results, but presents potential problems, particularly in developing countries, because of the high cost of the large number of HIV tests required. Thus, this *ad hoc* approach might be reduced to studies of sectors with only one or two high risk occupations and where the preliminary sociological studies showed high HIV levels. This would make funding more readily available and the workers concerned enough to cooperate.

The Prevalence of HIV Infection Among Other Occupations. For other occupations that are not high risk occupations the calculations of the prevalence of HIV infection will be based on the existence among the total labour force nationwide.

The number of HIV-infected employees in a sector. The number of HIV-infected employees in a sector is estimated by applying the sero-prevalence rates estimated for high risk occupations and other occupations to the number of employees in each category in that sector.

HIV-and AIDS-Related Expenses Borne by a Sector

The estimation of the HIV-and AIDS-related costs particular sector must bear, one must assess not only the actual costs, but also analyze how these costs will be shared among individuals, their employers, and the government. This will depend on many factors, such as the existence of a social security system in the country, corporate attitudes toward and policies for employee welfare in the sector and labour market conditions. AIDS-related costs to enterprises may be listed as follows.

Medical care costs, Sick leave costs, Death-related costs; Other costs related to the social security system (such as an increase in unemployment); Replacement costs; Costs of indirect impacts (global wage increase, prevention).

The AIDS epidemic may directly affect social security systems through:

The medical care costs of the insured person and the person's family; Benefits for loss of wages; Funeral and other death-related costs.

However, the epidemic may also have an indirect impact in a number of other areas:

- *unemployment benefits:* HIV infected people may lose their jobs and/or encounter difficulties in finding jobs because of this.
- *old-age pensions:* If the family of the AIDS-infected person is entitled to receive a pension after his or her death, it is a benefit for the family, but a cost for employers and the government.

If the overall effect of the AIDS epidemic results in a hefty increase in the social security system's costs, this may lead the government to increase social security contributions and/or limit or reduce social security benefits, probably medical care benefits, which normally cost the most.

Without a SSS, enterprises will directly bear the HIV-and AIDS-related costs of their infected employees. The more vulnerable to AIDS the sector, the higher the cost for its firms. With a comprehensive SSS, HIV-and AIDS-related costs will be shared nationwide among employees and employers of all sectors and the government. The costs for each firm will depend on the total number of infected employees nationwide, the type of amount of benefits covered by the SSS, and the total number of employees in the firm and their wages.

Medical Care Costs. The costs of treating sero-positive and AIDS patients is the highest HIV-and AIDS-related cost in most countries affected by the AIDS disease. Before developing serious infections or full-blown AIDS, HIV-positive persons may suffer from minor infections, such as fever, due to their weakened immune systems, and may also require counselling and psychological assistance. Although these costs may not be negligible, they are very difficult to assess. Therefore, this study considers only the medical care costs of AIDS patients. If a country has a comprehensive social security system comprising all HIV-and AIDS-related medical care costs, the only costs borne by firms will be their contribution to the system. The share of the total additional funds required at the country level that will be borne by firms will depend largely on government policy. The costs to enterprises will vary depending on the number of staff employed and their wages and the number of AIDS patients in the country.

In countries without a social security system, labour laws and/or corporate regulations may need employers to cover the costs of non-occupational diseases of their employees. Hence the HIV-and AIDS-related medical care cost borne by each enterprise in this case will depend on the number of AIDS-infected employees in the enterprise.

Sick Leave Costs. The remuneration of sick employees are generally paid in part or in full during a limited number of days of absence from work. Compensation for sick leave may be part of the social security system. In countries without a social security system, enterprises may give employees with disability insurance as part of their benefits package or continue to pay employees partial wages during sick leave. Again, the extent of sick leave benefits differ with a country's prosperity and may be very limited in developing countries.

Death-Related Costs. The major death-related costs is life insurance. Some employers give life insurance as an employee benefit. Sometimes it is given directly by enterprises, but more often by insurance companies that charge firms the premium. In other countries, particularly developing countries, death benefits may be limited to a wage-based family allowance or funeral costs. Social security system benefits generally did not include life insurance, but may provide other cash benefits.

Replacement Costs. Employers directly bear the costs of replacing employees who die from AIDS. Contrary the death of AIDS-infected employees may enhance an enterprise's productivity by limiting the number of employees in overstaffed enterprises or permitting a firm to replace the employees with a modern piece of equipment rather than other employees. On the contrary the death of an employee from AIDS will usually have the following negative effects:

(a) Loss of production if a replacement is not hired immediately;

(b) Costs of training a new employee which will be higher the greater the skill requirements and will also depend on labour market conditions;

(c) Payment of higher wages, which may be necessary to attract new staff.

The Effects of Market Conditions and Government Policy on firm's Costs

Enterprises will have to bear the costs of HIV infection and AIDS; provided market conditions may permit them to pass this cost on to their customers, for example, the transport sector may be able to increase transport tariffs. If the government decides to let each sector absorb its additional costs, it will not increase the transport budget. If the cost is to be absorbed by the budget, the transport ministry has two main options. Either to increase transport-related taxes that the ministry collects directly, such as fuel taxes, truck licenses and registration fees, which would increase the fixed costs of private enterprises or to reduce expenditures, which would perhaps mean holding off on infrastructure or other development projects. This would again affect private enterprises which rely on the government to give infrastructures such as roads.

Whatever option the government opts the, resultant will be to halting development of the transport and reduce its contribution to the gross domestic product.

If the government decides to raise the transport budget to cover the increased costs, these will be passed on to other sectors as their budgets would have to be curtailed to maintain the national budget at the same level or on to taxpayers if the national budget is to be increased.

If demand for transport is inelastic, that is, if an increase in tariffs has no effect on demand. Firms will probably increase their tariffs to cover their increased costs, which will finally be borne by the other sectors in proportion to their demand for transport services.

Application in the Transport Sector: Thailand's Trucking Industry

Behaviour Patterns of Thai Long-Haul Truck Drivers

High mobility and frequent several contacts are the behaviour patterns of Thai long-haul truck divers. To evaluate the Thai truck drivers' risk of HIV infection, the Institute for Population and Social Research of Mahidol University, Bangkok, undertook an ethnographic study, which reveals that long-haul truck drivers generally originate from rural areas. They were often rice farmers before becoming drivers. They take amphetamines (in pill form) as they are under pressure to complete as many trips as possible to earn more money. It is commonly believed that they should drink a small amount of alcohol and then have sexual intercourse to release the amphetamine effect. Truck drivers believe that sleeping with prostitutes is perfectly natural. They also believe that truck stop brothels are safe from the HIV because foreigners would not sleep with cheap, local prostitutes and because if a prostitute was infected she would not be allowed to continue to work in the brothel. As truck drivers generally visit prostitutes after taking amphetamine pills and drinking alcohol, it is very difficult for prostitutes to convince them to use condoms.

The study provided the following data on the long-haul truck drivers' sexual behaviour:

- All had had commercial sex at least once 60 per cent at truck stop brothels, 38 per cent at other brothels en route, and 2 per cent near cargo pick-up points.
- Eighty-six per cent of the single men and 63 per cent of the married men had had commercial sex in the past six months.
- Eighteen per cent had used condoms during commercial sex.
- Fifteen per cent had had a sexually transmitted disease in the past six months.

The study concluded that long-haul truck drivers' behaviour exposed them to a significant risk of contracting the HIV. The institute concluded that a targeted HIV prevention campaign for truckers was urgently needed. The institute's study has been criticized as not being representative enough of the whole group because of the limited sample used.

Background Information on HIV Infection and AIDS in Thailand

Two major sources of information and statistics on HIV infection are the AIDS/AIDS Related Complex (ARC) Voluntary Reporting System and the Biennial Sentinel Sero-Prevalence Surveillance. Each source gives different epidemiological information. The AIDS/ARC Voluntary Reporting System can, at a little cost, provide information about infected individuals and service and care planning. The Sentinel Sero-Prevalence Surveillance can monitor the trend of the epidemic in specific population groups and give information about the general population.

A working group comprised of various domestic and international AIDS surveillance and research agencies, the Thai Working Group, has been created to develop estimates of the total number of HIV-infected persons and to predict the number of HIV-infected persons and AIDS cases by the year 2000. Estimates and projections based on all the sources of information are as follows:

Estimates of the current situation (end of 1991):

- 997 reported AIDS/ARC cases (cumulative since 1984)
- 200,000 to 400,000 HIV-infected persons
- 561 new AIDS/ARC cases in 1991
- 700 living AIDS/ARC patients
- 200 deaths from AIDS/ARC in 1991
- 18 months average between the onset of AIDS and death
- 20.7 per cent average HIV-infection prevalence among cheap prostitutes
- 5.6 per cent average HIV-infection prevalence among male clients of clinics for sexually transmitted diseases
- 2.9 per cent average HIV-infection prevalence among young Thai army conscripts (considered as representative of the general population of rural origin)

Projections for the year 2000:

- 2 to 4 million HIV-infected persons (cumulative)
- 180,000 new AIDS cases in 2000 (high scenario)
- 260,000 living AIDS patients (high scenario)
- 560,000 total deaths from AIDS (high scenario, cumulative)
- 160,000 deaths from AIDS in 2000 (high scenario)

- Difference between the low and high scenarios for HIV-infected persons depends on how effectively transmission is slowed down
- High scenario for AIDS cases and deaths is based on a high estimate of the current number of sero-positive persons; future behaviour change will not improve the situation because of AIDS' long latency period, and only the discovery of an efficient treatment could reduce the estimate.

Sero-Prevalence among Long-Haul Truck Drivers

As the truck drivers are sexually active and their relationship with prostitutes is the main source of HIV infection. The prevalence among this group was compared with that among rural men in general and rural and urban men together of the same age. The sero-prevalence survey in May 1991 among twenty-and twenty-one-year-old Thai samples, considered as representative of the rural population, was 2.9 per cent. A study by the Thai Working Group calculated that the rate of sero-positivity of people aged twenty and thirty was almost the same. Thus, the sero-prevalence of thirty-year-old men of rural origin can also be assumed to be 2.9 per cent in 1991.

Comparing the sexual behaviour of truck drivers and other rural men, the prevalence of HIV infection among truck drivers can be calculated at 4.5 per cent based on the information that 64 per cent of rural men had had commercial sex on at least one occasion and 2.9 per cent are sero-positive and that 100 per cent of truck drivers had had commercial sex on at least one occasion and can be compared to rural men, thus 2.9 per cent/64 per cent × 100 per cent = 4.5 per cent.

The Thai Working Groups's study on the HIV epidemic estimated that about 90 per cent of sero-positive persons are older than fifteen and that in 1991 about two-thirds were men. Based on a study 200,000 to 400,000 sero-positive persons in late 1991, the total number of sero-positive men over the age of fifteen is 120,000 to 240,000. The estimated total male population aged fifteen and over in Thailand is about 30 per cent of the total population, that is, about 17 million people, which gives an average prevalence of HIV infection among men older than fifteen of 0.7 to 1.4 per cent.

A comparison of the sexual behaviour of truck drivers and other men older than fifteen gives a rough estimate of the existence of HIV among truck drivers of 0.9 per cent to 1.9 per cent based on the number who "had had commercial sex on at least one occasion" (0.7 per cent/75 per cent × 100 per cent = 0.9 per cent; 1.4 per cent/ 75 per cent × 100 per cent = 1.9 per cent), and of 3.3 to 6.6 per cent based on the number of men who "had had commercial sex in the past six months" (0.7 per cent/16 per cent × (86 per cent + 63 per cent)/2 = 3.3 per cent; 1.4 per cent/16 per cent × (86 per cent + 63 per cent)/2 = 6.6 per cent), presuming that the proportion of married and single men among truck drivers is the same as among the general male population.

Estimation by the Thai Working Group suggest that the number of HIV-infected people will reach 2 to 4 million by the year 2000, of which about 800,000 to 1.6 million will be men aged fifteen and more. The estimated total male population aged fifteen and over by the year 2000 will be about 20 million, which provides an average HIV existence rate among this group of 4 to 8 per cent, that is, a 470 per cent increase in ten years. If there is no dramatic change in long-haul truck drivers' sexual behaviour between now and the year 2000, the HIV prevalence rate among truck drivers will reach 17 to 29 per cent by the year 2000 presuming the same 470 per cent increase.

AIDS-Related Costs Borne by the Thai Trucking Industry

The Thai strategy is to introduce a comprehensive social security system under the aegis of (1990) Social Security argmentation in the following stage:

- First stage (1990) - injury and sickness benefits
  - maternity benefits
  - disability benefits
  - death benefits
- Second stage (1996) - family allowances
  - old-age pensions
- Third stage (later) - unemployment benefits

The system's main features are first, the SSS covers organizations with twenty employees or more and second, the government, employers, and employees must provide equally to the social security fund with contributions equal to 1.5 per cent of wages. Contributions will be raised to 3 per cent in the second phase and 5 per cent in the third phase. This application considers only those SSS benefits regarding to HIV infection and AIDS and applicable during 1991-2000.

Based on these figures, the HIV prevalence rate among Thai long-haul truck drivers has been calculated at 3 to 5 per cent in 1991.

TABLE 1

ESTIMATED NUMBER OF HIV-INFECTED PEOPLE IN THE TRUCKING INDUSTRY, 1991 AND 2000.

	1991		
Occupation	*Total number*	*HIV infected (%)*	*Total infected*
Long-haul drivers	200,000	3-5	6,000-10,000
Others	400,000	0.6-1.2	2,500-5,000
Total	**600,000**		**8,500-15,000**
	2000		
Occupation	*Total number*	*HIV infected (%)*	*Total infected*
Long-haul drivers	230,000	17-29	40,000-67,000
Others	460,000	5-10	23,000-46,000
Total	**690,000**		**63,000-113,000**

Source: Government data and interviews

Under the sickness benefits, the Social Security Act provides "Benefits for non-occupational sickness shall consist of medical examination expenses; medical treatment expenses; lodging, meals, and treatment expenses in hospital; medicine and pharmaceutical expenses; cost of ambulance or transportation for the patient and other necessary expenses in accordance with the rules and rates prescribed by the Medical Committee." This definition of sickness benefits comprises all HIV- and AIDS-related medical care costs. Later, in May 1991, the Medical Committee of the Social Security Organization established a list of cases where medical care costs will not be compensated, one of which is "treatment during a period of research and experiment."

The Social Security Act also gives for cash benefits for sick leave at the rate of 50 per cent of wages for absences from work not exceeding 180 days in a calendar year.

In relation to **death benefits**, the Social Security Act gives for a "death benefit as a funeral grant at the amount of one hundred times the highest rate of daily minimum wages under the Labour Protection Law," that is, about US$460 at the minimum wages rate.

The system gives for **family allowances** from 1996. The only HIV-related benefit included is the coverage of infected children's medical expenses and is limited to a maximum of two children per insured person.

Old-age pensions will be granted from 1996 for insured persons over fifty-five years of age who have paid contributions for at least fifteen years, thus, the first pensions will be paid in the year 2005. As this application only considers the years 1991 to 2000.

The Cost of Medical Care for AIDS Patients

It is not possible at present in deriving those costs covered by Thailand SSS from those not covered for AIDS-related medical care. Thus, this study presumes that social security will cover the total estimated cost US$1,000 per patient per year, and that enterprises will not face any direct medical care costs. Assuming that social security remittances will be equally shared between employees, employers, and the government and that the social security funds will balance each year during 1991-2000, the cost of medical care borne by the trucking industry can be estimated as shown below:

	1991	*2000*
(1) Total number of ARC/AIDS cases	700	260,000
(2) Average percentage of insured AIDS patients	10	25
(3) Medical care cost per AIDS patient per year	US$1,000	US$1000
(4) Cost per year to SSS [(1)x(2)x(3)/100]	US$70,000	US$65,000,000
(5) Total number of insured persons in the SSS	3,000,000	9,000,000
(6) Cost to SSS per insured person per year [(4)/(5)]	US$0.023	US$7.222
(7) Number of employees in the trucking industry	600,000	690,000
(8) Total trucking industry SSS contribution [(6) × (7)]	US$13,980	US$4,983,300
(9) Medical care cost borne by trucking enterprises through social security contributions [(8)/3]	US$4,700	US$1,661,100

Sick Leave Costs of AIDS Borne by the Trucking Industry

Likewise the AIDS-related sick leave of sero-positive persons will not be considered as it is very difficult to separate from non-AIDS-related sick leave. In early 1992, the average wage of insured employees in Thailand was around US$200 per month. The yearly cost of sick leave per AIDS patient to the SSS is thus about US$600. The cost to the trucking industry, through the SSS, for the sick leave can be calculated as shown below:

		1991	*2000*
(1)	Total number of ARC/AIDS cases	700	260,000
(2)	Average percentage of insured AIDS patients	10	25
(3)	Sick leave cost per AIDS patient per year	US$600	US$600
(4)	Cost per year to SSS [(1)x(2)x(3)/100]	US$42,000	US$39,000,000
(5)	Total number of insured persons in the SSS	3,000,000	9,000,000
(6)	Cost to SSS per insured person per year [(4)/(5)]	US$0.014	US$4.333
(7)	Number of employees in the trucking industry	600,000	690,000
(8)	Total trucking industry SSS contribution [(6)x(7)]	US$8,400	US$2,990,000
(9)	Sick leave cost borne by trucking enterprises through social security contributions [(8)/3]	US$2,800	US$996,700

Thailand is facing a shortage of long-haul truck drivers due to massive migration of truck drivers to Saudi Arabia, where wages are much higher. As per estimation Thailand needs 20 per cent more truck drivers than are now available. Thus, one must assume that trucking firms will not be able to hire temporary replacements while their employees are on sick leave unless they are willing to pay wages equal to those truckers receive in Saudi Arabia. Thus, they will suffer from a loss of production when trucks go unused. An accurate calculation of the costs associated with the loss of production would need a detailed analysis of trucking operations' costs and profit margins. This calculation gives only a spitchy estimate of these costs.

Thai long-haul trucks are heavy six-wheelers, ten-wheelers or articulated vehicles. Each truck usually operates for sixteen hours per day, which requires two drivers per truck. If one of the drivers is sick and cannot be changed the truck will only be used for 50 per cent of the time. The average "production" of one truck used full-time is about 600,000 tonne kilometers per year, or 300,000 tonne kilometers per year per driver. If an AIDS-infected driver is on sick leave for six months in a year, a truck's production will be curtailed by 150,000 tonne kilometers per year.

The average tariff for road freight is US$0.05 per tonne kilometer. Therefore, the loss per AIDS-infected driver per year amounts to US$7,500. If we assume a profit margin of 10 per cent, the cost to the trucking firms will be some US$750.

This study has not examined the costs of replacing sick workers in other occupations in the trucking industry and no shortage of labour exists for other occupations, and except for positions requiring highly skilled employees, temporary staff are already available. The cost of sick leave attributable to AIDS and directly borne by trucking enterprises can thus be calculated as shown below (high scenario):

	1991	*2000*
(1) Total number of HIV-infected people	400,000	4,000,000
(2) Total number of living AIDS/ARC cases	700	260,000
(3) Total number of HIV-infected long-haul truck drivers	10,000	67,000
(4) Number of AIDS-infected long-haul truck drivers [(2)x(3)/(1)]	18	4,355
(5) Cost per AIDS-infected truck driver per year	US$750	US$750
(6) Sick leave cost directly borne by trucking enterprises [(4) × (5)]	US$13,500	US$3,266,300

Death-Related Costs of AIDS Borne by the Trucking Industry

Life insurance is not generally provided to employees by the enterprises of trucking industry instead they are provided only with very limited cash as a contribution toward funeral costs, which in Thailand tend to be substantial. As, now the social security system contributes to these costs, this study assumes that no firm is paying direct death-related cash benefits to employees. Assuming that social security remittance are shared equally between employees, employers, and the government, the additional contribution due to death benefits borne by trucking industry enterprises can be calculated as follows (high scenario):

		1991	2000
(1)	Total number of ARC/AIDS deaths	200	160,000
(2)	Average percentage of insured AIDS patients[13]	10	25
(3)	Death-related cost per AIDS patient per year[14]	US$460	US$460
(4)	Cost per year to the SSS [(1)×(2)×(3)/100]	US$9,200	US$18,400,000
(5)	Total number of insured persons in the SSS	3,000,000	9,000,000
(6)	Cost to SSS per insured person per year [(4)/(5)]	US$0.003	US$2.044
(7)	Number of employees in the trucking industry	600,000	690,000
(8)	Total trucking industry SSS contribution [(6)x(7)]	US$1,860	US$1,410,700
(9)	Death-related costs borne by trucking enterprises through social secutiry contributions [(8)/3]	US$620	US$470,200

Replacement Cost Borne by the Trucking Industry for Long-Haul Truck Drivers

As mentioned earlier the massive migration of long-haul truck drivers to Saudi-Arabia and the deaths of employees will further exacerbate the situation.

The replacement cost of truck drivers consists of two main factors:

- Loss of production, as estimated for sick leave, amounts to US$750 per long-haul truck driver for six months. Thus, the loss of production during the one-year training period is US$1,500.
- Training costs, which are the helper's wages during the one-year training period, are generally some US$ 1,500 per year.

The total replacement cost is therefore about US$3,000 per long-haul truck driver. Long-haul truck drivers' wages range from US$3,000 to US$5,000 per year (Salary and allowances), double in Saudi Arabia. Thus, employers are more likely to bear the costs of training a new driver rather than paying a new driver more, particularly as this would mean raising the wages of the other drivers.

The total replacement cost of AIDS-infected long-haul truck drivers directly borne by trucking firms can be calculated as follows (high scenario):

	1991	2000
(1) Total number of HIV-infected people	400,000	4,000,000
(2) Total number of AIDS deaths (in that year)	200	160,000
(3) Total number of HIV-infected long-haul truck drivers	10,000	67,000
(4) Number of AIDS deaths among long-haul truck drivers [(2)x(3)/(1)]	5	2,680
(5) Replacement cost per long-haul truck driver	US$3,000	US$3,000
(6) Replacement cost directly borne by trucking enterprises [(4)x(5)]	US$15,000	US$8,040

Prevention and Information in the Transport Sector

Trucking industry is a high risk area primarily due to sexual behaviour but the trucking enterprises are not yet eager to provide funds for prevention and information campaigns among their employees. The Ministry of Transport and Communications has allocated US$80,000 to produce materials targeted at private enterprises in the transport sector. Hoping that the private sector will also initiate some action.

Total AIDS-Related Costs Borne by the Trucking Industry

The total costs of HIV infection and AIDS that trucking industry firms must bear, including both their direct costs and those paid through the social security system, are shown in table 2.

TABLE 2
TOTAL AIDS-RELATED COSTS BORNE BY THE TRUCKING INDUSTRY, 1991 AND 2000.

(US$)

Type of Cost	*1991*	*2000*
Costs borne through social security contributions		
Medical care cost	4,700	1,661,000
Sick leave costs (cash benefits)	2,800	996,700
Death-related costs	620	470,200
Subtotal	8,200	3,128,000
Costs directly borne by enterprises		
Sick leave costs (loss of production)	13,500	3,266,300
Replacement costs	15,000	8,040,000
Subtotal	28,500	11,306,300
Total	36,700	14,434,300
Rounded to	40,000	14,500,000

Based on predictions of how the epidemic is likely to develop and its annual costs, the annual cost each year from 1991 through the year 2000 is given in table 3.

TABLE 3
ANNUAL COSTS, 1991-2000

(US$ millions, constant costs, 1991 base year prices)

1991	*1992*	*1993*	*1994*	*1995*	*1996*	*1997*	*1998*	*1999*	*2000*	*Total*
0.04	0.56	1.2	2.1	2.8	4.6	6.4	8.5	11.3	14.5	52.0

We have seen that the Social Security Act has the strength to reduce substantially the economic consequences of the AIDS epidemic on trucking enterprises. However, if additional contributions become too high for individuals, the government may decide to change the contribution sharing arrangement and charge enterprises more. The current cost for trucking enterprises is little, which partly explains their lack of concern. However, truck drivers currently sero-positive will develop AIDS in the coming years and costs will increase dramatically during the decade.

If there is not marked change in the sexual behaviour of truck drivers, the cost of AIDS borne by trucking enterprises will continue to escalate dramatically, by more than US$3 million per year after the year 2000.

The Effect of Market Conditions on AIDS-Related Costs Borne by the Trucking Industry

Private truck operators carry most road freight in Thailand. Road transport is therefore a very competitive market, and each firm will probably have to bear the AIDS-related costs itself to avoid losing part of its market. However, as AIDS-related costs will affect all truck operators equally, they may abandon competing and reach an agreement so that they all increase tariffs. The AIDS-related costs will then be passed on to road transport users, that is, mainly the construction, agriculture, and mining sectors.

Outline of Cost-Effectiveness Analysis

This chapter is intended at sectoral analysis that can be used to assess the financial impact of the HIV and AIDS on enterprises.

To obtain the private sector's support for prevention efforts, merely showing the costs of AIDS may be insufficient. The private sector may required to be convinced of the cost-effectiveness of investing in HIV and AIDS prevention activities. This needs a standard cost-benefit analysis to proove that small costs incurred today may create enormous benefits in the form of costs avoided in the future. This cost-benefit analysis has four main elements:

1. Developing a cost estimate as in this chapter. Given that some of the data used here are very rough, use of a computerized model would allow users to test the senstitivity of the costs when the main parameters, such as sero-prevalence rates, are varied.
2. Selecting the prevention activities most appropriate for the enterprises in a particular sector and estimating the costs of these prevention measures.
3. Assessing the efficacy of the selected prevention activities in delimiting HIV and AIDS cases in enterprises. This task may be the most difficult because of the latency period of AIDS.
4. Discounting the costs and benefits. The cost of prevention must be borne today, but its benefits will not occur for several years due to AIDS' long latency period. Thus, the benefits have to be discounted to assess their present value and compared with the current costs.

Conclusion

The method by which AIDS related costs to be borne out by enterprises may convince them to undertake and finance prevention activities because the AIDS and transport sector are going to effect each other *vice-versa*.

Thus, the prevention activities by the government in the transport sector will not only benefit the sector, but also other sectors by reducing the number of sero-positive individuals that can spread the infection. Transport workers and enterprises may feel somewhat guilty about their role in the transmission of the virus. This can have a positive effect, in which case they will willingly participate in prevention efforts, or they may react negatively and avoid addressing the problem. The success of prevention campaigns will depend largely on the presentation to transport workers and employers and how well they are supervised. Finally, such vehicles as trucks and buses can themselves be used in prevention campaigns by replacing commercial advertisements with AIDS prevention advertisements. However, this will reduce the enterprises' profits unless the government chooses to compensate them.

Twenty Six

Economic Fallout of AIDS in Thailand

Introduction

In the preceding years, Thailand has witnessed growth in two diametrically opposite sectors. Since, 1987 the Thai economy has achieved impressive annual growth of 9 to 13 per cent in its G.D.P., growing unnoticed alongside this economic prosperity is the pandemic of AIDS. The human toll for the country in terms of death and spread is of considerable economic significance.

The direct cost and the indirect costs of AIDS in Thailand are estimated based on differing future paths of this epidemic. This analysis is important to demonstrate the magnitude of the financial burden of AIDS.

Feature of the AIDS Epidemic

AIDS is a disease with multi pronged effect. The HIV is transmitted by sexual contact, by blood contact, and by infected mothers to their children during pregnancy or birth. AIDS is eventually dangerous, but the causes of death among AIDS patients vary. A complicating feature of the epidemic is the long period of latency between the initial HIV infection and the onset of serious illness. During this latent period infected individuals appear healthy, but they can and do infect others. The epidemic thus spreads unnoticed and undetected. Some infected individuals are detected through routine blood screening and through special surveys in which blood tests for the presence of antibodies are conducted. However, those people who test positive for the HIV or who are found AIDS cases represent only a small proportion of the total number of infected people. The costs of testing and the logistics of large-scale testing prevent any country from knowing with certainty the exact number of HIV-positive individuals.

AIDS epidemics typically advance in waves of infection, beginning with those engaging in the highest risk behaviours, then spreading to the general population (Myers and Ashakul 1991). In Thailand the first and second routes were homosexuals and IDUs. The third route infected female prostitutes via IDUs and homosexuals. The fourth route infects the male clients of the female prostitutes. These infected men then pass the virus to their girlfriends and wives, who make up the fifth route. The sixth and final route involves the children who receive the infection from their mothers. Infected mothers have a 30 per cent chance of passing the virus to their children.

The Present Situation in Thailand

Widespread transmission of the HIV started in late 1980s. Because of the long latency period between infection and the development of AIDS symptoms, Thailand has experienced less (reported) AIDS-related illnesses or deaths. A major number of AIDS cases and deaths will begin to develop in the mid-to late-1990s. As described above, the first wave of infected male gays was followed over time by IDUs, female prostitutes, male clients of female prostitutes, partners of males infected by prostitutes, and finally the children of infected women. Each of these groups has its own AIDS epidemic with a specific start date, size of population at risk, and infection rates.

Thailand's Ministry of Public Health (MOPH) has been conducting testing of various groups engaging in high and low risk behaviours, to track the epidemics" spread since 1989. The MOPH is sampling, referred to as the National Sentinel Sero-prevalence Survey, every sex months. Currently, all seventy-three provinces are included in the bi-annual survey. The Division of Epidemiology (1991) summarizes the results of the surveys (table 1). The figures given are the national mean rate (the number tested HIV-positive divided by the total number tested), the national median rate (the midpoint rate of all the reporting provinces), the range of prevalence rates found among the provinces, and the number of provinces reporting prevalence rates for the respective test group.

The data shown the individual waves and the rapidly

progressing spread of the epidemic. Most notable is the high level and increasing rate of infection confirmed during the June 1991 survey. Of the groups sampled, 24 per cent of brothel prostitutes, 8 per cent of men attending MOPH sexually transmitted disease (STD) clinics, and 1 per cent of women attending MOPH antenatal clinics tested positive for the HIV. While there may be some discrepancies in the data, the initial results from the December 1991 survey continue to show major increases in infection in certain groups, particularly blood donors, men attending STD clinics, and prostitutes.

While the national rates are surprising, regional variation may signal even higher prevalence rates in the future. For example, in the June 1991 survey, infected rates among brothel prostitutes in the northern provinces of Chiang Rai, Chiang Mai, and Phayao were over 40 per cent. Infected rates for men attending STD clinics in those provinces were over 20 per cent, and for women attending antenatal clinics the rates were over 3 per cent (Division of Epidemiology 1991).

The data from the MOPH's sentinel survey are used to calculate the number of HIV-positive individuals (table 2). Preliminary analysis from the June 1991 sentinel survey shows that an additional 50,000 to100,000 Thais became infected in the first six months of 1991, raising the cumulative total to 250,000 to 300,000 infected (personal communications 1991).

Almost 90 per cent of the blood donors in Thailand are male. Using the June 1991 antenatal and blood donor rates, this method calculated that an additional 50,000 to100,000 people became infected in the first six months of 1991, raising the cumulative total to 300,000 to 350,000 infected.

The MOPH and other AIDS experts in Thailand have estimated that as of the end of 1991, between 200,000 and 400,000 people were infected with the AIDS virus. The trends in the survey infected rates indicate that the epidemic continues to grow at alarming rates and with the exception of the IDU population, shows no signs of slowing. Moreover, the epidemic has spread to the general population, implying that the behaviours of a large number of people need to change to reduce the spread of the epidemic.

TABLE 1
THAILAND: ESTIMATED NUMBER OF HIV-POSITIVE PEOPLE AS OF DECEMBER 1990.

Population Group	*Population size at risk for HIV*	*Prevalence rate (per cent)*[a]	*Number of HIV-infected people*
Injecting drug users	49,550-99,100	22-45	16,000-32,000
Prostitutes			
Brothel	41,665-58,331	6-20	5,200-7,200
Nonbrothel	66,452-93,033	1-8	3,300-4,600
High risk men	4.6-5.0 million	1-5	92,000-184,000
Partners of high risk men	3.6-4.0 million	0.3-0.5	12,300-15,000
Newborns	3,000-6,000	30	1,000-2,000
Total			**129,000-244,000**

a. The prevalence rates are the regional median rates. Each region consists of a number of reporting provinces.

Source: Ministry of Public Health.

The Imminent Situation in Thailand

It is indeed difficult to project the proliferation of HIV. Because the infection is unnoticed, even estimating the current situation to determine the epidemic's starting point is problematic. Furthermore, changes in social behaviour, medical breakthroughs, and other unpredictable factors could affect future growth. However, to study the potential magnitude of the problem and its consequence on the economy future scenarios must be developed.

HIV Infection

The projections for the spread of HIV infection in Thailand were done using the iwgAIDS model (Stanley and others 1990). This model was presented by the U.S. Department of State's Interagency Working Group on AIDS Models and Methods. A demographic model is used as a foundation for the iwgAIDS model with AIDS-related processes integrated into it. The paradigm projects the spread of the HIV by heterosexual sex between both casual and married partners, homosexual and bisexual sex, intravenous drug use, blood transfusions, and prenatal transmission. This is a behaviour based model that needs detailed data on demography, sexual and drug injecting behaviour, epidemiology, and blood banking. In March 1990 the Thai Working Group on HIV/AIDS Projections was developed to work with the U.S. team (Thai Working Group on HIV/AIDS Projections 1991). The Thai Working Group, consist of experts from the public, academic, and private sectors, compiled and reviewed the available data required by the iwgAIDS model. Figure 1 shows the projections for the spread of the HIV in Thailand.

Highlights from the iwgAIDS model of HIV projections for Thailand are as follows:

- The number of people infected with the HIV is projected to increase from 160,000 in 1990 to between 3.4 and 4.3 million by 2000.
- While more males are initially infected, by the year 2000 more women will be infected than men.
- People in the fifteen to thirty-four age group will be the most infected.
- Urban infected rates among the general population will increase from 0.9 to11.2 per cent and rural prevalence rates will increase from 0.12 to 2.50 per cent between 1991 and 2000.

AIDS Cases and Death Toll

As the iwgAIDS model is still under development with adjustments and revisions occurring, specially with respect to AIDS cases and AIDS deaths. Hence an another model, Epimodel (Chin and Lwanga 1990), was used to project AIDS cases and deaths for this analysis (figure 1). Epimodel is an extrapolation model that can be used for confirming AIDS cases and deaths once a given infection level has been determined. Epimodel duplicates the HIV infections created by the iwgAIDS model to match the infection curve for Thailand. Epimodel predicts that the mean time from infection to AIDS illness is 9.8 years and the time from AIDS illness to death is 1.5 years. Applying these predictions to the iwgAIDS mode HIV projections, Epimodel then creates the resulting number of AIDS cases and AIDS deaths. Note that the mean conversion time of 9.8 years applies only to adults. Conversion intervals for infants and children are much shorter. Thus, the AIDS cases and deaths creates by Epimodel are somewhat understated because the HIV infections from the iwgAIDS model include both children and adults.

Costs Involving AIDS: Direct

Direct costs can broadly be categorized in overall system costs of prevention and personal health care expenditures. Overall system costs of the epidemic that have been calculated include the costs of blood testing, education and prevention programmes, HIV testing by the Thai military and other groups, and training of health care workers. These costs are borne by many strata of society due to the spread of AIDS.

Personal health care expenditures involves the costs of health care for people with AIDS. At this point, the analysis does not cover asymptomatic HIV-positive individuals. The estimation is that these individuals consume very few health care resources. Furthermore, given the overwhelming needs of AIDS patients, it is unlikely that present drug therapies, namely, the anti-viral AZT, would be given prophylactically to HIV-positive individuals in Thailand.

Very little clinical data exist on AIDS patients' care and costs because of relatively late advent of AIDS in Thailand. Therefore, a variety of secondary sources were used to estimate personal health care expenditures. The first step was to confirm the unit cost of care for non-AIDS patients in Thailand. The Ministry of Public Health and others have undertaken several of these cost studies. The study, completed by the MOPH in July 1991, evaluates unit costs for eighty-nine provincial hospitals from 1988-90 (Health Planning Division 1991). This report gives information on material and labour costs for out-patient costs per visit and in-patient costs per day. The information is categorized by size and type of provincial hospital.

The next step was to determine the AIDS-specific cost variables, such as patient days per episode, drug costs per episode, episodes per year, and so on. This AIDS-specific data was calculated based on a study of AIDS patients at Bamrasnaradura Hospital

(Cameron and Schopper 1990a,b). The sample of patients was relatively small. A report on the costs of AIDS in Puerto Rico (Shepard 1990) supplemented the Bamrasnaradura data.

Health care services are delivered in a variety of settings in Thailand, involving private hospitals, Ministry of Public Health hospitals, and other ministry hospitals such as Military, Police, and the Interior. Each hospital setting has its own cost structure. The cost of care considered here pertains to hospitals run by the MOPH, whose facilities present make up more than 60 per cent of the total number of hospital beds in the country.

This analysis shows an initial attempt to collect and organize the information required to assess the cost of care for AIDS patients. Many of the key predictions need more empirical research to verify and refine the estimates.

System Costs

In last five years, Thailand has implemented a number of initiatives to try to contain the AIDS epidemic. System costs, not including personal health care costs, are those expenses incurred by governments, businesses, and individuals to reduce the spread of the disease. Table 2 summarizes the major expenditures identified to date, which in 1991 came to almost US$107 million or baht 2.7 billion.

Personal Health Care Costs

Personal Health Care expenditures are costs that a patient will incur as a result of seeking treatment for full-blown AIDS. These costs are paid by the individual, third party payer, or the government. In the case of Thailand, which has very few health insurance coverage, individuals or the government will bear the burden. The annual cost of AIDS treatment is calculated to be approximately US$1,000 or baht 25,000 per case. This figure represents over 50 per cent of the average annual household income, implying that the government will most likely bear the burden of the cost of AIDS care after households' assets are gone. With current per capita annual health expenditures at US$20, AIDS treatment costs will severely constrain the MOPH's budget.

TABLE 2
THAILAND: SYSTEMS COSTS OF THE AIDS EPIDEMIC, ESTIMATES FOR 1991-92

Category	*Item*	*Cost (US$)*	*Cost[a] (baht)*
Blood supply			
Annual units tested	800,000		
ELISA test cost	US$1		
Percentage tested, ELISA[b]	110%		
Western blot test cost	US$25		
Percentage tested, Western blot	5%		
Subtotal		1,880,000	47,000,000
Military recruits testing			
Annual number of recruits tested	40,000		
ELISA test cost	US$1		
Subtotal		40,000	1,000,000
Thai government AIDS program[c]			
Ministry of Public Health		9,560,000	239,000,000
Other ministries		10,000,000	250,000,000
International donor AIDS program[d]			
To Ministry of Public Health		1,500,000	37,500,000
To Nongovernmental organizations		2,750,000	68,750,000
To Private organizations		1,500,000	37,500,000
Private sector[e]			
AIDS education in businesses		32,000,000	800,000,000
Media air time for AIDS education		48,000,000	1,200,000,000
Total		107,230,000	2,680,750,000

a. Coversion rate US$1=B 25
b. Unites of blood that test positive for HIV are tested again using the ELISA test for confirmation.
c. Based on projections of theThai government's budget for fiscal year 1992.
d. Estimates from the World Health Organization.
e. Estimates from the Prime Minister's Office.

In-Patient Costs. Costs incurred during hospitalization are referred to as in-patient costs. Annual in-patient costs are driven by the type of treatment received (drugs, laboratory procedures, surgery, and so on), the length of hospitalization, and the number of episodes of hospitalization required in a year. Table 3, 4 and 5 begin the assumptions and the results of the health care cost analysis for personal expenditures. As very few data exist for many of the key assumptions, a low and a high scenario are developed.

In this analysis, an average cost per in-patient day of US$22 is used for the high scenario and US$18 for the low scenario. This cost includes all materials as well as direct and indirect labour. This estimate is based on a review of several cost studies for non-AIDS patients. There is no unanimity amongst the researchers in estimating the inpatients costs.

TABLE 3
THAILAND: PERSONAL HEALTH CARE EXPENDITURE ASSUMPTIONS

Health care assumptions	*High Scenario*	*Low Scenario*
In-patient costs		
Material and labour cost per patient day (US$)[a]	22.00	18.00
Capital costs per patient day (US$)	1.84	1.40
Total costs per patient day (US$)	23.84	19.40
Patient days per episode	25	20
Annual percentage reduction of in-patient days per episode[b] (%)	10	10
Drug costs per episode (US$)	60.00	40.00
Episodes per year	1.5	1.5
Percentage of AIDS cases receiving treatment (%)	30-70	20-60
Out-patient costs		
Total costs per visit (US$)	6.40	5.20
Number of visits per year	5	3
Annual percentage increase in out-patient visits(%)	10	10
Percentage of AIDS cases receiving treatment (%)	40-70	30-60
Discount rate (%)	5	5

a. Material costs exclude drug costs.

b. Over time strategies will likely be adopted to reduce the length of in-patient care as physicians gain experience treating AIDS cases and as alternative, out-patient treatment options become available. Thus, in-patient days per episode are projected to decrease annually, while out-patient visits are projected to increase.

TABLE 4

THAILAND: ESTIMATED AND PROJECTED PERSONAL HEALTH CARE EXPENDITURE, HIGH SCENARIO, 1991-2000

Item	1991	1992	1993	1994	1995	1996	1997	1998	1999	2000
In-patient costs										
Total cost per in-patient day (US$)	23.84	23.84	23.84	23.84	23.84	23.84	23.84	23.84	23.84	23.84
Patient days Per episode	25	23	20	18	16	15	13	12	11	10
Cost per episode (US$)	596.00	536.40	482.76	434.48	391.04	351.93	316.74	285.06	256.56	230.90
Drug cost per episode (US$)	60	60	60	60	60	60	60	60	60	60
Total cost per episode (US$)	656.00	596.40	542.76	494.48	451.04	411.93	376.74	345.06	316.56	290.90
Episodes per year	1.50	1.50	1.50	1.50	1.50	1.50	1.50	1.50	1.50	1.50
Total cost per year (US$)	984.00	894.00	814.14	741.73	676.55	617.90	565.11	517.60	474.84	436.35
AIDS cases per year	5691	9286	14827	24288	37199	54409	76438	104455	139310	181062
Percentage receiving Treatment	30	30	40	40	50	50	60	60	70	70
AIDS cases Treated per Year	1707	2786	5931	9715	18600	27205	45863	62673	97517	126743
Total in-patient Costs (US$)	1679983	2492177	4828502	7206016	12583555	16809608	25917447	32439384	46304747	55304979

Table 4 (continued)

Item	1991	1992	1993	1994	1995	1996	1997	1998	1999	2000
Out-patient costs										
Total cost per Visit (US$)	6.40	6.40	6.40	6.40	6.40	6.40	6.40	6.40	6.40	6.40
Visits per year	5	6	6	7	7	8	9	10	11	12
Total cost per year (US$)	32.00	35.20	38.72	42.59	46.85	51.54	56.69	62.36	68.59	75.45
AIDS cases per year	5691	9286	14827	24288	37199	54409	76438	104455	139310	181062
Percentage Receiving Treatment	40	40	50	50	60	60	70	70	70	70
AIDS cases Treated per year	2276	3714	7414	12144	22319	32645	53507	73119	97517	126743
Total out-patient Costs (US$)	72845	130747	287051	517237	1045691	1682424	3033287	4559593	6689163	9563338
Total Costs										
Total costs(US$)	1752828	2622924	5115552	7723254	13629246	18492032	28950733	36998976	52993910	64868317
Discounted costs (US$)[a]	1752828	2498022	4639957	6671637	11212814	14488991	21603483	26294482	35868364	41814695
Total discounted Costs (US$)	166845273									
In-patient costs as a percentage of total costs	95.8	95.0	94.4	93.3	92.3	90.9	89.5	87.7	87.4	85.3
Out-patient costs as a percentage of total costs	4.2	5.0	5.6	6.7	7.7	9.1	10.5	12.3	12.6	14.7

a. Costs discounted at real discount rate of 5 per cent
Source: Described in the text.

TABLE 5
THAILAND: ESTIMATED AND PROJECTED PERSONAL HEALTH CARE EXPENDITURE, LOW SCENARIO, 1991-2000

Item	*1991*	*1992*	*1993*	*1994*	*1995*	*1996*	*1997*	*1998*	*1999*	*2000*
In-patient costs										
Total cost per in-patient day (US$)	19.40	19.40	19.40	19.40	19.40	19.40	19.40	19.40	19.40	19.40
Patient days Per episode	20	18	16	15	13	12	11	10	5	5
Cost per episode (US$)	388.00	349.20	314.28	282.85	254.57	229.11	206.20	185.58	97.00	97.00
Drug cost per episode (US$)	40	40	40	40	40	40	40	40	40	40
Total cost per episode (US$)	428.00	389.20	354.28	322.85	294.57	269.11	246.20	225.58	137.00	137.00
Episodes per year	1.50	1.50	1.50	1.50	1.50	1.50	1.50	1.50	1.50	1.50
Total cost per year (US$)	642.00	583.80	531.42	484.28	441.85	403.67	369.30	338.37	205.50	205.50
AIDS cases per year	5,691	9,217	14,324	22,507	33,338	47,563	64,832	866.14	113,364	145,342
Percentage receiving Treatment	20	20	30	30	40	40	50	50	60	60
AIDS cases Treated per Year	1,138	1,843	4,297	6,752	13,335	19,025	32,416	43,307	68,018	87,205
Total in-patient Costs (US$)	730,724	1,076,177	2,283,618	3,269,893	5,892,161	7,679,811	11,971,185	14,653,737	13,977,781	17,920,669

Table 5 (continued)

Item	*1991*	*1992*	*1993*	*1994*	*1995*	*1996*	*1997*	*1998*	*1999*	*2000*
Out-patient costs										
Out-patient costs										
Total cost per visit (US$)	5.20	5.20	5.20	5.20	5.20	5.20	5.20	5.20	5.20	5.20
Visits per year	3	3	4	4	4	5	5	6	6	7
Total cost per year (US$)	15.60	17.16	18.88	20.76	22.84	25.12	27.64	30.40	33.44	36.78
AIDS cases per year	5691	9217	14324	22507	33338	47563	64832	86614	113364	145342
Percentage Receiving Treatment	30	30	40	40	50	50	60	60	60	60
AIDS cases Treated per year	1707	2765	5730	9003	16669	23782	38899	51968	68018	87205
Total out-patient Costs (US$)	26634	47449	108152	186931	380719	597485	1075032	1579839	2274534	3207755
Total costs										
Total costs (US$)	757358	1123626	2391770	3456824	6272880	8277296	13046217	16233576	16252316	21128423
Discounted costs (US$)[a]	757358	1070120	2169406	2986135	5160714	6485478	9735288	11536899	11000207	13619570
Total discounted costs (US$)	64521175									
In-patient costs as a percentage of total costs	96.5	95.8	95.5	94.6	93.9	92.8	91.8	90.3	86.0	84.8
Out-patient costs as a percentage of total costs	3.5	4.2	4.5	5.4	6.1	7.2	8.2	9.7	14.0	15.2

a. Costs discounted at real discount rate of 5 per cent

Source: Described in the text.

TABLE 6
THAILAND: INFRASTRUCTURE AND CAPACITY ANALYSIS, 1991-2000

Category	*1991*	*1992*	*1993*	*1994*	*1995*	*1996*	*1997*	*1998*	*1999*	*2000*
AIDS patients										
Patient days per episode	25	23	20	18	16	15	13	12	11	10
Episodes per year	1.5	1.5	1.5	1.5	1.5	1.5	1.5	1.5	1.5	1.5
Patient days per year	37.5	34.5	30.0	27.0	24.0	22.5	19.5	18.0	16.5	15.0
Number of AIDS in-patients per year high scenario	5691	9286	14827	24288	37199	54409	76438	104455	139310	181062
Total in-patient days required	213413	320367	444810	655776	892776	1224203	1490541	1880190	2298615	2715930
Current capacity										
Hospital beds available	75000	76875	78797	80767	82786	84856	86977	89151	91380	93665
Annual hospital days per bed	292	292	292	292	292	292	292	292	292	292
Total Hospital days available	21900000	22447500	230086888	23583905	24173502	24777840	25397286	26032218	26683023	27350099
Percentage of bed-days for AIDS patients	0.97	1.43	1.93	2.78	3.69	4.94	5.87	7.22	8.61	9.93
Additional capacity requirements										
Total patient days required	213413	320367	444810	655776	892776	1224203	1490541	1880190	2298615	2715930
Annual Hospital days per bed	292	292	292	292	292	292	292	292	292	292
Additional beds required	731	1097	1523	2246	3057	4192	5105	6439	7872	9301
Incremental beds required	731	366	426	722	812	1135	912	1334	1433	1429

Category	1991	1992	1993	1994	1995	1996	1997	1998	1999	2000
Additional capacity requirements (Continues)										
Capital cost per incremental bed (US$)	16000	16000	16000	16000	16000	16000	16000	16000	16000	16000
Total annual Capital cost (US$)	11693836	17554356	24373151	35932932	48919233	67079589	81673479	103024110	125951507	148818082
Discounted capital Cost (US$)	11693836	16718434	22107166	31040217	40245974	52558613	60946008	73217311	85248938	95929463
Total discounted Capital cost (US$)	489705960									
Discounted capital costs (US$) when bed-days for AIDS patients are at 5% of capacity	315341719									
Assumptions										
Annual growth in hospital beds	2.5%									
Optimal hospital capacity	80%									
Annual hospital days per bed at optimal utilization	292									
Average life of bed (years)	30									
Capital cost per bed (US$)	16000									
Capital cost per bed-day (US$) [16000/(292×30)]	1.84									
Real discount rate	5%									

More information on costs per in-patient day for AIDS patients needs to be collected and analyzed to improve the accuracy of estimates. Furthermore, some estimates of capital costs need to be included. For this analysis, capital costs per bed are calculated at US$16,000 with an average life of thirty years. Table 6 illustrates the predications and calculations used to arrive at a capital cost per in-patient day of US$1.84. Total cost per in-patient day, including capital labour, and materials, is estimated at US$23.84 for the high scenario and US$19.40 for the low scenario. The number of patient days per episode is calculated to be twenty-five days in 1991 in the high scenario and twenty days in the low scenario. (Cameron and Schopper 1990a.b.).

Due to the unavailability of alternative treatment the patient days per episode is more but after the method well be developed in the future, the analysis assumes an annual 10 per cent reduction in patient days per episode, both as a result of physician experience and of alternative care options. The result is that from 1991 to 2000 patient days per episode fall from twenty-five to ten days in the high scenario and from twenty to five days in the low scenario. An initial estimate, drug cost per episode is set at US$60 in the high scenario and US$40 in the low scenario. These initial drug cost estimates do not include the use of AZT, which would increase the cost substantially.

Out-Patient costs. The estimated total cost per out-patient visit is US$6.40 in the high scenario and US$5.20 in the low scenario based on sources and studies described in the cost per in-patient day section. The analysis assumes that AIDS patients frequent out-patient facilities five times per year to receive treatment in the high scenario and three times in the low scenario. Thailand has limited data on out-patient care.

AIDS cases per annum. Projections of the annual number of AIDS cases were discussed before (see figure 1). The figures are adjusted on the assumption that not all those infected will receive treatment. The high scenario assumes that for in-patient care, 30 per cent of AIDS cases are treated in 1991, growing to 70 per cent by 2000. The range of patients treated under the low scenario is 20 to 60 per cent. For out-patient care, 40 percent are treated in 1991, rising to 70 per cent by 2000 in the high scenario, and 30 per cent increasing to 60 per cent for the low scenario.

Infrastructure and Capacity Analysis. Table 6 illustrates the impact the epidemic is likely to have on the present health care infrastructure. AIDS patients will consume 1 percent of the bed-days in 1991, increasing to 12 per cent of the bed-days 2000 in the high scenario. If, however, hospital beds need to be added when the system find a certain level of capacity, the MOPH will have to build additional hospitals to care for AIDS patients. If capacity is not required until AIDS patients use 10 per cent of bed-days, then the cumulative, discounted capital costs amount to US$176 million.

Summary: Personal Health Care Expenditures. Per annum health care costs for AIDS patients amount to US$1,016 (in-patient annual cost of US$984 plus out-patient annual cost of US$32) per patient in the high scenario and US$658 (in-patient annual cost of US$642 plus out-patient annual cost of US$16) in the low scenario. These amounts accounts 50 and 30 per cent, respectively, of the annual household income of an average Thai family. The cost of AIDS treatment is ten times the amount of money families presently spend on health care per year. Given the high costs of care relative to family resources, most families will not be able to bear treatment. Assuming that patients live for one and a half years on average from the onset of AIDS, the lifetime cost per patient would be US$1,524 in the high scenario and US$987 in the low scenario. Figure 2 summarizes these personal health care expenditures. The MOPH" current annual per capita health expenditure is US$20. The cost of treatment for AIDS patients far extent this amount. In the high scenario, aggregate health care costs grow from US$1.7 million in 1991 to US$65.0 million by 2000. In the low scenario, costs increase from US$709,000 to US$20 million.

Indirect Costs of the AIDS

The indirect costs of the AIDS pandemic involves the burden on society of an increase and redistribution of mortality due to AIDS. In other words, the estimated economic costs of the illness and death of adults of working age include not only the cost of medical care, but also the foregone contribution these victims would have made to the economy and to society. Deaths from AIDS will rise among women in their twenties and thirties, men in their thirties and forties, and infants and young children of HIV-positive mothers. In the next decade, most AIDS deaths in Thailand will be of adults in their prime working years. Because the epidemic is mainly urban as estimated by the National Sentinel Seroprevalence Surveys, most of these deaths will be of adults in cities, whose marginal product is higher than that of their rural counterparts. In 1991 urban marginal product of labour (marketed and nonmarketed) is calculated at US$1,500. National average GDP per capita in 1991 was approximately US$1,250. The methodology used is to discount prime adult years lost. The present value of cumulative indirect costs is US$8.5 billion in the high scenario and US$7.3 billion in the low scenario. The loss per death of US$22,000 is similar to 17.6 times per capita income in 1991.

TABLE 7
THAILAND: INDIRECT COST ANALYSIS, 1991-2000

Year	*Annual Deaths*	*Discounted years*	*Annual loss (US$)*	*Cumulative loss(US$)*	*Loss per death (US$)*
High scenario					
1991	4457	14.45	96605475	96605475	21675
1992	7489	13.73	154235955	250841430	20595
1993	12056	13.04	235815360	486656790	19560
1994	19557	12.63	370507365	857164155	18945
1995	30743	11.77	542767665	1399931820	17655
1996	45804	11.18	768133080	2168064900	16770
1997	65423	10.63	1043169735	3211234635	15945
1998	90446	10.09	1368900210	4580134845	15135
1999	121882	9.59	1753272570	6333407415	14385
2000	160186	9.11	2188941690	8522349105	13665
Low scenario					
1991	4457	14.45	96605475	96605475	21675
1992	7454	13.73	153515130	250120605	20595
1993	11770	13.04	230221200	480341805	19560
1994	18415	12.63	348872175	829213980	19945
1995	27923	11.77	492980565	1322194545	17655
1996	40451	11.18	678363270	2000557815	16770
1997	56198	10.63	896077110	2896634925	15945
1998	75723	10.09	1146067605	4402702530	15135
1999	99989	9.59	1483341765	5481044295	14385
2000	129353	9.11	1767608745	7248653040	13665

Aggregated Costs

Figure 3 indicates total annual health care costs plus the value of lost income are projected to increase from US$100 million in 1991 to US$2.2 billion by 2000 in the high scenario, and from US$97 million to US$1.8 billion in the low scenario. Over the ten-year period, US$8.7 billion will be lost due to AIDS in the high case and US$7.3 billion in the low case. These annual costs, both direct and indirect, are similar to some sixteen to eighteen times the per capital GDP.

Other Macroeconomic Consequence

The AIDS epidemic is likely to alter the performance of the Thai economy unless there is any considerable charges in social behaviour. The health care costs and lost income examined above are not the only prospective costs of the epidemic. Domestically, a shortage of labour, both in quantity and quality, may happen with an increase in AIDS. High rates of absenteeism brought on by illness will certainly be disruptive to companies. Finding and retraining workers to change those that have died will be difficult and costly, especially if the unemployment rate remains at the current low of 3 to 4 per cent. Various business surveys researching foreign investment criteria quote a large supply of inexpensive labour as a key factor in selecting Thailand. For the past two years foreign direct investment has overcome US$2 billion yearly. A reduction in the supply and health of labour could increase both wage rates and production costs, making Thailand a less attractive place to invest in.

Approximately 70,000 Thai labourers travelled abroad to find employment in 1991. These workers remitted nearly US$1 billion in wages to their families. Already countries are screening prospective foreign workers for the HIV before permitting them to enter. If Thai workers are no longer able to work abroad a valuable source of income will be lost.

The nation's rate of saving may also decline as spending on medical care rises relative to income. The country's total investment may be further reduced as the government is required to devote more resources on social and health services, rather than investing in infrastructure and other productive projects. Thailand's US$5 billion per year tourism industry may already be feeling the effects of AIDS. Tourist arrivals are down for a variety of reasons, with the fear of AIDS certain to be a major factor in the future.

Investment Estimated for Prevention

The iwgAIDS model used to create the high and low scenarios can measure various interventions on the spread of the epidemic. The behavioural changes suggested to alter the scenario are Sexual contacts with different partners are reduced by one-half, condom use doubles from about 25 to 50 per cent, sexually transmitted diseases are treated quickly and effectively.

If this level of extensive behaviour change occurs in the very near future it results in dramatic savings of lives and costs: by the year 2000, 3.5 million fewer people would become infected and US$5.1 billion would be saved. Even if the AIDS prevention budget triples in the next several years, the cost of prevention yields a seventeen fold return on that investment in human life.

The challenge posed to the three sectors viz. Society, government and private, to devote adequate resources, people and money, to reduce the spread of the epidemic. Urgent action is the need of the hour for both financial and humanitarian reasons.

Twenty Seven

HIV/AIDS Laws in China

Introduction

The proliferation of AIDS globally has become an issue of serious concern. In the preceding years there has been a rapid increase in the AIDS cases in Asia-Pacific regions, where an estimated 2 million people are HIV infected.

China is a country of low HIV prevalence. However, the increase of HIV/AIDS cases detected in the country can not be bypassed. Since the first AIDS case found from among a foreign tourist group in this country in 1985, there have been reported 261 AIDS cases and 969 HIV infections by November 1992. Out of the 30 provinces/municipalities/autonomous regions of the country (not including Taiwan Province), HIV infections have been found in 18 provinces and autonomous regions.

After the Chinese policies of reforms and opening to the outside world, China's communication with foreign countries has been broadened in political, economic and cultural areas, etc. Consequently, there are more opportunities and routes for HIV to be transmitted into the country, China is a developing country with a large population of which 80 per cent is rural. If there is a rampant prevalence of HIV/AIDS in the country, it would have an inestimable bearing on the economic development of this country and the world as a whole. For this very reason the Chinese government has assigned a high priority to the prevention and control of HIV/AIDS by framing a national comprehensive programme comprising of therapeutic, administrative and economic measures, and by framing a plan of action for its implementation. The state legislative bodies have, at the same time, implemented relevant laws, legislations and regulations for its prevention and control with the hope to secure, by mandatory force of the state, the implementation of relevant laws and regulations. The legislative activities are the most significant link for the prevention and control of HIV/AIDS of the country. A brief introduction in this aspect is hereunder given.

Goals

China is a country with high population density. Hence, "putting prevention first" for the secure health of the broad masses of people has been the consistent bases of China's policy in health services, as well as in the prevention and control of HIV/AIDS. HIV/AIDS is a disease both with a medical and social nature. It has been, therefore, specified in the legislation that HIV/AIDS patients are subject to respect and security under the precondition of ensuring the interests of the vast majority of the population.

Contents of Legislation

China's legislation monitoring the prevention and control of HIV/AIDS covers the following contents, inter alia, quarantine services at the border, civil law concerning marriage and family, and criminal law. A brief description of relevant aspects and its background are given hereunder.

(i) A Public Health

As an infectious disease HIV occupies an important place in the state legislation concerning the control of infectious diseases. "The Law Governing the Control of Infectious Diseases in the People's Republic of China" adopted by the National People's Congress in February of 1989 and the process for its implementation as approved by the State Council in October of 1991 are of prime task to the prevention and control of infectious diseases of the state. Aspects related to the control of HIV include:

(i) It has been specified in the epidemiological reporting system that, whenever an AIDS case is found a report must be made to local health authorities within 6 hours from city/township and within 12 hours from rural areas.
(ii) Measures for the monitoring pathogen transmission include: establishment of strict managerial and operation

procedures in medical health institutions to stop iatrogenic infection; strict management is applied to the storage, delivery and transportation of virus strains of infectious diseases and establishment of strict hygienic managerial requirements for the disposal of water and solid wastes contaminated by HIV.

(ii) Primary Legislations Governing the Prevention and Control of AIDS

Since the identification of the first AIDS case in 1985 in this country, surveillance centres on AIDS have been set up by health authorities in all the provinces/municipalities/autonomous regions and the prefectures under its jurisdiction. In order to strengthen its activities, the State Council approved and made, in 1987, "Certain Regulations Relating to the Surveillance and Management of AIDS" as jointly suggested by nine departments concerned, including the Ministry of Public Health, the Ministry of Foreign Affairs, and the National Tourism Administration. This is the first legislation mainly formulated for the prevention and control of HIV/AIDS with the following main contents:

- Target persons for surveillance are specified;
- Serological tests are to be given, upon their entry into this country, to those foreigners applying for residence and/or for a stay more than one year, and appropriate measures are to be taken by health departments if HIV is found;
- Chinese citizens, having resided and/or having stayed outside the country for a period more than one year, are subject to physical examination by health departments concerned within a certain period of time after their return; and
- Strict management is applied to blood and blood products as a possible transmission route of HIV.

(iii) The Management of Blood and Blood Products

Blood and its products are known as a most prone route through which HIV is transmitted. Health authorities under the State Council have, since the identification of the first AIDS case in China, framed a series of regulations and notifications including, inter alia:

(iv) Quarantine Services at the Border

The rapid increase in the communication with the outside world has posed serious threat, because of the possibility of transmission of HIV. The quarantine services at the border is doing a yeomans service in early detection and consequent deportation of the HIV positive foreigners.

The Frontier Health and Quarantine Law of the People's Republic of China and its task for implementation specifies the following systems for the prevention of HIV/AIDS.

Epidemiological Reporting System

A system of mutual notification and reporting shall be established between the health departments and health and quarantine authorities.

Surveillance System of Infectious Disease

All incoming and outgoing passengers are subject to surveillance for infectious diseases. They are required to fill in the health declaration form and to make health certificates and other relevant documents.

Monitoring System

The health and quarantine authorities shall apply medical control measures, i.e., isolation of the infected passengers for observation, and shall refuse the entry of any AIDS patient.

(v) Gender

Owing to their specific status, women suffer the worst and encounter more difficulties. It is to this end that the state has framed legislation to ensure women's rights and interests and to protect the health of women and children.

Legislation of this country for the protection of women's rights and interests, of women's and children's health, and for the prevention of HIV infection include, inter alia:

(a) The state ensures women's equal rights and interests to that of men in political, economic cultural, social aspects, as well as in family life. This aspect has manifested itself to the complete in the Constitution

Law, the Law for the Protection of Women's Rights and Interests, the Marriage Law, and the Civil Law of this country.

(b) The state has established a series of systems to make sure the health of women and children. The Ministry of Public Health has framed "The Routine Regulations for Health" specifying the establishment of pre-marital health care, health care in the period of pregnancy and delivery, defining duties and responsibilities of health-care gives and its work performance requirements and provision of physical examination and medical treatment.

Control of HIV Infection

Sexual behaviour is the most significant causative factor for HIV infection of women, while venereal diseases constitute an important factor for women's vulnerability. Hence, the control of venereal diseases is an significant link to prevent women from being infected.

(vi) Criminal Legislation

Criminal sanction is the most severe feature the state adopts against unlawful practice. In order to make sure effectively the implementation of the systems and measures established for the prevention and control of HIV/AIDS, and to curb and crack down the malfeasance and criminal acts that cause the spread of HIV, Article 178 of "The Criminal Law of the People's Republic of China" promulgates that those in violation of the "Frontier Health and Quarantine Law of the People's Republic of China' are subject to a fixed term imprisonment up to three years and/or detention. Corresponding penal articles are promulgated also in the "Frontier Health and Quarantine Law of the People's Republic of China" and the "Law Governing the Prevention and monitoring of Infectious Diseases of the People's Republic of China."

Of the 969 HIV carriers, 585 are Chinese nationals, of which 537 are drug injectors living in the border areas of Yunnan Province. Hence, IV drug users constitute the most threat of the spread of HIV in this country. A most resolution was thus reached in December of 1990 by the National People's Congress that penal sentence is to be given to those who cajole, abet, deceive and/or compel others to take or inject narcotic drugs. Education, compulsive means and/or administrative sanction are to be given to those who take and/or inject the drugs. The National People's Congress adopted, in 1991, a resolution to strictly prohibit prostitution. A test for venereal diseases and their treatment through compulsive means are to be given to prostitutes, and administrative punishment or penal sanction is to be given depending on the seriousness of the wrong-doing.

Conclusion

The number of HIV/AIDS cases in China and its socio-economic consequence to the continental part of the country is not yet significant. However, with the increase of its continuity, more socio-economic problems can be foreseen, i.e., the increase of economic expenditure; the decrease of socio-productivity as the result of increases in the number of HIV carriers; and the protection of people with HIV and AIDS patients (their employment and medical care), etc.

The legislation regarding to the prevention and treatment of HIV/AIDS of this country is at its initial stage and with certain limitations. The established standards are incomprehensive, certainly concentrated on measures for its prevention and treatment. More exploration, investigation and proofing are required in a number of aspects in the legislation. It is imperative, therefore, to sum-up the experiences both of the positive and negative sides of other countries, and to further emphasise that preventive measures are far more significant than remedial measures.

Of prime importance for the framework of corresponding policies and legal measures is the better understanding of the specific features of HIV/AIDS, and by approaching it from medical, social, economic and legal points of view.

1. Steps desirable to strengthen and improve the legal and other related matters. Strengthening of health education to help cultivate a healthy life-style.

2. Revising legislation relating to the rights and obligations of people with HIV and AIDS. In special, the social status and basic rights and obligations of HIV/AIDS patients are to be defined further in order to prevent social discrimination of HIV/AIDS patients, and the fear of people with HIV among the society and community.
3. Managerial procedures shall be emphasised over the main causative factors for the spreading of HIV such as blood and iatrogenic infection.
4. Legislation relating to maternal health and delivery are to be perfected with an aim to reduce the suffering and adverse effects of HIV infection in women.

Twenty Eight

Research Studies from Uganda

HIV/AIDS is as much about social phenomena as it is about biological and medical concerns. All over the world, the global pandemic of HIV/AIDS has shown itself capable of triggering responses of compassion, solidarity and support, bringing out the best in people, their families and communities. But the disease is also related to stigma, ostracism, repression and discrimination, as individuals affected (or believed to be affected) by HIV have been rejected by their families, their loved ones and their communities.

This rejection holds as true in the rich countries of the north as it does in the poorer and developing countries of the south. All over the world, ignorance, of knowledge, afraid and denial have engendered serious and often tragic results, denying people living with HIV/AIDS access to treatments, services and support, as well as making it hard for prevention work to take place. The epidemic of fear, stigmatization and discrimination first described by Jonathan Mann (1987) has undermined the capability of individuals, families and societies to protect themselves and give support and reassurance to those infected (Merson, 1993).

The London Declaration on AIDS Prevention following the World Summit of Ministers of Health on Programmes for HIV Prevention in January 1988 was one of the first international statements to recognize that:

> *"Discrimination against, and stigmatization of, HIV-infected people and people with AIDS and population groups undermine public health and must be avoided." (para 6).*

In 1988, Resolution WHA 41.24 of the 41st World Health Assembly later on urged Member States to foster a spirit of understanding and compassion for HIV-infected people and those suffering from AIDS. Additionally, the resolution recommended Member States to protect the human rights and dignity of affected individuals and population groups to discourage discrimination and stigmatization in the provision of services, employment and travel.

In 1989, the United Nations Centre for Human Rights convened the first international consultation on HIV/AIDS and human rights. This forum reaffirmed the public health rationable for the prevention of HIV/AIDS- related discrimination and the promotion and protection of human rights in the context of HIV/AIDS-a view reaffirmed in United Nations General Assembly resolutions in 1990 and 1991.

In late 1996, for the human rights the second international consultation on HIV/AIDS and human rights was convened jointly by UNAIDS and the Office of the High Commissioner. Twelve international guidelines on HIV/AIDS and human rights were drafted at this meeting, the majority of which stressed, once again, the need to avoid HIV/AIDS-related discrimination and to ensure the promotion and protection of the human rights of people living with, and affected by, HIV/AIDS.

International human rights law wants to guarantee freedom from discrimination on various grounds including sex, race, language, religion, political opinion, birth or other status. In Resolutions 1995/44 and 1996/43, the UN Commission on Human Rights confirmed that the phrase "other status" is to be interpreted as incorporating health status, comprising HIV/AIDS. This implies that discrimination against people living with HIV/AIDS-or those perceived to be at higher risk of infection –is legally prohibited.

Resolution 49/1999 of the UN Commission on Human Rights reaffirms that:

> *"Discrimination on the ground of HIV or AIDS status, actual or presumed, is prohibited by existing international human rights standards, and that the term, 'or other status' in non-discrimination provisions in international human rights texts should be interpreted to cover health status, comprising HIV/AIDS."*

Among its several provisions, the resolution encourages states, UN agencies, non-governmental organizations, UN treaty bodies and inter-governmental organizations to combat HIV/AIDS-related discrimination, prejudice and stigma and to monitor and implement HIV/AIDS-related human rights. Visibility and openness about HIV/AIDS are prerequisites for the successful mobilization of government and community resources to respond to the epidemic. Since they fear stigma and discrimination, people living with HIV/AIDS may be deterred from being open about their serostatus. This makes the governments able and others to deny that there is a problem.

Consultations and meetings have already taken place designed particularly to review experiences and progress in combating the soons of stigmatization and discrimination that are serious obstacles to prevention and care. Objectives also comprise sharing best practices with respect to existing codes and legislative frameworks, and to further contribution to international endeavours ensuring that HIV/AIDS related discrimination is reduced and its effects ameliorated (see, for example, HRI, 1996).

Given this intensity of activity, it may be surprising to learn that comparatively little systematic research has taken place on the *forms* that HIV/AIDS-related stigmatization and discrimination take, the various *contexts* in which they occur and their varying factors. Indeed, a review of the abstracts from recent regional and international conferences on HIV/AIDS shows that the majority of papers dealing with such concerns concentrate either on individual cases or experiences, or on the role of non-governmental organizations in exerting pressure on governments and national authorities to act to prevent further discrimination.

Background to the Present Studies

In 1994, under the auspices of the World Health Organization's former Global Programme on AIDS (WHO/GPA), the first steps were taken to develop a general research protocol to explore these issues systematically and in some depth (WHO, 1994). Given the Comparatively uncharted nature of the field, this protocol was developed in two parts: the first offered guidelines for a country-level extended rapid assessment of the factors of HIV/AIDS-related discrimination, stigmatization and denial; the second provided guidelines for more in-depth study. Central to the issues highlighted were these research questions:

- How are HIV/AIDS-related stigmatization and

discrimination defined and perceived across various societies at the individual, institutional and policy levels?

- What forms do HIV/AIDS-related stigmatization and discrimination take at various stages of the epidemic and in what contexts do they occur?
- What are the chief sources of HIV/AIDS-related stigmatization and discrimination?
- What are the responses to HIV/AIDS-related stigmatization and discrimination?
- What are the most proper research methods for analysing and understanding HIV/AIDS-related discrimination, stigmatization and denial?

After consulation with WHO's regional offices, three countries - India, Uganda and Venezuela - were recognized as having the capacity and willingness to undertake extended rapid assessments along the lines outlined in the general research protocol. In all three countries the seriousness of the epidemic among all, or particular sections of, the population warranted the commissioning of such work. Potential principal investigators from each country were later invited to prepare local research proposals based on the general research protocol and to submit these to WHO/GPA for scientific evaluation and approval. The approval of national authorities and national or local ethical review committees was sought in each case. Two studies carried on by the Tata Institute of Social Sciences in India (Dr. Shalini Bharat, Principal Investigator) and by TASO in Uganda (Ms Sophia Mukasa Moniko, Principal Investigator) were later funded. With the support of UNAIDS, preparatory work commenced in 1997. Work was completed in late 1998.

This report brings together highlights from these investigations. It offers :

- a review of appropriate literature;
- a statement of research questions and methods prioritized by each of the local investigations;
- a description of importent findings from work conducted in Uganda and India;
- a thematic analysis of issues recurring in each study site; and

- recommendations for policy, programming, practice and further research.

Relevant Literature: A Review

Before the development of the general research protocol, a literature review was undertaken. Among other issues, the protocol examined the nature, sources and forms of HIV/AIDS-related stigmatization, discrimination and denial, key contexts in which it occurred (comprising the workplace, the health care system and with regard to travel and migration), and implications for intervention. An expanded and partially updated version of this review has later been published (Malcolm et al. 1998). It is this version that forms the basis of discussion here.

Stigma and HIV/AIDS

In a now classic statement, the sociologist Erving Goffman (1963) defined stigma as a "significantly discrediting:" attribute possessed by a person with an "undesired difference". Stigma is a powerful sources of social control applied by marginalizing, excluding and exercising power over individuals who display particular traits. It is a common response to perceived threat when escape from, or the destruction of, this threat is not possible. While the societal rejection of particular social groups (e.g. homosexuals" injecting drug users, sex workers and migrants) may predate HIV/AIDS, the disease has, in various cases, reinforced this stigmatization.

By attributing blame to particular individuals and groups, society can absolve itself from the liability of caring for and looking after such populations (McGrath, 1992). This is seen not only in the manner in which "outsider" groups are blamed for having brought HIV into a country or neighbourhood, but also in how such groups are later denied access to the services and treatment they need.

Gilmore and Somerville (1994) have described what they see as the four important features of any stigmatizing response: the problem that starts the reaction, the identification of the group or individual to be targeted, the assignment of stigma to this individual or group; and the development of the stigmatizing response. Other authors prevalent-feelings that individuals harbour about their condition and the likely reactions of others. Enacted stigma refers to actual experiences of stigmatization and discrimination (Scambler & Hopkins, 1986; Jacoby, 1994).

Felt stigma generally precedes enacted stigma and may limit the extent to which the latter is experienced. For instance, some people living with HIV, aware that several people with HIV/AIDS have been treated badly by others, may conceal their serostatus. To the extent that they are successful in "passing" as non-infected, such individuals may limit the amount of enacted stigma prevalent in a society or community- at least in the short term.

Sources of HIV/AIDS-related Stigmatization, Discrimination and Denial

An historical and sociocultural perspective may be helpful in the negative reactions triggered by HIV/AIDS. In previous epidemics, the real or supposed contagiousness of disease has resulted in the isolation and exclusion of infected people (Volinn, 1989; Gilmore & Somerville, 1994). Sexually transmitted diseases specially are notorious for triggering such socially divisive responses and reactions (Carrara, 1994; Goldin, 1994).

From early in the AIDS epidemic, a series of powerful metaphors were mobilized which serve to reinforce and legitimate stigmatization. These comprise HIV/AIDS as death (e.g., through imagery such as the Grim Reaper); HIV/AIDS as punishment (e.g., for immoral behaviour); HIV/AIDS as a crime (e.g., related to innocent and guilty victims); HIV/AIDS as war war (e.g., in relation to a virus which needs to be faught); HIV/AIDS as horror (e.g., in which infected people are demonized and feared) and HIV/AIDS as "otherness" (in which the disease is an affliction of those set apart). Together with universal belief that HIV/AIDS is shameful (Omangi, 1997), these metaphors constitute a series of "ready-made" but highly inaccurate explanations that provide a powerful ground for both stigmatizing and discriminatory responses. These stereotypes also enable some people to refuse that they personally are likely to be infected or affected.

People living with HIV/AIDS are seen as ignominious in various societies. Where the infection is associated with minority groups and behaviours (for example, homosexuality), HIV/AIDS may be linked to "perversion" and those infected punished (Mejia, 1988). In individualistic societies, HIV/AIDS may be seen as the result of personal irresponsibility (kegeles et. al., 1989). In yet other circumstances, HIV/AIDS is seen as bringing shame upon the family and community (Panos, 1990; Warwick et al., 1998).

The manner in which people respond to HIV/AIDS therefore different with the ideas and resources that society makes available to them. While negative responses to HIV/AIDS are by no means essential, they not infrequently feed upon and reinforce dominant ideologies of good and bad regarding to sex and illness, and proper and improper behaviours (Warwick et al., 1998).

De Bruyn (1999) has recently identified five factors as contributing to HIV/AIDS-related stigma:

- The fact that HIV/AIDS is a life-threatening disease;
- The fact that people are frightened of contracting HIV;
- The disease's association with behaviours (like sex between men and injecting drug use) that are already stigmatized in various societies;
- The fact that people living with HIV/AIDS are often thought of as being responsible for having contracted the disease;
- Religious or moral belief that lead some people to conclude that having HIV/AIDS is the outcome of a moral fault (like promiscuity or "deviant" sex) that deserves punishment.

HIV/AIDS-related stigmatization causes resources inevitable to preventing infection to be displaced. People are victimized and blamed, social divisons are reinforced and reproduced and new infections continue to emerge as long as people misread the nature of the epidemic and its reasons. More importantly, while negative responses of stigmatization and discrimination seemingly give cohesion to societies and communities, they lead to greater instability in the long term. The social categories and obstacles that have been constructed around it cannot contain HIV/AIDS. It needs a more effective means of prevention that this.

Forms of HIV/AIDS-related Stigmatization, Discrimination and Denial

There are several levels at which HIV/AIDS –related discrimination, stigmatization and denial may be experienced and felt. These comprise societal and community levels, besides to the experience of individuals.

Societal and Community Levels

Societally, laws, rules, policies and procedures may result in the stigmatization of people living with HIV/AIDS. A considerable number of countries have enacted legislation with a view to controlling the actions of HIV/AIDS-affected individuals and groups (Tomasevski et al., 1992). These laws comprise legislation for:

- The compulsory screening and testing of groups and individuals.
- The prohibition of people living with HIV/AIDS from particular occupations and types of employment;
- The medical examination, isolation, detention and compulsory treatment of infected persons;
- Limitations on international travel and migration;
- The restriction of certain behaviour like injecting drug use and prostitution (Gostin & Lazzarini, 1997).

International experience now shows that such kinds of measures serve only to increase and reinforce the stigmatization of people living with HIV/AIDS and those at greatest risk of contracting the virus. In several countries, discriminatory practices such as the compulsory screening of certain populations or "risk groups" cause both the further stigmatization of such groups and a misplaced sense of security among those who do not see themselves as belonging to these sections of the population. Moreover, a recent review has, moreover, pointed to the gaps between more liberal national policies and the application of these policies and principles in practice (Gruskin, Hendricks & Tomasevski, 1996). Even where supportive legislation is in prevalance, its application may be partial, uneven or ignored.

Restrictive and coercive measures-repeatedly enacted to "protect" society from infection-discriminate against, or exclude, those who are already infected. Laws that insist on the compulsory notification of HIV/AIDS cases and the restriction of a person's right to anonymity and confidentiality and as the right to movement of those infected, have been justified on the basis that the disease constitutes a public health emergency (Manuel et al, 1990). While with other infectious diseases such responses may be justifiable, in the case of an already highly stigmatized condition like HIV/AIDS disease they result in punitive measures that further discriminate against people living with HIV/AIDS and may drive those infected, and those most vulnerable, further underground (Gostin & Lazzarini, 1997).

Perhaps in consequence, several countries have now enacted legislation to protect the rights and freedoms of people living with HIV/AIDS and to safeguard them from discrimination (Mann, Tarantola & Netter, 1992; Mann, Tarantola & Netter, 1996). Much of this legislation has sought to make sure the right to employment, education, privacy and confidentiality, as well as the right to information access, treatment and support. However, the failure of governments to protect people living with HIV/ AIDS from discrimination, through legislation or through the active implementative of such legislation, is a violation of their human rights. The apathy of some governments in giving effective systems of prevention, treatment and care may also arise from more deep-seated stigmatization at a societal level.

Governments and national authorities contribute to HIV/AIDS-related stigmatization in other ways. They may, for instance, cover up and conceal cases or fail to maintain reliable and transparent reporting systems (Milner, 1991; Whiteside, 1993). Ignoring the existence of HIV/AIDS, neglecting to respond to the requirements of those living with HIV infection, and failing to accept burgeoning epidemics in the belief that HIV/AIDS "can never happen to us" are some of the most widely reported responses of denial (Daniel, 1991; Milner, 1991). This denial fuels stigmatization by making those few individuals accepted to have HIV/AIDS appear abnormal and exceptional. They do little to enable people to develop a more realistic appreciation of individual vulnerability, and contribute to a vulnerability to the epidemic (Mann, Tarantola & Netter, 1996; UNAIDS, 1997).

Stigma and discrimination, both real and perceived, may also arise from a kind of community-level responses to HIV/AIDS. The harassing and scapegoating of individual is suspected of being infected or of belonging to a special group has been widely reported. It is generally stimulated by the need to blame and punish and can, in extreme circumstances, extend to acts of violence and murder (Nardi & Bolton, 1991). Attacks on men who are presumed gay have increased in several parts of the world, and have been related to the growing HIV/AIDS epidemic. Sex workers and street children in Brazil have likewise been singled out for violence and abuse (Peterson, 1990 Byrne, 1992). HIV/

AIDS-related murders have been reported in countries as diverse as Brazil, Colombia, Ethiopia, India, South Africa and Thailand (Panos 1990; AFAO, 1997). In December 1998, Gugu Dhlamini was stoned and beaten to death by neighbours in her township near Durban, South Africa, after speaking out publicly on World AIDS Day about her HIV status.

Individual Experience

People's experience of HIV/AIDS-related stigmatization and discrimination is affected by common belief, forms of societal stigmatization, and factors like extent to which individuals are able to access supportive networks of peers, family and kin. It may also be influenced by the stage of the epidemic and whether individuals feel they can be open about their serostatus, age, gender, sexuality and social status-among a lot of other variables.

Overall, the negative depiction of people living with HIV/AIDS –reinforced by the language and metaphors used to talk and think about the disease-has reconfirmed fear, avoidance and the isolation of affected individuals and, in few cases, friends and families. In a highly stigmatizing enviornment, people may withdraw from society as a means of self-preservation. This isolation also means exclusion from social and sexual relationships and –in extreme circumstances-has led to premature death through suicide or euthanasia (Gilmore & Somerville, 1994; Hasan et al, 1994).

Who to tell, how and when, can be a potential source of fear and anxiety among a number of people living with HIV/AIDS and may prevent individuals from accessing treatment and care (Moynihan et al., 1995; Omangi, 1997). Even where laws have been enacted to protect the rights and confidentiality of people living with HIV/AIDS, some people are ready to litigate in case their identity will become widely known. Those who are recognized as belonging to marginalized and/or minority groups may also worry about the reactions of others, regardless of their serostatus. Fear of telling family members about their homosexuality has recently been cited by some Mexican men as amount to the fear of revealing their serostatus (Castro et al., 1998a; 1998b).

The impact of HIV/AIDS on women is especially acute. In various developing countries, women are already economically, culturally and socially backward and lack equal access to treatment, financial support and education. Being outside the structures of power and decision-making, they may be refused the opportunity to participate equally within the community and may be subject to punitive laws, norms and practices exercising control over their bodies and sexual relations. In many societies, women are erroneously perceived as the chief transmitters of sexually transmitted infections (STIs), which may be referred to as "women's disease" (de Bruyn, 1992). Together with conventional beliefs about sex, blood and other sorts of disease transmission, these perceptions provide a fertile ground for the further stigmatization of women within the context of HIV/AIDS (Ingstad, 1990; Peterson, 1990; Mushingeh, Chana & Mulikelela, 1991; Thant, 1993).

There is explicit evidence from recent UNAIDS-supported studies of household and community responses to HIV/AIDS in developing world (Warwick et al., 1998; Aggleton and Warwick, 1999 that seropositive women are likely to be treated very differently from men. Whereas men are likely to be "excused" for the behaviour that resulted in their infection, women are not. In India, for instance, the husbands who infected them may abandon women living with HIV/AIDS. Rejection by wider family members has also been reported as common (Bharat & Aggleton, 1999). In some African countries, women whose husbands have died of AIDS-related infections have been blamed for the death. Remaining relatives may also evict the surviving spouse from her home (Henny, 1990).

Perhaps in result, individual denial of risk and vulnerability is not an uncommon response to the epidemic. Such denial may manifest itself in self-distancing from the problem and in, extreme cases, can result in people misperceiving their vulnerability. Denial can also discourage voluntary testing among a large number of people, particularly among members of particularly vulnerable groups. This, in turn, may enhance the potential risk of HIV transmission within community (Lie & Biswalo, 1996).

Contexts of HIV/AIDS-related Stigmatization, Discrimination and Denial

HIV-related stigmatization, discrimination and denial may seem in a variety of contexts. Central among those are the family and local community, employment and the workplace, and the health care system.

The Family and Community

In the majority of developing countries, families are the chief care-givers to sick members. There is clear evidence of the important role that the family can play in supplying support and care for people living with HIV/AIDS (World Bank, 1997; Warwick et al., 1998; Aggleton & Warwick, 1999). However, response of all family is not positive. Infected and affected family members may still be stigmatized and discriminated against within the home. There is also mounting evidence that women (Bharat & Aggleton, 1999) and non-heterosexual family members (Castro et al., 1998a; 1998b) are more likely to be badly treated than children and men.

The family's attempts to "manage" stigmatization within the wider community also have consequences for quality of care. Families may shield affected members from the wider community by reserving them within the house or by protecting them from questioning (L wihula et al., 1993). The extent to which such policies are successful may depend upon the wealth of the household concerned and its capacity to provide care without calling upon other community members for support.

Afraid of rejection and stigmatization within the home and local community may prevent people living with HIV/AIDS disclosing their serostatus to family members (McGrath et al., 1993). Families may reject seropositive members not only due to the stigma related to HIV/AIDS, but also because of the connotations of homosexuality, drug use and promiscuity that HIV/AIDS carries (Panos, 1990, Misra, 1999; Mujeeb, 1999).

Employment and the Workplace

While HIV is not readily transmitted in the majority of workplace settings, the supposed risk of transmission has been used by a number of employers to terminate or refuse employment (see, for example, Barragan, 1992; Gostin, 1992; Panos, 1992. Shisam,

1993; Hasan et al., 1994; Omangi, 1997). There is also testimony that where people living with HIV/AIDS are open about their serostatus at work they are likely to experience stigmatization and ostracism by others (Panos, 1990; Gostin, 1992; Gostin & Lazzarini, 1997).

Pre-employment screening takes place in many industries – especially in countries where the resources for testing are readily available and affordable. In several poorer countries screening has also been reported as taking place, particularly in industries where health benefits are available to employees (Parker, 1991; Jackson & Pitts, 1991). Employer-sponsored insurance schemes providing medical help and pensions for employees have come under increasing pressure in countries that have been seriously affected by HIV/AIDS. Some employers have used this pressure to deny employment to people living with HIV/AIDS (Whiteside, 1993; Williams & Ray, 1993).

Only a very few companies in developing world appear to have developed strategies to combat fear, stigma and discrimination in the workplace (see Hughes, 1988, for instance, and an equally small number have begun to define the liabilities of employers towards employees with HIV/AIDS (Jackson & Pitts, 1991; Bezmalinovic, 1996).

The Heath Care System

Several reports reveal the extent to which individuals are stigmatized and discriminated against by the health care system. Several accounts also proliferate of withheld treatment (see , for example, AIDS Bhedbhan Virdhi Ándolan, 1993; Carvalho et al., 1993; Panebianco et al., 1994); non-attendance of hospital staff to patients left lying in their beds (see, for instance, Daniel & Parker, 1990; Ogola, 1990; Masini & Mwampeta, 1993); HIV testing without consent, breaches of confidentiality, and refusal of hospital facilities and medications (see, for example, Panebianco et al., 1994).

Contributing to such responses are ignorance and dearth of knowledge about HIV/AIDS transmission (Kegeles et al, 1989; Herek & Capitano, 1993; Herek et al., 1998); fear (Blendon & Donelan, 1988; Tesch, Simpson & Kirby, 1990; Rosasco Dulato, 1992); moralistic assumptions of guilt (Cole, Zhang & Chen, 1993,

Masini & Mwampeta, 1993); and the perceived incurability of HIV/AIDS. All of these conspire to make it seem pointless to offer good-quality care.

Lack of confidentiality has been frequently cited as a specific problem in health care settings. Wide variations in practice exist between countries, and between health care facilities within countries. In some settings signs have been placed near people living with HIV/AIDS with words like 'HIV-positive' and "AIDS" written on them. Elsewhere, registers of HIV-positive people have been compiled and their names released to media and police without permission (Panos, 1990; Singh, 1991).

Principles of confidentiality also vary between countries and cultures. In some places, for instance, confidentiality may be less an individual issue that, a community and collective concern. The term "shared confidentiality" describes a situation where family and community members realize they have the right to know the serostatus of family members, neighbours and friends (Campbell et al., 1997).

Implications for Enquiry

The above are not the only settings in which HIV/AIDS-related stigmatization and discrimination take place. It should be conspicuous that responses in one setting (e.g., the hospital and health care setting) may have results for the way in which people react in others (e.g., at work or at home). We require to examine more closely the fields in which stigmatization occurs; the forms the HIV/AIDS-related discrimination takes, individual, social and institutional factors, and the responses to which stigmatization gives rise. Only by understanding more about such processes will it be feasible to develop the kinds of programmes and interventions that will be successful in preventing HIV/AIDS-related stigma and the negative results to which it gives rise.

Research Questions

As stated earlier, a common core of research questions underpinned the investigation. To make sure that research remained sensitive to local priorities and requirements, these were modified according to issues of particular local relevance.

The study in **India** therefore examined:

- What are the different direct and indirect forms of expression of HIV/AIDS-related stigmatization, discrimination and denial in India, and how do these forms vary across different city locations?
- What are the various contexts namely kinship relations, work settings or caring settings, in which discrimination and stigmatization occur, and how do such expressions vary in accordance with the contexts and level at which they occur?
- What are the dominant individual, socio-economic or cultural determinate that influence or contribute to HIV/AIDS-linked stigmatization, discrimination and denial?
- What is the complete status of HIV/AIDS-related stigmatization and discrimination on the national agenda with regards to human rights debate, public health issues and existing social tensions and conflicts?
- What is the role played by policies, media and advertising to endorse or contain HIV/AIDS –related stigmatization and discrimination? What has been the role of non-governmental organizations?
- What are the results of HIV/AIDS related stigmatization, discrimination and denial, and can some of these experiences be used in interventions?

(Source: Tata Institute of Social Sciences application for funding, dated 25/10/95)

The study in **Uganda** aimed to give particular attention to :

- Analysing the different forms of HIV/AIDS –related stigmatization, discrimination and denial in contrasting sites within Uganda:

  What are the different kinds of HIV/AIDS-related stigmatization, discrimination and denial in specified study areas? How are these forms defined in different cultural, economic and social contexts? Do the different stages of the epidemic influence the forms of HIV/AIDS-related stigmatization, discrimination and denial?

How are these different forms manifested at the individual, family, institutional and policy levels?

- Establishing the determinants that influence different forms of HIV/AIDS-related stigmatization. Discrimination and denial:

  What are the births of HIV/AIDS-related stigmatization discrimination and denial? What are the specific factors liable for enhancing these forms? What is the relative impact of factors influencing HIV/AIDS-related stigmatization, discrimination and denial? How does the impact differ across different cultural, social and economic settings?
- Assessing the many responses to which HIV/AIDS-related stigmatization, discrimination and denial give rise:

  What has been the response of people living with HIV/AIDS to stigmatization, discrimination and denial? What has been the response of affected families and communities, and of institutions like education, health care and employment systems? How has the legal and judicial system addressed issues concerned to stigmatization, discrimination and denial?

(Source: TASO application for funding, dated 29/7/96.)

Set of Methods

Sites

India

Given that the forms and factors of HIV/AIDS-related stigmatization, discrimination and denial vary according to context, principal investigators in India and Uganda were encouraged to recognize two or more sites from which data might be collected.

In India, investigators aired at collecting data in three contrasting locations; Mumbai, where the impact of HIV/AIDS is particularly severe; and New Delhi in the north of the country and Bangalore in the south-both cities in which numbers of cases of HIV infection are rising incessantly. Given the tight time-frame for the preliminary work, it was feasible to conduct in-depth work in only two of these locations: Brihan Mumbai or Greater Mumbai in the state of Maharashtra and Bangalore in the state of Karnataka.

These cities differ dramatically from one another; Mumbai, well established as the financial capital of India, and Bangalore, rapidly developing due to the introduction of new technology. In the words of the Principal investigator :

> *"Referred to as the, metaphor for modern India; Mumbai (makes) one of the most considerable contributions to the Indian economy and (is) a major partner in the global process of development. With its ever growing population, the 'Dream City' is a breeding ground for drug peddlers, traders of flesh and people indulging in high risk behaviour."*
>
> *"(Bangalore) once a quaint cantonment town is today a vibrant metropolis with a cosmopolitan population.....Well known for the electronic and computer software industries, Bangalore is valued as the Silicon Valley of India and today has the distinction of being the fastest growing city in South Asia. But its expansion has brought in its wake unplanned development, discrepancies in living standards and large scale migration.. Unlike Mumbai, Bangalore has no well-demarcated red-light area. The sex trade is spread all over the city and is mainly street based."*

Following the prior reporting of significant levels of HIV/AIDS-related stigmatization, discrimination and denial in the workplace, in the health care system and within the home and community, a decision was taken to restrict the focus of the investigation to these three settings. Much valuable contextual data relevant to the latter two settings existed from an earlier study of household and community responses to HIV/AIDS supported by WHO/GPA (Bharat, 1995).

Uganda

In Uganda, the study took place in two contrasting locations: Kampala District and Mbarara District. Kampala District is the largest urban area in Uganda and houses the capital city of the country. It is an important centre endowed with social, professional, welfare and legal organizations and services active in the struggle against HIV/AIDS. The district contains a heterogeneous population of various cultures, ethnic groups and ways of life. In contrast, Mbarara District is a rural area that is comparatively homogeneous with respect to culture, behaviour and perceptions.

There are far fewer organizations providing HIV/AIDS-related services in this part of the country. It is generally believed that knowledge of, and awareness about, HIV/AIDS is lower in Mbarara than in Kampala.

In Uganda, TASO's prior experience providing care and support to people living with HIV/AIDS and their families had suggested that it would be beneficial to focus on three contrasting settings within which HIV/AIDS-related stigmatization, discrimination and denial might be expected to manifested itself. These are the individual and family level, the institutional and community level comprising the workplace, health care system and places of worship) and the policy level. It should be recognized, however, that these three settings to some extent overlapped, and the responses within one of these environments might be anticipated to influence those in others.

Methods

The general research protocol for the UNAIDS studies of the factors of HIV/AIDS-related stigmatization, discrimination and denial had identified the appropriateness of various different methods in the investigation of relevant issues. These included-both primary and secondary approaches to data collection and analysis.

Primary approaches comprised of key informant and in-depth interviews with individuals living with and affected by HIV/AIDS-related stigmatization, discrimination and denial, focus groups in communities and settings affected by HIV/AIDS-related stigmatization, discrimination and denial, and observation in workplace, health care and community settings where HIV/AIDS-related stigmatization, discrimination and denial might manifest itself.

Secondary approaches comprised the analysis of existing sources of information like newspaper, radio, and television reports describing examples of HIV/AIDS-related stigmatization, discrimination and denial; legal records and case notes concerning to relevant court cases, and national and local policies relating to HIV/AIDS-related stigmatization, discrimination and denial. Principal investigators were, however, given the option of choosing one method over the other (or stressing the use of certain approaches) depending upon local expertise and issues examined.

India

In India, key informant interviews, in-depth interviews and focus group discussions were the most important methods used to collect data. These were complemented by case studies of individuals who reported having been subjected to HIV/AIDS-related stigmatization, discrimination and denial; by observation of HIV/AIDS patients in health care and other settings; and by "dummy" patient interviews. Respondents were selected particularly so as to illuminate key issues and concerns. Given the nature of the enquiry (an extended rapid assessment) and the lack of relevant sampling frames, no effort was made to utilize more representative forms of sampling.

A total of 31 key informant interviews took place in Mumbai and a further 54 in Bangalore. They included voluntary sector workers active in HIV/AIDS prevention and care, deans and heads of hospitals, medical professionals from a range of specialties, the heads of personnel and social welfare departments in chosen industries and companies, and experts from the fields of insurance, law and consumer rights.

In-depth individual interviews took place with 31 HIV-positive people in Mumbai and nine of their household care-givers. In Bangalore, 13 interviews were made with people living with HIV/AIDS, and five with household care-givers. Additionally, six in-depth interviews were made with HIV-positive members of socially marginalized groups in Mumbai and three in Bangalore. These groups comprised *hijra*, gay men and women sex workers.

Twenty focus group discussions took place with hospital staff in Mumbai and 13 in Bangalore. Four focus group discussions were organized with women sex workers in Mumbai and one in Bangalore. One focus group discussion took place with *hijra* in Mumbai and one in Bangalore.

Twenty-seven private clinics were chosen for dummy patient interviews in Mumbai and 13 in Bangalore. In both sites, extra contextual data were collected from community support group members, community members, truck drivers (Bangalore) and other groups. For a full breakdown of the sampling, see Bharat (1999).

Uganda

In Uganda, researchers conducted an initial reconnaissance exercise in each of the districts in which they intended to conduct the study. They sought to recognize certain areas within each district in which the study might be conducted, establish the household concentration of people living with, and affected by, HIV/AIDS, and identify community leaders and obtain their consent for the study. In addition, researchers aimed to identify local organizations working with, and providing services for, people living with HIV/AIDS.

Eight potential categories of respondents were recognized: people living with HIV/AIDS, families affected by HIV/AIDS, counsellors, legal professionals, medical personnel, community leaders, religious leaders, and NGO and community-based organization (CBO) workers. This approach allowed the study to concentrate on the different determinants determining HIV/AIDS-related stigmatization, discrimination and denial.

Data were collected by the way of individual interviews, focus group discussions and observation. In-depth individual interviews were held with 22 people living with HIV/AIDS in Kampala, 20 in Mbarara, and 10 representatives of families affected by HIV/AIDS in each of these locations. Besides three counsellors, three medical personnel and two community leaders were interviewed in each site. Three religious leaders in Kampala and two in Mbarara, two legal professionals in Kampala and one in Mbarara, and three NGO/CBO representatives in Kampala and one in Mbarara were also interviewed.

Focus group discussions organised with two groups of people living with HIV/AIDS (one male and one female) in Kampala and Mbarara, respectively. One mixed focus group discussion comprising people living with HIV/AIDS was held in Kampala and two were held in Mbarara. Focus group discussions with counsellors also took place in Kampala(1) and Mbarara (2) and with community workers in Mbarara (1).

Observations took place in hospital environments where people living with HIV/AIDS received care. Attention focused not only on the way in which such individuals were received in reception areas, but also the way in which staff responded to their requirements. Additionally, it was possible to observe how relatives and care-givers within the home responded to people living with HIV/AIDS.

As was the case in India, sampling was carried out on the ground of awareness of the contexts and settings in which HIV/AIDS-related stigmatization, discrimination and denial has been documented to prevail. Further details of the sampling and data collection and analysis can be found in Mukasa Moniko, Otolok Tanga & Nuwagaba (1998).

Basic Findings

India

Forms

A wide range of different kinds of HIV/AIDS-related stigmatization, discrimination and denial were discerned in the study conducted within Mumbai and Bangalore. While the focus of the fieldwork was on stigmatization and its results within the health care and employment settings, stigmatization, discrimination and denial in intimate relationships at home, in the community and even after death with regard to the disposal of bodies and funeral arrangements) were also discussed. In each of these settings, felt and enacted stigma were identified, as well as HIV/AIDS-related stigmatization, discrimination and denial in both overt and covert forms.

The majority of people living with HIV/AIDS who were interviewed had learned about their serostatus either during an illness, surgery or pregnancy. Differential treatment was reported as occurring just after (and sometimes even before) disclosure was made. As Saroja, the 38-year old-HIV-positive wife of a man diagnosed in hospital in Bangalore, recounted.

> *"The staff were looking after my husband well, but after they tested his blood for HIV/their behaviour get changed and they*

separated our vessels, pushed him to a corner of the room and talked about us in hushed tones. I couldn't know why their behaviour had become so cold."

The experience of the following HIV-positive person getting treatment for tuberculosis was typical of several others in the same hospital in Bangalore.

"My blood was tested and from that day they stopped giving me injections. They did not tell my why."

In Bangalore, individuals diagnosed with HIV/AIDS in private hospitals were reportedly transferred to government hospitals where conditions and the quality of care are generally far worse. As a surgeon in a government hospital explained.

"In private hospitals the news of HIV-positive patients once discerned is closely guarded and the patient is conveniently transferred to a government hospital."

Likewise in Mumbai, a nephrologist attached to a private hospital said:

"We are not bound by any rule to give treatment to positive patients. Let the government hospitals take that liability. There is a great deal of risk of infection to my staff in the nephrology department, and I'm responsible for my staff's welfare and health."

Elsewhere in Mumbai, a few private hospitals were reported as accepting people living with HIV/AIDS as patients-although this acceptance came with a price. The costs of fumigating operating theatres and labour rooms, or liberally giving double and even triple hand gloves to staff, and an HIV-AIDS kit to all staff assisting in surgery, amounted in some medical professionals, eyes to an indirect form of discrimination against people living with HIV/AIDS.

During the course of the study, it was feasible to recognize some of the ways in which the identity of HIV-positive patients was marked. Medical files in the majority of hospitals in Mumbai are theoretically kept in the safe custody of the ward nurse, but in at least one private hospital the identity of HIV-positive patients on the general ward for economically poorer patients was plain for all to see. A ward boy says:.

"When the patient comes to our wards, it's written on the file

"HIV" in big letters. Anybody can see it. It's kept next to the patient. Anybody can see it".

Less obvious , but nevertheless stigmatizing, practices were noted in few Mumbai hospitals. In a private hospital, staff reported keeping tubs of disinfectant under the beds of HIV-positive patients in which eating vessels, clothes and linen were soaked before to being washed separately. As one care-giver says:

"The tub is the symbol for the staff. We don't use any board, etc., to declare AIDS but the tub lets us understand."

Other ways of letting staff know who is HIV-positive and who is not comprise shouting to ward boys "take this HIV-positive patient for X-ray". In a public hospital in Mumbai and in Bangalore beds are earmarked for HIV-positive patients to permit the staff to easily discern them. As a senior doctor put it:

"We never keep them in the middle of other patients since they may also contract the infection. But we do not tell other patients about positive patients."

In the course of the study, many accounts were elicited of medical and nursing staff breaking the confidentiality of an HIV-positive diagnosis and telling family members and relatives before the patient him/herself. A couple interviewed in Bangalore revealed these:

Husband: "The doctor didn't inform me. He informed my wife and asked her to inform me."

Wife: "I took my husband to the lab and got his blood tested. After two days they called me and informed me that my husband's blood test result was positive. My husband informed them he had illicit relationships with a woman three years back. The doctor told me the news."

In the case of less-educated or economically poor patients, other family members might be informed first so they could help explain the situation to their relatives.

"When a young woman who is first-time pregnant is found to be HIV positive we call her mother-in-law. We read the report to the mother-in-law and ask her to get the son also tested. These patients who come in here are from low-income groups, and if the girls are newly married they are really dumb and

don't understand anything, so mother-in-law is called."
(Gynaecologist, private hospital, Mumbai)

Sometimes doctors and nurses argued that this was done to protect the patient from shock and feasible self-destructive behaviour. As a nurse in Mumbai explained:

"The patient, as it is, is half-dead. If he is told of the test results, he might commit suicide."

That said, there was significant evidence that once the news had reached relatives the results were far from supportive. Young women in particular reported being blamed and rejected by in-laws and other family members. Men were dealt with far more supportively and positively. As Mary, a 25-year-old HIV-positive woman in Mumbai, explained:

"My in-laws blame me for their son's death. They have severed all relationships with me. They never made discrimination with their son but to me they say, "You also have AIDS. Stay happily wherever you are.' I took great care of their son—never felt dirty while cleaning him up. But they always say 'You married him and our son got bedridden'. I have lost faith in everybody."

And as Nigamma, a 40-year-old HIV-positive widow in Bangalore, recounted:

"My in-laws do not have a good opinion about me. They say that my husband got this disease from me. I sometimes feel why should I survive with the insult. It is better to die. But I am living for the sake of my children."

HIV-positive interviewees reported experiencing strong pressures to keep their serostatus secret within the workplace. The shame of accepting to colleagues and friends that you have HIV, coupled with the perceived likelihood of being dismissed on discovery, combined to silence the huge of respondents. As one HIV-positive 23-year-old man put it:

"You know how the society is. They want your reputation to be sullied. I know if my HIV-status comes to be known to them, they will call me names, laugh at me, jeer at me, and I'll have no other alternate than to commit suicide. I shudder at the very thought."

And as another HIV-positive respondent explained:

> *"And who will give me a job? My health will not be good. I will be unable to work so they will think. What will I do for my living? So it is better not to tell anybody."*

The experience of those few respondents who had disclosed their serostatus at work was far from reassuring:

> *"Those staff members who know about me talk about it. They point at me and say, 'Look, he is the HIV fellow.' They....keep their distance from me and remain aloof. I don't share my tiffin box with them any more. I don't feel like coming to work. I did not come to work for 10-15 days and then lose wages." (Tatya, 38-year-old hospital ward body)*
>
> *"My colleagues didn't openly say anything to me, but the environment was no longer the same. They avoided me. If I entered the room they would leave abruptly. Then they asked me to keep a separate glass for water. I decided to leave the job." (Daljit, 25-year-old factory worker).*

If there was a margin of security for hospital and some factory workers who were open about their serostatus, the same was certainly not true for those employed in more marginal occupations. Ram Niwas, for instance, used to sell bhel puri in an upper-middle-class residential neighbourhood in Mumbai. He used to consult his local doctor about his medical condition and when he came down with an STD was advised to take an HIV-antibody test as well. He showed the positive result to his doctor who briefed it to him but also alerted the local police inspector. The next day the police asked him to move out from the locality of the rich and influential people because he was said to pose a risk to their health.

In a number of businesses with whom contact was made, denial was the order of the day. Personnel managers and welfare officers refused to accept either that HIV infection was a problem or that it might be so in the future. A local transport company in Mumbai was reported as not having a written policy on HIV/AIDS since "there is not a single case of HIV reported in the company so far". The human resource development officer in a software company in Bangalore said in interview that:

> *"Our staff is very highly paid. They are drawn from the most reputed institutions and we are quite sure they do not have*

behaviour which makes them suspect for HIV. They are very well educated and have easy access to sources of information, so cannot easily fall for such things."

In a small –scale private box manufacturing company in Mumbai, the managing director, who reported keeping in view that HIV was spread by infected water and blood, said there were no medical facilities available for staff. If workers did not pack the needed number of boxes each day they were simply not taken on for work the next day. If they were sick, they were sent home soon.

Determinants

Clearly, several factors underpin the forms of stigmatization and discrimination described above. Several of these relate to the very real fear of HIV/AIDS that exists among both the general public and professionally qualified health care workers. The sources of these fears are complex and comprise lack of knowledge and understanding, as well as the manner in which AIDS has been reported in the national and local media (e.g. as being highly " contagious" when in fact it is not).

Other reasons of stigma and discrimination have their origins deep within Indian culture and the manner in which "sexual wrongdoing" is popularly understood. Others—especially those within the health care setting-appear to relate both to dearth of knowledge about HIV/AIDS, its routes of transmission and ways of protection, as well as to local beliefs about infection through closeness and proximity.

Long- standing opinions of gender that result in women being blamed for the transmission of sexually transmitted infections-either directly as the supposed "vectors" of transmission or indirectly through failing to "satisfy" their husbands-influence the ways in which families and communities react to the seropositivity of their members. While seropositive men may be offered support and care, the same is unlikely to be true for women-several of whom are blamed for the illnesses from which they and their husbands may suffer.

Processes of stigmatization, whereby people living with HIV/AIDS are rendered outsiders and "others", are also reinforced by the tendency for people living with HIV/AIDS to make themselves not visible and to disavow their condition. This enables employers and others to refuse that there is a problem.

Responses

Clearly, HIV/AIDS has evoked a number of responses in the Indian context, some of them positive, others considerably less so. At the positive end of the spectrum are the reactions of households and families who agreed to give care and support for affected members. These responses, it has to be said, were corporeatively infrequent, but were more likely to occur when male household members rather than women were affected.

Much more common were responses of ostracism and rejection. The predominant effects at the individual level were fear and withdrawal leading to secrecy about HIV status and self-imposed social isolation. In some cases, suicidal tendencies were noted, and in a few other examples people living with HIV/AIDS sought to avoid stigmatization by denying their serostatus, thereby risking transmission of infection to others.

Negative responses in the health care setting (or the belief that there will be negative responses) lead people to hide their HIV status in treatment facilities for fear of being refused care. Individuals who are sick may also delay seeking treatment until the last moment, harming their own health in the process.

Within the workplace, widespread denial that HIV/AIDS is a problem means the majority of companies and employers have no policies and procedures with which to respond to seropositive employees. The belief that HIV only affects promiscuous people, and that "such types" are unlikely to work in a given location further helps to institutional denial. Because of the social stigma related to keep their serostatus secret. This helps to the invisibility of the epidemic and makes life more difficult for those individuals affected.

Sometimes, however, HIV/AIDS-related stigma may trigger more positive responses such as the altruistic actions of those who carve roles for themselves as educators, counsellors and HIV/AIDS activists. Through their work, such individuals may evolve a collective identify and mobilize group support that results in a greater awareness of the epidemic and-more positive responses towards those affected.

Uganda

Forms

While the Ugandan Government has enacted a national multisectoral policy on HIV/AIDS which demands that:

> *"All Ugandans have individual and collective liability to be actively involved in AIDS control activities in a coordinated way. The fight against AIDS is not only directed at the prevention of the spread of HIV, but also addresses the active response to, and management of, all perceived results of the epidemic."*

While capacity-building and non-discrimination have been highlighted as central features of Uganda's response, there was explicit evidence from data collected in both sites that the rejection of people living with HIV/AIDS by family and community continues. Near bout the same number of people living with AIDS in each site reported having been rejected by their families as reported having been admitted a finding which initially surprised the principal investigators of the Uganda study.

Women in particular were often blamed for the death of a husband. As a member of an all-women focus group of people living with AIDS in Mbarara said:

> *"A large number of old men think that it is women who spread AIDS in families. Others think that to get AIDS one must have been promiscuous to others. It is (seen as) a curse on the family."*

In another focus group discussion undertaken in this same site, respondents suggested that:

> *"People would wish that a widow living with AIDS died sooner rather than later so that she does not spread AIDS after she has got treatment and looks health."*

Legal professionals interviewed as part of the study reported that:

> *"Widows have told us several times that, after the death of their husbands, among the results faced is ostracism, the children are taken away from them, property is grabbed by the in-laws, and people mock them that much...".*

Members of a women's focus group conducted in Mbarara explained how:

> *"One father-in-law sold land that belonged to his deceased son,*

comprising the plot where the widowed daughter-in-law lived. She was told to go where she got AIDS from!".

Perhaps due to fear of punitive actions, some women in Kampala were reported as deserting their sick husbands before the death as a means of avoiding reprisal afterwards. Men participating in a focus group conducted with people living with HIV/AIDS said:

"Kinship/relatives always blame their widowed in-law for having 'killed' their son in case he dies of AIDS. Other causes (for running away) are that the widow fears the likely reprisal but also running away is a demonstration of a kind of denial, not wanting to face the truth there and then."

Sometimes, more extreme responses were noted, as in the following story, told by other women in a focus group conducted with women infected with HIV in Mbarara.

"A 20-year-old woman had got results that she was HIV positive. She had to be put aside for crisis counselling. She was intended to kill her children as she had never gone with anybody else apart from her husband."

In spite of the fact that legal measures have been taken against companies that have attempted to make discrimination against people living with HIV/AIDS within their workforce, seropositive workers reported being fearful of disclosing their serostatus in the workplace. "Finger-pointing" was a frequently cited workplace response to people living with HIV/AIDS who were open about their condition at work.

"Even if your boss has not shown any indication of dismissing you, the fellow workmates talk behind your back. In this case, the boss may sack you and your job (is) given to a healthier person, judging from what was always talked about you".

There was also proof in the Uganda study of the mediating effects of relative affluence on the manner in which individuals with HIV/AIDS might anticipate to be treated by family and community. Particularly in rural areas, families were reported as giving support and care only as long as their livelihood and standard of living could be maintained. As a group of women living with HIV/AIDS interviewed in Mbarara explained.

"PWAs {people living with HIV or AIDS } live freely in families

in which they belong and experience love and care. But this is only as long as the family has enough resources. If the resources are depleted, then the PWA takes the blame since after all he has to die. "

Beyond the enacted stigma and discrimination evident in the examples described above was the felt or perceived stigma that led individuals to police their own behaviour to prevent their serostatus becoming known to others. As one interviewee explained:

"It is not good to disclose one's serostatus because once one's friends know, they start spreading rumours which may even reach schools where one's children study, and obviously such children get affected."

In few cases, this self-stigmatization resulted in an individual's avoidance of particular social settings and/or places of work. These comprised bars and clubs as well as other environments in which individuals felt they might be subjected to stigmatization and discrimination. Regarding employment, counsellors in a focus group discussion in Kampala stressed how they had.

"....encountered clients who have not been removed from their work but who have sort of dismissed themselves due to self-stigma."

Others also saw felt stigma as triggering an uncooperative approach as individuals declined to accept the help and support offered to them.

"Some people are not very supportive since the PWA him/herself may not be cooperative to other members (of the family). He/she may stigmatize him/herself, hence repelling the would-be help from other people." (Focus group discussion, Mbarara).

Determinants

The writers of the report on the Uganda study recognized a range of factors of HIV/AIDS-related stigmatization, discrimination and denial. Among the key individual and family determinants identified were dearth of knowledge coupled with the persistence of lay or popular faiths about HIV/AIDS. Despite years of government publicity and work by non-governmental and community organizations, and regardless of attempts to encourage non-discrimination and social solidarity, at family and community level, HIV/AIDS is still perceived as a condition linked to promiscuity and sexual wrongdoing.

Among some rural people, HIV/AIDS continues to be associated with witchcraft and curses, making ostracism and stigmatization seem legitimate, besides causing individuals to be singled out for condemnation within their own communities. As a man with HIV/AIDS participating in a focus group discussion in Mbarara explained:

> *"In my family I was the first to suffer from AIDS. At one time during funeral rites (for another person), an announcement was made that I had got AIDS and that I had brought a curse to the family."*

As highlighted above, the consequences of becoming infected are not the same for women and men. Long-held ideologies and beliefs make it seem logical that, while men may seek several partners (and receive social status for doing so), women should limit themselves to only one. To some limit, such practices are legitimized by the traditional marriage bond that denies women the opportunity to object when their husbands put them at risk. The authors of the Uganda report quote from Ngugi's (1996) work.

> *"I knew my husband was having sex outside our marriage with several partners but I have no right to refuse sex with him according to our tradition. He is my husband and had paid bride wealth. I tested HIV positive and I am bitter. And following of my socio-economic status I cannot just walk away".*

The resemblance between the above situation and respondents' accounts in the present study are striking. The origins of these behavioural discrepancies can be found in traditional values and beliefs.

> *"African cultural values and value systems increase the spread of HIV even within wedlock... Most women have continued to get HIV through such biased cultural norms and values that allow extra marital sexual relations for men."*

There was explicit evidence throughout the Uganda study that both socio economic status and contact with community-based organizations (CBOs) could mitigate the stigma related to HIV and AIDS. Wealther people were seen, for instance, as having the capacity to better manage both the flow of information concerning to affected family members and the care of affected persons at least until AIDS-related sickness starts impose hard financial burdens upon individuals and the household.

In relation to contact with CBOs, respondents in both Mbarara and Kampala reported some ambivalence to the assistance provided by CBO workers who arrived in vehicles with "TASO" (or an equivalent name) emblazoned on the side.

> *"We are happy with the services given to us...But I feel a bit uncomfortable when TASO staff come in their vehicles to visit me. I like to come to TASO but not TASO come to my home." (PWA focus group discussion, Kampala)*

Finger-pointing was not unknown in the self-help meetings organized by some CBOs.

> *"Although you could not clearly see them, whenever I went to CBO meetings people would point fingers at me saying my husband died of AIDS. I had to stop going to attend their meetings." (PWA focus group discussion, Mbarara)*

Clearly CBOs need to consider carefully the way in which they make their services available and the manner in which they work with clients if their endeavour are to have maximum profit.

Responses

Reported responses to the stigma, discrimination an denial of HIV/AIDS in the Uganda study were of three main kinds. First, there were responses of an individual nature. These comprised "coming out" to the family and community as having HIV/AIDS. Interestingly, revealing HIV/AIDS status was found in few cases to diminish the stigma related to the condition. As reported in a counsellors' focus group discussion in Mbarara,

> *"One lady who had AIDS had earlier been rejected by the relatives and the community, but after she went public and declared her serostatus, those who had deserted her now come for help and guidance on how to meet with AIDS."*

In this case, we can see how admitting one's serostatus

may reduce both the felt and enacted components of HIV/AIDS-related stigma. An additional perceived benefit for some women was that admitting their seropositivity reduced the likelihood that other men would approach them for unwanted sexual relationships.

The power of counselling to support people in confronting HIV/AIDS-related stigma and discrimination is a recurrent theme throughout the Uganda study. In a focus group discussion of people living with HIV and AIDS in Mbarara, it was reported that:

> *"Once you have been counselled, you don't mind about people's comments and reactions against you."*

However, there were others who did not gain the strength to be fully open about their condition. For them, a more alone and generally isolated life was the only alternate. The psychological rejection that derives from HIV/AIDS-related stigma can seriously neglect the individual's feeling of self-worth and self-esteem, and in extreme circumstances it can lead to individuals dying alone from treatable conditions like tuberculosis.

At the family and community levels, HIV/AIDS-related stigmatization and discrimination were reported as having lessened as more and more families wee affected, and as responses of support had been forthcoming. In a focus group discussion comprising men living with HIV/AIDS in Kampala, it was said that:

> *"Several people (families) have lost their dear ones. It is due to this reason that they come to help with the situation ad not to stigmatize and discriminate against PWAs."*

And in a similar group discussion in Mbarara, a man reported:

> *"My family and relatives from the time I disclosed my serostatus have been supportive, sympathetic and caring. I was happy that my family accepted me. They advised me to go to TASO for long life, care and support. One of them organized a TASO counsellor for me."*

However, as reported earlier, the responses women received were likely to be very different from those accorded to men.

"Self-stigmatization" could also be a problem for some:

"Some people are not supportive since the person with AIDS him/herself may not be cooperative with other (family) members. He/she may stigmatize him/herself hence repelling help from other people." (Mixed focus group discussion, Mbarara).

Within the institution, HIV / AIDS-related stigmatization and discrimination have influenced the responses of several health care staff, some of whom are now reported as taking active steps to challenge the sorts of stigma that existed early on in the epidemic. As a key informant interviewed in Kampala put it:

"The attitude of health workers towards people living with AIDS and HIV is positive (now) because almost everybody has been affected. Near about everyone has lost a relative, a friend or neighbour."

In Mbarara, some health workers were even planning to have money curtailed from their salaries every month to give support for people living with HIV / AIDS. As the administrator of the local hospital explained:

"Health workers in this area have a socio-medical committee particularly aimed at addressing the social aspects of persons living with AIDS. They are proposing to fund it by curtailing some money from their own monthly salaries."

As mentioned earlier, attempts have been made at government level to enact legislation to protect people living with HIV / AIDS from discrimination and to promote a more compassionate and caring response. While an evaluation of the impact and effectiveness of this legislation was well beyond the scope of the Uganda study, the authors come to conclusion that the existence of a clear legislative framework to promote the human and civil rights of people living with HIV / AIDS is a decisive component of any programme to lessen HIV / AIDS-related stigma and discrimination.

Subject Analysis

Throughout both of the studies many themes recur.

First, it is important to recognize that HIV / AIDS related stigmatization, discrimination and denial can appear in a number of forms, at a number of levels and in a variety of contexts. Mapping these forms is the first step towards being able to recognize their determinants. It may be important theoretically and practically to differentiate between individual, family-level, community and institutional factors.

Second, pre-existing local cultural practices and beliefs are both factors and legitimators for HIV/AIDS-related stigmatization, discrimination and denial. These faiths frequently establish categories of person or types of behaviour that are likely to be stigmatized (e.g. sexually "promiscuous" individuals, sex workers, drug users and homosexuals). The advent of HIV/AIDS repeatedly reinforces these already existing types of stigma, imbuing them with new and potent legitimacy.

Third, there is an important differentiation to be made between "felt" and "enacted" stigma. Felt stigma arises from the real or imagined stigmatizing responses of others. It has an important role to play in "policing" the behaviour of people living with HIV/AIDS, causing some to deny their serostatus, others to conceal it, and all to experience anxiety about telling others an seeking care. The results of both felt and enacted stigma undermine endeavours to challenge HIV/AIDS publicly admitting their serostatus and playing their full and proper role in prevention and care.

Fourth, socio-economic status and relative financial (and productive) security can influence the stigmatizing process. By enabling some families to "conceal" HIV/AIDS-affected members either within the home or in private medical facilities, some individuals are able to avoid being overtly stigmatized. At the same time, however, it may be particularly shameful for wealthy individuals and their families to admit being affected. More generally, socio-economic status and wealth permit people to better manage the flow of information concerning to HIV/AIDs and its impact upon family and household members.

Finally, it is explicit that there is a strong gender bias in HIV/AIDS related stigmatization, discrimination and denial. Women and men are not dealt with in the same way when they are infected—or believed to be affected—by HIV/AIDS. There is testimony that men and more likely to be admitted by family and community. Women, on the other hand, are more likely to be blamed, even when they have been infected by their husbands in what for them have been monogamous relationships. This double standard exacts a terrible toll on women as mothers, as daughters, as care-givers and as people living with HIV/AIDS. HIV/AIDS-related stigma, and the discrimination to which it leads, therefore plays an important role in intensifying gender inequalities.

Policy, Programme Development and Future Research

The local studies of the factors of HIV/AIDS-related stigmatization, discrimination and denial analyzed here took the form of extended rapid assessments of six months' duration. When originally planned, they were seen as the precursors to later inquiries involving larger numbers of respondents and a more in-depth approach. Given the scope and nature of the enquiry, therefore, it would be not reasonable to expect detailed policy and programming implications to be derived from the data. This was not the objective of the local investigations carried out.

However, regarding policy development the following general points can be made:

- Endeavours to tackle HIV/AIDS-related stigmatization, discrimination and denial appear doomed to fail in the absence of a supportive legal framework. In the words of the India report, "It is not enough to spread awareness about HIV/AIDS, its transmission matters or even about legal rights. What is urgently required is government anti-discrimination policy supported by a law that will ensure the protection of (HIV) positive people's rights."
- Even where these kinds of laws exist, or where governments make active endeavours to combat HIV/AIDS-related discrimination, it is important to challenge popular myths, stereotypes and judgements that provide the ground upon which HIV/AIDS-related stigma can grow. At the policy level, prevention programmes should foster tolerance and social solidarity using, wherever feasible, an approach which is non-judgemental and not based on fear.
- In both employment and health care, discriminatory policy requires to be developed to protect and safeguard the employment and health care rights of people living with

HIV/AIDS. Central to this must be principles of confidentiality and respect for human rights.

- Interventions targeting discrimination require to take place concurrent with the establishment of a supportive legal framework that comprises generic anti-discrimination laws covering health care, employment, education, housing and social security, and effective enforcement mechanisms. Other important and complementary activities must comprise efforts to change attitudes through communication campaigns in the media, education and training.

In future prevention, care and impact-mitigation programming:

- Interventions and activities should aim to move from providing only information to providing services and social support with a view to countering the prejudices and popular faiths about HIV/AIDS that seemingly justify stigmatization and discrimination.
- Greater attention requires to be given to the gender-biased nature of HIV/AIDS-related stigma. Endeavours should be made to address not only women's risks of HIV/AIDS infection but their heightened vulnerability to the social stigma related to HIV/AIDS. In the majority of societies, a double standard exists whereby men are allowed (and even encouraged) to have more than one partner, while women are blamed for the results of this behaviour. The effects of this double standard on women's health and well-being, property rights and rights of access to children are serious, and need to be addressed urgently.
- Endeavours must be made to tackle the forms of felt and enacted stigma that make it difficult for people living with HIV/AIDS to be open about their serostatus. This secrecy reasons them to withdraw from social life, and makes it difficult for them to play a full part in prevention and to benefit from care.

With respect to future research, more needs to be learned about:

- The overt and the more hidden and institutionalized forms

of HIV/AIDS-related stigmatization, discrimination and denial that exist in various settings and at different stages of the epidemic.

- The determinants of these different sorts of HIV/AIDS-related stigmatization, discrimination and denial, and the circumstances and determinants that lead to a reduction in stigmatization and its negative consequences.
- The pervasive discursive, cultural and structural frameworks that act as sources of HIV/AIDS-related stigmatization, discrimination and denial, the manner in which these are utilized and resisted, and their results for the social exclusion of certain categories of individual.
- The processes and dynamics of exclusion that accompany HIV/AIDS-related stigmatization, discrimination and denial, in comprising the self-exclusion related to felt stigma and the collective exclusion associated with institutionalized forms of discrimination.
- The positive responses to which HIV/AIDS-related stigmatization, discrimination and denial can give rise, the circumstances in which these occur, precipitating and supporting determinants and the key parties involved.
- The price that societies and communities pay for HIV/AIDS-related stigmatization, discrimination and denial, its impact upon family and community, health care systems labour and productivity.

References

AFAO (Australian Federation of AIDS Organizations) (1997) Human rights: from policy to practice, National AIDS Bulletin, 11 (5) 28.29.

Aggleton P. & Warwick, 1. (1999) Community responses to AIDS www.unaids org/publications/documents /children/children /sexandy youth 99. Html# Young.

AIDS Bhedbhan Virdhi Andolan (AIDS Anti-Discrimination Movement (1993) Hard times for positive travel. India, New Delhi.

Barragan, E.M. (1922) VIH/SIDA y trabajo-fragmentos a debate, Sociedad y SIDA, 21:1.4.

Bezmalinovic, B. (1996) The private sector, how are the corporations responding to HIV/AIDS? In: Mann, J. & Tarantola,

D.J.M. eds. AIDS in the world 11. New York, Oxford University Press.

Bharat , S (1995) Household and community responses to HIV and AIDS in India. Final Report to WHO/ GPA/ UNAIDS.

Bharat S. (1999) HIV/AIDS related discrimination, stigmatization and denial in India. Final Report to UNAIDS.

Bharat S. & Aggleton, P.J. (1999) Facing the challenge: household responses to AIDS in India. AIDS Care, 11:3.46.

Byrne, L. (1992) Heath risks of Rio's street children, British Medical Journal, 304: 1459-50.

Campbell, C.J. Marum, M.E, Alwano-Edyegu, M, Dillon, B.A, Moore, M.& Gumisiriza, E (1997) The role of HIV counselling and testing in the developing world, *AIDS Education and Prevention,* 9 (suppl. B) 92-104.

Carrara, S. (1994) A AIDS e a historia das doencas venereas no Brasil. In. Parker, R, Bastos, C, Galvao, J. & Pedrosa, J.S. eds. A AIDS no Brasil. Rio de Janeiro, Relume-Dumara Editores.

Carvalho, A.P. Barbara, V.A.L., Lacerda, M.C.R. Farha, J, Pedrosa, J.S. & Viera, W. (1993) *The fight against discrimination by private health insurers, report of Rio de Janeiro experience, abstract, IXth.*

International Conference on AIDS and Ivth STD World Congress, Berlin.

Castro R, Orozco, E, Aggleton, P.J. Eroza, E, Hernandez, J.J. & Manca , M.C. (1998a) family responses to HIV/AIDS in Mexico, *Social Science and Medicine,* 47 (10). 1473-1484.

Castro , R, Orozco, E, Eroza, E, Manca, M, Hernandez, J-J & Aggleton, P. 1998b) AIDS-related illness trajectories in Mexico; findings from a qualitative study in two marginalized communities, AIDS Care, 10.583-598.

Cole, B.L. Zhang, Z. & Chen C.Z (1993) HIV-related knowledge and attitudes among medical students in China, AIDS Care, 5 (3): 305-312.

Daniel, H. (1991) We are all people living with AIDS, myths and realities of AIDS in Brazil. International Journal of Health Services, 21 (3). 539-551.

Daniel, H. & Parker, R. (1990) Brazil, the goal of solidarity. In The 3rd epidemic, repercussions of the fear of AIDS. London, Panos Institute.

De Bruyn, M. (1992) Women and AIDS in developing countries, Social Science and Medicine, 34:249-262.

De Bruyn, T. (1999) HIV/AIDS and *discrimination 2. Stigma and discrimination. Definitions and concepts.* Ottawa, Canadian HIV/AIDS Legal Network and the Canadian AIDS Society.

Gilmore, N. & Somerville, M.A. (1994) Stigmatization, scapegoating and discrimination in sexually transmitted diseases, overcoming them and us Social Science and Medicine, 39. 1339-1358.

Goffman E. (1963) *Stigma: notes on the management of a spoiled identity.* New York, Simon and Schuster.

Goldin, C.S. (1994) Stigmatization and AIDS, critical issues in public health, *Social Science and Medicine,* 39:359-1366.

Gostin, L.O. & Lazzarani, Z. (1997) *Human rights and public health in the AIDS pandemic.* New York, Oxford University Press.

Gruskin, S, Hendricks, A. & Tamasevski, K. (1996) Human rights responses to HIV/AIDS In. Mann, J, & Tarantola, D.J.M. eds. AIDS. *In the world 11.* New York, Oxford University Press.

Hasan M.A. Farag, A.B. & Elkerdawi, M.M. (1994) *Human rights of HIV infected persons/PLAs* in Egypt, abstract, Xth International Conference on AIDS, Yokohama.

Henry, N. (1990) Africans, facing AIDS, haltingly talk of it, Tanzanian counsel service, *Washington Post*, 17 September: A 17-18.

Herek, G. M. & Capitano , J.P. (1993) Public reactions to AIDS in the United States a second decade of stigma, *American Journal of Public Health*, 83: 74-577.

Herek, G. Mitnick, L, Burris, S, Chesney, M. et al (1998) Workshop Report: AIDS & stigma: a conceptual framework and research agenda. AIDS & Public Policy Journal, 13 (1) 36-47.

HRI (Human Rights Internet) (1996) *Human rights and HIV/AIDS effective community responses.* Ottawa International Human Rights Documentation Network.

Hughes, H. (1998) Ze Cabra—macho does it safely, building on AIDS awareness campaign among Brazil's construction workers, AIDS Action , 4 September:2-3.

Ingstad, B. (1990) The cultural construction of AIDS and its consequences for prevention in *Batswana, Medical Anthropology* Quarterly, 4:28-40.

Jackson, H. & Pitts, M. (1991) Company policy and AIDS in Zimbabwe *Journal of Social Development in Africa*, 6. 53-70.

Jacoby, A. (1994) Felt versus enacted stigma, a concept revisited, *Social Science and Medicine*, 38: 269-274.

Kegeles, S.M. Coates, T.J. Christopher, T.A. & Lazarus, J.L. (1989) Perceptions of AIDS, the continuing saga of AIDS –related stigma, AIDS, 3 (suppl.) S253-S258.

Lie, G.T. & Biswalo, P.M. (1996) HIV-positive patients choice of a significant other to be informed about the HIV-test result, findings from an HIV/AIDS counselling programme in the regional hospitals of Arusha and Kilimanjaro Tanzania, AIDS Care, 8:285-296.

Lwihula, G, Dahlgren, L, Killewo, J.& Sandstrom, A. (1993) AIDS epidemic in Kagera Region, Tanzania-the experience of local people, AIDS Care, 5:347-357.

Malcolm, A, Aggleton, P.J. Bronfman, M, Galvao, J, Mane, P. & Verrall, J. (1998) HIV and AIDS-related stigmatization and discrimination: its form and contexts. *Critical Public Health*, 8 (4) 347-370.

Mann, J. (1987) Statement at an informal briefing on AIDS at the 42nd Session of the United Nations General Assembly, 20 October.

Mann, J, Tarantola, D.J.M. & Netter, T.W. (1992) eds. AIDS in the world. Boston, MA, Harvard University Press.

Mann, J, Tarantola D.J.M. & Netter, T.W. (1996) eds. *AIDS in the world 11*. New York., Oxford University Press.

Manuel, C, Enel, P, Charrel, J, Reviron, D, Larher, M.P. Thiron, x. & Sanmarco, J.L. (1990) The ethical approach to AIDS, a bibliographical review, *Journal of Medical Ethics*, 16. 14-27.

Masini, T. & Mwampeta, S. (1993) *Societal response-discrimination and stigmatization in Tanzania*, abstract, IXth International Conference on AIDS and IVth STD World Congress ,Berlin.

McGrath, J.W. (1992) The biological impact of social responses to the AIDS epidemic, *Medical Anthropology*. 15.63-79.

McGrath, J.W. Andrah, E.M. Schumman, D.A. Nkumbi, S. & Lubega, M. (1993), AIDS the urban family its impact in Kampala, Uganda, AIDS Care, 5:55-70.

Mejia, M. (1988) SIDA historia extraordinarias de siglo xx. In Gavan Diaz, F, ed. El SIDA en Mexico, los efectos sociales. Mexico City, Mexico, Universidad Autonoma Metropolitana.

Merson, M. (1993) *Discrimination against HIV infected people or people with AIDS*, WHO/GPA, Speech to Commission on Human Rights, Geneva, 18 August.

Milner, E. (1991) Thailand, piercing the social stigma, *South*, 123:24-25.

Misra, S. (1999) Social discrimination and rejection in Cambodia. Posting to SEA-AIDS www. Hivnet. ch. 8000/asia/sea-aids/.

Moynihan, L, Seals, B, Demi, A. Sowell, K, Cohan, L. & Guillory, J. (1995) *Living with HIV, issues of stigma and disclosure in women infected with HIV*, abstract, HIV International Women's Conference.

Mujeeb S. (1999) Human right violations of PLWA/HIV by their family violations of PLWA/HIV by their family members. Posting to SEA-AIDS, www.hivnet.ch:8000/asia/sea-aids/

Mukasa Moniko, S., Otolok Tanga, E., & Nuwagaba, A. (1998) *Determinants of AIDS-related discrimination, stigmatization and denial in Uganda*. Final Report to UNAIDS.

Mushingeh, C., Chana, W.K. & Mulikelela, D.M. (1991) *An investigation of high-risk situations and environments and their potential role in the transmission of HIV in Zambia, the case of the Copperbelt and Luapula Provinces* (unpublished report, Population Council of Zambia).

Nardi, P.M. & Bolton, R. (1991) Gay-bashing, violence and aggression against gay men and lesbians. In: Baenninger, R., ed. *Targets of violence and aggression*. North-Holland, Elsevier.

Ngugi, E., Wilson D., Sebstad, J. et al. (1996) Focused peer-mediated educational programs among female sex workers to reduce sexually transmitted disease and human immunodeficiency virus transmission in Kenya and Zimbabwe. Journal of Infectious Diseases, 174 (suppl.2): S240-S247.

Ogolo, H. (1990) Tanzania, hope in the extended family. In: *The 3rd epidemic*, repercussions of the fear of AIDS. London, Panos Institute.

Omangi, H.G. (1997) Stigmatization and discrimination in the context of HIV and AIDS in Kenya, *Newsletter of African Network on Ethics*, Law and HIV, 3:4-5.

Panebianco, S., del Rio, C., Baez-Villasenor J., Uribe, P. & Morales, G. (1994) *Human rights violations and AIDS, two parallel public health epidemics*, abstract submitted to Xth International Conference on AIDS and International Conference on STDs, Yokohama, 7-12 August.

Panos (1990) *The 3rd epidemic, repercussions of the fear of AIDS*. London, Panos Institute.

Panos (1992) *The hidden cost of AIDS, the challenge of HIV to development. London*, Panos Institute.

Parker, M. (1991) South Africa—undermined by AIDS, South, 123:17-18.

Peterson, C. (1990) Prostitutes and public health services co-operate on AIDS prevention in Brazil. Hygie, 9:29-31.

Rosasco Dulato, A.M. (1992), Conocimientos y actitudes sobre el Sida de trabajadores asistenciales en tres instituciones de salud en Lima, Peru. In;

Bond, L., ed. *A portfolio of AIDS./STD behavioural interventions and research.* Washington, DC, Pan-American Health Organization.

Scambler, G. & Hopkins, A. (1986) Being epileptic, coming to terms with stigma, *Sociology of Health and illness*, 8:26-43.

Shisam, K. (1993) What AIDS policy options does India require now *CARC Calling*, 6 (2): 29-32.

Singh, N.K. (1991) AIDS and Society, *Health for the millions*, 17:29-30.

Tesch, B.J. Simpson, D.E. & Kirby, B.D. (1990) Medical and nursing students' attitudes about AIDS issues, *Academic Medicine*, 65 (7): 467-469.

Thant, M. (1993) The economic implications of AIDS in Southeast Asia, equity considerations. In: Bloom, D.E. & Lyons, J.V., eds. *Economic Implications of AIDS in South East Asia*. New Delhi, UNDP.

Tomasevski, K., Gruskin, S., Lazzarini, Z. & Hendricks, A. (1992) AIDS and human rights. In: Mann, J., Tarantola, D.J.M. & Netter, T.W., eds. *AIDS in the World*. Boston, MA, Harvard University Press.

UNAIDS (1997) *Expanding the global response to HIV/AIDS through focused action.* Geneva, UNAIDS.

Volinn, I.J. (1989) Issues of definitions and their implications, AIDS and leprosy, *Social Science and Medicine*, 29(10): 1157-1162.

Warwick, I., Bharat, S., Castro, R., Garcia, R., Leshabari, M., Singhanetra Renard, A. & Aggleton, P. (1998) Household and community responses to AIDS in developing countries, *Critical Public Health*, 8(4):291-310.

Whiteside, A. (1993) The impact of AIDS on industry in Zimbabwe. In: Cross, S. & Whiteside, A., eds. *Facing up to AIDS, the socio-economic impact in Southern Africa*. New York, St Martin's Press.

WHO (1994) *General research protocol for the study of the determinants of HIV and AIDS-related discrimination, stigmatization and denial in developing countries.* Geneva, World Health Organization Global Programme on AIDS, Social and Behavioural Studies and Support Unit.

Williams, G. & Ray, S. (1993) *Work against AIDS, workplace-based AIDS Initiatives in Zimbabwe*, Strategies for Hope No. 8. London, ActionAid.

World Bank (1997) *Confronting AIDS: public priorities in a global epidemic*. New York, Oxford University Press.

Twenty Nine

AIDS Prevention: A Case Study of Senegal

Senegal is one of the poorer countries of the World. Per capital income is below US$600 a year, and life expectancy is low. Most men will not live to 50; women can expect to live to 52. While attempts are being made to increase access to education—primary school enrolment rose by 30 per cent for boys and twice that for girls between 1980 and 1995—literacy among adults is still the exception. Some 57 per cent of adult men and 77 per cent of women are illiterate.

Social Organization

Senegal is a religiously cohesive country. Some 93 per cent of the population is Moslem and another five per cent is Christian. Most of the people actively participate in religious activities. Both Moslem and Christian religious leaders actively promote family and sexual norms that would tend to reduce the transmission of HIV. But religious traditions undoubtedly help in other ways to limiting the rapid spread of HIV in Senegal. Firstly, circumcision is universal and circumcized men seem less likely than the uncircumcized to contract or pass on sexually transmitted infections, including HIV. Secondly, alcohol consumption in uncommon, according to Islamic tradition. In the behavioural study in Dakar in 1997, just three per cent of women and four per cent of men reported having any alcoholic drink in the previous month.

Much social activity is organized around religious associations, which are active in different fields of development, comprising health and education. Other community organizations, like women's groups and youth clubs also contribute to health and education campaigns. They get together to promote immunization, for instance, or to fight malaria.

The Health Sector

Senegal has long stressed prevention and primary health care as the most rational use of limited resources. Spending on health from public funds is around US$ 1 per capita. This is supplemented by donor funds, but at least 40 per cent of spending on health comes out of family budgets. Poor families in Senegal spend more on health than on anything else barring for food.

Reproductive health and child health are well established priorities, and are reflected in health indicators. Infant mortality and under-5 mortality rates both dropped dramatically between 1970 and 1996. In that time, infant deaths dropped from 135 to 60 per 1000 births, and the fall in under-5 mortality was greater still. Family planning services are getting expanded: modern contraceptive use doubled in the five years to 1997. The country's STD control programme will soon enter its fourth decade. Safe motherhood is actively promoted, with most pregnant women now going to clinics for care before child-bearing. This gives an important opportunity for sexual health education. With the advent of AIDS, it also gives a solid infrastructure for monitoring the spread of infection.

NGOs are particularly active in the field of health—at least a quarter of all NGOs nationwide invest in this field. This proved especially important in the 1980s and early 1990s, when an economic downturn and devaluation of the currency led to a collapse of much of the government-run infrastructure in health. The number of medical consultations reduced by eight per cent between 1978 and 1986, even though the population grew by 28 per cent over the same period NGOs were obliged to step in to take up much of this slack, and became very active in rallying public support for health campaigns.

It was against this background of economic distress—a background shared with several other countries on the continent—that the fight against AIDS was launched in Senegal.

Marriage Patterns

As in several West African countries, polygamy is common in Senegal. Over all,nearly half of all married women share their husband with other wives. In polygynous societies it is a general rule that men marry much later than women (since a small number of older, wealthier men are able to partner a much larger number of younger women). This is especially the case in Senegal, where half of all women are married by 20 but where half of men remain unmarried by age 31. In the 1997 behavioural survey in Dakar, half of all the female respondents were married, in comparison to less than one third of the male respondents.

Senegalese women tend to be comparatively old at first marriage compared to women in other countries in Africa. And the age of marriage has been rising in current years. Twenty years ago, of girls aged around 15 to 19, just over four in 10 were still single. By 1997, over seven out of 10 were unmarried in their late teens. The age at marriage is rising since more girls are spending longer at school than they used to. In fact, those with no schooling are still getting married young: half of unschooled girls are married by 18. For women with secondary education or above, the median age at marriage is a full 10 years more than that.

For men, education makes a difference to marriage patterns, too. The more educated a man, the less likely he is to have many wives. However there appears to be a kind of social compensation for formal monogamy: more educated men are also likely to have more sexual partners overall in their lives than less educated men.

Married women in Senegal rarely have partners beside their husband. In the 1997 Dakar study, 99 per cent of married women said they had not had sex with anyone barring their husband in the preceding 12 months. Among men, the proportion is much higher: some 12 per cent of married men said they had sexual partners other than their wives in the previous year. Unfortunately, these data do not exist for the pre-AIDS era. However, as discussed below, these rates of extramarital activity are low compared to those found in other countries.

Premarital Sex

For women, sex-before marriage was traditionally uncommon. However it is not unheard of in Senegal—women married some decades before report younger average ages at first sex than at first marriage, suggesting that some at least must have been sexually active before their marriage. In current years, the age at first sex and the age at first marriage have both been rising. But the age at marriage is rising faster than the age at first sex. This implies that, while they remain virgins for longer, Senegalese women are more likely to have premarital sex now than in the past.

Again, education is a determinant. For uneducated women, the gap between age at first sex and age at marriage remains small. More educated women wait prolong to have sex, but then have more years of premarital sex than those with less schooling. Women with at least secondary education are virgins for six years longer, on average, than women with no education, but they get married nine years subsequent than uneducated women.

Women are far less likely to have sex before marriage than men. In the Dakar behavioural study, 68 per cent of women said they had not had sex before marriage. Among men, less than 10 per cent were virgins at marriage. This is probably not surprising given the high average age at marriage for men.

Prostitution

In several countries, prostitution was ignored until the advent of AIDS, when it became explicit that sex workers were very vulnerable to HIV infection and could quickly pass the virus on to large numbers of other people.

In Senegal, however, services for prostitutes have existed since the profession was legalized in 1969. Registered sex workers have since then been needed to have continuous health checks, and are treated for curable STDs if essential. This system of registration provided a framework within which to approach sex workers with educational and health campaigns.

Advent of AIDS and Senegal's Response

The first reports of AIDS in Senegal came in 1986, when six cases were identified. The response was soon. A national AIDS programme was set up, and steps were quickly taken to protect the population from unnecessary exposure to the virus. By 1987, for instance, a system had been established in all ten regions of the country so that every blood unit for transfusion could be screened for HIV antibodies.

Strong interest from a well established scientific community contributed in solidifying the response. Senegalese researchers collaborated with partners from other countries in establishing research projects. These projects created credible data early on, data that could be used to create political support for a response in this difficult area.

Political Leadership

While politicians in few other countries ignored the threat of AIDS for fear of alienating conservative supporters by initiating a discussion about safe sex, politicians in Senegal supported efforts to confront the epidemic. The government in Dakar behind a declaration on AIDS made by the heads of state of members of the Organization of African Unity in June 1992. The declaration focused on the need for political, religious and community leadership in the fight against the epidemic.

The government has put money where its mouth is. In collaboration with international donors, it invested close to US$ 20 million in AIDS prevention programmes between 1992 and 1996. And it tackled hindrances to programme success. For instance, an excise tax which quadrupled the price of condoms to Senegalese consumers was dropped to help condom promotion campaigns. Political support for the leadership of the national AIDS programme, leadership that has been significantly consistent over time, has also contributed to a successful response.

Efforts have more recently been made to increase the scope of political support for AIDS prevention. Information campaigns to meet the requirements of members of parliament were designed, and in July 1996 the first parliamentary meeting on AIDS was held—a two day information session involving NGOs, people living with HIV and several other actors in the national response. Other influential groups, like as media owners, editors and journalists, have also been targeted with information and provided with training on HIV-related issues.

Religious Leadership

Perhaps the greatest hindrance to AIDS prevention activities in many countries has been opposition, or even just the fear of opposition, from religious authorities. The tendency for religious leaders to prescribe abstinence and mutual monogamy in the face of overwhelming testimony that these behaviours are not always the norm has been seen in almost every corner of the world. The fear of offending powerful religious constituencies has generated gridlock in some national governments, and for good reason. Conservative lobbies have shown that they can hinder everything from family life education to condom promotion if they choose.

Since almost all Senegalese are active practitioners of Islam or Christianity, religious leaders obviously have very important role in national life. Their support for AIDS prevention activities was vital if the activities were to succeed. And it was clear that religious leaders wanted to be involved in this important area. As early as 1989, a conservative Islamic organization, Jamra, approached the national AIDS programme to discuss HIV prevention strategies. Although initially quite hostile to condom promotion and some other aspects of AIDS prevention, the group became an important partner in a dialogue between public health officials and religious leaders.

In order to better understand the requirements of the religious constituency, the government supported a survey of Moslem and Christian leaders. The survey results showed that religious leaders realized they were poorly informed about HIV and AIDS, and wanted more information to enable them to give clear guidance to their followers. They also expressed reservations about what they were prepared to support. For instance, they were reluctant to support condom use between unmarried youngsters, but were prepared to support it within marriages.

In response, educational materials were designed to meet the requirements of religious leaders. They focused in part on testimonials from people living with AIDS—the human face of the epidemic, generally hidden where prevalence remains low. Training sessions about HIV were organized for Imams and teachers of Arabic, and brochures were produced to help them spread information. AIDS became a regular topic in Friday sermons in mosques throughout Senegal, and senior religious figures addressed the issue on television and radio.

In March 1995, 260 senior Islamic leaders gathered for a conference on AIDS. The outcome of the conference was clear support for AIDS prevention efforts. The religious leaders declared that HIV was not a divine retribution for immoral behaviour. They supported the rights of people living with AIDS, comprising the use of condoms to protect from infection within marriage if one partner is infected. And they stated that everyone should have access to full and proper information about HIV and AIDS.

Among Christians, and particularly Catholics opposed to the use of any contraception, there was substantial resistance to AIDS prevention at first. And yet Christian organizations are important providers of health services in Senegal, and AIDS clearly threatened to become a major health issue if it were not prevented. Led by a Catholic NGO, SIDA Service, the churches steadily developed a more supportive outlook towards prevention. They provided important counselling and psychosocial support, and frequently referred those in requirement to alternative providers where they could not meet needs, for instance for condom provision.

In January 1996 Christian leaders gathered in another conference on AIDS. Every bishop in Senegal was in attendance. Again, the outcome was a consensus that AIDS prevention was an important national activity.

The moral support for AIDS prevention given by religious leaders permitted secular and health authorities to work productively in imparting education and certain HIV prevention services.

Community Leadership

As mentioned, Senegalese society has a tradition of active community involvement in health and development issues. When it became explicit that AIDS was a substantial threat to national well-being, religious, women's, youth and other community groups were well placed to respond. By 1995, 200 NGOs were active in the fight against AIDS. Over 400 women's groups, with a total of half a million members, also supported AIDS-related activities, which ranged from national AIDS walks to puppet shows.

Explicitly, this was a new field for NGOs and community organizations, and many required support in developing skills for AIDS prevention work. An umbrella NGO organization was formed, providing support for members and acting as a liaison with the national AIDS programme. Training was imparted for more than 100 organizations that wanted to respond to the threat of HIV but felt they lacked the necessary skills.

Staying Safe: Young People

Policy makers quickly felt that young people needed information about HIV and safe behaviour before they became sexually active. Although sexual activity begins relatively late in Senegal, an effort was made to introduce sex education early. By 1992,sex education was part of the curriculum in both primary and secondary schools. Additionally, an effort was made to reach young people who were not in school, mostly through youth groups.

Young people get information from various sources, but parents can be especially influential. Through religious and community organizations, parents were actively encouraged to assume liability for protecting their children's sexual health by giving full information and support for safe behaviour.

Messages for young people have tended to throw light on increasing knowledge about the risks of unprotected sex and encouraging abstinence. But there is some concern that actual provision of services for young people who do choose to be sexually active has been not adequate.

Staying Safe: Sex Workers and their Partners

Registration of sex workers had been routine in Senegal for more than 15 years by the time AIDS arrived. Registered sex workers were needed to have regular health checks, and STDs were treated if necessary. This meant that sex workers were in incessant contact with the health services, and the spread of HIV infection could easily be monitored in this group.

It was soon clear that sex workers were at extremely high risk both of contracting HIV and of passing it on to their clients. Preventive interventions centering on the promotion of condom use with clients were soon put in place. Several sex workers began to join support groups to safeguard their health in the face of AIDS. Over 30 such groups have been set up. Members attend talks, films and other information sessions about HIV and AIDS—usually around five times a year. They also act as outreach educators for women who work in the sex trade but who have not joined support groups. These comprise women who have not registered as sex workers. It is hard to know accurately how many unregistered sex workers there are—by some estimates thee are as many again as there are registered sex workers. Little is known, too, about levels of infection or risk behaviour among these women. They will certainly become an increasing focus for future prevention efforts.

There are also renewed attempts to reach populations that may be regular suppliers or consumers of casual sex, whether or not in exchange for money. These comprise mobile populations such as migrant workers and transport workers. Locations where casual sex may take place, such as weekly markets, are also becoming targets for more active prevention efforts.

It has long been known that the presence of other STDs makes it easier to contract or pass on HIV infection. So regular and proper treatment of STDs move up the list of health priorities once the threat of an HIV epidemic became clear. The provision of STD services was strengthened both among sex workers and in the general population.

Senegal was one of the first countries in Africa to set up a national STD control programme, and one of the first to integrate STD care into its regular primary health services. In response to the threat of AIDS, the country carried on a massive training of health workers in the syndromic management of STDs. The quality of care improved greatly after the training compared with a baseline study before training. The provision of correct advice about future prevention and about partner notification rose even more dramatically.

The Outcome of Response

What difference, if any, have all these prevention activities made? This is sometimes difficult to tell, since it is impossible to know what would have happened without the prevention activities, or because we don't know enough about the situation before the HIV epidemic. In few areas, though, the effect is obvious. Condom use, for instance, rose from virtually nothing before the AIDS epidemic to 67 per cent among men having casual sex in 1997. Is it conceivable that this rise would have taken place without the education and condom promotion campaigns to which the men were exposed? Not really.

This section will examine the current status of knowledge, sexual activity, condom use, STD prevalence and HIV prevalence in Senegal. Where feasible, it will look at trends over time to try to condition what effect prevention activities may have had.

Knowledge about AIDS and How to Prevent it

AIDS awareness campaigns have well been doing their job. In repeat cross-sectional surveys in 1997 and 1998, over 95 per cent of secondary school pupils and 99 per cent of sex workers knew about AIDS and could name at least two correct ways of preventing it.

High proportions also knew about more complex issues like asymptotic infection. Four out of five students and close to 70 per cent of sex workers knew that HIV could be transmitted by some one who looks perfectly healthy.

In the general population in all over the country as a whole, more men than women know about sexual transmission of HIV (81 per cent of men versus 76 per cent of women). However, in urban areas there is no difference in knowledge between men and women. Nor is there any difference between men and women who have more than primary education.

Such high levels of knowledge exhibit the success of the relentless information campaigns that have reached the Senegalese people everywhere from the classroom to the mosque to the radio to the marketplace. These information campaigns have not, however, done such a great job of minimizing misconceptions. Up to a third of the various population groups questioned about knowledge and behaviour in 1997 and 1998 thought they could contract AIDS from a mosquito bite or from sharing a toilet with someone who had AIDS.

The campaigns have, on the other hand, clearly been

successful in fostering supportive attitudes to people living with HIV and AIDS. Three quarters of female students questioned in 1998 said they believed that HIV-positive students should be permitted to attend school.

Sexual Activity

There is only limited information about sexual activity before AIDS. What is explicit is that women are choosing to remain virgins for longer than they did in earlier decades. Most of the women who were in their early 20s in 1997 did not have sex until they were almost 19 or older. For their mother's generation, the median age at first sex was closer to16. Such a trend has not been found in other African countries. The more educated a girl is, the longer she is likely to wait before having sex. In a study of female students in 1998, 95 per cent revealed that they had never had sex.

Male students were far more sexually active than female students, but they still reported only sporadic sex, and a confined number of partners. While two thirds of male students questioned in 1998 said they were not virgins, only a quarter had had sex in the past year, and fewer than one in 10 had had more than one partner in the earlier 12 months.

And yet in the population as a whole, premarital sex is known. Some 14 per cent of unmarried women in a population-based study in Dakar said they had had sex in the past 12 months, and 38 per cent of men report the same. This is due to the rapidly increasing age at first marriage, described in greater detail earlier. It is worth repeating that, while premarital sex seems to be on the rise, it is happening at even later ages. Since younger women are more vulnerable to HIV infection than more mature women, it is likely that this increasing age at first sex provides added protection against HIV infection.

Young people do not appear to be engaging in one-night stands. In one study, the median time between first meeting and first sex was three months for men and five months for women, and casual relationships among people under 25 tended to last an average of 6 months for women and half that for men.

Among married people, casual sex is very rarer than among the unmarried. Some 99 per cent of married women and 88 per cent of married men in a study in Dakar in 1997 said they had not had sex with anyone other than their spouses in the previous 12 months. Of those who did have extramarital partners, the great majority of both men and women had only one.

Unfortunately, it is not feasible to know to what extent AIDS prevention campaigns have affected the comparatively low levels of sexual activity outside marriage recently recorded in Senegal. It appears likely that extramarital sex was never common in this cohesive and religiously active society. It is feasible, however, that AIDS prevention campaigns have reinforced these traditional patterns of behaviour, staving off an increase in extramarital sex at young ages which may otherwise result from increasing urbanization and social mobility, and probably also from economic changes which make access to cash increasingly important for young people.

Condom Use

The main channel for the spread of HIV in Senegal, as in most of sub-Saharan Africa and various other countries, is unprotected sex between men and women, at least one of whom has other, non-faithful partners. While most AIDS prevention campaigns intend to discourage sex with many partners, they also aim to increase condom use in partnerships that may be risky.

Before the HIV epidemic, condom use in Senegal was very low, less than one per cent. And indeed, it remains low as a method of contraception or between spouses. However, in casual sexual relationships-—exactly those targeted by the AIDS prevention campaign—condom use has risen significantly. In a 1997 population survey in Dakar, more than two thirds of men and close to half of women who had had casual sex in the past 12 months used a condom with their last casual partner. In studies of particular populations a year later the rates were even higher. Some 81 per cent of workers and 67 per cent of schoolboys said they had used a condom the last time they had casual sex (although the total number of sexually active schoolboys was small). And it appears that condom use is fairly consistent. Nearly two thirds of male students with non-regular partners said they had used a condom every time they had had sex with a non-regular partner over the last year. Just one in 10 said they never used condoms in casual encounters.

Information and condom promotion targeted at sex workers appears to have been even more effective. In a 1998 study of prostitutes, 99 per cent reported that they had used a condom with their most recent new client, and 97 per cent with their most recent regular client. It is common the world over for prostitutes to use condoms less repeatedly with non-paying partners than with their clients, and Senegal is no exception. However, even with men who are not clients, condom use remained a comparatively high 60 per cent, according to the study.

One of the factors known to increase the risk for sex workers is, logically enough, the number of partners they have. In a clinical study of sex workers in Dakar, the average number of partners reported by sex workers was quite low. 2.2 a week. Overall, 84 per cent of sex workers in this group reported that they used a condom with every client. However, of a small group of women who had several partners—seven a week or more—96 per cent said they used a condom with every partner. This suggests that women increase their levels of protection in line with their exposure to risk. It would be plausible to assume that they made this decision in response to information about the risks of unprotected sex with many more partners.

All the information on condom use relies on people reporting their behaviour accurately. Is it feasible that people are simply reporting more condom use in response to prevention campaigns, rather than actually using more condoms? It would seem unlikely, million in 1997. Efforts to improve condom distribution also seem to have paid off. Virtually all sex workers questioned reported that they could easily get hold of a condom if they wanted to. Over 85 per cent of secondary school girls said the same, even though this group was the least likely to report actual sexual activity.

Prevalence of Sexually Transmitted Diseases

The behavioural data suggest, then, than sexual activity with multiple partners other than spouses is comparatively low, and a high proportion of casual sex comprising virtually all commercial sex) is protected by condoms. But again, most of this information relies on people reporting their behaviour accurately. Is there any other evidence to support these claims?

Yes. Since STDs are spread in the same way as HIV, they are a good marker of risk activity. And because they are curable, they usually reflect risk activity in the comparatively recent past, whereas HIV infection may be caused by risk behaviour many years previously.

A study of sexually transmitted diseases among sex workers and pregnant women in 1991 and 1996 showed significant falls in infection rates for all STDs measured, and for both groups of women.

These clinical findings confirm low reported prevalence of STDs. In a national DHS survey in 1997, just 0.7 per cent of women and one per cent of men reported having any STD symptoms in the past year. Since several sexually transmitted infections in women are asymptomatic, it is to be expected that women report lower levels of STDs than are found in systematic screening programmes. In a population-based study in the capital the same year, 2.3 per cent of men reported any symptoms of STDs in the past year.

Fewer than half of all sex workers questioned in a 1998 study reported any STDs in the previous 12 months, and just eight per cent reported more than one episode. However, it is worth noting that even these levels seem comparatively high in the light of low levels of partner exchange and vary high levels of condom use reported by sex workers in surveys.

Prevalence of HIV

With such low rates of casual sex, falling rates of STD infection and high levels of condom use, it might be expected that HIV infection in Senegal has remained low. A feasible exception might be among sex workers, whose levels of STDs suggest a quite high cumulative risk of HIV infection, even when the majority of their sexual contacts are protected by condom use.

And indeed, the available HIV surveillance data bear out these expectations. National AIDS programme data demonstrate that HIV prevalence among pregnant women was 1.41 per cent at the end of 1996. There has been no considerable trend over time in this population. There are also sentinel surveillance sites at antenatal clinics in three other major urban regions—Saint-Louis, Kaolack and Ziguinchor; they all demonstrate much the same rates, with HIV infection below two per cent in pregnant women most yeas between 1989 and 1996, and no upward trend in HIV prevalence over time.

In male STD patients, generally thought to be a group representing high risk of infection, HIV infection rates have remained more or less consistently below 5 per cent over time in all sites. It is only among female sex workers, probably the group at highest risk of infection, that HIV prevalence levels have risen considerably over time. They are highest in the south of the country—HIV infection among registered sex workers in the southern city of Ziguinchor reached close to 35 per cent in 1996. In the capital, Dakar, HIV infection among sex workers seems to have remained stable at around 17 per cent since 1993.

Stable HIV prevalence does not, of course, mean there are no new infections. For every person who drops out of the group tested for HIV—since they have died, are too sick to present at health facilities, are no longer fertile or for any other reason—there must be one new infection to keep prevalence stable. But in the case of Senegal, it does not seem that stable prevalence is masking rising incidence. An incidence study of sex workers in Dakar registered new HIV infections at around 1.1 per 100 person years of observation in the decade between 1985 and 1995, with no considerable rise in infection levels over time.

Among pregnant women, too, there appears to be no evidence of high infection rates in the youngest age group—the age group where prevalence levels are most likely to reflect incidence, or new infections. Between 1989 and 1996, only one out of more than 400 pregnant teenagers screened for HIV was found to be infected with the virus.

Senegal's Response and its Importance

One of the great dilemmas for prevention programmes in public health is that it is not feasible to be sure what would have happened if the prevention programme were not in place. This is particularly true for national level programmes. If a prevention programme reaches the whole country, then there is no population within the country that can be used as a comparison group to show what would have happened without the programme. In this condition the best that can be done is to make comparisons with other countries with corresponding situations where no interventions took place. But even that is not as easy as it sounds. First, countries with no interventions rarely have monitoring and evaluation systems to gather data that would permit for the necessary comparisons to be made. Secondly there may be other factors moreover the intervention which differ from one country to the next. Having said that, much can still be learned from inter-country comparisons.

One of things that has changed over time in Senegal has been the age at first sex, which has risen gradually over the years. How does that compare with other countries? Age at first sex has risen faster and to higher levels in Senegal than in any of the other African countries for which data are available. Practically, that implies that fewer teenagers are sexually active and exposed to HIV infection in Senegal than elsewhere. This is confirmed by the data available, which demonstrates the proportion of 15-19 year-olds who are still virgins. Since the safest kind of sex is no sex this confirms that young Senegalese women are less vulnerable to HIV infection or other STDs than young women elsewhere.

Premarital sexual activity is also far lower in Senegal than in other countries with similar data at least for women. In Dakar in 1997 some 14 per cent of women said they had had sex with at least one person in the earlier year. In a DHS survey undertaken in Zambia a year earlier that proportion was a high as 40 per cent, while in Tanzania it was 35 per cent. Among married women too there was a difference although levels were low everywhere. Just one per cent of married women in Dakar had sex with someone other than their husband in the previous year, compared with twice that level in Zambia and five times that in Tanzania. In Cote d'Ivoire and Guinea Bissau, the proportion of men reporting two or more casual partners in the previous 12 months was between three and four times as high as in Dakar.

Although sexual activity outside marriage is far lower in Senegal than in other countries studied, condom use in extra-marital sex is far higher. Indeed, twice as a number of men and women used a condom at last non-regular sex in Dakar as in other African cities where similar studies have been undertaken. Indeed the only country in Africa that reports similar levels of condom use in casual sex in Uganda, where an active prevention campaign was put in place only after hundreds of thousands had died of AIDS, and millions more had watched the ravages of the disease at close quarters.

High levels of condom use are supported by comparatively good availability of condoms. In 1997, around seven million condoms were distributed in Senegal to meet the requirements of the four million people in the most sexually active age bracket of 15-49. That compares with two million condoms for five million people in the same age bracket in Burkina Faso. In Tanzania in the same year, just over 19 million condoms were imported to serve a population of 15.5 million people between 15 and 49.

How do these varied levels of sexual activity and condom use translate into HIV infection? UNAIDS estimates for the end of 1997 put HIV prevalence among adults in Senegal at 1.8 per cent, in Burkina Faso at 7.2 per cent, in Tanzania at 9.4 per cent and in Zambia at 19.1 per cent.

In terms of HIV infection measured among pregnant women at individual sentinel sites in major cities, the gap is similarly large.

Senegal

Much has been written about the requirement to intervene early to stop the spread of HIV before it gets a grip on a population. Obviously, however, if a country intervenes early and HIV infection rates stay low, it is difficult to say that the low rates were definitely the result of the intervention.

Nevertheless, Senegal's HIV prevention programme has been extensive and comprise the elements of an effective programme. There is good proof that Senegal has maintained one of the lowest rates of infection in sub-Saharan Africa by changing the behaviour of several of its citizens.

Like Uganda, Senegal is not a rich country. It has 9 million people, with 44 per cent living in towns. Per capita income is below US$600 a year. Total HIV prevalence among adults is estimated at about 1.8 per cent.

Senegal has long stressed prevention and primary health care. Reproductive health and child health are well-established priorities. In addition, registered sex workers are needed to have regular health checks, and are treated for any curable sexually transmitted infections (STIs) that are found.

What was the response in Senegal?

- As in Uganda, politicians in Senegal were quick to move against the epidemic once the first cases came to light in the second half of the 1980s.
- Since 93 per cent of Senegalese are Muslims, the government made efforts to involve religious leaders. HIV/AIDS became a regular topic in Friday sermons in mosques, and senior religious figures talked about it on television and radio.
- Various other levels of Senegalese society joined in. By 1995, 200 NGOs were active in the response, as were women's groups with about half a million members.
- HIV prevention was included when sex education was introduced in school.
- Parallel endeavours reached out to young people who are not in school.
- HIV voluntary and confidential counselling and testing were made available.
- Programmes were soon put in place to support sex workers to persuade their clients to use condoms.
- STIs moved up the list of health priorities. Senegal was one of the first countries in Africa to establish a national STI control programme that integrated STI care into incessant primary health services.

Those were the actions. What happened in epidemiological terms?

Again, sentinel surveillance was the best option for monitoring the disease, but with more groups than in Uganda. In the data available, the bottom line shows that HIV prevalence among pregnant women was jut over 1.4 per cent at the end of 1996, with no significant trend over time.

The next line represents male STI patients. Their HIV infection rates are higher, but remained under 6 per cent.

Female sex workers are probably at highest risk. The top line shows their HIV prevalence levels rising significantly after 1989. Since 1993, however, especially in the capital Dakar, they have remained stable at around 17 per cent.

Some changes in behaviours resemble the changes seen in Uganda.

Graph available tracks age at first sexual experience for women in five African countries. The line that falls most steeply is that representing women in Senegal. In 1997, most Senegalese women in their early 20s did not have sex until they were almost 19 or older. For their mother's generation—the women who were between 40 and 49 in 1997—the median age was closer to 16.

What about condom use? From virtually zero before the HIV/AIDS epidemic, consistent condom use with casual partners in Senegal increased to 68 per cent among men having casual sex in 1997.

The national HIV/AIDS programme has reduced the checks posed by some traditional religious teachings. The programme achieved a significant rise in condom sales and distribution.

Annual condom distribution increased from 800,000 in 1988 to 7 million in 1997. Most were distributed free but some were sold at a social marketing price.

It is unlikely that this increase would have happened without the education and condom promotion campaigns to which men were exposed.

In a study of STIs among pregnant women in 1991 and 1996, It shows big reduction in infection rates for all STIs measured, particularly trichomoniasis, from 30 per cent down to 18 per cent.

This shows that HIV infection has remained low in Senegal since the start of the epidemic and shows no signs of an upwards trend. But why?

Three major factors can be recognized, namely:

- People are choosing to have their first sexual experience at a later age (there is also evidence that extramarital sex is relatively limited).

- Condom use during extramarital sex, and especially during commercial sex, is high.
- STI control programmes are explicitly rather effective.

The first two factors are strongly linked to the country's HIV/AIDS prevention attempts. And the change in social norms, which is evident in delayed sexual activity, is probably being reinforced by the AIDS prevention programme.

Clearly, much in the social structure and health services of Senegal before AIDS favoured a successful response. Additionally, strong political commitment and the implementation of effective prevention activities helped keep Senegal's rates of HIV infection among the lowest in sub-Saharan Africa.

Thirty

Law in Papua New Guinea on HIV/AIDS

Introduction

Some 85 per cent of the population of near about 4 million lives in traditional village settings in rural areas, which may be extremely remote and inaccessible. Access is generally limited to poor bush roads, small plane airstrips or walking tracks only. In coastal and island regions, and on the major river systems, small boat and canoe transport is common. In spite of this, there is a high casual flow rate between rural and urban areas. Cash cropping and access to money have intruded to varying degrees into the subsistence economy.

Village societies are small homogenous groups characterized by face to face relationships and group allegiance conditioned by one of the very wide variety of kinship systems, ranging from patrilineal/patrilocal through bilateral to different types of matrilineal society. Traditional values, rights and obligations relate not to the individual but the group, from which the individual's status and position in society is derived.

Christianity is the professed religion of almost the whole population, with the Catholic, Anglican, Lutheran and United (Protestant) churches predominating, though a number of variety of fundamentalist churches are also present. Religious adherence tends to be conditioned by village or cultural group, rather than individual choice. In spite of the advent of Christianity, traditional religious beliefs, comprising those of good and evil spirits, sorcery (white and black), telepathy, etc. persist at all levels of society, side by side or even syncretised with the introduced religious systems.

The country is governed by a Westminister-style National parliament, elected by universal franchise, and Provincial

Assemblies for each of the 19 provinces. Government authority is relatively weak, which gives rise to incessant demands from various sectors of the society for the imposition of draconian measures to combat social problems.

The depressed economy and the low standard of national unity give rise to much violent crime, principally robbery, rape and murder. This is not confined to urban centers alone. Nation-wide cultural traditions of xeno-phobia and retaliation legitimize self-help measures for the removal of wrongs. This can take place on an individual or group level. Tribal clashes are frequent, even in "mixed" urban areas, and may continue for prolong periods.

Health services are offered mainly by the government. Private doctors practice in the larger urban centres, and missions operate their own services in remote rural areas. Large employers, like mining companies, are needed to provide medical facilities on site. Government health services, provided through the Department of Health and Provincial Governments, are comparatively inexpensive, but problems are repeatedly faced with funding, staffing and drug distribution, etc.

Legal System

Papua New Guinea's legal system is followed from the English common law adversarial system, with a typical appellate court hierarchy, principles of *stare decisis*, etc. Most overseas decisions have persuasive authority only. A substantial body of indigenous case law has developed since Independence in 1975.

The inferior courts comprised of: District Courts, each declared for its own area which is in practical terms a province, and limited jurisdictionally in other ways as well; Local Courts with a more limited jurisdiction still; and Village Courts, which introduce customary principles to village-level disputes and are subject only to the Constitution and to laws which are particularly applied to them. These courts operate with varying degrees of success and adherence to constitutional principles.

The formal courts are paying incessant attention to custom, which may be pleaded as a question of fact. Because of the diversity of cultures, however, a unified customary law is unlikely to develop, though general trends can be extracted.

The Constitution, adopted at Independence in 1975, is one of the world's lengthiest and most detailed. It is notable for its entrenchment of human rights, mainly due to upon the Universal Declaration of Human Rights. These are predicated on the concept of the rights (and obligations) of the individual, in contradistinction to traditional Papua New Guinea societies, whose mores are founded on the rights and obligations of the group.

Rights are divided into fundamental and qualified, with some of the latter applicable to citizens only. The independence of the judiciary and the comparative case of access by the literate and urban population to the courts has meant that rights are strenuously upheld, where adjudicated, and a considerable body of constitutional case law has already developed. The main prohibiting factors to this process have been widespread ignorance of constitutional rights and the legal process, and illiteracy and remoteness in the rural sector.

Fundamental Rights are:

- Right to Life (Section 35)
- Freedom from Inhuman Treatment (Section 36)
- Right to Protection of the Law (Section 37)

Other Rights are each defined comprehensively and at length, and may be qualified generally in the interests of defence, public safety, public order, public welfare, public health, the protection of children and persons under legal or practical disability, the development of underprivileged or less advanced groups or areas, or to protect the rights and freedoms of others, to the extent that the qualification is reasonably justifiable in a democratic society.

The HIV/AIDS epidemic has implications for nearly all human rights, but the primary operational right is the Fundamental Right to Life. AIDS threatens human life, and governments and the international community are obligated to take all measures to protect human life. Hence any action which inhibits or restricts an individual's ability to protect him or herself from contracting HIV contravenes this most fundamental of rights.

The most notable Qualified Right in the context of HIV/AIDS is Section 49, the Right to Privacy, with regard to personal and family life, communications and personal papers and effects.

Criminal law is codified, and is primarily governed by the

Criminal Code (Chapter 262), which was adopted from the Code of Queensland. Much of it persists in its original form, with no changes or adaptation to the country's circumstances.

Papua New Guinea's legal system, comprising a body of imported law which is generally paternalistic, outdated and inappropriate, a modern and detailed system of entrenched constitutional rights, and a growing recognition of general trends in customary law which are generally in conflict with both of the foregoing, contains fundamental tensions and conflicts, several of which remain to be resolved.

Dimensions of the Epidemic in Papua New Guinea

By late 1992, 127 HIV infections and 46 AIDS cases had been detected. The great majority of these were detected in the Capital. Slightly over half of infected persons are male, and the principal age category for both sexes is the 15-30 age group. A high rate of under-reporting is suspected for Papua New Guinea.

A Medium Term Plan was developed in 1989 by WHO and the Department of Health. A review in 1992 found that significant progress is being made, although much anticipated funding has not been forthcoming and the programme suffers lack of resources, staffing, etc.

Epidemic management is currently vested in the Department of Health, which has established a National AIDS committee (originally the National AIDS Surveillance Committee, set up in 1986) to advise the Departmental Secretary. Committee membership is drawn from the public and private sectors.

No public health legislation has yet been enacted particularly regarding HIV/AIDS. The existing Public Health Act (Chapter 226) contains separate Parts for: infectious diseases, with provision for proclamation of a disease; venereal diseases, which are only defined in the body of the Act; and other special provisions for typhoid, Hansen's Disease and malaria. The Part most appropriate as it stands at present for HIV/AIDS would be Part V- Venereal Diseases. Should it be considered appropriate to bring HIV/AIDS within the ambit of this Part of the Act, legislative intervention will be required. The decision to include or not will rely on the direction of policy formulation and the limit of its conformity with the existing provisions of the Act. For example, Part V includes provisions and procedures for treatment and cure which are not proper to HIV/AIDS, and some partner notification needs which may run contrary to policies on confidentiality. Some amendment may be necessary to take account of such matters. Consequently, references to the Act in this paper are made for information purposes only, and should not be taken to refer to HIV/AIDS.

(A) Public Health

1. Notification

There is no current legal need for notification of HIV infection. However, anonymous or coded test result reporting is collated at the STD/AIDS Unit of the Department of Health. Reporting is comparatively comprehensive, although substantial under-reporting is recognized. It is from these reports that the national database has been compiled, and a quarterly report has been distributed since late 1990.

Part V of the Public Health Act provides for the appointment by the Minister of a Commissioner for the purposes of the Part (Section 49). There have been several departmental reorganizations and redivisions since the Act was originally written, and the present-day equivalent of the position is Senior Medical Officer, STD/AIDS Unit.

Medical practitioners diagnosing a case of a venereal disease must notify the disease to the Commissioner (Section 52). The practitioner must also advise the sufferer of the dangers of infection and the "legal results" of infecting others, and warn him/her against contracting a marriage until cured (Section 53).

2. Testing

Under the Medical Code of Ethics, no-one may be needed to submit him/herself for medical examination unless the law needs it.

Test specimens are taken at STD clinics, provincial hospitals, health centres and sub-centres, special survey sites, and private practitioner surgeries. Serodia and ELISA tests are performed in Papua New Guinea; Western Blot confirmation is undertaken in Australia. Coding is used to detect specimens and other patient data are collected.

Mandatory nominal testing may infringe the Qualified Right to Privacy, unless it is carried out in an "optional" situation, e.g., for employment application. So far, such testing is performed in only three specific examples, on Defence Force servicemen, foreign work applicants and job applicants to one large mining company.

The Defence Force has made a policy of mandatory testing of all applicants for enlistment, and all servicemen as part of their Annual Medical Board. Voluntary testing of authorized civilians, and the families of servicemen, is encouraged. Alongside these testing policies, the Force has instituted strong awareness measures, comprising the promotion of its own brand of condom.

Where applicants for entry visas are required to undergo medical testing before entry (e.g., applicants for work visas), an HIV test is now needed as part of the medical.

Ok Tedi Mining needs a pre-employment medical examination for prospective employees. There is no obligation on existing employees to inform the company of their HIV status, nor are they needed to undergo testing.

3. Compulsory Treatment

Under the Code of Ethics, no-one is compelled to submit him/herself for treatment unless the law needs it. It is the patient's consent which makes it lawful for the doctor to examine or treat.

Section 56 of the Public Health Act needs a person becoming aware that he is suffering a venereal disease to consult and place himself under the treatment of a medical practitioner, clinic or hospital within 3 days for the purposes of treatment, and must continue to present for treatment at prescribed intervals until certified cured.

4. Quarantine

Part IV of the Public Health Act provides different anti-infection measures, including quarantine, for declared infectious diseases, although these have rarely been imposed in practice. In the light of the Constitutional Rights to Liberty of the Person mentioned in Section 42, and The Right of citizens to Freedom of Movement within the country in Section 52, the imposition of any legislative restrictions, like quarantine, on people with HIV would prove difficult. Even if such measures were to be attempted on the grounds of public health, they may feasibly be held unconstitutional.

(B) Confidentiality and Discrimination

1. Confidentiality

Under the Code of Ethics, a doctor owes his patient complete secrecy on all matters confided to him. There are some exceptions to the preservation of the bond of secrecy; where the patient gives consent; in the interest of all concerned; where needed by law; where there is a question of danger to society. On the other hand, in serious illness where the likelihood of recovery is slight or absent, the doctor may, acting in the patient's best interests, inform a near and responsible relative of the true state of affairs and discuss how far to go in informing the patient. However, the Code does not have the force of law, and any statutory or judicial needs of disclosure will override the Code's adjuration to preserve secrecy.

Under the Public Health Act, it is both an offence and professional misconduct on part of a medical practitioner to divulge personal particulars of a person suffering from a venereal disease other than in according to the Act. For other such medical matters, the imported legal system imposes the equitable duty of confidence on medical practitioners and so on, with the feasibility of a tortious or contractual action for breach. The Constitutional Right to Privacy would extend to communications between a patient and a health care worker. The only proven exception so far to this is a situation where the patient chooses to take the matter to law, in which case medical information should be subpoenaed and come within the custody of the court in the first example.

Ok Tedi Mining, which provides an industrial and a clinical medical facility in an isolated environment, specifically insists on a policy of confidentiality regarding medical records for all its employees.

2. Duty to Disclose/Rights to Medical Information

Under Section 19 of the Evidence Act, medical communications made by a patient to a medical practitioner or his delegate are privileged, barring criminal proceedings.

Section 51 of the Constitution, Right to Freedom of Information, guarantees to citizens the right of reasonable access to official documents, subject only to the requirement for secrecy in respect of, inter alia, the maintenance of personal privacy and security of the person. This is a Qualified Right and may be prohibited by a law made in the interests of public health, public welfare, etc.

3. Partner Notification

No partner notification is currently needed by law, although the presumption that a doctor has a liability to protect others from infection by tracing contacts probably operates. Positive test results are notified to the medical care provider or AIDS counsellor who ordered the test. Both are encouraged to involve the other in counselling, follow-up and partner notification.

A medical practitioner diagnosing a case of venereal disease as defined under the Public Health Act must warn the infected of the dangers of infecting others, and against contracting a marriage until cured. Where the practitioner has reason to believe that a person infected aims at to contract a marriage, he may, after intimating his intention to his patient, warn the intended spouse or his/her parents or guardian, and the Commissioner.

4. Discrimination

The Constitution in Section 55, Equality of Citizens, gives to all citizens "the same rights, privileges, obligations and duties regardlesas race, tribe, place of origin, political opinion, colour, creed, religion or sex." Laws may however, take affirmative action for females, children, youth and the under-privileged or less advanced.

The Defence Force policy is to refuse admission to the Force of applicants who test positive. Servicemen testing positive who show no evidence of progressive clinical illness are not discharged, but are confined to base duties only within the country, as far as feasible in non-combat roles. Those who demonstrate progressive clinical illness are downgraded accordingly and may be discharged for physical disability.

Ok Tedi Mining will employ HIV positive persons with no

symptoms, and only discontinues employment when AIDS develops, on the grounds of unfitness to work, as is the case with other diseases like kidney failure, terminal cancer, unstable diabetes, etc. Confidentiality is maintained and a policy of non-discrimination is followed.

(C) Women's Issues

1. Vulnerability to HIV

In spite of Constitutional guarantees of equality, the status of women in Papua New Guinea, as in several other developing countries, is depressed in various of the ways which increase vulnerability (e.g., fewer educational opportunities, higher illiteracy, less access to the cash economy).

Specifically, most women cannot need fidelity from their male partners. Customary polygyny is legal and still widely practiced. Even where monogamy is the overt ideal, promiscuity is unsanctioned but widespread, and double standards between sexes are common. Women cannot often compel condom use. Condoms are not always available, or affordable, in rural sectors. Some churches oppose their use, or even promotion for safe sex. Finally, in the modern Papua New Guinea context, women's vulnerability is increased by the very high incidence of pack rape.

2. Status within Families and Societies

National Goal No.1 (Integral Human Development) of the Constitution recognizes the family as the basic social unit, and equality is guaranteed for all citizens by Section 55. Conventional societies are based on extended family or clan lines. Within the traditional social units, however, defined in each culture group, women's status and roles are explicitly defined, as different and separate from men's, but not necessarily inferior. Modern reality, however, differs markedly, with society tending towards the nuclear family and concomitant weakening of women's family status.

3. Economic Rights

Within traditional society, women played a vital role in the subsistence economy as the principal food producers.

The Constitution in National Goal No.2 calls for equal participation by women citizens in political, economic and developmental activities, but again, fact is different. Urbanisation, the tendency to formation of nuclear family units and economic development strategies which are very targeted towards men, have depressed women's economic status.

(D) Information Law

1. Rights to Information

The Constitution in Section 46 gives Freedom of Expression. It is defined to include freedom to hold and communicate opinions and information and particularly guarantees freedom of the press and mass media. Papua New Guinea does in fact have a strong free press.

The Right to practice, manifest and propagate Conscience, Thought and Religion comprising traditional religious beliefs and customs) may be exercised, provided it does not disturb the freedom of others to do likewise, and there is no unsolicited intervention into another's religious affairs or religious harassment.

The spreading of HIV/AIDS information is a priority of the NAC and the Health Department, and the area in which most action has been taken so far.

2. Obstacles to Information

The major legal hindrance to information comes currently from the Censorship Board, which has put bans on information regarding condom use. Appeals to the Board have not yet been successful. This hindrance may be surmounted, however, by legal challenge on constitutional basis or by HIV/AIDS-specific legislative action.

By Section 228 of the Criminal Code, it is an offence to publish an item which is obscene or might otherwise tend to corrupt morals, unless it can be proved as a question of fact that it was for the public interest.

A major non-legal obstacle is presented by the churches, most of whom have so far refused to relate themselves with the spreading of epidemic-related information other than by the preaching of chastity and fidelity. Some of the minor religious movements are actively spreading totally inaccurate and inflammatory messages, and there is currently no legal mechanism by which this tendency can be arrested.

(E) Families and Carers

1. Marriage, Divorce and Separation

Family law in Papua New Guinea is in a very confused state, with imported and customary legal systems co-existing, and conventional constraints on the latter breaking down in the face of a changing social structure Detail reform has been not possible so far—even piecemeal improvement of the law has proved extremely difficult.

The National Goals of the Constitution recognize the family unit as the fundamental basis of society, and call for the promotion of the Melanesian family in every way.

Section 3 of the Marriage Act (Chapter 280) recognizes both statutory (registered) and customary marriages. Polygamy is legal where customary. Most, but not all, customs require payment of a brideprice. Confusion and conflict between legal regimes leads to various situations of voluntary and involuntary de facto relationships.

Statutory marriages are dissolved in accordance with the Matrimonial Causes Act (Chapter 282). Either party may petition on the old Anglo-Australian fault ground. It is a very expensive process and few nationals embark upon it. Customary marriages are left to be dissolved by customary procedure. Various societies have no such procedure, or are vague about the process, as the concept of marriage dissolution was largely alien to pre-modern societies.

The law's inability to resolve conflict between the imported legal regime and custom, and between different customary regimes in situations of "mixed marriage" is notable.

2. Non-consensual Sexual Intercourse

Forced sex, generally with multiple perpetrators, is becoming increasingly common in Papua New Guinea. In the village setting, though, it is sometimes not easy to define the element of force when a young man is expected to "force" his attentions on a prospective marriage partner, and the girl is expected submit to male demands on her sexual services.

In urban areas, though, where conventional social control mechanisms have been greatly weakened and economic and social depression are most prevalent, abduction and stranger-rape are common. It is a part of the on-going street crime situation, which is gradually worsening.

Rape offences under the Criminal Code applicable to females only, and there is no rape in marriage. An assault with intent to have anal intercourse carries a lesser penalty.

3. Termination of Pregnancy

By Sections 225 and 226 of the Criminal Code, all abortion is illegal. Although there is no Papua New Guinea case law directly on the matter, analogy may be drawn from Queensland verdicts on the interaction between the equivalent of these sections and that of Section 280, surgical operations, which make lawful operations for the patient's advantage, or on an unborn child for the preservation of the mother's life. The Queensland cases have held that this section must be negatived by the prosecution in order to prove an unlawful abortion. Practically, this principle is applied in Papua New Guinea.

(F) Prisons, Custodial Institutions and Welfare Homes

No specific laws have been enacted regarding to HIV and prisoners, though group testing is under discussion and counselling planned.

Although detailed provisions are laid down by law with respect to the operation of corrective institutions, prison discipline and management in Papua New Guinea is in fact by no means perfect. This should be borne in mind when examining the details of statutory needs laid out below.

1. Testing

The corrective Institutions Act (Chapter 63) needs that a medical officer "examine" all prisoners upon admission to, and discharge or removal from prison on a regular basis, and where a prisoner seems to require medical attention." He may also examine warders where he thinks it important and both warders and detainees must submit to any medical treatment ordered. Nominal medical records are kept on prisoners and warders.

Compulsory testing of prisoners may contravene the constitutional Right to privacy.

2. Segregation and Preventive Measures

There is a high incidence of homosexual activity, both consensual and forced, amongst male prisoners and probably warders as well. Secret self-circumcision and other genital mutilation practices have sprung up among male prisoners as a sub-culture ritual. They use whatever cutting implements are available, generally shared rusty razor blades, and general infection often results.

A prison should have an infirmary for sick prisoners. III prisoners may be shifted to hospital, but must be returned to prison if their sentences are not expired.

According to the Act, where a medical officer suspects a prisoner of having an infectious or quarantinable disease (not defined), he must inform as soon as the Commissioner and the Department of Health, and institute "all necessary measures" to make sure that other prisoners are not infected. Additionally, the common law duty of care owed by those in authority to their charges means that all prison authorities are bound to make sure that prisoners are protected from danger of infection.

Segregation of prisoners may contravene the fundamental Right to Liberty. It may, however, be the sole viable preventive measure available in a situation where behavioural change proves too slow, although in reality it may not be ecomically possible (recent calls for the establishment of a maximum security prison are defeated on financial grounds).

The illegality of all homosexual activity implies that it is hard to distinguish between consensual and non-consensual sex, and victims of forced sex may be not interested to complain, particularly in prison situations. It is also an impediment to condom distribution in prisons. Prison authorities could be held responsible for condoning illegal acts.

3. Early Release

Prisoners undergoing life sentence are to be reviewed after 12 years by the Visiting Justice who reports to a Reviewing Committee, and after 15 years by the Reviewing Committee itself. Where a life prisoner reaches 55 years of age, he is to be reviewed at every year. Health reasons constitute a ground for the Reviewing Committee to recommend to Cabinet that the life sentence be commute. Practically, though, the operations of the Reviewing Committee, like those of Visiting Justices, have largely lapsed.

A visiting medical officer must report to prison authorities any case of a prisoner whom he considers may not survive his detention, who is unfit for detention, or whose life may be jeopardized by imprisonment.

(G) Employment Issues

1. Workplace Testing

The Defence Force has made compulsory testing for servicemen as part of the Annual Medical Board. In the private sector, Ok Tedi Mining requires testing for employment applicants only, as does the Department of Foreign Affairs for non-citizen work visa applications.

2. Policies on Infected Employees

The Constitution is Section 48 gives to every person the Qualified Right to Freedom of Choice of Employment, subject only to laws regarding the employment of non-citizens. This Right refers to choice, not practice, of employment.

All employment is understand to be by contract unless otherwise regulated by statute, and basic employment is governed by the Employment Act (Chapter 373) which determine minimum standards for the contract of employment. The Act may be displaced by other legislation related to employment (e.g., Employment of Non-Citizens Act, the Public Services (Management) Act, etc.). The Act is supervised by the Department of Labour and Employment, via Labour Offices and Inspectors. Employees in urban centres are quick to seek recourse to the protection thus offered.

Unless displaced by the conditions of a contract or legislation, the Act makes provision that employment may be terminated according to the common law principle of the right to hire and fire in the employer, with a period of notice dependent on the method of salary payment.

No employment legislation has been made particularly for the protection of HIV infected employees.

In truth, paid employment is available to only a small section of the population, and unemployment is a potent contributing factor to the depressed economy, offset only by reliance on subsistence economy survival in rural areas. Even if laws were to be put in place preventing dismissal on the basis of infection alone, it is likely that they will be circumvented, by the use of real or spurious threats to force resignation. In most of the situations, though, the ease of termination offered by the Employment Act and the principles of common law will suffice.

Ok Tedi Mining follows a policy of confidentiality, no discrimination and no limitation on fitness to work unless HIV-related illness is present. An exclusion clause may be placed in the company-provided medical insurance plan, on the same ground as other medical conditions which do not impair fitness but show a high risk of a re-occurrence of a medical or surgical condition.

3. Disability Support

There is no system of social security in Papua New Guinea, nor is there likely to be one. Concern here centres on persuading rural dwellers to integrate people with HIV into the village community. There are reports that this has happened in some examples, but for other areas, discrimination and stigmatization have surfaced.

Both the Defence Force and Ok Tedi Mining will repatriate people with AIDS upon their becoming unfit for work.

Most of the employment contracts comprising Public Service do not appear to provide for the employee's right to terminate on disability grounds.

4. HIV Education in the Workplace

The Defence Force has made a rigorous system of HIV education and awareness amongst servicemen. Private enterprise is being encouraged to follow suit on a voluntary ground.

The Ok Tedi Mining policy stresses the requirement for information and education promotion with a view to ensure protection from discrimination and prejudice.

(H) Criminal Law

1. Transmission Offences

The Public Health Act provides for offences of marrying while suffering a venereal disease in an infectious stage (Section 64); knowingly infecting another person; or knowingly doing or allowing the doing of any act which is likely to lead to any other person's infection (Section 66). It is also an offence for the owner or occupier of premises to knowingly allow a female suffering a venereal disease to use the premises for prostitution besides to any other legal liability for keeping a brothel etc. Section 67).

The Criminal Code Part V, Division 1 codifies the common law range of offences against the person, ranging from murder to common assault. Some of these may be applicable to HIV transmission, depending on the resolution of matters of causation, *mens rea* in the accused and implied consent in the victim. The year and a day rule applies to unlawful killing by Section 297, so that the greatest offence chargeable for a deliberate act aimed at to transmit infection would be attempted murder. The act of unlawfully, and with intent to injure or annoy, administering poison or other noxious thing to a person, which may probably be extended to cover situations of malicious acts intended to transmit infection, is found under the offence of wounding in Section 322.

In the light of a recent report of a pack rape in a rural sector allegedly carried out with the expressed intention of transmitting HIV infection, the matter of transmission offences has assumed high significance in Papua New Guinea.

2. Sex Workers

Although prostitution *per se* is not an offence, it is against the law to live off the earnings of prostitution, or to keep a brothel, or to procure. The National court has construed the Summary Offences Act with a view to apply the offence of living on the earnings of prostitution to the prostitute herself. However, this interpretation was not applied in a subsequent case of receiving money for an isolated prostitution association, which was held not to constitute living, even partly, off earnings.

Both male and female prostitution are now common in towns, and female prostitution in rural areas also. However, it is generally difficult to define prostitution explicitly, along a continuum from casual sex given for favours to clear-cut commercial sale of sexual favours. Urban sex workers are not generally organized into brothel situations, but rather, free-lance around bars and discos. Organization is more prevalent in rural areas, for instance in the village drinking clubs established along the major highway artery to and through the highland region, and along the shores of the coasts and big rivers. Some villages in different regions of the country are renowned for the fact that the entire adult female population is available for sex work.

3. Homosexuality

Ritualized homosexuality occurs in a few societies in Papua New Guinea. More widespread, though, is homosexual activity as a transitional phase in the development of the individual. Thus, it can be said that bisexuality, and not the exclusive homosexuality, is the norm.

The Criminal Code in Part IV, Division 2 retains its original terms of outlawing all homosexual activity by making crimes of all "carnal knowledge against the order of nature" (anal intercourse), and "acts of gross indecency" between males. Although actual prosecutions are not common, the illegality condition gives rise to practices of blackmail and discrimination, e.g., threats of exposure and prosecution are used to force resignations in the workplace.

The Code provisions may well conflict with the constitutional Right to Privacy in Section 49, the Right to Equality of citizens in Section 55 (which comprises equality regardless of sex, although not particularly sexual preference). For those whose traditional cultures comprised ritualized homosexual practices (and there are several in the country) they may constitute an infringement of Freedom of Religion in Section 45.

4. Illegal Treatment and Advertising

Only a medical practitioner, or a person acting under his direct instructions, may prescribe for and treat a venereal disease.

The Public Health Act in Section 140 comprises a general offence of the publishing statements promoting the sale of any medicine, instrument or appliance for the alleviation or cure of venereal diseases, complaints or infirmities arising from or concerned to sexual intercourse, diseases affecting generative functions, etc. (this does not apply to publications with respect to medical research, and publications sent to medical practitioners or pharmacists for the purposes of their businesses, or advertisements, etc. approved by the Commissioner for Venereal Diseases). This provision is not limited to defined venereal diseases alone, and could therefore apply to the advertising of false cures for HIV/AIDS.

(I) The Legal Process

1. Legal Aid and Access to the Law

Section 37 of the Constitution gives to all persons the fundamental Right to Protection of the Law. No person may be charged with an offence that is not defined by a written law. Determination of civil rights and obligations must be made by a court or similar impartial authority, within a reasonable time.

In different situations, persons may obtain free legal representation from the Public Solicitor. However, the office is under-resourced and its first priority is criminal defence. Even this is only available at National and Supreme Court level. The Public Solicitor and the Law Society administer a means-tested legal help scheme for situations where the Public Solicitor is unable to act.

Where violations of Constitutional Rights are concerned, the National Court will act of its own initiative to protect them. The court has made simple procedures whereby rights violations may be brought quickly before the court.

2. Evidence

The Evidence Act Section 19 prohibits a medical practitioner (which has been held to comprise all persons) from divulging in any civil proceedings any communication made to him by a patient unless the patient consents. The privilege has also been held to attach to any information given to persons particularly or impliedly delegated by the practitioner to obtain information from the patient for the objective of medical treatment. On its wording, this protection may not extend to medical information the practitioner has about the patient.

Spouses are not compellable to reveal communications during the marriage in any legal proceedings barring divorce and matrimonial causes proceedings.

3. Courtroom Procedure

Under the Constitution, all court proceedings shall be held in public unless the parties agree otherwise. A court may be closed where it is empowered to do so by law in the interests of, *inter alia,* the protection of the private lives of persons concerned in the proceedings. Under the District Courts Act (Chapter 40) which was enacted prior to the Constitution, a court may be closed keeping in view "the interests of public morality."

The Judicial Proceedings (Regulation of Reports) Act (Chapter 51) prevents the publishing of any "indecent medical, surgical or physiological details the publication of which would be calculated to injure public morals." However, this does not apply to the communication of the content of pleadings, transcripts of testimony or similar documents to "a person concerned in the proceedings."

4. Sentencing

Judges take various factors into account in sentencing, including age, medical infirmity and likelihood of surviving a prison sentence. As no case involving a person known to be HIV-positive has yet come before the courts, no particular sentencing policy has evolved in relation to any crime. However, guidance may be drawn from the 1989 case of The State V. Thomas Pipon, in which the judge noted in sentencing that knowingly attempting to infect a victim of sexual assault with HIV would constitute an aggravating factor of more extreme seriouseness than infection with gonorrhoea, a curable disease.

Thirty One

Ethical and Legal HIV/AIDS in Indonesia

Background Information

The Republic of Indonesia, lies between the Asian and Australian continents, and is an archipelago comprising 13,000 islands. The unevenly distributed population lives in about 6,000 islands, especially in five big islands: Sumatera, Java, Kalimantan, Sulawesi and Irian Jaya. The total population in 1993 is about 187 million, with more than 60 per cent living in Java island, which is only 6 per cent of the total land area. As the fourth biggest nation in the world, Indonesia includes about 300 ethnic groups with their own languages, but nationally the Indonesian language (which is basically similar to Malayan language) is used. Administratively, the republic comprises 27 Provinces, covering 302 Regency/Districts and about 6000 subdistricts (the lowest official/governmental level of administration).

As a developing country, the Republic of Indonesia has to face a great deal of problems comprising health. Communicable diseases remain a major health problem, in particular. Malaria, Dengue, TB and sexually transmitted diseases are just some of the diseases whose propensity to affect the population is compounded by improper health awareness in certain segments of the population.

The first case of AIDS found in Indonesia was recorded as a foreign tourist who died in Bali, in 1987. Since then, cumulatively a total number of 31 AIDS cases involving 22 deaths, and 109 HIV (+) have been found and recorded (from 1987 up to 31 March 1993).

To respond to the HIV epidemic properly, an appropriate legal and ethical environment is required. But, bearing in mind that the introduction of HIV/AIDS to Indonesia is comparatively new, it is a fact that up to this date no special AIDS law has been made. Health-Legal approaches in Indonesia are based on the available 1945 Basic Constitution, Epidemic Law, Quarantine Law, The Health Law, etc., implemented administratively and/or operationally through Government Regulations, Presidential Decree/Instruction, and implemented technically through a Health Minister's Regulation and/or Decree, and through a Director General's Decree and/or Instruction.

The following issues are intended as background information for setting up a legal and ethical network to address HIV/AIDS in Asia and the Pacific.

Public Health Versus Individual Rights

Surveillance and Notification of AIDS has been carried out in Indonesia as soon as the first case of AIDS was found in 1987. The legal aspect of those activities are based on the Health Minister's Decree.

Testing, Counselling for AIDS are implemented voluntarily. Consent is required from each individual of the target group of a serological survey for HIV/AIDS.

Confidentiality of the HIV (+)/AIDS cases is given through the same Health Minister's Decree.

Compulsory treatment is not applied, barring in relation to control measures during/concerned to certain epidemic diseases.

Prevention measures, e.g., quarantine is not permitted for HIV(+) and or AIDS cases. But it could be conducted if necessary for cases of other epidemic diseases stated in the Health Minister's Decree with regard to the implementation of the Epidemic Law mentioned above.

Brothel laws, upto this date, have never been made because prostitution is illegal in Indonesia.

Partner notification is conducted based on the CDC Director General decision concerned to NAC policy.

Rights to medical information The issue had been recently discussed in a workshop held on "Medical Ethics and Rights of a Patient," held in Jakarta. Traditionally, doctors tend to keep the medical information confidential unless asked by the patients and/or their families.

There is no regulation on *Discontinuation of treatment* for non-communicable disease patients; it is considered as the right of the patient. But if it happened in cases of particular epidemic diseases (stipulated in the Health Minister's Decree) following their reluctance to follow the treatment programme, the patient concerned could be charged as trying to endanger other people and could be punished according to the regulation.

Discrimination of People Living with HIV

To date, there has been made no special law dealing with the right of people living with HIV in Indonesia. But according to the Epidemic Law, discrimination of people contracting certain epidemic diseases, if important, could be applied in endeavours such as isolation and/or quarantine.

Legally, there can be no discrimination against people living with HIV/AIDS. But factually, based on religious or cultural reasons, discrimination of people contracting particular diseases (not only HIV) postulated in those religions and/or specific cultures, to some extent, still exists in some communities.

The Duty to treat (AIDS cases) has been applied to all government hospitals under the strategy of the national AIDS control programme. All general hospitals must accept/admit the hospitalization of AIDS cases with no discrimination.

AIDS cases are subject to be treated as other infectious disease patients, for whom general precautions should be made. People living with HIV/AIDS have the same rights as other people in accommodation, employment, schools, and also have the same facilities as migrant workers and travellers.

International law is obeyed fully, and confidentiality is applied by the Indonesian Government.

Information Law

In Indonesia, there is no hindrance to HIV information, as long as it will not disturb the socio-cultural and or political stability and/or offend the ethnic-religious norms.

Broadcasting/censorship laws, obscenity law, advertising regulations are to some limit subject to the guidelines stated in the existing criminal law. However, these are applied only to prevent the ill use of "freedom to speak and/or dissemination of information."

Sex education is inevitably accepted by the community as long as it does not contradict ethics and/or religious norms.

Right to information is guaranteed by law and regulations, comprising the health aspect of information.

Family Law

Legal approaches to inheritance, divorce/separation, maintenance, custody/adoption, carer and survival support, age of marriage and sexual consent are enforced through the implementation of the civil law; legal approaches on non-consensual intercourse, termination of pregnancy (without medical reasons/judgement) are enforced through the implementation of the criminal law. The termination of pregnancy because of medical reasons/judgement, and conducted by the right health professional, is made feasible through the implementation of the health law (1993).

HIV/AIDS Policy in Prisons and Institutions

Principally, the HIV/AIDS policy in prisons and institutions in Indonesia is similar to the policy applied for the general population.

Testing, if needed, should be conducted voluntarily. Segregation of prisoners living with HIV/AIDS is not permitted, except for reasons other than their HIV status (e.g., criminality). If hospitalization is required, the prisoner should be admitted to the nearest hospital. The provision of condoms and bleach is legal, but provision of needles is prohibited with regard to the anti-narcotic regulation and/or safety reasons. Counselling, care and support is provided through collaborative endeavours among the Ministries of Health, Social Affairs and Justice.

HIV/AIDS Legal Policy at the Workplace

Legal policy on HIV/AIDS at the workplace, up to this date, has not been made, but is now in the process of being made.

Workplace testing may only be conducted with regard to a cross-sectional survey on STDs, to be conducted anonymously and voluntarily by the authorised health team.

Policies on HIV infected employees, comprising sick leave,

disability support, and occupational health safety are similar to the policies which govern people living with other diseases.

HIV education at the workplace to some extent has been given and will be extended in the near future through intersectoral collaborations, involving non-governmental organizations.

Criminal Law and HIV/AIDS

In the prevailing Criminal Law, there are no legal statements related to transmission offences. In few cases (e.g., where the activities of sex workers and homosexuals are made public held to be against ethics norms), the performer could be charged legally.

Thirty Two

The Existing Situation of HIV/AIDS in New Zealand

Although HIV infection is not notifiable in New Zealand, laboratory reports of non-recognizable information are available. Statistics need to be interpreted with caution: not all people at risk will have been tested and testing may not be requested until several years after infection has occurred. In last 10 years, about 90-100 persons each year in New Zealand have been found to be infected. In 1944, 89 people were found to be infected, bringing the total to 997. Of these:

- 57 per cent were homosexual/bisexual males
- 3 per cent were intravenous drug users
- 2.8 per cent were recipients of blood products (1.2 per cent transfusion related)
- 0.2 per cent were infected perinatally

In the fourth quarter of 1994, 26 people were newly-found to be infected with HIV. Of these 22 were male and 4 were female. No ethnicity data is available.

AIDS

AIDS is notificable in New Zealand. The total number notified since monitoring started (on 31 December 1994) is 473. Of these 387 (81.8 per cent) are known to have died, 68 (14.4 per cent) were alive on that date; 390 (82.5 per cent) were European/pakeha, 52 (11 per cent) were Maori and 2.5 per cent were Pacific islanders.

Risk Factors

Of the twelve people notified with AIDS in the fourth quarter of 1994, all were male, and all reported having had sexual relation with other men.

Of the twenty-two men found to be infected with HIV in the fourth quarter of 1994, information is available on twenty of them. Thirteen were reported to have had sex with men. One was reported as an injecting drug user. Six were considered to have been heterosexually infected, five from different parts of the world where heterosexual transmission is common.

Two of the four women were reported to have been heterosexually infected, one from a part of the world where this kind of transmission is common. One women was reported to be an injecting drug user.

Use of Sentinel Populations

Sentinel populations are those in which HIV is or might be spreading e.g., people attending STD clinics, injecting drug users. Prevalence surveys have been undertaken using anonymous unlinked methods. Transmission through male-to-male sexual intercourse remains the largest group. This comprises men who identify as gay or bisexual and others who do not identify as such but who have had sex with other men.

Although the number of those who have acquired HIV from hetrosexual intercourse remains low in New Zealand, the number of women infected continues to rise. In most of the cases, women are the sexual partners of men in other high-risk groups-bisexual men, injecting drug users, men from different countries where heterosexual transmission is common.

Injecting drug users are the third largest group, with transmission attributed to sharing injection equipment. No new cases of medically acquired HIV have been reported since blood donor screening was applied in 1985.

There has been one case reported of mother to infant (vertical) transmission.

Existing Legal Framework

Non-Discrimination Law

The Human Rights Act, 1933, specifies prohibited grounds of discrimination. These comprise discrimination on grounds of physical illness, the presence in the body of organisms capable of carrying disease and sexual orientation.

Privacy

The Privacy Act, 1993, and the Health Information Privacy Code, 1994, protect privacy interests, comprising those of people with HIV/AIDS. Rule 11 of the Code deals with limits on the disclosure of health information. One circumstance in which it is sometimes permissible to reveal information without the consent of a person with HIV/AIDS is where there is cause to believe that the disclosure is important to prevent or lessen a serious and imminent threat to public health or safety, or to the life or health of another.

Needle Exchange

The Health (Needles and Syringes) Regulations, 1987, make provisions for a needle exchange scheme.

Criminal Offences

The Crimes Act, 1961, contains different provisions which have a bearing on the intentional, reckless or negligent communication of HIV/AIDS. It is crime to wilfully and without lawful excuse cause or produce 'disease or sickness' in another person (Section 210), and, with reckless disregard for the safety of others, to cause 'actual bodily harm' to another person (Section 188(2)).

The Homosexual Law Reform Act, 1986, had the effect of decriminalizing anal intercourse between consenting persons over the age of 16 years.

Proposed Legal Reforms

These include:

Health and Disability Services Amendment Bill

This legislation disestablishes the Public Health Commission and returns the responsibility to enhance, promote and protect public health (defined as the health of all the people in New Zealand or the health of a special community) to the Ministry of Health. The Core Services Committee which has the liability for advising on national priorities for health will be expanded to ensure that public health and personal health needs are considered as a whole. The four regional health authorities will assume liability for purchasing services to address the prioritized health needs.

Review of the Health Act, 1956

This is currently underway and questions are being raised about the feasibility of moving from the communicable disease model to a health promotion model. The new regulations will have to mesh with other legislation particularly dealing with emergencies such as epidemic out-breaks. The progressive work on the harmonization of New Zealand's laws with those of Australia continues. Other legislation which has specifically been asked to be reviewed comprises the Health (Needles and Syringes) Regulations, 1987 and the Misuse of Drugs Act, 1987.

Prostitution

The government has announced that it does not aim at to proceed with legislation in this area.

Immigration

The Advisory Committee on STD/HIV/AIDS has suggested that there should be no move to introduce mandatory testing of immigrants.

Prospects

General

It would be proper to say that New Zealand is moving towards the maintenance mode with regard to HIV/AIDS. Efforts to provide personal health services for people diagnosed with AIDS, in ways which suit them and those close to them will continue. This comprises services for refugees who come to New Zealand. Voluntary testing related to appropriate counselling and support is also being encouraged. At the same time (within the health public policy framework) attempts are being made to link the work on HIV/AIDS to the wider setting of sexual health. A paper advising the Minister of Health on STDs is in preparation. This paper will clearly acknowledge the interface of HIV/AIDS with other sexually transmitted diseases. This in turn can be related to other work under way in the Ministry on unplanned pregnancy, cervical cancer and infertility. At the other end of the spectrum, work on bloodborne diseases, comprising hepatitis with regard to injecting drug users, transfused blood and blood products will be continuing.

It was recommended to the Minister in April 1994 that the Ministry of Health should undertake a review of the Health (Needless and Syringes) Regulations, 1987, and the Misuse of Drugs, 1978, in the context of the public health regulatory review. It was also advised that the Departments of Justice and Police, and the Ministries of Health and Women's Affairs should prepare policy papers on legislation and law enforcement policies affecting prostitution, and public health policies concerning to the sex industry, for consideration by the government.

Thirty Four

HIV/AIDS in the South-East Region - at a glance

REPORTED AIDS CASES AND PEOPLE LIVING WITH HIV/AIDS

South-East Asia Region, October 2000

Country	*Reported AIDS cases*	*Estimated no. of People with HIV/AIDS*	*Rate per 100,000 population*
Bangladesh	17	13000	10
Bhutan	1	<100	<5
DPR Korea	0	<100	<1
India	12239	3700000	370
Indonesia	411	52000	25
Maldives	5	<100	<50
Myanmar	3817	530000	1176
Nepal	383	34000	145
Sri Lanka	116	7500	40
Thailand	135950	755000	1240
Total	152939	~5091800	~338

**Source:* UNAIDS report on the global HIV/AIDS epidemic. June 2000.

INCIDENCE AND PROJECTIONS OF HIV INFECTION AND AIDS IN INDIA, INDONESIA, AND THAILAND

(number of people)

Country	*Reported incidence (cumulative)* AIDS	HIV+	*Estimated incidence (current)* HIV+	*Year 2000 projections (cumulative)* AIDS	HIV+
India	116[a]	7272[a]	1 million[e]	1 million	5-7 million
Indonesia	24[b]	46[b]	2500	5000	50000
Thailand	2135[c]	34545[d]	450000	500000	3 million

a. As of April 1992
b. As of October 1992.
c. As of September 30, 1992
d. As of October 1991, after which this statistic was no longer reported.
e. Expected incidence as of December 31, 1992

Sources: Reported incidence of HIV and AIDS for India: WHO(1992); estimated incidence and projections for India: private correspondence with James Chin; reported and estimated incidence of HIV and AIDS for Indonesia: *Jakarta Post* (1992) and correspondence with George Loth; projections for Indonesia; correspondence with George Loth; reported incidence of HIV and AIDS for Thailand; UNDP 1992) and private correspondence with Steven Kraus; estimated incidence and projections for Thailand: private correspondence with Steven Kraus and Ministry of Public Health, Thailand (1992).

ESTIMATED COSTS OF THE AIDS EPIDEMIC IN INDIA, INDONESIA, AND THAILAND

(1991 US$)

Country	*Direct Costs per case (A)*	*Indirect costs per case (B)*	*Total costs per case (A) + (B)*	*Projected AIDS cases by 2000 (see table 1) (C)*	*Aggregate cost C*(A+B)*
India	738a	10100	10838	1 million	11 billion
Indonesia	1490a	14680	16170	5000	81 million
Thailand	987-1524	34322	35309-35846	500000	18 billion

Note: These figures do not take into account direct costs associated with the prevention of HIV infection.

a. These direct cost figures are the arithmetic mean of the full cost of treatment in the public and private sectors in India and Indonesia, respectively.

Sources: Direct costs for India: World Bank (1992) and authors' calculations based on data from physicians at Madras Medical College (see table 4); direct costs for Idonesia: authors' calculations (see table 4); direct costs for Thailand: Viravaidya, Obremskey, and Myers (chapter 2 in this volume). Indirect costs are based on the following assumptions:

- On average individuals with AIDS leave the labour force at age thirty-five in all three countries.
- The social discount rate is 3 per cent;
- Individuals retire from the work force at age sixty;
- Average annual earnings equal GDP/adult (US$580 in India, US$843 in Indonesia, and US$1971 in Thailand (World Bank 1991).

THE COST OF DRUG THERAPIES TO TREAT OPPORTUNISTIC INFECTIONS ASSOCIATED WITH AIDS IN INDONESIA.

Infection	*Proportion of AIDS patients affected (per cent)*	*Episodes (length of treatment)*	*Drugs*	*Total drug cost per month (US$)*
Tuberculosis	61	1 (6 months)	INH	4.15
			Myambutol	5.40
			Rifamycine	40.50
			Thiacetazone	5.00
Oral Candidiasis	60	2-3	Acyclovoir	25.00 (per episode)
Chronic Fever	52	1 (1 month)	Tylenol	5.00
Chronic Diarrhea	25	1 (1 month)	Oral rehydration therapy solution	5.00
Cryptococcal Meningitis	13	1 (10 days)	Ampicillin or amoxycillin	30.00 (per episode)
Pneumocystis Carinii Pneumonia	6	1 (1 month)	Bactrim	40.00

Source: Correspondence with George Loth. The expected pattern of opportunistic infections is based upon the actual experience of a particular sample of individuals in Thailand.

COMPONENTS OF THE COST OF DIAGNOSING AND TREATING HIV INFECTION IN INDIA AND INDONESIA

Country and system	*Services provided (unit)*	*User cost as a percentage of full cost*	*Full cost per unit (1991 US$)*	*Number of units per case*	*Full cost per case (1991 US$)*
India					
Public Health Care System	Tests				
	ELISA	0	1.00-3.50	1	1-4
	Western Blot	0	24.80-35.50	1	25-36
	Consultation/visit	0	3.00[a,b]	20	60
	Drugs[c]	0	10.60-17.70	20	212-354
	Hospital (day)	0	2.00-16.00a,b	25	50-400
Private Health Care System	Tests				
	ELISA	100	10.60	1	11
	Western Blot	100	24.80-35.50	1	25-36
	Consultation/visit	100	1.00-9.00[b]	20	20-180
	Drugs	100	10.60-17.70	20	212-354
	Hospital (day)	100	4.00-32.00b	25	100-800
Indonesia					
Public Health Care System	Tests				
	ELISA	100	3.00	1	3
	Western Blot	100	40.00	1	40
	Consultation/visit	30-50	.30-8.20	12-15	4-123
	Drugs	10-50	-	-	249[d]
	Hospital (day)	20-50	5.00-59.00	30	150-1770
Private Health Care System	Tests				
	ELISA	100	5.00-7.00	1	5-7
	Western Blot	100	40.00	1	40
	Consultation/visit	100	2.50-12.00	12-15	30-180
	Drugs	100	-	-	249[d]
	Hospital (day)	100	25.00-59.00	30	750-1770

- = Not available

a. Based on private cost of treatment and our assumption that the full cost of hospitalization and treatment in the public sector is less than in the private sector.

b. We have assumed that these figures (from World Bank 1992 and from correspondence with Chandna Salgaocar and Sanjay Chaudhary) do not include drug costs.

c. The drugs administered provide treatment for symptoms of AIDS and do not include drugs that treat the actual HIV infection.

d. Expected drug costs based on table. 3.

Sources: India: Madras Medical College data; National AIDS Control Programme, India: World Bank (1992).

APPENDIX: BACKGROUND INFORMATION INDIA

System	*Description*
Public system	
Health centres	The Ministry of Health and Family Welfare operates a system of public health centres. The various health centres are organized in a hierarchical structure, ranging from community health centres that offer out-patient and limited in-patient care, to village health guides that offer primary health services and health education to the rural population. The community health centres each serve approximately 100,000 people. The primary health centres have a smaller medical staff than the community health centres and each serve 20,000 to 30,000 people. Subcentres, which are staffed by para-professional health workers, each serve roughly 3,000 to 5,000 individuals. The subcentres tend to be used by the poorer population, which would otherwise depend on traditional or Ayurvedic practitioners. Approximately 64 per cent of India's population has access to the public health care system. There are no user charges for the services offered at public health centres.
Hospitals	Approximately 75 per cent of all hospital beds are publicly administered. Most of the beds in public hospitals are used by low-income patients, and there is no charge for their use.
Private system	
Physicians	Private physicians (numbering 331,000 in 1987) practice mainly in large cities. General practitioners often price discriminate, charging rich patients more than poor patients. Specialists treat mainly wealthy patients in urban areas. Among all physicians, including those in the public sector, 60 per cent of physician time is spent treating private patients.
Central Government Health Insurance System (CGHIS)	The CGHIS provides health insurance for all central government employees. There were approximately 3.3 million government employees in 1987. The CGHIS operates its own health care facilities, which include 293 clinics.

Table (Contd...)

System	*Description*
Employee State Insurance Corporation (ESIC)	The ESIC provides health insurance for employees of firms with twenty or more workers. Employees who earn less than Rs. 1,600/month are eligible, but must contribute 2.25 per cent of their salaries, while employers must contribute 5 per cent of total wages payable. State governments contribute about 12.5 per cent of ESIC expenditures. Workers who earn less than Rs. 6 per day are not required to contribute but are entitled to all the benefits. The ESIC operates dispensaries and clinics that are staffed by physicians and offer out-patient treatment. The ESIC administers its own hospitals and reserves beds for its beneficiaries at public hospitals. As of 1987, approximately 28 million people were covered by the ESIC.
Hospitals	Private hospitals generally provide more amenities and have more modern medical equipment than do government hospitals. Approximately 25 per cent of the total hospital bed supply is administered by the private sector, which includes voluntary and religious hospitals. These hospitals serve predominantly wealthy patients, but do reserve some beds for poorer patients. Patients must pay for the services provided.

Sources: Bhatnagar (1985): Directorate General of Health Services (1990); Roemer (1991); Ron, Abel-Smith, and Tamburi (1990); correspondence with Chandana Salgaocar.

INDONESIA

System	Description
Public system	
Health Centres	There are two types of permanent public health facilities in Indonesia: *puskesmas* (health centres) and *puskesmas pembantu* (health subcentres). *Puskesmas* provide preventive, maternal and child health care, and out-patient health services. As of 1986, 14 per cent of the population had *access to puskesmas*. There are approximately 5,000 *puskesmas*, and fewer than 3 per cent of these offer in –patient services. The *puskesmas pembantu* consist of a small clinic, *Balai Pengobatan*, and a maternal and child health centre, *Kesehatan Ibu Dan Anak*. The *puskesmas pembantu* are usually headed by a nurse or midwife. The *puskesmas pembantu* provide more coverage to rural areas than do *puskesmas*. However, most people in rural areas do not use these facilities, depending instead on traditional healers, private physicians, and medication from private drug stores. *Puskesmas* and *puskesmas pembantu* charge user fees that vary considerably across the country.
Hospitals	Public hospitals are operated by the Ministry of Health and are divided into four classes that differ by the quality of the medical services they offer. There are user fees at the public hospitals. The poorer population generally uses these hospitals, as the fees are lower than in private hospitals. Even though the majority of the population is poor, the Ministry of Health Hospitals have low occupancy rates. The Ministry of Defense also operates certain public hospitals.
Service posts *(posyandu)*	These are not permanent facilities, but exist on a temporary basis as monthly clinics. The staff is comprised of village health volunteers (*kaders*) and aids from the *puskesmas*. The *posyandu* serve mainly populations in rural areas as *puskesmas* are often not able to serve these areas.

Table (Contd...)

System	*Description*
Private System	
Physicians	Seventy per cent of Indonesian physicians serve urban populations that constitute 25 per cent of the population. Most Indonesian doctors work for the government, but also practice privately. Medical school graduates are expected to fulfill a two-to five-year mandatory term of working for the government.
Hospitals	Approximately 23 per cent of hospitals are private nonprofit, while 47 per cent are private for profit. Private hospitals tend to provide higher quality care than public hospitals. The private sector is the predominant provider of in-patient health care. The government requires private hospitals to reserve 10 per cent of their beds at the lowest room rate for poorer patients.
ASKES	ASKES is a health insurance scheme for government employees and their families that covers an estimated 9 per cent of the Indonesian population. Government employees must use health facilities operated by the Ministry of Health, with ASKES covering all fees. The program is funded by a 2 per cent salary deduction from all government employees.
PKTK	PKTK is a voluntary health insurance scheme for private employees that requires participants to use the *puskesmas*. The scheme is funded by a 7 per cent salary deduction from all participating employees. Many employees are deterred from joining the program due to the relatively high cost.
Dana Sehat	This is a health insurance scheme for rural villagers to cover user charges at *puskesmas*. The premium is approximately Rs. 40-50 per month.

Sources: Kurina (1992); Roemer (1991); World Bank (1989).

THAILAND

System	Description
Public system	
Hospitals	There are two types of public hospitals in Thailand administered by the Ministry of Public Health: provincial and district hospitals. Provincial hospitals provide more advanced medical care than do district hospitals and are larger. All public hospitals charge user fees.
Health centres	Commune health centres are operated by the Ministry of Public Health and provide primary health care services to rural populations. In general, individuals tend to use private drug stores more than health centres. People from urban areas more frequently consult private physicians than health centres.
Village drug Cooperatives	These cooperatives are operated by the Ministry of Public Health to provide rural populations with drugs through the public health center structure. They are run by village health volunteers and village health communicators working for the ministry. The cooperatives are funded through private contributions of approximately US$1 per family.
Health Card Fund	This is an insurance scheme that provides up to four members of each enrolled family with free care at the health centres six times per year and a 10 per cent discount at the village drug cooperative. Enrollment costs US$12/year.
Private system	
Physicians	Only 10 per cent of Thailand's physicians are engaged in private practice full time. The remaining 90 per cent work for the Ministry of Public Health and most also engage in private practice. The urban poor and rural populations receive little private physician care.
Hospitals	There are 989 hospitals in Thailand, and approximately 25 per cent are privately run. Of all private hospitals, one-third are nonprofit and two-thirds are for profit. Private hospitals provide relatively high quality services to patients in terms of staffing, room conditions, and medical care.

Table (Contd...)

System	*Description*
Insurance schemes	A number of insurance schemes exist for public and private employees. Government employees are entitled to free medical care at facilities operated by the government. Private companies often offer their own medical services to employees or contract with public and private health facilities to serve their employees. Firms having more than 500 employees are required to provide a physician on call to their employees.
Social security system	As of March 1991, the Thai Government launched a social security system to provide health care for employees. Enterprises with twenty or more workers are covered. In the next few years, social security coverage will be extended to include smaller enterprises. This system is funded by the government and by a 1.5 per cent wage deduction from employers and from employees. As of 1991, 3 million people were covered.
Free Medical Care Project	This insurance scheme provides free services to the poorer population. Individuals earning less than US$66 per month and families earning less than US$87 per month are covered. As of 1985, there were 11 million members.

Sources: Giraud (chapter 5, this volume); Griffin (1990); Kurian (1992); Roemer (1991).

SELECTED SOCIAL INDICATORS IN SOME ASIAN DEVELOPING COUNTRIES

Country	Adult literacy rate, 1990 (per cent)			Female literacy index, 1990 (north=100)	Female labour force 1988-90 (as percentage of total	Rural-urban disparity in access to services, 1987-90 (rural-urban parity=100)[a]		Percentage of labour force in agriculture		Percentage of population below the poverty line 1980-89		Fertility rate 1990
	Total	Male	Female			Water	Sanitation	1965	1986-89	Total	Rural	
India	48	62	34	35	26	92	11	73	63	48	51	4.2
Indonesia	77	84	68	72	40	168	113	71	54	39	44	3.3
Lao PDR	44[b]	-	-	-	45	53	27	71	76	-	-	6.7
Malaysia	78	87	70	74	31	-	-	59	42	27	38	3.8
Myanmar	81	89	72	76	37	67	87	64	64	40	40	3.9
Philippines	90	90	90	94	37	75	87	58	42	58	64	4.1
Thailand	93	96	90	95	47	127	102	82	79	30	34	2.4
Viet Nam	88	92	84	88	47	94	115	79	68	-	-	3.9

- = Not available

a. Figures are expressed in relation to the urban average, indexed to equal 100. The smaller the rural figure, the bigger the gap; the closer the figure to 100, the smaller the gap; and a figure above 100 indicates that the rural average is higher than the urban average.

b. Data refer to 1989 overall literacy rate.

Source: UNDP (1992).

THE EUROPEAN REGION COUNTRY INFORMATION

	Total Popu-lation (thou-sands)[a]	Popu-lation 0-14 years (%)[a]	Popu-lation 15-49 years (%)[a]	Popu-lation >50 years (%)[a]	Annual growth rate (%)[a]	Urban popu-lation (thou-sands)[b]	Infant morta-lity rate[b,c]	Life expec-tancy Men[b]	Life expec-tancy women[b]	Gross national product per capita (US$)[d]	Male lite-racy rate in 1990[e]	Female lite-racy rate in 1990[e]
	(1)	(2)	(3)	(4)	(5)	(6)	(7)	(8)	(9)	(10)	(11)	(12)
Albania	3338	32	52	16	0.9	1223	23	71	77	-	-	-
Austria	7805	17	51	32	0.4	4658	8	73	79	19060	-	-
Azerbaijan	7337	33	-	-	0.8	3962	-	70	70	-	-	-
Belgium	10010	18	50	32	0.1	9656	8	73	79	15540	-	-
Denmark	5169	17	52	31	0.2	4407	7	73	79	22080	-	-
France	57379	20	51	29	0.4	41715	7	73	81	19490	-	-
Germany	80606	17	49	34	0.4	69243	7	73	79	22320	-	-
Hungary	10493	19	50	31	-0.1	6967	13	67	74	2780	-	-
Israel	5411	30	50	20	4.3	4944	9	75	79	10920	-	-
Italy	57826	16	51	33	0.1	40406	8	74	80	16830	98	96
Latvia	2669	22	48	31	-0.3	1924	10	67	76	-	-	-
Lithuania	3760	22	49	28	0.2	2656	10	68	78	-	-	-
Luxembourg	380	17	51	31	0.7	325	8	72	79	-	-	-
Netherlands	15270	18	54	28	0.7	13564	7	74	81	17320	-	-
Norway	4310	19	51	30	0.5	3285	7	74	81	23120	-	-
Romania	23377	23	50	27	0.3	12899	22	67	73	1640	-	-

(Contd.)

Table (Contd...)

	(1)	(2)	(3)	(4)	(5)	(6)	(7)	(8)	(9)	(10)	(11)	(12)
Russian Federation	149248	23	-	-	0.2	104474	-	70f	70f	-	-	-
Spain	39153	18	52	30	0.2	31219	6	75	81	11020	-	-
Sweden	8692	18	48	33	0.5	7337	5	75	81	23660	-	-
Switzerland	6862	17	51	32	0.7	4319	7	75	81	32680	-	-
Turkey	59577	34	52	14	2.0	39010	55	65	70	1630	90	71
Ukraine	52236	21	-	-	0.2	34998	-	71f	71f	-	-	-
United Kingdom	57826	19	49	31	0.2	51635	7	74	79	16100	-	-

a. Estimate for 1993. Source: UN Population Division 1992.

b. WHO estimate for 1993 based on data from UN Population Division 1992.

c. Per 1000 live births

d. Data for 1990. Source: World Bank (STARS) (April 1992).

e. Source: Statistical Yearbook (UNESCO, 1991)

f. Figure does not differentiate by sex.

REPORTING OF HIV AND AIDS

	HIV Infection first reported[a]	*No. of AIDS cases reported*		*Cumulative no. of AIDS cases reported By 1 July 1993b*
		1991[b]	*1992*[b]	
Albania	-	0	0	0
Austria	1985	176	170	943
Azerbaijan	1987	0	0	0
Belgium	1984	229	118	1364
Croatia	1986	10	7	49
Czech Republic	1985	2	9	36
Denmark	1978	204	196	1182
France	1982	4248	4151	24226
Germany	1980	1450	1286	9697
Hungary	1985	31	32	120
Israel	1981	28	27	234
Italy	1982[c]	3607	3812	16860
Latvia	1987	0	1	4
Lithuania	1988	0	0	3
Luxembourg	1984	12	12	62
Netherlands	1982	431	468	2575
Norway	1982	60	50	319
Romania	1985	360	408	2353
Russian Federation	1987	25	26	127
Slovakia	1985	0	0	6
Slovenia	1986	7	3	25
Spain	1981	3469	3469	18347
Sweden	1985	137	119	817
Switzerland	1985	432	445	3028
Turkey	1985	18	25	99
Ukraine	1987	3	4	14
United Kingdom	1982	1810	1268	7341

a. Compiled from answers by countries to the GPA questionnaire.

b. Based on other information reported to WHO/GPA by countries.

c. On stored sera, 1979.

THE NATIONAL AIDS COMMITTEE (NAC) AND THE NATIONAL AIDS PROGRAMME (NAP)[a]

	National AIDS Committee			*Full-time NAP manager (since)*
	Year Established	*Chairman's position*	*NGOs represented (since)*	
Albania	1987	Minister of Health	1990	1991
Austria	1983	-	1985	-
Azerbaijan	-	-	-	-
Belgium	1988	Member of Medical Faculty	-	-
Croatia	1989	Minister of Health	no	-
Czech Republic	1990	Chief Public Health Officer	1990	no
Denmark	1986	-	1986	1986
France	-	-	-	yes
Germany	-	-	-	-
Hungary	1987	Chief, Division of Public Health And Epidemiology	1988	no
Israel	1986	Director General, Ministry of Health	no	no
Italy	1987	Minister of Health	yes	no
Latvia	-	-	-	-
Lithuania	-	-	no	1989
Luxembourg	1984	Directeur de Sante	1984	no
Netherlands	1985	-	1985	1985
Norway	1985[b]	Professor of Theology	1987	1985
Romania	1990	Minister of Health	1990	no
Russian Federation	-	-	-	-
Slovakia	1986	-	no	no
Slovenia	1985	Director General of the University Institute of Public and Social Welfare	1985	no
Spain	1987	General Secretary for Health	1988	1992
Sweden	1985[c]	-	-	1986
Switzerland	1988	Chief, Infectious Diseases	1988	yes
Turkey	1987[d]	Minister of Health	1992	no
Ukraine	1991	Member of Academy	-	no
United Kingdom	1985	Deputy Chief Medical Officer	no	1985

a. Compiled from answers by countries to the GPA questionnaire, updated where possible by other information available to GPA in mid-1993.

b. Reference Group for the Social and Health Departments.

c. Abolished July 1992.

d. Reorganized in 1993.

GOVERNMENT DEPARTMENTS AND MINISTRIES IMPLEMENTING AIDS-RELATED ACTIVITIES[a]

	Health	*Education & culture*	*Social welfare & family affairs*	*Informa tion & media*	*Interior home affairs*	*Women & youth*	*Armed forces*	*Finance & planning*	*Labour*	*Other*
	(1)	(2)	(3)	(4)	(5)	(6)	(7)	(8)	(9)	(10)
Albania	x	x		x						
Austria	x									
Azerbaijan	x	-	-	-	-	-	-	-	-	
Belgium	x	-	-	-	-	-	-	-	-	
Croatia	x	x		x						
Czech Republic	x	x								
Denmark	x									
France	x	x					x			
Germany	x	x								countries, municipalities agriculture, justice, local government, tourism, economic cooperation, research and technology
Hungary	x									
Israel	x	x	x				x			
Italy	x	-	-	-	-	-	-	-	-	
Latvia	x	-	-	-	-	-	-	-	-	
Lithuania	x			x						

(Contd.)

Table (Contd...)

	(1)	(2)	(3)	(4)	(5)	(6)	(7)	(8)	(9)	(10)
Luxembourg	x	x	x							
Netherlands	x	x	x	x						justice, local government
Norway	x	x								
Romania	x	-	-	-	-	-	-	-	-	
Russian Federation	x	x	x	x						
Slovakia	x	x		x			x			
Slovenia	x	x		x						
Spain	x	x					x			justice
Sweden	x		x							
Switzerland	x	x								
Turkey	x	-	-	-	-	-	-	-	-	
Ukraine	x	-	-	-	-	-	-	-	-	
United Kingdom	x									local government

a. Compiled from answers by countries to the GPA questionnaire.

SUPPLY OF CONDOMS

	Contoms distributed (thousands)[a]		*Condom social marketing programme in 1992*[b]
	1990	*1991*	
Albania	-	-	no
Austria	-	-	no
Azerbaijan	2000	3000	no
Belgium	10000	10000	yes
Croatia	-	-	no
Czech Republic	3520	5231	no
Denmark	-	14000	yes
France	70000	92000	yes
Germany	-	-	no
Hungary	15000	18000	yes
Israel	-	-	yes
Italy	-	-	no
Latvia	-	1000	no
Lithuania	-	-	no
Luxembourg	-	-	no
Netherlands	390	350	no
Norway	9951	8937	yes
Romania	-	-	no
Russian Federation	-	-	yes
Slovakia	1500	2500	no
Slovenia	-	-	no
Spain	-	1000	yes
Sweden	22000	22000	yes
Switzerland	12700	13800	yes
Turkey	13452	12264	yes
Ukraine	-	-	no
United Kingdom	145000	148000	no

a. Compiled from answers by countries to the GPA questionnaire. The stated number of condoms distributed does not always include those sold by the private sector.

b. Compiled from answers by countries to the GPA questionnaire and other information available to GPA. Some of the replies concerning "condom social marketing" pertain to condom promotion activities in general.

c. 1990 and 1991.

AIDS INFORMATION, EDUCATION AND COMMUNICATION (IEC)a

	AIDS & STD education included in school Curricula (since)	Frequency of AIDS messages on:				Free air time given to AIDS messages			Promotion of condoms:	
		radio		television						
		more often than weekly	less often than weekly	more often than weekly	less often than weekly	yes	partly	no	through mass media	to vulnerable groups
	(1)	(2)	(3)	(4)	(5)	(6)	(7)	(8)	(9)	(10)
Albania	no		x		x	x			yes	yes
Austria	yes		x		x			x	yes	no
Azerbaijan	1990		x		x		x		no	yes
Belgium	yes		x		x		x		yes	yes
Croatia	1990		x		x		x		yes	no
Czech Republic	1991	x		x			x		yes	yes
Denmark	yes		x		x		x		yes	yes
France	1987		x		x		x		yes	yes
Germany	-		-	x		x			yes	yes
Hungary	no	x		x			x		yes	yes
Israel	yes		x		x	x			yes	yes
Italy	1993		x		x			x	yes	yes
Latvia	1990		x		x		x		yes	yes

(Contd.)

Table (Contd...)

	(1)	(2)	(3)	(4)	(5)	(6)	(7)	(8)	(9)	(10)
Lithuania	no	x		x				x	yes	yes
Luxembourg	1988		x		x		x		no	yes
Netherlands	1991	x		x			x		yes	yes
Norway	1986		x		x	x			yes	yes
Romania	no		x		x		x		no	no
Russian Federation	1989		x		x		x		yes	yes
Slovakia	no		x		x	x			yes	yes
Slovenia	1989		x		x		x		yes	yes
Spain	1992		-		-		x		yes	yes
Sweden	1977		x		x			x	yes	yes
Switzerland	[b]	x		x			x		yes	yes
Turkey	no		x		x		x		no	no
Ukraine	—	x			x		x		yes	yes
United Kingdom	1992		x		x			x	yes	yes

a. Compiled from answers by countries to the GPA questionnaire.

b. Different in each canton

HIV ANTIBODY TESTING[a]

	Laboratory testing facilities at		
	Central Level	*provincial level*	*district level*
Albania	x		
Austria	x	x	x
Azerbaijan	x	x	x
Belgium	x	x	x
Croatia	x	x	x
Czech Republic	x	x	x
Denmark	x	x	x
France	x	x	x
Germany	x	x	x
Hungary	x	x	x
Israel	x	x	x
Italy	x	x	x
Latvia	x	x	x
Lithuania	x	x	x
Luxembourg	x	x	x
Netherlands	x	x	x
Norway	x	x	
Romania	x	x	x
Russian Federation	x	x	x
Slovakia	x	x	x
Slovenia	x	x	
Spain	x	x	x
Sweden	x	x	x
Switzerland	x	x	x
Turkey	x	x	
Ukraine	x	x	x
United Kingdom	x	x	x

a. Compiled from answers by countries to the GPA questionnaire.

Index

O

P

T

ENCYCLOPAEDIA OF AIDS

ENCYCLOPAEDIA
OF
AIDS

(In 7 Volumes)

(Volume 3)

Editor

G.C. Satpathy

KALPAZ PUBLICATIONS
DELHI–110 052

ENCYCLOPAEDIA OF AIDS
(Health, Reference)

Rs. 7000 (Set)
Rs. 1000 each volume

ISBN: 81-7835-112-9 (Set)
ISBN: 81-7835-134-X (Vol. 3)

Published in 2003 in India by
Kalpaz Publications
C-30, Satyawati Nagar
Delhi-110 052
e-mail: kalpaz@hotmail.com

Laser Typeset at: Varsha Graphics, Delhi
Printed at: Mehra Offset Press, Delhi

Contents

Preface

The later half of the twentieth century will be remembered in the history of medicine for two remarkable events, one good, that is the eradication of smallpox, and the other one bad, when the world was alerted to the first case AIDS in 1981, now running in a pandemic proportion. In a little over two decades it is estimated that over 36 million people are now infected with HIV/AIDS with 5.3 million being infected every year. India alone has about 4 million HIV/AIDS patients, the second highest number among all nations. Now it is well perceived as a serious threat to humanity, and the control of this epidemic lies not only in the hands of physicians alone but the entire society must involve to the task. No cure or vaccine is yet in sight. So the only mode of controlling it is prevention. The key to prevention lies in information, education and communication.

Twenty years of observation and study of the syndrome has generated profound interest among all branches of medicine, social activists, research workers, public health issues, health and sex education strategies, with innumerable clinical and pharmacological research being conducted on it all over the world. It is not possible to compile the whole saga of AIDS, which is unique in many ways and not yet fully understood. We have tried to accumulate as much information as possible in this seven-volume encyclopaedia, probably the first such attempt made ever. Since the process of acquiring information is never-ending, we hope to provide more and more information in future.

It has been a herculean task to compile the huge materials systematically, besides being an unique experience. In spite of the best efforts for accuracy and perfection, there may be shortcomings, which may be excused. It will be a success story for us if by this work the society to which the work is dedicated is benefited at large. The study does not end here. It shall be a continuous series in future with comprehensive details having a deep bearing on the subject.

Guwahati-23
Rathyatra-2002

Dr. G.C. Satpathy
MD, IPM

Acknowledgements

During the course of this research work, I happened to visit several academic fora which willingly afforded their support and facilitated my work. These are the Ministry of Health, Govt. of India, World Health Organisation, health departments of the States and academic institutions of higher learning. I have used the material from published works including scholarly journals and magazines to fill up the gaps in these volumes.

I have also taken academic support from several sources, which include universities, institutes, centres for higher learning, Acts passed in this direction, Statistical Year Book (UNESCO), voluntary organisations, legal luminaries, social activists, prison management, legal issues of AIDS, Legislation Enquiry Commission on HIV Law, Sri Lanka, Prevention of Brothels Act, Myanmar, Laws of HIV/AIDS in Pakistan, Documents in sub-Saharan, Africa, European Council Recommendations, UNESCO Courier, Philippines Overseas Employment Agency, Foreign Exchange Regulations Deptt., Central Bank of the Philippines, National Advisory Committee on AIDS in Singapore, Vietnamese National AIDS Committee, National Blood Transfusion Centre in Cambodia, Infectious Diseases Act, Thailand, AIDS Prevention Act in Korea, Labour Protection Law, Thailand, Social Security Act, Thailand, Homosexual Law Reform Act, 1986, Universities of Nairobi, Manitola (in Canada) and Washington, Institute of Systemic Therapy, Harare, Zimbabwe, The AIDS Service Organisation, Kampala, Uganda, Health Economics and HIV/AIDS Research Division, University of Natal, Durban, School of

Public Health, University of Natal, South Africa Institute for Medical Research, Johannesburg, Centre for African Family Studies, Nairobi, Kenya, Malwai Institute of Management, Malwai.

I feel much grateful to these institutions and learned authors whose writings have proved useful in the texts of these seven volumes.

The publisher and myself feel much beholden to the panel of highly qualified and experienced advisers who are distinguished in their respective fields, for their valuable and timely guidelines, contributions and encouragement in making this work an epoch-making one.

I am grateful to several other research institutes and NGOs etc., scholars whose writings have been used in these volumes.

I am extremely grateful to my wife, son Anurag and daughter Anamika for their consistent encouragement to me during this stupendous research work.

Dr. G.C. Satpathy

Our Distinguished Panel of Advisers

1. Dr. A.K. Das, MD, MNAMS, Ph.D., FICA	Dean and Director-Prof. Dept. of Medicine, JIMPER, Pondicherry
2. Mr. D.K. Arya IPS (Retd.)	Former Director General, BSF
3. Dr. K.V. Dakhina Murty MD, DM, DNB, FISN	Prof. & Head, Deptt. of Nephrology, Nizam's Instt. of Medical Sciences, Panjagutta, Hyderabad
4. Maj. Gen. K.K. Ganguly	VSM (Retd.)
5. Col. M.K. Bhandari MD, FICA	Asso. Prof. of Medicine, Armed Forces Medical College, Pune
6. Dr. M.C. Dash	Vice Chancellor, Sambalpur University, P.O.: Jyoti Vihar, Orissa
7. Dr. N.C. Borah MD, DM	C.M.D. GNRC Hospitals Ltd. Dispur, Guwahati
8. Dr. P.C. Bhattacharya MD	Sr. Consultant, downtown hospital Dispur, Guwahati
9. Dr. S.B. Gupta MD	Physician and Cardiologist Central Railway Hospital, Mumbai

Introduction

The HIV / AIDS epidemic is inextricably associated with the social and cultural values and economic relationships between individuals and within communities. HIV is a virus that can infect a person regardless of sex, race or social status. HIV virus is also not random in its spread and impact. In its impact, the poor and marginalised people and communities are the most affected. This is because social inequalities facilitate the transmission of the virus and the virus in turn reflects and reinforces those inequalities. The virus differentiates not only in its medical manifestations but also in its disproportionate impact on those who are socially, sexually and economically vulnerable.

Absence of defences makes people vulnerable. In the context of HIV, it can be taken to mean absence of choices. As HIV transmission is preventable, this consists of a series of choices at the systemic and personal levels, whether it is the choice to provide uninfected blood or the choice to use a condom or even have sex. Vulnerable are those individuals and societies whose capacities to make the necessary choices are limited by obstacles which include:

(a) **for individuals:** lack of knowledge and awareness, their social and economic position within societies, lack of personal freedom resulting from cultural, social and legal structures and even physical location.

(b) **for societies:** lack of political will, lack of resources, lack of knowledge and skills, lack of implementing capacity and denial.

The statistics of HIV / AIDS demonstrate the magnitude of the problem. Surveillance systems tell us where the virus has been but we need to better understand where it is likely to go. Assessment of vulnerability provides some of these road maps. HIV infection differs among different groups of people, including between the rich and poor, between men and women, between different ethnic and marginalised groups. The epidemic problem is specific in its association with the disease, death and the rising numbers of people, infected by HIV. In pervasiveness, it affects every aspect of human life and national development. The causes and consequences of the virus embrace poverty, livelihoods, gender, governance, rights and ethical issues.

The important risk factors for HIV infection in the times to come may not be sexual activity or drug use as such but rather social and economic dependency. HIV/AIDS being preventable, people who have access to information and choices, will in the future be able to protect themselves against infection. An improved understanding of the factors that make people vulnerable to HIV is necessary. This will generate the conditions in which all individuals may be empowered to exercise choice for their protection against infection.

Some socio-economic issues related to poverty and livelihood, mobility, gender and rights need to be addressed to meet the challenges posed by the epidemic. The uneven distribution of wealth and power between people, structural poverty and lack of sustainable livelihoods give the main impetus for the accelerated spread of HIV. Poverty reduces the power of people to control their circumstances and make informed choices. Families affected by illness and death from HIV/AIDS suffer from the loss of livelihoods of both those who fall sick and those who care for them while simultaneously expenses for treatment increase. As a result, children may be neglected, malnourished and withdrawn from school. Rich, powerful and mobile people too encounter the risk of infection.

Migration in itself is not a risk factor for HIV, it can generate conditions in which people are most vulnerable. Separated from spouse, family and socio-cultural norms, isolated and lonely and a sense of anonymity can lead to sexual practices which make migrant workers more susceptible to HIV. It is then carried back to their families. As men migrate in search of work, women become the *defacto* heads of households, resulting often in social, economic and sexual exploitations.

Poor women and children migrants are particularly vulnerable to abuse and exploitation. The lack of safe, secure and legal channels for migration drive women and girls into the hands of traffickers who promise them 'lucrative jobs' and 'safe travel' to location of work. Caught in the web of trafficking, those affected face an increased risk of HIV/AIDS as they are unable to control their working and living conditions. For many women sexual intercourse is not a question of choice but rather a question of survival and duty unless the interaction between HIV infection, cultural values and the rights and needs of women are recognised, the fundamental changes necessary to stem the epidemic will be unattainable. Where women are denied dignity and respect, HIV/AIDS spread. One of the worst ironies of the epidemic in India is that younger girls are being forced into sexual relations and sex trade in the attempt by men to avoid infections and even from a mistaken belief that intercourse with a virgin can cure the virus.

One thing is obvious that respect for human rights is critical in the context of the epidemic as human rights matters most when they are most under threat. The fact that those under threat most are those who are already socially and economically vulnerable means that the need to incorporate human rights concerns in HIV policy becomes an imperative. Similar issues arise in relation to drug users, gay men and sex workers and people living with HIV/AIDS for whom discrimination and social stigmatisation are daily realities. People need protection against the abuse of their rights threatened by the epidemic.

The most important and urgent need at hand is to contain the epidemic through reconciliation rather than conflict including when dealing for example with issues related to individual *vs* public rights/interests. Alienation of people with HIV from society does not help to contain the epidemic. A protective and supportive legal framework is essential complemented by careful and informed ethical considerations. Policies and laws that reduce stigma and build self-esteem of affected people generate the environment for mutual trust. The general lack of understanding of a human right approach is due in large part to lack of involvement, participation and ownership of infected and affected communities and groups in HIV strategies.

Last, but not the least, there is the urgent need of human rights standards, systems to document and monitor legal, ethical and human right, practices, supportive policies and law, education and information dissemination and strengthened partnerships and voices. Human rights should not merely provide the backdrop against which HIV/AIDS strategies should be planned but rather act as a powerful tool that can be actively used to assist people to protect themselves from HIV/AIDS.

This requires that human rights considerations must address the immediate and important concerns such as stigma and discrimination against people with HIV and access to health care and employment. It must also address the fundamentally unequal social economic position of women and poor marginalised people within societies. Those living with the epidemic, those at the forefront of change must be persuaded to come out and make visible the unvisible.... the realities of life in the post-HIV era.

1

HIV/AIDS: Global Scenario

International Situation (1998)

Expanding at an accelerated rate, in every country, there are 16,000 new HIV infections daily in India. Approximately six million new infections were noticed in 1998 alone and at the end of the year, 33.4 million people were living with HIV.

Young people below 25 years are the victims of new infections. Ten per cent of the newly infected are below 15 years of age. Rate of infection is increasing in women. They now constitute 43 per cent of all those over 15 with AIDS. Ninety per cent of infected women currently live in third world countries. AIDS is among the five top killer diseases throughout the world. Two and a half million people died of AIDS in 1998.

Overview—Regional

The worst affected is the sub-Saharan Africa and the increasing infections are concentrated in east and southern Africa. Eastern Europe noted a 6-fold increase in HIV infections over the last four years. Latin America and Caribbean infections still concentrated in marginalised groups.

In the Asia-Pacific region infection rate is low and spread is rapid. South and East Asia, Cambodia, Myanmar, Thailand and Vietnam have high levels of HIV. In Bangladesh, Pakistan and Sri Lanka, infection ratio has not yet reached 1 adult : 1000. Proportionate growth rate is the highest in the world in India and China, with over 7 million already infected in the Asia Pacific region.

Situation in India

The largest HIV-positive population in the world with 4 million adults infected is in India. Infection is spreading from urban to rural areas and from groups practising risk behaviour to the general population. One per cent of all pregnant women are infected in 5 states. Eighty-nine per cent of reported cases are in the sexually active and economically productive age group of 18-40 years. The infection is increasing among women and young people and half of these occur among adolescents. Estimated 25 per cent of infections are currently among women and the female to male ratio of infection is increasing sharply. Approximately 30,000 new born children are infected and the country may have 120,000 AIDS orphans. Seventy-five per cent of infections are through sexual transmission, 8 per cent through intravenous drug use and 8 per cent through blood transfusion, etc. The percentage of mother-to-child transmission could be on the rise as indicated by increasing infection rates in pregnant women. The worst is being awaited. By the year 2000, approximately 1.2 per cent of the adult population could be infected. Factors governing the spread of AIDS are listed below:

(a) Lack of general awareness and knowledge of prevention practices among the rural population and in the most vulnerable groups.
(b) Prevalence of sexually transmitted diseases (STDs) and reproductive tract infections.
(c) Unsafe sexual intercourse without use of condoms and sex relations with several partners.
(d) Injecting drug use in all major cities.
(e) Low social status of women, different standards of morality which increase risk of infections for women.
(f) Illiteracy, limited buying and negotiating power with limited access to supportive services for the large number of marginalised populations as women, slum dwellers, street and working children, prostitutes.
(g) Mobility of population is a key factor—nearly 180 million migrant workers, thousands of truck-drivers uniformed personnel, all men, are on the move in India.

Effects

(a) AIDS declarated the life expectancy the world over.
(b) Under-five mortality rates have been doubled.
(c) There are 8.2 million orphans since the epidemic stated in 1986.
(d) Retardation in the growth and economic development of the

country due to increased morbidity and mortality in young adults between 20 and 40.

(e) Increased national health care expenditures because of increased demand for health care services. More people become ill due to AIDS. Increase in the onset of opportunistic infections like TB adding to the strain on the health care system due to AIDS. People living below the poverty line are worst affected as revealed by a survey made in New Delhi.

(f) People living with AIDS (PLWAs) suffer emotional trauma and are ostracised and denied their basic human rights.

Recommendations

Preventive interventions can overcome the epidemic. HIV cases have been drastically reduced by joint efforts in Thailand. A sharp decline in the rate of new infections among young have taken place in Uganda in the last two years. Approximately 40 per cent reduction in new infections is achieved in Tanzania due to STD prevention. In India, a project for prostitutes in Kolkata revealed that the incidence of STDs can be reduced and the levels of HIV infections can be kept low. Safe sex practices and sex education can drastically reduce the percentage of infections.

Present Trends

The first case of AIDS was reported in 1987 and since then, the epidemic has spread sharply. Due to heterosexual transmission, active sex industry, and interacting with less studied patterns of bisexual or injecting behaviour, WHO/UNAIDS estimates show that India has the largest number of HIV positive cases in the South and South East Asian region. India is expected to have the largest concentration of AIDS patients in the world if the current rate of transmission continues as it has a large and increasing population.

Variable Trends

Seventy-three per cent of the country's 930 million people, were thought to be relatively spared by the epidemic in rural areas. It has been revealed that in some areas, HIV has become common in villages as well as in cities. A recent survey in Tamil Nadu shows that 2.1 per cent of the adult population living in the rural areas had HIV, as compared to 0.7 per cent of the urban population. It was commonly assumed that HIV infection in India was concentrated among urban prostitutes and their clients and in drug injectors in a few states. It is now evident that the virus is firmly embedded in the general population, among women whose only risk behaviour is having sex with their own husbands. It has been established that in at least five states, more than one per cent women in urban areas are now infected.

Accounting Factors

(a) Abject poverty and low economic status are the conditions responsible for the spread of HIV/AIDS.

(a) AIDS incidence is highest among the developing countries.

(b) People with low incomes cannot afford treatment for STDs. They cannot buy even condoms. 320 million people or 36 per cent of the population of India live below the poverty line.

(c) Commercial sex as a lucrative occupation for young and poorly educated daughters in poor families. There are approximately 100,000 prostitutes in each of the metropolitan cities in India. Due to the clandestine nature of the trade, the majority of the sex workers lack legal provisions, suffer discrimination, and have little means of protecting themselves.

(d) The poor and illiterate individuals in a society are more likely to contract STDs and other infectious diseases. Those are deprived of their right to information on risk behaviour and are too illiterate to understand prevention messages and with no access to quality services. The average literacy rate is 43 per cent for women and 57 per cent for men.

(e) Untreated STDs raise the risk of HIV infection per sexual intercourse episode.

(f) It is evident that people with current or past STDs are 2 to 9 times more likely to get infected with HIV. The lesions caused by untreated ulcerative STDs such as herpes, syphilis and chancroid provide an easy entry for HIV. Our country has a very high prevalence of sexually transmitted diseases.

(g) Estimates reveal that the annual incidence of STDs in India might be as high as 5 per cent of the population with over 40 million new infections per year.

(h) STD baseline surveys conducted in Chennai and Jaipur, as well as among sex workers in Kolkata and in a rural area of Tamil Nadu show that STDs are not an exclusively urban problem. Prevalence rates range from 1.2 to 10 per cent for urban population and up to 7 per cent for rural population.

(i) Different standards of morality and gender bias lead to conditions where women are not given the same rights as men, are important elements in the spread of HIV/AIDS. Women have little or no control over decisions relating to sexuality, nor over the sexual behaviour of the male partners or the use of condoms for the prevention of pregnancy or STD/AIDS. A study in India illustrates a situation common to many societies. Of a sample of nearly 400 women attending the city's STI clinics, 93 per cent were married and 91 per cent never had sex with anyone but their husbands. All these women were infected with a Sexually Transmitted Infection (STI) and 13.6 per cent tested positive for HIV.

(j) Migration of population is an important key factor in the spread of HIV in India. Over 180 million migrant workers in India, many of whom are single men, live apart from their wives. The armed forces personnel, and long route truck drivers are more likely to have unsafe sex. Due to this mobility of the male population the virus, has been brought to the aerial areas. The migrant men comprise 30 to 40 per cent of the population of large cities and account for much of the clientele of the 'red light' areas. In a study of 5722 male truck drivers in Assam, 82 per cent of the men reported regular sex with commercial sex workers (CWSs) along the national highways without the use of condoms; 15 per cent reported a history of sex with men; 36 per cent had been treated for an STD; 40 per cent used cannabis and 2.4 per cent had injected heroin.

(k) Rapid urbanisation is the outcome of economic growth resulting in large slum populations and an increase in the unorganised labour such as construction workers, casual landless labourers and child workers. Some 100 million people were estimated to be living in urban slums in 1996, expected to rise to 110 million in 2001. Two-thirds of these are children, youth and women who are less literatee, lack basic knowledge of safe health practices, and have little or no access to information, or health and other supportive services. The spread of AIDS is facilitated by poverty, ignorance and violation of basic rights in these areas.

(l) Sexual behaviour and desire to discuss sex and sexuality affects the chances of transmission. Behavioural studies by NACO revealed that sexual risk behaviour is well established in India. Unprotected sex and frequent partner exchange through casual and commercial sex is prevalent resulting in the increased risk of infection. It has also been revealed that knowledge of prevention practices is low in the rural areas and where knowledge levels are high as in some of the major cities, misconceptions have still not been dispelled. More than 90 per cent of those infected are unaware of their HIV status. The belief that condom use leads to loss of pleasure, cultural sensitivity, association with birth control, powerlessness of women and lack of assurance of quality are the important reasons for low condom use especially with irregular partners. It is reluctance to address sex and sex-related issues, and the denial of the existence of risk behaviour, in particular among youth. The topic of sex is taboo in general and is closely associated with morals and promiscuity. Homosexuality is a morally proscribed behaviour that forces those men who have sex with men underground. All this leads to inadequate policy support for sex education in schools youth and for-out-of school and to a denial of the right to information and services.

(m) Injecting drug use (IDU) is potentially a major cause for HIV transmission which is evident by the extremely high prevalence rates in north-eastern states like Manipur, Mizoram and Nagaland where some sites have reported prevalence at 85.6 per cent. The pattern of sexual networking and sexual mixing of injecting drug users who select sexual partners from people who shared needles, traded sex for money increases the infection rates among them. The five city survey, conducted by the NGO SHARAN in 1997-98 indicates that in the last few years, injecting drug use has become tradition and the number of IDUs is increasing, majority being from the poor sections of the society. Most IDUs are sexually active, but intercourse is unprotected. The needles/syringes were found to be freely available in pharmacies, these were not procured by IDUs. The sharing of injecting equipment was high in spite of the IDUs with a little knowledge of the consequences like AIDS, abscesses, etc. Injecting drug use is a legal offence and this drives users underground preventing them from accessing information. India has a large population of young people, about 400 million below the age of 18. Studies and field experience give evidence of early onset of sexual activity and low levels of awareness among young people. There is also a comparatively large population of children living in difficult circumstances such as street children and child labourers, many of whom are vulnerable to sexual abuse. As the epidemic matures, there is an increasing pool of potential sexual partners who are already infected. This is true for both young men, who in many countries tend to have their first sexual experiences with sex workers, and for young women who tied to have sex with older men. Young people can also be made more vulnerable to HIV by several other taboos ideologies and social norms. This is in particular the case where voting people are denied knowledge and skills on sexual and reproductive matters, barred from reproductive health services alongwith HIV prevention and STD care and counselling and homosexually ostracized. Adolescents are in general left alone to deal with the biological and social transformation of adolescence, at times with no caring adults to talk to.

(n) Discrimination and curtailing of human rights of women and children of marginalised populations such as commercial sex workers and men who have sex with men have resulted in their lack of access to information and acceptable services. This can also heighten the risk of infection and the further spread of the virus.

(o) Infected blood is also a major source of HIV infection. Of about 2 million bottles of blood that are transfused each year in India, more than half reportedly were supplied by people who sell their blood. Although the government has made HIV screening mandatory, not all blood banks comply. The main issue is one of supply—the demand exceeds the supply and at present, only 60 per cent of the demand is being met which has implications for HIV transmission.

Future Challenges

The major challenge will be to reach large numbers of vulnerable populations, in particular in the countryside. Specific challenges include:

(a) Taking action from project scale best practices to large-scale activities.

(b) Strengthening state level capacity in all aspects of programming.

(c) Generating a wide network of voluntary counselling and testing centres to make infected persons aware of their status in a supportive and conducive environment.
(d) Care and support for large numbers of people living with AIDS.
(e) Ensure sustainability and multi-sectoral ownership by integrating the HIV/AIDS prevention and care programme into the development agenda.
(f) Preventing infantile transmission and giving care for affected children.
(g) Ensuring that prevention and care take place within a human rights framework.

Impact

The long-term implications of HIV/AIDS are only just being recognised, it is obvious that it will have a multiplier effect which will leave a profound impact not only on individuals; households and communities, but also on life expectancy, per capita income, school enrolments and health. In India, the impact is still not visible. Studies in Africa show that impact is clearly evident only two decades after the onset of epidemic in a country.

Effect of HIV/AIDS on Population

AIDS will not stop population growth but the rate may slow down, which may result in smaller populations over time. For example, in Zambia, the population is predicted to be 7 per cent smaller in 2005 than it would have been without the epidemic. The population structure may vary because of the increased mortality in the 20-40 year age group. Gender proportions may shift in some age groups due to higher infection rates and mortality in women. AIDS sharply reduced life expectancy in some countries. For example, life expectations in Burkina Faso has been reduced by 11 years and in Zimbabwe by 22.2 years.

As the epidemic is spreading, HIV will result in an increased share of total deaths from infectious diseases in developing countries. In 1990 it accounted for 2.0 per cent of all infectious diseases deaths. In 2020, it is expected to account for 13.6 per cent. In Africa HIV/AIDS will account for approximately one-third of infectious diseases deaths. In 2010, AIDS may increase the infant mortality rate by 75 per cent and under-five mortality rate by 100 per cent in worst affected regions as most women will complete their child bearing before falling ill. The number of orphans will rise.

Effects on Economy

Macro-economic impact is uncertain-HIV may reduce the rate of economic growth. It will reverse hard-earned achievements in development. The increased mortality in the 20-40 year age group can reduce the working population, which contributes to the growth and economic development of the nation. There could be productivity loss due to morbidity and premature mortality of People Living with AIDS (PLWAs) and due to time spent by care givers of these patients. There is the loss due to chance in the skilled workforce and the expenditure incurred in re-training the new workforce.

A recent study of the economic consequences of HIV / AIDS in the country reveals that AIDS imposes a major burden on the economic front especially when costs of treatment of PLWAs, prevention programmes, and labour costs are also taken into consideration. A study on AIDS and industry opines that AIDS will have direct effects on productivity, increasing absenteeism, leave and medical care. Educational staff will probably experience levels of illness and death as the general population at all levels thus affecting the provision and quality of education.

Families and the Household

Death of adult earner leads to profound emotional loss and medical and funeral expenses are also borne alongwith loss of income. If both parents die from AIDS household composition and roles may change and in various cases leads to the dissolution of households, grandparents are left to raise young children or dependent children are sent away, as witnessed in the Kagera district, Tanzania. A household with an infected member will find that expenditure increases as the person requires medical care, special diet, etc. AIDS places new, often unaffordable demands on resources and time which could have been spent on productive activities. In poorer households death of the prime carrier results in a drop in food expenditure and consumption as evidenced in Kagera household where per capita consumption fell by 15 per cent. Low income households are more severely affected by an AIDS death which tend to worsen poverty and increase inequality. In Delhi, India, a study conducted using major illness and death as a proxy for AIDS-related morbidity and mortality shows that the household expenditure on health care in India is four to five times the level of state expenditure on the same.

Women being the prime care givers, are likely to be worst affected in a family. A Mumbai-based study of the household and community responses to AIDS reveals that the household responses were more supportive in case of HIV-positive males than females. The psychological trauma experienced by PLWAs cannot be calculated. Denied their basic rights, the social stigma and ostracisation of these families by the society further exacerbates their economic difficulties that lead to increasing poverty. The most devastating effect is the discrimination and refection suffered at the hands of the health care workers and hospitals who deny people living with AIDS treatment and care.

The Health Sector

AIDS will increase demand for health care and reduce supply at the same time which has two related impacts. First, health care becomes more scarce and more expensive. Second, national health care expenditure rises. As several studies suggest, adults with AIDS use more health care prior to death than those who die of other causes. In worst hit nations, HIV-infected make up large percentage of patients in the hospital. In Chiang Mai, Thailand, 50 per cent of the beds are occupied by HIV-positive patients. Statistics from Kenyatta hospital, Nairobi, on admissions and mortality, suggest that the increased need to care for the people with HIV has squeezed out some HIV-negative people who would otherwise have received care.

HIV/AIDS increases cost greatly as it requires additional safety measures for medical procedures and for blood screening to maintain the quality of care and to avoid infection. AIDS may reduce the supply of health care through sickness of health care professionals. HIV infection will increase the onset of opportunistic infections like tuberculosis, one of the leading factors of adult death in the region. Studies have indicated that 60 per cent of AIDS cases in India manifest themselves as TB cases. These increased levels of TB will sharply increase the medical expenses of the individuals and families affected, and that of health care. Increased medical expenditure strains the already fragile and overburdened health care system. According to the World Bank estimates, if India maintains its current level of health care subsidies at 21 per cent of total health care expenditure, a severe AIDS epidemic would increase government health care expenditure by about $ 2 billion every year by 2010. If subsidies are increased by 50 per cent level, the same size epidemic would increase annual government health by an additional $ 30 billion expenditure.

Prevention—Declining Rate of Positivity

The Sonagachi project in Kolkata, India shows how some workers as young as 13 years old learn to protect themselves against HIV/STDs when empowered with knowledge, skills and supportive services. The use of condom accompanied by STD care and an effort to build preventive skills, resulted in a drop in STD cases from 80.6 to 59.3 per cent. HIV prevalence remained at virtually the same level. Girls mostly enter the sex trade because they lack the education and skills for other employment. The Sonagachi project has responded to the sex worker's expressed need for literacy, other kinds of education and skills training. To promote further empowerment, the project has helped them in forming a collective through which they protect themselves from violence and harassment, leading to greater self respect and dignity.

In a randomized study in Mwanza, Tanzania, approximately 40 per cent reduction in new HIV infections was attained through the implementation of a comprehensive public health STD prevention and care programme. Recent trends in HIV infection in women attending several antenatal clinics in Uganda show great declines in HIV prevalence. Between 1990 and 1993 and 1994-1995, HIV prevalence in pregnant women at sentinel sites decreased 29 per cent overall. Even more encouraging, prevalence declined by 35 per cent in young women aged 15-19 and 20-24. As infection levels in these young age groups reflect more recent patterns, the data suggest that there has been a large reduction in the rate of new infections among young Ugandans over time. According to the surveys of such populations, behaviour change may account for the reported declines. In Thailand, AIDS was given a due consideration, by widely publicizing the results of a national survey that the country was heading for a major epidemic. The Thai government by integrating AIDS into other sectors such as the Ministry of the Interior, Ministry of Education, Office of the Prime Minister, Ministries of Health and Defence ensured that prevention of HIV infection is a collective effort. Due to these indications, these efforts are taking effect. HIV prevalence in military conscripts declined from 3.6 per cent in 1993 to 2.5 per cent in 1995. In national surveys conducted in 1990 and 1993, the percentage of men visiting prostitutes fell from 22 to 10 per cent. Condom use in commercial sex-transactions is now the norm. Rates of STIs and HIV among men aged less than 21 were dramatically lower than recorded in 1991.

Prevention Works with Young People

There is ample evidence that sex education reduces sexual risk taking behaviour. Young people in Uganda are increasingly abstaining from sex in the face of HIV. In 1995 over half of men and 46 per cent of women aged 15-19 said that they never had sex, an increase of 75 per cent since 1989 for both sexes. Various studies conducted globally, in different cultures examined the age of first sexual intercourse. The findings revealed low levels of sexual activity among students who were given sex education and found that sex education either delayed the onset of sexual activity or reduced its frequency and increased the adoption of safer practices by sexually active youth. More alternatives are at hand now due to the availability of new techniques. The female condom enables women to have an option. It is being made available through price negotiations. In India, pilot studies in acceptability and availability are being conducted by non-governmental organisations. The regimen or antretrovirals, a short one which is less expensive reduces mother to child transmission as shown in studies in Thailand.

Realities

Half of all new infections the world over are in young people below 25 years. As per UNAIDS estimates, more than 3 million children and young people worldwide became infected with HIV in 1998. This included about 590,000 children under 15 and over 2.5 million 15-24 year olds. During 1998, more than 8500 children and young people became infected with HIV every day—six each minute. Approximately, 700,000 young people get infected with HIV every year in Asia and the Pacific.

In India, current statistics indicate that youth will increasingly be at the centre of the epidemic both in terms of transmission and impact. The statistics provided are, however, limited. Children and youth in all socio-economic groups are especially vulnerable to HIV infection as is evident by outcomes of recent studies :

1. Adolescents are sexually active before marriage and outside of marriage, more than was previously thought, and boys are

more sexually active than girls. On the basis of various studies conducted in India, it was obvious that one out of 10 boys below 16 years has had sexual experiences. A study of unmarried urban college students of low socio-economic status in Mumbai has shown that 26.4 per cent of boys had engaged in premarital sex as has 3 per cent of the girls. A study done among married adolescents reported 48 per cent of boys and 3 per cent of girls as having premarital sex in rural Maharashtra. According to a recent survey by a marketing and research group in 5 Mumbai schools, out of 430 students, at least 13 per cent between the ages of 12 and 15 had sexual experiences. Of these, 75 per cent had more than one partner.

2. The prevalence of Reproductive Tract Infections (RTIs) and gynaecological morbidities was alarmingly high. In Chandigarh, an opinion poll of 100 teenagers aged between 14 and 16 disclosed that 38 per cent of boys and 27 per cent of girls had experimented with sex. Above 10 per cent of them had sexually transmitted diseases. In rural Maharashtra, it was found that one in every two women was infected with RTIs. According to a study conducted in Ahmednagar, Maharashtra, it was found that 51 per cent adolescents reported at least one type of gynaecological morbidity such as menstrual disorders and prolapsed uterus.

3. Adolescents, both boys and girls, lack information on sex and HIV/AIDS prevention. Girls have almost no information, and boys have misinformation. According to a 1993-94 study of urban educated youth close to 40 per cent of girls were unaware that condom use could prevent transmission of HIV and STDs, and about 50 per cent of youth were unaware of infected needles as a mode of HIV transmission. Several young people start experimenting with sex earlier than believed and without knowing concepts like safe sex, contraception and other health issues. Many of the adolescents knew a little about AIDS, but it was not useful information as they had not context to place it in leading to serious implications for reproductive health because lack of information can result in unintended pregnancies, STDs or HIV. Sex education is not available widely to children and is still an issue despite findings to the contrary that sex education delays onset of sexual activity and promotes safer sex. Underlying all the above findings is a lack

of power and participation in decision making by adolescents, especially among girls, and even more so among unmarried girls.

4. Existing reproductive health service do not serve adolescents and there is an under-utilisation of services by adolescents for gynaecological conditions such as RTIs. Statistics from a recent study in Maharashtra revealed that 82 per cent of married adolescent women did not use health services for post-natal care and 51 per cent did not use services for gynaecological problems. According to a research study by the NGO Butterflies, a large number of street children had genital lesions, suggestions of secondary syphilis. One out of ten tested positive on a VDRL test. None went for proper medical treatment.
5. Street children and child labourers are particularly vulnerable due to high incidence of sexual abuse and exploitation. These children have little or no family support, no access to services without the welfare and social safety nets of the organised sector. There are approximately 100,000 street children in the metropolitan cities like Mumbai, Delhi and Kolkata and the numbers are on an increase because of rapid urbanisation. Street children are particularly vulnerable to HIV infection because of lack of awareness and an absence of safety nets. As young as 8, many of them report having sex for companionship or as being victims of regular sexual abuse. Some are dragged into sex trade as a means of survival. Approximately 60-90 per cent street children in Mumbai are sexually active. About 20 per cent of street boys in the 16-20 age group visit commercial prostitutes regularly and 80 per cent periodically. According to a study conducted in the slums in Chennai, 80 per cent of youth engaged in pre-marital sex; 85 per cent of the same group reported never using condoms.

Our government admits that 17.5 million children in the 5-14 age group are in the labour force. Other studies range from 40-100 million. The most exploitative forms of child labour and child prostitution, forced and bonded labour. These child labourers work and some live in conditions of extreme poverty and fall prey to sexual exploitation increasing their vulnerability to HIV/AIDS. In this scenario, the situation of the girl child labourer calls for particular attention. Life on the street for the girl child is double as oppressive an de-exploitative than that of a boy. Girl children at about nine and ten are forced into consuming drugs and then sexually abused.

6. Child prostitution, child trafficking and sexual abuse leading to forced and coerced sex increase the vulnerability of children to HIV. A 1990 study conducted by the Central Social Welfare Board in six metros reported that approximately 40 per cent of the total commercial sex worker population is below 18 years of age, many of them as young as 8 or 9 years. Each year, about 50,000 more are forced into sex-trade. The average age of children in brothels is as low as 13. Commercial child sex workers increase at the rate of 8-10 per cent every year. Approximately four hundred thousand are the minors, of which 20,000 are annually trafficked into India from Nepal. The children of sex workers numbering about 53 lakh throughout the country are an especially vulnerable group since they fall easy prey of the sex trade. Studies show that the incidence of rape in the under-10 age group has increased by 84 per cent between 1990 and 1994. The general incidence of reported rape in all age group has increased from 20,194 in 1990 to 21,500 in October 1995. These data show only the tip of the iceberg. A study in 1993 shows that 15 per cent of secondary school girls have been sexually abused. The Social Welfare Board reports increased molestation, rape, sexual abuse of progressively younger children more within the family than outside. Increasingly, adult males are targeting younger children for sex in the belief that they are free from HIV and STDs or that sex with a virgin will increase their virility or cure of them of STIs.

7. In many countries children resort to drug use for recreational purposes. As per the UNDCP report, the drug users to a large extent are in the age group of 16 to 30 years. Drug use increases the chances of engaging, in risk taking behaviour and as a result increase their vulnerability to HIV infection. There is little or no use of condoms among drug users. The UNDCP reports of a close relationship between living on the street and use of drugs.

8. *Mother to Child Transmission.* The rising prevalence of HIV among women attending antenatal clinics increases the chances of more children being boric with HIV. Above 4.5 per cent of women attending antenatal clinics in Mumbai were

tested positive. It is approximately that at the end of 1997, 30,000 newborns were infected and 20,000 have died from their infection in India.

Impact on Children

There is a large increase in the number of children who lose one or both parents. Illness or death of parents or guardians robs a child of emotional and physical support which is worst in poor households. Very young motherless orphans have a higher mortality rate than other orphans because about one-third of them are themselves infected at or around the time of birth. The fear, discrimination, ignorance and social stigma associated with AIDS leave affected children completely isolated. Orphans particularly disadvantaged in terms of school enrollment due to reduced ability of families to pay fees, are withdrawn from school to earn, help in family chores or care for ailing family members as indicated in statistics from seven African countries, Haiti and Brazil. Child malnutrition is the severest and lasting consequence of death of the adult earner through reduced household income, which result in reduced food expenditure and consequently a drop in food consumption. In poorer households in Kagera, stunting among children under 5 is substantially higher for orphans (51 per cent) than for children whose parents are alive (39 per cent). Childhood malnutrition can declerate intellectual development and thus reduce productivity in the long run.

The Rights of the Children

The United Nations Convention on the Rights of the Child (CRC) drafted in 1989 is a global covenant on the rights of children. According to it, the countries are morally and ethically bound to honour the rights of children as outlined by the convention, including protection from HIV/AIDS and to take concrete steps to ensure their implementation. All but two countries in the world are signatories to this landmark covenant. India acceded to this Convention in 1992. As regards HIV/AIDS, the CRC has spelt out principles for reducing children's vulnerability to infection and to protect them from discrimination because of their real or perceived HIV/AIDS status. Children should have access to HIV/AIDS prevention education, information and to the means of prevention. Steps should be taken to remove social, cultural, political or religious constraints that block children's access to these. Children's right to confidentiality and privacy pertaining to their HIV status should be recognized. This includes the recognition that HIV testing should be voluntary and done with the informed consent of the person involved which should be obtained in the context of pre-test counselling. If the child's legal guardians are involved, they should pay due regard to the child's opinion. All children should receive sufficient care and treatment for HIV / AIDS, including those children for whom this may require additional sums due to their circumstances, such as orphans. States should include HIV/AIDS as a disability, if disability laws are there to strengthen the protection of people living with HIV / AIDS against discrimination.

Children should have access to HIV/AIDS prevention education and information both in school and out of school, irrespective of their HIV / AIDS status. No discrimination should be suffered by children in leisure, recreational, sport and cultural activities due to their HIV/AIDS status. Special steps should be taken by government to lessen and prevent the impact of HIV / AIDS caused by trafficking, forced prostitution, sexual exploitation. inability to negotiate safe sex, sexual abuse, use of injecting drugs and harmful traditional practices.

Tasks for the Reduction of Children's and Young People's Vulnerability to HIV

(a) The most important challenge in India would be to reach the maximum of young people outside the school system who constitute unorganised and informal labour force.

(b) To implement youth-oriented programmes for the prevention of not only HIV / AIDS but to promote general development of young people by complete participation of young individuals themselves in every stage of programming.

(c) Upscale current best practices, for example, School-based HIV / AIDS education already implemented in several schools, and the UTA programme in colleges, these need to be scaled up to increase the limit of coverage.

(d) Reorientation and strengthening of available services to become 'youth friendly' services to ensure accessibility and acceptability to adolescents and children.

(e) Promotion and development of programmes that ensure that the rights of young people are respected, protected and fulfilled.

(f) Ensuring care and support of orphans and young people living with HIV/AIDS.

(g) Increasing rates of infection in women in developed and developing countries alike.

Women now account for 43 per cent of approximately 33 million people living with AIDS throughout the world. Women's share of reported AIDS cases increased from 12 per cent in 1985 to ten years later in France. The proportion of women infected rose from just 1 per cent in 1984 to 25 per ten years later in Brazil. Today, they account for 25 per cent of all those infected. In Africa, the risk for girls aged 15-24 is two to one, in comparison to boys, in countries where the majority of infections are among the young. In sub-Saharan Africa, infected women now outnumber men six to five. In western Kenya, approximately one in four girls between 15 and 19 is living with HIV, as compared to only one in 25 boys in the same age group. In Zambia, 16 times as many girls are infected as boys.

The ratio is still 4:1 in India but there is evidence that rates of infection in women are increasing since mid-1990. More and more women attending antenatal clinics are testing positive. More than 1 per cent pregnant women in some cities are now HIV positive.

Risk Factors

Physiological vulnerability. For women, risk of HIV infection during unprotected sex is two or four times that of men. Semen has higher concentrations of virus than the vaginal secretions of women. Male to female transmission is more efficient due to the bigger surface area of mucous membrane which is exposed to the partner's sexual secretion in the vagina and on the cervix from where the virus may pass. Adolescent girls are at greater risk due to the immature genital tract and scant vaginal secretions are less of a constraint to HIV.

As with HIV, women often acquire STDs at an earlier age than men. Gonorrhea and syphilis are asymptomatic 50-80 per cent of women as against less than 10 per cent of men. In women they often go untreated. In India, reproductive tract infections and STIs in women have remained a neglected health issue. Bang and Bang's 1989 study in a village in Maharashtra revealed that 92 per cent of women examined had RTI and only 7.8 per cent had ever sought treatment. More recent evidence from demographic studies suggest that rates of RTIs/STDs among women are as high as 20-30 per cent in some parts of the country. This problem is further aggravated by neglect and limited access to health care and opportunities to be informed about the functioning of their bodies, sexuality and health. Women are more likely to suffer from anemia and might require more blood transfusions as compared to the men.

Gender-related vulnerability and barriers to prevention and coping. Girls face discrimination have less access to education, information and skills training than boys' which handicaps them for life. 73 million girls the world over are denied the right to education and the right to participate in their societies as equal to men. In India, 60 per cent of the 110 million school dropouts are girls. As per the Human Development Report 1998, approximately 57 per cent of Indian women are illiterate. As adults they have less opportunity for employment, often no right to work or to own or inherit land and property in their own names. In extreme cases, where women lack alternative work opportunities they may be induced to turn to prostitution. Therefore, the number of sexual partners a women has and the decision to practise safer sex is frequently determined by her low economic status. A study conducted in Thailand revealed that female prostitutes who were in debt to their employers were three times more likely to be infected. Global data indicates that more than 60 per cent of women live below the poverty line. No statistics are available in India but NGOs with field experience report that the percentage of women below the poverty line generally exceeds that of men in both urban and rural areas.

Socio-cultural elements that allow little or no control over sexual relations within and outside marriage. It is throughout indecent for a woman to take the initiative in sexual encounters. So they are inhibited from seeking out information on HIV or buying condom. Many of them dare not bring up the subject of safe sex even with regular partners due to the fear of violence or rejection. Infidelity in women is strictly censored but they are expected to tolerate infidelity in men. Men seek out younger female partners in the belief that they are least likely to be infected which is most risky as a group more likely to have HIV already (older men) transmits the virus to a group with low levels of infection (young girls). In India, women's social status depends on bearing children. Safer sex, in particular, the use of a condom is incompatible with pregnancy.

Violence and rape. Increased violence against women, especially rape, is a risk factor. Women and girls who are raped may contract life-threatening sexually transmitted diseases, including infection with HIV. If a women is a reluctant partner, the risk of damage to the genital mucosa is great, which is the cause of increasing risk of HIV infection. Researches established that non-consensual sex is a pervasive reality in women's lives. Innumerable girls and women are sold into marriage, sex trade and slavery every year. Girls in sex trade may lack knowledge about HIV or of how to protect themselves. Even if well informed, they may find it hard to insist on safer sex for fear of violence or loss of business. According to a study conducted by the NGO Sakshi reveals that 60 per cent of 13-15 year olds in schools have been victims of sexual abuse, 40 per cent within the family and 25 per cent are victims of serious abuse such as rape.

Tasks ahead for the reduction of girls and women's vulnerability are to:

(a) improve access to information, education and skills regarding HIV/AIDS, sexuality, reproduction,
(b) provide services and technologies to lessen women's individual risk and improve women's access to them,
(c) improve understanding of how gender influences men's knowledge, attitudes and sexual behaviour,
(d) design and implement prevention programmes that more effectively address the gender-related elements that influence personal and societal vulnerability to HIV,
(e) advocate for and provide more resources for gender-sensitive care and support,
(f) advocate for laws and policies against gender-related discrimination,
(g) for public commitment to gender and to a participatory approach to developing mechanisms for addressing gender, and the incorporation of gender across programmes.

In various countries, HIV has already become the single greatest cause of child death. Since the beginning of the epidemic, approximately three million children have died of AIDS. In India, it has been established that about 30,000 children are born infected and 20,000 die every year from AIDS. Babies acquire the virus from their mothers either while still in the uterus, most commonly during the last three months of pregnancy, during labour and delivery, or through breast milk.

Element Enhancing the Risk of Transmission

The risk of MTCT, including transmission through breast milk, is increased by :

(a) recent infection with HIV—a woman who has been infected with HIV during pregnancy or while breastfeeding is more likely to transmit the virus to her infant. Unprotected sex during pregnancy and lactation not only exposes a woman herself at risk of HIV but also increases the risk to her infant;

(b) the progression to AIDS—a woman is more likely, to transmit HIV infection to her infant when she develops AIDS;

(c) infection with certain sexuality transmitted diseases (STDs)-maternal STD infection during pregnancy may increase the risk of transmission to the unborn child;

(d) vitamin A deficiency—the risk of MTCT appears to be greater if an HIV positive woman is deficient in vitamin A, and increases with the severity of her deficiency;

(e) breast conditions—cracked or bleeding nipples, or breast abscesses, may increase the risk of HIV transmission through breastfeeding;

(f) duration of breastfasting—an infant continues to be exposed to the risk of HIV transmission for as long as he or she is breastfeeding. The longer the duration of breastfeeding, the longer the infant is exposed to the risk of HIV infection.

Prevention and Reduction MTCT

Specific measures to prevent HIV infection in women and their partners include:

(a) prevention education and counselling to children and youth especially girls;

(b) providing information about transmission of HIV and STDs;

(c) promoting safer sex and making condoms widely available;

(d) providing early detection and appropriate treatment of STDs;

(e) to ensure the safety of medical procedures such as blood transfusion and ensuring that universal precautions as implemented in all health facilities;

(f) accessibility to acceptable voluntary counselling and testing and other supportive services.

Proven strategies to reduce or prevent MTCT when a woman is known to be infected with HIV include:

(a) Counselling of HIV positive mother in early pregnancy alongwith offer of termination of pregnancy.
(b) Anti-retroviral therapy. Revealations from a recent study in Thailand show that a shorter regimen, where AZT is given orally during the last four weeks of pregnancy and during labour reduced MTCT by 50 per cent. None of the infants were breast-fed.
(c) Restricting the use of invasive obstetric procedures, e.g., artificial rupture of membranes and episotomy to reduce the exposure of the infant to the blood of an infected mother.
(d) Replacement feeding for the infant.

Strategies which may reduce MTCT, to a large extent but where further studies are needed, include:

(a) Vitamin A supplementation during pregnancy.
(b) Cleansing of the birth canal with a microbicide during labour and delivery.
(c) Detection and treatment of STDs.
(d) The breast-feeding dilemma.
(e) In populations where the breast-feeding is the norm, infected breast milk may account for up to one-third of all cases of MTCT.
(f) For mother in developing countries, this risk poses an agonising dilemma. Artificial feeding may help avoid passing on HIV to the infant, but where the water supply is unsafe, the child may be exposed to other deadly diseases. Another formidable barrier is cost. For example, a year's supply of artificial milk for an infant will cost a Vietnamese family more than the country's per capita annual income. Prolonged breast-feeding has a naturally contraceptive effect, and a woman who does not breast-feed may become pregnant again. If bottle feeding becomes a badge of HIV status, a woman who decides not to breast-feed may risk loss of confidentiality and social rejection.

However, drafting correct guidelines on breast-feeding for HIV-positive mothers has proved difficult. Most mothers are not aware of thier HIV status. It becomes inadvisable to promote bottle-feeding in such a situation. It is still not possible to compare the risk of HIV acquisition from breast-feeding with the risk of infant and child morbidity and mortality from unsafe artificial feeding in various settings.

UNAIDS Recommendations

(a) Supports breast-feeding as the best method of feeding only for infants whose mothers do not know their HIV status.

(b) Mothers who decide not to breast-feed must be ensured access to safe and sufficient quantities of nutritionally adequate breast milk substitutes.

(c) Priority should be accorded to Primary prevention: Improve access to antenatal services and voluntary, confidential IAIV Counselling and testing for pregnant women.

HIV/AIDS has brought in its wake blatant violation of the rights of people in both developed and in developing countries. The key rights to information, education, health and non-discrimination are among the first to be violated in the panic surrounding a growing HIV infection rate. Respect for human rights is necessary to protect public health. In the same way, it has been recognised that protection of human rights is necessary for preventing the spread of HIV and for ensuring care and support to people living with AIDS. Human rights abuses pertaining to HIV/AIDS are as below:

1. Calls for mandatory testing by persons who mistakenly think that it can contribute to public health. There is no public health reason for requiring testing, besides it is too expensive. The knowledge acquired is outdated in six months. There is a time interval when a person may be infected but not test positive.
2. Demands for detention or isolation, or other attacks on the liberty and freedom of movement of HIV-infected persons and their families. There is not public health necessity to restrict their movement or freedom.
3. Violation of rights of marriage and bearing children. Persons living with HIV and those who rare for them have a right to marry and bear children. They have a right to make informed selections about that risks they wish to take.
4. Attempts to deny social security, assistance and welfare to HIV-infected persons. They deserve care and support, just like anyone else.
5. Denying the right to education of HIV-infected persons. They

should be able to complete their studies and make their contribution to education while they are still able.

6. Denying HIV infected persons, the right to work. HIV cannot be passed on through casual contact, and there is no reason to try to keep a person from making a productive contribution to the workforce while he or she is still healthy.

There is a active debate in India on mandatory testing for HIV infection. The government feels that there is no public health rationale for the mandatory testing of a person for HIV / AIDS. Such an opinion could be counter-productive because it may scare away a large number of suspected cases from getting detected and treated. HIV testing carried out on a voluntary base with appropriate pretest and post-test counselling is thought to be a better strategy and is in line with the VMOIUNAIDS guidelines on HIV testing.

The Government of India's policy is that:

1. No individual should be made to undergo mandatory testing for HIV.
2. No mandatory HIV testing should be imposed as a precondition for employment or for providing health care during employment.

Attempts to deny or reduce access to health care services to HIV-infected persons. Health care workers often refuse to care for HIV-infected patients especially at the beginning of the epidemic. Afterwards, policy makers who face excessive cost in the health budget try to blame HIV-infected persons for their condition and deny them health care. Both are flagrant violations of medical ethics and basic human rights.

Invasions of privacy, including publication of the names, addresses of persons suspected to be infected with HIV. This destroys lives and families. It has no public health benefit whatsoever, because people with HIV are not contagious to the general public. Also, breaches of confidentiality of HIV status during testing, treatment and notification, as well as in employment and health care settings are in violation of the rights of people. Unless people feel that their right to privacy is assured, they will not seek testing, counselling or care.

Denial of access to available information, health services and prevention methods that will enable persons to reduce vulnerability to transmission of infection and 1'CCC]vc counselling and care, if infected.

Discrimination against children, minorities, migrants, refugees, poor and disadvantaged classes, men having sex with men, sex workers and injecting drug users. This is often done with a sense of moral superiority. It should be exposed for the basic violation of human rights that it is.

AIDS—A Differentiation with Other Ailments

One of the crucial elements that has been made about the HIV/AIDS epidemic is that it is different from most other epidemics and diseases, and as a result requires a different and much broader response—one which goes beyond the health sector. The elements that make it different are:

1. HIV does not occur randomly as in malaria through the bite of a mosquito but through specific risk behaviours that are mostly within the realm of private life which is the most common mode of HIV transmission, is unprotected sex one which is intimate and private and not open to public debate.
2. Unlike other infectious diseases, HIV selectively and disproportionately targets two groops : the voting adults and the very poor, poor populations. 80-90 per cent of those infected with HIV are young adults at the prime of their productive and reproductive lives.
3. Unlike other diseases, AIDS retains a long period of 'invisibility' with opportunistic infections appearing years later. It takes between 5 to 10 years or even longer between the initial infection and the onset of clinical symptoms of AIDS. Persons who are infected may have many years of productive normal life. However, the danger is that most are unaware that they are infected with the virus and can continue to spread it to others.
4. The prognosis for people infected with the virus is bleak. There is no vaccine against HIV and no effective medical cure for HIV infection. Treatment options are prohibitively expensive. HIV/AIDS is essentially, an incurable and fatal disease.

HIV accelerate the present health problems. The weakend immune system falls prey to a number of infections, especially tuberculosis.

HIV destabilises society because of the fear, blame, and stigma attached to it. It threatens basic human rights and invades even the rights to privacy and human dignity. No other disease affects human society in this way, or to this extent.

The scale of the epidemic is also different from most other diseases. Virtually every country in the world has seen new infections. HIV infections have been reported in every state in India and some states have seen a doubling of infections. Malaria causes over a million deaths a year. In 1998, AIDS death totalled some 2.5 million.

The epidemic's visible and less-visible consequences constitute an urgent and massive threat to development: deteriorating child survival, reduced life expectancy, increasing number of orphans, loss of the most productive section of the population.

AIDS—Primary Facts

AIDS stands for Acquired (A) Immune (I) Deficiency (D) Syndrome (S). The immune system defends the body against infections and diseases. AIDS is a medical diagnosis for a combination of symptoms which result from a breakdown of the immune system. The immune deficiency is caused by virus. This deficiency is 'acquired', which means that it is obtained or received by a person and is something which does not ordinarily exist within one's body. 'Immune deficiency' means that there is a deficiency in the immune system or that the immune system is weakend. AIDS is a 'Syndrome' which means it is not one particular isolated disease but one which has a variety of symptoms leading to various disorders and a set of diseases.

Causes

AIDS is caused by a virus known as Human (H) Immunodeficiency (I) Virus (V). HIV weakens the body's defence system or immune system.

The Immune System

In healthy individuals, infections are kept at a distance, due to an array of defenders which constitute the immune system in the body. The most important elements of the immune system are white blood cells which are present in the blood. These cells fight and destroy any infection-causing bacteria and viruses that may enter the body, and thus protect the body against disease.

HIV Immunity

HIV directly attacks the white blood cells. It enters and stays inside the basic genetic material (DNA) of the cells. It multiplies and attacks other white blood cells. Slowly, the number of white blood cells in the body is reduced and the immune system is paralyzed. HIV remains practically immune to counter attacks, since it hides inside the very cells that are supposed to attack the viruses.

Meaning of HIV Positive

When an individual is said to be HIV-positive, it means that the person is infected with HIV. However, the person may not have AIDS, that is, he/she may not have developed the signs and symptoms of AIDS.

When a person is infected with HIV, he/she does not show any external signs of the infection until the progression to AIDS which can take anything from six months to 10 years or more. Approximately 50 per cent of those infected take about 8 years to progress to AIDS. Till such time, he/she may continue to appear normal and healty but can infect others. A person infected with HIV may initially be perfectly healthy but will eventually develop AIDS. A person infected with HIV is said to have AIDS when his/her immune system is totally destroyed; he/she does not respond to treatment and opportunistic infections invade his/her body. It is not possible to identify an HIV-positive person by looking at his/her face. It takes about six weeks to three months to detect the presence of HIV infection in the body. HIV is known to be present in all the body fluids and blood. It is present in small (non-infective) quantities in body fluids other than semen, vaginal and cervical secretions. HIV is transmitted through the blood or sexual secretions (semen, vaginal or cervical secretions). There are four ways or routes of transmission of the virus:

(a) Penetrative sexual intercourse with an infected person. This is the commonest route of transmission.

(b) Transfusion of infected blood. The chances of getting infected are 90 per cent. Infected blood directly transfers HIV into the blood stream.

(c) Use of non-sterile, HIV-infected or contaminated syringes and needles. This is common among drug users.

(d) An infected mother to her unborn child. There is a 30 per cent chance that the child will be infected.

The most common route of HIV is through heterosexual sex. It accounts for nearly eighty per cent of the world's AIDS cases. The next important route is injecting drug use. HIV can be spread through unprotected sexual intercourse. The ranking in order of risk is as follows:

1. Anal intercourse carries the highest risk. During such an act, the possibility of wear and tear is great. This gives an opportunity for the virus to enter the body easily. Also, the risk of condom breakage is high during anal sex.
2. Vaginal intercourse.
3. Oral intercourse has minimal risk.

Babies acquire the virus from their mother while still in the uterus, most commonly during the last three months of pregnancy, during labour and delivery, or through breast milk. HIV cannot transmitted by:

(a) Casual contacts such as kissing, shaking hands, sharing cups, etc.
(b) Donating blood.
(c) Masturbation.
(d) Using public toilets, swimming pools, community showers, saunas.
(e) Medical treatment is hospitals, in doctor's and dental clinics and in all therapy situations where normal rules of hygiene and infection control are maintained.
(f) Caring for people living with AIDS victims.

Protection from AIDS

Since a major route of transmission is sexual intercourse, one can protect oneself from HIV/AIDS in the following ways;

(a) Have sexual intercourse with only one faithful, uninfected partner.
(b) Use a condom in all types of penetrative sex.
(c) If one uses needles, syringes or other instruments that pierce the skin, make sure they are sterile.
(d) Make sure blood is tested before transfusion. Use blood that is certified anti HIV non-reactive.
(e) Avoid pregnancy if infected with HIV.

Presence of HIV

There are different tests to detect the presence of HIV. The ELISA test was till recently the simplest and least expensive. There are now easy simple and rapid (ESR) test such as saliva and finger prick tests which enable almost immediate results. All test results should be confirmed either through 3 ELISA tests or through the Western Blot test.

Results of the Tests

The tests confirm whether antibodies against HIV are present in the blood at the time of testing. However, they cannot establish whether the person can get infected or not in the future. This means that even if the test is negative, the person still has to take preventive steps.

Limitations

Generally, the body requires six weeks to six months to produce antibodies after the entry of HIV. Hence, if the blood is tested before antibodies have been formed, the test results would show a 'false negative', i.e., the antibodies are not detected. This period is called the 'window period'. In such situation the test will have to be repeated after three months to confirm the presence or absence of HIV.

Origin

No one knows for sure about the origin of HIV. What is important is that it is now present in India and is spreading at an accelerated rate to learn to protect ourselves from HIV.

AIDS Terminology

AIDS is Acquired Immunodeficiency Syndrome, an incurable condition of a body's weakened immune system or complete lack of ability to fight infections. People suffer from AIDS when they are infected by HIV. People with AIDS die from a variety of infections which attack the body in its weakened state.

Asymptomatic HIV Infection. The state of HIV infection in which an individual is infected with HIV, but shows or feels no signs or symptoms indicating the illness.

Azidothymidine (AZT). It is also known as zidovudine, retrovir or 3'azido-3'-deoxy-thyone. The drug interferes with one of the HIV enzymes responsible for replication of the virus. The drug has side effects, including severe anaemia.

Blood product. Substances that can be produced from human blood to treat a variety of medical conditions such as haemophilia.

Body fluid. Any fluid or secretion that comes from the body. HIV can be present in blood, semen, breast milk and vaginal fluids.

Condom. A thin latex rubber sheath which is designed to cover a man's penis from tip to base. A condom is used during sexual intercourse to prevent skin to skin contact or passing of semen. It is known to act as an effective check against the transmission of HIV and other sexually transmitted diseases. It protects both persons involved in the sex act.

Confidentiality. The protection of personal data and test results to ensure the rights and welfare of the individual from whom such data are collected. Only the individual and the health professionals directly involved in the care of the person are aware that certain tests were performed and can have access to test results. This information is not given out under any circumstances to any other person without the individual's explicit agreement.

CSW. Commercial Sex Worker. Also called a prostitute, a term that is considered offensive to some. A CSW is a man, woman or child who engages in sex for the purpose of receiving payment.

ELISA Test. Enzyme-Linked Inimuno-Sorbent Assay test. This test is used to detect the presence of HIV in a person's body. It actually detects antibodies to HIV, and not HIV itself, but this is a very accurate way of determining that HIV is present.

Epidemic. Spread of a disease in a population.

Epidemiology. The study of how and why diseases spread and how to control this spread.

HIV. Human Immunodeficiency Virus. This is the virus that causes HIV infection, whose final stage is known as AIDS. Three types of HIV are found in the world: HIV I, II and III. There are several subtypes and strains.

HIV infected. The condition of being infected with the Human immunodeficiency virus. Persons with HIV are referred to as HIV-positive. A more neutral term is 'Person with HIV.'

HIV Positive (HIV +). The condition of having been tested for the presence of IRV in the blood and having it confirmed that the virus is present.

HIV Test. The blood test which finds out the presence of antibodies to HIV in a sample of a person's blood. The presence of antibodies reveals that the person has been infected with HIV. The most common tests are the ELISA and the Western Blot.

Human Rights. The basic rights to which every human being is entitled. These include the right to food, shelter, education, health, property, employment and freedom of movement.

Immunodeficiency. The inability of the body's immune system to protect the body from infection.

Incidence. Incidence of HIV is the number of new cases, i.e., the number of people who became infected during a specified period of time, usually over a 12 month interval.

Incubation period. The time interval between infection and the ability of a blood test to detect infection. This term is also used to describe the time interval between infection and the onset of the clinical signs and symptoms associated with AIDS.

Pandemic. A global epidemic.

PLWA. People living with HIV/AIDS.

Prevalence. The number of people currently infected with HIV at a given point in time. Because there is no cure for HIV/AIDS, HIV prevalence reflects the cumulative numbers of infection from the past and the mortality rate of those infected.

RTI. Reproductive Tract Infections.

Safer sex. Sexual behaviour and practices which can lessen the risk of passing on HIV from one sexual partner to another. These practices include having only one faithful partner and using a latex condom in every act of sexual intercourse.

Sero-conversion. The change from HIV negative to HIV positive in an individual. This occurs within 6 to 12 week after infection with HIV. During this period the individual may have flu-like symptoms. After a few weeks he or she may feel and look healthy, but will remain infected and infectious STI.

STI. Sexually Transmitted Infections

STD. Sexually transmitted disease. A disease that can be contracted by having sexual intercourse with a person who is infected with the organism that causes the disease. STDs can also be transmitted through blood and blood products.

Syndrome. A collection of signs and symptoms that result from a single cause. Syndromes typically occur making diagnosis of the illness easier.

Transmission. Passing of it virus from one person to another.

Vaccine. A substance that increases a person's immunity to a certain disease. Dead germs or weakened live ones or parts of germ cells are put into the body to cause the immune system to fight them. The resulting increased immunity can last for years.

Virus. A virus is a tiny infectious particle; it is so small (20 to 300 nanometers) that it can only be seen with an electron microscope. Viruses attack the cells of living things. They grow and reproduce inside the cells. And then burst out, killing the host cell and seeking out new cells to infect and kill.

Western Blot Test. A test that confirms the presence of HIV antibodies in a person's blood sample.

Window period. The time period between which an individual contracts HIV and the time a blood test confirms the presence of the virus. This period is usually from 6 to 12 weeks.

2

Significant Issues, Outputs and Future Challenges

Major Issues: The Epidemic in India

In India, the challenges posed by HIV/AIDS, despite interventions by government agencies, civil society organisations as well as non-governmental organisation, in the past 15 years, remain formidable. The epidemic is one of the most serious public health hazards in India. Prevalence of infection throughout the country reveals the spread from urban to rural areas and from groups of high risk to the general public. Migration of labour, low literacy rates leading to low awareness, gender discrimination, prevalence of sexually transmitted diseases (STDs) and reproductive tract infections are the major factors attributed to this rapid spread. Detected for the first time in 1986, India had approximately 3.86 million HIV affected people at the end of year 2000. HIV infections have been reported in all the states and union territories. Still driven predominantly by heterosexual transmission, HIV is expanding rapidly into the general public. The scale of prevalence is now shifting towards woman and adolescents with an accompanying increase in vertical transmission and pediatric HIV.

As gender disparities are on increase, the epidemic affects more and more women who end up bearing the brunt of its negative results. It is estimated that women now constitute nearly 25 per cent of new HIV infections. The tendency to stigmatize women in such circumstances aggravates the problem further. The infection is also spreading rapidly in the informal sector, which accounts for as much as 95 per cent of the workforce in the country. Low productivity, poor living conditions, inadequate social protection and poverty are some of the factors that lead to this scenario. HIV/AIDS goes beyond the boundaries of public health and raises fundamental questions of human rights and threatens key development achievements in many fields. Protection of human rights is necessary to safeguard human dignity. When rights are protected, less number of people get infected, and those living with HIV/AIDS and their families can cope better with the disease.

The complexity of the problem is being accentuated because of its effect on the whole scenario—societies, communities, families and individuals. It has thrown open a whole range of issues in social and health care support. The increase in AIDS cases is reducing the ability of families and communities to support and take care of their children, resulting in new challenges. At present the weight of AIDS is becoming more and more evident. The epidemic is in a voluminous stage in Maharashtra, Tamil Nadu and Manipur. In Maharashtra, for example, 60 per cent of sex workers tested were found to be infected. HIV has reached 14–60 per cent in Sentinel STD clinics and is seen in over 2 per cent of women attending antenatal clinics. As the problem in these states was detected early, it is becoming more obvious. Of the total bed occupancy in Imphal and Mumbai hospitals, HIV-associated illnesses account for 24–40 per cent cases. In the last 4 years, the epidemic has spread rapidly across other southern and western states, and in the north-east which has a high prevalence of HIV injecting drug users.

Due to the rapid rise of HIV infections in Andhra Pradesh and Karnataka, the two states have overtaken Tamil Nadu. While HIV prevalence is still low in several other states, the presence of high rates of Sexually Transmitted Diseases (STDs) as well as the presence of sexual networks and migration are all indicators of high vulnerability. According to a study conducted in 1999, it has been revealed that injecting drug use is on increase, about 45 per cent of attendees, linked to an IDU treatment centre in New Delhi, tested positive. Though the epidemic has spread far beyond its initial focus on persons engaging themselves in risk behaviour, trends of sub-epidemics are becoming more than visible in these very groups. The necessity to closely check this trend, amongst commercial sex workers (CSWs) or injecting drug users (IDUs) and men having sex with men (MSM), is imperative due to the implications it has for a wider heterosexual epidemic. According to these epidemiological observations, the programme has been oriented on preventive measures in states with low level epidemics, while the dual strategy of prevention and control will be initiated in other states.

Indian Response

India is one of the few nations where HIV prevention activities were initiated at a very early stage of the epidemic. Government response to the epidemic was initiated in 1986 and the National AIDS Control Organisation (NACO) was established in 1991. First phase of the programme was initiated with the help of the World Bank. NACO was formed within the Ministry of Health and Family Welfare with a senior IAS official, of the rank of Additional Secretary to the Government of India, to facilitate quick decision making. The setting up of NACO witnessed many achievements, which included an increased level of awareness, setting up of infrastructure at the state level for programme implementation and improvements in blood safety. There was an evident necessity to create a sense of ownership amongst states, particularly by involving non-governmental organisations in the programme. The perspective of the programme tended to be medical—a health issue, with the necessity for more emphasis on social and developmental implications.

Main Assumptions

The mode of transmission in India is heterosexual in more than 90 per cent of cases. The 15–49 year age group has the highest prevalence of sexually transmitted diseases (STDs) and HIV infection. The chances of patients getting infected by HIV is 5–10 times more than among those without STDs. Based on the following definitions, state epidemics can be categorized as generalised, concentrated and low:

Generalised. States where HIV prevalence is one per cent or more in antenatal women.

Concentrated. Where HIV prevalence in antenatal women in less than one per cent and the prevalence in STD and other high-risk groups is five per cent or more.

Low. States where the HIV prevalence in antenatal women is less than one per cent and the prevalence in STD and other high risk groups is less than five per cent.

According to the lesson learnt in first phase of the programme, the second phase response has adopted a twin approach. While it is apparent that groups with high-risk behaviour cannot be neglected, it is also important to adopt a multisectoral approach. The present phase of the national programme sees a more de-centralised approach and building up capacities at state level, with the states taking on larger responsibilities for implementation. NACO has promoted State AIDS Control Societies (SACS) with mechanisms for programme management at the state level.

Every state has drawn up a programme implementation plan (PIP) based on extensive consultations with different sectors in the state alongwith non-governmental organisations, community groups and different ministries.

SACS include a strong NGO component on targeted interventions and community mobilization on STD/RTIs. In the past two years, there has been a major effort to support the state programmes by mobilizing technical resources within the country, particularly with the setting up of Technical Resource Groups (TRGs). Surveillance has also been strengthened. Issuses of Care and Support, including home based care and continuum of care has been taken up as an integral component of the National AIDS Prevention Policy. Some steps that can be taken in this direction are: voluntary blood-testing centres, drugs for management of opportunistic infections and setting up of more counselling centres.

Priorities and Planning (2000)

Priorities for the year 2000. Working closely with NACO, the Theme Group set itself the following objectives for the year 2000:

(a) Support further development of collaborative framework
(b) Support and strengthen TRGs
(c) Support build up of state capacities
(d) Facilitate formation of Theme Group
(e) Work within Human Rights framework

Programme Management. In August 2000, the second UNAIDS strategic planning retreat was organised in Bangalore, the first retreat being organised earlier in 1999. These retreats offer a platform for planning a concerted efforts in defining roles and responsibilities of collaborating agencies alongwith the UN system, the government and bilateral donors. The retreats have played a major role in helping the UN agencies develop strategies in their own fields of strength, which could be taken to scale by the national programme. The Bangalore retreat addressed issues core to the current stage of the national response to the epidemic. Other important areas for discussion that were identified here are:

(a) making decentralisation a reality
(b) builidng stronger partnership at the state level
(c) addressing stigma, and
(d) growing concern on the IDU problem in the north-east.

Organised jointly by UNAIDS and NACO, the retreat aimed at the implementation of second phase of the national programme. With the emphasis on decentralisation, focus was on planning interventions in the states, building capacities at state level and addressing the issue of absorptive capacities. Five major areas of challenge were also reorganised. These were:

(a) necessity to build capacities within states
(b) to ensure that targeted interventions achieve desired impact
(c) achievement of behaviour change outside the 'high-risk' groups
(d) necessity to comfort discrimination and stigma, and
(e) addressing the urgency of care and support.

Strategy meetings have encouraged to lay stress on the overall national strategy and gaps that UNAIDS, as a support organisation, can address. The strategic planning retreat was followed by Theme Group meetings. These meetings have been critical in defining the role expectations from UNAIDS by stakeholder institutions. This also resulted in the formulation of a work plan for UNAIDS.

Joint UN Programme

(a) The UN system has the aim to facilitate a multisectoral response to HIV by joint programming.
(b) The UN system encourages active involvement of NACO and bilaterals in the Theme Group which is the supreme body governing UN response in India.

The UN system has various inherent strengths owing to its structure and worldwide mandate. UN agencies have close working relationships with the government through various ministries and departments and therefore, have possibilities to engage in policy dialogue. It has partnerships with civil society which provide for grassroot experiences and education. Therefore, the UN system is uniquely positioned to address a mandate that cuts across a range of important issues like gender and human rights, health, poverty alleviation and wide development strategies. It supports government efforts to develop partnerships with all representatives of civil society. Because resources to combat HIV/AIDS epidemic are generally limited, UN agencies leverage these advantages to develop focussed and well-defined fields of contribution, falling within the mandate of each agency. Some of these strategies would include developing partnerships around HIV with ministries and civil society; mainstreaming HIV within their own agency programmes; supporting efforts in mainstreaming human rights, gender and approaches to poverty alleviation.

Upto 1986, World Health Organisation (WHO) was the UN agency which had the lead responsibility on AIDS by its Global Programme on AIDS (GPA). After the rapid spread of the infection by mid-1990s made it clear that the need for a more concerted and expanded UN effort beyond health to tackle the serious impact that it was causing on human lives. It was also evident that it would be difficult for one UN agency to take on the mandate of addressing the HIV/AIDS epidemic. The necessity for more coordination in an effort to maximise the impact was needed.

To meet this challenge, the United Nations adopted an innovative approach in 1996 by involving six organisations together in a joint and cosponsored programme—the Joint United Nations Programme on HIV/AIDS or UNAIDS. The six original cosponsors of UNAIDS – UNICEF, UNDP, UNFPA, UNESCO, WHO and the World Bank—were joined by UNDCP in 1999. Working at one platform through UNAIDS, the cosponsors expand their outreach with other UN agencies, with the governments, with civil society organisations and regional and country level networks of people living with AIDS.

UNAIDS in India performs four key functions:

(a) Coordinating the UN system's HIV/AIDS response
(b) Advocacy
(c) Building/strengthening partnerships, and
(d) Providing information.

The aim of the organisation, under the larger umbrella of its global mandate, is to catalyze, strengthen and orchestrate the unique expertise, resources and networks of influence from other UN agencies. Its recognition lies in the fact that it is a cosponsored institution, within the UN system, created specifically and exclusively to respond to the HIV epidemic. It facilitates cosponsor engagement in significant fields as per Indian's requirements.

UNAIDS cosponsors from within the UN system are: UNICEF, UNDP, UNFPA, UNESCO, UNDCP, WHO and the World Bank. Besides these, other agencies actively working in the Indian UN Theme Group include ILO and UNIFEM. In addition, bilateral agencies such as DFID, USAID, CIDA, SIDA and AUSAID have given the programme firm and committed support through journey in the Theme Group.

In recent past, there has been a greater stress on decentralisation and better inter-institutional coordination. In working at a single platform, the agencies have been able to expand and strengthen their outreach through strategic alliances with other UN agencies, bilateral agencies, regional and country networks of people living with HIV/AIDS and other non-governmental organisations (NGOs). To augment its global mandate of addressing AIDS by ploughing back lessons from the countries in which it is engaged, UNAIDS India has adapted its global strategies to specific socio-economic needs of India. These strategies are contingent on various factors like the government response to the problem, its policies, economic situation, and so on. These are also governed by social factors, values and norms that exist at a particular point of time. To some extent, it also depends on the response of other agencies working on the issue. The response of the civil society organisations, for example, is well acknowledged in addressing the HIV/AIDS. Accordingly UNAIDS India has set its goals and Priorities. The Herculean task at hand includes a measured look at the resource available. The roles have been decided by taking into consideration the cosponsor requirements as well.

Tasks Ahead

To match the broader mandate of UNAIDS and the response to the epidemic in India, UNAIDS in India recognised the following roles.

1. ***Coordination.*** For the whole UN system, extended to other bilateral agencies.

2. ***Support.*** For National HIV/AIDS programme.

3. ***Service.*** For several cosponsors and stakeholders by providing information, best practices, for example, and providing technical inputs, such as a monitoring and evaluation framework.

4. ***Institutional capacity building.*** For local level organisations, at the national and state level, around programme planning and implementation.

5. ***Advocacy.*** Impacting socio-political perspectives on how the epidemic is viewed in India.

However, these roles can feed into each other, they have different constituencies and call for careful planning ensuring effective implementation.

The priority for UNAIDS lies in the fact that it works within a complex web of institutions. UNAIDS India has various stakeholders who are its constituencies. The organisation works in close association with other agencies in the UN system, with the National Programme, with bilaterals, with SACS and civil society organisations. These institutions, being the stakeholders of UNAIDS, also have their own structure, agenda and programme. They work on their commitment to the epidemic through their own programme and resources. From UNAIDS, they seek complementary inputs to arrive at their priorities. The organisation has framed institutional techniques to enhance its key roles of support and coordination. The effort has been to avoid a large and vertical programme structure. A few of these innovations include setting up of an inter-institutional Theme Group, a Virtual Team (VT) of specialists in various UN organisations and Technical Resource Groups (TRGs), which are created to give technical support to the national programme on a comprehensive set of issues related to HIV/AIDS.

The cosponsors have identified the following two roles specifically for UNAIDS India:

(a) Assisting in the capacity building process of NACO and the SACS that includes the development of and assistance in formulating a strong monitoring and evaluation system for the National Programme.

(b) Be a technical group ensuring dissemination of global best practices and their adoption within the National Programme.

One important priority of UNAIDS India has been to facilitate more cosponsor involvement in the programme. The strategy has been to strengthen the Theme Group process and support the cosponsors in formulating their own work plans. UNAIDS assisted this process through its secretariat ensuring effective outputs from each Theme Group meeting. The Theme Group met three times in a year and gave strategic directions to the national programme. This year, ILO also joined the Theme Group. Focal points on HIV, within each agency, have also been meeting regularly. Individual agencies have made major staff sensitization efforts for HIV/AIDS.

The Theme Group emerged in 1998 and has since played the key role in steering the activities of the secretariat. It has been strengthened with the involvement of cosponsors, bilateral partners and the government. The Theme Group meets thrice in a year to review progress and plays an important monitoring role for the secretariat and cosponsor involvement. The Theme Group identifies the objectives and the plan of action of the secretariat. The focus in the year 2000 was on operationalising the workplans that were developed by cosponsors. These workplans have been finalized after a review by the Theme Group. The plan to operationalise was further strengthened with the formation of the Virtual Team.

Virtual Team

One of the mechanisms created by UNAIDS to deliver outputs/inputs from cosponsors into the National response is the Virtual Team (VT). The UNAIDS secretariat plays a key facilitative role in supporting the UN cosponsors to mainstream HIV in their task. This has been planned through the Virtual Team members. With effect from this year, Virtual Team has been in place and functional.

Objective of V +

To strengthen the multi-sectored responses to HIV/AIDS on national and state levels, using agency expertise and promotion of counterpart collaboration.

Till now, the Virtual Teams have been working more or less within the programme of their agencies. An important role that has been added to the Virtual Team is that of giving support at state level. Therefore, the VT is placed in a strategic situation to give support at state level so that the policy decisions at Theme Group level can be directly discussed with the states and can be supported during implementation. The main driving force of this activity is the necessities of the state. The major factor in the opportunity for strengthening state responses lies in the fact that:

(a) NACO has invited the Virtual Team to offer support at state level, and
(b) The state have been requesting for technical support on various issues.

At present, Virtual Team consists of three different member categories that have various roles and functions in their support to the National Response. All Virtual Teams meet at regular intervals facilitating information sharing and co-ordination. Virtual Teams follow strategies suitable to their multiple modes of functioning. A document which clearly delineates VT strategies, state linkages, strengths and aims has now been finalised by the Theme Group.

The Virtual Team leader is the UNAIDS India Country Programme Adviser, who leads the team in close co-operation with the Project Director, NACO. Though a relatively new venture, the Virtual Team brings with it a wide range of issues and programme-related expertise, includes women's skill, youth programme, issues related to drug abuse, targeted interventions, communication and programme-related experience and expertise.

Internal Strategy and Review

UNAIDS India reviewed organization's achievements and expectations. This review offered an opportunity for UNAIDS to ponder over its roles, opportunities, strengths and weaknesses, both in relation to internal strategies and expectations of the stakeholders. The review also pointed out restructuring and redesigning of various innovations to further strengthen the processes which are already operational. One such restructuring has been done with various TRGs.

Sensitization of the UN Staff

As a first step towards mainstreaming HIV, a number of sensitization workshops were held by UNICEF, UNFPA and UNDP for the members of their staff. As a result several staff members have commenced a dialogue with their programme partners to determine the HIV-associated issues and their impact on the related sectors.

With the emphasis on decentralisation gaining importance, UNAIDS facilitated a process of focussed and need-based capacity building for the states. The states achieved more support in programme planning and implementation. The necessity to support SACS by accurate strategic planning was given crucial significance. Part of this capacity building exercise also meant developing state-appropriate Targeted Interventions (TI). For the achievement of this, the TRG on TIs was strengthened and other agencies such as NGOs and CBOs were also included in this process. To ensure some level of accountability and quality control, UNAIDS supported NACO to develop a monitoring and evaluation framework based on global experience and local needs. As a part of this, monitoring tools were developed. UNAIDS also developed tools for strategic planning. A TI manual was developed and field-tested. It is now handy as a best practice tool. All officials (about 120) of SACs were imparted training on TI planning. A TI consultant has also been appointed to support NACO State AIDS Societies are empowered to offer funding support to non-governmental organisations.

NACO and Targeted Interventions

The fundamental purpose of targeted interventions is to lesson the rate of transmission amongst the most vulnerable and marginalised sections of society. Being one of the most important components of second phase of the national programme, TI envisages a comprehensive and integrated effort for addressing these groups in an effort to reduce their vulnerabilities and alleviate the impact of HIV/AIDS, thus preventing the disease from spreading further. Targeted interventions offer a basis for comprehensive intervention in marginal groups. Programme Implementation Plans (PIPs) developed by the states in the preparation of second phase provided a framework for initiating activities. A working group on M&E has been established and includes representatives from NACO, UNAIDS, DFID, USAID and the World Bank. UNAIDS supported the formulation of the M&E framework including Behavioural Sentimental Surveillance (BSS) and providing the tools for monitoring. The M&E framework is being executed in association with the global indicators group at Laussane University, MERG and UNAIDS headquarters. The monitoring and evaluation framework has been developed jointly ensuring greater programme coordination and efficiency.

Major Outputs

The development of a sustainable technical support network and efforts to build long-term capacities in the country for strengthening state capacities is one of the important interventions supported by UNAIDS.

TRGs were set up to provide technical support to state programme/SACS through improved programme design, by imparting state-of-the-art knowledge in technical fields, by transferring the knowhow to enhance programme implementation and by identifying best practices. The TRG initiative picked up significant momentum in the year 2000. UNAIDS supported strengthening of systems for TRG-state links by playing a key role in facilitating linkages between the national programme, state level programme as well as TRGs. To facilitate the transition towards a more state driver programme, UNAIDS supported NACO in establishing systems for connectivity and TRG management. Subsequently, a TRG management cell was set up in NACO, with two senior scientists appointed to facilitate TRG-state linkages and peer review of best practices.

Technical Support Groups (TRGs)

To provide technical support to states, TRGs have been constituted and TRG covers a different thematic area:

(a) Clinical management
(b) Research and Development in HIV/AIDS
(c) Counselling
(d) STDs
(e) Women, Children and AIDS
(f) Targeted Interventions
(g) Law and Ethics
(h) IDUs
(i) Surveillance
(j) Blood Safety

Based on a technical needs assessment in three states, TRGs were reconstituted to reflect state's necessities. All the TRG chairs, members, and SACS were joined electronically and trained in Information Technology. At the Bangalore Retreat, UNAIDS gave a hands-on interactive session on the Internet, thus linking up on-line with the NACO information centre, to which 35 state AIDS societies, all TRGs, UNAIDS and their cosponsors are joined. Furthermore, discussions on programme themes are at present weekly events led by NACO. These link-ups between TRG members and SACS have made communication faster and effective. TRGs have also finalized their workplans. At present, they have a *state-of-the-art paper* and several of them have been invited by SACS to provide technical assistance.

In the year 2000, the portal site, youandaids.org was initiated. IT applications function under this umbrella. The portal provides a discussion forum for youth, women, positive people, common messaging system, chat groups, MIS linkages with Geographical Information System and e-surveillance. A one-day workshop on connectivity was also held. The portal has improved information exchange at all levels. UNAIDS has facilitated the sharing of best practices by developing TRG-global network linkages. It has developed global and national best practices guides, strategies in partnership with NACO, TRGs, SACS and the UNAIDS headquarters. UNAIDS has also ensured dissemination of these global best practices.

Social responses of fear, denial and stigmatization have been long standing barriers in tackling the HIV epidemic in India, just as in several other parts of the world. This has had serious impact on prevention programmes and more importantly undermined the ability of individuals and societies to protect themselves and provide support and reassurance to those infected.

UNAIDS in India has considered tackling stigma and discrimination a priority issue. In the Bangalore retreat on strategic planning, stigma was the main issue discussed. Presentations on the complexity of the issue highlighted the necessity for all partners to sit together in tackling the issue.

UNAIDS India took serious measures for keeping in step with the worldwide mandate to ensure more involvement of people with AIDS. The measure encouraged meaningful greater involvement of people with HIV/AIDS (GIPA) initiatives amongst all of its collaborators—governments, private sector, bilaterals and community partners. At the strategic planning retreat in the year 2000, positive peoples networks reiterated the necessity to evolve an enabling environment in which widespread discrimination could be curbed by lifting the veil of ignorance around HIV and PLWAs. This would encourage HIV counselling testing, treatment and opportunities for positive people to merge into the folds of society. Following suggestions were made at the retreat:

(a) Urgent necessity for organising workshops for media orientation to HIV issues and involving cable networks and regional print media as well.
(b) Sensitizing private and public health systems through coalition with positive people.
(c) Involving HIV-positive national level UN volunteers in lecture tours around the country, for giving HIV a 'face' and de-stigmatizing the issue.

Alongwith these suggestions, meetings involving positive groups, media and communication agencies were also held. Presentations by different groups were made on intervention experiences in India. Workshops were also held on sensitization of the judiciary. Another initiative has been the photo-documentation 'People Plus' initiated by INP + networks. An exhibition of these photographs was held on World AIDS day. UNAIDS supported a National non-governmental organisation convention which brought together non-governmental organisations from all over India and helped identify their role within the national programme. It offered a platform for discussion with the primary objective of supporting and strengthening the formation of networks of persons living with HIV/AIDS (PLWAs), Non-governmental Organisations (NGOs), Community-based Organisations (CBOs) and men having sex wtih men (MSM).

To develop and strengthen the response within the human rights framework, UNAIDS worked on a joint project on advocacy with the National Human Rights Commission (NHRC) this year. The 1st 'National Conference on Human Rights and HIV/AIDS' was held in New Delhi, in November 2000. The conference stressed at initiating a discussion between concerned agencies and groups on the linkage between human rights and HIV/AIDS prevention and management. National Human Rights Commission (NHRC), in collaboration wth National AIDS Control Organisation (NACO), Lawyers Collective, UNICEF and UNAIDS organised a conference and brought together major stakeholders including the NHRC, law enforcement agencies and NACO to identify the important problems and recommend an action plan. The priorities of the conference were to:

(a) discuss and identify major issues in the HIV/AIDS related Human Rights framework;

(b) build linkages between State Human Rights Commissions and the State AIDS Control Societies;
(c) identify future interventions to evolve an enabling environment at various levels, and
(d) identify measures to expand the response within a rights based approach.

The conference was part of a number of meetings planned by the core group on human rights and public health established by National Human Rights Commission. This initiative provided a forum and momentum to select the role of human rights in its response to HIV/AIDS. It gave all partners the opportunity to consider the significance of recognising, promoting and protecting human rights, implementing an enabling environment and identifying the central role of law as a necessary component of the response strategies to prevent and manage HIV/AIDS in India.

To strengthen marginalised groups and in promoting their capacities to mainstream HIV, UNAIDS India supported the set up of a National Sex Workers Forum. A strategic plan addressing problems of stigma and discrimination was also developed. MSM networks were supported to determine the networks of community-based groups and their strategic necessities. This, in turn, encouraged development of technical support systems.

The key strategy to strengthen behaviour change beyond high-risk groups has been to address populations at risk by broadbasing the response and mainstreaming HIV into the prevailing structures such as the local self government. While second phase of the national programme has stressed on targeted interventions, there is also immediate necessity to address the bridge populations in the Indian situation. At present the government is focussing more concertedly on young people and migrant groups. Non-commercial sex is now seen to constitute vital source of infection with half of all new infections occurring in the age group of less than 25 years. The effort has been to encourage the people to protect themselves. Innovative approaches were employed to reach the population at large.

UNAIDS supported NACO's efforts at community mobilization through the Family Health Awareness Week. Started with the idea of increasing awareness among and reaching out to communities at large, a third phase of the FHAW took place in the first and second week of June 2000 throughout the country. The population targeted to be covered by the campaign is approximately 600 million, of which 34 million attended the camps. Family Health Awareness Week was initiated by NACO in 1999 with the following priorities:

(a) Creating awareness on HIV/AIDS and other STIs by involving the Primary Health Care structure.

(b) Early detection and treatment of Reproductive Tract Infections (RTIs)

Training was imparted to medical officers and para-medical staff to choose 100 districts where the programme was to be piloted. The training enabled detection of STI cases and referring them to PHCs. The FHAW programme was encouraging because a large number of people attended many of these centres seeking treatment for RTIs and STIs besides initial apprehension. It also validated the possibilities of reaching the awareness programme among rural communities and helped more access to health care. It was an important step in bringing about a firm linkage between NACP and the primary health care centres, thus encouraging the decentralization approach. UNAIDS and cosponsors actively supported this venture of NACO. The evaluation of FHAW is being done and results are expected to be available soon. It is hoped that FHAW experiences and lessons for community involvement be documented as best practices in the Indian scenario.

Of the worldwide estimated 16,000 new infections everyday about 1,600 are in children below the age of 15 years. Young people between the ages of 10 and 24 constitute more than half of new post-infancy infections throughout the world. Investing in HIV prevention among young people is, it is hoped, to contribute significantly to a more sustainable response to HIV/AIDS. It is apparent that the rising number of infections occur among the young people in India. The vulnerability of the youth to the infection becomes more severe because of different changing norms of society.

Young people are being appreciated as a resource for changing the course of the epidemic at an increasing rate. They are responsive to HIV prevention programmes as well as are effective promoters of HIV prevention process. Keeping it in consideration, UNAIDS has supported early interventions by targeting adolescents with information on HIV/AIDS and the skills to improve their self-confidence enabling them to make effective decisions. They have helped the formation of an inter-agency group for promoting and piloting of a strategy for young people and out-of-the-school youth. This working group includes representatives from UNICEF, UNESCO and UNFPA. UNICEF has also framed adolescent health and education guidelines along with NACO and make them available to the public at large.

UNAIDS is encouraging the development of a policy on non-discrimination at the workplace. In its planning process, the project is a tripartite response to HIV intervention at the workplace. The project will be executed by ILO next year in close collaboration with UNAIDS, in full consultation with representatives of the Theme Group on HIV/AIDS in the country. The project proposes to introduce activities which would be systemic, cost-effective and properly targeted to mobilize the world to work for prevention of HIV/AIDS throughout the country.

Efforts in Association with Panchayats

The year 2000 witnessed various innovative efforts in reaching out to the general public, right up to the village level via existing democratic institutions like 'Panchayats' or local governments. UNDP is working to strengthen the local self governments in an effort to include them in responding to the epidemic. This also follows in with the decentralization efforts of the government in the second phase of the national programme. Local self governments, municipalities and zila parishads have been included in this programme. The priority of the programme is to strengthen local initiatives and offer an enabling environment to reduce stigma and discrimination. The first round of sensitization started in Tamil Nadu in the Gandhigram Rural Institute. Meetings were also held in Udupi and Gulbarga districts of Karnataka.

Development Priority

An important priority of UNAIDS India has been to put HIV/AIDS as an objective issue on the national and state agenda. It has played an important role in sensitizing opinion leaders and policy makers on HIV/AIDS issues in an effort to place it as a development priority. With the changing socio-political circumstances, ongoing advocacy efforts were strengthened with policy makers. International exposure and interaction has led to more political support to the programme.

At the level of policy and political support, there has been a deviation in the momentum at both the highest level and in the states which are experiencing the most extensive spread of the epidemic. Political advocacy received impetus with the prime minister of India urging parliamentarians in December 1998 to accept the existing situation as a threat to India's development rather than only a health issue. Chief ministers from different states have taken interest in mobilising their administration and in raising public awareness. To encourage the momentum, UNAIDS has approached policy makers for tackling the epidemic.

A meeting of 25 young parliamentarians with the UNAIDS executive director, Dr. Peter Piots, in March 2000, brought together renowned political leaders to address issues of HIV. The team alongwith executive director and the country programme advisor of UNAIDS, consulted with parliamentarians the role they could play in controlling the epidemic. At the time of discussion, it was suggested that the parliamentarians could take the issue to their constituencies and focus on important people involved in local governance who, obviously could reach out to the representatives of parliament in the field, with an effort to draw a political commitment from them. Representatives from various political parties of India, namely, Bhartiya Janata Party (BJP), Congress, CPI-M and DMK were present at this meeting. The meeting generated an enthusiastic response and the group members also expressed their apprehensions. Issues of how to discuss sexuality or condom use in a public domain, and of the overwhelming prospect of caring for children orphaned by AIDS-affected parents were raised. The meeting had an overwhelming response. Many members of parliament expressed their interest in carrying the issue forward. Some of them, for instance in Sivaganga District of Tamil Nadu, even organised meetings at the zila parishad level in their own constituencies.

The initial success led to more meetings with chief ministers and a video conference between chief ministers of three States—Maharashtra, Tamil Nadu and Andhra Pradesh (states with high prevalence) as well as union minister of health, Dr Thakur, in November 2000. All the representatives in the conference agreed for a necessity to break the 'silence'. They also made commitments and offered suggestions of national importance. The issues raised in the conference were: trafficking, initiation of sex education in schools, and the urgency to discuss the issues at a political level. A meeting with leaders at the national level also gave way to more advocacy with political leaders throughout the country. Many discussions and video conferences have followed these initiatives. Meetings and discussions held with chief ministers from 10 states on HIV / AIDS have resulted in their including HIV in their political agenda. A 12-member team of programme managers and policy makers also visited Uganda and key lessons were exposed in the state responses.

UNAIDS has also developed and disseminated advocacy implements to sensitize policy makers and programme implemeters on the effect of HIV on development goals. A multimedia presentation kit on the AIDS epidemic in India is at hand now.

Issues of Mother-to-Child Transmission (MTCT)

There are approximately 12 million women of childbearing age who are HIV-positive worldwide. The number of infants who acquire the virus from their mothers is rapidly rising in a number of places, notably India and Southeast Asia. Mother-to-Child transmission (MTCT) is by far the biggest source of HIV infection in children below the age of 15 years. NACO and UNICEF have been collaborating on the MTCT issue. The project implementation commenced in March 2000. UNAIDS supported this initiative of UNICEF in sensitizing the policy makers on the necessity for MTCT prevention. An 18-member team visited Thailand in 2000 to identify key lessons on MTCT so that they could include those lessons in programme designs.

For the first time, India launched a worldwide theme on the World AIDS Day, 2000. This was also a first time for a country in the global south region. This years' theme of 'Greater Male Involvement' encouraged identifying key issues and strategies for male involvement and offered an opportunity for public debate and discussions on the issue. This year's theme was also selected in an effort to encourage participation by men in adopting safer behaviours and playing a major role in caring.

According to Men and AIDS a Gendered Approach, 2000 World AIDS Campaign, Geneva, there are five important reasons for focussing the World AIDS Day Campaign on men which are stated as below:

1. Men's health is important but receives inadequate attention
2. Men's behaviour puts them at risk of HIV
3. Men's behaviour put women at risk of HIV
4. Unprotected sex between men endangers both men and women, and
5. Men need to give greater consideration to AIDS as it affects their families.

The campaign was initiated in March 2000, during the visit of the executive director UNAIDs, Dr Peter Piot, at Vigyan Bhavan, New Delhi. Amongst those present at the launch were the union health minister president of the Malaysian AIDS Council and president of the Positive Women's Network. The campaign had three main priorities.

1. Raise awareness of the relationship between men's behaviour and HIV.
2. Encourage men and adolescent boys to make a commitment to prevent the spread of HIV infection.
3. Promote programme that respond to the necessities of both men and women.

Participation of Corporate Sector

UNAIDS has been working in the process of strengthening and sensitizing the corporate sector in HIV/AIDS and has actively supported the necessity for interventions in the workplace. The Theme Group has been actively working in advocating the issue. A meeting was held with members from the corporate sector and the prime minister's office. After that, in a meeting with key business representatives, the Prime Minister of India called for the formation of business coalition on World AIDS Day.

International Day for Alleviation of Poverty

Every year, 17th October is celebrated as the International Day for Alleviation of Poverty by UNDP. The Theme for the year 2000 was 'HIV/AIDS—Breaking the Silence'. UNDP and UNAIDS jointly organized a short commemorative event to rethink and rededicate efforts towards poverty eradication programmes and to place emphasis on the link between HIV/AIDS and issues of poverty. For creating public interest, activities like talks and street play marked the day. AIDS activists, working in association with HIV positive people for several years, spoke to the people gathered at the function. The event was well attended by members of non-governmental organisations and CBOs working on the issue and programme staff from other UN agencies.

A rise in the number of people living with HIV generated the necessity to provide adequate care and support, both medical and social. With limited treatment facilities and no cure available, India could face a dilemma with major consequences for productive human resource.

The government recognizes the urgency to provide care and support that is appropriate and feasible. Providing for these needs in circumstances where resources are limited and the numbers are large is a Herculean task. With its major partners, WHO and the International Alliance on HIV/AIDS, UNAIDS has planned a strategy paper on care and support. Work has been started in association with UNCTAD on compulsory licensing of HIV drugs in India. In a preliminary meeting, UNAIDS brought together representatives from the ministry of commerce, NACO, the drug controller general and the ministry of patents. The objective of the meeting was to evolve a policy paper on the issue.

UNAIDS is at work to enlist best practices on HIV care and support in the country. The points of reference for this have been prepared. The programme is already underway under the aegis of International Alliance on HIV/AIDS. UNAIDS will build on these efforts. UNAIDS has also encouraged the formulation of legal and ethical guidelines for health care settings. The guidelines have been approved by NACO. UNAIDS and WHO, also supported a meeting held at the Asia region level on vaccine development and ethics.

Future Challenges

UNAIDS is at the heart of a complex net of institutions. As this strategic positioning has been a strength, it has also generated challenging situations for the programme's functioning. Effective management of this network has been critical in evaluating the strengths and limitations of the organisation. Working through a non-vertical structure and by developing mechanisms such as the Virtual Team has allowed the programme to integrate perspective from various organisations. UNAIDS has achieved major success in putting systems into place in several areas of intervention keeping the main aim of de-centralization in perspective. It has, because of its position in the global scenario, been able to integrate the resources and information in the form of global best practices. Being a part of the VN system puts UNAIDS at an advantage of taking many advocacy stands, which it might not have been able to do under several circumstances.

Having come thus far into tackling the epidemic, UNAIDS has now to evaluate carefully its future decisions keeping in view the present approach of the government, particularly because the main purpose of developing a collaborative framework is to ensure that inputs are fed into the national response appropriately. In this regard, some of the priorities that lie ahead for organisation include the following:

1. Scaling up interventions. While a long aim of the organisation would be to support and strengthen the national programme to make an effective national response to the HIV epidemic, the challenges and risks to achieve the perceived aim are many. Numbers in India and its diversity are serious issues which lay impact on the strategy and planning of HIV/AIDS interventions. The challenge lies in scaling up interventions while maintaining their quality ensuring effective behaviour change. Because many efforts have been made to combat the rising epidemic, there is still an enormous requirement for continued attention to programme design and implementation throughout the country.

2. Strengthening Advocacy. Although a major emphasis of the present programme is on decentralization, the differential characteristic of the epidemic across several states makes it difficult to maintain a common strategy. UNAIDS has a major responsibility in strengthening linkages between states and TRGs so that the differential necessities can be met appropriately. The plans must include the private sector more substantially in this field. It is to be seen if the corporate sector is willing to accept the HIV/AIDS issue as a development threat. Therefore, concerted advocacy will have to be undertaken on this issue.

3. Strengthening a Co-ordinated Response. UNAIDS plays an important role in coordinating the response of the UN system to the epidemic. Because the UN Agencies have responded well to the initiatives and support of UNAIDS, the response of the national machinery to this coordinated effort will have to be strengthened further. For example, efforts would have to be made to test how other ministries can integrate HIV into their present structures.

4. Multisectoral Response. Another important objective of UNAIDS is to strengthen a multisectoral, scaled up decentralised response to HIV/AIDS. This aim is again contingent on various factors. Many of the initiatives like Virtual Team, and introduction of a more IT educated system are new and the response of the states and SACS will have to be measured carefully. Following are only some of the many issues which need to be carefully addressed:

Would SACS be willing to accept inputs from TRGs? Would they be in agreement with VT recommendations?

Would they have capacities to use a proposed M&E framework and analyse the data?

Would TRGs be able to adquately respond to the state needs?

Last, but not the least, although UNAIDS has made concerted efforts in meeting its objectives, the fact remains that HIV/AIDS raises social, ethical, moral and personal issues that are difficult to bring to the public domain. UNAIDS India will continue to work hard through these challenges and many more to strengthen a coordinated response, encouraging innovative efforts of its stakeholders and to ensure more involvement of positive people in tackling the HIV epidemic. It will work to build a common and evolving understanding of the epidemic in India within a wide framework of the development challenges India continues to face, in order to help maintain an effective national response.

3

Crisis, Vaccine Development, New Diagnostics and Strategies for Hope

Health Crisis

AIDS is not new to India. For several years the epidemic was limited mostly to drug users and sex workers, which made it more easy for the rest of the population of India to pretend it did not exist. With a raging tuberculosis epidemic and frequent outbreaks of the bubonic plague, there has been no shortage of health crisis. But while nobody was looking, AIDS crept into the general public. At present 0.7 per cent of the whole adult population are thought to carry the virus. Health officials consider 1 per cent an epidemic. New India is at a cross-roads. Public health officials are happy to contemplate a mere six-fold increase in infections by 2004, about 20 million adults. The alternative is even grimmer. If infections are allowed to go beyond 5 per cent of the adult population, scientists believe the probabilities of keeping the epidemic from accelerating greatly, at the cost of millions of human lives, would be slim. India, in other words, is teetering on the brink of becoming another sub-Saharan Africa. 'It is like a fire,' says Dr Salim Habayeb, the World Bank's lead public-health specialist for South Asia. 'In the start it is easy to control as you can go to the source. We are trying to put out the fire before it is too late.' But what if we keep that source under wraps? We may be the land of the *Kama Sutra,* but sex is not a topic for discussion. Public-health officials have long despaired of this taboo as it makes the aim of raising the people's awareness of sexually transmitted diseases all the more difficult. But in the big cities, in truck stops that dot the country and in towns where migrant labourers toil far away from their families, an underworld of illicit sex supports 2 million to 5 million sex workers. Indians to a large extent prefer to ignore it. Thus, when the first AIDS case detected in Chennai in 1986, the government argued that AIDS was a western epidemic which would not affect their uniquely moral society.

It proved false. Insidiously, the disease spread into high-risk populations—sex workers, intravenous drug users and patients with sexually transmitted diseases. It spread from brothel to brothel, through the blood supply and shared needles. It spread from the cities to the country. As a result, it spread to innocent women like Vineeta. Her in-laws rejected her and her two-year-old son to the streets after the expiry of her husband. She discovered five months later that he had died of AIDS—and had passed it on to her and her son, Many (not their real names). The in-laws had hidden not only her husband's illness from her but also the results of her own blood test, which showed positive for HIV. 'I felt as if a Himalaya had fallen on my shoulders,' says the tiny, dark-eyed woman, 'I cursed my husband. If he was aware he had AIDS, he had no business runing my life and his child's.'

There were warnings of the disease to come. In the north-east region of Manipur in India, the number of HIV-positive drug users went from 5 to 50 per cent during a two year period in the late 1980s. 'Back then I barely knew anything about HIV,' says Tuanz, a former addict from Manipur who is HIV-positive. 'By the time we knew about AIDS it was too late to mend'. In Mumbai, about 40 per cent of the city's sex workers were infected with the virus by 1991. In Tamil Nadu, in 1992, tests showed that only one quarter of blood supplies were tested for the virus, and that 15 per cent of local cases reported were caused by contaminated blood.

International Assistance

That year the government began accepting help from abroad. The World Health Organization and the US Centres for Disease Control assisted design a programme to combat the epidemic, and the World Bank gave $85 million. The Indian government began lobbying each of the country's 32 states and territories to take part.

The efforts showed some achievements. After a period of six years, a national infrastructure of state-run cells came at fore to fight the menace out of virtually nothing. In provinces and territories throughout the country, local units of the newly established National AIDS Control Organisation (NACO) set to work distributing kits to test donated blood. The commercial practice of blood selling was stopped and thousands of unregulated, privately run blood banks were closed. Parliament passed laws fixing standards for condom manufacurers. Thousands of public health professionals were trained in identify the infected persons and to carry out the awareness programmes about the epidemic.

In some parts of India today the problem looks almost on the verge of control. Awareness programmes targeted at sex workers in Kolkata's Sonagachi district in 1992 caused condom use to soar from almost nil to 70 per cent in two years. HIV infection among sex workers touched high at only five per cent. (By comparing, 70 per cent of Mumbai's sex workers are now HIV-positive). Andhra Pradesh's chief minister Chandrababu Naidu has driven home the message by putting his imprimatur on a Chocolates and Condoms stand and distributing every wedding couple a gift of condoms and AIDS prevention leaflets.

Awareness Programmes

In rural areas, where 80 per cent of Indians live, many still have not heard of AIDS. Part of the reason is India's culture of denial. While big epidemic-stricken cities worked furiously to stanch the spread, one-third of the country's provinces and territories chose to use only a small proportion, if any, of the funds allocated by NACO. Another one-third used scarcely more than half. Many people downplayed the importance of the epidemic and even blamed World Bank of exaggerating the threat to justify its projects. Others went so far as to challenge the existence of AIDS. Even at present, many public officials still argue that measles, tuberculosis or hunger are more pressing problems. Meanwhile, more and more people contract HIV. 'I'm very worried and disillusioned,' says Subhash Hira, a University of Texas professor and director of Mumbai-based AIDS Research and Control Centre. 'State-level heads have no sense of urgency.'

The problem will soon become impossible to tolerate, and not just in the big cities. Among women seeking neonatal care (generally considered the best indicator of infection among the general population), the proportion who carry HIV in some regions is already four per cent. 'They are on the edge of a pretty big disaster,' says Michael Sweat, a professor of international health at Johns Hopkins Medical School.

The World Bank Efforts

The World Bank and the Indian government have already increased their efforts enormously. In 1999, India commenced the second phase of its programme tripling the budget to more than $300 million. In the second phase, public-health professionals will open hundreds of new clinics and will run TV and radio ads. The aim now is just to forestall the worst: to keep HIV from reaching 5 per cent of-India's adults. When sub-Saharan Africa reached this threshold, says the World Bank's Habayeb, the infection rate took off: the graph of new cases was 'almost vertical'. 'When it exceeds 5 per cent, you need not millions but billions', he says. 'It's not that far to 20 per cent. And the only way to stop it is to go on war footing.'

It is difficult to think how the disease will be curtailed with anything less. The barriers are legion: illiteracy, poverty and a ruling class that has shown little interest in this epidemic of the poor. Immunologists point to places like Botswana, where AIDS deaths have created a shortage of teachers, decimated the service sector and shattered the local economies. 'Imagine if one in five people you know suddenly died,' said Ken Mayer, a professor of medicine and community at Brown University who has studied AIDS in India. In Karnataka, locals have erected a shrine to India's only AIDS goddess—'Aidsamma'—at a temple near Mysore. Let it not be India's only hope of staying off the epidemic.

AVERT

Prevention of AIDS is an important objective for the US Agency for International Development (USAID). The 10-year, $10-million programme in Tamil Nadu, begun in 1995 and spearheaded by AIDS Prevention and Control (APAC) in Chennai was the first state-level HIV prevention programme in India. It is aided by USAID through the National AIDS Control Organisation (NACO). Annual behavioural surveys reveal that a lot of strides have been made toward raising awareness about HIV transmission, sexually transmitted disease (STD) prevention and condom use among target groups in Tamil Nadu. Now a similar project, AVERT, has been initiated in Maharashtra. Forty-one and a half million dollars will be spent over seven years in a bilateral programme, the largest AIDS prevention project sponsored by USAID anywhere in the world. Maharashtra has the highest number of people living with HIV in

India, almost half of the reported cases in the country. Utilizing the lessons learned in Tamil Nadu, a comprehensive plan to reduce the transmission of HIV/AIDS in Maharashtra has been tailored in collaboration with the Government of India, NACO, the state government and other bilateral donors.

For achieving the goal, AVERT aims to increase availability and improve the quality of information, products and services that help to reduce the HIV/AIDS transmission in Maharashtra; strengthen state and municipal capacity for HIV/AIDS prevention and control alongwith strategic planning, implementation of programme, monitoring and evaluation; and increase availability and use of epidemiological statistics or advocacy, strategy development and decision-making—statistics which will, in time, be generated within the project itself. Like the APAC programme, upon which AVERT is modelled, USAID works with the state government, private health-care providers, community-based groups and non-governmental organisations to promote prevention of HIV/ AIDS and other sexually transmitted diseases through outreach programmes. These programmes target high-risk groups such as sex workers and their clients and migrant workers.

'Issues in Maharashtra differ from Tamil Nadu and are more complex. The sex industry is different,' says Bethanne Moskov, team head, infetious diseases, at USAID, New Delhi. She adds: 'We want to go to the next level, with a multi-sector approach.' It means broader programs that encompass more of the community. Targeted intervention programme will be made in equilibrium with those promoting community awareness. Educating young people is part of it, as is sustainability. AIDS is a fatal, incurable disease, and the message must continue to go out.

USAID has other priorities related to HIV/AIDS prevention and control. One specifically aimed at children affected by AIDS involves development of community care centres for HIV-positive children, drop-in centres and shelters for street children and education. At present, USAID-aided projects for children affected by AIDS are run by Salaam Baalak Trust and Project Concern International in New Delhi; Committed Communities Development Trust and Prerana in Mumbai; Community Health and Education Society in Chennai; and Society for Development Research and Training in Pondicherry. All these urban centres show a high rate of

HIV infection. Coverage is being expanded throughout India. Other initiatives include an HIV Business. Coalition, a Ports Project and media sensitization. Another initiative raises awareness in men about their responsibilities in prevention. The Leadership and Investment in Fighting an Epidemic (LIFE) initiative is a $100-million programme that supports prevention, care and treatment, care for children affected by AIDS and capacity and infrastructure development, including surveillance systems.

Developing the Vaccine

Researchers are looking for answers: treatment, prevention, or remedy for HIV / AIDS, a disease which today affects more than 36 million persons around the world. About 70 per cent of the infected population live in sub-Saharan Africa, but the number of AIDS cases are growing in South Asia. India alone constitutes more than 3.7 million, as per the reports of United Nations Programme on HIV / AIDS (UNAIDS) and World Health Organization (WHO) data. The disease is spreading rapidly than anticipated, and 95 per cent of new HIV infections now occur in economically poor countries—which makes these countries important stations for scientific research and development. India, with its already sophisticated pharmaceutical industry, was recently welcomed as a strong partner in this global war against HIV / AIDS. While the introduction of antiretroviral drugs in 1996 dramatically cut the death rate due to AIDS in rich countries, these drugs are palliative and not a cure. Prevention is much better. That is exactly the aim of researchers who are working overtime to develop an HIV / AIDS vaccine. However, global spending on developing an AIDS vaccine is about $300 million annually—just 10 per cent of what Europe and the US spend every year on drugs to treat HIV / AIDS. To change this skewed scenario, the Rockefeller Foundation commenced a programme in 1994 which was spun off two years later as the International AIDS Vaccine Initiative (IAVI). It is being run as a 'social venture capital' fund. The big donors include the Bill & Melinda Gates Foundation, the Rockefeller Foundation, the Sloan Foundation and the Starr Foundation; the governments of the UK, the US, the Netherlands, Canada and Ireland; and the World Bank.

IAVI's mission is to accelerate development, manufacture and distribution of AIDS vaccines at affordable prices in developing countries. This can be achieved through partnerships between scientists, industry and public sector. The aim is to develop about a dozen candidate vaccines, and get two or three of them into major clinical trials very soon. Strict observance of medical ethics is mandatory when a vaccine comes to human, or even animal trials, and is of paramount concern. In January 2001, clinical trials started in Kenya to test IAVI's first AIDS vaccine. 'An AIDS vaccine for the world's poorest countries is an international public good that is not likely to happen without innovative public-private collaboration,' says Seth Berkley, president and CEO of IAVI. International collaboration and partnership with industry is perhaps the only way a successful AIDS vaccine can be developed. 'A safe and effective HIV vaccine will not come from one laboratory or even one country, but from the worldwide effort currently underway in dozens of countries, involving hundreds of laboratories, each planning work that came before,' feels Charles A. Gardner, science attache at the US Embassy in New Delhi.

Till now, more than 60 HIV vaccine trials have taken place all over, more than half of them in the US. These were just the first steps on a long path toward an eventual vaccine. At present there is a necessity to test vaccines under various conditions, and especially wherever the incidence of disease is very high. 'This will necessitate collaboration between high-tech laboratories in the US, Europe, India and elsewhere with clinicians and health professionals in field sites in Asia and Africa. If we want a vaccine that is safe and effective in India, it must eventually be tested in India,' points out Gardner. It is in this scenario that the AIDS vaccine development projects of Indian laboratories, in partnership with US companies and institutions, assume great significance. Indian researchers have been working on HIV for a few years now and have developed high degree of skill. IAVI has decided to build upon this work, bring in industrial partners and develop vaccines in India. In March this year, IAVI signed an agreement with the Indian Council for Medical Research (ICMR) to develop and evaluate one or more vaccines suitable for use in India. The joint efforts will include collaborative research on different approaches to vaccines, building capacity to conduct vaccine testing, technology transfers and, eventually, clinical trials of jointly developed AIDS vaccines.

Research

In a separate venture, IAVI has concluded a Vaccine

Development Partnership that integrates researchers from India and Therion Biologics, Cambridge, Massachusetts, to build preventive AIDS vaccines meant specifically for India. IAVI will aid Therion to design, engineer, and manufacture a vaccine for HIV subtype C—the most prevalent strain of the virus in India. Most AIDS vaccines at present being developed are based on subtype B, which is the predominant strain in the US and Europe. Therion will work in close association of a team of Indian scientists from the National Institute for Cholera and Enteric Diseases (NICED), Kolkata. They will jointly develop a preventive AIDS vaccine based on the Modified Vaccinia Ankara (MVA) pox virus vector. Vijay Mehra, programme director, applied vaccine research, IAVI, who did the basic work for the partnership with Indian institutions states that the first discussion with Indians started almost three years ago. The Indian research institutes were chosen on the basis of the work already done there. 'NICED scientist Sekhar Chakrabarti commenced the research on developing MVA for the delivery of foreign antigens at the NIH [National Institutes of Health] and has continued to work on that. Thus he was the most obvious choice for constructing the MVA-based vaccine in collaboration with Therion. Ramesh S. Paranjape of National AIDS Research Institute (NARI), Pune, is obtaining HIV isolates from recent sero-converters, characterizing the isolates, subcloning and sequencing the genes. NICED's Chakrabarti will bring these DNA clones to Therion to develop the HIV vaccine,' Mehra said.

The partnership is of the hope that pending regulatory approval, the vaccine may be ready for human testing within two years. 'Our aim is to support India in moving forward a number of candidates and to mobilize Indian researchers and institutions to join the global effort. If appropriate, we will work with Indian vaccine manufacturer to help production of the vaccine for India and perhaps more broadly,' said Berkley. 'One critical problem is to assure whatever work goes on in India is built upon the state of the science globally—assuring that Indian scientists do not 'reinvent the wheel',' he added. Berkley is of the opinion that the partnership will benefit both sides. 'Therion is a biotechnology research company. If there is an agreement between Therion, ICMR and IAVI, it should permit Therion to share in the learning involved in preparing a vaccine and the patents of any eventual vaccine. The agreement will be specific that the vaccine must be provided near cost price for developing countries especially India (this is a standard provision in any venture into which IAVI puts any aid) but the vaccine may also be sold (or licensed to others to be sold) at a profit in rich countries. Therion will share in these profits.' However, the partnership will boost India's vaccine research capabilities and vaccine manufacturing industry. Both should be heavily involved in the search for an HIV vaccine and the IAVI partnership will help and supplement existing national efforts.

Another Indian partnership with an American company for developing an AIDS vaccine is in progress at the Department of Biotechnology (DBT). Recently, DBT has sponsored several programmes related to HIV/AIDS. Studies were conducted to assess the genotype of HIV-1 in circulation in the community. This was done to understand the type of strains HIV-1 virus necessitated for development of AIDS vaccine. The study clearly indicated that HIV-1 subtype C is the predominant type. A large number of HIV-1 and 2 isolates have been well characterized and a repository has been done at NARI. It has also aided a programme on developing HIV-DNA candidate vaccines at the All India Institute of Medical Sciences (AIIMS), New Delhi, the three ICMR institutes namely National Institute of Virology (NIV), Pune; NARI and NICED, and Jawaharlal Nehru Centre for Advanced Scientific Research, Bangalore. Now DBT is talking to an American company, Chiron Corporation, for a possible collaboration to develop an AIDS vaccine. Chiron, headquartered in Emeryville, California, is a biotechnology company that has stakes in three global healthcare markets: bio-pharmaceuticals, blood testing and vaccines. In order to move speedily so that an affordable vaccine is available, DBT is negotiating with Chiron for developing candidate AIDS vaccines, in addition to Indian institutes—AIIMS and the National Institute of Immunology (NII), Delhi, an Indian pharmaceutical company may also be one of the partners in joint development of a candidate vaccine,' says V.K. Vinayak, advisor (medical) at DBT.

The partnership with American research and vaccine manufacturing companies is going to be mutually beneficial. 'Training of Indian researchers and transfer of the technologies to the Indian pharmaceutical companies would be an integral part of the collaboration if it will be agreed to,' points out Vinayak. 'Indian institutions will get an exposure to the advanced technologies developed by Chiron. We would like the vaccine to be manufactured in India, so that it can be provided at an affordable cost to the health-care system. This unique technology will then be available in the country, which could be utilized for developing other vaccines or improve existing vaccines.' Both IAVI and ICMR have recognised working groups who will cooperate in monitoring the programmes on a regular basis, through project meetings and teleconferences. In addition, IAVI has quarterly meetings of a project management committee of outside exports, who review all vaccine development partnerships and advise on several issues.

Both the US and India have well-established ethical guidelines for research, involving human subjects. The ethical guidelines prepared by the ICMR have been 'deemed comparable' by the US-Department of Health and Human Services (DHHS). Each US institution is required to establish an ethical review committee, and has to get the same approved by the DHHS. For a typical vaccine clinical trial, it can take eight to nine months to write, review, modify, rewrite and remodify the informed consent farms and research protocol enabling it to meet all the requirements. Informed consent must be given in the participant's own language, and explained orally by a qualified professional. IAVI is also working on the ethical issues. It has already initiated a dialogue with Indian non-governmental organisations and has commissioned the Social and Rural Research Institute, a unit of IMRB, a Delhi-based market research firm, to conduct one-on-one interviews with a representative sample of a broad range of NGO leaders on ethical and social issues. At present, IAVI plans to have similar meetings with professional groups and elected members. Inputs from this exercise will go into preparing a document summarizing the social and individual implications of vaccine research and trials in India. The document will then be released to media and the public. "Some issues do pose a real challenge. For instance, we must be absolutely sure that participation in clinical trials is truely informed and truely voluntary, 'says Berkley. While IAVI will bring in its international experience in this field from earlier trials in Africa, 'at the end of the day, it is India who will assure that the appropriate ethical standards are in place," the IAVI chief added.

New HIV Diagnostics

Appropriate diagnosis has always been a prerequisite for treatment of any disease. This also is the case with AIDS that is threatening life and society in dozens of poor nations and spreading its tentacles across the world with pounding impunity. But thanks to medical research, most known strains of the AIDS-causing human immunodeficiency virus (HIV) globally can now be detected. After the detection of the first AIDS case in Chennai in 1986, India has been wholly dependent on imported diagnostic kits until the mid-1990s. But these were expensive by Indian standards. The concern for cheaper indigenous kits and self-reliance encouraged the Indian Department of Biotechnology (DBT) to commence three independent projects in 1993-94 to develop HIV diagnostic kits. It was part of a special programme to aid indigenous research in diagnostics, says V.K. Vinayak, adviser (medical) in DBI. At present more than 20 MNCs and Indian companies are marketing these kits including Dr. Reddy's Laboratories, Johnson & Johnson, Ranbaxy Laboratories, Transasia, Bayer Diagnostics', Quick Diagnostics, Rashmi Diagnostics, Glaxo (India) Limited and Infar (India) Limited.

HIV-1 and HIV-2 are the two agents of AIDS, the former being the predominant. While HIV-1 is divided into group M (11 subtypes A to K) and Group O (9 subtypes), HIV-2 has five subtypes (A to E). HIV-2 is mainly found in West Africa but subsequently has been detected in western United States, Europe, Canada, Central Africa, Brazil and India. Of the various subtypes of HIV-1, subtype C rules the roost in India, South Africa, Zambia and other central African countries.

Detection of the Presence of Common Antibodies

An infection is detected in two ways. Either the pathogen components are directly detected from any appropriate tissue (generally blood, as it is the easiest to probe) or from any measurable alteration in a biochemical trait because of body's response to the infection. The second approach is generally used for diagnosing HIV. Proteins called antibodies, generated by the body's immune system in response to invading HIV, are identified. Antibodies reflect the activity of various pathogens and are present in blood as part of blood that remains liquid when blood cells form a clot. Though it is possible to diagnose HIV infection by separating the virus from a blood sample or by demonstrating the presence of viral antigens (substances that stimulate the body to produce anti-bodies) in blood, viral culture is expensive, not readily available and slow—it takes about a month to complete the viral culture test. More common are blood tests, which are comparatively inexpensive, widely available, and accurate in detecting infection when used to screen patients and confirm diagnosis. Most indigenous kits work on the same fundamental principle—they detect the presence of some or the most common antibodies present in serum. The end-point formats, sources of proteins, their sequences and methods of purification, however, change.

All the three DBT-sponsored kits have been developed and two of them commercialized. The one perfected by a team led by Vijay Chaudhury of Delhi University South Campus (DUSC) has a lot of molecular biology inputs. No special equipment is required for this screening test which takes three to five minutes to perform, says Chaudhury. His team joined together two genes, one from an antigen protein present on the surface of red blood cells, and the second from the HIV virus itself. The genetically-engineered stuff was put inside a bacterium that produced hundreds of copies, resulting in a watery material containing both the genes. The first gene links with the antigen on red blood cells, while the second joins with the antibodies produced against HIV. The end result is that the red blood cells clump together, which can be detected by the naked eye, indicating whether the blood is infected or not. The kit is free of any potentially infectious material and hence is non-hazardous. It is a field-level rapid test, according to Bakulesh Khamar, director research of Ahmedabad-based Cadila Pharmaceuticals Limited, which has commercialized the technology. It hit the market this August as NEVA HIV (naked eye visible agglutination assay) kit.

Work on the Delhi Unversity kit was commenced about 90 years back and the technology was transferred to Cadila in February 1999. The company is now enhancing the product and its newer version will detect subtype 'O,' which is found in Africa and is yet to be detected in India, Cadila scientist R.V. Bhatt said. NEVA HIV costs a mere Rs. 39 per test. The company plans to export the kit and is in the process of registering the product in various countries.

Another kit originated at the National Institute of Immunology (NII) in Delhi. It is an enzyme linked immunosorbent assay ELISA kit that uses synthetic peptides (small selective stretches of proteins) as representatives of viral proteins as the major system components. It works by attaching HIV antigens to a plastic well or beads. A second antibody joined to an enzyme is added followed by addition of a substance that makes the enzyme to react by forming a colour, which is measured by an instrument called a spectrophotometer, explains NII's Satish Gupta, whose team has developed the kit. The kit was taken up for commercialization by Delhi-based ACE Diagnostics Limited in 1998, but unfortunately, the company closed down before the product could reach the market. Now Biotech Consortium of India Limited (BCIL), a DBT body that assists commercializing biotechnology, is looking for another firm which can market the kit.

Research for a third ELISA kit was done at Indian Institute of Science (IISC) in Bangalore. The kit is manufactured and marketed by Bangalore-based XCyton Diagnostics Limited under the brand name HIV Chex and has been available since 1997. IISc helped optimize the commercially viable synthesis of HIV peptides, modify the peptides to improve yield and research the structural aspects of HIV-1 C peptides. A group led by microbiologist Pradeep K. Seth at the All India Institute of Medical Sciences (AIIMS) in New Delhi also came out with an enzyme immunoassay for screening those infected with HIV-1 and HIV-2 in 1999 after four years of research, but it is yet to be marketed. If ELISA test results are reactive, the test is again done on the same blood sample. If the sample is repeatedly reactive, the results are confirmed using a Western Blot antibody screening test, discovered in 1979. It is more expensive, specific and can differentiate between HIV antibodies and other antibodies that react to the ELISA, which gives positive results even when a person is not actually infected with HIV.

The only indigenous Western Blot kit has been developed at Cancer Research Institute (CRI) of Tata Memorial Centre, Mumbai. Financed by the DBT, the kit uses virus proteins (viruses are grown in cell culture systems) separated on the basis of their molecular size and trapped on a synthetic membrane, which reacts with serum. All or some of the viral proteins demonstrate colour development in the form of discreet bands on the white membrane background only if the serum is infected. The colour forms because of strong binding of the antibodies present in the serum and the viral proteins. The kit is being marketed by Delhi-based J. Mitra & Company under the brand name HIV W.Blot. J. Mitra is also selling a rapid test kit called HIV TRI-DOT as well as an ELISA kit under the name Microlisa-HIV, both developed inhouse. J. Mitra's kits detect HIV-2 and both subgroup 'O' and subgroup 'C' of HIV-1.

All the indigenous kits have been independently assessed by

several organizations including the World Health Organization (WHO), Institute of Tropical Medicine in Antwerp, Belgium, National AIDS Research Institute (NARI), Pune, Christian Medical College and Hospital (CMC), Vellore, and National Institute of Communicable Diseases (NICD) Delhi for their specificity and sensitivity which varies from approximately 98 to 100 per cent. Rapid tests cost between Rs. 40 and Rs. 100 per test. The price of screening ELISA tests ranges from Rs. 30 to Rs. 100 per test. Confirmatory Western Blot test costs Rs. 700–1500 per test. The kits by Cadila and XCyton are also procured by NACO to be used in government hospitals and centres in the country.

India and WHO accept positive results from three successive ELISA tests with various kits as 'confirmed' as Western Blot tests are an expensive affair. Western Blot was considered for a long time as the gold standard, but not anymore. WHO, based on studies, says that three ELISA tests of various antigen type (or one could be a rapid test) can give results like those of Western Blot for diagnosis of HIV infection at a much lower cost. Thus, WHO recommends Western Blot only in situations where, based on the ELISA, the tests remain indeterminate or inconclusive. A new step in this direction is a project initiated recently by Department of Science and Technology (DST) under which the Jawaharlal Nehru Centre for Advanced Scientific Research (JNCASR) in Bangalore is working to develop an HIV antigen capture assay to identify the viral antigen—different from the other existing kits which identify antibodies. Hyderabad-based Bharat Biotech Limited (BBL), a co-partner, will fine tune and commercialize the technology.

But what would be this assay's advantages? A major drawback of antibody detection is that the human body needs weeks to months to react to HIV attack and develop antibodies. During this 'window period' there are large quantities of virus and viral antigen in the body fluids but little antibody. Hence antigen detection during this early phase is more advantageous. Detection of antibodies in the first 6–12 months in HIV-infected infants is not reliable either as maternal antibodies interfere with the assay. This assay is as effective as other confirmatory tests used globally.

The HIV-1 antigen capture assay was added as an interim measure by the US Food and Drug Administration (FDA) in 1996 to HIV antibody testing to save blood supply further until other tests became available to detect early HIV infection. The expensive assay has its shortcomings, however, presence of viral antigen in body fluids is remarkably variable in individuals. So results can be unreliable. But where antibody assay fails, this is the best alternative. Thus, this assay can be used to monitor the growth of the virus in labs and validate therapeutic strategies in clinics, thus helping fundamental and applied research.

According to BCIL, approximately 2.1 million HIV diagnostic kits worth Rs 115 million were sold in 1997-98 which increased by 80 per cent to 3.85 million kits worth Rs 290 million in the following fiscal year, probably due to HIV screening in blood banks became mandatory. In 1999-2000, the sales increased extra by about 20 per cent to 4.7 million kits amounting to Rs 289 million (the decrease in value is due to a drop in the price of kits), three-fifths of which were rapid kits and the rest ELISA. An annual growth rate of 20 per cent in the consumption of kits is hoped over the next four years. National AIDS Control Organization (NACO) procures about 3.5 million ELISA kits, 0.85 million rapid kits and 7,000 Western Blot kits for its programmes every year.

Experts say the indigenous HIV diagnostics kits can now cater to the country's demand and compete with imported kits. There are also kits manufactured by Indian companies with technology transferred from abroad. Morepen Laboratories of India and US diagnostics firm Ameritek Inc. agreed to collaborate in manufacturing rapid diagnostics kits. Morepen plans to make the kits from next January at its unit in Parwanoo in Himachal Pradesh. Many foreign pharmaceutical companies are coming up with diagnostic products based on HIV isolates from specific Indian strains. For instance, Princeton, New Jersey-based Premier Medical Corporation (PMC) announced a rapid test kit named Bio Sign HIV 1-2 that is specially made for Indian conditions. The product has been introduced in India by the Mumbai-based subsidiary PMC Medical (India) Private Limited.

The market for such kits is expected to increase with the accelerated growth rate of HIV infection and more serious efforts to track and contain the epidemic. This is clearly reflected in a recent announcement by the Health Minister C.P. Thakur that HIV diagnostic centres will be established in every district.

4

Expanding the Horizon

The present Chapter discusses the pioneering job of seven Indian non-governmental organisations (NGOs) in anticipation to the HIV epidemic in India. These are by no means the only Indian NGOs doing innovative work in this area, but programmes of this kind are still the exception rather than the rule. Most Indian NGOs do not yet offer a high priority to HIV and AIDS. Perhaps this is not surprising. India has many large seemingly interactable health problems. Diseases such as malnutrition, malaria, diarrhoea and pneumonia claim the lives of millions annually, especially of young children. Among adults, Tuberculosis is still a major killer epidemic. The HIV disease in comparison, is still virtually invisible. At the present early stage of the epidemic the numbers of people who have been identified as HIV-infected or who have clinical symptoms of AIDS are still very small. Most Indian NGOs—including most of those discussed in this chapter—have had little or no direct contact with people living with HIV/AIDS. Many NGOs see AIDS programmes with little scepticism, or even as a diversion from health and development problems which seem to be more important. NGOs that give AIDS a priority concern are sometimes criticized for pandering to the whims and fashions of donors abroad and international agencies. There are strong reasons, however, for Indian NGOs to provide HIV/AIDS awareness and prevention an integral part of their activities; and in the times to come, there will also be an urgent priority for NGOs to give care and support to people with AIDS and their families. This discussion demonstrates how seven Indian NGOs in five states have successfully integrated HIV/AIDS into their task. In so doing, they are not only widening the front against the HIV epidemic, but are also offering an important contribution to the development process itself.

Indian Perspective

Stretching in a diamond shape from the snowy Himalayas to the warm waters of the Indian Ocean, India is the world's seventh largest country in area and the second most populous. It has a strategic position in South Asia, bordering with several other countries: China, Nepal and Bhutan in the North; Bangladesh and Myanmar (Burma) in the East, and Pakistan on the West. Populated with approximately one billion people India has 18 regional languages and more than 1,600 spoken dialects. Over 80 per cent of Indians follow the Hindu religion and about 10 per cent Muslims; the rest of the population are Christians, Sikhs, Buddhists; Jains or Parsis, etc.

With a federal system of government, India is the world's largest democracy. The central government headquarters are located in the capital city of New Delhi, but responsibility for key areas such as health, education and transport lies with the governments of 28 states and 7 union territories. The country is criss-crossed by a vast network of surface transport facilitating the movement of goods and people to and from every corner of the country. Since her independence from Britain in 1947, India has become self-sufficient in food and has achieved large industrial growth. The country's main exports are coffee, tea, fish, machinery, iron and steel, transport equipment, textiles, leather goods, clothing, polished diamonds and handicrafts. Economic reforms in the past have boosted exports, foreign trade and investment. As a result a sharp rise in incomes was noted mainly among the country's middle and upper socio-economic groups. Besides these achievements, average GNP per person is only $310 at present. Adult literacy is a modest 62 per cent and among women only 34 per cent can read and write. Radio is the most popular medium of mass communication, but television also has a huge outreach and the cinema is significantly popular. The print media reach over 200 million people covering most towns and cities.

Non-governmental Organisations (NGOs)

Among India's greatest assets are its many non-governmental organisations (NGOs) involved in promoting health, development, education and social welfare. The social reform movements which commenced to challenge feudalism in the late 19th century were followed in the 1920s and 1930s, by the independence movement inspired by Mahatma Gandhi and his philosophy of non-violence, self-reliance, and non-discrimination. In the 1950s and 1960s new generation of Gandhian-inspired NGOs came at fore, often in response to natural calamities such as droughts and floods; many continued to work with communities on health and development activities.

The early 1970s witnessed the rise of another wave of NGOs, generally known as 'social action groups'. Starting with an analysis of the local socio-economic and political situation, these small and highly localised groups help the poor and disadvantaged to form their own organisations to work for their human rights. These rights include, for instance, minimum wages, the liberation of bonded labour, the protection of their environment and their entitlement to land rights, education, bank loans, health care and food for work schemes in times of natural calamities. Women's organisations form a distinctive strand within the social action group movement. They have taken the stand in campaigns against sexual abuse, the dowry system and violence against women. Many also offer health services for women and help women achieve self-independence through vocational training and income generating plans. These NGOs and community groups are many traditional charities which make grants for social work or directly provide services such as hospitals, schools, orphanages and homes for handicapped people.

The so-called 'intermediary' or 'support' NGOs have begun providing those working at base with training, evaluation, research, documentation and opportunities for networking with one another. Alongwith many other kinds of Indian NGOs and community groups, these have achieved a lot of practical experience of working with the poorest and most disadvantaged groups in society. They are also a major priceless asset in India's struggle against HIV/AIDS.

The Disease

HIV is expected to have reached India in the early 1980s, but it was only in March 1986 that the first case of HIV infection was detected. The virus spread with great rapidity to reach all parts of the country. The epidemic varies widely from one region to the other, reflecting the country's great diversity. In the north-eastern state of Manipur, HIV has already reached epidemic scale among injecting drug users. In some other states, in comparison, only a few cases of HIV—and no case of AIDS—have yet been found.

India's first case of AIDS was reported in Mumbai in May 1987, and by October 1995 a total of 2,095 cases had been reported, but it is identified that the actual total is much more. As in other developing nations, most HIV infections and cases of AIDS in India go undetected and unreported, because of a lack of HIV testing facilities and insufficient systems for diagnosis and reporting. By October 1995, mere 21,131 HIV infections had been officially reported, with Maharashtra, Tamil Nadu and Manipur accounting for most of these cases, largely due to better HIV diagnosis and reporting systems in these states. As per the estimates of the Government of India, in association with the World Health Organization (WHO), 1.75 million people in India had become infected with HIV by the year ending 1994. Since then thousands of new infections have occurred. However, as per Dr. Shiv Lal of National AIDS Control Organisation, by the year 2000 up to 7 million people were infected with HIV and 2 million are likely to develop AIDS in the country. Most information on the HIV epidemic in India comes from limited studies of groups such as truck drivers, sex workers and injecting drug users, who are regarded as most vulnerable to HIV. For instance, studies of Mumbai's female sex workers, who number at least 50,000, estimated that more than 50 per cent were infected with HIV by 1994. As the first to bear the brunt of the epidemic, such groups are often mistakenly seen simply as reservoirs of infection, and stigmatised as the only groups likely to transmit the virus to other sections of the population. HIV is now spreading within the rural areas of India as well, mostly due to sex between people who do not know they may be passing on or receiving the virus during unprotected sexual intercourse.

Differentiation

The HIV epidemic differs from other major infectious diseases in different ways:

(a) Because of the long time lag—from 5 to 10 years or even longer—between the initial infection with HIV and the onset of clinical symptoms of AIDS, most HIV-positive persons feel quite normal. Not knowing that they are infected with HIV, they continue to spread the virus to others. To prevent millions of infections and premature deaths in India, HIV awareness and prevention programmes must begin well before the impact of the epidemic becomes a menace.

(b) HIV greatly exacerbates existing health problems, particularly the spread of tuberculosis, resulting in more human grief and misery, and placing even greater strain on already overburdened health services. TB and HIV form a deadly combination, each multiplying the impact of the other. When people are infected with both TB and HIV, TB is much more likely to become active due to the person's weakened immune system. As more TB cases become infectious, huge numbers of people carry and spread TB to healthy people. In India, where 50 to 60 per cent of the population are already carriers of the tuberculosis bacillus, the HIV epidemic is likely to lead to an alarming increase in active tuberculosis cases.

(c) There is no vaccine against HIV and no effective medical treatment for HIV infection. Most HIV-related illnesses can be cured effectively with standard medicines, but when HIV disease reaches the climax known as AIDS, it is inevitably fatal. Preventing the initial infection with HIV is thus the only way of preventing AIDS deaths.

(d) Unlike other infections 80-90 per cent of those infected with HIV are young adults at the top of their productive and reproductive lives. They generally have young children, who are still dependent on them for sustenance, education, social support and moral guidance. They also have elderly dependents who, after their premature deaths, will be left to fend for themselves while trying to raise a generation of orphaned grandchildren.

(e) HIV destabilises society as it brings fear, blame and stigma into families, neighbourhood, workplaces, schools and places of worship. It exacerbates long-standing prejudices against stigmatised groups like prostitutes, homosexuals and injecting drug users. It threatens basic human rights such as medical confidentiality, security of employment, the right to education, and even the right to privacy and human dignity. No other disease affects human society in such a big way or to this extent.

Primary Facts

Acquired Immune Deficiency Syndrome (AIDS) was first recognised in 1981. It is caused by the virus Human Immunodeficiency Virus (HIV), which reduces the capacity of the body's defences (or immune system) to combat infections. There is a time lag of several years—even 10 years or more – between the initial infection and the commencement of AIDS. Without a blood test, it is generally not possible to be certain whether a person has HIV. Most people with HIV do not know they are infected; they look and feel absolutely normal. There is still no vaccine against HIV and no remedy for AIDS. Although most AIDS-related diseases can generally be treated with standard medicines, the advance stage of AIDS inevitably leads to death. HIV spreads in three ways: through sexual intercourse, through blood, and from mother to child:

Sexual intercourse. Globally, approximately 75 per cent of all HIV infections occur through sexual intercourse when one or other partner has HIV. The risk of spreading HIV is much increased when other sexually transmitted diseases (STDs) prevail. Women are physically more vulnerable than men to STDs, alongwith HIV.

Blood. The use of blood contaminated with HIV for transfusions carries a very high risk of spreading the virus. HIV can also spread easily when people share needles and syringes to inject themselves with drugs. If one user has HIV, the small amount of blood which he or she leaves in the needle or syringe will be injected into the bloodstream of the next user, who may also get HIV.

Mother to child. HIV can be passed on from a mother to her child during pregnancy, at the time of delivery or through breastfeeding. However, in countries with high infant mortality, where bottle feeding carries a high risk of disease and death, WHO and UNICEF recommend that mothers with HIV should still be encouraged to breastfeed their babies.

Sexual Behaviour

HIV cannot be transmitted through coughing or sneezing; through saliva, tears or sweat; by shaking hands; by sharing eating and drinking utensils, telephones, bathrooms or toilets; by mosquitoes or other insects; by walking barefoot where people have spat; or by living or working with a person who has AIDS or HIV infection. Sexual intercourse between two persons who do not have HIV and are completely faithful to each other carries no risk at all of spreading HIV. If one partner has HIV, sex in which the penis enters the vagina or the anus carries a high risk of spreading the virus. (Oral sex carries a lower risk.) This risk can be greatly lessened by using a condom every time. HIV is not spread by other forms of physical contact such as kissing, cuddling, fondling, caressing, or massaging.

Issues at Hand

A crucial factor in the spread of HIV in the country is high prevalence of sexually transmitted diseases. In Tamil Nadu state, for instance, Dr. K. Kantharaj, deputy director of the state AIDS cell, has estimated that 20 per cent of adult men suffer from an STD at any particular time. People with STDs, especially if genital sores are involved, are at much higher risk of spreading — or being infected by — HIV through sex.

A study conducted in a town in Tamil Nadu by Dr Sunithi Solomon the strong link between HIV and other STDs. In her study carried out in 1995, Dr Solomon found that 90 per cent of truck drivers (all men) who had experienced an STD and requested an HIV test also had HIV. These data are not representative of all truck drivers—or of the male population in general — in the state of Tamil Nadu, but they offer grounds for major concern.

Migration is a key factor in the spread of HIV in India. The country's highly developed network of roads and railways has encouraged a massive movement of people from rural to urban areas in search of employment. As per to the Indian government's ministry of labour, there are approximately 80 million migrants in India, most of whom are men who are either single or living apart from their wives and families. They comprise 30–40 per cent of the population of large cities at any given time, where they also constitute for much of the clientele of the 'red light' areas.

The double standard of sexual morality which, as in several other nations, is practised by large number of people in India, is an important element in the spread of HIV. Women are expected to retain their virginity until married, while men often desire to visit a sex worker to gain sexual experience before marriage. Even after marriage, it is not unusual for men to have sexual partners other than their wives. Women, who are biologically more vulnerable to HIV infection in comparison to men, pay the price for the sexual freedom of their husbands. Growing number of Indian women who had sex only with their husbands are now being infected with HIV. In Pune, a study in 1994 revealed that 14 per cent of married women with STDs—none of whom reported sexual contacts outside their marriages—were HIV-positive. Increasing numbers of pregnant women are testing positive for HIV. For instance, at the HIV sentinel surveillance centre in Salem District, Tamil Nadu, HIV prevalence among pregnant women rose from 0.1 per cent in September 1954 to 0.9 per cent in October 1995.

HIV is also transmitted through sex between men, many of whom may be married and continue to have sex with their wives. Amongst male sex workers, HIV infection is now reaching proportionately high levels. In one such group in Maharashtra state, 50 per cent were found to be HIV-infected in 1995. In India, the problem of HIV transmission among men who have sex with men cannot simply be dismissed as a problem of a 'minority' group. In such a large country as India, a 'minority' group may have millions of people spread over a wide geographical region. In some parts of the country, particularly in the slums of many big cities and in the north-eastern states, HIV is spreading through the sharing of drug-injecting equipment. In Manipur state, HIV has spread at an alarming rate amongst injecting drug users, estimated to number about 15,000. In 1989 there were no HIV infections reported within this group. And in 1994, as per Dr Swarup Sarkar of the Indian Council for Medical Research, the HIV infection rate had reached an estimated 90 per cent.

Contaminated blood is also an important factor of HIV infection. Of about 2 million bottles of blood that are transfused annually in India, more than 50 per cent are supplied by people who sell their blood. Many do so out of abject poverty; some also sell sex. In 1992, 86 per cent of a group of commercial blood donors screened in Mumbai were detected to be HIV-infected. The government, however, had made HIV screening mandatory, not all blood banks comply. By 1994, 12 per cent of all HIV infections in the country were estimated to have been acquired through HIV-contaminated blood.

In India, like many other countries, the HIV epidemic has been perceived largely as a medical problem. Yet the epidemic has its roots in India's patterns of economic and social development, and in the attitudes, beliefs and values that determine people's sexual behaviour. It is crystal clear that the HIV epidemic is indeed a development problem, requiring a multiplicity of responses from individuals, communities, government agencies and innumerable of non-governmental organisations.

Severity and Extent

India is perhaps, to have the largest HIV-positive population in the world. However, as people living with HIV generally feel quite normal and look no different from those who are uninfected, the epidemic is largely unseen. This makes it difficult for people even to accept the prevalence of the epidemic, let alone understand its severity and extent. Not surprisingly, misunderstandings about HIV and AIDS are a lot. Many people believe that AIDS is a phenomenon of large cities like Mumbai and Chennai. Others think it to be a disease of prostitutes, not their clients. Some people are of the opinion that AIDS was well-known to ancient Indian practitioners of traditional medicine, as *megavettai* (syphilis), and that it can be treated by traditional medicine. Many newspapers carry a mind-boggling variety of advertisements from quacks offering treatment for AIDS. People who take these medicines sometimes believe they do not need to use condoms during sex, making them (and their sexual partners) more vulnerable to HIV.

The states of Tamil Nadu, Maharashtra and Manipur, which have reported the most cases of HIV infection and AIDS, have also attracted the most media attention. Local AIDS service organisations and HIV-positive persons and government officials in these states have helped to sensitise the mass media to the gravity of the epidemic. Simultaneously, however, some mass media stories about AIDS have created alarm and spread misconceptions amidst the general public. Due to this, many people who know they are HIV-positive hide the fact since they fear rejection by their families and friends, and the loss of their jobs and their standing in their societies.

Even among health workers knowledge of how to cope with HIV/AIDS has been limited, at least until recently. A study conducted among medical students and physicians in 1992, for instance, found that 27 per cent of students and 40 per cent of doctors did not know that HIV is the cause of AIDS; 15 per cent of students and 35 per cent of physicians said that HIV-positive patients should be denied first aid; and 81 per cent of physicians felt that a syringe could be re-used without sterilisation if the needle was changed. The situation has since changed for the better, but many private clinics and hospitals still test for HIV without the knowledge of their patients and refuse medical treatment to those who are diagnosed HIV-positive.

Efforts of Government

When the first cases of HIV infection were reported in India, the government responded by passing an HIV quarantine law. This was followed by calls from some government officials to ban sex with foreign tourists and to send HIV-positive African students back home. The government also appealed for a return to the nation's 'pristine values' and offered to pay sex workers to retire. Other efforts to prevent HIV transmission consisted of refusing HIV-infected people access to health care. Many of these early reactions to the epidemic were responsible for creating great fear and rejection of people with HIV/AIDS. The National AIDS Control Programme was organised in 1987, and in 1992 the National AIDS Control Organization (NACO) was set up. The important objective of NACO is to help the implementation of the National AIDS Control Programme through co-ordinating bodies—state AIDS cells, empowered committees and technical advisory committees—at the national and state level. Different international agencies as World Health Organisation, the World Bank, the ODA, NORAD, USAID, UNDP, SIDA and the Ford Foundation have offered technical and financial help for the implementation of the national programme.

NACO is developing a national HIV sentinel surveillance system to monitor the spread of HIV across the country, working through specially appointed medical professionals in every state. It has also made a big effort to disseminate basic information about HIV and AIDS through print media, radio, television, posters, roadside billboards and other means of mass communication. NACO also makes an important contribution to STD control, particularly by providing government STD clinics with trained workers, laboratory facilities and an extra room to ensure that patients have privacy to discuss their problems. However, it trains private practitioners in the diagnosis and treatment of various STDs. Condoms of questionable quality are a major barrier to HIV/AIDS prevention in India, and NACO has given a directive to condom manufacturers to enhance condom quality. To reduce HIV transmission through infected blood in hospitals, it is at present mandatory to test each bottle of blood for HIV prior to transfusion. NACO supplies HIV test kits to blood banks and has also set up zonal blood testing centres.

Besides, NACO seeks to involve other government institutions in the prevention of HIV/AIDS. The National Council of Educational Research and Training (NCERT) under the Ministry of Education, has worked in association with NACO on the production of an AIDS information package for government schools. (The emphasis of these materials is on delaying the first sexual encounter to avoid becoming infected with HIV; condoms are not mentioned.) The National Social Service Scheme also works with NACO to make information about HIV/AIDS available to university students across the country through its 'Universities Talk AIDS' programme. NACO is also collaborating with the World Health Organisation, OXFAM and several local NGOs on the Continuum of Care project. This priority begun in Manipur state and now being extended to other parts of India, aims to provide primary care and support to people with HIV/AIDS within the home and the society and through the different levels of the health care system. Given India's federal system of government however, NACO's powers are limited mainly to guiding and supporting the different State AIDS cells and other coordinating bodies. Since various State health departments are already burdened by more immediate health problems such as cholera and malaria, the funding and implementation of AIDS programmes is often delayed.

Legal Barriers

An important part of NACO's agenda is to combat discrimination against people with HIV and AIDS and to evolve a socially supportive environment for groups living on the margins of 'normal' society. Yet many of the sexual and drug-injecting behaviours that make people more vulnerable to HIV infection are either illegal, or are widely treated as socially unacceptable, and thus, are pushed underground or tolerated. As a result, organisations working amongst marginalised or stigmatised groups, who are often the most vulnerable to HIV infection, face immunerable difficulties in their work. For instance, the supply of condoms to prisoners in an all-male prison in Delhi was stopped by a public petition, as Indian laws make homosexuality illegal. Moreover, anyone identified as an injecting drug user can be imprisoned or put into a rehabilitation centre. Indian government agencies are not thus permitted to carry out needle exchange programmes or even supply bleach to disinfect drug-injecting equipment and therefore reduce the probability of injecting drug users becoming infected with HIV. However, the central government has recently given the green light to a limited pilot project, which will permit NGOs to distribute needles and syringes to drug users in Manipur state.

Non-governmental Efforts

A number of organisations have emerged in response to the HIV epidemic in India. Among the first were the Indian Health Organisation, in Mumbai, the Gujarat AIDS Awareness and Prevention Unit, in Ahmedabad; the NGO AIDS Cell at the All India Institute of Medical Sciences, in New Delhi; and in Chennai, the South India AIDS Action Programme, the Community Action Network and the AIDS Research Foundation of India. These and other organisations have played a significant role in raising awareness of the epidemic, and have also assured to precipitate government action. Equally importantly, they have assisted to remove the veil of secrecy and hypocrisy surrounding sexual attitudes and behaviour. The pioneering work of these organisations has also assisted to inform and inspire a small but growing number of NGOs and community groups, who now regard HIV/AIDS work as an integral part of their task. The programmes listed in this chapter demonstrate the work of seven such organisations. Their experiences reveal the potential of NGOs and community groups to respond in a constructive way to the multiangular challenges and problems posed by the HIV epidemic. India's HIV epidemic still being at an early stage, most of the organisations discussed here are concerned with AIDS prevention, rather than with care and support for HIV-positive persons and their families. Many communities, however, will soon begin to experience AIDS-related illnesses and deaths. NGOs will require thus, to develop new skills like counselling before and after HIV testing, developing home-based care for people with AIDS, and support for children orphaned by AIDS. Nor are Indian NGOs themselves immune from HIV: their staff will have to learn how to protect themselves against HIV; besides this, they will need to develop humane, non-discriminatory regulations for staff who are HIV-positive.

Mahila Sarvangeen Utkarsh Mandal (MASUM), Pune

A few kilometres outside the lush greenery of Pune, the drought zone starts. The arid landscape is dotted with remnants of farming people eking out a precarious existence from the parched soil. Many men have long since left to seek work in urban cities like Mumbai, returning home frequently with some of their little earnings.

In recent years, local men have been contracting HIV in the urban areas and bringing the virus back to their native villages, where they have sex with their wives and other partners. Some people in the area know that they are HIV-positive and even some more have developed AIDS, but the virus has almost certainly penetrated into many communities already. It is at present only a matter of time before HIV infection and AIDS come out as great health and social problems.

***Streewadi Arogya Kendra* (The Feminist Health Centre)**

In the centre of this seemingly backward area, a narrow dirt road winds its way to the collection of tumble-down mud huts that form the village of Saswad. Outside one mud hut an incongruous-looking sign announces the existence of the *Streewadi Arogya Kendra* — the Feminist Health Centre. Inside, a nurse and a village health worker are busy tending to the local women's health needs. Biweekly a gynaecologist and a counsellor also visit the clinic. Most of the women have gynaecological disorders such as vaginitis, white discharge and pelvic inflammatory diseases and more general problems such as depression. The centre was set up in February 1994 by MASUM, the *Mahila Sarvangeen Utkarsh Mandal* (Rural Women's Association), which grew out of an action research project recommended by the Indian Council of Medical Research. Setup in 1987 at the request of local women, MASUM is engaged in identifying the various forms of exploitation and abuse faced by women, and assist them organise themselves to deal with these problems.

The women using the Feminist Health Centre earn barely enough to feed their families from their small plots of land and part-time work on other farms. Most belong to oppressed castes and minority religions, and are plagued by problems such as alcoholism among men, and sexual exploitation within the home and the community. Few young women are unable to refuse the sexual advances of fathers-in-law or brothers-in-law. Sexual abuse of young girls is also common and many mothers are silent witnesses to this form of exploitation. Although there is no organised sex trade in the area some women sell sex frequently. The Centre imparts education to sexually transmitted diseases (STDs) which are common to a large extent and also offers primary treatment for these infections. Women requiring further diagnostic tests and more specialist care are advised to visit primary health centres or hospitals. Few women also bring their husbands to get information and treatment for STDs. Besides this, the Centre offers many allopathic medicines and herbal remedies for common diseases, and dispenses condoms to couples and individual women. All clinical tests information, medicines and condoms given by the Centre are free of charge.

Sexual Health

MASUM aims to promote women's sexual health in the widest sense. The Centre offers women with primary sex education and assists them to understand various sexual practices. With guidance from the health worker, each woman examines her own genitals with a speculum and a mirror. Women also learnt how they can protect themselves from STDs through condom use and non-penetrative sex. According to Manisha Gupta, Chairperson of MASUM, the goal is to help women define their own sexuality from a woman's view-point and assist them to know that there are safer ways of enjoying sex. Women are advised to talk about their sexuality, to place their ailments in the context of their domestic and working lives, and also to relate their physical problems to their emotions and feelings. Small sets of women with identical physical, sexual and emotional problems meet at the centre to share their experiences of ill-health and sexuality with one another. Only rarely are they reluctant to state frankly with one another about sex. To describe their feelings and provoke discussion, groups of women perform role plays about the different forms of sexual and economic exploitation which they and their daughters face everyday. Groups of adolescent girls also meet to discuss problems related to reproduction, sexuality and self-assertion. Young girls who have suffered sexual abuse, generally within the home, are offered counselling and emotional support.

The Latent Threat

The women's close contact, through their menfolk, with Mumbai has made them aware of the huge but largely invisible threat posed by HIV to their own health and existense. Women often come to the Feminist Health Centre to seek an HIV test. MASUM does not actively promote HIV testing, but woman wishing to know their HIV status are given counselling and are advised about places where they can have an HIV test carried out. MASUM's information is that everyone, regardless of whether or not they are HIV-positive, needs to behave responsibly—not only to avoid becoming infected, but also to avoid passing HIV and other STDs on to others.

Media reports have already generated widespread fear of AIDS across the region, generating a social environment in which people infected with HIV are likely to suffer stigmatisation and rejection. With great foresight, MASUM thus advises non-discrimination and support for people with HIV and their families. When cases of HIV infection and AIDS begin to come at fore in local communities, the women will be able to make an informed, compassionate response. Most significantly, MASUM does not cure HIV / AIDS as a separate issue, but as a health, social and economic problem generated by double standards in sexuality.

Manisha Gupta says "The problem is to do with how we have constructed sexuality. If we were able to handle relationships transparently, more honestly; if sex was not bought and sold in the markets; if sex was not coerced... There is a total lack of concern for women's sexual and reproductive rights, and I think that AIDS is a symptom of that problem.

It is extremely difficult for women to negotiate with their husbands after safer sexual behaviour. In practice, women find it not easy subject even to discuss sex with their husbands, let alone encourage them to adopt safer practices such as the use of condoms (except perhaps as a method of contraception) The threat of HIV and AIDS has led MASUM to alter the emphasis in the way sexual issues are debated. In the past, according to MASUM, great emphasis was placed on women as the hapless victims of sexual abuse and exploitation by men, thus reinforcing their feelings of helplessness. MASUM now advises women to insist on their sexual rights within the family and the wider community, and to negotiate with their sexual partners about the most suitable and safest forms of sexual behaviour. MASUM encourages women to be assertive (without being aggressive), not submissive in the face of male exploitation and abuse. Manisha Gupta says, 'The major emphasis in all our projects are a means to that end.'

Development Priorities

MASUM at present works among women from the poorest communities in about 30 villages. All its programmes are oriented to help women overcome social, economic and sexual exploitation. A

Savings and Credit Scheme makes loans to women not considered credit-worthy by banks, who otherwise would have to borrow money from moneylenders at high interest rates. A handloom centre and two tailoring courses provide groups of women with a regular source of income. MASUM also arranges monthly meetings with the women, few of whom are accompanied by their husbands, to debate issues such as changes in economic and agricultural policies that will affect their lives. Such issues include, for instance, the effects of patenting seeds and medicines by MNCs. Women also learn about how the government is structured and how it works, how elections are held, and their voting rights. Once a month, 25 college students come from Pune and work as volunteers for MASUM, for instance, by conducting slide shows on sexual and reproductive health for groups of women. The volunteers also help women to defend their human rights, for instance, by filing court cases on behalf of women who have suffered sexual violence from men. In the village of Malshiras, about two hours drive from the Health Centre in Saswad, MASUM runs a Rational Drugs Counter, the *Lokseva Aushadhalay*, which sells primary drugs under their generic names. Prices are kept low—about 20 per cent of the market price. Condoms are also given free. Attached to the drugs counter is a Pregnancy Care Centre, which assists women to prepare for childbirth; traditional birth attendants and teachers from children's day care centres are also imported training in reproductive health and safe, aseptic methods of delivering babies.

Alcohol is way of village life and its misuse often leads to the sexual exploitation of the women, exposing them to the risk of STDs and HIV infection. Over-consumption of alcohol also mars the economic base of the household, forcing women to turn to sex trade and to risk becoming infected with HIV. To counter this menace, MASUM members organised a complete ban on the sale of alcohol in their villages for a period of three years. However, when compaigning for elections started, the candidates and party members started selling alcohol again and sales have continued since. Whenever the occasion arises, groups of women from MASUM also organise hunger strikes, protest marches and public meetings to support particular causes, for instance, in favour of better pay for women farm workers and against sexual molestation of women working in the fields. These activities have not endeared MASUM to local landowners, who consider the new assertiveness of local women as a threat to their interests. All these activities are run by local women themselves, support by a 10-member executive committee with the assistance of local people (including MASUM staff). None of MASUM's running costs are funded by foreign donors. The handloom unit and tailoring courses are financed from the sales of the products they make and by the state government. The savings and credit scheme was initiated with a donation from a private company in Mumbai. Income from the scheme supports the Drug Counter, the Pregnancy Care Centre and the Feminist Health Centre.

Behavioural Changes

Despite the many problems they face, the women of MASUM are starting to have an influence on community attitudes. One positive sign is the outcome of a group of local young men who perform street plays about the problems of deserted women, violence against women, illiteracy and (most recently) AIDS. In 1994 the group won first prize from the Indian Health Organisation for an instructive play about HIV and AIDS. 'We asked ourselves,' says Vasanth, a member of the street theatre group, "what was new about AIDS. We felt it was the hysteria, the putting of people into various categories and saying that they had this or that bad habit. So we thought to write a play which would raise those things.'

Besides winning the prize for their play, the group felt dissatisfied. 'We felt happy about winning the prize, but had we in fact assisted anyone with AIDS? We did not want to just cash in on other people's sorrow. So we thought to upgrade our own social consciousness,' explains Vasanth. The group visited a drug-de-addiction centre to understand the problems surrounding drug addiction, and then spent a day with a group of commercial sex workers trying to know the difficulties in the climate in which they work. The next day they spent with AIDS patients in a hospital in Mumbai.

'That assisted us to understand the people we were talking about in the play,' says Vasanth. 'In the end, those people are more important than the prize we won. Now we feel closer to understanding AIDS from the inside.' To avoid adverse reactions from the villagers, the performers do not hand out condoms at their performances, but advise the participants to ask for them from MASUM staff and government health centres. They plan to distribute condoms, however, when HIV / AIDS is an issue of less controversy.

Since MASUM's inception approximately 10 years ago, its members have been able to initiate and sustain a sometimes painstaking process of social and economic development among rural populations. Their activities are assisting to promote new attitudes and forms of behaviour leading to a social climate in which women are more assertive, and less open to exploitation and abuse. In this new environment, women are also becoming less vulnerable to HIV, as they are gaining greater power to select and to insist on safer sexual behaviour.

The Lawyers' Collective, Mumbai

When human rights lawyer Anand Grover decided to take up the case of Dominic D'Souza, he had no opinion that he was about to become involved in an important piece of legal history. D' Souza, a young man from Goa, was detected as HIV-positive in February 1989, after donating blood to a local hospital. Due to his HIV status, he was arrested and placed in a separate cell by the police, who were acting in accordance with the Goa Public Health Act. The Indian Health Organisation, a Mumbai-based NGO which has played an important role in AIDS awareness and prevention, asked Grover to challenge the terms of Goa Public Health Act, which required anyone considered a public health threat to be placed in isolation. As an eminent member of the Lawyers' Collective—a small group of practising lawyers involved in 'public interest litigation' —Grover had sufficient experience of human rights issues related to housing, the climate, gender and labour relations. On his own admission, however, he knew very little about AIDS at that time, and took up the case with curiosity and apprehension. D'Souza's case, the first of its kind in India, attracted widespread media coverage and soon become a controversy for AIDS activists in India. After 64 days in isolation, D'Souza was allowed to return home, but had to remain there while awaiting the verdict of the court proceedings. Two months after the judges handed down the verdict: the Act would be amended so that it was no longer mandatory to detain people with HIV, but the authorities would still retain the right to do so in 'justifiable cases'. It was a victory of sorts, but it still left the government with the power to detain HIV-infected people. For D'Souza, the probabilities of being imprisoned again for being HIV-positive remained a real threat. Grover took D'Souza's case to the High Court, but the judges ruled to uphold the provisions of the amended Act.

Publicity and Advocacy

The case of Dominic D'Souza opened up a new vista of public service litigation in India. People began coming to the Lawyers' Collective for help with human rights problems pertaining to HIV and AIDS. These included, for instance, issues such as HIV testing and medical confidentiality, and discrimination against HIV-infected people with regard to employment and the custody of children. The Collective also realised that AIDS prevention efforts were being impeded by the fact that certain activities—such as homosexuality, sex trade and injecting drug use—are treated as criminal offences in India. 'We recognised," says Grover, 'that there was little legal experience in these fields. We felt a necessity to share perceptions and experiences with others who would face the responsibility of taking up legal issues arising from the epidemic in the times to come epidemic in the times to come.

Grover and his colleagues also became convinced that there was a dire necessity for new, comprehensive legislation to deal with the multi-faceted human rights issues arising from the HIV epidemic in the country. To place such laws on the statute books, however, is a long and painstaking process. In the meantime, says Grover, 'If no laws are at hand, the lawyer has to be motivated and creative enough to go to the courts and articulate the necessities of HIV-infected people.' The Collective has, thus, set itself the long-term goal of promoting new laws related to HIV and AIDS, which are widely supported by the general public. To help generate a climate of public opinion in favour of such changes, representatives of the Collective compaign persistently, especially through the mass media; they are also involved in lobbying eminent political leaders. Simultaneously, members of the Collective work on several fronts to protect the rights of people with HIV, and also offer them the legal advice and support. The Collective's main HIV/AIDS-related activities consist of:

(a) developing and training a country-wide network of lawyers to take individual cases to court: the Collective trained 25 lawyers throughout the country in 1994, and plans to train at least another 100 during 1995 and 1996;

(b) carrying out court cases on behalf of individuals. Members of the Collective do not charge fees for legal help given to people with HIV or those who are not aware of their sero-status but are compelled to undergo an HIV test—for instance, prior to surgery, or to being appointed in a new job;

(c) organising workshops to frame policies aimed at protecting the rights of people with HIV and their families. The first 'National Workshop on HIV/AIDS Ethics and the Law', held in April 1994, produced a 10-point programme of legal and social reforms aimed at protecting the basic rights of those infected with HIV, and preventing the further spread of the virus;

(d) campaigning for the decriminalisation of homosexuality and sex trade and for the enactment of laws covering issues such as HIV testing, confidentiality of HIV test results, and discrimination against people with HIV.

Few of these efforts have already borne fruit. The Collective's lobbying of political leaders at national level, for instance, helped persuade the government to leave its plans for mandatory testing and the confinement of people with HIV.

Offices

The Lawyers' Collective works from two offices—one in Mumbai and the other in Delhi—with a combined staff of twelve practising lawyers and several law students, journalists and administrative personnel. Routine running costs are covered by income from members. The Collective publishes a journal, *The Lawyers*, which is sent to its representatives in various parts of the country. The cost of producing and distributing the journal is supported by subscriptions.

The Collective is acutely aware of the need for allies and partners in trying to influence the legal system's approach to the HIV epidemic. Its members therefore collaborate with government agencies at national and state level. For instance, a member of the Collective is on the National Legal and Ethical Committee on HIV and AIDS of the National AIDS Control Organisation. The Collective also works in close association with NGOs such as the Pune-based Association for People with AIDS and HIV, and with international organisations such as WHO and UNDP. The Collective's public interest activities (including those not related to HIV and AIDS) are financed completely from the personal resources of the members concerned.

However, as the amount of HIV/AIDS-related work increases

and staff have to travel to other parts of the country to deal with cases, the Collective will have to look for other source of income. The Lawyers' Collective is the first body of professionals in India who have begun jointly to examine how they can use their particular professional skills to respond the challenges of the HIV epidemic. They have set an example for people in other strata of life whose professional skills can also play an important role in preparing Indian society to cope with the effect of the epidemic on health, education, the workplace, the family and other important fields of national life.

Seva Mandir, Udaipur

Every day, about 8,000 trucks ply up and down National Highway No. 8 between Delhi and Mumbai. At different points along the way, rustic tea stalls known as *dhabbas* line the roadside. Day and night, weary truckers pull up for tea, food and a chat, and also to purchase sexual favours from local women. This highway, like others across the country, is therefore major route not only for goods, but also for the spread of STDs alongwith HIV. The truck stop near Udaipur, in southern Rajasthan, is extremely popular with truckers. But the *dhabbas* here now display colourful stickers on the safer sex, and have eye-catching condom dispensers with a ready supply of free condoms. The *dhabba* workers also hand out pamphlets on AIDS to the truckers, and talk with them about protecting themselves against STDs and AIDS.

The AIDS prevention activities at the *dhabbas* near Udaipur were initiated by a local NGO, Seva Mandir, meaning 'Temple of Service': the name exposes the Gandhian thoughts which underlie the organisation's approach to development. For the past 25 years, Seva Mandir has been working with the local tribal people, the Bhil, in a wide variety of rural development priorities. There are not yet many known cases of HIV infection or AIDS in the zone but social, economic and geographical elements combine to make the local population vulnerable to STDs, alongwith HIV. Much of the region has been ravaged by deforestation, climatic degradation and drought. With little or no income from the fields, many of the zone's men have left their families behind and gone to big cities like Ahmedabad in search of work. In the cities, they are increasingly likely to contract HIV and then bring the virus back to their families and communities.

Near the highway, tribal women sell sex to the truckers in order to survive, exposing themselves at risk of contracting HIV, and then passing the virus to their husbands and other sexual partners. Most of these women are not full-time sex workers, but sell sex whenever in need of cash. *Dhabba* workers or other brokers generally negotiate with the women's clients. Besides, this pre-marital and extra-marital sex is common — and widely accepted — among the Bhils themselves. 'STDs are common and condoms are not yet widely used, so HIV infection is bound to exist and spreading', says Ajay Mehta, Seva Mandir's Programme Director. 'We proceeded on that assumption, and we do not think that verifying the presence of HIV is a priority. For Sewa Mandir, however, HIV / AIDS is not just a health issue, but a social malady joined with the endemic development problems of the area. 'We are trying to address both the question of abject poverty and the lack of health awareness, in the hope that the spread of HIV can be decelerated before it assumes epidemic proportions in this area,' says Ajay Mehta.

Conferences

Seva Mandir's AIDS programme commenced in April 1992, with a conference in Udaipur aimed at giving 400 governmental and non-governmental grassroots workers a primary knowledge of HIV and AIDS. To gain public support for the programme, the staff organised rallies in Udaipur and the villages where they worked, holding aloft banners with AIDS messages. Films were shown using an audiovisual van to attract crowds of people, who were then given pamphlets on HIV / AIDS. The following month, Seva Mandir gave new responsibilities to its different cadres of village-based health and development workers, most of whom are part-time volunteers, although some get a monthly stipend for working on a full-time scale. The cadres normally work on a variety of projects, including health, adult literacy, and water conservation through the construction of anicuts (mini-dams) across the rivers and streams. First, six highway contact teams were formed to contact local women, *dhabba* workers and other sex brokers. Each team is headed by a community health worker who lives near the highway and enjoys a good rapport with the *dhabba* workers, brokers and prostitutes. Four village level health workers make up the rest of the team. At the same time, 14 village contact teams', consisting of village level health workers, were formed to visit communities living more than 25 kilometres from the highway.

The team members were trained to debate on the primary facts about HIV/AIDS and STDs, to distribute condoms, and to refer villagers to Seva Mandir's Health Officer for STD remedies. They were then assigned five villages each to visit on a regular basis. Team members travel from village to village, staying for two or three days in each, and discussing HIV/AIDS and other health issues with village leaders and groups of families. They also give small supplies of condoms to those who request them. At night, the team performs a *bhajanmandali* (a kind of traditional folk theatre with music and songs), which they themselves have scripted, explaining how HIV spreads and what one needs to do to protect oneself. They often go to the local *dhabba* and talk to the employees about HIV, AIDS and other STDs.

Team members carry out these and other health or development activities for a few days each month, and resume farming at other days. They are thus always available to their communities for help and guidance.

Programme Coordination

To bring the factor of HIV/AIDS awareness into all its programmes, Seva Mandir has trained all its staff and volunteers in the basic facts about the HIV epidemic. Among the first to be trained were family planning workers and traditional birth attendants (TBAs) who then present talk with people about protecting themselves by abstaining from sex before marriage and fidelity within marriage. They also promote condoms as having different advantages, ensuring contraception and preventing the spread of STDs and HIV, without side effects. We also train the TBA ensuring aseptic conditions during delivery," says Assistant Health Officer Dr Rupshri Bakshi. They now take extra care to protect themselves when mopping up blood spills after delivery and disinfecting the area completely. Most of the women in the villages where Seva Mandir works suffer from STDs.

'We have to strengthen women's capacity and boost their confidence so that they can reduce their vulnerability to sexual exploitation unwanted pregnancy, STDs and AIDS,' says Dr Chandra Bhandari, coordinator of the women and children's development projects. As a first step towards advising women to discuss their problems and share experiences, local women have organised themselves into about 80 groups which meet at regular time intervals. Young people are also being reached with information about HIV/AIDS through Seva Mandir's school health education programmes. Health workers debate problems related to puberty discuss, personal hygiene and sexual responsibility with older students. A workshop for adolescents from the villages as well as those out of school was used to train boys and girls on sex, pregnancy, STDs and HIV/AIDS. Seva Mandir also uses its water conservation and adult literacy projects to convey information about HIV/AIDS to the villagers. 'We knew that AIDS awareness could not work in isolation,' says Ajay Mehta, 'so we have made it an important feature of our economic development programmes. We explain in simple terms how falling ill with AIDS will endanger people's productivity in the field and so reduce their incomes.'

Seva Mandir's AIDS programme at present covers about 200 villages and is carried out by project workers as part of their normal duties. The formation of the highway contact teams and village contact teams has helped to sharpen the focus on HIV/AIDS and to ensure that condoms are available for the villagers whenever needed.

Constraints and Their Removal

The first difficulty in starting the programme was in convincing Seva Mandir's own staff that HIV/AIDS would soon generate huge problems in the communities where they were working. It was not surprising that this was difficult, since nobody from Seva Mandir had ever seen anyone with HIV and AIDS: 'It took a great deal of motivating on our part to convince them that they owed it to their communities to act before it was too late,' says Seva Mandir's Health Officer, Dr. Lodha. Seva Mandir thus included HIV/AIDS literacy in its STD prevention, family planning and reproductive health priorities. The workers taking part in these programmes had seen and were familiar with STDs and understood that the same behaviours were responsible for spreading HIV. Workshop were held to help workers open up to the prospect of having to talk about sex in very explicit terms.

The programme also faced other difficulties. Prostitutes and their brokers, who felt that Seva Mandir's AIDS programme threatened their profession, were initially hostile. With skilful handling, however, an uneasy truce has been reached. There was no problem, however, with the *dhabba* owners and their workers, who were soon convinced of the vital role they could play in preventing the spread of HIV and other STDs. Every three or four months, Seva Mandir's community health workers take out questionnaires to the villages where they work and complete them, based on debates with village people. This helps Seva Mandir evaluate the efficacy of its HIV/AIDS priorities. So far, the responses are usually encouraging: 'People now are aware of AIDS, and know the dangers of high risk behaviour', says Dr Lodha. 'Group debates with the villagers and *dhabba* workes reveal that condoms are being demanded and used increasingly. In the beginning, there were problems with the disposal of condoms after use, but villagers are learning to discard used condoms into pits.'

Seva Mandir's AIDS programme is not separately financed, but utilizes small amounts from the money allocated for its other purposes. Plans are underway to extend the programme to all 500 villages covered by Seva Mandir's development projects. It is hoped that approximately 1,000 part-time workers, all of them inhabit in the villages and 200 full-time workers will be included in the programme. Seva Mandir has used its long-standing relationship of mutual trust with the communities through its AIDS programme where it works to promote more responsible sexual attitudes and safer sexual behaviour. The programme is associated with the Mandir's development projects, which have helped rural population to achieve a lot of economic and social progress. The staff and village-based volunteers carrying out the HIV/AIDS literacy programme are the same as those involved in Seva Mandir's other health and development projects. The varying social climate brought about through the programme is helping to give individuals and communities the choice of breaking away from high-risk sexual behaviour, and to choose other forms of sexual expression which greatly lessen their probabilities of becoming infected with HIV.

SHARAN as well as SAHARA

In a Nizamuddin slum in New Delhi Mushtaq's hands move swiftly over the wall, fingers searching frantically in the dark crevices between the old bricks. He pulls at something, a plastic syringe with no needle. Cursing, he replaces it. The next crevice proves lucky. The much used, blood-stained, but intact needle and syringe trembles in his hand. Mushtaq pulls out a vial from his hip pocket and fills the syringe. Picking up a dirty rag from the rubbish heap nearby, he rubs it over the veins on his left hand and injects himself. Withdrawing blood back into the syringe a couple of times in order not to waste a drop of the drug, he mops up the bleeding with the rag and thrusts syringe, needle and rag into the nearest crevice he can find and vanishes into the darkness. In 1986 SHARAN (sanctuary), an urban development NGO which runs a health clinic in Nizammudin discovered there were a number of heroin users in the neighbourhood. Low-grade heroin had become readily available in the slums and large numbers of slum dwellers were smoking the drug. By 1990 the scenario had begun to show even more serious trends. Unable to buy expensive heroin, slum dwellers were switching to an injectable painkiller, Buprenorphine (trade name Tidigesic) that was only one-fifth of the cost. Often Buprenorphine was mixed with anti-allergy drugs or sedatives. Few of these drugs are frequently prescribed and can readily bought over the counter with no questions asked. Similar epidemics of injecting drug use were occurring in other large Indian cities such as Kolkata, Chennai and Bangalore as well as in other slums in Delhi. In the Northeastern state of Manipur, media reports reveal of an HIV/AIDS epidemic amongst injecting drug users.

Programme Initiation

In 1990, SHARAN decided to become involved in HIV prevention, after a needs assessment survey in Nizamuddin revealed an alarmingly high level of injecting drug use and a very low level of HIV/AIDS knowledge and awareness within the community. Scenes of desperate drug users picking up discarded syringes from rubbish dumps were common. Many had sores, thick scar tissue and blocked or collapsed veins, and few did not carry their injecting equipment with them for fear of arrest or harassment. Syringes were hidden in nooks and crannies wrapped in polythene packs or bloodstained pieces of cloth and were frequently shared. At first, however, SHARAN's own workers felt that integrating HIV prevention into the organisation's health and community development programmes, at such an early phase of the epidemic in India, was uncalled for. There were criticisms too that the organisation was pandering to the interests and agendas of international donors. 'It took lengthy sessions along with courage of conviction born out of our own experiences, especially in Manipur, to convince ourfellow workers', says Project Director Luke Samson.

SHARAN commenced to conduct detoxification camps, in association with a sister organisation, SAHARA (shelter) which already had significant experience of running a rehabilitation and de-addiction centre. Some ex-injecting drug users joined SAHARA House, a totally drug free climate where they were usually successful in overcoming their addiction. For those who returned directly to society, however, the theme was very different: We found that the people we were sending back to society after seven days of detoxification were still highly vulnerable to injecting drugs, and to HIV,' says Jimmy Dorabjee, manager of SHARAN's Drugs and AIDS Programme.

SHARAN's purpose was to promote oral maintenance therapy in which a drug in tablet form is kept under the tongue and slowly absorbed as it dissolves. Research had already shown that Buprenorphine was an effective alternative for heroin and might really assist in the management of heroin addiction. SHARAN started providing injecting drug users with Buprenorphine tablets, taken sub-lingually (kept under the tongue), as a means of weaning them off the injecting practice. The outcomes have been very encouraging: 'We have found sub-linguals to be an effective way of getting people off injections, while providing them with a safe substitute,' says Jimmy Dorabjee.

By March 1996 the project was helping 544 drug users, few of whom were 'chasing' (inhaling) heroin when they joined the programme. Of the 181 who had been injecting drugs, 40 per cent were injecting less occasionally and 45 per cent had given up the habit completely. Those still injecting drugs used their own syringes generally and needles (which they either purchased themselves or got free from SHARAN's drop-in-centre), reducing the risk of transmitting or contracting HIV to a large extent. Of the 53 injecting drug users who joined the programme in early 1993, more than 70 per cent were on oral maintenance therapy or had completely stopped taking drugs.

SHARAN works in close association with the drug rehabilitation centre, SAHARA, which offers residential care for drug users who want to leave the habit, but are in necessity of the social, emotional and practical support which a small, highly committed community can give. A core group of 9 volunteers, 7 of whom are themselves ex-drug users, assists in the every day running of the centre. 'When our first HIV-positive member joined SAHARA, he was very apprehensive that he might not be welcomed by us,' says Harsha, one of the SAHARA's volunteers. 'I shared a cup of tea with him from the same cup. He was taken aback.... After that there was no problem.' At start, SAHARA set aside a whole floor for HIV-positive residents. This policy was soon abandoned as it meant that people with HIV, simply by living in a certain part of the building, were in effect obliged to reveal their HIV-positive status. Residents known to be HIV-infected are now cured differently from others, besides receiving a special diet if they wish.'

The SAHARA volunteers and other residents write and produce plays on AIDS, which portray people with HIV in a positive, non-discriminatory manner and also perform these at local schools. The base of SAHARA's programme is spiritual. The day begins with a prayer and ends with devotional songs. Although SAHARA is primarily a Christian organisation, residents are not advised or obliged to adopt Christianity. Sex education promotes abstinence before marriage and mutual fidelity within marriage, but also includes safer sex (including condom use). Soul-searching sessions are carried out to identify issues such as dishonesty to oneself, development of will power and explore areas of strength to give footholds for sustaining safer, more responsible behaviour.

Expanding the Concentration

SHARAN's clinic attends to the primary health necessities of people in Nizamuddin, and is backed up by links to more specialised treatments at hospitals. Besides giving free immunisation to women and children, SHARAN also offers basic primary school education for few children, and assists others gain admission to government schools. Community members play an important role in all SHARAN's activities with staff working mainly as motivators and helpers, rather than as instructors. In the past, SHARAN has widened and intensified the HIV/AIDS programme to include men and women from the general public of the slum area, focussing especially on STD cure and use of condom. (The presence of an STD, especially when there is an open sore greatly increases the probabilities of transmitting or being infected by HIV.)

With encouragement from SHARAN workers, more persons at present seek treatment for STDs at SHARAN's clinic, where staff also advise about the need to use condoms to lessen the chances of becoming infected with HIV or another STD. The clinic gives condoms and SHARAN's outreach workers advise the people within the community — individually and in groups — about their effectiveness in preventing infections and as a method of contraception. These efforts are assisting, albeit in a quiet, low-key way, to overcome resistance to condom use. SHARAN staff reported the increased demand for condoms, from women in particular. In addition, SHARAN counsellors have started a tuberculosis detection and treatment programme, by talking with patients and members of the community about the links between AIDS and tuberculosis.

Challenges Ahead and Outcomes

The controversial nature of SHARAN's oral maintenance therapy programme for injecting drug users has prevented its legal endorsement by the Government of India. This is not easy now for SHARAN to obtain finance for the programme, or to replicate it in other communities where drug injecting behaviour is a grave problem. 'Another problem is that people in these communities find it very difficult to understand HIV/AIDS,' says Project Director Luke Samson. 'They have not come across anyone with AIDS, and people they know with HIV-related diseases seem different to them from someone with tuberculosis or even underfed. Thus, it was initially very difficult for SHARAN to encourage people to change their drug-using and sexual behaviour. The problem has been partly overcome by concentrating on the problem of STDs, which are a common experience within the slums. By encouraging community members to seek STD cure, to use condoms and to avoid injecting drugs, the probabilities of HIV transmission are being reduced.'

Growing numbers of community members know that the HIV epidemic is not a vague threat, but an imminent reality. During the periodic discussions within the community, SHARAN staff have found people increasingly interested in asking about HIV/AIDS, and in discussing the likely effects of the epidemic. Most importantly, peoples are starting to realise that, through individual and community action, they can protect themselves against HIV and assist others to cope with its effect on their lives.

Social Awareness Service Organisation (SASO)

'We already have an epidemic of AIDS, and we are seeing children are now exposed who have got HIV from their mothers,' says Umesh Sharma' a representative of the Social Awareness Service Organisation (SASO), in the north-eastern state of Manipur. This small state borders northern Myanmar and the region which is the world's largest supplier of opium and heroin. Home to 33 tribes who traditionally smoke these drugs for medicinal and recreational purposes, who inject heroin, approximately 90 per cent of whom are estimated to be infected with HIV. SASO was set up in February 1992 by a group of committed volunteers with the following objectives:

(a) To achieve the social upliftment of its members and their communities.
(b) To engender discipline and courtesy amongst its members to create a healthy image.
(c) To help relief work during natural calamities like flood, famine and drought by providing volunteers and contributing financial help.
(d) To share the grief of its members in case of sickness and accidents.
(e) To promote culture, education, science, sports and other social activities.

As part of its programmes, SASO assists to create public awareness of the dangers of drug addiction, alcoholism and AIDS, to remove discrimination and to provide health care and psychological support to those in need.

Introduction

Manipur's HIV epidemic takes place against the background of ethnic unrest that exists in the state since 1980. Existing political instabilities, inter-tribal disputes and shortage of monetary resources allow limited options to young people. Large-scale heroin trafficking from Myanmar via Manipur to other parts of India has increased the vulnerability of young people to drug abuse.

In 1990, approximately 54 per cent injecting drug users in Manipur were HIV-positive, the state was promptly dubbed the 'AIDS Capital of India.' The government of Manipur responded by incarcerating injecting drug users, many of whom were brought to prison by their own parents. It also banned the sale of hypodermic syringes, prompting drug users to resort to riskier selections such as needles attached to ink droppers. But these make-shift syringes expelled merely one-third of the drug they were loaded with. As a result, users had to pump the droppers several times to inject the full dose. In the process, blood was repeatedly sucked back into the droppers, which were then handed to the next user without sterilisation.

Herculean Task

Discrimination against injecting drug users intensified in 1990, when newspapers reported attacks on them by terrorists. 'Many of us were afraid to come out into the open and seek advice or help,' says Chandra Babu, a former injecting drug user. 'But we wanted to be accepted and show that we ourselves could alter the manner we were being perceived.' To get exposed a healthier image of former drug users and win public support for their cause, SASO commenced to organise concerts and sporting events. In July 1992, for instance, SASO organised a concert with the theme 'Say No To Drugs', which started with advice on drug use, alcoholism and the problems associated with it.

A little later, with finance raised from previous concerts, and with support from the Manipur State Social Welfare Board and and the Government of Manipur, SASO conducted a seven-day programme on drug use and AIDS for youth and parents in various districts of the state. The programme used the expertise of the prevailing de-addiction and rehabilitation centres in Imphal, the capital city. In 1993, SASO obtained support from OXFAM for a one-year project on HIV/AIDS. The members developed a street play about the problems of drug use and AIDS, which was staged every fortnight and drew large audiences. After the play, members advised the audience of the necessity to avoid stigmatising people with AIDS. Members of SASO have also written articles on drugs and AIDS in print media.

One SASO member says, 'In the play, we question the attitudes of people. Many people with HIV have died as they were refused medical cure. We try to tell the people that drug addiction is not a crime, but a habit that can be changed with help' he adds. Every year, during Holi—the spring festival which is celebrated in North India—SASO conducts a marathon race and an arm-wrestling tournament in memory of their friends who have died. Other particular events have included a 73 kilometre cycle rally with the theme 'Cycling—Better than injecting drugs', and a musical production on the theme 'Fight AIDS—not people with AIDS.' The funds raised were used to buy medicines and food for drug users in prisons and people with AIDS.

Advice and Encouragement

SASO offers a counselling service at its office for injecting drug users, HIV-infected people and their families. Persons are given the telephone numbers and addresses of SASO volunteers, or the names of hotels and restaurants where volunteers can be contracted at the time of need. SASO staff and volunteers also go to clients and their families at home to give practical, moral and social support. In the Sajiwa Central Jail in Imphal, where several injecting drug users and HIV-positive people are imprisoned, SASO workers are busy with counselling the inmates. 'We talk about the necessity for injecting users, whether infected with HIV or not, to support one another,' says one volunteer. 'We advise them to adopt safer behaviour, such as using bleach to clean their injecting equipment, to avoid sharing needles and to adopt safer sexual practices.' Since March 1994, SASO has also operated a round the clock telephone line. The service is run by workers who answer queries on drug use and HIV, and advise the callers to come to the SASO office for counselling and further help.

Structure

SASO has about 100 workers, 30 of whom work full-time, in various parts of Manipur. A managing committee of 11 workers handles the everyday activities of the organisation. Which finance from OXFAM, volunteers have been trained to debate HIV/AIDS and to offer primary nursing care for people with AIDS.

Inside the confinement ward of the Jawaharlal Nehru Hospital in Imphal, SASO workers counsel patients with HIV infection and help the nursing staff take care for them. Once the patients are discharged, volunteers see them at home every week. 'At times we pay for the medicines, X-rays or blood tests they require if the family is too poor,' say Umesh Sharma. 'But we are facing the problem of growing numbers of people with AIDS who need to be cared for in their own homes, but are too poor to meet the costs.'

To take care of people with AIDS, SASO seeks the assistance of government doctors as well as some private practitioners. In 1994, the organisation became an associate NGO in the Continuum of Care Project. This initiative is a joint venture of WHO, the National AIDS Control Organisation, local hospitals and NGOs, to initiate a care and suport system spanning health care networks homes and the community.

In a very short time, SASO has proved that it is possible for persons with HIV to initiate and sustain programmes to assist themselves.

Besides this, by reaching out to the general public, they are assisting to lessen the stigma attached to HIV/AIDS. They are thus helping to generate social climate in which all sections of society are mobilised to respond to the HIV epidemic in a spirit of mutual solidarity, rather than with ill-informed panic, blame and fear.

The Mother Saradadevi Social Service Society

The hilltop temple of Lord Muruga, the presiding deity of the town of Palani, near Madurai is thronged by innumerable pilgrims, as the day breaks over the town. The popularmost pilgrimage centre in Tamil Nadu, Palani is the heart of old and new. The burgeoning influx of pilgrims responds to a wide variety of shops, hotels, restaurants, lodges and tourist cottages near the temple.

At the same time, like many other temple towns, sex trade in Palani has boomed. Although sex trade is officially illegal in Tamil Nadu, women from the vicinity come into the town to sell sex in the evenings. To be safe from the vigilance of the local police, they do flesh trade in places that are deserted at night.

The number of people in Palani infected with HIV is not known. However, as a temple town and the centre of a huge vegetable producing area, Palani is a centre for many thousands of temple visitors, traders, truckers and agricultural labourers. HIV is definite to be present and likely to be spreading rapidly within the public.

Prasanna Raja, secretary of the Mother Saradadevi Social Service Society in Oddanchatram, a small town an hour's drive from Palani says, 'We are aware that hospitals in the towns of Madurai and Dindigul were seeing large number of persons with HIV infection and AIDS'. 'We know that we had to do something amongst the communities we were working with. What we had thought a problem of Chennai really came at our own doorstep.' he adds.

Established by Prasanna and her husband Raja in 1988, the Society is named after the wife of the well-known Hindu spiritual leader, Ramakrishna Paramahamsa, who attracted a large following in the early part of the twentieth century. Saradadevi was a leader in her own right, who carried out progressive work in promoting women's education and the rights of widows. The Society works on a variety of health, climate and economic development activities for women of various religious faiths.

The Project

The Society's AIDS project was set up in Palani and the village of Porulur 90 kilometres away, in January 1994 at the same time. Its objectives are:

(a) To enhance the level of information about STD/HIV/AIDS among women in sex trade and women living in the slums.

(b) To increase the women's awareness about safer sex.

(c) To increase the women's utilization of condoms.

(d) To uplift the women's consciousness regarding their health.

(e) To offer the women with STD/HIV/AIDS prevention and support services like STD treatment facilities.

The project is co-ordinated by Prasanna and Raja, with two counsellors, who are professional nurses. A group of twenty 'animators', mostly women, complete the team. 'All the animators have completed primary school,' says Prasanna, and as all are married, they are less inhibited about debate on STDs and HIV. Also, they have greater credibility. People accept advice on sexual matters from married men and women more than from single young people, whom they find easy to dismiss.'

Elementary Structure

The two coordinators started after training the animators in manners of communicating programmes about HIV/AIDS and STDs. The week-long training course also included debates that assisted the animators to enhance their understanding of their own sexual behaviour, their behaviours to sex, and the specific problems women face pertaining to exercising influence over sexuality and reproduction. The coordinators also emphasised to maintain a non-judgemental attitude while working with women in sex trade. The coordinators began by selecting low-income women, especially women who spent at lest part of the year in sex trade setting up a good rapport with them and befriending few who became 'key' informants. The animators visited the women daily to understand the types and extent of risky sexual behaviour that were prevalent and existing beliefs and attitudes to HIV/AIDS. At the same time, they tried to understand the manners in which the women were vulnerable to STDs as well as HIV.

The animators came to know that several women from both urban and countryside areas had more than one sexual partner. Few of them, also had sexually transmitted diseases. A significant number sold sex due to poverty. Few of the women who sold sex were 'family women': they lived with their families and sold sex without the awareness of other family members to supplement family's tiny income. Wives were occasionally the target of physical and sexual abuse by their husbands, few of whom also had sex with other women, including prostitutes.

Though the animators were initially met with doubt, their non-judgement behaviour to the women's sexual lifestyles, alongwith their persistence, eventually paid off. Besides this many of the women were already familiar with the work of the Society, whose income-generating schemes and other programmes for women had won it enough respect in the area.

At weekly staff meetings, the animators shared their experiences, documenting their progress by recording the numbers of women they had visited and the STD cases they had detected. Using locally available materials such as tamarind seeds, flowers of food grains, each animator kept a visual record of the women they conversed with and the STD cases they came to know.

The animators explained their work during the previous week, including the problems they encountered. Other animators then put questions and the group tried to find out the possible solutions. This overcame the difficulties of transferring 'solutions' given by superiors directly to the field, which is fairly common with many NGOs. It also provided the animators more confidence in their own strength to identify and solve problems in implementation.

After some initial reticence, the animators became comfortable about discussing sexual activities that helped spead of HIV. They also found it easier to exchange about how both men and women could alter their behaviour to protect one another from HIV and other STDs. 'We found the staff gaining in confidence,' says Raja. 'They valued their work and became responsive to the difficulties of the women. This encouraged them to overcome these difficulties in an environment of healthy competition.'

Participatory Rural Appraisal

The society's main operational strategy is the establishment of women's group, which enable women to work together to have more say in the decisions affecting their lives. 'The setting up of women's group is the primary task of our work,' says Raja. 'Implementing a project without this factor would be like setting a boat on the river without oars.' Within the first six months of the project, 50 women's groups each with 20 to 25 members — were set up. Each group now meets regularly to discuss problems related to income, health, children, sexuality and the attitudes and sexual behaviour of their husbands and other sexual partners.

In assisting women's groups to get started, the Society realised that Participatory Rural Appraisal (PRA) approach was very useful. PRA is method of enabling communities themselves to define, evaluate and influence their economic, climatic, health, and educational status. To do so, it employs tools which display information visually. 'We extended this tried and tested approach to our AIDS work and it has been very significant,' says Prasanna. The following PRA exercises have been particularly useful:

Mapping

This exercise helped the women to understand what facilities were available in their area, and also assisted to motivate women to set up their own groups. The women drew a map of their town or village on the ground with powdered chalk and added features such as schools, houses, temples, hospitals and water pumps. Using neem or tamarind seeds, they counted the number of men, women and children in their area and discussed the work done by each.

The exercise led the Society to identify women in sex trade and to verify their findings by cross-checking with key members of the community.

Seasonal Analysis

This exercise assisted the women understand how seasonal variations in their income affect their sexual vulnerability. In urban areas, during the festival months, a large part of the women's earning comes from selling fruits, flowers, pictures and *pooja* articles to pilgrims. Between festivals, many women adopt prostitution to maintain their income. In countryside, women earn sufficient during the months when there is lot of work for both men and women in the fields. During the dry months from April to September, there is little agricultural work left to do, so the men go to the adjoining state of Kerala, where extra labour is needed in the fields. The women are left behind in the villages and many of them adopt prostitution to sustain the household till September. 'This analysis greatly assisted us anticipate and plan for STD treatment and condom distribution as per the requirement of the seasons.' says Satyabhama, an animator.

Trend Change

In this exercise, the women analysed the changes they had experienced in their lives pertaining to work, illness, family planning, child bearing and sexual relationships. The exercise was done in small groups of two to three persons to help the free exchange of information related to sex. These laid the foundation for one-to-one debates between animators and women in sex trade. Through the exercise, the women found the underlying reasons for the spread of STDs and HIV as well as the impact of male sexual behaviour, the influence of cinema and the role played by modern transport facilities. However, they also understood that preventing an HIV epidemic would necessitate cooperation of the whole community, in particular of the men.

This encouraged many women to try to discuss HIV, AIDS and STDs with their husbands and other sexual partners and to cure their STDs. Few of them began to try to encourage their husbands and other sexual partners to use condoms.

Timeline

The aim of this exercise was to assist women and the Society members to be aware of the history of their village or town, religion, festivals, customs and beliefs. The process was useful in understanding the relationships between sex trade and caste, religion and local politics resulting in the discussion that cleared up some misunderstandings about women in sex trade and also assisted to promote caring attitudes and better self-esteem among the participants.

Wealth Ranking

In this exercise, the women laid down the criteria for rich, middle class and poor families and classified themselves into these groups. It was revealed that amongst the poorer families, there were more women who turned to prostitution and Society staff decided to spend spare time with these women. STDs were also detected to be the highest amongst these women and their husbands. The exercise also assisted the society to give the most vulnerable women opportunities and training for other means of livelihood.

Venn Diagram

This exercise was used to understand the women's relationships with the police and health facilities. The women debated over police harassment, and their reluctance to seek STD cure at government-run primary health centres, where the staff often subjected them to ridicule and humiliation. This prompted the Society to intensify the STD services offered by its own health centre and to send one of its nurses to help part-time at the STD clinic of the Palani government hospital.

Matrix

The decision-making matrix exercise helped the women and the staff of the Society to recognise the decision-makers within the women's families and why. The exercise also assisted the women to discuss inequalities in their sexual relationships with men and to identify manners of persuading their sexual partners to seek STD treatment, if need arises, and to use condoms regularly. The PRA approach enabled the women—who are illiterate to understand their economic, social and physical vulnerability to HIV and AIDS in about six months. The exercises had a profound effect on the women's attitude towards themselves:

'When they know that STDs did not originate in their bodies, but were passed to them by their husbands or clients, they realised there was no need to feel guilty or ashamed,' says Raja. 'They became confident when they learnt that STDs could be easily and inexpensively cured, or, better still, prevented by using condoms. Many of them had never seen a condom before.'

The Approach

Using the PRA theory, the Society identified neighbourhoods where the men needed to be sensitised to HIV/AIDS. The staff visited these neighbourhoods frequently holding video shows of popular films to attract crowds. They talked about HIV/AIDS and issued pamphlets and condoms. Members of the women's groups reported that these meetings were assisting to make local men aware of the dangers of risky sexual behaviour, and of the necessity to use condoms to protect themselves, their wives and other sexual partners. Home visits by the animators and counsellors have also assisted to motivate women who are not group members to seek cure for their STDs. The Society's workers also explain how condoms can prevent STDs and emphasise their importance in protecting people from HIV infection. Using a banana as a model, the animators showed how condoms should be worn. 'Some of the women attempt the demonstration themselves,' says Usharani, an animator. 'The 250 women in sex trade here in the town take about 25 to 30 condoms every week. The members of the rural groups take about 10 to 15 condoms each every week from us, but still shy away from talking about condoms in the group meetings.

The number of condoms distributed each month is rising gradually. After a year of the project, women involved in sex trade started coming to the animators' homes to take condoms whenever the need arises. A women's group in one area also took a joint decision to follow a 'no condom — no sex' policy with their clients. With finance from the South India AIDS Action Programme, the Society has also set up a truckers project at the Oddanchatram check post, which covers Gandhi Market, famous for its vegetables and butter. Truck drivers now take about 1,000 condoms every month from the iron pots placed in the area's petrol stations. Besides this, an animator from the Society visits the groups of truck drivers early each evening to discuss about STDs, HIV/AIDS and condom use. Using a banana, he shows how to use condoms; he also gives condoms and replenishes the supplies in the iron pots. It is not yet possible to identify people with HIV/AIDS in Palani Taluk (sub-district) but it is only a matter of time before the burden of sick and dying people starts to make its presence felt. Plans are being made to provide home- and community-based counselling, alongwith care and support for women with HIV and their children in Oddanchatram.

Confronting the Resistance

First, the project faced a lot of resistance from local political leaders, who thought the Society was encouraging the formation of women's groups in order to weaken the influence of the political parties. The problem was overcome when the project staff visited local political leaders to explain their plans and to seek their cooperation. Initial reluctance on the part of the animators to talk about specific sexual matters had to be overcome through special training sessions. In few cases meetings with their parents or husbands were also necessary. The animators also had to put up with taunts from men in the areas where they worked, who nicknamed them 'balloon sellers' as they regularly distributed condoms. To overcome this problem, the Society obtained the cooperation of the police, and also introduced uniforms and identity cards for the animators to make their work more official.

Outcomes

The Society also assists women to overcome their vulnerability to social and economic exploitation by helping them to increase their earnings. In association with the state government, the Society has distributed 35,000 fruit tree seedlings to women farmers and has enabled 45 women to be trained as radio, television and computer mechanics. The Society also imparted vocational training to 20 women sex workers who did not want to remain in the trade. These women now do tailoring, manufacture leather goods and make knit wear garments for export in the adjoining town of Thirupur.

The representatives of the women's groups have recently started to reach out to others like themselves, to make one another aware of the sexual dangers to which they are exposed to have their STDs cured and to encourage their husbands and other sexual partners to use condoms. The Society's aim is for the 50 womens' groups that have been set up to be registered as societies in their own right, which will enable them for government finance. Each member at present contributes 100 rupees per month to her group. If a group collects 15,000 the state government will contribute equal amount. This will qualify the members together to start small income generation programmes like poultry farming:

'Money will assist to align them together,' says Prasanna, 'and in the times to come it will also make them self-dependent and less vulnerable to HIV.'

Lessons Learnt

AIDS is a preventable medical phenomenon. People may become safe from HIV virus which is the cause of AIDS through behaviour which prevents or minimises the risk of HIV transmission. In essence, this behaviour can be summarised as follows:

(a) Sexual transmission of HIV can be eliminated in a number of ways: by completely avoiding the sex, by mutual fidelity between uninfected partners, by non-penetrative sex, or by the use of a condom with every act of sexual intercourse. It can also be reduced to a large extent through the prompt and effective cure of other STDs which greatly increase the occurrence of HIV transmission.

(b) HIV transmission through drug use can be eliminated by not injecting drugs, by not sharing drug-injecting equipment with others, or by disinfecting equipment before re-use thoroughly.

(c) HIV transmission within medical institutions can be overcome by the screening of all blood products used in transfusions, by limiting blood transfusions to essential cases only and by global infection control techniques. These techniques include, for instance, the use of latex gloves, washing the hands before and after attending a patient, and the safe disposal of needles and syringes.

There is no doubt that suitable information about how to overcome HIV, a reliable supply of qualitative condoms (free or at low cost), accessible STD cure services, and safe alternatives to shared drug-injecting equipment are important to a large extent in any HIV prevention strategy.

The availability only of suitable advisory services does not necessarily mean that people will use them. Until people feel that the *desire* to protect themselves and those they love from AIDS and simultaneously feel *empowered* to change their behaviour, simply giving information and services will not make a great difference to the spread of HIV. For people engaged in uncontrolled economic, social or sexual relationships the mere availability of free condoms may be totally in significant.

Environment

For non-governmental organisations, the important questions are how they can help to generate the individual and collective will for behaviour change and also help to encourage individuals and communities so that they can avoid the social, economic and cultural issues which eliminate such behaviour change.

The organisations discussed in this work are addressing these questions by assisting to generate a social climate in which safe (or safer) behaviour is encouraged and supported and unsafe behaviour is discouraged. To attain these objectives, they are going beyond the provision of information and services and working with communities to change the prevailing attitudes, values and the manners in which relationships in society are structured. It has been identified that disadvantaged and marginalised groups are most vulnerable to HIV. Women, who are biologically more vulnerable to HIV as compared to men, are also less able to protect themselves from the virus by insisting on condom use or deny to have sex with their husbands or other partners. A major proportion of Indian women are thus at high risk of becoming infected with HIV through their husbands, who are likely to have other sexual partners working in the nearby towns and cities. Many Indian non-governmental organisations are experienced at reaching and supporting disadvantaged groups, offering them advisory services, and also assisting them to organise themselves to express their needs, insist on their rights and improve their well-being. These skills can also be used to help empower disadvantaged groups like low-income women, migrant workers, refugees, injecting drug users, prostitutes and HIV-infected people — to organise themselves, improve their economic position and protect themselves from HIV. Such AIDS programmes are not a diversion from more urgent health or development issues. On the contrary, they are a positive contribution to development by assisting to empower the poor and the disadvantaged with at least some of the information, framing services, self-confidence and bargaining power they require to take greater control of their own lives.

Other Priorities

Indian NGOs vary to a large extent in their purposes, objectives, size, strategies, geographical scope and fields of activity. The types of programmes they can organise in support of HIV / AIDS awareness and prevention are also many and varied:

(a) ***Women's organisations*** can give primary health care services (as well as STD cure and the supply of condoms): run income generation and vocational training activities: set up savings and loan schemes: campaign against the physical and sexual abuse of women; and assist to set up and sustain local women's groups to promote the concerns and rights of their members.

(b) ***Legal aid agencies*** can use the existing legal system to defend the basic human rights of people with HIV and their families, working simultaneously for changes in legislation (e.g., the repeal of laws which criminalise homo-sexuality) to promote HIV prevention and outlaw discrimination against HIV-intected people (e.g., within

the workplace).

(c) ***Development organisations*** may offer a wide variety of health, social and educational services; set up employment and income generating schemes; campaign against the stigmatisation of people with HIV; and assist local people resist activities (such as the destruction of forests) which result in marginalised groups (like tribal people) losing their main source of income, and having to go to urban areas or turn to sex work to survive.

(d) ***Intermediary or support organisations*** can impart training, research, advocacy, documentation, information dissemination and networking for non-governmental organisations carrying out HIV/AIDS awareness, elementary care at community level.

(e) ***Hospitals and health centres*** can ensure that all their services involve the absolute minimum of risk of transmitting HIV to patients and staff. They can also give confidential, voluntary HIV counselling and testing; train their own workers to cure HIV-infected persons without discrimination; disseminate information about HIV and AIDS to patients and members of the community, provide patients with prompt treatment for STDs and HIV-related illnesses and train family members to look after the people with AIDS within the home.

(f) ***Trade unions*** (not, strictly speaking, non-governmental organisations but similar to them in many respects) can train educators from among their own members; campaign for medical secrecy, job security and non-discrimination with HIV-infected persons at the workplace; lobby for a reliable supply of free (or low cost) condoms at the workplace and organise workshops and training schedules on HIV/AIDS, sexuality and the workplace.

(g) ***Professional groups*** like associations of teachers, employers, health workers, advocates, film producers and mediamen can draw up codes of professional conduct for their members; they can also organise workshops and seminars to develop practical programmes in support of HIV/AIDS awareness elimination, care and support, both within their workplaces and in the society at large.

(h) ***Community-based organisations*** such as people's committees, associations of stigmatised persons like sex workers, homosexuals and injecting drug users as well as groups of disadvantaged people like Scheduled Tribes and Castes may associate with other non-governmental organisations to advise their members about HIV and AIDS; lobby the government for programmes as STD cure and access to condoms; resist physical and sexual abuse of women; campaign for respect and acceptance of their members; and fight economic exploitation by campaigning for the payment of minimum wages to both women and men, and the regulation of traditional land rights.

(i) ***Social welfare agencies*** may offer economic and social support to marginalised groups like refugees, old people who have lost their relatives, injecting drug users, and children orphaned by AIDS.

(j) ***Support groups*** may enable people with HIV to give mutual, emotional, social and practical support; to educate the population about HIV/AIDS; to campaign through the mass media against the stigmatisation of persons with HIV; and to lobby political leaders for legislative amendment to remove discrimination against HIV-infected persons.

Infected Population

Experience abroad has revealed that people living with HIV are potentially society's most effective AIDS campaigners, educators, counsellors and care-givers. Even without publicly declaring their HIV-positive status, they can contribute their uniquely valuable insights to AIDS elimination programmes, and to self-help care and support groups. If they are able to declare their HIV-positive status frankly the effect of their work can be even greater. Though 'coming out' in this manner is not a decision to be taken lightly: the outcomes can be serious, not just for the person concerned but also for his or her family, neighbours, workmates and friends. As in most countries, some people living with HIV in India have started to organise themselves into support groups. The first such group—the Association for People Living with AIDS and HIV Infection—was set up in Pune in August 1992. The Association gives its members with group therapy and legal advice, and members see one another at home in the event of illness. It also conducts a telephone help line, and carries out networking among similar support groups in India and other countries too.

Such support groups in India still suffer from financial barriers and managerial difficulties. To a large extent this is due to the reluctance of donor agencies to finance care and support work. The primary problem is the stigma attached to AIDS and the discrimination to which persons with HIV are subjected. A large number of people in India who know themselves to be HIV-infected are reluctant to join a support organisation because they are afraid this will lead their HIV-positive status exposed. They remain cut off from the information, care, counselling and support they need, and may continue practising high-risk behaviour. In India, HIV prevention thus necessitates to fight stigma and discrimination.

Programme Initiation

When starting a new programme or activity, there is the need to have a clear understanding of the purpose and objectives of their task and the strategies required to achieve these. In some of the programmes discussed in this chapter, it was necessary first to convince, a sceptical board of trustees of the significance of starting HIV/AIDS work. Generally the programme leaders began by sensitising their own workers to the social and development implications of the disease. This was not always easy: few staff members were initially unconvinced of the significance of HIV/AIDS as a health and development issue in India; others were reluctant to describe sensitive issues such as sexual behaviour, or nervous about distributing condoms and showing their use in public. Few were also uneasy about working with stigmatised groups such as women in sex trade, homosexual men and injecting drug users. Their behaviours changed as they learned more through special workshops, training sessions, role plays, participatory exercises, videos and the sharing of personal experiences. At community level, workers confronted the problem of how to convince people of the necessity for behaviour change, besides Manipur state, AIDS in India is a virtually invisible epidemic at present. Some have overcome this problem by keeping in mind the widespread and readily acknowledged problem of STDs; any form of safe or safer sexual behaviour such as abstinence, mutual fidelity, condom use, non-penetrative sex, etc. that offers protection against STDs is also an effective form of HIV elimination.

Others have used 'respectable' issues such as family planning or gynaecological problems as initiating factors for discussions about sexuality and safer sexual behaviour. Where community workers felt reluctant to distribute condoms, other arrangements like installing condom dispensers or iron pots at *dhabbas* and health centres, or promoting links with health centres that have a reliable supply of condoms were made. Few organisations held open discussions within women's groups on crisis situations as rape, in order to discuss sexuality and devise measures through which women can protect themselves from sexual abuse and infection. Some NGO staff and community volunteers have also written and performed plays that explore social and sexual relationships, injecting a note of humour to break down the visitors resistance to becoming involved. A strategy has been the use by women's groups of participatory rural appraisal exercises to assist members understand their social, sexual and economic situation enabling them to develop their own strategies and activities for changing their lives and protecting their health.

Expanding the Scope

All the programmes discussed in this chapter are new and are growing and changing according to new situations and necessities. Nobody would claim to have developed a perfect strategy; they welcome suggestions about how to make their efforts more effective. A remarkable feature of these programmes is the manner in which NGO staff members readily admit to having experienced 'personal growth', in other words, a marked development of their own understanding of sexuality and human behaviour. All these programmes are in need of a more systematic approach to planning, monitoring and evaluation. They have already succeeded, however, in three important ways:

(a) They have shown how to reach and support sections of the general public like women in sex trade and injecting drug users who fall between the cracks of official AIDS activities because they are stigmatised or living on the margins of 'normal' society and the legal system.

(b) They have shown how community-based organisations.

such as women's groups, can assist economically and socially disadvantaged persons gain greater control over their lives, and so protect their health and well-being.

(c) They have illustrated that NGOs working in different fields as legal aid, rural development and women's health have a common interest in the HIV epidemic as a development issue. Not only have they widened the front against the epidemic, but they have demonstrated how HIV/AIDS programmes can promote development by enabling the poor and disadvantaged to have some control of at least some important aspect of their lives.

In the times to come, broadening the scope against HIV and underdevelopment in India will mean more new collaboration, unlikely alliances and mutual support among a wide variety of NGOs, community groups and other strata of society. It will mean learning from the experiences of others, sharing information and expertise, and replicating successful strategies or adapting them to local circumstances. It will also mean the involvement of sections of society that are not directly health oriented: businesses, government departments, religious leaders, artists, entertainers and political leaders. The HIV epidemic will exert a dangerous toll of pain, suffering and grief on individuals, families and communities globally. But there is no cause for resignation, defeatism or despair. Unlike other fatal diseases, the HIV epidemic gives a unique opportunity for positive social change. The epidemic is teaching us new lessons about sexual behviour, gender relations, human rights, individual and collective responsibility, and community involvement in health care and development. It is also helping to build bridges and forge alliance between the health departments and several other groups, organisations and institutions outside the health sector. When the historians of the 21st century analyse the HIV epidemic, they may well conclude that, paradoxically, HIV has helped to make human society more open and honest about sexuality, more responsible about sexual attitudes and behaviour, more ignorant of social differences and sexual orientation and less exploitative of women and other disadvantaged persons. Whether these inferences can be drawn later in the times to come will depend on the human response to the HIV epidemic at present — in short, on the extent to which stigma, fear, blame and defeatism are replaced by acceptance, caring, solidarity and hope. 'I look at life as an opportunity,' says Shekhar, an HIV-infected man from Chennai, 'an opportunity to leave the world a better place than when I came into it. AIDS cannot steal that opportunity away from me.'

AIDS Bhedbhav Virodhi Andolan (ABVA), New Delhi

ABVA was set up in 1998 by professionals from the fields of education, health, law, etc. Its first priority was to stop the forcible HIV detection of prostitutes in Delhi. Following are a few published reports of ABVA.

(a) *Less than Gay—A Citizen's Report on the Status of Homosexuality in India*
(b) *Needle of Suspicion*
(c) *This Sugar is Bitter*
(d) *Women and AIDS.*

ABVA fought successfully for the withdrawal of the proposed AIDS legislations. In 1992, the first protest was made before the Police Headquarters by ABVA and other organisations to rise against the Delhi Police harassment of homosexuals in Delhi Central Park.

In 1994, media gave attention on Tihar jail where the then Inspector General of Prisons, Kiran Bedi to denied distribute condoms to the male prisoners on the grounds that no homosexual activity prevailed in the prisons, and even if there was, the prison officials would be persuading a crime. ABVA used this incident to file a public interest litigation for the repeal of Section 377 of the Indian Penal Code.

Documentation. Archive. Research. Education. (DARE), New Delhi

A Resource Centre for Lesbians, Gays and Bisexuals. First of its kind in India DARE is a resource centre to create, document and keep handy the information on the same-sex love in a friendly and safe environment to all those interested in the subject. This includes lesbians, gay men, bisexuals and anyone who is associated with it and wants to seek information on it.

As a group of people, DARE cares and hopes to:

(1) create awareness on lesbian and bisexual history in India;
(2) fight negative stereotyping, especially the opinion that homosexuality is a western phenomenon;
(3) inform on legal, health and psychological issues;
(4) persuade research in several fields by offering

bibliographies, source materials and guidelines to scholars; and

5. shape an archive to maintain and visibilise our history.

People's Union of Civil Liberties (PUCL), Bangalore

PUCL is an organisation which, like Citizens for Democracy (CFD) was set up by J.P. Narayan with the primary intention of promoting participatory democracy. The main important task of the organisation is on the social and economic issues of the rural labourers and minorities. The important focus is on women's participation in panchayats and combating the increase in communalism in Bangalore.

Till now, lesbian, gay and bisexual rights have not been on the agenda of PUCl, Mr. Ramdas, a member of the organisation at this workshop stressed that since it was a question of human rights violation, it was within the purview of PUCL's mandate.

5

Indian Response and United Nations

Collaboration and Integration

In 1999, HIV infection affected approximately 3.5 million persons in India. With no state touched, HIV/AIDS continues to illustrate itself to be one of India's most complex epidemics, a Herculean task that goes beyond public health raising fundamental questions of human rights and threatening development achievements in several fields. The necessity to eliminate the epidemic and provide care and support for those infected or affected calls for an unprecedented response from the whole society. The nature of the national response, its urgency, scale and quality, has changed to large extent over time. For an initial late period in the late 1980s and early 1990s, the increasing presence of HIV was met largely with denial or indifference from most political areas. In the mid-1990s, the widespread HIV in the most affected states started to bring about a much greater recognition of the necessity to work in a determined fashion. It has taken until the most recent period, coinciding with the set up of the new phase of the programme for a much greater openness and realism to emerge in facing the difficult problems posed in developing a strong and broadly-based national response to the epidemic.

The formulation of the new national programme places the country on the threshold of a new theory, one marked by a focus on persuading and enabling states themselves to take responsibility to respond to the epidemic. All states are initiating to mobilise, as part of the preparation of the second phase of the national programme. It is also leading to growing partnerships between government, NGOs and civil society. There are still, however, formidable challenges in the times to come, especially in the field of implementation. Emergence of a joint framework for external collaboration in support of national efforts took shape first in May 1998. Debates among all stakeholders stressed the value of evolving a collaborative framework in which each agency could join and yet feel their individual approaches and different contributions find a place. This was followed up in June 1999 by the Mussoorie UN Strategic Planning Retreat where NACO and major bilateral partners participated with the UN system to initiate a joint programme platform for all agencies to work within.

This chapters is based on the outputs of the Mussoorie Retreat. It carries those discussions further in discussing national response as well as the strategic theories that were in agreement with government should shape the external response. It also coordinates specific action plans of the various agencies as part of an 'integrated' workplan for 1999–2001. Recognising the significance of persuading various approaches to meet the diversity of local settings, the framework is deliberately kept wide and flexible as a first step towards harmonising approaches to the HIV epidemic by external partners. It aims to identify the common strategic theories on which plans can be built, encouraging a process of sharing of information and mapping the work of the several agencies. For the UN system, there is a major attempt to focus their collective inputs towards supporting the development of concrete operational 'models' in the fields of the agency's comparative advantage.

The development of this external partnership framework is grounded in the worldwide experience that prevention of HIV works, if any, only if:

(a) effective partnerships among government, NGOs and civil society are at the centre of the response and continually evaluated and refined, and
(b) interventions are based on respect for and maintain the dignity of both vulnerable and affected individuals.

This joint effort by NACO, external partners and the UN system in India is a direct contribution towards these objectives.

Accelerating Pace of Epidemic

The setting in the late 1990s, an epidemic accelerating rapidly and often unpredictably:

Now well into its second decade, India's epidemic is marked by heterogeneity—not a single epidemic but alongwith a number of other epidemics, often co-existing in the same state. Primarily driven by heterosexual transmission, HIV infection is going to increase beyond its initial focus among prostitutes and their sex partners into the general population at large. Simultaneously important sub-epidemics are emerging with potentially explosive expansion among groups of injecting drug users (IDUs), and among Men having Sex with Men (MSM). These have a crucial role associated to the wider heterosexual epidemic and necessitates careful monitoring. The most recent approximation of HIV infection for the country is of 3.5 millions. Aggregate figures for India, however, conceal widely contrasted levels of existence throughout the states:

At peak in the state of Maharashtra HIV has reached 60 per cent in Mumbai's sex workers (SWs), 14–16 per cent in sentinel STD clinics and more than 2 per cent among women attending ante-natal clinics (ANCs). The last four years has seen a broadening of the epidemic throughout the southern and western states of India and the continued concentration of HIV through Injecting Drug users in the north-east. The sharp increases witnessed in Andhra Pradesh and Karnataka disclose that these two states have overtaken Tamil Nadu as states with the highest existing rates. In other parts of India the overall levels of HIV are still low (in few cases nearly zero reporting). High levels of other sexually transmitted diseases (STDs), the evident presence of sexual networks and presence of migration and severe gender discrimination all point to a significant vulnerability. Differences in current levels of HIV prevalence across states are largely a matter of time.

The epidemic also continues to shift towards women and towards the young people with 25 per cent of all HIV infections in India now approximated to be women with an accompanying rise in vertical transmission and pediatric HIV. Such tendencies underline the significance of structural factors in generating vulnerability to infection including:

(a) migration both within and between states as a major (but still poorly studied and understood) source of expansion of HIV between urban and rural populations;
(b) gender discrimination (especially unequal power in

decision making between men and women and the latter's inability to negotiate after sex), alongwith the difficulties faced in communicating openly on sexual matters between generations represent and remain major barriers to prevention;

(c) indications are that a rapid use in injecting drug use is underway with drug users switching from inhaling to over-the-counter injecting drugs. In a recent study conducted in 1999 of 200 injectors linked to a treatment centre in New Delhi, 45 per cent were detected HIV-infected. On HIV among MSM groups, little reliable statistics are available. Informal approximations suggest rapid increases may be taking place in this particularly vulnerable community.

Form and Expansion

India's epidemic seems to be following the so-called Type 4 Pattern, first discussed in Thailand. The epidemic shifts from the highest risk groups (prostitues, drug users) to bridge populations (sex partners of sex workers, STD patients, partners of drug users) and then to the general public. The shift generally occurs where the existence in the first group reaches 5 per cent. There is a time-lag of 2-3 years between the shift from one group to another.

Forecasting the future of an epidemic as complex as HIV will always be difficult especially at the low levels of infection currently prevailing in India. Behavioural surveys (BSS) track behaviours in groups whom the programme is targeting with interventions. Major gaps continue, however, in available knowledge of risk behaviours amongst other important groups especially adolescents or men having sex with men, either as identified gay individuals or understanding the extent of bisexual behaviours. It is obvious that in a country such as ours, even low levels of infection in a population with relatively low risk behaviour can turn into very large numbers of new infections. Significant new elements are on the scene. The burden of AIDS cases is going to be felt in states affected early on in the epidemic. Mumbai in Maharashtra and Manipur report hospital bed occupancy rates from HIV-linked illness ranging from 24–40 per cent in certain referral hospitals. Home-based care is still in its infancy in different parts of the country. Simultaneously, greater visibility and awareness of

HIV has triggered a mixed response from society. While individual examples of support and care are increasingly seen, HIV-positive persons in general have been poorly received by communities. Access to health care is emerging as a critical first point of contact with public and private service for HIV-infected persons and their families and a site of frequent, occasionally blatant, discrimination. Mass campaigns initiated to bring awareness on HIV have inadvertently at times triggered fear and concern among the population.

Countrywide Response

The national response encompasses the efforts of both government and of civil society. These have moved at different speeds at different times in the country. Any evaluation has to take into consideration both the geographical diversity of response and the critical element of time. Broadly though, since its start in 1987, the national HIV programme has moved through three phases:

1986–1992: marked by denial of the threat of HIV to India. This was a time which witnessed the beginning of a largely research-based programme. Surveillance programmes were started in 55 sites in 3 states only, but remained fragmented, programme activities were left to the states to take up without strong central guidance.

1992–1997: First acceleration of the programme, backed by World Bank finance and strong WHO GPA support. This phase witnessed the emergence of the National AIDS Control Organisation (NACO). Achievements included much higher levels of awareness generation, the putting in place of state level structures for programme implementation and improvements in blood safety. The start up of successful individual projects such as the innovative intervention in Sonagachi amongst prostitutes in Kolkata and breakthroughs in reaching out to college youth in University Talks AIDS (UTA), were amongst its achievements. The area of these efforts remained on a limited scale. Political acceptance was weak and 'ownership' of the programme by the states proved difficult to establish. Involvement of NGOs in the numbers and quality needed for sustained interventions proved difficult to get. While an emphasis on blood safety and strengthening of infrastructure yielded some gains, the approach remained primarily medical, with HIV being seen largely as a health issue.

1998 onwards: giving a major focus to targeted interventions. Building on the experience of the first phase, there was a big drive to focus on coverage amongst groups with the highest risk behaviours sex workers (SWs), truck drivers, injecting drug users (IDUs) while widening the approach to a multi-sectoral one. As the current phase of the national programme, has witnessed outcome of a strongly de-centralised programme with responsibility for implementation placed on the shoulders of the states. New more elastic state structures of the State AIDS Societies have been set up with stronger mechanisms for programme magagement at state level, including a strong NGO component of targeted interventions, supported by efforts to mobilise the community around awareness and treatment of STD/RTIs. An innovative approach to providing technical support to state programmes has been started by setting up a network of 12 Technical Resource Groups (TRGs), each covering different thematic fields of the epidemic and mandated to give technical support to the states. Surveillance has been both widened and strengthened. A new national HIV programme has been submitted to the cabinet. With a new round of resources mobilised from Government of India, the IDA, major bilateral donors and the UN system, the programme is moving into a significant dimension of 'implementation'.

The setting up of the new programme has contributed to a growing momentum behind the national response indicated by the prime minister's strong statement to parliamentarians in December 1998 calling for renewed efforts to combat HIV not as a health problem but as a threat to India's development. The country has clearly moved beyond denial, into a new phase of response.

Several challenges remain to be faced. These include building the capacities needed to implement and the strategies of prevention on the scale of a country the size and complexity of India, building a genuinely multi-sectoral response that is sustainable. It also has a major task of mobilising and co-ordinating a wide range of partners, including the private sector. Confronting the many new legal and ethical problems that HIV raises calls for involvement of new actors and strategies alongwith those that can lead to the involvement of affected groups themselves. They underline the necessity for a continuous learning of what works in different settings throughout the country, refinement of strategies and course correction.

Second Phase of National AIDS Control Programme

Building on the lessons from the first National AIDS Control Project, the second phase has five key components:

1. Targeted interventions for communities at highest risk
2. Prevention of HIV transmission among the general population
3. Provision of low cost care
4. Strengthening institutional capacities
5. Intersectoral collaboration.

The project will be implemented under the National AIDS Control Policy which has been framed and approved by the National AIDS Committee. The policy aims to set up an enabling framework to mobilise the capacity of the private sector and of civil society; and laws stress on specific objective of ensuring the protection and promotion of human rights of people living with HIV/AIDS alongwith their rights to equal access to the health care system, education, employment, privacy and other fundamental rights.

The second phase has been started through a participatory process with Government of India, state governments, UNAIDS and bilaterals working in collaboration with community members, PLWAs, industry and labour organisations, NGOs and civil society. Every state and union territory has registered a State AIDS Control Society (SACS) which will be accountable for implementation of the programme at the state level. The cities of Mumbai, Chennai and Ahmedabad have formed the Municipal AIDS control societies to effectively implement the AIDS control programme in these metropolitan cities. Each SACS developed a Project Implementation Plan (PIP) as part of preparation for addressing the second phase which allows for addressing the specific necessities of the state and the epidemic. Key features of the second phase are:

(a) Special delegation of financial and administrative authority to NACO

(b) A greater 'Ownership' of the decentralized programme plans by the states

(c) A criteria for NGOs/CBOs in the implementation of intervention programme with marginalised populations
(d) Involvement of democratic institutions (Panchayati Raj) and youth organisations at the district, block and village level
(e) Involvement of the community in social mobilization and awareness at grassroot levels

Future Challenges

Determination of the big challenges that still face the national programme as it goes into its implementation phase in 1999/2001 was the topic of various focused group discussions among many stakeholders in mid-1999 taking place alongside interviews with key individuals, preceding and culminating in the Mussoorie Strategic Retreat in June 1999. It was a process that led to the recognition of 5 areas that were thought to be crucial or in some way pivotal for the future of the programme, and without which other efforts are likely to be much less effective. This included:

1. The need to build capacities within states rapidly. All states, whether facing advanced or still early epidemics, will require greatly enlarged capacities for programme management, especially in building capacities amongst NGOs and Community Based Organisations (CBOs) to carry out intervention projects in the scale needed. This will necessitate a massive training and capacity building effort throughout the country as well as development of support systems for the implementation of programmes. Technical resources and collaborations to support such an effort to such an extent are not yet available and need to be generated in manners that will be sustainable for the programme period and beyond. New models of collaboration between NGOs/CBOs and government need to be identified and developed.

2. Toensure targeted interventions achieve impact. If the focus on targeted interventions are to succeed, very high levels of coverage and saturation among high risk groups will also need to be achieved. This indicates that information, services and support must reach a very high proportion of the population with the risk behaviour in question and a high percentage of those reached actually adopt safer behaviours. The approaches choosen, however, need to be carefully designed so as not to further contribute to the marginalisation that generates vulnerability to HIV infection. One of the striking lessons of the first phase was that only delivery of services or HIV awareness is not going to be successful in reaching marginalised groups. Unless supportive inputs are given, including policy adjustment, to generate space for self-organisation and persuading more negotiating power of marginalised populations, STD and IEC services alone will not bring behaviour change. The generation of such an 'enabling' climate also includes empowerment processes of the marginalised groups themselves. Ensuring such frameworks are put rapidly in place becomes a major object in itself.

While focusing on people involving the highest risk behaviour, there is increasing need to work with 'bridge' populations, reaching groups such as male sex partners of prostitutes. Such populations at high risk are at times difficult to define or react with interventions and call for different and innovative strategies.

3. Achieving behaviour change beyond the 'high risk'. In the increasing number of states where HIV existence among women attending antenatal clinics is significant and rising, there is a need to go beyond high risk groups and address behaviour change in the general reproductive age-group. This necessary widening of the net includes young people, women, disadvantaged slum populations, migrant labourers, etc. all of whom need to be empowered to protect themselves. The challenge lies in setting up a behaviour change programme that is not limited to awareness generation and fully covers the 'at risk' population. The very size and heterogeneity of these population groups add to the problem of this task. It is also critical that states with presently low epidemics put in place identical programme efforts as present, so they can yield lessons later when the time comes for expansion of such efforts in the general population. The same theories of targeted interventions apply—early intervention; sub-population specific messages; services tailored for sub-population; an enabling policy climate; and involvement of the community. There are as yet however, few tangible strategies at hand in India for reaching these large, often difficult to reach populations.

Innovative efforts are being tried for reaching the population at large through social mobilisation up to the village level for generating awareness and discussion on STD, HIV and sexual health themes and provision of STD services on a 'pulse' approach. Prevalent democratic institutions such as 'panchayats' are playing an important part in such programmes, with important lesson to be drawn for community mobilisation and service demand creation.

4. The need to confront discrimination and stigma. The arguments to handle the stigma that surrounds HIV/AIDS come both from the public health and human rights domains. Stigma discourages persons at risk from seeking HIV testing status to a large extent, thus creating missed opportunities to better target counselling efforts and prevent further transmission. Fear of HIV also translates into overt discrimination against individuals or families infected or believed to be infected with HIV. Stigma related with HIV also unconsciously shaped the IEC strategy in the first phase of the programme emphasising the fear of contact and infection. Against this climate, it is crucial that interventions are initiated that counter such misconceptions and 'normalise' the presence of HIV-infected individuals in the community. Supportive efforts and models are also required to tackle discrimination in health and other primary services. A policy on non-discrimination in the workplace of the private sector is also urgently felt.

5. Addressing the urgency of care and support. The need for care and support services is often only perceived many years after the epidemic has made its entry into a population. Uptil now, this is one of the obvious consequences of the epidemic. With the large numbers already infected in the country, providing large scale non-institutional care becomes one of the greatest challenges of the unfolding epidemic. Piloting such approaches and finding manners so they can meet future needs across the states is urgently felt. If the speed of HIV goes unchecked, there is a risk that India's large investment in and infrastructure of health services will be overwhelmed by the burden of HIV care. It is also unlikely to be able to give the kind and level of care and support needed. There is a need to experiment with alternative theories; in doing so expand community and home-based care, wherever possible involving HIV-positive groups in the dialogue and planning of such interventions.

The above 5 challenges aim to capture what are considered to be critical questions at present. They are also connected to each other, with progress on challenge often contributing to or forming the necessary base for movement on others. They also require to be set within the wider development challenges that the country is facing, and linked to efforts to reduce poverty and expand service provision to disadvantaged groups. These are all areas however where external partners could help national efforts in the recognition of effective strategies and in strengthening the national response. Ensuring that these efforts are collaborative and sharing experiences will shorten the learning curve and the lead-time required to mount effective interventions.

Joint Strategy

The challenges recognised above cut across the work of all external partners. And while each partner is supporting the national programme with their own mandate and modalities of action, they are also playing several roles:

(a) the central government and the IDA loan providing core finance to the states,

(b) major bilaterals (USAID, DFID, CIDA, Ausaid) centering on capacity building at state level and modelling collaboration with non-governmental and other implementing agencies.

(c) the UN agencies largely focussing on specific contributions related to their mandates and mainstreaming HIV with their development partners.

(d) UNAIDS giving support in technical resources to the national programme and working with the cosponsors to deepen their involvement in addressing the epidemic.

An important aim of the national programme is that these various roles and inputs are supplementary and synergistic to each other and continue to be focused in support of the national programme.

Making a common platform for all external stakeholders is a central part of the strategic response. Three components of this common platform are:

(a) ***Each agency defining in their own programmes, suitable response to the five challenges identified.*** Over the last decade, a number of examples of best practices have come at fore. While many of them provide guidelines for the response, the need to be able to scale up to meet the challenges of the epidemic remains. The need also exists for sharing of the lessons learned and for each partner to adapt approaches that suit the programmatic requirements.

By working closely with individual states, major bilaterals are at times in a position to facilitate the adaptation of national policy strategies to state level encouraging innovation and ensuring lessons are drawn out from these experiences. Refining strategies, documenting successes and sharing these lessons learned across states will be a great contribution of the bilaterals. Agencies like UNDP, WHO and UNDCP are working in support of specific aspects targeted interventions. UNICEF/UNFPA/UNESCO work on issues pertaining to behaviour change will also give critical inputs to this process of applying and refining strategies in these 5 areas.

(b) ***Focusing the efforts of the UN system.*** The strengths of the UN system lie in

(i) its programmes of cooperation and links with other ministries and departments;
(ii) in the partnerships it has with civil society and in their access to ideas and experience, both globally and locally;
(iii) in the UN's work in critical crosscutting areas of gender, human rights and broader development strategies such as poverty elimination; and
(iv) the support to the governments efforts to develop partnerships with all members of civil society.

Challenge	*Response/Opportunities*
1. Focussing on strengthening capacities with states	Strengthen state specific surveillance systems Support states in strategic planning and evolving evidence based responses to the

(Contd.)

Challenge	*Response/Opportunities*
	particular stage of epidemic faced Strengthen programme management capacity in states Build capacities to work with non-governmental organisations and civil society Link technical resources in states with the relevant National Technical Resource Group TRGs
2. Ensuring Impact of Targeted Intervention	Evolve common principles of programme design that are shared across all partners (viz. Common conceptual frameworks/ definitions of Targeted Interventions, etc.) Recognise these groups Interventions Evolve lessons from successful approaches to working with marginalised groups, rights and potential for shaping programme actions Ensure sustainability of interventions through community ownership and participation Provide support to scaling up of successful interventions Generate an enabling environment for targeted interventions, addressing wider structural and policy issues
3. Achieving Behaviour change beyond High risk	Pilot new large scale approaches to groups such as youth, migrant workers, etc. Encourage participation of young people and involve them as a programme Evaluate promising approaches and support scaling up Social mobilisation up to the village level to create awareness using, grass root health professionals and prevailing democratic institutions such as 'panchayats' Carry out systematic behavioural surveys

(Contd.)

Challenge	*Response/Opportunities*
	to track behaviour changes, especially among youth
4. Tackling Discrimination and stigma	Develop strong law and ethics components of each state programmes Sensitisation of the media and judiciary Develop innovative interventions against stigma as a programme activity Pilot models in selective public and private services Mount efforts to tackle the double stigma of MSM and HIV Challenge discrimination in language and/or media
5. Addressing the urgency of care and support	Develop and expand home-care models and build links with primary and care Pilot alternative low cost community-based models, evaluate and scale up Create space for involvement of people with HIV infection in planning intervention, of care and support programmes

The UN system is increasingly addressing issues that are not easily addressed by other partners, specifically focussing on issues that have not been (and do not easily get) taken up by larger development efforts. Taking these into consideration and recognising that financial resources of the UN system for HIV are limited in comparison to the larger funding of the programme, the UN agencies are seeking to focus on some well-defined concrete areas of contributions specially those falling within the mandate of each agency. This includes efforts to:

(a) frame and evaluate operational programme approaches so that lessons learned can be scaled-up by government in the national programme,

(b) develop partnerships around HIV with ministries and civil society organisations with whom they are already working in other areas,

(c) offer access to worldwide knowledge on HIV and

networks in the area of each agencies mandate and strength,

(d) mainstream HIV within their own agency programmes and organisations,

(e) support efforts in mainstreaming human rights, gender and approaches to poverty elimination,

(f) specifically working to reduce overlap in areas where a number of UN agencies are working (like 'adolescents')

Strategic Focus

(a) WHO will continue to focus on surveillance, blood safety; clinical care; and STDs (especially on syndromic management), covering up to the continuum of care and ensuring that analysis of epidemiological and behavioural statistics informs all the agency responses, working closely with NACO and UNICEF on MCT.

(b) UNDCP will concentrate on introducing HIV/AIDS issues into prevailing national drug demand reduction projects at present planned to be supported by UNDCP (especially in the north-eastern states of India), setting up linkages between the two programmes and identifying strategic gaps in drug-related HIV programmes.

(c) UNIFEM will help in building capacities of women's organisations, bringing in gender perspectives to the national HIV policy and programme, and assist forge a collaboration between government and the women's organisations in addressing problems of HIV/AIDS.

(d) UNESCO will take the lead in reaching young people out of school in non-formal education and include HIV in curricula across the spectrum of educational programmes.

(e) UNDP will assist empowerment of vulnerable and marginalised populations, making HIV an integral part of its Human Development aims, working with non-governmental organisations and partnerships with civil society including people living with AIDS (PLWAs)

(f) UNFPA will work within important areas of support related to HIV in condom programming, reproductive health and adolescent reproductive health. Specifically drawing on its 38 district level projects in 6 states to frame and define approaches to integrate HIV/STD control into RCH and the primary health care system, and undertake research on population projections on HIV and operational research on the female condom, and microbicides.

(g) UNICEF will take a lead with WHO in demonstrating feasible strategies for Mother to Child Transmission; and within its CRC mandate, develop strategies for involvement of youth especially tackling discrimination; and supporting formative research on areas related to vulnerability of children (street children/orphans, etc.).

(h) ILO will act in promoting the active involvement of its social partners (employers and unions) in tackling HIV-especially in workplace interventions and protecting rights of HIV infected workers.

(c) Technical Resource Groups and Theme Group support. To build long-term capacities in the country, the necessity to set up thematic technical resource networks was identified. This led to the set up of Technical Resource Groups (TRGs) in 12 thematic fields. The TRGs bring together-diverse skills and expertise in the given thematic field and give suitable and timely technical support to SACS. The TRGs are developing medium and long-term plans based on the necessities identified by the national programme. Each theme group member will also support the Technical Resources Network (TRGs) in the field nearest to their mandate and strengthen technical capacities at state level.

(d) Supporting areas of common support shared by all parties. All partners will be working in support of the national programme in:

(a) actively build a common and emerging understanding of India's HIV epidemic. Strengthening this understanding at both the national and state levels and offering a common pool of analysis among all stakeholders necessitates ample investment and yet will contribute greatly across the programme. Together aim to greatly expand the number and quality of community-based surveys, and seek to fill gaps in awareness of behavioural patterns of risk behaviour,

(b) persuading innovation and experimentation,

(c) ensuring that 'cross-cutting' approaches of gender, community action and rights are built into all interventions in a sensitive and effective way.

(d) involving as far as possible HIV-infected groups in the planning of any interventions that directly or indirectly affect them. Strengthening the capacities of group able to voice the concerns of positive groups still recognisably weak at the moment is an important aspect for the future shape of the programme.

Planning with NACO

A major objective of developing the collaborative framework is to more closely relate external inputs to national priorities. To make this a regular feature of future work it is proposed to:

(a) regularly revise this collaborative framework in terms of relevance of the strategy outlined. This may emerge as the epidemic emerges,

(b) work together with NACO towards a joint monitoring and evaluation framework, and a joint approach to programme review/evaluation,

(c) fully support NACO initiative of regular donor's coordination,

(d) keep agency workplans as rolling plans covering 18 month 2 years periods, updated and refined each year,

(e) common participation in the planning, debriefing of missions and field visits

(f) when and where suitable, support action in a regional context supporting interventions on specific cross-border action that will support the national programme.

The success of such a collaborative effort will be scaled by its contribution to the national response. Strengthening, broadening and sustaining the response in future is the target of all the partners in this venture.

6

Persons Living with HIV/AIDS: A Case Study in Mumbai and Bangalore

Introduction

Few diseases in human history are perhaps as feared—and as despised—as the disease, better known by the acronym, AIDS (Acquired Immuno Deficiency Syndrome). Not only the disease, but also persons infected or affected by it, are feared and disapproved because AIDS is invested with different meanings. AIDS has been largely thought as a 'queer' disease, an 'abnormal' illness and described using military metaphors of wars and weapons. Labels and descriptions like these indicate that AIDS is a disease of 'others', of persons living on the margins of society, of those whose lifestyles are dismissed as 'perverted, and morally sinful. It is this concept of AIDS as the disease of the 'others'—who are 'queer' and 'different' and whose behaviour is shameful—which has proved AIDS a stigmatised and loathsome disease. The gravity of AIDS and its transmission through intimate sexual behaviour makes it a fatal disease as well. Underlying the labelling and metaphorical descriptions is the core of 'sex' in AIDS—sex that is non-conventional, socially disapproved and morally condemned. Isolation, stigmatisation, denial and all other shapes of discrimination are natural results of this strong sexual connotation, posing problems for positive persons in sharing their HIV/AIDS status with others and in accessing treatment and support. The present discussion is concerned with these negative consequences of living with HIV/AIDS, i.e., discrimination, stigmatisation and denial in India.

The AIDS Scenario

As per available UNAIDS/WHO reports, south and south-east Asia is the epicentre of the HIV epidemic with the majority of new infections expected to be occurring here. Within this region, India is approximated to have the largest impact of the epidemic with about 3–5 million HIV infections. From 1986, when the first HIV infection case was reported in a female prostitute in Chennai, Tamil Nadu, the sero-positivity has risen from 2.5 per 1000 in 1986 to 11.2 per 1000 in 1992 to 16.3 per 1000 by end 1996. As of March, 1998, it was 22.73 per 1000 or about 2.2 per cent. At end July 1998, 78904 HIV positive persons and 6386 AIDS cases were detected from all states of the country.

These data do not reflect the reality adequately. Weakness in sero-surveillance system, bias in selecting the target groups for surveillance and unavailability of testing services in many parts of India are the few reasons for under-reporting and for the discrepancy between official data the and real scene. Maharashtra and Tamil Nadu with better infrastructure, therefore, continue to reveal higher rates, and many rural areas and a few states like Arunachal Pradesh reveal about zero prevalence rate. In the same way, while commercial sex workers (CSWs) and injecting drug users are shown to have high HIV infection rate, women in the general population remain under-reported. For instance, while HIV rates are reported to be increasing among women attendees at STD and maternal clinics, women who have completed their family size or are not married, or who do not come forward to attend STD or other clinics for many reasons, have little probability of being represented in the official statistics. A stronger evidence of a wider spread of HIV infection across income groups, comes from a study conducted in 1998 in New Delhi. Of the total 167 HIV infected individuals interviewed, 53 per cent had at least a bachelor's degree and the mean earnings of the sample were above the national per capita earnings, a majority of them being salaried employees, with a few owning private businesses. Even as the individual cases of HIV infections reveal a steady rise, notwithstanding a weak and inadequate sero-surveillance system, the social, psychological, and economic implications of the epidemic reach beyond the infected individuals to affect millions of households and their native communities. The challenge to give care and support to these individuals and their households has hardly been addressed. What has also not been addressed is the problem of discrimination and stigmatisation faced by people with HIV/AIDS and their household members.

Discrimination and Stigmatisation

The aspects in which discrimination and stigmatisation in HIV/AIDS are experienced vary to a large extent. Discrimination and stigmatisation also take on various forms and are expressed sometimes openly and sometimes in latent manners.

Context here refers to both physical/spatial settings (health care, work, household, community) and relational aspects of it (care giving, earning, familial and social relations, and death).

The discrimination and stigmatisation were mainly experienced in the care-giving and to a little extent in the familial and social relationships. Another context was death or post-life discrimination. The employment context did not evolve as a major context of negative experiences for positive workers, but as is described later this is mainly because of secrecy maintained about one's HIV/AIDS status in the work context.

The Care-giving Context. The care-giving context consists both household and hospital care-giving, and the latter was the focus of most discussions and interviews with HIV positive people. The hospital care-giving context assumes main significance for them. It is the context they cannot avoid and have to interact with over an extended period of time. A majority of the PLWH/A first encountered their sero-status within this context, either during an illness episode or during surgery/blood transfusion/pregnancy. Fewer learned of their sero-status in comparison in the context of blood donation or in the context of travel abroad (mainly to gulf nations for employment. Differential treatment, labelling and social/emotional distancing were encountered by HIV positive people in this very care-giving context, almost soon after the revelation of their sero-status by hospital staff. Most of the PLWH/AIDS explained that their problems started soon after they learnt of their sero-positivity in the hospital. The experience of HIV positive persons receiving TB treatment was identical to many others in the same hospital. Oral medicines were given instead of injections for TB once patients detected to be sero-positive. No consent was taken for HIV tests and no explanations given for change in treatment mode.

Doctors in various specialities and non-governmental organisation workers acknowledged that health care settings were a big source of discrimination and stigmatisation. But fixation of responsibility was always on others. For instance, doctors in public hospitals alleged that they were the more committed lot around and the only ones to give treatment and care to infected patients, while the private hospitals pushed them and conveniently transferred their responsibility to government hospitals. Doctors and staff in private hospitals, on the other hand, blamed the government hospitals for shirking their responsibility and giving shoddy and substandard treatment to infected persons.

The small private clinics, it was pointed out, by both positive patients and doctors across different hospitals, blatantly denied care and treatment to infected persons (statistics from private clinics confirm these observations).

The government hospitals are reportedly 'under orders' to give suitable health care facilities to HIV-infected persons. In Bangalore the Bowring Hospital is said to be 'specially' designated for AIDS care. Staff at this hospital were of the opinion that because of this, all city hospitals were 'dumping' their AIDS patients on them. In reality HIV/AIDS patients from Corporation Hospitals, Trust run hospitals and some private hospitals are regularly asked to seek treatment in Bowring Hospital. This was not only reported by the patients but doctors too at these hospitals admitted transferring sero-positive patients to Bowring Hospital. Catholic Church run hospitals and some other private hospitals gave all treatment facilities to persons with HIV and AIDS. In fact, Catholic hospitals have a written policy on AIDS. These are the only hospitals clearly stipulating unconditional care to patients with HIV/AIDS. Besides the issue of whether or not hospitals accepted sero-positive patients, two other issues were observed to be major. First, the quality of care given and the other the attitude of individual doctors and health care staff (both these aspects are described under 'Discrimination in Hospital Settings'). Generally, the perception was that care in government hospitals was of substandard quality with poor facilities. A majority of the hospital staff in Bangalore explained that while they provided 'proper and adequate' care to HIV-infected patients, the families of the patients did not do so.

'Family discriminates the most' was a common refrain heard from many of the patients. Family members, it was alleged, generally left the patient with HIV infection in their care and left or when they were near, kept a lot of distance from the patients. The patients themselves did not, in such overwhelming manner, report neglect and discrimination from their family members except that they did take precautions by keeping their vessels and personal items separate. The NGO staff and doctors attributed the families' uncaring response to lack of adequate knowledge and wrong conceptions about AIDS. Once these were cleared, family members gave support to their members with HIV/AIDS. Some kind of discrimination was also reported in care settings managed by NGOs. Assumption by some NGO staff that their HIV positive women clients were perhaps into sex trade and a casual attitude towards their rights and necessities suggested judgemental opinions of the staff. HIV patients who had once been inmates at one of the centres in Bangalore, said that they were provided care with an 'attitude'. One HIV infected woman, who was photographed for an AIDS programme without her knowledge, was rebuked for questioning the staff on the issue.

At the time of a group debate, commercial sex workers who were accessing support from a local NGO reported being talked to in derogatory words by the NGO staff and denied services when they required them the most. When there were conflicts of interests among NGOs, HIV infected persons took the brunt as services were stopped or denied to them.

In Mumbai too, the hospital care-giving context was the basic context where many of the positive people had experienced discrimination and stigmatisation. Here too one government hospital, the J.J. Hospital, was usually named as the hospital for HIV/AIDS care and many sero-positive persons were regularly asked to seek treatment there. The reality, as revealed by a public hospital doctor, is that all hospitals alongwith the Mumbai Corporation hospitals are expected to give care but many of them, as it was alleged by patients, subjected them to hardships and harassment when accessing health services. Recently some private hospitals are reported to have started accepting positive patients. This development has come about with the realisation that HIV/AIDS is not a class specific disease. With many HIV-positive patients coming from the upper income group, private hospitals have had to open their doors. This has benefited the positive patients but not without a hefty price. Private hospitals are providing quality service but the cost is passed on to the patients. Much of the cost is for fumigating operation theatres or labour rooms used for HIV-infected persons, for liberally providing double and triple hand gloves to staff and AIDS kit to all staff helping in surgeries. According to senior medical professionals, such precautions and irrational use of safety gears are not needed and amount to discriminatory practices towards HIV/AIDS patients. As will be discussed later, positive patients felt stigmatised due to such 'unnecessary' and selectively followed precautions by staff.

The employment context. The employment context did not evolve as a major context of discrimination and stigmatisation for positive people. The explanation, however, is that a majority of the patients said that they had not revealed their HIV/AIDS status in their place of work. Many of them expressed a heightened fear of social isolation and stigmatisation from fellow workers and loss of employment from management if they were to disclose their HIV status at their job setting. This fear was substantiated by the experiences of those patients whose HIV/AIDS reports were shared with fellow workers and management. Many of them said they faced resistance from management and very often from their own colleagues too. It is evident that the employment sector is a likely context of discrimination and bias towards positive people, even though there was more of perceived discrimination reported than real discrimination.

The relationship context. The relationship context of discrimination was tempered by sero-status revelation. A majority of the respondents had revealed their sero-positive status only within close relationship, i.e., parent child, spousal or sibling relationship. Within each of these relationship contexts, gender played a major part in mitigating the effect of the disease. Therefore, daughters, wives and daughters-in-law felt greater discrimination as compared to sons, husbands and sons-in-law. The relationship that was put to greatest stress following HIV positivity was the parents-in-law and daughter-in-law relationship. This was followed by spousal relationship. These observations were found true everywhere. Discrimination for daughter-in-law was blatant even as the son of the house was well cared for. On the one hand, women were supposed to provide care to their husbands, on the other they were stigmatised as women of loose character and the source of infection to their husbands. There was blame and abuse directed at women who were unable to defend themselves.

In majority of the cases, after the death of the son, parents do not take the responsibility of the daughter-in-law and ask her to leave. She either returns to her natal family or ekes out a living all by herself. In an extreme care of rejection and shrinking of responsibility, parents-in-law abandoned the sick daughter-in-law and her child, both of whom were HIV-positive.

The situation of HIV-positive women was no different in the country. Blame, anger, rejection and aspersions cast on the woman's character were admitted by a large number of the female patients. Even in cases where parents knew their son visited prostitutes, the wife was blamed for not keeping her husband uncontrol 'control', for that is a 'good/traditional' wife's role, implying that it was she who had failed in her role as a wife thereby justifying family's rejection of her. The parents knew it very well that even before marriage, their son used to visit the prostitutes.

Within the spousal relationship most men admitted that their wives were the main caregivers. Many of them felt guilty and repented for putting their wife's life to danger by their 'wrong deeds'. In the rare cases where wives left home, at times temporarily, out of anger and frustration, husbands were terribly hurt that they were deserted.

In the community/societal context, social separation and labelling were commonly reported wherever the individual's HIV status was public knowledge. Often it took extreme forms.

Discrimination and stigmatisation at the time of death. Differential treatment and fear of contagion expressed at the time of death is a major source of anguish and distress to positive people. Dead bodies of AIDS patients are packed in black plastic bags/ sheets and handled with disrespect and a casual attitude because the mortuary and ambulance staff are full of fear and anxiety. During a debate with male HIV-positive persons, many spoke agitatedly and with great concern and anguish about what they called 'stigma in death'. They spoke of the irony of maintaining great secrecy in life to protect their identity and reputation while after death, their plastic cover wrapped body proclaims to the world their AIDS status. Following is an excerpt from HIV-positive member of a support group.

> Today everybody tries to keep HIV cases a secret and great care is taken to keep names secret. But when we die a plastic bag is used to declare to the world that this person has died of AIDS. So, everybody in the neighbourhood comes to know and then they talk ill about the family, and do not visit them. Why, why is this being done? The ambulance man refuses to take the body till we have paid him more. Our relatives refuse to give shoulder to the body.

The plastic sheet is viewed as a symbol of shame and stigma related with AIDS. It is a stigma to wrap the bodies in black plastic sheets. There is a strong demand from positive persons that this practice be stopped. Though plastic sheets are used for dead bodies only in some hospitals, it was not referred to by any of the positive patients as a means of distress and stigma. Nor was it described at the time of community group discussions as an indication of AIDS death. But it was instructed that bodies were taken straight for cremation/burial because doctors advised against rituals. The same advice was being given everywhere in the hospitals. Positive persons expressed sorrow that they were not found worthy of the last rituals at the time of death.

Two other aspects, one in which AIDS related discrimination was actually experienced and the other in which it was more feared than really experienced by respondents, were children's education and life insurance. The school as a setting for discrimination with children of HIV-positive parents or those who are themselves HIV-positive is beginning to get acknowledged by NGOs. One HIV-positive couple and one widow of an HIV-positive man were emphasised to withdraw their children from school. Both these cases the children were between 5–7½ years and were themselves HIV-negative. The HIV/AIDS status of the parents was known to some teachers which went against the children to remain in their school. No reasons were given by the school management and the affected parents were too nervous to insist, and in one case, not keen to encourage the matter lest their identity got known to others as well.

In a foster care programme run by a child adoption agency, Mumbai a foster mother looking after an orphan, aged 5½ whose parents died of AIDS, told her experiences with the child's school. The school authorities, showed ignorance about HIV transmission routes, when they insisted that the child's presence in their school would severely affect other children. The child though himself HIV-negative carried the stigma of being born to HIV infected parents. In yet another case an HIV-positive widow was assisted by social workers to get her son aged 6 years admitted to a boarding school, which had initially been worried about possible effect on other children. In case of children who are HIV-positive, school staff are not only biased but also worried over probable transmission of the virus to others, should the child have cuts or wounds following fights with other school children or in the event of an accident. Such fears expressed by staff of a municipal school has made one NGO, that gives care to children with HIV, hide their sero-status in the school. One NGO that offers shelter to children of HIV-positive parents or those who are HIV-positive themselves, have been successful in educating the staff of a neighbouring municipal school about transmission routes and precautionary measures. All school-aged children in their home, as a result, are admitted into the said school.

Childcare institutions are another setting with potential to discriminate with a child who is HIV-positive. In a few institutions, destitute children (found abandoned or relinquished by the mother) are tested for HIV at the time of admission to the institute and when found HIV-positive are either segregated to a separate room or transferred to an NGO with shelter programme for these children. The institute officials not only fear virus transmission but also manifest a trend to transfer responsibility of such children to other NGOs despite adequate staff and space. Denial of life insurance to HIV-positive persons is yet another major issue brought up during debates. The Life Insurance Corporation (LIC) of India has pleaded that HIV test to the list of medical tests required at the time of applying for a policy. A person with HIV-positive test result is denied a policy on the basis that life insurance covers 'risk of loss' as against actual loss. Since there is no cure at present available for HIV, the risk to loss of life is taken to be 'definite' in comparison to that for cancer or heart diseases for which timely/ suitable medical intervention is known to lessen the risk to a large extent. HIV positive individuals, however, feel frustrated and discriminated at not being able to take LIC policy for their family's future security. One senior LIC official defended the LIC decision and explained it as being no more discriminatory for positive persons as for other patients of terminal diseases. Policyholders who test HIV-positive after obtaining the policy have no reason to worry, yet a large number of the respondents expressed worry that their premature death due to AIDS may result in the policy being not honoured. These fears were dispelled by the LIC representative, yet some were found to have stopped payment of their LIC premium following their positive HIV test results, thus incurring loss and feeling insecure. While the LIC rules are clear on HIV/AIDS, even as they are termed discriminatory, especially by healthy and asymptomatic HIV-positive individuals, there are inummerable misconceptions and anxieties among positive persons pertaining to their existing LIC policies. Fear of disclosure and stigmatisation stops them from seeking clarification from LIC directly, with the result that a few infected persons are likely to forego their claims to their policies. More statistics is needed to find out the impact of life insurance policy on HIV positive individuals.

Forms of Discrimination and Stigmatisation. Both overt and covert forms of discrimination and stigmatisation were reported; the latter more difficult to challenge and question, especially by people who are emotionally and physically weakened by their sero-positivity. Overt forms of discrimination and stigmatisation include behaviours that are direct and carried out openly following knowledge of one's sero-status. Few of the overt forms of discrimination experienced by respondents are as below:

(A) At Home and in the Community

1. Sever relationships, desertion, separation
2. Deny property share, access to finance
3. Block access to ones spouse or children, or other relatives
4. Physical separation at home, separate sleeping arrangement
5. Block entry to common areas, facilities like toilet, etc.
6. Block entry to common places like village or a neighbourhood area

7. Deny last rituals
8. Give labels, call names.

(B) In Hospitals

1. Refusal by hospitals/doctors to provide treatment for HIV/AIDS related illness
2. Refusal to admit in the hospital for care/treatment
3. Refusal to operate or help in operation/surgeries/ dressing of wounds
4. Blocking access to facilities like common toilet and common vessels
5. Physical separation of the person in the ward, separate arrangements for bed outside the ward in a gallery/ corridor
6. Stoppage of ongoing treatment/medication/injections
7. Early discharge from the hospital
8. Mandatory testing for HIV in surgery and pregnancy cases
9. Limiting the positive person's movements within the ward/room
10. Selective use of protective gears like gloves, masks, etc. only for HIV/AIDS patients
11. Refusal to lift/touch dead body of positive person
12. Covering the body with plastic sheet
13. Reluctance in giving services of ambulance/hearse.

(C) At Work Place

1. Remove from employment
2. Compel to resign
3. Stoppage of health/insurance facilities
4. Maintain social distance
5. Give labels, call names
6. Make fun/jeer at.

Covert forms of discrimination and stigmatisation include those behaviours that are indirect, hidden and more subtle. These are:

(A) At Home/in the Community

1. Pass remarks/saying disparagingly about the positive member (for example 'he is paying for past sins')

2. Arouse guilt feeling for jeopardising the family economy and for degrading family prestige.

(B) In Hospitals

1. Delay in treatment/slow service (e.g., made to wait in queues, asked to come again)
2. Excuses/explanations for non-admission of patients (but not direct refusal)
3. Shunt the patients between wards/doctors/ hospitals
4. Keep under observation (without any treatment plan)
5. Stop treatment/operations
6. Advise repeat HIV tests/other diagnostic reports
7. Conditional treatment (e.g., treatment given only on the condition that patient will come for follow up or join a drug trial programme).

Expression of Discrimination and Stigmatisation. HIV/ AIDS related discrimination and stigma can be expressed verbally or non-verbally. Saying of insulting terms (e.g., lowly people, gutter worms, bad men), insulting language (e.g., men who are used to being in the gutter, 'such' people), fear based sayings (dreadful disease, worms eat them away), labelling ('the one with AIDS' — AIDS *wala/wali*), are a few of the manners in which discrimination and stigmatisation are expressed verbally. Non-verbal expressions consist of behavioural practices such as, putting up 'AIDS' board on hospital beds, writing HIV/AIDS in red ink on files, sequence of beds to isolate patients or to inconvenience them, not taking permission for HIV test, lack of discretion in sero-status revelation, mandatory HIV testing, lack of pre- and post-test counselling services, withholding access to children or other relatives, etc. Many respondents reported experiencing discrimination and stigmatisation directly and blatantly, but equally at times some forms of discrimination and stigmatisation were perceived and apprehended. They were based on the experiences of other infected people or conveyed by media messages. For instance, messages that induced fear (AIDS equals death). They were also based on their own inner fears, anxieties and insecurities within past relationships with many others. Few ways of discrimination were very subtle and difficult to pinpoint like 'a smirk' on the face of a hospital stuff, or the washing of hands after touching a HIV positive person's file or clothing. These experiences harass positive people emotionally but they were unable to challenge them.

The perceived and the subtle forms of discrimination and stigmatisation are very crippling and disabling, affecting infected person's desire to live, to reveal sero-positive status and seek adequate cure and support.

Results of Discrimination, Stigmatisation and Denial. Results of discrimination and stigmatisation are discernible at both the individual and societal levels, a majority being destructive or less productive rather than constructive, which is not surprising. As is obvious there are connections between results at individuals and societal levels resulting in an overall social burden of the epidemic. The most widely reported individual level results are the fear of social isolation, judgmental attitude, severing of relationships and denial of support and care contributing to an environment of fear and distrust at the societal levels. As negative experiences increase HIV positive persons became more and more distrustful of relationships, both personal and social.

Depression, anxiety, self-isolation and suicidal thoughts/self-harming trends are recurrent themes in individual interviews. The fear of others keeps positive persons from accessing help and support. Self-isolation and the trend to hide and withhold sharing of HIV status with others is not only burdensome to the individuals but also contributes to a 'latent epidemic' rendering it faceless and nameless. The most worrisome outcome of this is the high probability of the silent spread of the epidemic as many HIV-positive persons, in their desire to remain undetected, fail to learn to adopt safer methods of sexual and injecting drug use behaviour. Another result with identical consequences for a silent spread of the virus is the trend of some healthy, asymptotic positive patients to hide their HIV status in health settings in their efforts to receive unbiased treatment and care.

A few of those who are unable to conceal their sero-positive identity, avoid visiting doctors or hospitals or delay treatment seeking to the limit they can, harming their health and immunity levels in the process. Over the counter drug buying is also reported for recurring problems like fever, diarrhoea, etc. to prevent hospital based discrimination.

Anger is also one of the outcomes that is directed mainly at care givers and the government/policy makers but frequent outbursts are targeted towards household members and the general public. Cases of duping and exploiting positive members for monetary gains in the name of 'wonder drug', 'vaccine trials', 'AIDS cure' have led to frustration and rage. The government is held responsible for not checking malpractices and the dubious ways of quacks and self proclaimed doctors.

Among the more constructive outcomes is the individual level acceptance of one's sero-positive identity and bravity to challenge discrimination. Although this type of outcome is still limited to a small proportion of the positive people's population, it is slowly gaining in numbers. At the societal level it is taking the form of a positive people's support group movement. The Indian Network of Positive People (INP+) and its state branches are undertaking the task of mobilising support. The movement is still in its rudimentary stages and is yet to set up itself as a visible social movement articulating its demands. While the basis of the support group mobilisation is Human Rights and AIDS, there is still a significant level of secrecy and distrust shown by members. State and national level conferences of the support groups, for instance, are restricted to its own members with limited and invited participation of HIV 'negative' people, mainly a select group of legal and health workers.

Health Care Settings

The one aspect that was the central point of debates held with HIV-positive people and their family care givers, health workers and NGO staff, pertaining to HIV/AIDS associated discrimination and stigmatisation, was the health care setting. This consisted of private, public, municipal corporation and charitable trust run hospitals, Catholic hospitals and NGO run services. To protect the identity of hospitals, the discussion where will be with reference to public and private hospitals (Public hospitals will consist municipal corporation hospitals, government TB sanatorium and hospitals for factory workers; private wil consist, privately managed, charitable trust run and Catholic hospitals). With HIV-positive persons, most of the discussion on discrimination started at the same time with reference to problems confronted while accessing treatment and care, and ended, sometimes with despair and helplessness, but sometimes with several suggestions to improve the condition. Unequivocally, the health care setting was where, they said, their negative experiences with HIV/AIDS started, and should end.

The health care setting is the only aspect where HIV-positive persons interact, if at all, maximally with others, consisting of health professionals (mainly doctors) and para-professionals. For many positive persons this is the only setting in which they relate to others about their sero-positive identity. It is also the setting, which they would like to avoid, but are unable to, because of their deteriorating health condition, or for the necessity to maintain it at a stable level.

The discussion here is confined on the following three topics:

(a) Hospital practices for cure and care of persons living with HIV/AIDS.
(b) Attitudes of health professionals and workers involved in providing services to persons living with HIV/AIDS.
(c) Experiences of persons living with HIV/AIDS in accessing health care.

Hospital Practices

An evaluation of the practices followed at the health care settings for HIV-positive people is significant as they expose the extent to which there is acceptance of HIV/AIDS as a health problem that needs responding to, the level to which there is concern for the health of the positive persons and respect for positive people's right to lead their lives with dignity, and the extent to which there is commitment to improving their quality of life. Hospital practices persisting to the HIV epidemic were evaluated for the following:

(a) Hospital policy on HIV testing, patient consent, pre- and post-test counselling.
(b) Hospital practices, with special reference to HIV as the basis for admission for select groups.
(c) Hospital management of persons living with HIV/AIDS, use of precautionary measures, use of signs/symbols for HIV patients, practices for indoor patients, care giving (physical and emotional).

Testing for HIV and Related Issues

In all hospitals HIV test is done for patients who do not respond to treatment for TB, STDs, diarrhoea, lymph nodes, what are called as the 'marker diseases'. Blood is also tested on 'suspicion' for patients who seem to have HIV, based on symptoms like thin physique, dark skin, weight loss, skin problems, or those belonging to risk groups like truck drivers and commercial sex workers (CSWs) as disclosed by their history of exposure. As a rule pregnant women, wives of HIV-positive men and patients for surgery are subjected to mandatory testing in private hospitals. In both the study, sites hospitals in general did not have the concept of patient consent for HIV test. Patient consent for HIV test is not taken before drawing their blood for HIV test or before sending them for HIV test to an outside laboratory. Doctors act on the assumption that patients will comply with the advice given by the doctor or will be willing to co-operate for any test that the doctor desires to get conducted. A patient's consent is implied when the HIV test and its likely outcomes are informed during 'counselling'.

The 'verbal consent' meant a 'yes' from the patient when asked if he understood what HIV test meant. His affirmative reply is taken to indicate his consent. In reality, the practice of written consent is a rarity. In fact, pre-test counselling is also not uniformly adopted. Usually, the patient is first required to get the HIV test done from the microbiology laboratory of the hospital or an outside laboratory before any further course of action can be framed.

Approximately all public and private hospitals can provide the services of AIDS counsellors through a local counselling centre for AIDS. There are fixed days for the counsellors to visit these hospitals. In one private hospital, counselling is given by the doctors. In these hospitals where there are no especially appointed/ visiting counsellors, counselling is only done after the HIV reports are received, in other words it is only post-test counselling that is made handy to the patients.

Everywhere, AIDS counsellors are conspicuously absent in all the hospitals. Doctors attending to the patients do most of the counselling depending upon time availability. In several hospitals, this counselling was more in the shape of giving information about AIDS than anything else. As the patients' experiences reveal, post-test counselling is chiefly about informing them of the HIV test outcomes and the likely future problems. In few hospitals post-test counselling induced more fear than support.

Private hospitals adopt the policy of mandatory testing for a select group of patients. These are patients brought for surgery (major or minor) and pregnant women. Spouses of all HIV infected persons are advised/subjected to HIV tests irrespective of whether or not they need any medical services. The process of patient consent, pre-and post-test counselling are as a rule not followed in their case. Doctors across hospitals defended HIV tests for surgeries and labour on the bases that they were invasive in nature and involved large blood spillage and they thus, necessitate to take precautions. But in many of the cases, as the patients' experiences reveal, these tests were conducted to refuse treatment/health services to HIV patients and not just to take precautions. Many of the pregnant women and patients requiring surgery were refused hospital services following their HIV positive test outcomes. Another serious problem pertaining to HIV testing is the demand for repeat testing of blood for HIV, by hospitals and doctors even if the patients possessed test reports from another laboratory/ hospital. Discussions with few respondents in Mumbai showed that the practice of demanding fresh HIV test done at particular laboratories, thus putting the patient to larger emotional and monetary difficulties. For patients necessitating immediate medical attention this also meant delay in starting treatment. AIDS patients were not started on treatment till a new HIV test report had been submitted even if that meant delay treatment. There was a clear tendency on the part of these hospital doctors to disbelieve the authenticity of HIV reports from other hospital/laboratories, the consequences of which were borne by the patients, financially and psychologically too.

How the HIV test reports are made open, and to whom, is an issue related to *confidentiality*. The doctors alone have the right to reveal the HIV test results. Hospitals having the services of AIDS counsellors, however, may also depend on them to inform the patient with his/her HIV test outcomes. But across hospitals *what* is informed and to *whom* shows a great deal of variation and a clear violation of patients' right to 'confidentiality'. In private hospitals, the most often *quoted* policy is that test outcomes are only revealed to the patient and to nobody else. But, in reality in about all hospitals, with a few exceptions, results are also shared with the person accompanying the patient. Although doctors would like to believe that confidentiality is maintained, in reality quite some people come to know of a patient's HIV status.

If there is no one accompanying the patient, relatives are especially called, at times from the native village, to receive the HIV test outcomes. The parent(s), wife, or a sibling are called to receive the test results. Close relatives are given the results in many hospitals ostensibly 'to save the patient from shock and possible self-harm'.

Confidentiality is usually not kept with married patients for he is at times accompanied by the spouce and doctors in the practice of sharing diagnosis with the wife. Pertaining to unmarried young men, it is generally left to their discretion unless they are accompanied by a friend or a relative in which case the results are often shared with them too. It is obvious that the theory of confidentiality is at times confused with sharing of HIV results with a few 'select' groups of persons including hospital staff and 'close' attendees of the patient. Among the hospital staff even those not directly related with care, for instance, the technical staff, are kept aware of the identity of the patient. The blood sample is not unlinked, anonymous. The attendees may be understood as parents, spouse or whoever is accompanying the patient in the hospital. What is not kept in mind, however, is that the theory of confidentiality involves informing HIV test report to the patient alone and to nobody else, unless (s)he gives consent to do so and names the person to be informed. However, it is significant to note here that confidentiality is most often and easily broken in the case of women, the less educated and the economically weaker persons living with HIV/AIDS. In the case of a pregnant woman, confidentiality of her HIV status does not look to be an issue at all. She is often not even told of her own HIV status; the decision to inform her husband is already taken by the doctor on the assumption that it is the husband who will decide the future course of action—whether or not to continue with the pregnancy and whether or not to himself get diagnosed for HIV.

Therefore, policy regarding patient confidentiality is especially discriminatory towards positive people belonging to the semi-literate and economically poor sections of the society. In the case of educated and economically better persons living with HIV/

AIDS, however, confidentiality of HIV test outcomes is strictly observed.

Hospital Admission Policy. In all the hospitals included in this study the management admitted that HIV-positive patients were admitted for treatment in the wards. Also, that a patient found to test HIV positive after admission was permitted to continue to remain in the ward and seek cure. While this was largely true as a stated policy, there were denies by individual consultants related with the private hospitals, staff protests to help in surgeries related with HIV-positive persons, and examples of transferring patients to other hospitals. In Mumbai, one private hospital included in this study, until two months ago did not admit HIV/AIDS patients under pressure from the hospital workers.

Admission/treatment plan for HIV patients varied across departments within a hospital. For instance, in the above said public hospital of Bangalore, the skin and STD department admitted and treated various positive patients. In the similar way, a Mumbai-based private hospital, though the management stated that patients with HIV/AIDS were admitted, there were exceptions. A nephrologist attached to the hospital strongly defended her policy of denying treatment and admission to HIV-positive patients necessitating kidney transplant or a dialysis.

The Medical Director of a private hospital in Mumbai agreed that even if the hospital policy was favourable towards positive patients, it was untimately the decision of individual doctors whether or not to treat infected persons. Attitude of individual health care professionals were major factors affecting their decision to give care for infected persons.

Athough most hospitals report non-discriminatory admission and treatment 'policy' (unwritten) for HIV/AIDS persons, many discriminatory 'practices' continue without being challenged by the management. For instance, doctors at few hospitals give early discharge to patients detected HIV positive even though the patient has still to cover the full course of treatment.

In few hospitals patients for surgery are advised against surgery for once their HIV test outcome is positive. The earlier decision for surgery is reversed pleading that it may not be of much significance to the patient.

Similarly, invasive procedures like injections are stopped and replaced by oral medicines as was observed in the case of TB patients with HIV. Such decisions of the medical workers may be justified in few cases but to a large extent they remain to be discussed as they are not regularly followed as norms by other doctors and even more subjective than objective. In any case, HIV infected persons consider such decisions discriminatory and biased as will be revealed later from their personal experiences.

Management of patients with HIV/AIDS. In their efforts to manage patients with HIV/AIDS, hospitals have recommended many precautionary measures to be followed exclusively with infected persons. These are:

(a) Use of rubber gloves, at times double and triple gloves, for giving care and treatment.
(b) Use of 'AIDS kits' (gloves, masks, apron, boots, cap and eye goggles made of rubber), for surgeries.
(c) Use of chemical solution for soaking patient's clothing/bed linen.
(d) Fumigation of operation theatre/labour room/ward meant for infected person.
(e) Use of bleaching powder for disinfecting all used materials (e.g., bed pan).
(f) Use of black plastic sheets/bags for packing dead bodies.

The use of gloves, chemical solution, disposable syringes and needles are widely practised as safety measures in several hospitals. However, few other measures like use of multiple gloves, AIDS kit, fumigation of rooms, etc, are followed chiefly in private hospitals, where the cost is borne by the HIV/AIDS patients. Some of these costly practices are followed in one Mumbai public hospital as well, if the patients can afford in order to get services.

If patients cannot pay for such measures they have per force to shift to other public hospitals where the staff has no 'choice' but to 'manage' without the costly gears. Issues of discrimination and stigmatisation regarding these practices arise when these are selectively used with patients only when their HIV test outcome is positive and when few practices are dismissed as unnecessary by fellow workers. None of the hospitals followed global precautions in managing patient care. When precautions such as double gloves and masks suddenly begin to be used for patients for whom care otherwise was being carried out the same way as for other patients in the ward, the effect is quite dramatic both on the patient concerned and on other inmates of the ward. As will be observed from the patients, experiences, hospital practices such as these are sources of stigma for patients during hospitalisation. Some senior gynaecologists and surgeons are of the opinion that some of the practices, for example, fumigation of room and AIDS kit for all staff during surgery are necessary. Good quality gloves, mask and goggles are sufficient.

In public hospitals such elaborate procedures and materials are unaffordable. In fact, gloves are the only protective gears at hand to nurses in a public hospital. They too are in short supply and usually big sized and of low quality through blood seeped in at the time of invasive procedures like child delivery. Private hospitals were able to take most precautions and AIDS kits of good quality, supplied in sufficient number too. But in public hospitals the conditions were sadistic.

The former way of isolating and identifying HIV-infected persons in the wards by using boards proclaiming their status were reported to have been done away with in many hospitals. Hospitals usually have medical files of patients marked 'HIV positive' in bold red ink. These files are maintained in safe custody of the ward nurse and no one can gain access to these, so claimed the nurse and ward workers, in both private and public hospitals. But in a private hospital, as revealed by the ward staff, the identity of a positive patient in the general ward (chiefly for poorer patients) is public knowledge.

By the same indication the HIV positive status of hospital staff too becomes common knowledge very easily. During debates, in a private hospital, staff members freely referred to ward and bed numbers of their HIV-infected colleagues admitted there for treatment. It is probably difficult to avoid such identification in a close hospital setting, but what is important to note here is the lack of the 'culture of patient confidentiality' among hospital staff. Breaking confidentiality in the case of AIDS patients is a part of the same culture.

Within a hospital, departments differ in the practice of detecting HIV positive patients. For instance, in a public hospital the skin and STD department follows the practice of writing

Immuno-compromise patient' and keeps 2 empty beds between the HIV infected and the other patients as a barrier. But the conjested, labour ward of the same hospital uses a symbol (a cross within a circle) to recognise the HIV patient's bed because 'in a congested gynaecology ward where there are patients kept on the floor too. Staff have to quickly recognise the positive patient to take precautions' In other departments of the same hospital, the use of any symbols/boards is taboo. However, in yet another department of this same hospital a separate small room, inside the ward is used to separate HIV-positive patients. The staff explained that the room is meant for patients with any infection like gangrene, but now it is being used to keep HIV-infected persons. Behind all such practices, the unstated intention is to warn the related ward staff about the necessity to take special precautions with patients with HIV/AIDS. It is sought to be done in an unobtrusive way so that other patients do not come to know of the person's HIV/AIDS status. But in congested public hospitals, the behaviour of individual staff workers is perhaps difficult to control.

Marking 'HIV positive' on files and case sheets in red ink is followed in other private hospitals too and these are kept only with the ward nurse-in-charge.

Steps are being taken in the hospitals to overcome labelling of positive patients but, as is evident from the discussion above, many other practices followed in the hospitals defeat this objective. The most prominent is the use of precautionary measures, especially gloves (double gloves often) very selectively in wards, creating suspicion among other patients, and a feeling of being discriminated among the positive patients. The personal experiences of some positive patients also show that hospital practices are not always respectful and non-discriminatory towards them.

Discrimination and stigmatisation towards HIV/AIDS and PLWH/A are at times exposed in people's practices and attitudes — what they believe and think about these problems, and how they behave in situations involving positive people.

HIV/AIDS Knowledge. In all hospitals in India, the nurses, the technical staff and doctors are well informed about HIV/AIDS. Many of them have attended training programmes on AIDS. However, the ward staff in most hospitals lacked sufficient information. They knew of the primary facts but various misconceptions and fears about modes of infection and transmission prevailed even among the staff of a well-known private hospital in Mumbai. For example, despite working in a health care setting of the staff cannot differentiate between HIV and AIDS.

Usually, the staff knew about the various modes of transmission of HIV/AIDS. Few of them concentrated more on the sexual transmission and some on the parental (through blood), though they mentioned the other routes as well. The staff in some hospitals was curious as to 'how a new born/infant acquires AIDS'. Needles, syringes and blood were stated to be definite sources of infection probably because in a hospital setting the staff are asked to take precautions chiefly with these. It was perhaps also to drive home the point to the researcher that these put great risk to them in their employment. Most of the staff knew that they require to take care with needles, blood and other fluids of a positive patient and many other precautions they mentioned looked exaggerated and based on their fear.

A majority of the staff in hospitals was aware that casual contact and sharing meals/vessels/clothes were not the infection carriers. Yet, in practice, as will be seen later in a discussion in this chapter, a great deal of anxiety and fears were expressed pertaining to sharing of food, casual contact, etc, when they asked to determine their risk of infection to HIV.

The management and senior doctors in many hospitals emphasised the need of periodic programmes for staff. However, ward boys, *ayas* (female helpers) and sweepers usually said that no special lectures had been arranged for them so far. For the staff in a private and a public hospital of Mumbai, the arrival of the researcher was the first time where they were involved in any debate on AIDS. At the end of debates, the researcher was asked for AIDS-related realities and various clarifications were sought. This, however, was contested by senior doctors. As an explanation, it is possible that not all staff have been covered by special AIDS lectures in hospitals because of time inconvenience or the barriers in catering to a large staff population. But, what is disappointing is the large size of the half-or ill-informed staff. Worse, in few hospitals there was a deliberate attempt made to withhold information from the staff lest they begin demanding safety kits, compensation and the like.

Practices of Staff and Risk Determination. Usually, staff members in both hospital types had a very healthy acceptance of their work even though they all were of the opinion that there was always a fear of some infection. They admitted that their work involved contact with wounds, and fluids of patients and that it was 'unclean' and 'hazardous' job. Many of them had internalised their job-related fears and risks and left matters to fate and to God.

Even with healthy work attitudes there was a lot of fear of infection when it came to discussing HIV infection. Most of the technical staff, sweepers, ward, boys and *ayas* said they were at high risk of infection with the virus. This risk determination was significantly higher among the staff of hospitals in Bangalore in comparison to Mumbai. In Mumbai an interesting feature was the difference in risk determination between ward staff and sweepers and nurses. It seems that staff who give maximum close care such as nurses and those who handle body fluids such as, sweepers, have a lower risk determination and fear than ward staff who provide more distant or superficial care. Their job description shown that ward staff is involved in making the beds, giving food and wheeling the patients from one service (X-ray, for instance) to another. It was the sweepers and *ayas* who worked most of the times with the fluids, blood, sputum, urine, etc. Even then, the ward staff feared infection the most and offered the greatest resistance.

But this is not a common feature everywhere in hospitals. In some public as well as private hospitals, staff members in few departments know that HIV does not pose a major risk to them if sufficient precautions are taken. Doctors who are proactive and supportive seem to have a model effect on them.

Attitudes of staff. Hospital staff who had various anxieties and fears were usually also those who had a derogatory attitude towards persons living with HIV/AIDS. In Bangalore, staff members across hospitals, targeted and commercial sex workers truck drivers are the big sources of HIV transmission in their city/ state. Labelling them as 'bad men/women' who have 'dirty' habits and who are 'not satisfied with what they have at home'. The poor, the slum dwellers and the illiterates were largely believed to be

AIDS 'infected' in larger proportions. Typically migrant population from neighbouring states were targeted more.

For few staff workers, cases of AIDS patients seem to introduce an element of curiosity and interest in their otherwise humdrum employment with a curiosity to learn all about how infection may have occurred. A large proportion of staff members, fewer nurses though, from various city sites confirmed the idea of a separate hospital/ward for positive patients. The arguments in favour were:

(a) Better patient management since all patients suffer from the same disease.
(b) Better infection control for patients.
(c) More easy to handle safety precautions.
(d) No threat of infection to other patients.
(e) Better mental preparedness of staff.

Simultaneously, there was agreement that no one from among them would want to go to the separate ward/hospital, due to the fear and the risk of infection. As a counter measure, thus, they argued for mandatory testing for all patients in all hospitals so that precautions may be taken from the start eradicating the needless worry with individual AIDS patients. Another strong demand made was for extra benefits/salary/risk allowance/compensation/insurance, for risking their life in taking care of infected persons. These demands were more loud and forceful in all hospitals in Bangalore as compared to Mumbai.

Attitudes of doctors. In Mumbai doctors usually favoured the right of persons living with HIV/AIDS to sufficient care and treatment and disapproved of separate hospital services for them. Although there were exceptions such as the nephrologist in a private hospital, there was usually a more supportive response. Some young resident doctors were confident of the situation changing for the better.

In contrast, in Bangalore, like the hospital staff, doctors expressed attitudes that can be said to be biased towards positive persons. The usual perception shared was that HIV positive people have bad habits of visiting commercial sex workers, of smoking and drinking, are promiscuous and 'immoral'. Certain sections of the general public were specially blamed. People's fear and bias towards persons living with HIV/AIDS were largely justified.

Most of the medical professionals justified the necessity to know the mode of infection for a patient, in order to take better precautions. They also justified a doctor's fear of infection saying that 'doctors too are human beings'.

Displaying solidarity with fellow professionals, most of the doctors rated nurses, surgeons and gynaecologists especially high on risk of HIV infection and their fears and apprehensions, and refusal to treat AIDS patients, were largely justified.

Experiences of Infected Persons

The limit and impact of AIDS-related discrimination and stigmatisation in health care setting can be seen through the personal testimonies of infected persons. These encompass a gamut of experiences in the health care sector—beginning with HIV testing without consent, to sero-status revelation, lack of proper 'counselling', problems in accepting health services, difficulties in seeking admission in wards, dying uncare, to post-death ignonimity.

Patient Consent and Pre- and Post-HIV Test Counselling

Patient consent for HIV test is an alien concept in many hospitals. None of the patients knew that they have the right to decide whether or not they desire to have the HIV test done. As many of the patients disclosed HIV test is ordered either without their knowledge or without sufficient explanation.

In both private and government hospitals post-test conselling chiefly involved announcing the results of the HIV test, or mostly giving AIDS information. There was no element of counselling in it, rather more of fear and phobia inducement.

Successive Testing for HIV

Several patients in Mumbai reported underlying repeat testing for HIV—twice, thrice or more than three times. It is a general practice with infected persons to repeat the HIV test at various laboratories because they tend to deny their status and hope for a negative report. But many patients stated that they were pressurised to get repeat tests conducted on the insistence of their doctor or to comply with the hospital requirements. Women care givers of HIV-positive husbands and children found themselves helpless as blood was drawn repeatedly for certain tests, one of these HIV.

The above revelations give a hint of unhealthy practices in HIV testing probably in connivance with HIV test laboratories. Also, some latent researches being conducted on blood and blood products drawn from HIV-positive patients in some hospitals, without their consent cannot be ruled out. These observations, however, need to be confirmed. Repeat testing for HIV was not reported to such an extent by HIV-infected persons except when they did it themselves to confirm reports.

HIV Status Disclosure/Confidentiality

HIV status revelation for many positive patients is stated to have occurred within the doctor-patient relationship. But more often than not it lacks in discretion that is morally needed. Many patients reported that their results were disclosed to their parent(s), sibling, spouse or other relatives. It is a common practice in Indian hospitals to inform the diagnosis first to close relatives to save the patient from possible emotional stress. Thus, in HIV/AIDS too confidentiality matters no more than it does in other diseases.

However, confidentiality looks to be breached in public hospitals mainly with semi-literate and poor patients. In all private hospitals, rich patients were respected to their necessity for confidentiality although there too the outcome may be made to close relatives (parents, spouse) as suggested by staff in a private Mumbai hospital. But since no rich patient was directly interviewed for the study, this cannot be emphatically stated. The reality that private hospital doctors did not agree to the researcher's request to seek co-operation from their well placed clients confirms this to a large extent.

Refusal for Admission/Treatment

Government and municipal corporation hospitals, by order, cannot refuse admission or treatment to HIV-positive patients. But, this is not always the case, as disclosed by many patients. HIV test outcome time and again became the basis for refusing admission or treatment, or for giving early discharge from hospitals or for stopping treatment halfway through.

Quality of Hospital Care for Persons Living with HIV/AIDS

When care and treatment is handy in health care services, it is the quality of that care that ultimately matters. If quality of care were taken as index, the most government hospitals would score low, more so for patient with HIV/AIDS.

Experiences of some HIV/AIDS patients disclose the substandard facilities made available to them, the attitude of staff in giving services and the less than human conditions of their stay in wards. Patients who were currently receiving/or had received care, etc. at a government hospital recounted the uncaring and callous attitude of staff and management towards them.

There is a desire among hospital staff to serve these patients and to provide close care. Women patients, especially commercial sex workers are treated still more miserably. Use of derogatory language and treating them, as 'different' classes of patients are other manners of stigmatising them.

Subtle forms of discrimination on part of ward staff in a private hospital consisted minimal care giving in an effort to minimise contact with patient/clothing, etc, a careless attitude to their necessities resulting in slow services, and a display of anxiety through use of precautionary gears selectively. During debates, staff in a private hospital admitted to a notable change in their attitude whenever a patient is found to be HIV positive. Ironically when one of the ward staff finds himself on the other side of hospital care and treatment, he too goes through the same experience.

Private Clinics

Besides the several big and small government/private hospitals, the Indian metros are dotted with several small private clinics that either run as single medical specialisation facilities or as polyclinics. All these are registered health facilities and are usually preferred over government hospitals, even by patients from lower income groups, for their prompt service. Patient population also perceives these as offering better quality care. An added attraction of going these private clinics is that they give anonymity and confidentiality much more than the public hospitals. Because of this, STD patients and those requiring abortion services prefer these clinics. To make a more comprehensive and holistic understanding of discrimination and stigmatisation in the health care setting, a quick survey was made of a small number of private clinics by using a variation of the 'dummy patient interview method'. In the original method, the researcher or volunteer of the researcher seeks medical treatment in the guise of a patient. The intention is to determine the quality of medical services offered. For the purpose of the present discussion, the original technique was varied such that a research staff visited the clinics posing as a community worker and referred fictitious cases of HIV-positive patients for treatment to the doctor at the clinic. The intention was to determine the response of private clinicians to health care needs of HIV-positive patients. Doctors at six types of clinics/specialities were visited.

The staff member, posing as community worker, would say that (s)he wishes to refer one HIV/AIDS patient to the clinic from the community in which (s)he works. The details of the patient varied depending on the type of clinic visited. For instance, the HIV patient was described as a pregnant woman (for the maternity clinic), a young man (for the dental clinic), a middle aged man (for the general physician), a child (for the children's centre), a young man (for surgery), a young man (for dermatology clinic). The responses were evaluated in terms of whether the doctors at the clinics accepted/refused/conditionally accepted to treat the patient. The research staff noted down the response and the reasons given as soon as (s)he left the clinic.

Many doctors denied to accept the patient with HIV/AIDS for the treatment at their clinic. In Bangalore, of the 13 clinics visited, doctors in 9 clinics denied and 4 accepted on specific conditions. In Mumbai, of the 24 clinics visited, 15 denied, 8 accepted on specific conditions and only 1 accepted unconditionally. Gynaecologists at all the maternity homes in both cities denied except for 3 in Mumbai who agreed on specified conditions. The other groups of doctors who refused in large numbers were dentists and general physicians. Children's specialists–(3) in Mumbai were the only doctors who accepted (2 conditionally) on sympathetic bases since the child was described as a thalassemic child who was infected through blood transfusion. Evaluation of the stated reasons revealed a high degree of fear among the doctors of risk of infection, loss of business as regular patients will refuse to come, loss of 'reputation' of the clinic, and lack of required equipments to ensure safety.

Those who agreed to accept the patient unconditionally put the following conditions:

In Bangalore

(a) Will give tablets for symptomatic condition, will not touch or physically examine the patient (1).

(b) Will treat in a different nursing home (to protect 'reputation' of own clinic and will charge more (for disposables, etc.) (1).
(c) Will treat only if mode of infection is not sex (i.e., will treat if other modes of infection)
(d) Will accept only if government makes it compulsory to accept (i.e., till he has choice he will not accept) (1):

In Mumbai

(a) Will only do filling and cap fixing (will not do any job with bleeding) (2).
(b) Will charge more (20–30 per cent) (3).
(c) Will depend on patients economic condition (i.e., will do only if the patient can pay) (1).
(d) Will see health of the patient (i.e., if health very bad, will not take the case) (1).
(e) Will not take the child in advanced stage and will charge more (for the child's condition) (1).

Vicious Circle

Discrimination and stigmatisation in the workplace present serious implications for the HIV-infected persons, as these responses, among others, are associated with their source of livelihood. The very existence of positive people and their families is at risk when HIV/AIDS threatens to rob them of their right to safety and dignity in their work environment, to earn for their family and to enjoy benefits given to workers in any work set-up. The work place, where an individual spends the maximum time outside the home, is a microcosm of the community outside; it reflects the societal attitudes and biases. Thus, it is no surprise that the work setting is the least likely among all settings for an HIV-infected person to share his/her sero-status. Various respondents said that they had not, and would not, reveal their health status to their fellow workers/employers. Fear of social discrimination and separation lowering of one's dignity and above all possible loss of employment were given as causes reasonable for their silence. Even patients who had disclosed their sero-status at home were afraid of rejection and stigmatisation in their work settings. Majority of the patients had these fears in their minds. These were probabilities that could happen to them, that could make them 'untouchables' among their fellow workers. The apprehensions of a young factory worker in Mumbai exposes the fears of many in a similar situation.

An adolescent boy shuddered at the very thought of others coming to know of his sero-positivity in his work environment.

Scenarios such as these make HIV positive workers hide their difficulty from their fellow workers and friends. In a society hung up on social image, the prospect of damaging one's social prestige and dignity, family name and honour, play on their minds.

Such fears and doubts were usual to patients in both the study locations. As in Mumbai, in Bangalore also anxiety about possible social discrimination and isolation and loss of employment were given as reasons for not sharing one's sero-status among fellow workers. Most of the positive workers interviewed in Bangalore have either kept silent or have moved out of their employments in anticipation of the social rejection at their work place. Job loss and ensuing financial difficulties is among worst feared results of AIDS, especially among the poor population.

Most of the asymptomatic HIV-infected persons think there is no need for them to disclose their sero-status at their work place till they are physically healthy because no tangible gains will accrue from it. Organisations/industries by and large do not have any AIDS policies yet and no extra or special benefits are given to those found HIV-positive. 'Is there any benefit, are they giving me any special support?' is what positive people seem to ask when thinking of disclosure at workplace. But, the fear that their sero-status may be found out one day weighs heavily on their minds as they invent excuses each time they take leave for medical treatment or when they have to remain absent for long periods because of opportunistic infections. Such confidentiality interferes with their treatment schedule (for example, taking tablets at scheduled hours in the presence of fellow workers) or with observing simple health precautions in front of others as these are likely to call unnecessary attention from others.

Not only that there is a great fear and anxiety among persons living with HIV/AIDS, the degree of sensitivity to people's comments and remarks is also high. This results partly from the fact that AIDS, a serious problem, has also become a topic of joke among some. 'Lean and thin looking people are made fun of as 'AIDS sufferers' in poor communities. At times AIDS is the topic of casual talk among factory workers and office goers and generally it is in a lighter vein.

The Enemy Within

The fears and anxieties of positive people are not entirely unfounded. Personal experiences of those few patients whose sero-status was public knowledge in their organisation, provided support to their fears. Discrimination in the form of social separation, hostility, and attempts to terminate the services of the infected worker from their midst were reported from both the study sites.

It is clear that the management alone is not thought as a threat. At times the hostility comes from within the worker's own community. Colleagues and other staff sometimes put pressure on the management to terminate the services of a positive worker.

Spread of the virus through casual contact during work hours is a general anxiety shared by the workers. Sharing utensils in the canteen, drinking water from the same glass, sitting in close proximity while operating machines or having infected people as group members, were few of the likely routes described for the 'AIDS virus' to spread in the entire 'factory area' in Mumbai. Anxieties such as these made some positive workers leave their job rather than face the humiliation of being removed by the employers or by fellow-workers.

Physical distance maintained by colleagues at lunch times or during work hours was particularly stigmatising, making it stressful for HIV-infected persons to tolerate the situation. During Focus Group Discussion's hospital staff, also admitted that they no longer felt very comfortable being as close to their HIV-positive colleagues as before.

Labelling and isolation sometimes force HIV-positive workers to quit their present jobs. Some of them settle for less paying jobs or shunt between jobs to escape being stigmatised at their successive work places.

Hostility from workers sometimes forces management to terminate the services of positive workers. In one case it was the denial of workers to work alongside an HIV-infected member that forced the management to ask the worker to sit at home while drawing full pay. The doctor who intervened on behalf of the person said, 'My patient was highly disturbed at this insult but as he needed rest, I advised him to accept the situation and earn while sitting at home.'

The level of discrimination and stigmatisation can be imagined to be greater in the unorganised work sector where illiterate or semi-literate workers are anyway powerless and lack rights. The case of a HIV-positive barber employed in a shop highlights the fact that in the unorganised sector loss of business due to the presence of an HIV positive employee is a strong barrier in retaining them.

Discrimination from Top

When it is not the fellow workers, it is the management that discriminates through its biased attitudes towards positive workers, or because of lack of sufficient knowledge of the issues associated with AIDS or through lack of AIDS associated policies. Discrimination and stigmatisation from the top leave individual workers helpless and alone in fighting for their rights to earn their livelihood. In some cases, HIV-positive workers lost their employments or were forced to seek early retirement because of ignorant and incaring employees and lack of organisational plans or AIDS.

This is not an isolated case in the transport department as is evident from the cases of two other respondents both of whom are finding it hard to work as conductors in the moving buses through polluted areas of the city. They keep falling sick because of throat infections and asthmatic condition. Both of them have pleaded for lighter jobs, but like N.K, are not confident of an affirmative response from the management.

Denial

The response of the organised work sector to the AIDS epidemic in the country can be said to be one of 'denial' of the epidemic to a large extent. In India, the industrial sector was not only unreachable for research but also in a state of classic 'denial'.

In Mumbai, 50 small/medium/large public and private industries were sent out a questionnaire seeking information about their AIDS associated policy, if any, and the precautions taken to deal with the cases of HIV/AIDS in their work force. Only 4 questionnaires were returned from 2 medium, 2 large; of these 2 were private and 1 public sector industries. None of these four industries had a written policy on AIDS. In response to the question about policy for staff found to be HIV-infected, one private company reported; 'No known cases of HIV and thus no need felt so far.' One public sector company reported that it allowed infected workers to remain in their job positions, 1 private sector accepted requests for change in job positions. Besides this dismal scene, the welfare departments in two eminent Mumbai based private industries are involved in responding to the epidemic in major ways. The welfare officers in both these industries spoke about a supportive management that acknowledged the fear of the epidemic in the work sector. However, one of them was hopeful about the whole-hearted commitment of the corporate world in fighting the challenge of AIDS.

In 1996, these two eminent industries in Mumbai had started the process of bringing the corporate world to face the challenge of AIDS. This initiative was named Industrial Response to AIDS (IRTA). A follow up of the IRTA, considerably supports the scepticism shown by the welfare officer. Out of the 13 companies that pledged support to the formulation of an AIDS policy in the corporate sector, and donate finances for it, only two took interest in taking forward the initiative. After 2 years all that the IRTA has finally culminated into is a corporate regulation policy on AIDS. Initial attempts to collect information on AIDS associated policies and programmes from the local industries drew a blank. Of the 9 small and large-scale industries contacted from both the private and public sector, three gave small significance to the subject. This is displayed from the unsuccessful attempts made by research staff to gather relevant information from the respective personnel departments. Among these, two were large manufacturing units, one each in the government and private sector and a third was a state government owned unit.

Denial of the epidemic and low HIV threat perception among staff members were not unique to small/medium sized industries employing semi-skilled and semi-literate workers only. In a software industry (Bangalore is known as the 'Silicon valley' due to several computer industries coming up here) the Human Resource Development officer hoped that their staff, being among the highest paid professionals in the country, has very low risk of AIDS.

In one large scale private manufacturing company that employs about 5000 employees, the HRM chief said that there was no written policy on AIDS in the company. Till now no cases of HIV/AIDS had been reported among the staff. The social counsellor and medical officer of the company confirmed this. The company, according to them, is welfare focussed, offers free meals, good working conditions, good medical facilities and the workers are among the highest paid in the city. The HRM chief was quite sure that the workers would have no hesitation in reporting their sero-status to the company, should they test positive for it. He also hoped that HIV/AIDS cases could not be kept confidential and latent in the company since any long term absence of workers is easily noticed.

Denial of HIV/AIDS as a threat to the private industrial sector seems to emerge from two basic reasons:

(a) No reported cases of HIV/AIDS among the staff, and
(b) The belief that workers who are well educated/better paid/well covered by company health insurance schemes will not have risk behaviour.

In the government owned industrial sector, however, the reasons are, pressure from union, fear of adverse publicity and a wish to sweep such problems under the carpet until encountered.

Acknowledgement

Acceptance of HIV/AIDS as a problem among the industrial sector workforce came from a public and a private sector company in Bangalore. However, the concerns and the concentration in the two companies differed markedly. In the Public Sector Company, a large manufacturing unit, the threat of the epidemic was more seen from the workers' perspective. The management recognised the significance of organising AIDS awareness workshops, providing counselling services, and making handy free condoms to the workers. The top management supported these measures of the personnel department. There were 10 reported HIV-positive cases in the staff. HIV test was included in the annual medical check-up of workers for which pre/post-test counselling was given and secrecy of cases was preserved. The stated objective of such annual check-ups was 'to detect positive workers and for them to know their HIV status so that they do not spread the infection'. However, there was no need felt for a written policy on AIDS 'when the labour laws were silent on it and the central government had not issued any guidelines yet'. There was no pre-employment testing for HIV, but the chief of personnel was strongly against employing a HIV-positive worker.

In comparison to the above public sector company, in a large scale private company the focus and concern with AIDS primarily seemed to be a class phenomenon. The perception of AIDS as a threat to the company came about after the identification of two HIV-positive cases in the senior executive cadre. The acknowledgement of the possibility of the threat of HIV to the workforce of the company followed from this. The company did everything to keep secrecy of the two cases and took care of the emotional needs of the persons concerned. But the major problem before the company was to protect its market sales. Thus, in the industrial world it is a vicious circle of non-visibility of the HEV-epidemic in numerical strength and its consequent denial as a real threat.

Because HIV positive workers do not reveal their HIV/AIDS status at the workplace because of the fear of discrimination, the threat of job loss, lack of support and benefits in the absence of AIDS policy, the epidemic is not visible as a real problem. Consequently, because it is not visible, there is denial of the risk posed by the epidemic. This vicious circle needs to be broken and a good start has been made by the production of a corporate policy guidelines on AIDS by the Bombay Chamber of Commerce and Industry but its outcome remains to be seen.

Gender

Sero-positive men and women are bound together by a common fate. Neither is in a privileged position; both are vulnerable to physical, emotional and social discrimination and yet, both experience the epidemic in somewhat different manners, and in somewhat varying intensities.

For both men and women, the contexts and forms of HIV/AIDS associated discrimination and stigmatisation would seem to be identical but it is the context of 'relationships' that sets apart their experiences from those of the men. Women are wives, mothers, daughters and daughter-in-law before they are HIV-positive women. Their pain and trauma as positive women are not in a vacuum but stationed within various sets of relationships.

This is not to say that men's experiences are in a vaccum. They are not, but to the extent that familial and social, relationships are governed by societal and sexual norms, the effect of HIV/AIDS for men gets blunted and shared; for women it gets sharper and more concentrated in her.

In pregnancy women are discriminated on their 'assumed' HIV status. They are wives of men who are suspect for high-risk sexual behaviour and, therefore, should be screened for HIV before delivery can be undertaken. There is a high possibility that if found HIV-positive they will be denied services at the hospital. Denying labour services to a full term pregnant woman, because of her HIV status, is the most extreme form of discrimination. No such case was reported in this study but in Mumbai many women, and even men whose wives were pregnant, spoke of their harassment running between hospitals and nursing homes to register for delivery. Within the marital relationshiop, women who left their husband because of his HIV/AIDS status were criticised for their behaviour and suspected of marital infidelity and of being the cause of infection. Many of the married women were forced into having sexual intercourse even as the husband's HIV status was known to them. A wife spoke of her helplessness in the situation. Some men, even while taking treatment for AIDS associated problems seem to be in the state of denial of their sero status, as they spoke about their marriage plans. But a young girl, who was widowed soon after her marriage. When her husband died of AIDS, it incarcerated for life although she herself is HIV negative. Her marriage seems difficult as neighbours warn the prospective grooms of her previous husband's death due to AIDS. Some mothers are pressurised to refuse to themselves the pleasures of motherhood because they are too weak to look after the child and hope that the child's HIV status will turn negative and that the child's future may get secured though adoption.

Much of the discrimination and stigmatisation that women suffer occurs after the husband's death and mainly from the in-laws. There is clear discrimination made between the son and the daughter-in-law even as both share their HIV identity. Many positive women spoke about denial of medical assistance, share in husband's property or in pension amount or insurance amount due to him. There was discrimination in food quality and distancing within the home. The widow is at times blamed for the son's death and asked to leave the home, but few of them are not welcome in their natal homes also. And then they are faced with the prospect of being without a roof over their head.

Such support and care was seen in homes where husband was open in admitting his risk behaviour to the wife and where the in-laws and other family members were counselled about HIV/AIDS. The fear of infection did not generate a gap between the infected daughter-in-law and others and the acceptance that the daughter-in-law was not accountable for the disease absolved her of the blame. However, not all HIV-positive women were so fortunate. Many were blamed for the son's ill-health and were refused food. In fact, some were doubtedly blamed.

As HIV-positive widows, not only that women are refused the right to live in the marital home, they are also denied share in husband's property. In Bangalore two cases of property disputes were reported.

Marginalised Infected Persons

Among the population of those living with HIV/AIDS, the sub-populations of female commercial sex workers, eunuchs and homosexuals experience AIDS associated discrimination and stigmatisation in manners that marginalise them not only from the society at large but also from their own community. Indeed, with HIV/AIDS, their marginalisation seems complete.

For the CSWs social discrimination and stigmatisation are not novel experiences. The everyday business of living and earning through their bodies stigmatises them as 'loose women', 'dirty women', 'women who break homes/families'. In the scenario of AIDS they are perceived as the 'carriers of the AIDS virus' and the 'main source' of HIV infection in the general community with intervention targeted basically at them. Documentation of sex workers' experiences of seeking medical assistance exposes the biases and prejudices of the medical workers towards them. Sex workers interviewed for this study talked about their preference for private doctors because treatment was assured on payment, even though the prejudices prevailed there too. In the public hospitals, on the other hand, they not only were discriminated and stigmatised but denied treatment also, or given un-satisfactory treatment. They reported how the medical staff made fun of them, and remarked upon their dress or makeup. The staff generally made them wait longer. In one public hospital there were separate lines for commercial sex workers and 'housewives'. The discrimination is made loud and clear when clinic staff instructs the sex workers to 'sit on one side. Let these women from 'decent' homes come first they need to go back home in time what is your hurry?' Commercial sex workers typically advised to abort pregnancies with the moralistic warning that they will be bad examples to their progeny.

The experiences of commercial sex workers living with HIV/AIDS need to be examined against this background of their general and ongoing experience in society and especially in the health care setting. Debates with two HIV-positive commercial sex workers and 4 focus group discussions with commercial sex workers who worked as peer educators in 2 AIDS prevention programmes (some of whom were HIV-infected but not recognised as such in the group), disclosed discrimination and stigmatisation experienced in the health care setting and from within their own community of commercial sex workers. Interviews with 3 HIV-positive sex workers and one FGD with a group of peer educator commercial sex workers (whose HIV status was not known) supported much of these outcomes.

Among the commercial sex workers, as in other groups of sero-positive individuals, HIV test is advised by health care professionals whenever there is recurrent fever, TB, diarrhoea or an STD. Although these are indicators used for HIV testing in the general community as well, for the commercial sex workers any single episode of a disease is taken as suggestive of HIV infection. This, the commercial sex workers in Mumbai alleged makes them feel stigmatised and stressed. One of them explained, even before asking me what health problem I had, the doctor asked me, 'Do you have AIDS? Go for an HIV test first'. Physically weak and thin looking commercial sex workers are often subjected to such questioning in medical setting and suspected for HIV by their own follow-workers also.

In one of the women's hospitals frequented by commercial sex workers, blood sample is taken from every treatment seeking sex worker without explaining the purpose and nature of the test. When test outcomes are demanded, the staff, sometimes explain, 'there is some mistake in the blood, do not worry'. And when HIV test results are shown there is no post-test counselling and the manner of disclosing test outcomes itself lacks in discretion.

Several commercial sex workers during a FGD said that usually doctors avoid touching the commercial sex worker, more so when she is HIV-infected. On insisting admissions for destitute and very ill commercial sex workers, doctors argue, 'if we start admitting everyone who comes, how will we function?' Of the three public hospitals, close to the red light area, only one was named as giving sufficient services to commercial sex workers both in terms of treatment and admission. Few of the problems faced by commercial sex workers are identical to those experienced by the general population seeking health care services in the government hospital. However, what differentiates their experiences from those of the general population is the stigmatising attitude of health workers that singles them out from the others.

It is not uncommon, for instance, for HIV-positive commercial sex workers to be told by doctors that they are 'scourge' of society and the root cause (*jad*) of the epidemic. One HIV-positive commercial sex worker, who insisted on admission in the hospital, because she had no place to go and was very sick, was told by the nurse, 'you do the sins *(paap)* and then burden us by coming to the hospital'. Labelling is easy when it comes to referring them and they are simply referred to as, 'hey, you with HIV, (HIV *wali*)', as though this was their job.

The general perception that commercial sex workers are carriers of the AIDS virus is shared by many doctors. The research staff of this project was told by a female doctor at the women's hospital in the red light area that as more and more sex workers are becoming HIV-positive, more and more men were getting infected and dying of AIDS.

Revelations of their HIV status in their own community of sex workers and with *'gharwalis'* (Literally house owner; but in regard to sex workers it means the woman who owns them because she has purchased them for a price) is very rare. The reasons are much the same as in the general community namely, fear of isolation, ostracisation, loss of income and destitution. The first reaction of most commercial sex workers to their HIV test outcome is one of denial. They do not accept the report and stop taking treatment in the hope of forgetting all about it. Peer educators said they come to know of positive sex workers only when they began falling sick. The fear of social rejection from the other sex workers is powerful even among the peer educators who are expected to be more knowledgeable and attitudinally more aware. As per the incharge of a local AIDS NGO, despite being a part of the AIDS awareness and education programme, the HIV-infected peer educators are unable to discard their own fears and keep their HIV status confidential from the other peer educators. But it is the *gharwali* who is feared the most by the HIV-infected commercial workers since she controls their access to their male customers and thereby to their income source.

Much as the *gharwalis* would like to deny AIDS as a problem, they are encountered with the problem of HIV-infected sex workers with an alarming rate at present. But 'only about one in ten would have a supportive attitude'. The descriptions of the peer educators and of the positive sex workers disclosed the rejecting behaviour of the *gharwalis* towards sex worker with HIV / AIDS working under their control. Commercial sex workers suffering from AIDS and dying on the street of the red light area is a common sight, so the research staff was told. The form of destitution is the worst fear among women in the sex business. Therefore, sex workers with HIV / AIDS suffer discrimination many times over.

Homosexuals

In Mumbai and Bangalore, it was a Herculean task to interview HIV-positive homosexuals. Homosexuals are not only a marginalised, but also a latent population in the Indian society. In the metros a few support groups have emerged but these too work confidentially and are open only to some select heterosexuals, mainly professionals such as social counsellors. Efforts to elicit voluntary participation of HIV-positive homosexuals in this study proved unsuccessful despite perseverance of months. In Mumbai two gay groups, i.e., Humsafar Trust and Udaan were contacted. At Humsafar Trust a meeting of the Principal Investigator with the gay members was arranged during a festival party at which the research purpose was explained and participation of eligible members requested. In addition to this, an Appeal Letter was put up on the notice board of the office for members to approach the PI individually over the phone. But none called. At Udaan despite assurances given by its co-ordinator to co-operate, meetings with potential respondents proved difficult. In Bangalore the gay group

'Good as You' and a group called 'SABRANG', which is a meeting point for members from all sexual orientations, who wish to promote people's right to choice of alternative sexuality and their social acceptance, were approached. But, none of the members volunteered to participate in the study.

The following discussion, highlighting pertinent problems with regard to homosexuals in the context of HIV/AIDS, is based on interviews/conversations with two gay activists in Bangalore, and one gay activist and one social counsellor working with a gay support group in Mumbai. Besides, relevant information collected from 2 HIV-positive homosexuals during the previous study of the PI titled 'Household and Community Response to HIV/AIDS in Mumbai', was also consisted. One of the two positive gays continued as a participant for the current study also, to give a sequel to his discriminatory experiences in the household and health care settings. In the two cities HIV-positive homosexuals were hard to recognise as a group or a community. According to a gay activist, they look to take on the heterosexual identity once they find their sero-positive status. They are thus lost to the gay community as they seek to merge with the mainstream community of heterosexuals to escape being 'found out' as gays. Coping with two stigmatised identities—one the gay identity and the other sero-positive identity-is difficult for the homosexuals, in a closed homophobic society. There is a far greater stigma connected with homosexuality than to AIDS in India.

A gay activist in Mumbai confirms this. According to him, once a gay finds out that he is HIV-positive, he stops coming to the Counselling Centre and perhaps joins a positive people's group instead, where he latents his gay status. Gay positives thus start to identify themselves more with the HIV-positive persons and their struggles. As health complications mount this identification intensifies.

In Bangalore too the gay positives are a latent population. One gay activist said, 'In Bangalore I do not know a single person who is gay and who is HIV-positive. I do not think any one can have any data on this'. It is in fact an issue. There are no data on gay positives because they are masked by the fact that they do not own up to their gay identities. In Mumbai, there is an indication of a high number of gay HIV-positives based on a recent survey and the number of men who come for AIDS counselling, but who do not come for follow up after confirming their HIV status (Ashok Row Kari, personal communication). Besides, some of them start aligning themselves with other sero-positive men and tend to sever their association with gay groups or keep their HIV status latest from other homosexuals. Social prejudices and attitudes towards the gays explain their behaviour. Gays in India are targeted as, 'sexually deviant' and 'pervert men' whose only preoccupation is with sex. They have no space in society 'to be themselves', to live their individual lives in their own terms, and be able to own up their gay identity. There are many fears that trouble gays—the fear of being socially ridiculed and ostracised, the fear of rejection from family, the fear of violence and aggression from the police and general population, the fear of losing employment, etc. Elaborating on the problems encountered by homosexuals in India, a gay activist in Bangalore talked about the lack of emotional support and understanding in family and society for them. It is a 'heterosexualised' world he said, in which issues concerning the homosexuals find no place. At the personal level homosexuals are unable to form long, sustained relationships because, there are no mechanisms in society that will help them work towards this. The narrow definition of the family, both sociologically and legally, limits it to one's relatives by blood or marriage or adoption. Persons deemed 'close' to you are not considered family. Homosexuals therefore, find inheritance laws unfavourable to them.

Similar problems confront them in a big variety of social situations, he pointed out. Homosexuals couples, for example, are denied the benefit of concessional couple memberships at club, etc. because a gay couple is not considered to be the same as a heterosexual couple. Against this usual background of a homophobic 'heterosexualised' society, the gays find the health care setting in India also highly 'hetrosexualised'. Health practitioners, staff and the whole system is oriented to give services only to those who fit the traditional definitions of 'sexuality'. The questioning done by medical practitioners, for example, is highly offending to gays who have consulted them for STDs, as reported by a counsellor for homosexuals. STDs among men are usually thought to be an outcome of sex with female sex workers. Therefore, all STD patients are asked standard questions such as, 'when did you last go to a woman' (implying a female commercial sex worker) or 'how often have you been visiting those women (in sex business)? For homosexuals, as per the counsellor, such questions are deeply disturbing because they feel repulsed by the very thought of having sex with a woman. Many gays are thus put off by the assumption on the part of the doctors that all men are heterosexuals. Because many doctors are not aware or pretend to tolerate the reality that several married men in India lead double lives as bisexuals, they stop further questioning after finding out that the patient is married. As a result, homosexuals as a vulnerable group in the HIV epidemic do not get recognised.

This blindness to the prevalence of homosexuals has led to ignorance among city doctors about the STD profile of homosexuals. An incident that occurred sometimes back in Mumbai is quoted to make the point. The story goes that, in a Mumbai hospital a homosexual with a STD in his mouth drew laughter from the doctor as he had never seen anybody with a STD in the mouth. As per gay activists this is because our medical education discriminates with homosexuals. It is a way of ignoring the fact of their presence in society. For all these reasons gays feel discouraged to consult doctors in the health care settings, especially in the government hospitals. For them discrimination and stigmatisation start from the very questions that are put to them by medical professionals.

Eunuchs

For the eunuchs or *hijras* (the third gender) discrimination and stigmatisation stem chiefly from their sexual identity (or a lack of it). Those in the sex business (some live through begging) are further oppressed and despised for earning through 'unnatural sex'. The AIDS epidemic has only added to their sense of isolation and marginalisation. In Mumbai interviews with two eunuchs living with HIV/AIDS and a group of seven eunuchs (some of them HIV-infected, but identity not disclosed to research staff), and in Bangalore with a group of four eunuchs (sero status unknown), give testimony to their negative social experiences.

Injections are usually perceived as more superior forms of treatment among communities. They are considered to be quick and more effective remedies over oral medicines. But medical professionals have reduced the use of injections to prevent infection through needle. This is being perceived as discrimination by those, such as sex workers, who were till now very used to taking injections, especially for STDs. In small private clinics, however, injections are still given for a higher fee.

Insiders' Perspective

For individuals living with HIV/AIDS people in the general community are either friends or foes depending on how they are 'perceived' to be treating them and how they are assessed along the support dimension. It is often argued that infected people's assessment is likely to be subjective and biased, influenced as it is, by their enhanced sense of vulnerability and persecution. To balance the scene, therefore, a perspective from the 'other' side is also necessitated. Since the health care setting is where a majority of the persons living with HIV/AIDS reported having experienced discrimination and stigmatisation in accessing health services, medical professionals were interviewed to consider the 'other side' of the story, or to gain the 'insiders' perspective, as it were.

Seventeen medical professionals, 11 from government and 6 from private hospitals, were interviewed in-depth to assess the phenomena of discrimination and stigmatisation in the hospital setting 'through their eyes'. These consisted 9 senior doctors, 2 resident doctors, 2 medical directors of hospitals (Total = 13), in Mumbai and 2 senior doctors and 2 medical superintendents in Bangalore. All of them were told to assess HIV/AIDS associated discrimination and stigmatisation in the hospitals as seen/ perceived by them and their opinions for the same. Many medical professionals affirmed the prevalence of discrimination and stigmatisation of people with HIV/AIDS in the medical setting, quoting events they had seen, of their neglect and harassment. There is an almost hystorical kind of fear . . . at all levels, starting from the bumblest, the sweeper or the ward boy upto the heads of departments which make them pathologically feared of having to deal with an HIV infected patient, and whenever they have an HIV patient, the responses are shameful.

Such behaviours are not limited to government hospitals alone. A senior and well known gynaecologist attached to both government and private hospitals reported that her fellow doctors from private hospitals routinely send their cases of HIV-positive pregnant woman to her at the government hospital because they cannot undertake these deliveries at their own hospitals. Although, the private hospitals named by her have recently relaxed their policies for HIV/AIDS patients, elaborate precautions like fumigating the labour rooms and keeping them isolated for 3–8 days are reported indicating the exaggerated fear of staff and doctors at those hospitals.

Speaking with a senior gynaecologist at one such private hospital, the fear of infection as justification for the necessity for elaborate precautions including the complete AIDS kits for all labour room staff, fumigation of the room and early discharge to the mother and baby were brought out amply. Other stories of a discriminatory nature cited by few doctors included, delays in surgical procedures, shunting the patients between OPDs or between government hospitals, refusal to undertake pathological analysis, isolation in the ward and substandard services. Interviews with many doctors revealed that it is not only the positive patients, but at times their consulting doctors too, who face problems getting them admitted for treatment at clinics. One doctor, associated with positive people's support group in Mumbai, recalled several cases when he struggled to ensure medical care for his patients. Doctors giving treatment to positive patients are now getting identified as 'AIDS doctors' and acquiring the status of a specialist. This in a way is making it easy for the non-willing doctors to shirk their professional accountability.

In Bangalore, one private doctor to whom many cases of infected persons are referred, both from the private and government hospitals, supported the observations made by doctors in Mumbai. He referred to the irrational fear of AIDS among doctors who tended to transfer their fear to their patients also. One of the many ways in which doctors across the board tried to ignore their professional duty was by referring their patients to a few 'HIV/AIDS' specialists in the city.

However, doctors in private hospitals in both the cities usually tended to defend their professional colleagues. The recent opening-up of some private hospitals to HIV/AIDS patients was cited by them as a big event in the medical field. The doctors showed humanitarian concern for HIV patients but while elaborating on the precautions taken to treat such patients, justified their fears and anxieties about infection and safety of their junior staff. According to a doctor the usual practice of wearing gloves was significant precaution complemented with a pair of ordinary eyeglasses and mask during surgery. The rest, he said were unrealistic and unaffordable in the government hospitals. There is a great necessity, the doctor said, of using scarce resources judiciously given our state of hospitals.

This is in contrast with the large-scale disposal of gloves, etc. in many private hospitals that ultimately is a substantial economic burden for HIV-positive patients in private hospitals. Here patients are expected to provide AIDS kits for attendant workers during surgery and child deliveries. Such fears were partly attributed to the doctors' unwillingness to have an open mind and partly to the loss of culture of 'care' among the medical professionals for whom patient's health was always to come before their own safety. Confirming the above point of view, some young medical residents in Mumbai discussed the tendency among present dayds medical practitioners of avoiding unnecessary risk to the extent possible and in the process becoming obsessed with their own health rather than their patient's.

This strong 'self preservation' trend and obsession with fear of infection was quite evident among health care professionals and workers at all levels. Statistics presented in an earlier discussion on 'discrimination in medical setting' confirms this. Among all health care professionals it was the doctors, and among them the senior doctors, who were held more responsible for being discriminatory towards HIV-infected persons.

The apprehensions of senior doctors, were attributed to the fear of the 'unknown' as they had no exposure to patients with HIV at the time of their training period. And hence the attitude 'why take unnecessary risk'? The young doctors, because of greater exposure to AIDS cases, it was argued would be more open and non-prejudiced in their approach. Pragmatically too, the doctors (both senior and junior) felt that 'very soon it will be a matter of their bread and butter if doctors continued to refuse positive patients in their medical facility'. Among the specialists, the surgeons and gynaecologists were termed as being more rigid and biased towards HIV/AIDS infected persons. In Bangalore, like Mumbai, mandatory testing for HIV was reported for both surgeries and child deliveries at all private hospitals and a few government hospitals too.

While the surgeons and gynaecologists were recognised to have a higher risk of infection in comparison to other medical professionals due to the invasive nature of their work, they were also treated as the major source of differential behaviour towards positive patients. An important observation made was that medical care to positive patients seemed to depend on doctors' freedom to exercise 'choice'. Here there is necessarily a divide between doctors in the private and the government health care sectors. Physicians in the private health care sector have the 'choice' and the freedom to deny care and whenever possible they choose to exercise that 'freedom'. The private health care culture, it is alleged, places no emphasis on health professionals, especially on the 'specialists' to accept HIV/AIDS patients. Administrators and doctors at private hospitals agreed that there were individual variations in doctor's decision to test all patients for HIV or to refuse them altogether. Consultants are not under compulsion by hospital policies. Physicians in the public health settings, in contrast, have no such choice; they are bound to accept all classes of patients irrespective of the degree of risk (although as reported earlier, some doctors in public care settings also manage to refuse care to positive patients). This privilege to exercise 'choice' on the part of private practitioners was a major issue identified in explaining their behaviour towards patients with HIV/AIDS.

An identical observation was made by another doctor who explained 'indeed no hospital (doctors) should or can refuse (positive patients) but private hospital doctors get off by the hook by staying they frame their own policies'. In fact, this was the message conveyed by one of the leading doctors at a private hospital who was clear in her mind that 'AIDS was the sole responsibility of the government and the public health sector'. It, therefore, seems that AIDS associated discrimination by doctors is individual specific, but 'system aided' where individual doctors with biased attitudes are 'tolerated' and in a way 'persuaded' to continue with their behaviour unnoticed. Few doctors sought to explain 'patient behaviour' as well and defended certain behaviours on part of the doctors. For instance, 'isolation' or the practice of keeping AIDS patients separately in wards was explained more in terms of protecting the patients from getting infections from others, or in terms of insulating them from feeling discriminated.

In a public maternity hospital the practice of mandatory HIV testing, for all pregnant women without their will, is explained with pro-patient arguments. The gynaecologist explained that she was more worried about preventing parental transmission of HIV and so began gynaecological intervention by putting those HIV-positive pregnant women, who could afford, on AZT early on in their pregnancy. For this she required to test all pregnant women for HIV. She argued that while surgeons were testing all patients for HIV to protect themselves, she was doing it to prevent further transmission to babies.

The gynaecologist discounted the argument that testing for HIV without patient consent was any violation of medical ethics. Many other practices 'perceived' to be anti HIV positive patients were sought to be logically explained. For instance, genuine problems of shortage of instruments and protective gears like gloves, etc. in government hospitals were pointed out by some junior doctors as likely causes for delays in giving services to positive patients.

But senior doctors did not purchase these arguments as they felt these were mere excuses because there was no lack of such supplies, only poor management. A common argument has been that all patients coming to the public health facility usually are subjected to substandard services and that positive patients are not the only exceptions. This was met by a strong disapproval.

At public hospitals, the non-availability of items of primary importance like gloves and masks was reported widely. Nurses and ward staff at times worked without any protection to hands and expressed fear of getting infected. In one government hospital nurses admitted sending their own blood samples for HIV testing to the hospital laboratory in order to check their sero status without the knowledge of their superiors. However, positive patients were seen as being extra sensitive to doctors' behaviour towards them.

But the situation was seen to be improving, albeit gradually. Increasingly greater exposure to HIV-positive cases was assisting in orienting the younger generation doctors to the epidemic and reducing their fears about it. In fact in each of the selected hospitals, government or private, there were a significant number of doctors, nurses and supportive staff who were unbiased, free of irrational fear and prejudices, and committed to their profession of patient care. HIV/AIDS has not led to a disregard of their moral duty to treat the sick.

In both the cities, the research staff met a number of doctors who worked along with AIDS NGOs offering free medical consultation to AIDS patients, helping in framing guidelines for care and treatment at short stay homes, being part of community based AIDS education programmes and serving on the panel of national or the state level government programmes. Their involvement, therefore, varied from AIDS awareness programmes to treatment of AIDS patients to training for AIDS care to research. Many NGO functionaries and HIV-positive people spoke highly of these doctors calling them 'doctors in the true sense'. Doctors who thus led from front had model effect on the nursing and ward staff who were in turn able to discard their fear of the virus.

One main question that was posed to the doctors was how do they explain the supportive and favourable response to HIV/AIDS from a section of medical professionals while a majority seems to be driven with fear and prejudice. In conclusion, it is these doctors who alone will give medical leadership in confronting the challenge of the epidemic.

Fear and Prejudice

Two important themes emerge powerfully from the evaluation of the phenomena of discrimination and stigmatisation in HIV and AIDS are 'fear' and 'prejudice'. It is the fear, almost a paralysing fear, of having a disease like AIDS, of being negatively judged for one's behaviour, of degradation of one's personal and social dignity, of being 'found out', of dying a stigmatised death that explains the silence and confidentiality about one's HIV/AIDS identity. And what explains the fear is the 'prejudice' in society towards behaviour that is thought 'deviant' or 'unacceptable' and towards people associated with those behaviours.

Prejudice leads to biased attitudes and rigid ways of thinking and behaving towards 'others' who are the object of prejudice. It results in stigmatisation, rejection, isolation and marginalisation of the objects of prejudice. These behaviours—their actual occurrence or the probability of their occurrence—lead to a fear response that can be very crippling. To understand the phenomenon of prejudice as a reason of the fear response, the attitudes of people—in the care giving setting, in the household, and in the general population, towards people with HIV/AIDS and towards the disease itself, needs to be analysed. Whether in Mumbai or in Bangalore, AIDS was most strongly related with sexual deviance—mainly associated to sex with prostitutes. Statements like the following are common when discussion is about AIDS.

Usually AIDS is compared with death and justified as punishment for people's sinful behaviour (*paap*). It was referred to as a 'dirty' (*gandi*), dreaded (*bhayanak*) disease which brought shame and disgrace to infected people and their family members—so, people ought to feel ashamed and hide the disease. Shirking a difference with the western perspective, AIDS is also seen as a result of one's past acts or sins (*pichle karmon/paapon ka phal*) and one's fate (*bhagya ki baat hai*). In various discussions with community members and hospital staff; the 'othering' of AIDS is evident. AIDS 'happens' to others who are unlike 'us' in behaviour and thoughts and this 'othering' phenomenon explains low risk perception of HIV for self.

Infected people are usually referred to in the third person with little emotional closeness shown towards them. In much of the conversation AIDS is also witnessed as an 'invited problem' not deserving people's sympathy and support. Prejudices and opinionated statements like these give rise to fear. Discussions and conversation with positive people brought out many types of fears. These are listed below in the order of their apparent intensity and salience as reflected from discussions held with many groups of respondents.

(i) Fear of AIDS stigma.
(ii) Fear of loss of one's image in family and society.
(iii) Fear of loss of family's name and social reputation, of being instrumental in damaging family's social reputation.
(iv) Fear of being found out, of one's sero status revelation of getting detected as sexually deviant.
(v) Fear of social discrimination and isolation, of being avoided, shunned by others.
(vi) Fear of being viewed and classified as members of deviant groups such as promiscuous people and homosexuals.
(vii) Fear of death, of dying early, in prime of youth.
(viii) Fear of dying pitiably, dying with stigma, dying uncared, without the last rituals.

(ix) Fear of inviting social ridicule, mock, laughter, and hatred.

(x) Fear of several illnesses, debilitating ill health, of painful conditions, not receiving medical attention and denial of admission to hospital.

(xi) Fear of being deserted, of loss of significant relationships, and loss of their trust and confidence.

(xii) Fear of losing one's employment or income source.

(xiii) Fear of passing the infection to others, to spouse, children, other family members.

Some fears are displayed by both the infected persons and those around him/her, for instance those providing care. The greatest concern of caregivers is with 'contagion' — that is the fear of contracting the virus, and of being'misunderstood' as to its 'source' should they contract the virus. Health staff constantly talk about the fear of 'getting' AIDS, and of encountering discrimination thereafter, were they to catch the infection through patient care. Others fears shown are the fear of getting associated with 'AIDS patients care' and the loss of one's employment. The 'others' around the 'infected' person fear the probability of being in the infected person's shoes, as it were. This fear appears very real to them, because it stems from their own prejudices and biased attitudes. And these prejudices feed fear among the infected one the one hand, and produce unsupportive responses like rejection and discrimination and isolation from health care givers and friends, on the other. These negative responses in turn generate fear and anxiety and so the cycle is in progress. In those social scenarios where fear and prejudice both overlap, their interaction can give rise to extreme forms of discrimination. For instance, in the health care setting, staff showed both fear and biased attitudes, were more vociferous in demanding isolation for HIV-positive patients and more resistant to give care.

Fear and prejudice result from insufficient awareness and misconception about AIDS, but only partly. Among the doctors and nurses, for instance, AIDS-related knowledge was significant, yet many of them were ambivalent about care to HIV patients. While fear, prejudice and inadequate knowledge explain discrimination and stigmatisation to a large extent, there are many other reasons also that contribute to unsupportive responses towards people with HIV/AIDS. As shown below, these factors are arranged in stepwise fashion to suggest their cumulative negative impact. While the lower end factors are more psychological in nature necessitating attitudinal change, the reasons at the higher end need systemetic and structural changes in the care giving sector.

Personal and Systematic Factors in Discrimination

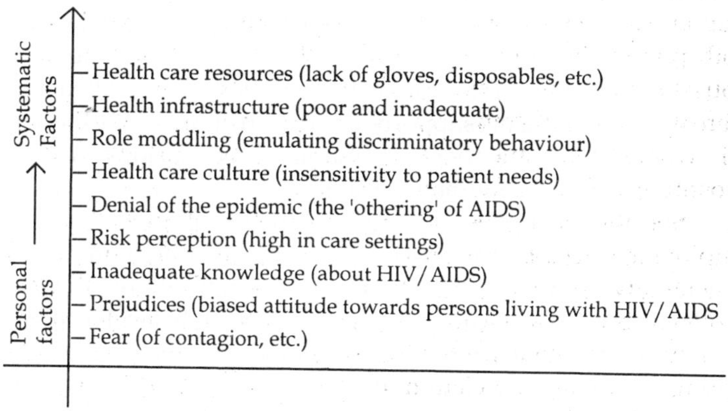

To summarise, epidemics of feared and despised diseases bring out the worst in human behaviour. And as Sontag writes... 'it is not suffering as such that is most deeply feared but suffering that degrades.' In fact, most HIV-positive patients felt 'it is not AIDS, but it is the stigma that kills'.

Conclusion and Suggestions

The study lists widespread existence of HIV/AIDS associated discrimination, stigmatisation and denial in a variety of contexts including health care, community, household and employment; and in many forms, both blatant and subtle, in two metropolitan cities of India. Seven broad themes are identified that describe the contexts, content and expressions of these negative experiences. These are, the health care setting as the major context reported pertaining to discrimination and denial of care services or substandard treatment; confidentiality and denial of the epidemic in the employment sector; the gendered nature of household response; the further marginalisation of vulnerable group members living with HIV/AIDS; the social prejudices and biases underlying HIV/AIDS associated segregationist trends and fear as the most widespread response to it; and finally a perspective from health care professionals on discrimination in HIV/AIDS. Discrimination due to HIV/AIDS is manifested in all walks of life but the context that was many times and at times spontaneously reported was the health care context. A majority of the respondents of the study recounted many examples direct, as well as, indirect rejection, refusal and resistance from health professionals, at all levels, in response to their necessity for care and treatment at health facilities, both public and private. Instead of the health care context, the household and the community contexts were other contexts that were witnessed to be un-supportive and even oppressive especially for women and members of marginalised groups namely, prostitutes, eunuchs and homosexuals.

Specific examples of discrimination reported from the employment sector were fewer in this study as compared to what is generally reported in the media, or is usually thought to be a problem, but what clearly emerged was a high level fear and anxiety about potential job loss and social separation in one's work setting following revelation of HIV/AIDS identity. Personal discussions with a few physicians who have, on request from many HIV-positive patients, issued certificates of fitness to assist them save their jobs, give indirect but strong support that threat to their job security is quite real (G. Bhave, personal communication). Thus, although the employment context is not mainly reported as a context of discrimination, it is the one context that possibly has the heaviest weight of the latent epidemic with grave consequences for a silent spread of the virus undermining any efforts towards normalizing the epidemic and giving it a human face. Another significant outcome pertaining to the workplace is the widespread denial on part of corporate heads of the threat of the epidemic to industry. Other contexts of discrimination that caused concern to people with HIV/AIDS are life insurance and education of children. With the listing of HIV test life in the Insurance Forms, fears about their policies not being honoured because of their HIV status are keeping the positive people from claiming insurance and also from exploring with other long term monetary gain plans. Some of them see Insurance Policies as discriminatory towards them. Problems in getting children admitted to school/boarding due to their parent's HIV/AIDS status are also emerging. Voices that are difficult to hear and likely to go unheard are those of destitute infants, tested for HIV in child care institutions with those revealed to be HIV-positive shifted to other select institutions for so called better care and management.

Various direct, blatant and extreme forms of discrimination are reported but many more are very subtle, insidious and sophisticated. Much of the stigmatization is reported to be real and experienced at first hand, as contained in the personal testimonies of positive people, but equally often much of it is perceived and apprehended. These subtle and indirect ways of discrimination and the 'perceived' and 'felt' stigma prove to be more crippling and disabling, affecting the HIV infected person's desire to live, to reveal HIV status and to seek treatment. What makes the situation particularly difficult is that such subtle and sophisticated forms of discrimination are hard to substantiate and even harder to challenge. The fact that the public health system in the country is anyway less than satisfactory and usually insufficient for a great majority of the treatment seekers, makes it even more difficult for the comparatively smaller and powerless segment of HIV-infected population to demand services and fight for their rights. Regarding HIV/AIDS knowledge and beliefs, the health care sector is not greatly different from the general community. Knowledge about routes of HIV transmission is accompanied by beliefs in casual and minor contacts made during patient care as risk factors for transmission. As a result, there exists a generalized and somewhat diffused sense of personal risk among health care workers. Further, this risk perception cuts across all level of health workers irrespective of professional knowledge base and competence. It is important to note that beliefs about transmission risk via needle stick injury and wounds of infected persons are generally high within the hospital scenario even though during discussion the sexual route of transmission is what is more readily and widely reported. There is thus an irrational and seemingly unrealistic perception of personal risk that is neither questioned nor reflected upon by professionals.

One of explanation is people's fear of the 'chance' factor, that is, the 'what if...' factor. There is a common apprehension among health functionaries of things going wrong 'just by chance' resulting in infection. Beliefs in casual ways of HIV transmission, particularly in the health care setting, need to be addressed through education and training to correct the unrealistic perception of personal risk and prevent discrimination of HIV/AIDS patients. The extent and nature of discrimination in the health care context ranges from denial of services (hospital admission, treatment and care), and poor quality of services to mandatory testing for HIV for cases of child delivery and surgeries, lack of informed consent before HIV testing, lack of counselling services and breach of secrecy of information about patients HIV/AIDS status.

The refusal of services for care and treatment represents the most immediate and pressing concerns of the positive patients and thus, these had spontaneity in their narratives, and were the most widely reported ways of discrimination by them. The ways of discrimination that are located within the Human Rights framework, were, not among their concerns and problems, at least 'not in the face of more critical and life threatening situations and therefore, evaluated from a more deeper probing on the issue. Many of the medical staff/physician practices and hospital policies can be seen as discriminatory towards HIV/AIDS patients. These are summarized below:

Many of the medical staff/physician practices and hospital policies can be seen as discriminatory towards HIV/AIDS patients as summarized below:

(a) Testing for HIV is at times routinely done for all patients seeking hospital admission and in some hospitals done selectively for patients necessitating invasive procedures such as, surgeries and child deliveries. This is more the case in private hospitals than in government hospitals, although surgeries necessitate mandatory testing in some public hospitals also.

(b) In approximately all hospital departments, besides a very few, HIV testing is done without seeking informed consent from the patient. Written informed consent is nowhere a practice.

(c) Where informed consent is taken, it is mostly with male patients and taken verbally. Female patients are advised to get themselves tested or are emphasised to undergo HIV test without their consent, following positive test results of their husband. HIV testing in their case is done without considering their asymptotic status, and without any immediate benefits accruing to them.

(d) Informed consent for HIV test is rarely thought important for members of vulnerable groups such as prostitutes and eunuchs.

(e) Testing for HIV is done with the express aim of ensuring the safety of professionals/staff and/or for exercising the power to deny or withhold care and treatment. It is remotely, if at all, related with public health safety and almost never with the purpose of benefiting the HIV-positive individuals regarding counselling, information and/or better care and support.

(f) Universal precautions are absent in all hospitals and they are replaced by selective, irrational and even greater use of precautionary equipments like gloves, and AIDS kits; pertaining to care giving to HIV positive patients. These practices are not only discriminatory towards positive individuals as they identify them as 'special' needs or 'risk' patients; they also put the attending staff on a false sense of security since they do not know about the HIV status of other patients, and neglect the need to take universal precautions.

(g) Confidentiality and privacy of HIV patients are lacking in medical care setting forcing some patients of HIV to delay or avoid treatment to the extent they can, jeopardizing their health concerns in the process.

(h) Confidentiality is breached not because there is a sense of duty to warn and protect spouse or to inform members in the spirit of great responsibility but more to shift the patient care to the family. Other cause why confidentiality is not respected is due to the lack of such culture in the hospital set up.

(i) Although concepts such as 'barrier nursing' and 'immuno-compromise patients' are adopted, it is ironical that they have become synonymous with HIV and thus at present serve the purpose of HIV/AIDS label that is again stigmatizing.

(j) Several hospitals lack counselling services, especially pre-test counselling services and in many others where post-test counselling is at home it serves only the purpose of information giving and is handled without sensitivity, creating more fear than support.

(k) In several hospitals doctors double-up as counsellors even as some of them do not know the professional skills or orientation and almost all are hard pressed for time.

(l) Pregnant women face double discrimination when they are emphasised to undergo mandatory testing for HIV and in the event of testing positive, are refused child delivery services/or advised abortion without counselling for other alternatives.

(m) Hospital staff usually have incomplete knowledge about HIV/AIDS because there are not sufficient training programmes for them. In some hospitals information is deliberately withheld from them to stop them from learning about methods of prevention and then demanding protective gears.

(n) The most disturbing discriminatory practice is the mention of AIDS in the death certificate in some hospitals and of disposing the dead body covered in black plastic sheets. These are big sources of worry and anxiety to positive persons.

The above stated practices and policies imply the violation of patient rights and human rights. These are partly because of inadequate knowledge about HIV/AIDS and many misconceptions and partly because of irrational fear of the virus and prejudices towards people with AIDS. However, it is to be noted that much of this is also done without any knowledge of the principles of human rights. The staff and physicians seem to be unaware of how greatly they violate the principles of informed consent and of secrecy. There is also a big gap in terms of legal education and sensitivity to issues associated with HIV/AIDS among hospital staff. In other words, general insensitivity and apathy characterizes care in hospital setting. The reality on the other hand is that HIV patients do not usually challenge these violations because they themselves lack knowledge about their rights as patients and also because more serious and life threatening problems encounter them forcing them to depend on the very medical community that discriminates with them. Another strong reason is the philosophy of medical practice in India and its authoritarian culture. The doctor patient relationship even in the best of circumstances is unequal and it is many times so when the patients are from the socially and economically disadvantaged groups. The doctor's judgment, decision and behaviour, thus, remain unchallenged by patients. Indian medical practice is also guided by the philosophy that professional knowledge is not for patient's consumption and, therefore, there is general disregard for the need for informed consent and counselling and patients right to information and confidentiality about his/her diagnosis.

In the employment context positive people usually maintain secrecy and silence. In those cases where revelation is made, discrimination and resistance are displayed at times from the employers and at times from their own fellow-workers. Employers refuse to employ or continue to have HIV-infected workers, due to their fear and ignorance about how HIV is transmitted. Equally often it is due to their unwillingness to bear increased burden of medical expenses and liability on the company. But in many instances the management is forced to bow under the pressure from the infected person's fellow workers. Thus, colleagues and the general community of workers single out positive workers and demand their removal in a bid to distance themselves. A major issue that encounter positive people is the lack of industrial policy guidelines on AIDS, preventing them from accessing any concession or services to take care of special health necessities in HIV/AIDS. In the want of any policy or government direction there is rigidity and elasticity in medical rules and service conditions of many organisations disallowing positive people to seek a shift to less cumbersome jobs or seek early retirement with benefits. As a result, many young, permanently employed positive people, with comparatively less serious medical conditions (such as, physical weakness, respiratory infections) but with the physical ability to work on less strenuous jobs, get dismissed because of lack of leave benefits or are emphasised to take premature retirement. The economic consequences for the family of such individuals are serious even as they lower the morale of the young, as yet asymptomatic HIV-positive individuals.

The management in organisations and industries is in a state of denial of the epidemic. There is great reluctance to acknowledge that the epidemic is for real and quite close to them. The invisibility of HIV infections in the work force due to silence and secrecy encourages the top management deny it as a major health problem. There is also significant amount of ignorance about HIV risk assessment such that well paid educated and upwardly mobile staff are discussed as being immune to HIV. Clearly AIDS is perceived as an illness of the very poor, the illiterate and the marginalised. There is thus a vicious cycle of silence and denial in the industrial sector waiting for the epidemic to explode. Current discourses in HIV/AIDS tend to promote the 'equal-opportunity' disease concept but as the results of this study reveal, women and members of marginalised groups are affected more negatively and discriminated more harshly than others. Discrimination for women very often commences from home within intimate relationships. And it goes to many other spheres including health care and right to share in property. For members of victimized groups, like sex workers, gays and eunuchs, HIV/AIDS implies two stigmatized identities compounding the prevailing forms of discrimination towards them and intensifying their sense of alienation in society. For all HIV positive sex workers and eunuchs, the extreme manner of discrimination occurs with loss of sex business and their complete destitution and death on the streets.

In the heterosexualised society as in this country the HIV-positive homosexuals encounter discrimination in all walks of life. Handling two deviant 'selves' becomes difficult and most of them find it less traumatic to accept their positive status than their gay identity. Fear of discrimination and stigmatization pressurises several of them to remain hidden posing grave risk to the silent spread of infection. In sum, those who are already on the periphery of society are further edged out by AIDS associated discrimination and stigmatization. The results of discrimination and stigmatization and denial related with HIV/AIDS are various and largely negative. The pre-dominant results at the individual level are fear leading to privacy of one's HIV status and self-imposed separation and social withdrawal. Depression, anxiety and a sense of helplessness are common. Suicidal trends are harboured by many. In a few cases there is denial of their sero-positivity due to fear of rejection resulting in a careless attitude to their health and to sex with other partners. On falling sick many asymptomatic positive individuals conceal their HIV status in treatment facilities to avoid being refused care. There is grave danger of spread of HIV-infection from latent positive patients. Many patients delay or avoid taking treatment till the time they can, harming their health in the process.

One of the consequences is great economic cost to infected individuals and to their families when they lose employment or are forced to quit job or work on a lesser paid job. There is not only frustration but also a great deal of discontentment at society's callous attitude towards them and anger at discrimination from the health professionals. In a few cases, however, stigmatization is internalized. Shame and prejudices related with AIDS are justified on moralistic grounds, and considered as their fate. Individuals also feel to powerless to question the perpetrators of discrimination. At times the results are constructive as well. A few positive individuals accept their sero-status and work towards living with the virus. Some of them carve altruistic works for themselves as educators; counsellors and as AIDS activists to develop a collective identity and mobilize group support for a greater visibility of the epidemic. These are the effects that require to be promoted and supported for encountering the threat of AIDS. To conclude, HIV/AIDS related discrimination and stigmatization and denial is pervasive and extensive affecting people's desire to fight and survive HIV. Several of the outcomes are probably well known by now but this research gives the much necessitated empirical support to the 'observations' made so far only in anecdotal reports and media. These revelations are screaming evidence of the discrimination and stigmatization of people living with HIV/AIDS and a grim confirmation of the violation of their rights to care, safety and dignity in life.

Suggestions

Following are the several recommendations to reduce discrimination and stigmatization related to HIV/AIDS.

Persons Living with HIV/AIDS

(a) Persons living with HIV/AIDS need to be better educated about their rights as patients and about how to avail justice for discrimination and stigmatization encountered in treatment settings. They need support and awareness pertaining to their primary needs.

(b) Persons living with HIV/AIDS also require legal education and access to justice system for violation of their rights in the context of employment and education.

(c) A more enabling climate needs to be generated for positive people to increase their visibility, to develop a collective identity and form support groups so that discrimination, stigmatization and denial because of their HIV/AIDS can be challenged collectively.

Members of Marginalised Groups

(a) Social marginalisation of members of infected minority groups will only assist intensify the risk of HIV infection. It is thus imperative to protect the rights of minority group members and address their issues in HIV/AIDS distinctively so that they do not get missed out in generic approaches to reduction of HIV/AIDS discrimination and stigmatization.

(b) Discrimination and stigmatization of women who are wives of positive men or who are pregnant must be given specific consideration as they are forced to undergo HIV tests, are ill informed of theirs and their husbands HIV status, and are not given choices on matters of pregnancy, abortion and breast feeding. Discrimination in terms of their early discharge or denial of services based on their gender must be strongly challenged.

Health Care Sector

(a) In the health care sector, the concept of universal precautions needs to be promoted and the irrational and selective use of safety measures minimized as these not only generate a false sense of security among health care professionals, but also adversely affect the emotional health of HIV patients.

(b) Human rights theories of informed consent and confidentiality need to be incorporated in medical practice so that health care staff and professionals do not violate HIV patient's rights to informed choices, privacy and counselling.

(c) Newer concepts and labels such as, 'barrier nursing', 'immune compromise patient' are becoming synonymous with HIV/AIDS and thus serve the same function, as did the labels of 'AIDS'. These concepts need to be used for all types of infections without disclosing the nature of infection to staff involved in treating.

(d) There is an urgent necessity to impart legal education and knowledge among medical professionals and staff about their duties and responsibility towards patient population generally and towards patients with HIV/AIDS in particular. It is important that they know when and how they breach morality principles of health care and the law that ensures patients rights to care and treatment.

(e) Universal precautions that are reasonable and appropriate for the type of medical facility must be applied for all patients (for example, use of gloves for care of all patients and the full safety kit with masks, etc. for all cases necessitating invasive procedures) to eradicate their selective and irrational use only for patients with HIV/AIDS. This will not only assist lessen discrimination but also the risk of infection to staff who work with a false sense of security when they use protective gears only with positive patients.

(f) Minimal protective gears like good quality gloves must be supplied in sufficient numbers to all staff in public hospitals so that the non-availability of such items is not given as an excuse to refuse care to positive patients.

(g) Mandatory testing must be strongly discouraged for individuals including pregnant women regardless of what treatment (invasive or otherwise) they seek, as it at times leads to denial of services to those found positive.

(h) Counselling services must be made available in all health facilities to take care of the psychosocial necessities of positive patients.

(i) To assist individuals who wish to learn of their HIV status without the fear of revelation to others, voluntary testing services alongwith counselling services must be set up in all cities/districts.

(j) Lack of sufficient AIDS education gives rise to irrational fear based on misconceptions and to inappropriate care practices. Hospital staff, under all categories and at all levels, must be given complete and appropriate HIV/AIDS education. No medical institution should be permitted to withhold or limit HIV/AIDS education to any groups of staff under any circumstances.

(k) HIV testing should not be conducted without informed consent of the patient and without pre- and post-test counselling. Treatment and care, as required, must follow HIV-positive test outcomes and efforts must be made to ensure that these are not refused.

(l) It is very important to challenge beliefs in casual ways of HIV transmission and address the diffused and irrational sense of personal risk to HIV infection among health professional to reduce levels of discrimination of HIV/AIDS patients within the health care sector.

Anti-Discrimination Legislation/Measures

(a) Efforts are required to lessen discrimination and stigmatization of persons living with HIV/AIDS in all walks of their lives, notably health care and employment.

(b) An effective mechanism like a grievance cell should be put in place in health care sector for infected people to seek protection of their rights as patients.

(c) Fear based AIDS messages and biased social attitudes towards positive people must be tackled urgently as fear and prejudices lie at the core of segregating tendencies.

(d) It is not sufficient to spread knowledge about HIV/AIDS, its transmitted routes, or even about legal rights. What is urgently required is the government anti-discrimination policy on AIDS supported by a law that will ensure protection of positive people's rights.

Others

(a) Employment sector must develop policy guidelines on AIDS to address the issues of HIV positive workers sensitively and within the human rights framework.

HIV test at the time of seeking employment or as part of routine medical check-ups for permanent staff must be discouraged as these prevent individuals from earning their livelihood and lead to social isolation and rejection for those found HIV-infected.

(b) Childcare institutions must not be permitted to shift their responsibility of care and protection of HIV-infected children to other institutions. Special facilities must be added to the existing ones to give all necessary care and treatment to infected and sick children.

(c) Life Insurance policies must be expanded in appropriate manners to address the needs of HIV-positive people wishing insurance cover and efforts must be made to dispel misconceptions and fears about claims to prevailing insurance policies.

(d) Research on drug trials or any aspect of HIV patients lives within the health care sector must be done only after informed consent of the patient.

It is suggested that there be more proactive responses that address the root causes of discrimination and stigmatization namely AIDS-related misconceptions, ignorance, prejudices and biases; that seek to give equal and better approach to health services; that promote development of policy guidelines in the employment sector and support legislative responses in the form of anti-discrimination bill and a law on AIDS. Reactive responses that seek legal redresses after discrimination is experienced, and that put people to great deal of inconvenience must be recommended to, only as last measures.

7

Governing Legislations

India has the second largest population in the world of approximately one billion persons, out of which 74.3 per cent reside in the rural areas and 25.7 per cent reside in the urban areas. The decedal rate of growth recorded in the 1991 census was 23.6 per cent. The majority of the working population is engaged in agriculture and allied activities (68.8 per cent). Mining and manufacturing constituted 13.5 per cent and services for about 17.7 per cent of the working population. The overall literacy is 52.1 per cent, 63.9 per cent for males and 39.4 per cent for females. The majority of children, more than 90 per cent attend primary education. India is a multi-lingual, multi-ethnic, multi-religious and a multi-cultural country. Though a large proportion of people are Hindi-speaking (39.9 per cent), there are more than 16 different recognised languages and 250 regional dialects. The largest religious group, the Hindus, form the vast majority (82.6 per cent). The other religious groups form a significant minority – Muslims 11.4 per cent, Christian 2.4 per cent, Sikhs 2.0 per cent, Buddhist 0.7 per cent and Jains 0.5 per cent. The historically oppressed castes and tribes recognised by the Constitution as Scheduled Castes and Scheduled Tribes form 23.6 per cent of the population. India is divided administratively into 28 States (based on languages) and 7 Union Territories (as per 2001 census) which are administered by the central government. Each state and union territory is divided into districts, totalling 593 (as per 2001 census) districts in the country.

Fundamental Rights

Being a sovereign, socialist and secular democratic republic, India is governed by a written constitution, the longest constitutional document in the world. The most important chapter in the Constitution is Chapter III, the fundamental rights chapter. These rights include, among others, equality before law (Article 14), prohibition of discrimination on bases of religion, race, caste, sex or place of birth (Article 15), equality of opportunity in matters of public employment (Article 16), protection of certain rights regarding freedom of speech, etc. (Article 19), Protection in respect of conviction for offences (Article 20), protection of life and personal liberty (Article 21), protection against arrest and detention in certain cases (Article 22), freedom of conscience and free profession, practice and propagation of religion (Article 25), and protection of interest of minorities (Article 29). There are several sources of law in India: the constitution, customary law, common law, statutory law and rules and regulations framed under various statutes.

Customary Law

Customary law differs in various parts of the country, even amongst the same religious group. This was superseded to a large extent by religious laws. Therefore, with the setting up of Moghul empire in India, Muslim came to be governed by Muslim Law and Hindus by Hindu Law. This was not limited to personal relations but was also extended to the sphere of contractual relations and crime. The British, through their political rule, left some arenas of law untouched, but legislated on some other spheres. Thus, we had the Indian Penal Code, 1860; the Transfer of Property Act, 1860; the Indian Contract Act, 1872; the Indian Evidence Act, 1872; and the Code of Civil Procedure, 1908. All these laws were to assist trade and commerce for the exploitation of the resources in India. However, laws pertaining to marriage, divorce, succession, guardianship, custody, etc., known as family law or personal law, remained unchanged. There are different personal laws, for different religions. After independence, Hindu law was significantly codified and 'secularised,' as was the Parsi law, though much later. All other religious groups continue to be governed by their 'non-secular' personal laws.

HIV/AIDS : The Indian Scene

The first HIV-infected person was detected in 1986 in Chennai. From the surveillance conducted, the HIV prevalence rate was 1.3 per cent in 1990 amongst those screened. High prevalence rates were seen in sex workers in Mumbai (27 per cent), sex workers forced out of Mumbai to Tamil Nadu (more than 70 per cent) and amongst intravenous drug users in Imphal in Manipur state (more than 43 per cent). The first AIDS case was reported in May, 1986. Until

December 1991, about 104 AIDS cases had been reported. It is estimated that there were approximately 400,000 HIV-positive person in India in 1990. The projection for the year 2000 is 5 million.

Public Health

Notification

There is only one law which provides for the notification of AIDS (Section 51, Public Health Act). Besides this, local municipal laws necessitate every medical practitioner who treats or becomes cognisant of any dangerous disease to give information of the same to the Executive Health Officer (Section 421, Bombay Municipal Corporation Act). Section 2 of the Epidemic Diseases Act also confers powers on an officer of the state government, in case of threat of an outbreak of a dangerous epidemic disease, when general provisions of law are inadequate to tackle the disease, to take such steps including prescribing temporary regulations to be observed by the public or any class of persons that may be deemed necessary to eliminate the outbreak and/or spread of any such epidemic diseases.

Testing, Counselling, Consent

The Goa Public Health Act provides that no person, including a foreigner, shall refuse the collection of blood for investigation of HIV or other communicable/infectious diseases if the health officer has reasonable grounds to suspect that such person is infected with HIV or other infectious diseases (Section 53, (1) (vi) Goa Public Health Act). Though other statutes do not empower testing for HIV specifically, the Epidemic Diseases Act confers the power to frame regulations for such a purpose (Section 2, Epidemic Diseases Act). These powers are amenable to challenge under Articles 14 and 21 of the constitution and remain untested. In states of India where there is no specific statute, consent will be needed before any testing can be done. There is no statutory provision pertaining consent for testing. A combined application of the doctrine of unconscionable contracts, Article 14 (equality clause) and Article 21 of the Constitution (no person shall be deprived of his or her liberty except by procedure established by law) may assist in developing the argument that consent has to be informed and supported by counselling services.

Confidentiality

There is no specific statute providing for medical confidentiality in India. Section 126 of the Evidence Act safeguards from disclosure, professional communications between advocates and their clients. No such provision prevails in the case of doctors. However, the common law doctrine would apply, under which due to the relationship between doctor and patient, the patient reposes confidence in the doctor and passes on all personal and confidential information to the doctor; the law safeguards it from revelation to third parties.

Preventive Measures

Preventive measures are detailed in local municipal laws, local public health laws and in Epidemic Diseases Act, 1897. The state government is empowered, if it is satisfied that the state or any part thereof is visited or threatened with an outbreak of any dangerous epidemic disease if it is satisfied that ordinary provisions of law are adequate for the purpose, to take steps which it thinks necessary and prescribe temporary regulations that would be needed to be observed by the public or any class of persons necessary to prevent the outbreak and expansion of such disease (Section 2, Epidemic Diseases Act). It further provides for the inspection of persons travelling by railway or otherwise and the segregation in hospital or temporary accommodation or otherwise of persons suspected by the inspecting officer of being infected with any such disease. Under local municipal laws, every medical practitioner is needed to notify the existence of any dangerous disease to the executive health officer (Section 421, Bombay Municipal Corporation (BMC) Act). Persons infected with a dangerous disease can be removed to hospital or other places where other patients suffering from the same disease are received for medical treatment (Section 424, BMC Act). Person suffering from dangerous diseases can be prohibited from entering public conveyances without notice (Sections 428 and 430, BMC Act). There are no specific brothel laws or laws affiliating to partner notification in respect of diseases or HIV.

Rights to Medical Information

Article 19(1)(a) of the Constitution gives the right to free speech to all citizens. It has been held that this right includes the right to impart and acquire information.

Since this right is available against the state and public authorities, the right to medical information is available against medical establishments and officers controlled by the state. There is, however, no specific statute conferring the right to medical information.

Discrimination

The constitution of India is anti-discriminatory and anti-arbitrary in its content. These provisions are detailed in the fundamental rights chapter, including equal protection of laws (Article 14), prohibition of discrimination (Article 15) and equal opportunity in matters of public employment (Article 16).

However, Articles 14, 15 and 16 are only applicable to the state and all the local or other authorities controlled by the state, which are considered to be 'state' within the meaning of Article 12 of the Constitution. They do not compel 'purely private institutions performing private functions' to comply with the equality provisions.

Duty to Treat

Doctors in India have refused to treat HIV and AIDS patients in some institutions, alongwith the All India Institute of Medical Sciences, the premier public medical institute in India. There is no specific statute or rules or regulations obliging the doctors to treat HIV patients. However, all doctors and medical personnel have a common law duty to treat patients who are brought to them. The Supreme Court has held that a doctor in a government hospital has an absolute duty to treat a patient to save his or her life (*Parmanand Kataria* verses *Union of India, A 89 SC 2039*). But refusal on various bases is commonplace. In India, besides this bases, in public hospitals, Article 14 will oblige a doctor not to deny the patient on account of his specific illness and the doctor would be bound to treat the particular person, including an HIV-positive person.

Accommodation and Employment

The vast majority of the housing in India is in the private sector. There are no specific laws prohibiting discrimination against any particular individuals on any particular ground in the private sector. However, in the public sector, i.e., where housing is built and/or allotted by the government or public sector corporations or local authorities, the equality and anti-discriminatory provisions of Article 14 would apply. In private sector employment, there are hardly any statutory conditions of service which prohibit discrimination against individuals on the basis of ill health. However, arguments may be developed against the refusal of treating persons with particular ailments unfavourably if they are otherwise fit to carry out their duties. Vis-a-vis employment by the state, the public sector and other authorities governed by the state, the equality and anti-discriminatory provisions of Articles 14, 15 and 16 would be applicable.

Migrant Population

With the increased opportunities of employment in various parts of the country, there is large scale migration of population from different parts of the country to the others. So far as citizens are concerned, they have the right to move freely across the territory of India (Article 19(1)(d)) and to reside and settle in any part of the territory of India (Article 19(1)(e)). These are fundamental rights. However, they are not absolute. So far as international travel is concerned, immigration into India of non-citizens is only subject to the non-arbitrary provisions of Article 14. However, besides this, long-term immigrants and students from overseas, unlike short-term tourists, are obliged to produce HIV-free certificates.

Women's Issues

Status within the Family and Society

Traditionally, in Indian families, irrespective of the community, women have had an inferior status to men. India is primarily a patriarchal and matrilineal society, besides some parts of south India, particularly Kerala, where there has traditionally been a matrilineal society. Traditionally, in all Indian communities polygamy was common and continues to be so in the rural areas. In the case of Muslims, the law still sanctions polygamy and entitles a man to have four wives. The position regarding the right to inherit is discussed later. After independence, the Constitution guaranteed equal rights to women in all walks of public life. Indeed, the Constitution sanctions law which may favour women. However, in practice, the situation is not much better for women. Inequality in public employment has been upheld (*Nergish Mirza* verses *Air India, A 81 SC 1829*).

Besides this, women in India have traditionally been subject to a number of derogatory practices such as dowry, *sati*, domestic violence and cruelty which in modern society have assumed new forms. Cruelty by a husband or his relatives against the wife has been made a punishable offence (Section 498 A, Indian Penal Code). Cruelty has been defined as: (a) any wilful conduct of a nature which is likely to drive a woman to commit suicide or to cause severe injury to life, limb or health (mental or physical) of a women; or (b) harassment of the woman when such harassment is with an intention to coercing her or any of her relatives to meet any unlawful demand or on account of failure to meet such a demand. The offence is cognisable, i.e., the police have the authority to arrest a person against whom a complaint is lodged, without a warrant of a magistrate. Increasing incidents of rape, particularly in custodial conditions, led to the law being amended significantly to provide for enhanced punishment in cases of custodial rape. Moreover, a rebuttable presumption is generated to the effect that no consent was taken when sexual intercourse is proved and the woman says that there was no consent (Section 114, A: Indian Penal Code).

Economic Rights

Though about 50 per cent of the population consists of women, they have much lower access than men to the job market. As per the 1991 census, the work force constituted 39.68 per cent of the total population on an all-India basis. While 35.56 per cent of the male population is in the workforce, only 22.73 per cent of the female population is in the workforce. Economic rights of women in the family set up is discussed elsewhere. However, there is no right to the matrimonial property on the dissolution of marriage. The woman has the right to reside in the matrimonial home only during the subsistence of the marriage.

As Carers

Though women are the primary carers in the family perspective, their rights as carers are not recognised in law to the fullest extent. An indication in this behalf in the law is the rights of women as natural guardians. In all personal laws, women are not the natural guardians of the children throughout their minority. Amongst Hindus, the natural guardian of the male and the female child is the father. The same position occurs in laws applicable to Christians, Parsis and Jews. Under Muslim law, the mother is the natural guardian of a female child up to the age of puberty and male child only up to the age of seven years; the father is the guardian thereafter.

Strategy of Empowerment

The government has recognised that the critical factor in hindering development is the illiteracy of women. In this context, the total literacy programme has been undertaken by the central government and state governments with the help of NGOs to combat illiteracy. Market success has been reported in few areas, whereas the programme has not taken off in other areas. However, in the realm of law, instead of progressing, the law appears to be taking a step backward, such as in the case of Muslims. Maintenance which was available to Muslim women under the ordinary law has been taken away under the Muslim Women's (Protection of Rights on Divorce) Act. It is thus necessary that, apart from social mobilisation through programmes such as the total literacy programme, laws under which women are treated as second class citizens, in particular in the sphere of personal law, be amended as quickly as possible to give effect to the fundamental right of equality under the Constitution.

Information Law

Right to Information. The Constitution of India guarantees the right to freedom of speech and expression to all citizens (Article 19(1)(a)). It is available only to citizens and against state action but not against private persons.

Barriers

There are as yet no specific statutes, rules or regulations governing HIV information. Barriers to the general right to information would obviously be relevant in this behalf. In this context, it may be pointed out that the right guaranteed under Article 19(1)(a) is not an absolute right. Article 19(2) of the Constitution makes it clear that the right to free speech guaranteed under Article 19(1)(a) is subject to reasonable restrictions that may be imposed by a law in the interests of the sovereignty and integrity of India, the security of the state, friendly relations with foreign states, public order, decency or morality, or pertaining to contempt of court, defamation or incitement to an offence. For our purpose, i.e. regarding the law relating to HIV/AIDS information, a law against 'moral indecency' may be protected under this clause. The specific statutes which restrict the freedom of information are stated below :

(a) Under the Official Secrets (OS) Act, 1923, wrongful

communications in respect of information which is classified as an offence.

(b) Under the Industrial Disputes Act, 1947, confidential information given during the course of adjudication proceedings is protected from being published to any other person, if a party supplying the information makes a request in this behalf.

(c) Under the Indian Penal Code, a person is prohibited from publishing anything which would reveal the identity of a rape victim.

(d) Sections 123 to 125 and 162 of the Indian Evidence Act protect the state from disclosure of documents and communications which are privileged, and publication of which would be prejudicial to public interest.

Broadcasting/Censorship Laws

In India, all radio broadcasting is under direct state control. Unit recently All India Radio was the only radio broadcasting corporation and is bound by its own rules and regulations. These are not publicly available. However, criticism against the government and anything considered to be immoral or indecent is shunned. The television media, until recently, was also completely state controlled. Of late, satellite television has made a major entry, and functions to a large extent outside state control. India has the distinction of having the largest film industry in the world. All films before exhibition are subject to certification under the Cinematograph Act, 1952. A film shall not be certified if, in the opinion of the authority, the film or any part of it is against the interests of the sovereignty and integrity of India, the security of the state, friendly relations with foreign states, public order, decency or morality or involves defamation or contempt of court or is likely to incite the commission of an offence. Regulation have been framed by the central government alongwith a guideline stating that visuals or words depicting women in ignoble servility to many or glorifying such servility as a praiseworthy quality shall not be allowed. Moreover, the authority is to ensure that the film is evaluated in the light of contemporary standards of the country and the people to which the film relates.

Obscenity Laws

Section 292 of the Indian Penal Code makes the sale, hire, distribution, exhibition or circulation of obscene books, pamphlets, paper writings, drawings, paintings, representations, figures or any other objects and for that purpose possession of the same a punishable offence. Import or export for the aforesaid purposes, receiving profits from such ventures, advertising for such purposes or attempting to do such acts is also punishable. 'Obscene' is defined as that which is lascivious or appeals to the carnal interest or tends to deprave or corrupt those to whom it is addressed. However, exceptions are made if the publication is for scientific, literary, higher learning, or bonafide religious purposes or that which is sculpted, painted, depicted or represented on ancient monuments or temples. Section 293 of the Indian Penal Code makes the sale of obscene objects to young people punishable, while Section 294 of the Indian Penal Code makes the commission of an obscene act and/or singing or reciting or uttering of an obscene song, balldd or words in or near a public place punishable.

Sex Education

There is no specific law pertaining to sex education. However, the *Strategic Plan For The Prevention And Control of AIDS* of the Government of India talks of the development of teaching material on sexuality and responsible behaviour for school children, youth in colleges and outside, as well as adult learners. The challenge, it states, is to initiate a debate among teachers, parents and children on sex without moral overtones and without simultaneously appearing to be supporting promiscuous or permissive behaviour.

Family and Carers

Family laws and law relating to care and custody of children in India is governed by different personal laws. These are primarily laws of several communities such as Hindus (Buddhists, Jains and Sikhs are also clubbed as Hindus), Christians, Muslims and Jews. All such communities have different laws relating to inheritance, marriage and divorce, maintenance, guardianship, custody, adoption, etc., i.e., family law or personal law.

Inheritance

Hindu Law. In traditional Hindu law, a woman had a limited right to property. Although she could receive property either by gift or inheritance, she had no right to transfer it on by will or any other means. This was changed under the Hindu Succession Act, which stipulates that any property held by a female Hindu, whether acquired before or after the commencement of the Act, shall be held by her as a full owner and not as a limited owner (Section 14, Hindu Succession Act).

Christians, Jews and Parsis. In India, Christian, Jews and Parsis are governed by the Indian Succession Act, 1925. There are separate rules for Parsis, Christians and Jews. In the law regarding to Christians and Jews, there is a distinction when a person dies intestate and has left a widow with lineal descendants or a widow and kindred or widow and no kindred. Specifically, when an intestate leaves a widow and lineal descendants, she gets one-third share and the two-third share goes to the lineal descendants. When there are no lineal descendants, the whole of the property goes to the widow. A widower has the same rights as a widow.

Parsis. For all purposes there is a distinction in devolution of property intestate amongst the male and female heirs. In cases of male intestate leaving behind a widow and children or leaving behind no widow, but only children, the widow and the sons get double the share of the daughter, if the widow survives. On the other hand, in the case of a female Parsi dying intestate, the widower and the sons and the daughters get equal shares. In other words, the property of the male Parsi preferentially devolves on to male lineal descendants.

Testamentary Succession. Personal laws of all communities provide for the devolution of property by will. The whole of the property of the deceased can be willed away. However, the will has to be in writing and attested in accordance with the rules. In the case of Muslims, no Muslim can dispose of more than one-third of the estate by a will.

Divorce and Separation

Again, various personal laws apply to various communities.

Hindus. The law regarding marriage, divorce and separation is governed by the Hindu Marriage Act, 1955, (HMA). The conditions for valid Hindu marriage include that the two parties must be Hindus, that neither is incapable of giving valid consent, and the man is at least 21 years and the woman 18 years of age. Divorce and separation is available both to the husband and wife on various bases, which consists adultery or cruelty or desertion for a period of not less than two years or conversion to another religion; or if the party is incurably of unsound mind, or suffers from a mental disorder such that the other party cannot reasonably be expected to live with him or her; or if one party suffers from a virulent and incurable form of epilepsy or has been suffering from a venereal disease in a communicable form; or if one party has renounced the world by entering a religious order or has not been heard of being alive for a period of seven years (Section 13 HMA). The wife has some other additional bases, viz. if her husband has been guilty of rape, sodomy, bestiality, or that an order of maintenance passed under various statutes has not been honoured, or the parties are living apart and cohabitation has not been resumed for a period of one year after the order. Both parties can also obtain divorce on the ground of mutual consent (Section 13-B, HMA).

Christians. The law for divorce and separation of Christians is based on the antiquated English law of the 19th century. Whereas the husband can obtain divorce on the sole ground of adultery, the wife cannot obtain divorce only on that ground. The ground of adultery for a woman has to be coupled with one of the grounds which by itself is adequate for a man to get divorce, viz. bigancy, incestual relationship, desertion, cruelty, change of religion, or rape, sodomy or bestiality (Section 10, Indian Divorce Act, 1869). However, legal separation can be obtained both by the husband or the wife on the basis of adultery or cruelty or desertion without reasonable excuse for two years or more (Section 22, Indian Divorce Act, 1869).

Parsis. Parsi marriages and divorces are governed under the Parsi Marriages and Divorce Act, 1936.

Marriages can be annulled on the basis of impossibility of consummation of the marriage. Divorce is available on grounds identical to those under the Hindu Marriage Act. Like in the Hindu Marriage Act, a party can sue for divorce if the spouse is suffering from an incurable venereal disease. Alongwith, refusal to have marital intercourse for a period of two years after a Magistrate's award for maintenance is a basis for divorce.

Muslims. Marriage and divorce under Muslim law in India is according to the Shariyat. Marriage in Muslim law is a contractual relationship for which a deed, a *nikahnama,* is drawn up setting out the conditions for the marriage. A Muslim man can divorce his wife unilaterally; the presence of the wife is not material. Divorce or *talaq* can be oral or in writing. Divorce by mutual consent is also recognised. Conversion to another religion *ipso facto* dissolves the marriage.

A woman can get a divorce under the Muslim Dissolution of Marriage Act, 1937. The bases available consist, among others, the whereabouts of the husband not being known for a period of four years, the husband neglecting or failing to provide maintenance, the husband being impotent at the time of marriage and at the time of the petition, or the husband being insane or contracting a venereal disease.

Special Marriage Act, 1956. Persons of various religions in India can marry under the Special Marriage Act. The bases for divorce are practically similar to the grounds available under the Hindu Marriage Act. The main difference is the conditions of a valid marriage. Both parties need not be Hindus. The Act provides, like the Hindu Marriage Act, for the marriage to be declared void or viodable as well as for judicial separation. Divorce can also be obtained on the basis of mutual consent. Significantly, divorce is also available on the ground of the spouse suffering from a venereal disease in a communicable form.

Maintenance

Maintenance is available for both the spouses, i.e., husband and the wife, during the pendency of the marriage as well as on and after the dissolution of the marriage. It also depends on the religion that one belongs to. Apart from Muslim personal law, all the other personal laws mandate maintenance during the pendency of the marriage as well as on and after the dissolution of the marriage. In addition to maintenance provided under various marriage and divorce and maintenance laws, under Section 125 of the Codes of Criminal Procedure, 1973, old parents, women and children of a person having adequate means who are unable to provide for themselves are entitled to maintenance from that person. The idea is to prevent vagrancy. By virtue of the passing of the Muslim Women (Protection on Divorce), Act, Muslims were taken out of the ambit of these provisions.

Age of Marriage

All laws pertaining to marriage provide for a minimum age for marriage; the woman is required to be 18 years of age and the man 21 years of age. There is no statutory law which needs a minimum age for a Muslim man or woman to get married. Under Muslim law the parties have to be able to have the capacity to enter into a contract of marriage, i.e., attaining puberty.

Age of Consent and Non-consensual Sexual Intercourse

There is no legally defined age for consent to sexual intercourse under different personal laws. However, statutorily, under the Indian Penal Code, it is an offence of rape if a man has sexual intercourse with a woman under 16 years of age. However, if she happens to be his wife, it is not rape to have sexual intercourse with her after she attains the age of 15 years. Punishment has now been increased for custodial rape. Moreover, under the Indian Evidence Act, a rebuttable presumption is generated whereby in a prosecution for rape, when sexual intercourse by the accused is proved and the question is whether she has consented or not, if a woman states that she did not consent, the court is required to presume that the sexual intercourse took place without her consent (Section 114-A).

Medical Termination of Pregnancy (MTP)

Until 1971, the law relating to abortions was exclusively governed by the Indian Penal Code. Under that Act, anyone causing a miscarriage is, unless it is done in good faith to save the life of a pregnant woman, liable to imprisonment for three years. Under the Medical Termination of Pregnancy (MTP) Act, 1971, the position changed radically, the effect being to legalise abortions done under the conditions specified under the MTP Act. Pregnancy under the MTP Act is permitted to be terminated:

(a) if it is less than 12 weeks old on a certificate of one registered gynaecologist or obstetrician;

(b) between 12 and 20 weeks, on a certificate of two registered gynaecologists or obstetricians;

(c) the pregnancy would involve a risk to the life of the pregnant woman or cause severe injury to her physical or mental health; or

(d) there is an adequate risk that the child, if born, would suffer from physical or mental abnormalities so as to be seriously handicapped.

Anguish, either caused by pregnancy because of rape of a woman or caused by a failure of contraception by a married woman, is presumed to constitute severe injury to the mental health of a pregnant woman.

Prisons and Institutions

Testing

There are no specific provisions for testing of HIV in prisons. However, as soon as possible after admission the prisoner is needed to be tested medically. A record of the state of the prisoner's health is needed to be kept in a register meant for the purpose. It is not known how many prisons have the facilities to carry out testing of HIV. A question may arise, in view of the statutory provision (Section 24, Prisons Act), whether a non-consensual HIV test can be conducted in prisons. In this respect, great advances have been made in the law by decisions, particularly of the Supreme Court, which lay down that :

(a) prisoners retain all rights enjoyed by free citizens except those lost necessarily as an incident of confinement;
(b) a prisoner wears the armour of basic freedom, even behind bars, and on, breach. . . . the law will respond to his distress;
(c) the right to life enshrined in Article 21 cannot be limited to mere animal existence and includes the right to live with human dignity and the bare needs of life such as sufficient nutrition, clothing and shelter over the head and facilities for reading, writing and expressing themselves in diverse forms, freely mixing and co-mingling with fellow human beings.

Segregation

Several prison manuals provide for segregation of prisoners who are suspected of having skin infections, or a contagious disease. Some prison manuals also necessitate that certain categories of prisoners be kept together in a group to enable daily medical checks. These include:

(a) permanently infirm prisoners;
(b) prisoners discharged from hospitals and who are convalescing;
(c) prisoners usually in poor health;
(d) prisoners losing weight without any apparent reasons.

Counselling, Care and Support

All prisons have visitors. These include magistrates or district and sessions judges who have the right and duty to visit prisons and inspect them. They also hear prisoner grievances. However, it is difficult to say whether the system works effectively. Prisoners also have access to the High Court and the Supreme Court through public interest petitions, mostly in the form of letters, ventilating their grievances. These worked quite well in the late 1970s and early 1980s when the Supreme Court had an activist judiciary. Most of the cases stated above developed in this manner. Apart from counselling, care and support that may be bestowed by the medical officer and the medical team, few jails have institutionalised systems of counselling, care and support. Some jails have developed informal liaisons with social welfare and academic institutions whose visitors give some counselling, care and support. However, this tends to be an exception rather than a rule.

Employment Factors

Terms and conditions of employment in India are, in fact, contractual. However, they are largely superseded by terms and conditions of service imposed by statute. In areas where statutes are silent, common law applies. The precise terms and conditions depend on whether an employee is in government, the public sector, the private sector, in an industry or in other sectors. For government servants, the terms and conditions are controlled by statutory and non-statutory rules framed under Articles 309 and 311 of the Constitution. Industrial establishments employing more than 100 workmen are governed by the Industrial Employment (Standing Orders) Act, 1946. Employees employed in an 'industry' are covered under the Industrial Disputes Act, 1947. Maharashtra has an additional Act, viz. the MRTU & PULP Act which permits both the employer and the employee to file a complaint in the labour Court and Industrial Court alleging an unfair labour practice on the part of the other.

Work Place Testing

There is no statutory requirement for testing of HIV. However, an employee is required to be medically fit to carry on his or her job. In reality, terminating the services of a workman on the basis of continued ill-health does not constitute retrenchment under the Industrial Disputes Act (Section 2(oo) (c) of the Industrial Disputes Act). Under the general requirement of medical fitness, employers may test persons for HIV. However, there is no clear-cut policy being followed in this behalf. At present, only defence personnel are being 'regularly' checked for HIV infection.

Plans for HIV Infected Employees

There are no specific policies for HIV-positive employees. The strategic plan for 1992-96 of the central government reveals that the general policy is for the prevention of stigmatisation and discrimination of persons with HIV through protection of confidentiality and partner notification. Under this general rubric it is presumed that the policy at the work place would be to not discriminate against HIV-infected persons. However, unless there is a separate statute mandating this, it cannot be enforced.

Occupational Health

Both the Workmen's Compensation Act (Section 3) and the Employees State Insurance Act (Section 52-A) provide that if employees in employments specified in the schedules to the Acts contract a disease peculiar to the employment after being engaged in such employment for a specified period, the disease is deemed to be an 'employment injury' arising out of the course of employment for which compensation is payable. However, the rates of compensation are still low.

Criminal Law

Under the Constitution of India, no person (citizen or non-citizen) shall be deprived of his life or liberty except according to procedure established by law (Article 21). Further, no person can be detained in custody without being informed as soon as may be of the grounds of his arrest (Article 22 and Section 50, Code of Criminal Procedure). The person is entitled to be consulted and to be defended by an advocate of his choice (Article 22). He or she is further entitled to be informed by the police of his or her right to bail in case of arrest in connection with a bailable offence (Section 50, Code of Criminal Procedure). Criminal law (substantive and procedural) in India, like in all common law countries, is based on the accusatory system as opposed to the inquisitorial system. The burden is wholly upon the prosecution to prove its case beyond reasonable doubt. Unlike other common law countries, confessions to the police officer or made in police custody are not admissible in evidence and cannot be proved against the accused (Section 25 and 26,

Evidence Act). However, confessions which lead to a discovery of fact but only to the extent that they relate to the discovery of the fact are admissible (Section 27, Evidence Act). Confessions admissible are those made before a magistrate and made in the established manner.

Transmission Offences

There are no specific offences for transmitting HIV. However, innumerable offences ranging from murder and hurt to nuisance may be attracted depending on the facts and circumstances of the case. As transmission of HIV may lead to death or hurt (grievous or simple), transmitting HIV with intention of causing death or hurt, or with the knowledge that it is likely to cause death or hurt, may attract the offence of murder (Section 302, Indian Penal Code), voluntarily causing hurt (Section 323, Indian Penal Code) or voluntarily causing grievous hurt (Section 325, Indian Penal Code). On the other hand, if the transmission is caused rashly and/or negligently, another set of offences may be attracted, viz., Section 304 A, Indian Penal Code (causing death by a rash or negligent act), Section 336, Indian Penal Code (any act done rashly or negligently endangering human life or personal safety of others), Sections 337, and 338 IPC (causing hurt or grievous hurt to a person by any act so rashly or negligently done as to endanger human life or the personal safety of others). Moreover, under Section 133, Code of Criminal Procedure (for removal of nuisance), any person conducting any trade or occupation injurious to the health of the community can be prohibited from doing so by an order of a magistrate.

IVDU

There is significant intravenous drug use in India, particularly in the north-eastern states, bordering Myanmar. A large number of drug injectors have been found to have also contracted HIV.

The *Narcotics Drugs and Psychotropic Substances (NDPS) Act*, 1985 control and prohibits certain operations, viz. the cultivation, production, manufacture, possession, sale, purchase, transport, warehousing, use, consumption, inter-state movement, import into and export out of India and the trans-shipment of drugs and narcotic substances. Unlike under ordinary criminal procedure, the NDPS Act, provides that a statement made and signed by a person before a competent officer during investigation is admissible in evidence if the court finds that it would be 'in the interest of law' to do so. Also, a rebuttable presumption arises that the accused has committed an offence of possession if the accused is found in possession of a drug or a psychotropic substance.

Sex Workers

The Prevention of Immoral Traffic (PIT) Act, 1956 deals with sex workers. The Act was enacted in 1956 and dealt only with women and girl prostitution. However, major changes were brought in by the 1986 amendment. The Act now covers the sexual abuse and exploitation of both females and males, adult and children. Brothel keeping and abatement of brothel keeping are offences. Sex business by itself is not an offence. However, living off the earnings of a prostitute, carrying on sex business in a public place, abetting sex trade, soliciting or reducing for the purposes of sex business are all punishable offences. Stringent punishments are liable to be meted out in the case of use of minors in sex trade. The presence of children in a brothel creates a rebuttable presumption that an offence of detention is committed. And if on examination the child is found to have been sexually abused, a rebuttable presumption is again generated that the minor is detained for the purposes of prostitution.

Homosexuals

Traditionally, in India, homosexuality has been ignored. The *Kama Sutra* contains an entire chapter entitled *Auparishtaka* (oral congress) on the subject. Vatsayana, its author, contends that the practice is permitted by the *Dharma Shastras* (religious scriptures). On the other hand, the Manu's *Smritis* (Manu's laws) prescribed severe punishment for male and female homosexuality. One of the forms that Shiva is worshipped is *Ardhanarishwara* (half-female god) containing both the male and female forms of energies.

The British with their Christian values obviously did not take kindly to the practice. Section 377 of the Indian Penal Code was enacted, dealing with 'unnatural offences' and provides that 'whoever voluntarily has carnal intercourse against the order of nature with any man, woman or animal' is punishable with imprisonment for life or ten years with or without a fine. The explanation to the section provides 'penetration' is sufficient to constitute carnal intercourse. Though the vague definition of 'carnal intercourse against the order of nature' has been a subject matter of great debate, it has been held to include acts of oral as well as anal sex. Consent, of course, is not relevant. Though the section applies both to homosexual and heterosexual anal and oral sex, there are no reported cases of heterosexual and or oral sex under this provision. A fair body of case law that exists shows that a large majority of persons have been convicted for non-consensual acts of sodomy. Very few cases of consensual sodomy and none of oral sex between gay men have been brought to trial. However, the provision gives the police enormous powers to harass and blackmail the already stigmatised homosexual community.

The Legal Procedure

India is a common law country. The adversarial system exists in civil litigation. The procedure followed in civil courts is laid down in the Code of Civil Procedure. The accusatory, instead of the inquisitorial system, exists in the criminal field. It is entirely up to the prosecution to prove its case beyond reasonable doubt. However, the burden shifts according to the evidence led or on the basis of rebuttable presumptions that are statutorily created under the Evidence Act. The accused has the right to remain silent and is always presumed to be innocent until proved guilty.

The Legal Assistance

The vast majority of the Indian population do not have access to the legal system. However, they are affected, more often than not adversely, by the legal system. Under the Advocate's Act, lawyers have a right to practice in all courts, tribunals and authorities to represent their client (Section 30, Advocate's Act, 1961). Though parties can appear in person, with complex substantive laws and even more complicated procedural laws and rules, it is advisable for litigants to be represented by lawyers. However, good lawyers are always available at a high price. Therefore, the poor are priced out of good lawyering. The need for legal aid has been recognised by the Constitution (Article 39A). The right to legal aid has also been recognised as a fundamental right under Article 21 in several decisions of the supreme court. However, except for criminal cases, there is no statutory right to legal aid.

Parliament has enacted the Legal Services Authority Act, 1987 to provide for legal aid and advice. However, that Act has not been brought into force. A public interest litigation filed in the Supreme Court has also not come up for hearing till today.

Acting for Somebody with HIV

Very few HIV-infected persons have gone to court. On the limited experience available, no guidelines can be worked out. However, given that a person with HIV is always conscious of the terminal nature of the illness, the positive person is very often demoralised, despondent and not very responsive or enthusiastic about his/her case. Therefore, an HIV client has to be handled in a more sensitive and empathetic manner than an ordinary client would be handled. These are qualities that are necessary in somebody acting for somebody with HIV. Moreover, the person acting for the person with HIV will also be required to take more initiative than an ordinary advocate.

8

AIDS Control: Indian Perspective

In India the HIV/AIDS epidemic is at present 16 years old. Within this short period it has evolved as one of the most serious public health problem across the whole country. The initial cases of HIV/AIDS were detected among commercial sex workers in Mumbai and Chennai and injecting drug users in the north-eastern state of Manipur. The disease spread rapidly in the areas adjoining these epicentres and by 1996 Maharashtra, Tamil Nadu and Manipur together constituted 77 per cent of the total AIDS cases with Maharashtra reporting almost half the number of cases throughout the country. Even though the officially reported cases of HIV infections and full-blown AIDS cases are in lakhs, it is realised that there is a wide gap between the reported and estimated figures due to the absence of epidemiological statistics in major parts of the country. The overall existence in the country for a population of approximately one billion is still, however, very low, a rate much lower than many other countries in the Asia-Pacific region.

(a) Almost all parts of the available surveillance statistics clearly reveals that HIV is prevalent in the country. In the recent years it has spread from urban to rural areas and from individuals practising risk behaviour to the general public. Studies indicate that more and more women attending ante-natal clinics are testing HIV-positive thereby increasing the risk of perinatal transmission. Approximately, 75 per cent of the infections occur from the sexual route (both heterosexual and homosexual), about 8 per cent through blood transfusion and another 8 per cent through injecting drug use. About 89 per cent of the reported cases are occurring in sexually active and economically productive age group of 18-40 years. One in every four cases reported is a woman.

The attributable reasons for such accelerated spread of the epidemic in the country at present is labour migration and mobility in search of employment from economically backward to more advanced areas, low literacy levels leading to low awareness among the potential high risk groups, gender disparity, sexually transmitted infections and reproductive tract infections both among men and women. The social stigma attached to sexually transmitted infection also hold good for HIV/AIDS, even in a much more serious way. This, along with lack of awareness, results in reporting of full-blown AIDS cases in cities like Mumbai and Chennai resulting into severe strain on the hospital infrastructure. There have been cases of denial of AIDS patients in hospitals and nursing homes both in government and private sectors. This has manifolded the misery of the AIDS patients. At times it is mistaken to be a contagious disease and patients are isolated in the wards generating a scare among the general patients. In the workplace there were cases of discrimination leading, in some instances to loss of employment. The active part played by some non-governmental orgnisations in bringing out public interest litigations against such cases of discrimination and the judicial pronouncements by courts in support of the rights of such people has assisted in eliminating the misery of the affected persons. The treatment options are still in the initial trial stage and are highly expensive. While there is no vaccine in sight at least till the year 2000 AD, multi-drug protease inhibitor therapy, widely known as 'cocktail-therapy', is not a cure to the disease and may assist only in prolonging the life of the patient. Therapeutic trials of these drugs are still in primary stage and there are fears of patients developing drug resistance and side effects if the therapy is not done under proper medical supervision. There were instances of quacks taking advantage of the situation and promising cure through so-called herbal treatment and defrauding unsuspecting persons who are infected with the virus of large sums of money.

(b) Limited to 8 per cent of the cases, is also a serious transmission of the disease through blood, though issue as unsuspecting persons can get infected through this route if safe blood is not ensured. Prevalence of a large number of small and medium blood banks, many being in the private sector, also complicates the problem. The Supreme Court directive of May 1996 has assisted in phasing out unlicensed blood banks by May, 1997 and the prospective phasing out of professional blood donors by December, 1997. Compulsory testing of blood for HIV as well as

Syphilis, Malaria and Hepatitis-B, which has now been introduced across the whole country will assist in checking transmission of HIV virus through blood transfusion.

(c) The problem of injecting drug users is not global and is limited to the north-eastern states and the urban phases of metropolitan cities. The injecting needles which are the main cause of transmission in such cases are used repeatedly by the drug users. The twin problem of drug addiction and HIV transmission pose a serious ethical and moral problem in the HIV elimination programme. Needle exchange programmes which have been taken up in other countries to ensure availability of sterile needles for drug users are frowned upon in India due to ethical and moral implications.

(d) Although transmission of HIV through use of needles, razors and other cutting instruments in the innumerable beauty parlours, hair-cutting saloons and dental is insignificant, lack of hygienic practices in majority of these establishments also poses a health risk to the unsuspecting general public who visit these places everyday. There is a great necessity in bringing these establishments to acceptable standards of hygiene to minimise and almost eradicate the probabilities of HIV transmission through the use of needles and sharp cutting instruments.

(e) With about 14 million TB cases prevalent in India, HIV/AIDS also poses a twin challenge of HIV/TB co-infection. Approximately 60 per cent of the AIDS cases are reported to be opportunistic TB infection cases. Treatment of TB among the HIV-infected persons is a new threat to the National TB Control Programme which has now adopted DOTS strategy for control of TB infection. Some of the drugs which are referred for TB treatment pose complications in cases of HIV-infected persons and had to be withdrawn in areas of high HIV prevalence. Simultaneously looking for HIV among TB-infected persons will also create the problem of scaring away of innumerable TB-infected cases in India from seeking treatment under the DOTS strategy. There is no risk of any TB patient getting infected with HIV unless he or she practises high risk behaviour or gets infected from transfusion of HIV-infected blood.

(f) HIV/AIDS is not a disease which spreads randomly and is transmitted as a result of a specific behavioural pattern and has strong socio-economic impact. It not only costs huge funds in terms of controlling the opportunistic infections such as TB, pneumonia and cryptococcal meningitis, but seriously affects individuals in their prime productive years causing grave economic loss to them and their families.

(g) All these aspects provide an unusual task of HIV infection through many routes which comes with its long period of invisibility and does not reveal with opportunistic infections till a few years. In India with a large population and population density, low literacy levels and the resultant low levels of awareness, HIV/AIDS is one of the most challenging health problems ever faced by the country.

Gravity of the Problem

Soon after reporting of the first HIV/AIDS case in India, the government recognised the gravity of the problem and took several important measures to tackle the epidemic. A high-powered National AIDS Committee was set up in 1986 itself and a National AIDS Control Programme was commenced a year later. In the initial years the programme concentrated on generation of public awareness through mass communication programmes, introduction of blood screening for transfusion purposes and conducting surveillance activities in the epicentres of the epidemic. In 1992, the government framed a multi-sectoral strategy for the elimination and control of AIDS in India. It is implemented through the National AIDS Control Organisation at the national level and state AIDS cells/societies at the state/UT levels. The programme focussed on the following areas which conform to the global AIDS prevention and control strategy:

(a) Programme management
(b) Surveillance and research
(c) Information, education and communication alongwith social mobilisation through non-governmental organisations
(d) Control of sexually transmitted diseases
(e) Condom programming
(f) Blood safety; and
(g) Reduction of impact.

After five years the government can look back with a definite measure of satisfaction for its success in important spheres like creation of awareness about HIV/AIDS among the urban and rural population of the country. Awareness levels which were almost negligible have gone to about 70-80 per cent in urban areas even though the level of awareness in rural areas remains low at about 30 per cent.

Many important actions have been taken to ensure safe blood by modernisation and strengthening of blood banks, introduction of licensing system of blood banks continuous phasing out of professional blood donors. Introduction of component separation facilities has also assisted in reducing the use of whole blood for transfusion. Some very successful intervention activities among the high risk groups like commercial sex workers in the Sonagachi area of Kolkata, men having sex with men in Chennai and injecting drug users in Manipur were carried out through the dedicated role of non-governmental organisations. Availability of good quality condoms through social marketing has made a significant increase in the last three years.

There are still many gaps left in the programme and many lessons have been learnt during the last 16 years. The accelerated spread of the disease from the initial epicentre to the rest of the country underscores the immediate necessity to have a paradigm deviation in the response against HIV/AIDS at all levels making it imperative to frame a comprehensive national policy on HIV/AIDS to cope effectively with the changed nature of the HIV/AIDS problem. The whole programme of prevention and control of HIV/AIDS necessitates a deviation towards a more holistic approach looking at AIDS as a developmental problem instead of a mere public health issue. For this, innumerable debates have been held with representatives of doctors, scientists, social workers, non-governmental organisations and other eminent personalities working in the HIV/AIDS elimination and control. Technical working groups were set up to address several aspects of HIV/AIDS prevention and control strategy have given valuable output. Finally the National AIDS Committee held deliberations on the policy guidelines and given their valuable input towards formulation of the policy document.

Main Priority

The main priority of the programme is to eliminate the epidemic from spreading further and to lessen the impact of the epidemic not only upon the infected persons but upon the health and socio-economic status of the general population at all levels. The specific priorities of the policy are:

(a) to reiterate strongly the government's firm commitment to eliminate the spread of HIV infection and lessen personal and social impact;

(b) to create a feeling of ownership among all the participants both at the government and non-government levels, like the central ministries and agencies of the Government of India, state governments, city corporations, industrial undertakings in public and private sectors, panchayat institutions and local bodies to make it a truly national effort;

(c) to get support of a large number of non-governmental organisations for an enlarged community initiative for prevention and eradication of the AIDS problem;

(d) to develop a more supportive socio-economic environment for elimination of HIV/AIDS;

(e) to prevent women, children and other socially weak groups from becoming vulnerable to HIV infection by improving health education, legal status and economic prospects;

(f) to give adequate and equitable provision of health care to the HIV-positive people and to draw attention to the compelling public health rationale for overcoming stigmatisation and discrimination against them in general public;

(g) to promote better understanding of HIV infection among the people at large, to create knowledge about the nature of its transmission and to adopt safe behavioural practices to prevent the disease from spreading;

(h) to provide proper health care both in the hospitals and at homes for the care and support of people living with AIDS; and

(i) to constantly interact with global and bilateral agencies for support and cooperation in the field of research in vaccines, drugs, evolving systems of health care and other and managerial inputs.

National AIDS Control Policy

The national AIDS control policy mainly aims at the following strategy for prevention and control of the epidemic:

(a) Prevention of further spread of the diseases by making the people at large and specially the high risk groups, aware of its implications and provide them with the required tools for protecting themselves from getting infected. Control of sexually transmitted diseases among sexually active, economically productive groups along with promotion of condom use a measure of prevention from HIV infection will be the most important component of the prevention strategy.

(b) To give an enabling socio-economic climate so that individuals and families affected with HIV/AIDS can manage the problem themselves with their family and community support.

(c) Improving services for the care of people living with AIDS during sickness both in hospitals and at homes through community health care.

(d) For this purpose the policy addresses the following components of the national AIDS control programme for bringing in a paradigm diversion in the response of HIV/AIDS at all levels both within and outside the government.

Managing the Issue

(a) AIDS control programme has hitherto been witnessed as a public health matter dealt by the Ministry of Health and Family Welfare. However, due to the behavioural nature and the strong socio-economic implications, the disease needs to be treated as a developmental issue which impinges on several economic and social sectors of governmental and non-governmental programmes. As economically productive sections of the population are the most susceptible to the illness, participation of ministries like railways, heavy industry, steel, coal and other government undertakings employing large workforce necessitate to be actively involved in the programme. Organised and unorganised sector of industry required to be mobilised for taking care of the health of the productive sections of their workforce. Social ministries like welfare, women and child welfare, education, etc. should devise and own up the HIV/AIDS control programmes within their own sectoral jurisdiction. There should be strong finance and managerial support to these sectoral programmes from within these ministries.

(b) The state governments at their levels should develop strong ownership of the HIV/AIDS prevention and control programme. As the existence of the disease and its implications vary from state to state, the state governments should formulate their own strategies and action programmes for tackling the disease keeping the national objectives in consideration. It has been witnessed that wherever there is strong ownership of the programme from the state government side, it has been largely successful. As high existence of the disease is directly associated with the degree of urbanisation and the resultant high risk behaviour among groups like prostitutes, drug users, men having sex with men in these communities, the municipal corporations of large metropolitan cities should be persuaded to devise their own programme strategy for AIDS prevention and control. Direct funding of programmes undertaken by the municipal corporations can go a long way in lessening the administrative barriers and assist in effective control of the disease.

(c) As HIV/AIDS is relatively new to the country, there has been no effective field organisation at the district or sub-district level to tackle the problem. In diseases like leprosy, TB, etc. the district level societies play a significant role in implementing the programmes and receive funds directly from the national programmes. There is an urgent necessity to generate a similar infrastructure at the district level for prevention and control of HIV/AIDS. This will not only assist in quick channelisation of resources but bring in participation of elected representatives of the people from the 3-tier *panchayati raj* system and urban municipalities. The district administration headed by the district magistrate/collector and the chief medical officer of health should be able to give the required administrative and technical infrastructure for supporting the programme.

(d) It is felt that only a large scale mobilisation at the centre, state, district and sub-district levels through organised sections of the community alongwith non-governmental organisation can assist in effectively prevent further expansion of the disease. There is also a significant necessity to strengthen the AIDS control organization at the national and the state levels by providing more number of qualified technical and managerial personnel.

General Awareness

(a) Besides strong IEC campaign of HIV/AIDS, there is still insufficient understanding of the grave implications of the disease among the legislators, political and social leaders, bureaucracy, media, leaders of trade and industry and professional agencies not to speak of the medical and paramedical professionals involved in health care delivery system. A strong advocacy campaign is required to be initiated at all levels for these opinion leaders, policy makers and service providers to make them understand and feel motivated about the need for immediate prevention of the disease and also for adopting a human approach towards those who have already been affected with HIV/AIDS. The government emphasises the necessity to start advocacy from the topmost level in government and spread it down across the country.

(b) There is still a serious information gap about the reasons of spread of the disease even among a large number of medical and paramedical professionals both within the government and outside. This at times leads to situations of discrimination of HIV/AIDS-infected persons in hospitals, dispensaries and workplaces, not to speak of the general public. There is a strong necessity for advocacy at all levels to eliminate such discrimination and overreaction by the public against HIV/AIDS-infected persons.

(c) In educational institutions AIDS education should be given through curricular and extracurricular approach. The programme of AIDS education in schools and the 'Universities Talk AIDS' (UTA) programme should have global applicability throughout the country to mobilise large sections of the student community to bring in awareness among themselves and as peer educators to the rest of the community. Non-student youth should also be addressed through the large network of youth organizations, sports clubs and Nehru Yuvak Kendras spread throughout the country. AIDS prevention education should also be integrated into the programmes of worker education and schemes of social development.

(d) Electronic and print media has almost reached global coverage for dissemination of information in the country. The impressive increase in the levels of awareness about HIV/AIDS in the general community can be partly attributed to the electronic media which has taken this message right up to the village level.

While there is general awareness about the disease, specific aspects like manners of transmission, method of protecting oneself from getting infected, etc. are still not known to a large section of the population. There is thus an urgent need to have tailor-made programmes for targeted sections of the populations like students, youth, women, children, migrant workers, etc. The electronic media should formulate a well-coordinated media policy for dissemination of information on all aspects of HIV/AIDS alongwith reinforcement of positive cultural values and social values like love, warmth and affection within the family. The print media should be used for developing campaigns for social mobilisation to generate awareness about prevention and for sharing information and expertise. The media should usually play a positive role in the creation of an enabling environment for AIDS prevention and control and care of the HIV-infected people. The best communication talents available in government and private sector should be utilised in designing these media campaigns which should be developed in local dialect and in tune with the local needs and ethos. Media campaigns in rural areas should lay emphasis on local cultural values and should be conducted through folk dances, jatras, puppet shows, etc.

(e) The corporate sector should be persuaded to undertake AIDS prevention programmes including provision of services for their employees both at the workplace and outside as a part of their social responsibility. The large network of ESI hospitals and dispensaries under the Employees State Insurance Scheme should be effectively used for spreading the message of prevention of the disease and providing services to HIV/AIDS-infected workers and families.

Involvement of Non-governmental Organisations, etc.

(a) Non-governmental organisations have made a great contribution in the health sector by their innovative genius in the fields of health, family welfare and in preventing the spread of communicable diseases. It is necessary to continue to encourage the involvement of the voluntary sector in HIV/AIDS. The National AIDS Control Programme has identified the importance of NGO participation in the programme for giving community support to people living with AIDS and their families and for giving the required care and counselling. NGOs bring with them their experience of community level work in enhancing people's participation, interpersonal approach and sensitivity, creativity and feasibility and therefore benefit the HIV/AIDS programme tremendously, NACO has framed specific guidelines for the involvement of non-governmental organisations in the NACP.

(b) In view of the need to expand the responses to the new challenges due to the spread of the disease in the country, it is necessary to update and revise the guidelines for participation of non-governmental organisations in the programme. The experience of both sides has been mixed so long. While there have been a number of successful programmes undertaken by non-governmental organisations for generation of awareness, provision of counselling facilities and intervention projects among prostitutes and other groups, there have also been occasions of failures by newly-formed non-governmental organisations because of lack of proper perspective. Very few grassroots non-governmental organisations are coming forward to involve themselves in the AIDS control programme.

(c) On the government side non-governmental organisations have been encountering the problem of structural and other barriers like lack of reciprocation from officials at several levels. There is also lack of uniformity in the approach and performance of various state governments and sufficient orientation among government officials towards the role of non-governmental organisations in the NACP. There are delays in handling non-governmental organisations cases which at times leads to decline of interest and withdrawal on the part of the non-governmental organisations. Delay in disbursement of funds and over-emphasis on utilisation of finance rather than on impact assessment of the work done are also few of the serious flaws in the system of non-governmental organisation financing.

(d) Government identifies all these barriers and commits itself to large scale participation and involvement of NGOs/CBOs in NACP in the following ways :

1. Participation of NGOs at the policy making level through regular interaction and sufficient representation at the National AIDS Committee.
2. Enlarging their involvement to new fields like provision of medical assistance including home-based care, opening of

hospices, etc. besides the conventional areas of awareness and counselling.

3. Government will put in big efforts to undertake training and capacity building programmes for the NGOs to strengthen them to take up these additional responsibilities.
4. Guidelines issued by NACO for participation of NGOs will be revised and updated to assist greater participation of NGOs in NACO programmes and for lessening of bureaucratic delays in NGO financing.
5. Government will persuade networking among non-governmental organisations to avoid duplication of efforts in few of the areas. Efforts will be made to identify nodal non-governmental organisations in different states for coordinating the work of all the non-governmental organisations working in that area. Governments also need to address the problem of motivation among government officials towards participation of non-governmental organisations in the programme.

(e) Government will address all these issues to ensure and upgrade collaboration between non-governmental organisations and the government at the central levels to ensure greater involvement of non-governmental sector in the NACP.

Diagnosis

(a) There is an active debate in India on the issue as to whether should be mandatory testing of people suspected of carrying HIV infection. A due consideration has been given to this issue. The government feels that there is no public health rationale for mandatory testing of a person for HIV/AIDS. On the other hand, such an approach could be counter-productive as it may scare away a large number of suspected cases from getting identified and treated. HIV testing conducted on a voluntary basis with appropriate pre-test and post-test counselling is thought to be a better strategy and is in accordance with the WHO guidelines on HIV testing. Government of India has earlier issued a comprehensive HIV testing policy and the following issues are reiterated here:

1. No individual should be made to undergo a mandatory testing for HIV.

2. No mandatory HIV testing should be imposed as a precondition for employment or for providing health care facilities during employment.
3. Sufficient voluntary testing facilities with pre-and post test counselling should be made at hand across the whole country in a phased manner. There should be at least one HIV testing centre in each district in the country which can be done in a phased way.
4. In case a person likes to get his HIV status confirmed through testing, all necessary facilities should be given to that person and the outcomes should be kept strictly confidential and should be given out to the person and with his consent to the members of his family. Revelation of the HIV status to the spouse of the person will wholly depend on the person's willingness to share the information. However, the person should be persuaded to share this information with the spouse and family as it helps the person in getting proper home-based care when he is afflicted with AIDS.
5. In case of marriage, if one of the partners insists on a test to check the HIV status of the other partner, such tests should be carried out by the contracting party to the satisfaction of the person concerned.

(b) The HIV testing policy adopted in the NACO is found to be appropriate for the various types of testing that have to be done. At present people are tested for:

1. Screening in blood banks
2. Epidemiological surveys; and
3. Confirmatory testing for clinical management and voluntary testing.

(c) In the case of screening for blood donation, a single test by Rapid/ELISA is done to remove the possibility of HIV-positive blood. In the case of epidemiological surveys also the same procedure is followed, i.e., with one or two tests either with ELISA or Rapid or Simple with high sensitivity. In both the above conditions the testing is anonymous and the result is not given to the person concerned unless asked for. In the case of clinical management and for confirmatory testing of HIV status of persons who voluntarily ask for it, the sample will be tested with at least two ELISA and one Rapid/Simple by a different antigen preparation. The result is given out with appropriate pre- and post-test counselling.

Counselling

Counselling services for suspected cases of HIV infection and for persons living with HIV/AIDS (PLWAs) should be expanded to increase their reach to those who require them. All hospitals, HIV testing centres, blood banks, STD clinics and organisations set up by PLWAs should have counselling services manned by trained and professional counsellors. Government will extend all necessary help in training counsellors in large numbers to manage these counselling centres and also for generating necessary infrastructure for set up of these centres. Group counselling among PLWAs which has proved to be very effective will be persuaded by giving necessary financial and other incentives.

People Living with AIDS (PLWAs)

(a) With the rapid spread of the infection throughout the country, there will be a sharp increase in the number of HIV-infected persons in the society. They will be belonging to various social strata and from different economic backgrounds. Besides providing counselling before declaring the HIV status, the government would try to ensure the social and economic well being of these persons by ensuring (i) protection of their right to confidentiality and other human rights, and (ii) proper care and support in the hospitals and in the community.

(b) The HIV-infected person should be guaranteed equal rights to education and employment as other members of the society. HIV status of a person should be kept confidential and should not in any way affect the rights of the person to employment, his or her position at the workplace, marital relationship and other fundamental rights.

(c) HIV-positive women should have complete choice in making decisions regarding pregnancy and child birth. There should be no forcible abortion or even sterilisation on the basis of HIV status of women. Appropriate counselling should be given to the pregnant women for enabling her to take a proper decision either to go ahead with or terminate the pregnancy.

(d) The government would actively persuade and support formation of self-help groups among the HIV-infected persons for group counselling, home care and support of their members and their families. Social action through involvement of non-governmental organisations would be persuaded and supported for this purpose.

(e) Pertaining to the treatment, care and support for persons living with AIDS, the policy is to prepare a continuum of comprehensive care consisting of clinical management, nursing care, counselling and socio-economic support through home-based care. Resources from government and private sectors will be mobilised for this purpose.

(f) Government would initiate intensive advocacy and sensitisation among doctors, nurses and other paramedical workers so that persons living with AIDS are not discriminated, stigmatised or denied of services. Government expresses grave concern at instances of denial of medical treatment by doctors in the clinics, nursing homes and in hospitals which is generating enhanced stigmatisation to the persons living with AIDS. With updated knowledge available on the risks or absence of risk of HIV transmission, such denial of medical care to needy victims is regrettable. The government would hope the health service sector to rise to the occasion and show necessary concern for the welfare of the community of persons living with AIDS and ensure proper medical care and attention. The professional organisations of medical and paramedical health professionals should disseminate information about HIV/AIDS to their members up to the field level. Training of health personnel in diagnosis, rational treatment and for follow up of HIV-associated illness should continue with greater vigour. An efficient referral system would be set up starting from testing centres and counselling sites to hospitals or clinics, community-based services and home-based care. Persons living with AIDS would be provided sufficient information for home care in the shape of books and documents to enable them to lead a healthier life and promote self-help.

(g) Clinical management of HIV/AIDS needs strict enforcement of biosafety and infection control measures in the hospitals in accordance with the universal safety precaution guidelines. Treatment of AIDS cases do not need any specialised equipment than what is required for treatment of the opportunistic infections arising out of HIV/AIDS. Hospitals are required to keep sufficient supply of biosafety equipments to be used by medical and paramedical professionals while treating HIV-infected persons.

Government would ensure sufficient supply of these equipments and also essential drugs for treatment of the opportunistic infections. Adequate facilities would also be generated for appropriate disposal of plastic and other wastes and injecting needles used for treatment of HIV-infected persons.

Surveillance and Monitoring

To adopt the right strategy for prevention and control of HIV, it is necessary to set up an appropriate system of monitoring of the epidemic through surveillance programmes. The government would enlarge and refine the sentinel surveillance system for obtaining statistics on HIV infection rates both in high risk as well as low risk groups of the population and for watching the trends. A quality control mechanism through an independent agency will be evolved and adopted to have good quality statistics. Government is aware of the inadequacy of a comprehensive epidemiological statistics on the existence of HIV/AIDS in the country. This gap in information would soon be filled through a proper sentinel survey mechanism covering both the high risk groups and general population. Special surveys, indicator survey and study of the risk behaviour of targeted groups will be undertaken for specified information on the existence of HIV/AIDS in the community.

Control of Sexually Transmitted Diseases (STDs)

The large existence of sexually transmitted diseases, in Indian population is cause for concern as presence of sexually transmitted diseases, specially with ulcer or discharge, assists transmission of HIV infection. The risk of transmission is 8 to 10 times higher in case of persons with sexually transmitted diseases compared with others. As the risk behaviour of persons with sexually transmitted diseases and HIV is the same, Government of India attaches top priority to the prevention and control of sexually transmitted diseases as a strategy controlling the expansion of HIV/AIDS in India. The following approach will be adopted by the government for sexually transmitted diseases control:

1. Management of sexually transmitted diseases through syndromic approach would be incorporated into the general health service. Once the sexually transmitted disease case management

is integrated in peripheral health system, unnecessary referral could be avoided leaving the specialised services free for management of complicated cases and operational research and supervision of sites where sexually transmitted disease patients are treated.

2. Sexually transmitted disease among women though highly prevalent, is suppressed due to the social stigma associated with the disease. It has therefore been decided to incorporate services for treatment of reproductive tract infections (RTIs) and sexually transmitted infections (STIs) at all levels. Department of Family Welfare and the NACO would coordinate for an effective implementation of such integration. Sexually transmitted disease clinics at district/block/FRU level would work as referral centres for treatment of sexually transmitted diseases referred from peripheries. Sexually transmitted diseases clinics in all district hospitals, medical colleges and other centres would be strengthened by giving technical equipment, reagents and drugs. A massive orientation training programme would be undertaken to train all the medical and paramedical workers engaged in providing STI/RTI services through a syndromic approach. All sexually transmitted disease clinics would also give counselling services and good quality condoms to the sexually transmitted disease patients. Services of non-governmental organisations would be used for giving such counselling services at the sexually transmitted disease clinics.

Condoms as a Control Device

In the absence of proper cure or prevention by vaccination, the only effective physical obstacle against transmission of HIV is the use of condoms. Condoms have been advocated earlier as a safe method of population control under the family welfare programme. Use of condoms now takes special importance in the AIDS associated scenario as it is the only effective way of prevention of HIV/AIDS through the sexual route apart from total abstinence. Government feels that there should be no moral, ethical or religious inhibition towards propagating the use of condoms amongst sexually active people specially those who practise high risk behaviour.

The government has adopted a conscious policy of use of condoms through the social marketing and community-based distribution network. It has been found that the social marketing strategy has assisted in increasing use of condoms in the country at large. There is greater need to ensure availability of condoms at places and times where they are required. Hospitals, STD clinics, counselling centres, nursing homes and even private clinics of medical practitioners should have sufficient supply of condoms for use of the patients. General availability of condoms in the community drug stores, important road and railway junctions, public places, luxury hotels, etc. should also be ensured for use among sexually active people. This will help in achieving the big purposes of control and prevention of HIV and as a useful equipment for promoting the small family norm. Government would promote development of culturally acceptable information packages about the efficacy of condoms to achieve both these objectives.

While ensuring availability of condoms, it is equally necessary to see that the quality and reliability is also guaranteed. Schedule 'R' of the Drugs and Cosmetics Act has been amended recently to include condoms for ensuring sufficient quality control in their production and distribution. There are sufficient number of manufacturers both in the government and private sectors in India to take care of the widespread demand for condoms among sexually active people.

Policy on Blood Safety

(a) In the past, about 6-8 per cent of HIV infections occurred through transfusion of blood and blood products in India. To minimise the risk of transmission of HIV through blood, government has taken several measures mentioned below:

1. Testing of all blood units used in the blood banks for HIV, Hepatitis-B, malaria and syphilis has been made mandatory.
2. Under the Supreme Court's order an appropriate licensing system has been introduced for licensing of all blood banks and stopping operation of all unlicensed ones.
3. Government has undertaken large scale mobilisation efforts to increase voluntary blood donation through participation of governmental and non-governmental agencies. At the same time, the system of collection of blood through professional blood donors will be phased out by December 1997 under the Supreme Court directive.
4. Government would ensure set up of sufficient blood banking

services at the state/district levels including provision of trained manpower.

5. To ensure rational use of blood, more and more blood component separation facilities would be set up in the country for availability of blood products besides whole blood.
6. Government has established national and state blood transfusion councils to oversee blood transfusion services as independent autonomous bodies. The facility of tax-exemption for contributions to these councils has also been given. These councils will play a very significant role in augmenting blood transfusion services in the country and to ensure safe blood to the people. To ensure creation of adequate medical and paramedical professionals specialised in blood banks, States are required to open separate departments of haematology and transfusion medicine in the medical colleges.

(b) With the modernisation of blood bank services, it is hoped that the necessity for blood will be fully met through the small but more modernised and efficient system of blood banks in the government, private and voluntary sectors thus minimising the risk of HIV transmission through blood.

R & D

(a) The research and development efforts in the field of HIV/AIDS have been very limited in the country. With the probability of a vaccine evolving by the turn of the century, government recognises the need to persuade and support research and development in the following areas:

1. The government will look out for collaborative research with scientific groups in developed countries for development of vaccines suitable for the strains of HIV virus existent in India. It is also necessary to develop protocols for vaccine trials in the country. At present R&D in HIV vaccine is thought as an expensive proposition but due to the enormity of the problem involved, the effort is worth the investment.
2. Development of anti-retroviral drugs in USA and other developed countries has also given hope to the large number of HIV-infected persons for greater longevity and a probable cure for the disease. However, these drugs are highly expensive even by the standard of the developed world. The

government is at present following a policy of permitting these drugs to be imported freely into the country to ensure their free availability to those who can afford. Efforts will be made to indigenise manufacture of these drugs by persuading the private sector drug industry to get into joint ventures. The efficacy of anti-retrovirals like AZT in prevention of perinatal transmission from mother to the child has also raised the hope of saving children from getting the infection from their mothers. However, pilot studies have to be conducted on the utilisation of these drugs on expectant mothers before they can be officially introduced for treatment at the pre-natal stage. Government will be sponsoring pilot studies on the efficacy of anti-retrovirals for clinical trials among HIV-infected persons alongwith pregnant women.

(b) Government would also persuade indigenisation of the HIV-associated equipment like test kits which will assist in lessening the cost of service to a great extent.

Indigenous Systems of Medicine (ISM)

(a) In a scenario where anti-retroviral drugs are extremely expensive, there is a considerable need to look into the indigenous system of medicine like Ayurveda, Unani and Siddha apart from Homoeopathy. Some of the medicines in these systems have the capacity of reducing the viral load in the body of the patient thus ensuring a healthier and longer life with the infection. The government has sponsored research projects in Homoeopathic and Siddha systems of medicines and is receiving encouraging response. It will pursue a policy of sponsoring research in ISM and Homoeopathy for development of drugs which can serve the purpose of anti-retrovirals, if not for a total cure from the infection.

(b) Simultaneously it is necessary to be vigilant against unscrupulous persons claiming to have invented a cure for HIV/AIDS by magic herbs. Any medicine or system of treatment which cannot stand the test of scrutiny by the professional organisations like the Ayurveda Council or the Homoeopathic Council cannot be accepted as a drug or a system of treatment in India. The Drugs and Magic Remedies Act necessitates amendments to stringently deal with cases of unscrupulous persons taking advantage of the misery of HIV-infected persons and defrauding them of huge sums of money. A massive awareness campaign has also been conducted to make people aware of the consequences of such medication by unqualified persons indulging in quackery.

Bilateral and Global Cooperation

Government notes with satisfaction the active support given by global agencies of the UN system and bilateral agencies from various countries in the developed world. The World Bank has participated in funding a major part of the national AIDS control programme during the past five years. It has also shown interest in continuing this policy of active participation in the times to come. The organisations which are constituents of the UNAIDS Theme Group have all done work in India on several sectoral programmes for quite some time. These organisations will have to take a relook at their programmes and priorities in the context of the increase prevalence of HIV/AIDS among the economically productive and socially exploited sections of the population. The Joint United Nations programme on HIV/AIDS known as UNAIDS will be needed to assume a larger role both in terms of providing financial as well as technical expertise to the programme. The Theme Group of UNAIDS consisting of six UN-based organisations will have to play a very effective role in acting as a coordinating agency between the government and the UN agencies in formulation and implementation of programmes for elimination of HIV/AIDS. Government's policy is to promote international cooperation to ensure optimal utilisation of funds to avoid unproductive duplication of efforts. Bilateral cooperation which has been developed with countries like USA, UK, European Union and others will be extended further to take up specific intervention programmes where the technical and managerial input from these countries can be put to maximum use. Government will promote mutual information sharing with these countries as well as the neighbouring nations in the South Asia region on their national AIDS control plans. Areas of interest which are common to the neighbouring countries like drug use, labour migration, socio-economic status of women and socially handicapped persons, etc. could be the common basis for regional cooperation among the neighbouring countries. Government will be actively looking for technical inputs for development of vaccines, drugs and equipment for elimination and control of HIV/AIDS and would search bilateral and multilateral collaboration towards this end.

Just as the HIV infection is transcending the dimensions of high risk population and spreading into the general public, prevention and care programmes have also reached a critical phase. Government of India is fully dedicated to prevent the HIV/AIDS epidemic at the initial state itself before it emerges into a catastrophic epidemic. Instead of a simple public health measure, the government looks at HIV/AIDS prevention and control programme as a socio-economic problem touching all sections of the population irrespective of their regional, economic or social status. A concerted effort will be made to expand the national programme through larger participation, ownership and involvement both at the governmental and societal level. Government of India reiterates its firm resolve to confront the key issues by committing sufficient funds and other resources for this important national programme. By following a concerted policy and an action programme that evolves out of it, government hopes to control the epidemic and arrest its spread within the next five years. Government hopes that all collaborating agencies whether in the governmental or non-governmental sectors, international and bilateral agencies, would adopt policies and programmes in conformity with this national policy in their effort to prevent and control HIV/AIDS in the country.

Policy on Diagnosis

HIV testing conducted on a voluntary basis with proper pre-test and post-test counselling is thought to be a better strategy and is in confirmity with the WHO guidelines on HIV testing. The basis and objectives of testing are to:

(a) watch the trend of HIV infection in a population or subgroup for facilitation of intervention using unliked anonymous testing;
(b) test blood or organs or tissue for ensuring safety of the recipients;
(c) detect an individual with HIV infection for diagnosing or voluntary testing aims.

There is an active debate in the country on the issue as to whether there should be mandatory testing of people suspected of carrying HIV infection. Considerable thought has been given to this issue. Testing for HIV is more than a mere biological test for it consists of ethical, human and legal boundaries. The government feels that there is no public health rationale for mandatory testing of a person for HIV/AIDS. On the other hand, such a theory could be counter-productive as it may cause fear to a large number of suspected cases from getting detected and counselled to take appropriate measure to improve his quality of life and prevent expansion of infection to other persons in the community. HIV testing done on a voluntary basis with appropriate pre-test and post-test counselling is considered to be a better strategy and is in accordance with the national policy on HIV testing and also the WHO guidelines.

Principles of HIV Diagnosis

It should be a part of the overall comprehensive preventive and promotive programme. Testing by itself does not result in behavioural changes that limit transmission of HIV to others and thus, testing should be a part of the whole control programme which is conducive for behavioural change of the individual by giving social support, means and skills to reduce or eliminate risk behaviour. Testing without 'explicit' consent of the patients (mandatory testing) has proved to be counter productive in the long run in the control of HIV epidemic. Social support and intervention must be directed to anybody vulnerable to risk behaviour irrespective of whether an individual or group join in testing procedure or not. Otherwise such testing can drive the target people underground and make it more complicated for starting intervention.

Any health programme which does not keep the dignity of a patient or deprives him of his prime right to employment or access to medical care or social support is dangerous on a long term basis. The question which must be asked before a testing procedure is undertaken is how this outcome will be used for the benefit of individual or of the community; if there is a policy and means to support the group under testing following the test outcome; and does the same principle of intervention apply even if people deny testing?

Affirmation

Sound and appropriate testing. No test in biological system is foolproof even under the best laboratory conditions. For instance, if we wish to detect an asymptomatic HIV-positive person by using ELISA (2nd ELISA done on sera reactive to first ELISA) in a population where the existence of infection is one per cent, that a person detected positive is really positive (positive predictive value) is only 50 per cent after one ELISA test and 99 per cent truly after two tests. This means one result will be falsely positive in every 100 tests, even by two tests if we use a western blot as supplemental test besides 2nd ELISA, the probability of detecting truly positive increased to 99.998 per cent which means there will be one false positive out of 10,000 declared positive. If we appreciate the limitation of any test which could measure the HIV status the cheaper test could be considered (for example, three ERS instead of ELISA and Western Blot) to get yield. Today three types of tests are at hand on similar principle to ELISA which have been widely classified, as one which can be completed within half an hour.

(a) Dip stick rapid test—similar to that conducted for examination of sugar in urine for diabetic.

(b) A simple test is one which does not consist any sophisticated instrument and even could be conducted in conditions without electricity.

Appropriate Test Procedure

Places where electricity is not available for large part of the working hours, use of techniques dependent on a sophisticated procedures will not be suitable. Rapid or simple tests are recommended where infrastructure is minimal or where quick screening of sample is required.

Cost Effective Test Procedure

It is usually witnessed that costly mass screening programme at times spread a false sense of security without any public health impact and at times delays the proper intervention measures. For instance, mass screening for HIV patient seeking hospital admission can only delay implementation of measures for hospital infection control methods that could have stopped more infective disease like hepatitis 'B' and 'C'.

Transfusion Safety

A single ERS test is sufficient to ensure transfusion safety with the provision of simple tests in places without electricity. The aim of the transfusion safety does not need identification of donor of the infected unit of blood and in low prevalence settings of HIV single ERS would detect at least 50 per cent SAMPLES FALSELY POSITIVE. However, the same test gives more than 99.9 per cent surety that blood found negative is in fact free of infection. Thus, while we can label blood as safe it is risky to label any donor HIV-positive on such test result and employees of blood bank must be well aware of interpretation of the test. Often employees of blood bank are encountered with situation where a donor might ask why his blood has been rejected. In such situation the donor could be referred to the voluntary HIV testing centre with pre- and post-test counselling and supplemental test facilities for HIV (3 ERS).

Surveillance

The aim of surveillance is best contained by annual cross-sectional survey of same risk group in the same place over few years by unlined anonymous testing, following test methods by 2 ERS. The main objective of the survey is to watch the trend of infection of HIV. Unlinked anonymous tests are only probable if blood is drawn for some other purpose and a part of it is tested for HIV without identification statistics.

Detection

This testing procedure must offer pre- and post-test counselling of the person and require explicit consent. Voluntary HIV testing and counselling when given to any asymptomatic person must have any of the following objectives:

(a) To allow early institution of an specific drug therapy if found to be effective (however today no such therapy has proved to be beneficial including anti-retroviral drugs or chemo-prophylaxis).

(b) To help infected or non-infected persons be more aware of their health status and prognosis to take decisions of child bearing, breast feeding and lessen or eliminate risk behaviour.

Increasing number of AIDS cases in the country calls for availability of diagnostic services for clinically suspected cases of AIDS. However, such testing method must be of highest specificity, accuracy and coupled with trained manpower for counselling. The outcome of the test must be kept confidential and even health care workers who are not directly involved in care of the patient should not be told about the outcome. Surveillance of AIDS cases in India does not necessitate reporting of the identification statistics of the patient. In the case of diagnosis of clinically suspected cases and for voluntary testing, the testing is conducted with 3 ERS using HIV kits with several antigens.

Research

Testing procedure for research are formulated in accordance with specific purposes and could be decided by the researcher. However, all the studies undertaken must follow ethical standards which primarily consists full explicit consent of the patient and pre-decided mutually agreed terms for any eventuality of the patient because of research activities. Government of India has earlier issued a comprehensive HIV testing policy and the following issues are reiterated here:

(a) No individual should be forced to undergo a mandatory testing for HIV.
(b) No mandatory HIV testing should be imposed as a precondition for employment or for giving health care facilities during employment.
(c) Sufficient voluntary testing facilities with pre- and post-test counselling should be made available across the whole country in a phased manner. There should be minimum one HIV testing centre in each district in the country for voluntary testing in the public sector.

National AIDS Control Programme—Second Phase (1999-2004)

The second phase of the National AIDS Control Programme has become effective from 9th November, 1999. It is a 100 per cent centrally sponsored scheme implemented in 32 states/union territories and 3 municipal corporations, i.e., Ahmedabad, Chennai and Mumbai through AIDS control societies. Project formulation for second phase National AIDS Control Programme followed a truly participatory process at the state and municipal corporation levels. Between April and June 1998, the Technical Liaison Officers (TLOs) of NACO, in collaboration with state AIDS control programme officers, conducted state level planning workshops in all the states and the cities of Mumbai, Chennai and Ahmedabad. Each of these workshops was organised for 2 days in which all major stakeholders such as senior officials of the government departments, non-governmental organisations, private sector, medical professionals and district level officials participated. On an average, about 100 stakeholders participated in each of these workshops. In addition to serving as a tool preparation, these workshops also turned out to be a major advocacy effort. In the formulation of the state implementation plan, the following steps were taken:

(a) Organisation of state level workshops (in which participants from government departments, non-governmental organisations, etc. debated the various issues under various components and came out with suggestions.
(b) Set up of core team to finalise the specific programmes for AIDS control project II based on the suggestions made under seven components.
(c) Core team held three meetings in June-July 1998, evaluated the recommendation to identify and select programmes/ activities which required to be given priority and focus.
(d) The activities suggested were listed and prioritized by the core team based on the suggestions at the workshop.
(e) In end July, 1998, the World Bank-laid down cost codes were received. A special task force was set up and the activities were classified under five components in accordance with the revised guidelines from NACO and World Bank.
(f) The several activities were divided into sub-activities, cost codes were assigned for each sub-activity. The implementation plan was made indicating the process, sub-process, activities, implementing agency, assessment parameters and risk.
(g) The unit cost and the number of units under each activity were finalised by the special task force and the outlay was drawn. Discussions were held with officials of USAID and VHS-APAC to evaluate the extent of the bilateral's participation in Tamil Nadu.
(h) The technical liaison officers, World Bank consultants and the PD, NACO, evaluated the draft project implementation plan prepared and suggest scaling down of outlay, taking into consideration the past and present expenditure and the absorptive capacity funds in the times to come. At this juncture, the procurement plan and the training action plan were prepared simultaneously.

(i) The special task force held various meetings to evaluate the number of interventions and units of various activities. After the southern states project implementation plan workshop at Bangalore in the first week of September 1998, it was decided to limit the interventions and the number of other units/activities and the outlay was revised. The procurement plan was finalised after excluding the cost of equipment to be procured and supplied by NACO. The training action plan was also revised the finalised on the basis of modified outlay.

In the month of September-October, 1998, National AIDS Control Organisation organised regional workshops for state AIDS programme officers for finalisation of the state project implementation plan. On the basis of the state project implementation plan, the national project implementation plan was prepared.

The mission of the International Development Association (IDA) visited during December 14-22, 1998 and appraised the project in collaboration with officials of the Government of India. The Mission assured funds of US $ 191 million with Government of India's share of US $ 38.8 million. The total project cost was approximately at US $ 229.8 million (Rs. 1155 crore). The detailed project document was considered by the Expenditure Finance Committee (EFC) in its conference held on 29th April, 1999 along with USAID and DFID assisted projects. The EFC suggested 3 projects for approval – NACP II (National AIDS Control Project) for Rs. 1155 crore, US-assisted AVERT project in Maharashtra for Rs. 166 crore and DFID project for AP, Orissa, Kerala and Gujarat for Rs. 104 crore for the period of 5 years from 1999-2004 except US assisted AVERT Project which will be for a period of 7 years. The World Bank and DFID projects are for a duration of 5 years (1999-2004), while US assisted AVERT project for 7 years (1999-2006). The negotiations for an IDA Project NACP II were held between the members of the Government of India and IDA in Washington from 7-12th May 1999. The second AIDS project was approved by IDA Board in its conference dated June 15 1999. The second NACP project was approved by the cabinet on 26th August 1999.

Important Objectives

(i) To shift the concentration from raising awareness to changing behaviour through interventions, particularly for groups at high risk of contracting and spreading HIV;

(ii) To support decentralisation of service delivery to the state and municipalities and a new facilitating role for National AIDS Control Organisation. Programme delivery would be elastical, evidence-based, participatory and to rely on local programme implementation plans;

(iii) To protect human rights by persuading voluntary counselling and testing and discouraging mandatory testing;

(iv) To support structured and evidence-based annual evaluations and ongoing operational research; and

(v) To encourage management reforms, such as better managed state level AIDS control societies and improved drug and equipment procurement practices. These reforms are proposed with an opinion to bring about a sense of 'ownership' of the programme among the states, municipal corporations, non-governmental organisations and other implementing agencies.

The National AIDS Control Project has two key important aims namely.

1. To reduce the spread of HIV infection in India; and
2. Strengthen India's capacity to respond to HIV/AIDS on a long term basis.

Operationally, the project interventions would seek to get the following by the end of the project:

(a) to keep HIV prevalence rate below 5 per cent of adult population in Maharashtra, below 3 per cent in Andhra Pradesh, Karnataka, Manipur, Tamil Nadu where the HIV prevalence is moderate and below 1 per cent in remaining states, where the epidemic is still at a nascent stage;

(b) to lessen blood borne transmission of HIV to less than 1 per cent.

(c) to attain awareness level of not less than 90 per cent among the youth and others in the reproductive age group; and

(d) to achieve condom use of not less than 90 per cent among high risk categories like commercial sex workers.

The Project

The project would adopt a multi-pronged approach that would concentrate on the most crucial intervention to begin limiting HIV transmission. Project activities are grouped into two components and five sub-components. Both components reflect activities at national, state and municipal levels.

Cost-effective Interventions

1. Priority targeted intervention for groups at high risk. The project proposes to reduce the spread of HIV in groups at high risk by recognising target populations and providing peer counselling, condom promotion, treatment of STIs and enabling environment. These would be locally modified and delivered largely through non-governmental organisations, community based organisations (CBOs) and the public sector using generic protocols.

(a) Identify those groups at higher risk. This would involve:

(i) participatory approaches;

(ii) locating groups at highest risk, chiefly commercial sex workers, truck drivers, injecting drug users, migrant labourers, men having sex with men;

(iii) evaluating the access and demand for health services among the groups of high risk; and

(iv) developing strategies based on outreach, peer education and partnerships.

(b) Provide integrated peer counselling, condoms, and treatment for sexually transmitted infections for those at high risk. Representatives of groups at high risk would be trained to give peer education aimed at changing high risk behaviours. Besides them, these interventions would:

(i) train primary health care providers in syndromic case management and counselling in condom use;

(ii) strengthening sexually transmitted infections clinics in each district hospital and medical college hospitals; and

(iii) improve referral services for sexually transmitted infections treatment. Besides this, client programme would aim to deliver targeted IEC, condom promotion and sexually transmitted infection treatment and counselling to clients of commercial sex workers.

2. ***Preventive intervention for the general community.*** This includes the following activities :

(a) IEC and awareness campaigns. Activities include:

(i) conducting mass media campaign at the state and municipal levels;

(ii) conducting local IEC campaign, use traditional media such as folk arts and street theatre;

(iii) promoting advocacy campaigns;

(iv) conducting awareness programme geared towards youth and college students; and

(v) organising family health awareness campaigns on a regular basis to create awareness and provide service delivery for control of STI and RTI infections.

(b) Voluntary testing and counselling. This involves

(i) increasing availability of and demand for voluntary testing, especially joint testing of couples;

(ii) training grass root level health care professionals in HIV/AIDS counselling;

(iii) providing counselling services through all blood banks in India and through STI clinics. It is envisaged that one voluntary testing centre would be set up in each district.

(c) Transmission by blood transfusion and occupational exposure. This activity would include:

(i) setting up of 10 new modern blood banks, upgrading 20 existing major blood banks and setting of 80 new district level blood banks;

(ii) establishing another 40 components separation units;

(iii) establishing mandatory screening of all blood units for Hepatitis C virus;

(iv) mobilising voluntary blood donation;

(v) training providers in the rational use of blood products;

(vi) assisting communications among blood banking services;

(vii) providing trained counsellers for blood banks in public and private sectors; and

(viii) training health care workers at all levels in universal precautions, including provision of post exposure prophylaxis drugs.

3. ***AIDS Care.*** These activities would provide finance for home-based and community-based care, including increasing the availability of cost effective interventions for common opportunistic infections. Specific activity would include:

(i) set up of best practice guidelines and providing appropriate drugs for treating common opportunistic infections at district hospitals;

(ii) training at selected state level hospitals for the provision of referral services.

(a) improve the quality and cost effectiveness of interventions provided by existing procedures;

(b) set up new support services for care for persons with AIDS in collaboration with NGOs and CBOs setting up small community based hospitals, hospice programmes, drop-in-centres and home-based care would be taken up.

Enhancing Capacity

1. Institutional strengthening. This component proposes to strengthen effectiveness and technical, managerial and financial sustainability at national, state and municipal levels.

(a) Building implementation capacity at the states and municipal levels by:

(i) ensuring sufficient staff and skills in AIDS control societies;

(ii) transferring implementation responsibilities to the state and municipal levels;

(iii) emphasizing management and implementation capacity at all levels.

There would be an enhanced emphasis in the second project, on setting up of blood banking services, blood testing centres and STD clinics in all district hospitals.

Accounts and Finance Unit. The World Bank has decided that for all IDA assisted projects stating after July, 1998, a 'Loan Administration Change Initiative' (LACI) is to be set up. The important objects of LACI is to assist the project to perform better by reducing delays and financial barriers through accelerated disbursement and facilitating project monitoring and control by linking expenditure with real physical progress. This system visualises a project financial management system at NACO and an accounts and finance unit in each state and municipal corporation.

(b) Strengthening leadership capacity of NACO. NACO would enhance :

(i) strategic planning skills;
(ii) concentrate on disseminating best practices for targeted interventions;
(iii) set up and manage network of technical expertise through technical resource groups in STI/HIV/AIDS and other important issues;
(iv) conduct operation research; and
(v) oversee research and development activities nation-wise.

NACO would be in overall charge of the financial management of the project and would be responsible for effective and efficient use of financial and other resources for the project.

(c) Expand and improve country-wide STI/HIV/AIDS sentinel surveillance. Specific activities include:

(i) sentinel surveillance in every state;
(ii) STI surveillance through specific surveys;
(iii) behaviour surveillance surveys; and
(iv) AIDS cases surveillance.

(d) Training. A training action plan has been finalised after convening four regional and one national workshop of various states with major objectives of:

(i) eliminating the spread of epidemic and strengthening the local capacity to respond to the epidemic in the times to come; and
(ii) to address the training needs identified in the various components of the project. Keeping in view the overall objectives of the proposed project, a two pronged approach have been adopted for training activities under the proposed project; at the national level, the activities

are of generic nature addressing the technical necessities development of curriculum and training/training materials, continual evaluation of the orientation/ training activities and incorporating the local best practices, orientation/training of trainers/training co-ordinators, periodic evaluation of effect of the training project activities and inputs for completing training infrastructure. At the state level the activities concentrate on implementation—development of training phase/ calendars as part of the state project implementation plan, organising training programmes, evaluation of the training activity to improve their quality and training for the non-governmental organisations.

(e) Build capacity for watching and evaluation programme activities. An independent National M&E agency would be selected in the first year of the project. Each AIDS Control Society would have a M&E officer. M&E would be conducted by an outside agency at baseline, interim, and final year. The performance and expenditure annual review would involve NACO, AIDS control societies and IDA jointly evaluating project expenditure, financial flows, annual action plans, PMRs and project input, output and outcome and process indicators.

(f) Increase India's capacity for research on HIV/AIDS. Most operational research, policy development studies; research and development (R&D) and cause of death and other studies would be organised by NACO, states and municipal corporations keeping in consideration the guidelines from an expert working group composed of NACO, state and associated officials. A research advisory committee has been set up to find out research needs of the country in the field of HIV/AIDS to promote research capability of Indian scientist/institutions. Initiative will be taken to develop a HIV vaccine programme in India. Mother to child transmission prevention programme has been introduced as an operation research.

2. ***Intersectoral Collaboration.*** This component would promote collaboration among the public, private and voluntary sectors. Activities would be coordinated with other programmes within the Ministry of Health and Family Welfare and other central

ministries and departments. collaboration would concentrate on:

(i) learning from the innovative HIV/AIDS programmes that prevail in other sectors; and

(ii) sharing in the work of creating awareness, advocacy at delivering interventions.

Various central ministers and some public sector organisations with very large workforce have developed their own programme and have funded under the NACP II. Few of these are, Ministry of Sports and Youth Affairs, Ministry of Labour (Employees State Insurance Corporation), the Indian Railways, the Ministry of Defence and the Steel Industry. Similarly, the private sector has also shown interest in getting actual participation in the fight against HIV/AIDS in India.

Procurement

NACO would be responsible for procurement of HIV test kits, equipment and certain drugs as central component through the National Thermal Power Corporation Limited (NTPC), the procurement agent appointed under the project.

Project Targets

The programme has the following rigid objectives to be achieved during project duration:

(i) To lessen blood-borne transmission of HIV to less than one per cent of the total transmissions.

(ii) To introduce Hepatitis C as the fifth mandatory test for blood screening.

(iii) To establish 10 new modern blood banks in uncovered areas, upgrading of 20 major blood banks, setting up of 80 new district level blood banks in uncovered districts, setting up another 40 blood component separation units, promotion of voluntary blood donation and increase its share in total blood collected to at least 60 per cent. The total blood collection in the country which is now about 3-3.5 million units is sought to be increased to 5-5.5 million units by the end of the project.

(iv) To attain awareness level of not less than 90 per cent among the youth and those in the reproductive age group.

(v) To train up at least 600 non-governmental organisations in the country in conducting targeted intervention programmes among high-risk groups and through them promote condom use of not less than 90 per cent among these groups and control of sexually transmitted diseases.

(vi) To conduct annual family health awareness campaigns among the general public and provide service-delivery in terms of medical advice and provision of drugs for control of sexually transmitted diseases and reproductive tract infections. These campaigns will be conducted jointly by NACO and RHC programme managers at the state level.

(vii) Promotion of voluntary testing facilities throughout the country at the end of the project. It is witnessed that every district in the country would have at least one voluntary testing facility.

(viii) Awareness campaigns will at present be more interactive and use of traditional media such as folk arts and street theatre will be given greater importance in the rural areas. It is proposed to cover all the schools in the country targeting students studying in class IX and class XI through school education programmes and all the universities through the "universities talk AIDS" programme during the project period.

(ix) Promotion of organisations of people living with HIV/AIDS and giving them financial assistance to form self-help groups.

Monitoring and Evaluation

For the effective monitoring and evaluation to evaluate the implementation of the second phase of the National AIDS Control Project at national and state level, the following mechanism has been envisaged.

(i) Generating a computerised management information system (CMIS) at the national and state levels.

(ii) Training NACO staff and health specialists in evidence based health programme management.

(iii) Conducting base line, mid-term and final evaluation.

(iv) Conducting the annual performance and expenditure review; and

(v) Conducting the national performance review under the National AIDS Control Board.

A national level independent outside agency is being identified who would be assigned the responsibility of development of CMIS, conduct of base line, mid-term and end term evaluation.

Financial Management System

It is envisaged to maintain an adequate project financial management system to provide correct and timely information regarding project resources and expenditure to facilitate efficient project management. For this purpose a consultancy agency is being selected for developing a project financial management system for NACP-II. The financial management system would be integrated one for the whole project. A common set of policies and procedures would apply to the whole project and a consolidated set of financial reports for the project would be prepared from the FMS.

Outlay for Second Phase

There are three funding agencies for second phase of National AIDS Control Programme. These are:

(a) International Development Agency (IDA): World Bank has provided funds to the tune of US $ 191.00 million as soft loan for the project and the domestic budgetary support is US $ 38.8 million. The total outlay is US $ 229.8 million (Rs. 11550.00 million).

(b) United States Agency for International Development (USAID): United State Agency for International Development has extended its assistance to the government of Maharashtra for implementation of 'AVERT' project based on their earlier experience of working in the state of Tamil Nadu under the AIDS prevention and AIDS Control (APAC) project. The allocation for USAID assisted 'AVERT' project is Rs. 1660.00 million.

(c) Department for International Development (DFID) of U.K. government: Department For International Development has extended its assistance for implementation of Sexual Health Projects in the states of Andhra Pradesh, Gujarat, Kerala and Orissa in continuation of their earlier projects in West Bengal. The outlay for this project is Rs. 1040.00 million.

Outlay for NACO Project Second Phase	*Rupees in Million*
IDA credit (1999-2004)	11550

USAID assistance for AVERT project in Maharashtra	1660
DFID assistance for sexual health projects for the states of Andhra Pradesh, Gujarat, Kerala and Orissa	1040
Total	**14250**

9

Women and AIDS

Background

Since the outcome of HIV/AIDS in the 1980s, which continues to spread at an accelerating rate, debates and research on bio-medical issues and on human rights/legal issues have gained significance. In the popular conception, medicine, and not the law, plays a leading role. But in the absence of a cure, and clear cut medical responses to HIV infection, prevention through education and behaviour modification is the only way for combating and controlling the expansion of epidemic. Therefore, legal interventions, as a mechanism for persuading social change, occupy the main importance. The legal response, which is more moralistic than rational, has paved the way for amendment of public health legislation in order to strengthen the coercive power to deal with HIV-infected persons or to find scapegoats to take the blame for society's own limitations. However, various studies have proved the fallacy of the belief that HIV/AIDS is the disease of the depraved and the deviants. The large number of women being infected through heterosexual activity proves that the virus is no more limited to the so-called 'High Risk' class of sex workers, their clients and blood donors. There are many infected men, who because of their high-risk activity are unknowingly transferring the virus to their wives and other sexual partners.

HIV Infection in Women

Several studies in the late 1980s and early 1990s have established that HIV/AIDS is greatly affecting the poor and women, who because of their socio-economic dependency are unable to take steps to safeguard themselves against the risk of infection. The race and gender pattern of HIV infection is confirmed in the 1991 WHO estimate that the cumulative total of persons affected with HIV globally was to the extent of 8-10 million. Of this, more than seven million infections were estimated to have occurred in developing countries of sub-Saharan Africa, the Caribbean, and South-East Asia. These patterns imply that the socio-economic element is a driving force behind HIV transmission. Poverty is the cause of breakdown in rural communities and migration of labour. Besides this, the lack of alternate economic opportunities at times forces women into sex business as the only available means of economic support. HIV infection is preventable by all those who have access to information and preventive measures and the means to implement these measures. Hence, factors such as low level of education and literacy, lack of access to sufficient medical care, the low status of women and the corresponding powerlessness to control the basis upon which their sexual relationships with men take place, enlarge the transmission risk. Women's risk factors consists of poor health care (even at the time of pregnancy), insufficient treatment of sexually transmitted diseases, lack of awareness or inaccessibility of preventive measures like condoms, lack of power to insist on the use of condoms, and other measures that are only within the control of women.

In India, apart from targeting prostitutes, there is a total lack of concentration on women in the context of HIV infection. Commercial sex workers at times identified as the chief cause for infections. Of late, there is a demand for the legalisation of sex business, not due to concern or compassion to safeguard such women, but due to concern for public health and as a strategy which gives compulsory health checks and screening of such women to combat the expansion of HIV. Though HIV infection has reached private homes, women, due to their easy visibility, are identified as being responsible for spreading the infection. Women are thought to be the 'reservoir' of the disease, as 'vectors' of transmission to their children and male sexual partners rather than individuals who are themselves infected or are at risk of HIV infection. They are in urgent necessity of information and education to safeguard themselves. However, mere knowledge about AIDS and knowledge of law will not ensure security and protection of oneself. Enforcing such measures is not easy in a relationship based on inequality. It is necessary to recognise that the policies and strategies for combating HIV/AIDS require considering not only HIV-specific issues but also the underlying structural inequilibriums and the politics of physical and economic vulnerability which is an important factor to increase women's risk to infection.

Because of the peculiarity of the transmission of the virus through sexual contact, and the moral stigma related with 'promiscuous' behaviour, several women are unwilling to be tested for the fear of being labelled as 'Loose Women.' They remain unidentified, suffering silently without any care and treatment. Thus, besides the lack of concentration on women, it is a Herculean task to ascertain the number of women already infected. Thus, the issue of women and AIDS necessitates to be placed in a broader social and cultural perspective. Women's vulnerability to HIV is increased by the inequalities and discrimination they encounter in the society. Women are the subordinate sex, relegated to second-class status, kept semi-literate or illiterate, dependent, isolated and confined within the boundary barriers of their homes. They are at times denied access to education, healthy independent income and property rights. All these factors as a whole increase women's vulnerability and obstruct any effective prevention campaign. There is a need to understand the interaction between HIV infection and cultural norms, the rights and needs of women and socio-economic patterns in the society which render women vulnerable to HIV infection.

The dilemma of bringing in equilibrium the individual human rights and public rights has revealed the importance of the legal response to HIV/AIDS. But what should the legal response be? What are the experiences of a decade of different legal response to HIV/AIDS? What are the modules by which law can be incorporated into HIV/AIDS policy? Can law, as a tool for social change, bring about the required changes in the behavioural pattern and value systems? Clear cut responses to several such questions are still latent. A deep analysis of the various roles of the law and the interaction between them is necessary if law is to be used effectively to reinforce HIV/AIDS policy. Analysing the decade's experiences of many countries we can identify three main models:

1. ***Prescriptive Model.*** In this model the coercive laws has proved ineffective and necessitate to be deleted.
2. ***Protective Model.*** Here the concentration is on human rights issues where one has to discover a balanced approach between individualism and collectivism.

3. Instrumental Model. Here the law concentrates on combating subordination and seeks to change underlying values and patterns of social interaction.

The critical point here is to find out to what extent the policies in the public spheres could enter and influence the behaviour in the private sphere of the family to bring about the required changes.

At many times, laws are framed in response to specific problems, viz. dowry, rape, sex business, etc. But at times it is found that such laws are insufficient to deal with the problem because various social structures and accompanying patriarchal norms and attitudes are not tackled and mere cosmetic changes are no remedies to the problem of power structure and gender inequality. Therefore, it is desirable to bring about a social change in a wider social context. AIDS also presents a unique opportunity for effecting such a change, particularly for women, since it forces society to face issues that had hitherto been largely ignored, such as the relationship between poverty and sex business, etc. AIDS is also offering the impetus to evaluate issues of sexuality and personal relations, and thus there is scope for women to be able to take a more assertive role in personal relationship, to enable them to set up relationships based on mutual trust and respect. It highlights the need for men and women to take equal responsibilities in their sexual behaviour and concern for their children rather than placing this responsibility on women alone.

The preventive strategies offered till now provide very small protection for women from HIV infection. Enforcement of these strategies (such as monogamy and fidelity, safe sexual practice and usage of condoms) is governed by male behaviour. Where the discussion about sex is still a taboo, it is not easy to educate women about safe sexual practices, and enforcement of such strategies is practically not possible. Law cannot necessarily resolve this dilemma. Thus, there is a necessity to address the wider socio-economic structure in the society and to strengthen women through legal intervention and policies. Several social structures and cultural elements like religion, type of family structure and the institution of marriage ascribe secondary status to women and influence the perception about women in all other fields. A lack of priority in respect of health and education for women, lack of property rights, lack of access to finance and credit facilities, lack of supportive services in domestic chores, and the existing discrimination in all walks of life, deny women several rights which together constitute the greatest impediment in access to health care, education and employment opportunities. These, *inter alia*, enlarge a women's susceptibility to the risk of HIV infection.

The Indian constitution guarantees liberty, justice, and equality to all citizens of the country and prohibits discrimination on grounds of religion, race, caste and sex. It denounces practices that are derogatory to the dignity and status of women; nevertheless, sexual equality remains a far-too-distant objective. Sexual inequality and the spirit of patriarchy still pervade our personal laws which confer lower status on women. Indian personal laws are still based on religion, but religion itself is a tool often used to victimise, separate and dehumanise women. Moreover, the diversity of personal laws for several communities is an obstacle for the democratic advancement of the country. Secularism cannot be achieved by recognising a variety of conflicting laws on the same subject. This affects the status of women because various reforms and policies are not implemented for fear of annoying communal sentiments.

Many of the prevailing legislations require to be amended to ameliorate the status of women. These include laws regarding marriage and divorce, age at marriage, maintenance, matrimonial home and matrimonial property, inheritance and succession rights, sexual crimes under criminal law (such as rape, adultery, sex business, kidnapping, enticing and seducing a married woman), employment associated laws, etc. Women perform a wide variety of roles in society. They are helped or hindered in these roles as per their status and rights in society and in their family, their literacy levels and access to training, technology and professional activities, their standard of living and access to financial resources. The interaction between law and economic dependency is well established in a legal regime where women are deprived or discriminated against regarding property rights and the right to independent ownership of property. Elimination of such legal obstacles to economic independence through effective legislative reform can enhance the status of women within the family and in the society.

Law can be used to enhance the status of women within marriage and other sexual relationships. The double standards of sexual morality incorporated in law should be deleted. A woman's sexuality is suppressed, and control over her body is denied because she is looked upon as the property of her father or her husband. In several Commonwealth countries, fidelity of a woman is a legal pre-requisite for claiming maintenance from her husband. The absence of any criminal sanctions for marital rape further reinforces attitudes about the sexual subordination of women. Similarly, woman do not have any freedom or right to control their reproductive functions. Thus, there is a need for enacting laws that recognise the rights of women to make their own decisions about sexual relations at par with their male counterparts. Law has a definite role to play even in broad community-based empowerment programmes, especially legal literacy. Legal literacy brings about an increased awareness amongst women and a change in their outlook which may lead to the assertion of their rights. One effective method to ensure the improved status for women is to involve more women in the political process and in the formulation of policies for women. Though several policies are framed for women, they are lacking in content because they have failed to incorporate women's experiences. Thus, more women should be involved in the process of policy formulation. It is also imperative that more women participated at the implementation level to ensure that the development benefits reach the needy. Besides this, women must form collectives to overcome their individual powerlessness and demand enforcement of their rights and changes in the prevailing social structures in the society. In addition to empowering women though law, many other social structures and attitudes in the society need to be changed, especially literacy levels and the health infrastructure. There is an urgency to ensure the equality of the sexes in the educational process and to prioritise the issue of women's health, often neglected by women themselves and by the society. Women encounter several problems that are acute in their own way. The HIV epidemic accentuates these prevailing problems. Mere knowledge of what has to be done in order to protect oneself from HIV transmission is meaningless if one has no power over the circumstances that give rise to the risk. Hence the short-term goal is that women should take greater control of their lives and make use of the existing preventive strategies that are available immediately. However, the long-term goal has to be minimising and eliminating women's subordination and to enhance the status of women. For this, an elementary change in socio-cultural values requiring reorientation of the values, beliefs, customs and the law that shape the perception and roles of women within the family and the society has to occur.

It is true that legislation alone cannot change the norms in society. However, an effective legislative policy is a necessary pre-requisite for bringing about a change in socio-economic scenario. In order to eliminate vulnerability to HIV, human rights considerations must look beyond the immediate concern to minimise and eradicate discrimination for the infected and address the unequal socio-economic position of women. In this scenario, support can be drawn from several international human rights instruments that offer scope to promote the human rights of women which have been neglected so far, and which are clearly revealed by the HIV epidemic. Formal legal recognition of such international human rights instruments must be attempted by bringing about the necessary changes in domestic laws. And if such rights already prevail in the domestic laws, there is an urgency to amend them suitably so as to make them implementable.

10

AIDS: Delhi at Forefront

Geographical Details

Delhi finds prominent reference in ancient times right from the epic *Mahabharata*. In the late of the eighteenth century and early nineteenth century, the British rule engulfed Delhi and on December 12, 1911 it was made the capital city of India and was made a union territory in 1956. Situated in the northern part of the country, Delhi is surrounded by Haryana on all sides except east where Uttar Pradesh touches it. The union territory of Delhi has been renamed as National Capital Territory of Delhi with effect from 1st February, 1992. Delhi is not only the biggest commercial centre in northern India but also the biggest centre of small industries. Since 1947, a large number of industrial units have been set up. Delhi is well connected by roads, rail and air with all sides in India. Being a cosmopolitan city, all major festivals of India are celebrated here.

Geographically Delhi is located in the heart of northern India surrounded by the states of Haryana and Uttar Pradesh. It covers an area of 1483 square kilometres of which 798 square kilometres is rural and 685 square kilometres is urban. The increase in population has been highest in comparison to all India statistics. During the period 1971-91 the growth of population has been 54.4 per cent on all India basis whereas in respect of Delhi the growth was 131.7 per cent. The growth rate during the last 7-8 years has been of the order of 150 per cent. The increase in Delhi's population is mainly attributable to large scale migration from neighbouring and other states. Main languages of Delhi are Hindi, Punjabi and Urdu. It lies between 28°25′ and 28°53′ northern latitude and 76°50′ and 77°22′ east longitude. Yamuna river flows by the side of its eastern border in north-south direction. It has an area of 1483 square kilometres, i.e., about 0.05 per cent of the total area of the country.

It possesses the most central geographical position being situated 1400 kilometres from Mumbai, 1442 kilometres from Kolkata and 2157 kilometres from Chennai. Protected by the ridge and river Yamuna, it occupies an unrivalled strategic position. As New Delhi is the capital city of the Republic of India, the National Capital Territory of Delhi enjoys an important position in the country as well as in the international arena.

Enhancement of Status

Till November 1983, Delhi was an union territory without legislature when the lieutenant governor was assisted by two bodies, namely the metropolitan council and the executive council. The main function of the metropolitan council was to discuss and make recommendations on the subjects in the state list and the concurrent list in the 7th Schedule of the Constitution. The executive council was set up on the lines of the council of ministers in states but unlike the latter, all members of the council were nominated by the President of India. The status of union territory of Delhi has been enhanced from December 1973 by setting up a legislative assembly and council of ministers. By virtue of implementation of the government of National Capital Territory of Delhi Act, 1991 exacted by the Parliament. Delhi is now known as the National Capital Territory of Delhi. Its council of ministers headed by the chief minister advise the lieutenant governor in exercise of his functions. The council of ministers are also collectively responsible to the legislative assembly.

Population

The present population of Delhi is about 13 million. As per approximation there is an increase of 0.5 million persons every year. More than half a million of population is floating and visiting Delhi every day for business, service and other activities.

Medical Care

The medical care facility in the NCT of Delhi are provided by multiplicity of agencies each operating a number of hospitals, dispensaries, special clinics and nursing homes. These agencies consist Delhi government, central government, local bodies, statutory bodies, voluntary organisations and private institutions. There are about 1300 hospitals, dispensaries, and nursing homes, etc., having about 25,000 beds. Delhi is implementing the National AIDS Control Programme since 1992 in order to control HIV / AIDS in Delhi. With the implementation of the HIV/AIDS control programme a significant amount of awareness has been generated among all sections of population in Delhi. As per un-official report, about 95 per cent of people had the knowledge of AIDS during 1998. This kind of awareness has been only to the extent of the severity of the disease of AIDS and the majority of the population particularly in the J.J. clusters and re-settlement colonies are not aware as to how the disease spreads and as to how it could be prevented. The awareness in respect of the highly vulnerable groups like commercial sex workers, drivers and street children has been much lower which is estimated between 75 to 90 per cent.

Hospitals—Common Scene

In Delhi all the hospitals are over-burdened because of alarming growth in population. A large number of patients coming from neighbouring states are also treated in Delhi's hospitals. Un-official reports suggest that about 25 per cent of patients seeking treatment in Delhi are from the adjoining states of Uttar Pradesh, Haryana, Punjab and Rajasthan and also from other states where the friends and relatives of such persons are settled in Delhi. There are in all 35 blood banks, of which 14 blood banks have been modernized by NACO directly. There are 10 regional blood testing centres. As at present, about 2.5 lakh units of blood are collected every year in Delhi against a demand of approximately 3.5 lakh units. Efforts have been made over the last 5 years that the blood safety norms of the highest order are followed. The HIV suspected blood is destroyed immediately. The AIDS prevention and control activities have been taken up in right earnest now and a society has been established in the form of Delhi AIDS Control Society under a senior IAS officer as its project director. At present, there is a clear understanding of the gravity of the situation and a high level of political commitment has been witnessed for the implementation of the programme for control of HIV/AIDS in Delhi. The officers and staff are getting sufficient training with a view to counter the menace of the AIDS in the capital city of Delhi. It will be the firm commitment of the city government to ensure that the HIV/AIDS do not invade the NCT of Delhi in the manner it has happened in few of the other states in India.

Prevention of Transmission

Admittedly, so far, the implementation of the HIV/AIDS Control Programmes in Delhi could not be taken with the desired intensity and level of seriousness because of the reason that adequate manpower was not available. As a result of that it has not been possible to fully take up the programmes and spend the allocations provided by the NACO. Hence, a large number of issues are to be dealt with during the second AIDS control project. The transmission of infection among the poor and vulnerable sections of population has to be addressed more effectively by making participation of the community in general and non-governmental organisations in particular. There is a need to find out hot spots and sensitive fields for suitable intervention. As at present, there are only 10 STD clinics which have not been utilised very effectively. The STD/STI centres and its services need to be expanded and treatment seeking persuaded alongwith promoting safer behaviour through increased use of condoms. Efforts will have to be made to prevent the transmission of HIV infection in the general population through awareness generation with emphasis on targeted IEC and inter-personal communication. Blood safety initiatives also must be strengthened. The surveillance system has to be further expanded and strengthened to evaluate growing trend of the epidemic more frequently. The training of the field functionaries will be given priority and intensified to cover all employees in various public sector departments and related agencies.

The State AIDS Control Society

A special and peculiar characteristic of Delhi is that it is not only required to cater to the needs of its own population of about 130 lakh but is also required to meet the needs of the floating and migrant population which seeks treatment and assistance from the adjoining states. It is a well known reality that Delhi offers a better medical infrastructure as compared to the neighbouring states and as a result of it, there is financial and physical pressure on the resources of NCT of Delhi. In reality a large number of patients who ought to have got the treatment in their respective states, rush to Delhi and generate an over-burdening effect on the medical and other resources of the city of Delhi. The State AIDS Control Society plans to make all out efforts to lessen the transmission of HIV infection among all sections of general public. It will make efforts to involve public sector undertakings both of the central government and that of the Delhi government and seek their co-operation in strengthening the implementation machinery both in physical and financial terms. It also intends to seek assistance from private sector in its effort to control and prevent HIV/AIDS transmission.

Second Phase

1. The second phase of the project commenced from June 1999 and will continue till 2004. The main aims of the programme will be:

(a) reduction of spread of HIV infection among the poor, marginalised and vulnerable groups at higher risk of HIV infection such as commercial sex workers, truckers, etc., so that the adverse effects of morbidity, mortality and socio-economic consequences can be minimised;

(b) awareness generation about the transmission of HIV among population at lower risk of the infection through proper communication strategies including mass media campaigns, interpersonal communication, targeted IEC, promoting safe blood and extension of voluntary testing, expansion and strengthening of STD/STI centres.

2. To strengthen Delhi's capacity to respond to future challenges posed by the epidemic :

(a) by enhancing the technical, managerial and financial sustainability of the programme both at state level and local levels such as municipal corporations/NDMC and civil districts, etc.;

(b) by building capacities for promoting low-cost community based care and provide for cost effective treatment of opportunistic infections.

(c) by promoting partnership with public, private and voluntary sectors.

The process of implementation of the programme will consist involvement and participation of different departments of government of NCT of Delhi, sensitization of public representatives like members of parliament and members of legislative assemblies and municipal counsellors and senior officers in the education department including the principals and vice-principals of colleges and schools. It is also proposed to develop communication strategies and programme for youths in educational institutions and non-student youths in J.J. clusters, re-settlement colonies and unauthorised colonies. It is also proposed to conduct HIV/AIDS sustainable intervention programmes in the red light areas and also develop specific programmes for floating and migrant workers. There is a proposal to install 'automatic voice response system' for information to the general population and also install condom vending machines at public places like railway stations, ISBTs, cinema halls, clubs and restaurants, entry points at national highways, institution of social welfare department and other public places in a phased manner. It is also proposed to install traffic signs and boards and hoarding in various parts of the capital and develop specific material for street children, prostitutes, truck drivers and other vulnerable sections of the society separately.

At present there are 35 blood banks with a proposal to increase the number to 50 by the end of 2004. Voluntary blood donation camps are to be arranged on a large scale by involving non-governmental organisations and other voluntary organisations. It is also proposed to establish a central blood bank which will give integrated information pertaining to all the blood banks through computers/telephones.

Media Coverage

Electronic media such as Doordarshan and private channels are to be used to generate awareness among the population at lower risk level of HIV. It is also proposed to establish 5 mobile STD clinics which will periodically visit the sensitive, underserved and affected areas. The above mentioned are few of the main processes of implementation of the programme. There will be other processes and strategies too, being detailed in other chapters. The main strategies and activities would involve promotion of safer behaviour and treatment seeking for STDs, among population at highest risk to lessen the risk of spread of infection not only among themselves but also to the population at low risk. This will be achieved by undertaking targeted intervention through non-governmental organisations, improving the facilities for clinical management of sexually transmitted diseases by expanding and modernising the same including introducing syndromic case management at the level of general treatment facilities. To prevent the risk of HIV infections among population at low risk, IEC will be targeted with concentration on adolescent and youth groups to promote 'responsible behaviour'. While mass media campaign will be continued for general awareness, health/HIV education will be undertaken in universities, colleges and secondary schools. Blood banks will be modernized and enforcement of standards including mandatory tests made effective for ensuring safe blood. Voluntary blood donation will be promoted by establishing blood donor clubs and rational use of blood will be persuaded through advocacy and training of health functionaries. Public representatives will be involved extensively to enhance voluntary blood donations.

Testing Facilities

Voluntary testing facilities will be expanded with provision for pre- and post-test counselling to enable safe behaviour and prevent transmission of infection. The surveillance system will be strengthened by enhancing the number of Sentinel Sites to evaluate the prevalence level frequently apart from undertaking behaviour sentinel surveillance. The capacity of Delhi AIDS Control Society and the field staff will be increased by means of technical and management support, imparting training and developing infrastructure. Operations research will be taken up to develop best practices for interventions, etc. Research and development will be undertaken, particularly for evaluating the effectiveness of indigenous, alternative therapies and systems of medicine for treatment of HIV associated illnesses. For impact reduction among persons living with HIV/AIDS, the facilities for treatment of opportunities infections will be offered in government hospitals apart from encouraging home and community based care to make it more sustainable. Pilot projects will be taken up for therapeutic intervention with AZT among antenatal mothers to prevent vertical transmission of HIV infection.

For tackling the epidemic effectively partnerships will be developed with many sectors and stakeholders by establishing inter-sectoral coordination committee at the state level and bringing them together for establishing linkages such as TB control, RTI and RCH programmes. An effective 'monitoring and evaluation system' will be developed and implemented which would include MIS, periodic evaluation studies, etc. The total outlay for the second AIDS control project is Rs. 61.40 crore, which will be spread over five years. In fact, the inputs for the programme will be much more in view of the contribution to be extended by the government of Delhi. Such a contribution will be in the form of making available the prevailing infrastructure facilities (hospital beds, STD clinics, Gynec and maternity centres, blood banks, TB wards, etc.) and the services of the whole team of medical and paramedical professionals in all health facilities from sub-centre to the medical colleges. Moreover, the infrastructure facilities and the manpower in the department of education, social welfare (including nutrition) and urban basic services will also be available for the programme.

Allocation of Funds

The entire investment under second AIDS control project and the facilities of the government, will be used to achieve the aim of reducing and preventing the risk of HIV infection and minimizing its impact in the state. With the active participation of several sectors in the programme and enhancing the capacity of the institutions, the state will be able to meet the future challenges posed by the epidemic.

Analysis

Because of the strategic and commercial prominence in the northern India and being the national capital, the growth rate in population has already reached the stage of explosion in the city of Delhi. The increase in population has been highest in comparison to all India statistics. The population of Delhi rose about 40 lakh in 1971 to about 94 lakh in 1991. The percentage growth in population during the above mentioned period was 131.7 per cent compared to all India figures of 54.4 per cent. By the end 2000 Delhi's population went to a staggering figure of 135 lakh. According to 1991 census, the sex ratio is 827 females per 1000 males. More than 90 per cent of the population is in the urban areas. The literacy rate is 75.29 per cent. It is 82.01 per cent among males and 66.99 per cent among females. The medical care facilities in the NCT of Delhi are offered by a number of governmental and the private agencies. As per 1997-98 figures there are 86 large hospitals with 20392 beds. Besides, there are 24 primary health centres, 740 dispensaries, 193 maternity homes, 11 polyclinics, 43 special clinics and 136 private nursing homes. The total beds availability is 24025. Bed population ratio achieved by 2000 was 5 per thousand. Today, it is 2.36. In rural areas this ratio is only 0.38 per thousand.

Present Trends

The first AIDS case was reported in Delhi in the year 1988. The number of AIDS cases have reached from 45 in 1993 to 286 in 1998. Statistics from the surveillance centres functioning in Delhi has demonstrated a steadily rising rate of prevalence of HIV infection. The prevalence was 2.25 per 1000 in 1993, 12.53 per 1000 in 1996 and 13.15 per 1000 in 1997. An analysis has demonstrated that a higher percentage of drug users are HIV-positive. Based on statistics from sentinal surveillance, there could be about 35000 HIV-infected cases in Delhi. Of about 6607 AIDS cases in India, 286 cases have been reported in Delhi which is about 4 per cent of AIDS cases in the country. Delhi stands as the fourth worst state in terms of AIDS cases with Maharashtra being at first, Tamil Nadu at second and Manipur at third place. Therefore, Delhi has more cases and is more prone to the disease even compared to larger states like Uttar Pradesh, Bihar, Karnataka, Gujarat, West Bengal and Rajasthan. The following elements make Delhi highly vulnerable to the HIV/AIDS:

(a) Expanding population of the capital with increasing numbers of migrant workers, street children, prostitutes, 42 resettlement colonies and slum population.

(b) Approximately 45 per cent population lives in 42 resettlement colonies and 1200 J.J. clusters. Large number of single males are living away from families. The sex ratio is about 800.

(c) Poor living conditions and poverty make women vulnerable to sexual exploitation.

(d) At least 5 lakh street children have no access to any health service and are prone to the disease of HIV/AIDS – due to adult exploitation, drug use, etc.

(e) There is high level of STDs among street children. Large number of men and women suffering from STDs feel hesitant to effective treatment.

(f) There are about 45,000 persons who are using intravenous drug.

After the verdict of the Supreme Court, the professional blood donation has been banned since 1st January 1998. At present the replacement donation is mandatory except in special circumstances. The NCT of Delhi has already established a state blood transfusion council (SBTC). There are 35 licenced blood banks in Delhi. In order to ensure 100 per cent blood safety every unit of the blood collected in Delhi is tested for HIV. There are regional blood testing centres and all the 35 banks have been linked to ZBTCs. The blood units which are sero-reactive for HIV are destroyed immediately. In spite of efforts, Elisa Reactivity rate has gone up as given in the table below :

Sero-Positive Rate among Donors

Particulars	*Annual Year*						
	Upto 1992	*1993*	*1994*	*1995*	*1996*	*1997*	*1998*
No. of Blood Units Tested	380114	119464	181846	235007	272028	272426	246778
No. of Elisa Reactive	772	628	1190	1323	222	1413	1209
Rate per 1000	2.03	5.26	6.54	5.63	4.49	5.19	4.90

The table reveals that the sero-reactivity rate which was 2.03 per 1000 in 1992 increased to 5.63 per 1000 in the year 1995. However, it decreased to 4.90 per 1000 during the year 1998 which can perhaps be due to the total ban on professional blood donations from January 1, 1998.

11

Sonagachi Project: Kolkata

Being a well-known project, the Sonagachi Project had large media, coverage in recognition of its effect on the lives of prostitutes and the social change approach it has added to standard public health strategies. As an HIV intervention it has had many evaluations, both internal and external. It was started by the All India Institute of Hygiene and Public Health (AIIH&PH) in 1992 as the STD/ HIV Intervention Programme (SHIP), in arrangement with the National AIDS Control Organization (NACO) of India, the ministry of health and family welfare of West Bengal, and WHO. Other donors consisted NORAD, DFID and HORIZONS/USAID. It also consists of two NGO partners, the Health and Eco-Defence Society and the Human Development and Research Institute. As a relatively mature project, it has widened its support base in the area since 1994 by enlisting a women's organization (*Sramajibi Mahila Sangha*) and a legal aid agency (Socio-legal Aid Research and Training Centre). Most significantly the Sonagachi sex workers, established their own organization in 1995, the *Durbar Mahila Samanwaya Committee* (DMSC), which is the major mover of the programme. Gradually, what started as a narrowly conceived HIV prevention project, has become a social movement in West Bengal of no less importance, and is drawing in prostitutes and women's rights organisations from all over India and abroad. As about one-quarter of the prostitutes in the Sonagachi area are from Nepal and Bangladesh, linkages to sex worker projects in those countries have also been developed. The capacity to move sex trade out of its feudal social and economic bases to new alternative forms of service provision underlies the project's growing vision, articulated by the prostitutes themselves in so doing, sex business could become an industry-regulated business with mechanisms to sustain safer sex practices. Such a vision is far beyond what most HIV prevention projects with sex workers, particularly in developing countries, are ready to conceive. There are instances, however, of government policies in Thailand and Senegal that set up some of the same aims and mechanisms. The essential difference between the process that has taken place in Sonagachi and elsewhere in the developing world is that the prostitutes themselves, alongwith their families and friends, have taken the lead and carry out the work of the intervention. This consists of support of the behavioural, clinical, financial, political and legal aspects of the project.

Thus, it provides a remarkable example of powerless women moving into the 21st century with an altered image of what they can perform for themselves and a lesson for those participating in the women's movement, poverty eradication and public health in general. It requires that thorough consideration is given to society's stance on sex business and that prostitutes can have a voice in the ensuing debate. The project is complex with various components and is well documented in both English and Bengali. Its basic specific aims were simple: to lessen levels of STDs, enhance condom use, and to develop an effective strategy that could be replicated else-where. In this the Sonagachi project has succeeded. In terms of HIV and sexual health, present syphilis infections and clinically detected genital ulcers have diminished. HIV infection rates in eastern India are generally lower than elsewhere in the country. Among the sex workers at Sonagachi they also remain comparatively low at approximately 6 per cent (as of 1998). The project is at present expanded to several other areas in Kolkata and West Bengal. Of greatest importance is the emphasis on meeting the felt needs of sex workers and enabling them solve their own problems. Hence, this is the final goal, one appreciated by sex workers themselves from around the world. The project has had contentious moments dealing with a large array of actors, sensitivities, and conflicting interests. It has also had some difficulties in techniques and modes of monitoring and evaluation. Until now, it has not been able to deal with all the factors that place the Sonagachi sex workers at risk. These imperfections, however, have not marred its obvious effectiveness or credibility. There is little doubt that the Sonagachi project is one of the best examples of an HIV elimination project that addresses the short-term needs to control the epidemic and the longer-term necessities to reduce vulnerability of women in the sex trade.

Local Scenario

Kolkata at times called 'the city of joy' is also a city of poverty, of Mother Theresa's domain, and the historical seat of the British Raj. It is a crowded and underserved city, fighting to clean itself up and modernize. It is also the traditional centre of Bengali culture and society, a culture that takes big pride in its poetry, arts, music and political thought and action.

The relentless oppression of women in India is powerful precisely because it is deeply integrated into class, caste, and ethnic hierarchies. Resistance to class exploitation and social denigration has fuelled several movements in modern Bengali history. It is within this cultural and historical scenario that the Sonagachi project has come up. Surrounding West Bengal are the states of Bihar and Uttar Pradesh in India and the adjoining countries of Nepal and Bangladesh, all of which are substantially poor and disadvantaged, both ecologically and socially. From these areas hail a large minority of Sonagachi's resident sex workers. Sonagachi is the derived pronunciation of a lane called Sanah Ghazi, named a dacoit or hoodlum, recast after as a religious teacher. The Sonagachi area was first identified as a major red light district of Kolkata when the British enacted the Indian Contagious Diseases Act in 1868. This was done to control STDs reaching England via British soldiers serving in India. At that time, approximately 30,000 sex workers were estimated to operate in the area. According to survey conducted in the late 1800s, there were three major reasons why women entered sex trade. These were seduction and abandonment, running away from the cruelty of husbands and in-laws, and becoming a family outcast because of personal attempts to break through the intense restrictions on the lives of young women. To this list today we must add poverty from birth, fake marriages and sale, situational poverty because of family losses, trickery and trafficking, abduction and sale. Besides this, some family traditions of dancers and entertainers, e.g., Agrawalis, have steadily become family lines of sex workers.

The pattern of recruitment into the sex trade consists cross-border movements and a large number of young girls, about 15 per cent under the age of 15 at the time the project began, entered in that way. The sex business is controlled by police, politicians, local hoodlum gangs, brothel owners, madams and pimps. While some sex workers are independent, others, particularly those newer to the business have madams and/or pimps. Some madam-controlled sex workers known as *Chhukris* are completely bonded and each one is obliged to earn enough to pay off an advance given to her or, at many times, to the person who 'sold' her into the trade. Another madam-controlled system is called the *adhia* system, in which the sex-worker turns over 50 per cent of her income to the madam. Pimps take 25 per cent sex worker's income and are organized in a hierarchical and regulated system headed by *mukia*, or political headman. Rooms are rented at high rates. The sale of sex is legal in India if it takes place 'within a room'.

To avoid arrest, freelance or 'flying' sex workers must also rent rooms at high hourly rates. The Prevention of Immoral Traffic Act, aimed to control the flow of new women into the business, in fact simply makes it easier for sex workers to be harassed, extorted, beaten, raped, and otherwise abused, when the Act is used to raid brothels on the excuse of removing younger women. The attitude of the surrounding society is generally to despise and stigmatize sex workers on moral and social grounds.

Besides this, many sex workers have *babus*, men who begin as clients and then form longer-term relationships. While few of these men in reality care for their women lovers and contribute to their expenses, many are abusive and exploitative. Nonetheless, many women need these companions for emotional and practical reasons, and are tied to these relationships. The Sonagachi project area consists four important colonies of brothels, located comparatively close to each other, known as Sonagachi, Rambagan and Sethbagan, Jorabagan, and Rabindra Sarani. Collectively, this is the largest red light area in Kolkata with approximately 370 separate brothels housing about 4000 prostitutes. The total number goes to about 5000 in September and October during the Durga Puja season, a time of revelry and greater earnings for prostitutes. Besides this, on the crowded streets and tiny lanes below the multi-storey tenement brothel buildings, about 1500 freelance sex workers do their work. The whole neighbourhood is served by several small shops, itinerant traders, vegetable hawkers, youth clubs, wine shops, and medical clinics, a few operated by quacks. Prices at these establishments are higher than in other neighbourhoods in Kolkata of similar class. Hordes of people can be witnessed at any time of day and night travelling on bicycles, scooters, rickshaws and on foot. It is a crowded, dirty, lively, and dangerous area where daily about 20,000 men come to drink and purchase sex. Not only the sex workers, but their clients too, are preyed upon by hoodlums. As in most such areas, the police either ignore or are involved in the ambient violence.

Every building has many brothels in it consisting of 5 to 25 rooms. Sex workers fall into several classes as per income, which is mainly based on age and attractiveness. Higher-income women have pleasant rooms, sometimes with air conditioning, while the lower-income group may share a single room among up to five women, with beds separated by curtains. Ages vary from 13 to 45 with incomes from Rs. 10 to 2,000 per night (50 Rs. = 1 US dollar). Despite crowded quarters, the women live their lives in considerable isolation from each other and from the larger society. Madams and pimps impose rules that keep sex workers from visiting each other. Older sex workers, unless they become madams, are unable to get many clients and many work at housekeeping chores or babysitting to make a living. Eventually, many become destitute.

Relevance

The AIDS epidemic in India is a rapidly rising one. As one of the world's most populated countries, its absolute numbers of HIV-infected and affected people are likely to become staggering in the coming decade. With high proportions of very poor people and cultural patterns dictating very low status for women, Indian women are increasingly becoming the bearers of the HIV burden. Sex workers represent those with the lowest status and the highest risk, among all women. The All India Institute of Hygiene and Public Health (AIIH&PH) has been known for its various health interventions and thus, has been able to lead in the development of a major support system for the project. This support mechanism is known as the conglomerate, and consists NGOs, community-based organization (CBOs), and government institutions. When the project was started the prevalence of HIV was very low in West Bengal, providing an opportunity for a creative and flexible intervention.

Formative Stages

The first baseline survey, conducted by personnel from the

AIIH&PH with the assistance of an NGO that had been operating in the area, the Society for Community Development, was carried out from April to June 1992. The survey covered STD epidemiology, socio-demographics and behaviour. Freelance sex workers were excluded. After an initial count of 362 brothels housing 3,664 prostitutes, the sampling methods were formulated. Sex workers were classified into those with charges higher than Rs. 100 per client (Class A), those with charges between Rs. 50 and Rs. 100 (Class B) and those with charges less than Rs. 50 (Class C). Sex workers were sampled randomly in proportion to the number in each class. Sixty-five brothels were randomly selected out of the possible 362 and approximately 6-7 sex workers interviewed in each (with non-responder replacement), for a total sample size of 450 (12 per cent of the possible total). Besides this, 360 women from this sample were willing to undergo an STD examination conducted at a two-room clinic set up in a volunteer local club in the centre of the red light district. STD specialists from the Calcutta Medical College attended the clinic, and laboratory work was undertaken at the Bacteriology Department of the Calcutta School of Tropical Medicine.

In short, the social survey discovered that 85 per cent of the sex workers were between 15 and 29 years old. Most advanced they entered the business because of poverty (49.1 per cent), family disputes (21.6 per cent) or being misguided (15.6 per cent). Also, 85 per cent were illiterate and many were heavily dependent on alcohol, and 9.3 per cent were newcomers, having been in the business for less than one year. In this sample 43 per cent of the women visited and worked in other areas of the city as well, staying there for some weeks or months before coming back to Sonagachi. The majority had 3 to 4 clients each day for weekly incomes that varied between less than Rs. 300 to more than Rs. 5,000. Many women (27 per cent) reported that men hired them in a group, a situation that seriously diminishes the woman's control. About 40 per cent of the women had children, but the proportion with *babus* was not determined; 45 per cent of the women used some form of contraception but only 27 per cent did so consistently. Condoms were always used by only 1.1 per cent and often used by another 1.6 per cent of women. At that time in 1992, 90.6 per cent of sex workers had never used condoms and merely 31 per cent had heard of AIDS. More, 69 per cent knew something about other STDs.

Endocervical smears identified 10.5 per cent positive for gonorrhoea, with 4.9 per cent confirmed by culture, although, for technical causes, it later appeared that the methods used were insensitive and underestimated the exact rate of gonorrhea. *Trichomonas vaginalis* infection was found in 11.1 per cent. Genital ulcer were seen in 6.2 per cent of the women. Serological testing for syphilis detected 25.4 per cent positive by VDRL (dilution = >1 : 8). The HIV positivity rate was 1 : 1 per cent.

A client survey was conducted in 1993 by 193 sex workers, as they had the easiest access to these men. Sex workers from each class of income were selected to conduct a brief questionnaire-based interview with one client each. As these women were largely illiterate, they had to memorize the questions and answers. Social workers visited them in the mornings and filled the form in with their help. Literate clients filled in their own questionnaires. The sample was biased towards men they knew, men who were spending the night, and fixed clients and, while useful, cannot be considered representative of all clients. Those clients who entered and left the brothel rather quickly were underrepresented. Thirty-seven clients of sex workers of class A, the highest income group, were interviewed, as were 75 and 81 of class B and C, respectively. Results showed an age range of 15 to over 40, with a trend of younger clients to visit less expensive sex workers and more educated clients to visit the more expensive women. The mean ages of clients by sex worker class were: A-42, B-39, and C-34. Of the clients 87 per cent were literate and 44 per cent were businessmen. Others were wage-earners, professionals, drivers, students and police. The proportion of students (8.8 per cent) was as high as that of drivers (8.3 per cent). Slightly over half (52.3 per cent) visited the brothels once or twice a week and 9.3 per cent visited everyday. Most were alcohol drinkers and spent time entertaining themselves in wine bars. While vaginal intercourse was most common, 47 per cent also enjoyed oral sex. Anal sex was reported as rare, and 4 per cent paid to be masturbated. Another survey of 200 *babus* was conducted, revealing that 26 per cent were illiterate, but 9 per cent were graduates of universities. Similarly, 46 per cent had low incomes, less than Rs. 1,000 per month, and 4 per cent had incomes over Rs. 2,500 per month. Although half had heard of AIDS, 73 per cent had never used condoms. Only 4.5 per cent admitted using condoms regularly. Besides this, in 1993 the project undertook another survey of sex workers to learn about their situations and aspirations regarding their children. Some 2,338 women were interviewed, 47 per cent of whom had children under 14 years old. Despite the considerable felt need for children, largely for emotional and social reasons, pregnancy was a serious risk for these women, with 14 per cent stating they had deliberately terminated their pregnancies, many more than once. A total of 768 abortions had been experienced by 330 women, or an average of 2.3 abortions per woman. One woman had had 15 abortions and one live birth. An even greater problem is the future of those born. About half were bought up in the brothel with little in the way of decent care. Few sex workers paid older sex workers to raise their children, but the majority kept their children with them, arranging makeshift creches when working. The others were brought up outside the brothel, either with family members or in orphanage homes, with 90 per cent of the fund, supplied by the mother. Less than 5 per cent were raised in government or NGO-run homes. About half of the children had received some form of education, but drop-out rates from primary to secondary school were very high. None managed to go beyond secondary school. The mothers stressed their need for hostel or boarding facilities with proper schooling and supportive environments for their children.

Functioning

The project started with a philosophy based on reliance, respect and recognition, i.e. giving due respect to the women, relying on their knowledge and recognizing their work. The project team members had to make it clear to all that they would not disturb the prevailing power structure or seek to remove women from prostitution. Throughout the project's life, all those who influence the sex business, even if in a negative way, have been drawn into its activities. Simultaneously, abuse by thugs, power brokers, unethical researchers, and others has been resisted by the sex workers and their supporters.

The project itself has become a sentinel of resistance through organization and affiliation, in order to create a platform upon which sex workers could personally and collectively grow. Thus, allies among government agencies, NGOs, CBOs, academic institutions, and several other organizations have been incorporated in one way or another. Publicity in newspapers, dozens of public appearances, conferences, workshops, and visible campaigning have been used to draw attention to the issues necessitating reform. These issues are those most associated with the safety and well-being of sex workers, as defined by themselves. They include their rights as workers, the rights of their children, the safety of their neighbourhoods, their concern over the trafficking of children in the sex business, and their legal and constitutional rights. For project workers, misgivings had to be overcome. Some felt endangered by being close to prostitutes, and feared catching diseases. Others felt embarrassed having to deal straight with sex. Hoodlums were a very real threat. Steadily, they overcame their fears and have become true supporters of the women. Police raids have been a major problem in this project, keeping the sex workers insecure and feared. After each raid, staff believed that condom use declined and STDs rose among clinic attendees. Thus, the AIIH&PH in cooperation with the Kolkata Police Department managed a training programme for police personnel. By April 1996, 180 police officers had undergone this training.

Health care. A clinic known as the Health Service Centre, was set up in 1992 on the premises of a local youth club, Palatak, in the heart of the Sonagachi area. The Health Service Centre is staffed by one of two rotating STD specialist doctors and is working 6 days a week from 11:00 to 14:00 to prostitutes and members of their families. Treatment is free and serum samples are collected opportunistically for syphilis screening. Sex workers are persuaded by their peers to go to the clinic for screening even when asymptomatic. Follow-up on treatment is conducted through the work of peer educators. On average, in 1998, 730 women attended the morning clinic every month. In 1993 another clinic was set up for evening sessions 5 days a week adjoining another club, specifically for clients. Demand has risen to a large extent and the clinic is at present crowded; other clinic days are the urgent need of the hour.

Steadily, throughout the life of the project, because of the demand of sex workers additional clinics of identical nature have been set up. In 1994, one in Sethbagan and another outside the project area in Bowbazar, another red light district in Kolkata. These are functioning, on behalf of the AIIH&PH, by the project with an NGO conglomerate. Between 1994 and 1998, nine other clinics were opened in red light districts in Kolkata specifically for prostitutes and their families.

As the years have passed, the women have witnessed the value of good-quality health services and have noted the poorer quality and disrespectful treatment in other facilities in the city. In 1995, the peer educators, undertook a fast evaluation of the situation of prostitutes in the rest of West Bengal. They discovered 254 red light districts and spots throughout the state. After prioritizing 30, they started organizing and, as of late 1999, 14 new projects had been set up. New clinics were erected, peer education begun and condom sales carried out. This effort is financed by the project and managed by the DMSC. Technical aspects of STD care like resistance to antibiotics and verification of cure, remain to be handled. Aggressive screening and more referral and follow-up of *babus* and other clients are needed in the next phase of growth.

Education. Peer educators were selected and trained, starting with an initial group of 12. By 1997 there were 65 trained peer educators who were given US$ 1 each day. These women were given 6 weeks of training and utilized specially tailored flip charts, requiring little literacy, to explain the primary facts of sexual health and safer sex to their peers. The Sonagachi area was divided into 11 zones that were covered by the 65 peer educators with 7 supervisors. From 10:00 until 13:00 each day, every group contacts 40 to 50 sex workers and 10 to 15 madams.

They persuade the women to go for regular check-ups and seeking care when they have symptoms. Leaflets are provided to those who are literate. Besides video shows, slide presentations, small group meetings and ventriloquist performances have been used to reach larger groups of sex workers and clients. They have also developed a performing group Komol Gandhar, that consists male and transgender prostitutes and perform at several cultural events. They perform plays about STD/HIV elimination and the issues surrounding sex business. This dance/theatre troupe has become significant medium by which the prostitutes can express themselves, forge a public identity and reach a large number of persons of all walks of life. It won first prize at a National Cultural Competition for Sex Workers, held in Benares in mid-1997 and, in 1998, it performed at the Twelfth World AIDS Conference in Geneva. After expanding to other brothels in Kolkata, the number of trained peer educators has reached 200 with a coverage of about

20,000 prostitutes and *babus*. As the project has expanded, it has become difficult to continue to pay all the peer educators needed in order to maintain ratio of one peer educators to 50 sex workers reached. At present the ratio is 1 : 160. In order to tackle this problem, the project has developed an additional cadre of volunteers to assist the peer educators reach women. Monitoring the quality of work of these volunteers represents a challenge in scaling-up, typical of most trainer-of-trainer-like projects. In 1998 the Positive Hotline was set up and maintained by the sex workers in response to hearing about the sad situation of an HIV-positive woman who was not a sex worker.

It has started with a single phone at one of the field offices and is staffed at night by the children of sex workers. This service to the larger community emerged from recognition of the necessity for counselling and support for HIV-infected persons, whether sex workers or not. A core team has been formed of volunteers, a doctor, a nurse and a counsellor. Besides medical care, the service offers psycho-social and legal aid support and the team can be sent to the homes of HIV-infected persons. As the number of HIV-infected persons grows in the country the aim is to develop a model of community-based care for West Bengal.

Contraceptives

In the beginning, the peer educators distributed free condoms and enquired about the extent of condom usage. Demand for the high-quality, imported condoms distributed by the project grew faster than the supply. During the first month of the project, 3592 condoms were distributed; by 1994, during the month of December, 79420 condoms were distributed. This rose to 110328 in December 1996. Due to budgetary obstacles, the project was unable to meet demands. In July 1995, the sex workers of Sonagachi set up a registered society called the Usha Multipurpose Cooperative Society Ltd., a consumers' cooperative which would help them save money and avoid the exorbitant interest charged on small loans by moneylenders in the area. Registering as sex workers, instead of 'housewives', required a long struggle with authorities, but with a growing capacity for advocacy and publicity, DMSC was successful. Starting with only 13 members, it now has over 1000 and regularly gives loans at low-interest rates to prostitutes. Small investment schemes utilizing bank deposits have also been developed. Its funds provide a creche for sex workers' children during working hours and it gives employment to older out-of industry prostitutes. In April 1997, it developed its first for-profit business, the marketing of condoms. Bought in bulk, the condoms were sold to any group wishing to buy. Recorded sales increased from a total of 213056 in 1997 to 443805 in 1998 and 730656 in 1999. The project still distributes free condoms too for newcomers to the brothel, to men who attend the STD clinics and to very poor sex workers. Simultaneously, condoms manufactured in India have improved and importing is no longer thought necessary. An activist-cum-sales arm of the Usha Cooperative, Besanti Sena, now markets condoms in 40 red light districts of West Bengal. With the profits made, they have purchased a piece of land outside of Kolkata at which they have been able to construct a training centre where they conduct most of their training. The older prostitute produce handicrafts there when specific market opportunities come at fore.

Persuasion

Organization has been the key to persuade the sex workers of Sonagachi. Several influences converged to encourage the sex workers of Sonagachi to organize themselves. First, a previous organization of sex workers, called Mahila Sangha, was set up in the Sethbagan area in the 1970s, to fight against the regular and violent extortion of money from sex workers by a local mafia. After gaining victory, they moved on to literacy and health programmes. As a result, one of the leaders moved over to the Sonagachi project and led the Sonagachi sex workers in their first appearance at the Calcutta Book Fair in 1992. Second, regular meetings of the peer educators started to knit them together and, to resolve conflicts, they formed an Advisory Board and a committee to handle grievances. In 1993, the peer educators and supervisors held a candlelight procession against AIDS which made the headlines. Step by step, new elements were added. The peers were given a green uniform jacket with a printed red cross on it and an identity card. With this they could feel like real health workers. Women started to take their clients into the clinic to have their STDs treated and were sought after for advice and information. It was discovered that, in the start, women with children were the most enthusiastic about becoming peer educators as it gave them a more respectable status in the eyes of their children. Running their own project and organizations required that few of the women, at least, were literate. The women wanted a literacy project for themselves. One of the supervisors agreed to teach and they began, but soon it became apparent that adult learners with special life experiences could do better if the literacy lessons grew from their own discourses. A new method of learning evolved which is participatory and has its own primer. A small newsletter with an attractive glossy format, *Namaskar*, was started, in which they can tell of their experiences. These are sold by the peer educators at fairs and meetings, particularly the annual prestigious. Kolkata Book Fair. Four editions have been produced so far. In addition, daughters of sex workers were recruited to be teachers of literacy and there are 14 such teachers so far. This strategy has had the advantage of giving pride to the mothers and to the daughters, and helping them gain status in society. Indirectly, their new identities may make it easier to negotiate better positions with regard to dowry and marriage at a later age.

DMSC started to develop cultural sports and artistic programmes for sex workers' children and, with the help of the project, placed at first 50, and now 100 children in mainstream boarding schools every year. A creche now operates for brothel children and several other activities sponsored by donors and operated by collaborating NGOs/CBOs. In 1994, researchers, with the assistance of an NGO and police, collected blood samples from 50 Sonagachi women without their consent. This generated panic in the area and the Institute registered its protest. Eventually, the situation calmed down but left the women with determination to set up an organization that could tackle local issues, such as that one, which directly affected their lives. In 1995, the DMSC Committee led a group of 1,000 sex workers to protest against police raids in the Sonagachi area. They joined rallies against the eviction of sex workers in other parts of Kolkata and demonstrated against the unethical and illegal testing of an unqualified AIDS vaccine.

They collected money to give to the state for flood victims and by 1996, began touring other areas of West Bengal to evaluate the situation of sex workers, which, in several cases, they found shocking. They visited sex worker projects in Bangladesh and Nepal. Not long afterwards, representatives of the Committee attended international meetings of prostitutes, meetings on the trafficking of children in the sex trade, and national and international congress on AIDS. In late 1997, the Committee brought together several thousand prostitutes including males and transvestites, for the First National Conference of Sex Workers in Kolkata. They have taken on the role of the Secretariat for the Asia/Pacific Sex Workers' Network. In March 1998, they held another conference, the Follow-up Phase of the First National Conference of Sex Workers. This conference was attended by 2,000 sex workers from 48 red light areas all over India. At this conference they were able to attain several of their objectives particularly those associated with networking. They now have a vision and a platform of objectives, aims at integrating themselves into a worker's world of rights and responsibilities. The Committee now has over 250 male and transgender members.

Three hundred sex workers have received legal training. As some wanted more than the short course primarily given, another 60 had additional legal training. One vexing issue has been the presence of young sex workers in the brothel. This is both against the law, causing the police to make repeated raids, and a problem to older sex workers. The younger women have less capacity to insist on safer sex, are biologically more vulnerable to HIV infection and draw clients away from the older ones. The members of DMSC have taken the stand that they can better regulate the entry of young women into the brothels themselves than can the police or other agencies. They established a system through which they could watch new arrivals and counsel them before they in fact enter the brothel industry. At first they were attempting to send them back to their homes but the majority simply denied to go, having run away from abusive or difficult situations. With the assistance of the social welfare department, they now have an arrangement whereby most of the girls are sent to boarding schools sponsored by the social welfare department. Over the years this process seems to have reduced the proportion of bonded sex workers, usually the youngest, entering the brothel, although indicators have not been recorded for this.

With the aim spreading this type of self-regulatory action, DMSC established in 1999 three more Self-regulatory Boards at Sethbagan, Tollygunge and Rambagan in Kolkata. These boards are comprised of members from the state government, women's rights groups, other local persons and prostitutes. Members of

DMSC at times take part in meetings and debates on trafficking, an issue of intense concern in the South Asian region. Helping sex workers leave the sex industry has never been an objective of the project but, inevitably, growth in self-esteem and a sense of control over one's own life has led some women to choose to leave the business. About one-third of the peer educators who have been active for at least several years have moved out of the brothels. They return daily to do their work; about 60 women have left sex business completely. The small salaries they receive from the project must be supplemented by other income and many of these women at present sell saris and other small merchandise. Besides this, the number of pimps and madams seems to be dropping. At Sonagachi, as elsewhere, the AIDS epidemic has led to the realization by many sex workers that they can avoid the repressive and unsafe conditions in illegal brothels by diversifying their work modes. Many have moved into residential or hotel-based sex work, a situation having implications for future HIV elimination and the evolving nature of the relations between the state and the sex business.

Clients and lovers. For clients, a clinic has been set up with free treatment, free condoms and counselling, but no clear mode of establishing client-targeted programmes has emerged. Police, youth groups and the general public have received many awareness programmes. Few clients have been reached at wine shops and through forms of 'edutainment', such as ventriloquist shows. *Babus*, however, represent a special problem and, as fixed clients, have received special consideration. A meeting in the local Botanical Gardens was held in June 1997, attended by about 150 *babus*, which discussed the problems of the Sonagachi area and the role of *babus* in the set up of safer sex norms. This was followed by four more such meetings. As a result, a *babu* committee and a collective, known as Sathi Sangathan (Companion's Collective), were formed. The aim is to work with DMSC to fight against all forms of harassment and violence against prostitutes and their clients. One of their services of has been to escort clients past the bands of *gundas*, or hoodlums that operate on the streets Sonagachi.

Monitoring and Evaluation

The project collects statistics on several different monitoring indicators both at the clinics and through the peer educators. It also relies on periodic cross-sectional surveys for feedback on effectiveness, with one completed at the end of 1993, another in mid-year 1995 and the latest in 1999. The first external evaluation took place in 1996 and another in 1999. One important suggestion made by these teams was that the project should develop different indicators. Instead of focusing narrowly on effectiveness in STD control, it should find a way to enlist the emerging strength and self-esteem of prostitutes. By 1998 several new indicators were added. The attendance of clients at the project's clinics had been difficult to monitor as men sought treatment who may not have been clients. A referral card given by the sex worker to the client (and later handed in at the clinic) now makes it possible to monitor how many clinic attendees are clients referred by sex workers. The duration of self-recognized symptoms when the sex worker presents to the clinic is now recorded. Despite continuing to ask how many sex acts were covered by condoms, the project now monitors how many condoms were sold, on the assumption that women will buy what they will in fact use. Levels of empowerment and engagement in the community movement are now measured by asking how many times the sex worker manages to negotiate with landlords, police and other power brokers, and how many sex worker organization meetings or conferences she attends. Changing the indicators for monitoring the success of an evolving intervention is necessary but must be done with care so that continuity with the past is minimally affected.

Effectiveness

At the end of 1993, 14 months after the intervention was implemented, the first follow-up survey was done. Sampling methods were necessarily the same as the baseline survey and 612 women were interviewed. Age distribution was similar to the first survey and the literacy rate remained very low. The proportion of new sex workers (in the trade less than one year) was enough higher (22.6 per cent) than as baseline (9.3 per cent). The median number of clients the previous day was 3. Group sex appeared to increase from 27.3 per cent baseline to 48.7 per cent. The proportion of women reporting oral sex appeared to decrease from 74.4 to 38.1 per cent. It is not unlikely that the questions were asked in different manners in every survey, leading to this puzzling result. The proportion of women reporting some knowledge of AIDS rose from

30.7 to 85.8 per cent. The percentage of clients using condoms always or often increased from 2.7 per cent at baseline to 69 per cent, a considerable increase. By 1998, this percentage rose to 90.3. Though the methods used to detect gonorrhoea were too insensitive to detect all cases, these same methods were used for the baseline and first follow-up surveys. This showed a decrease in gonorrhoea from 13.2 to 3.9 per cent. Neither HIV nor recent syphilis infections showed any major change in prevalence. To improve the survey methods, decisions were made for the second follow-up survey conducted in July-August 1995 to alter the sampling and STD detection techniques.

This decision meant sacrificing some of the past statistics in order to have improved measurement capacity in the times to come. However, the hoped-for improved random sampling methods did not materialise. True randomization is very difficult without identifying the women in some way, especially because the prostitutes were interviewed at the brothels and had to go voluntarily to the clinic for examination and testing. In fact, more went to the clinic than were randomly selected and it was hard to know who had really been interviewed. Besides this, although the laboratory methods to detect gonorrhoea were improved, laboratory capacity was not enhanced, and only 10 samples could be handled per day. In November 1995, when an external team of experts evaluated the project, it was recommended that in the future the laboratory work should be managed by a commercial laboratory with more capacity and that a reference laboratory be utilized for quality control. Nonetheless, clear evidence exists of a reduction in levels of recent syphilis and the presence of genital ulcers. Measures of current syphilis are higher for those who have more clients than others, are illiterate and have not attended any meetings organized by sex workers. Although the rates of HIV among sex workers in most parts of the country had, by then, shown dramatic increases, by 1998, among 503 randomly sampled women at Sonagachi, only 5.5 per cent discovered to be HIV-positive.

While condom use has increased rapidly it has not reached total or near-total coverage. Only about 50 per cent of the sex workers use condoms all the time with clients and, as is typical in sex worker projects, the greatest proportion of this level was reached early in the project. The project has not placed a big emphasis till now on specific negotiation skills or materials. Options that would enhance usage rates, such as female condoms and lubrication, are not yet incorporated. Measures of condoms use with *babus* are collected within cross-sectional *babu* surveys and show a reported rise in use at last sex from 4 to 30 per cent between 1995 and 1999. *Babus* continue to exercise enough control over their relationships with the women and denying risk for themselves and their own wives. Despite enormous changes in levels of self-esteem for several women at Sonagachi, these effects have not reached all. Passivity, fear, and desperate necessity for money militate against the assertiveness essential to make demands on a man who may be drunk and potentially violent.

One important manner in which *babus* can exert power is the giving of their name to sex workers' children so that the children can be enrolled in school. As they can repudiate this assignment at a later date with the school system, this gives them continuing leverage and power over the women. In addition, madams and pimps can demand that their workers take clients without condoms and many young women share single rooms with other women, making assertiveness embarrassing and difficult. There are some victories too. For instance, one of the most resistant groups, the Nepalese women, has started to demand condoms. Although the change in proportions is not very big, the trend is statistically significant.

One important facet of this project has been the way in which new entrants to the sex business are reached, with 48 per cent of sex episodes covered by condoms on the previous day by women who entered the brothel only 2 months ago or less. This compares to 63 per cent of acts covered by those working for 6 months at the brothel. This success is attributed to peer pressure and improved self-control among prostitutes. In the 14 clinic catchment areas now run by DMSC in West Bengal, survey statistics between 1996 and 1998 reveal a rise in condom use from 28.8 to 52.2 per cent. The project has relied so far on the ability of sex workers to convince each other of the value of using condoms and obtaining STD treatment. The main tool of communication has been the original flip chart developed early in the project.

Although some sex workers have learned how to present a slide show on STDs, the majority of peer educators have not been equipped with materials that could expand their messages and assist them to present them to others, alongwith other sex workers and clients. Investment in materials for behaviour change communication has been quite meagre compared to many other projects. Police violence, a major obstacle to the sex workers' ability to control their own lives, has diminished to a little extent but few objective indicators prevail to measure this. It is easier to show that sex workers are more able to confront the police than before the intervention.

Capabilities

Initially the project was financed by WHO, followed by NORAD for two years. In October, 1994, DfID started its financing. The number of worker working for the Sonagachi project is 49 full-time, 216 part-time and 25 volunteers. The project at present costs about US$ 90 000 each year to run. The salary of the project director has, until recently, been paid by the Government of India. There is a central office and two field offices in Rambagan and Chetla, alongwith 3 rented cars. Given the high level of activity, everybody seems overworked and space is at a premium and often shared by different project programmes. Some university students are conducting their own research on the project, which assists in documentation. Overall direction and management is conducted through a large group of partners called the Conglomerate. Although this might add some burdens to decision-making, it ensures greater spread of responsibility and strategic thinking. The World Bank evaluated the cost of the project, though a full-scale economic study has not taken place. A rough approximation, expressing the reductions in STDs as DALYs (disability adjusted life years), revealed cost per DALY saved to be Rs. 30 to Rs. 50. An impact-oriented cost-effectiveness study would necessitate knowing how many HIV infections were averted in the intervention and control groups, an expensive, prospective study of questionable ethics. Instead a cost-effectiveness evaluation was completed in 1999 that calculated the cost per service. It discovered that the cost per condom sold was Rs. 9.2 (US$ 0.22), per interpersonal contact for behaviour change communications was Rs. 35.3 (US$ 0.84) and per STD patient treated was Rs. 560 (US$ 13.3). The latter cost in the community-based STD programme in Mwanza, United Republic of Tanzania was US$ 10.8. Overall, the project invests 12 per cent of its expenditures in advocacy, a much higher level than most HIV intervention projects. Cost recovery has not in fact initiated, although a fee for service has been instituted in the extension clinics outside of Sonagachi.

Moral Empowerment

Ethical concerns permeate throughout the project's programme. Standard procedures for confidentiality and de-linking of HIV specimens were used at the time of the survey work. While sex workers are steadily gaining more pride in themselves, the surrounding society still greatly stigmatizes them and their children. Many do not wish to have their names attached to printed statements or in any way admit to their families that they are sex workers. This concern is respected by the project. Special consideration is given to protect the identity of STD and HIV-infected women. Generally, the project takes a very strong stance on ethics with regard to treatment of sex workers.

Replicability and Sustainability

The project has already started replicating itself in several ways, with clinics, outreach activities and peer education training for other brothel areas and flying and freelance sex workers in and around Kolkata. Fourteen clinics are now run by the DMSC. As of July 1997, 34 peer educators were selected and trained from among approximately 1,500 flying sex workers in the vicinity. The intervention has reached out to cover about 8,000 of an approximately 12,000 freelance sex workers in Kolkata too. The Usha Multipurpose Cooperative Society has begun the marketing of condoms and has plans for developing a department store. As most consumer goods are overpriced in the Sonagachi area, this would enable the sex workers to make basic commodities available to themselves at a lower cost. A registered organization, the Society for Human Development and Social Action, has been set up composed of the project partners, including NGOs and sex worker organizations. The new project director is the son of a sex worker who has been active in the project since its inception. Such an organization has the potential to offer the basis for the maintenance and growth of future efforts to provide sexual health and many other basic services, as well as a platform for advocacy where the sex workers can play the driving role. Skills, such as basic accountancy and literacy, are needed and steadily these needs are being addressed. English language skills are also generally lacking, requiring the use of interpreters when interacting with most outsiders. The capacity of Sonagachi's women to give the basis of a regional network of sex workers has been recognized and such a network was started in 1998. Six sex workers are receiving computer training which should help them maintain networks via e-mail, though language obstacles still remain. The peer educators themselves have trained 600 other sex workers, 200 each at 3 workshops for brothel-based sex workers.

Outcomes

The Sonagachi project has shown the great value of steadily placing the control of a community-based health intervention into the hands of the community. It has been possible to meet the costs of expansion, incorporating new components, and staffing them due to enthusiastic voluntarism on the part of the sex workers. Whether an HIV or malaria intervention, this approach is one of the most sustainable, if not biomedically perfect, in the reality of an imperfect world. Impact and effectiveness in such behavioural change interventions are difficult to achieve and to measure, but are far more likely to be sustained, once achieved, if the target group itself takes over. This has been accomplished to a greater extent in Sonagachi than elsewhere in the Asia-Pacific region. This project has had a remarkable emergence, even if sex workers are not yet ready to staff and completely manage their own clinics. A great deal of investment has been made in building capacity of staff and sex workers. The project often has had detractors and critics, but its basic soundness is reflected, not merely in impact indicators or the views of experts, but in the commitment and active participation of sex workers themselves. This could only be accomplished by treating the sex worker as a whole person, persuading her to recognise and express her needs and treating her in a fully ethical manner. Meeting the felt needs of the sex workers has persuaded them to commit themselves to HIV prevention. It was unfortunate that the laboratory STD work and sampling has, often been unreliable. Such projects have wide scope to recruit more expertise. A scientific research and training centre is envisaged for the future of Sonagachi, which is one way of assuring greater participation of scientists. Nonetheless, biomedical and self-reported behavioural statistics from repeated surveys ensured adequate replication to show effectiveness.

In the times to come, monitoring and evaluation in Sonagachi should be able to correct past mistakes and incorporate measures and documentation of personal growth and social empowerment among the women. The fuller participation in HIV prevention is needed of important men and women who strongly influence the safety of the sex industry, e.g., police, madams, pimps, *babus*. Again mentioning this project has spawned various organizations that provide a democratic basis for sharing decision-making power. Reforming the sex trade without involving police, madams, pimps and hoodlums will be very difficult, and they need to be included. Recently, as the number of pimps and madams declines, landlords have started to harass sex workers more directly. The future direction and management of the project through the HARD Trust has the potential to include all players and stakeholders. India and the rest of the world will have to reckon with the awakened women of Sonagachi as they move towards greater outreach to other sex workers in their region and around the world. The main remaining barrier is the attitude of society to sex work and sex workers. HIV infection, while a serious and sad disease problem globally, is also an opportunity to set right many of the abuses of the past. The Sonagachi project has started to wed prevention and cure in the best traditions of public health activism.

Index

I

S

O

P

R

S

T

ENCYCLOPAEDIA OF AIDS

ENCYCLOPAEDIA OF AIDS

(In 7 Volumes)

(Volume 4)

Editor

Dr. G.C. Satpathy

PUBLICATIONS

KALPAZ PUBLICATIONS

DELHI - 110052

ENCYCLOPAEDIA OF AIDS
(*Health, Reference*)

Rs. 7000 (Set)
Rs. 1000 (each volume)

ISBN: 81-7835-112-9 (Set)
ISBN: 81-7835-135-8 (Vol. 4)

Published in 2003 in India by
Kalpaz Publications
C-30, Satyawati Nagar
Delhi-110052
e-mail: kalpaz@hotmail.com

Laser Typeset at: Alphabet, Delhi
Printed at: Mehra Offset Press, Delhi

Contents

Preface

The later half of the twentieth century will be remembered in the history of medicine for two remarkable events, one good, that is the eradication of smallpox, and the other one bad, when the world was alerted to the first case AIDS in 1981, now running in a pandemic proportion. In a little over two decades it is estimated that over 36 million people are now infected with HIV/AIDS with 5.3 million being infected every year. India alone has about 4 million HIV/AIDS patients, the second highest number among all nations. Now it is well perceived as a serious threat to humanity, and the control of this epidemic lies not only in the hands of physicians alone but the entire society must involve to the task. No cure or vaccine is yet in sight. So the only mode of controlling it is prevention. The key to prevention lies in information, education and communication.

Twenty years of observation and study of the syndrome has generated profound interest among all branches of medicine, social activists, research workers, public health issues, health and sex education strategies, with innumerable clinical and pharmacological research being conducted on it all over the world. It is not possible to compile the whole saga of AIDS, which is unique in many ways and not yet fully understood. We have tried to accumulate as much information as possible in this seven-volume encyclopaedia, probably the first such attempt made ever. Since the process of acquiring information is never-ending, we hope to provide more and more information in future.

It has been a herculean task to compile the huge materials systematically, besides being an unique experience. In spite of the best efforts for accuracy and perfection, there may be shortcomings, which may be excused. It will be a success story for us if by this work the society to which the work is dedicated is benefited at large. The study does not end here. It shall be a continuous series in future with comprehensive details having a deep bearing on the subject.

Guwahati-23
Rathyatra-2002

Dr. G.C. Satpathy
MD, IPM

Acknowledgements

During the course of this research work, I happened to visit several academic fora which willingly afforded their support and facilitated my work. These are the Ministry of Health, Govt. of India, World Health Organisation, health departments of the States and academic institutions of higher learning. I have used the material from published works including scholarly journals and magazines to fill up the gaps in these volumes.

I have also taken academic support from several sources, which include universities, institutes, centres for higher learning, Acts passed in this direction, Statistical Year Book (UNESCO), voluntary organisations, legal luminaries, social activists, prison management, legal issues of AIDS, Legislation Enquiry Commission on HIV Law, Sri Lanka, Prevention of Brothels Act, Myanmar, Laws of HIV/AIDS in Pakistan, Documents in sub-Saharan, Africa, European Council Recommendations, UNESCO Courier, Philippines Overseas Employment Agency, Foreign Exchange Regulations Deptt., Central Bank of the Philippines, National Advisory Committee on AIDS in Singapore, Vietnamese National AIDS Committee, National Blood Transfusion Centre in Cambodia, Infectious Diseases Act, Thailand, AIDS Prevention Act in Korea, Labour Protection Law, Thailand, Social Security Act, Thailand, Homosexual Law Reform Act, 1986, Universities of Nairobi, Manitola (in Canada) and Washington, Institute of Systemic Therapy, Harare, Zimbabwe, The AIDS Service Organisation, Kampala, Uganda, Health Economics and HIV/AIDS Research Division, University of Natal, Durban, School of

Public Health, University of Natal, South Africa Institute for Medical Research, Johannesburg, Centre for African Family Studies, Nairobi, Kenya, Malwai Institute of Management, Malwai.

I feel much grateful to these institutions and learned authors whose writings have proved useful in the texts of these seven volumes.

The publisher and myself feel much beholden to the panel of highly qualified and experienced advisers who are distinguished in their respective fields, for their valuable and timely guidelines, contributions and encouragement in making this work an epoch-making one.

I am grateful to several other research institutes and NGOs etc., scholars whose writings have been used in these volumes.

I am extremely grateful to my wife, son Anurag and daughter Anamika for their consistent encouragement to me during this stupendous research work.

Dr. G.C. Satpathy

Our Distinguished Panel of Advisers

1. Dr. A.K. Das, MD, MNAMS, Ph.D., FICA	Dean and Director-Prof. Dept. of Medicine, JIMPER, Pondicherry
2. Mr. D.K. Arya IPS (Retd.)	Former Director General, BSF
3. Dr. K.V. Dakhina Murty MD, DM, DNB, FISN	Prof. & Head, Deptt. of Nephrology, Nizam's Instt. of Medical Sciences, Panjagutta, Hyderabad
4. Maj. Gen. K.K. Ganguly	VSM (Retd.)
5. Col. M.K. Bhandari MD, FICA	Asso. Prof. of Medicine, Armed Forces Medical College, Pune
6. Dr. M.C. Dash	Vice Chancellor, Sambalpur University, P.O.: Jyoti Vihar, Orissa
7. Dr. N.C. Borah MD, DM	C.M.D. GNRC Hospitals Ltd. Dispur, Guwahati
8. Dr. P.C. Bhattacharya MD	Sr. Consultant, downtown hospital Dispur, Guwahati
9. Dr. S.B. Gupta MD	Physician and Cardiologist Central Railway Hospital, Mumbai

Introduction

Approximately half of the global population who acquire HIV become infected in their mid-twenties. Thus, it is crucial that work be undertaken to help young people protect their sexual health. However, there has been a lot of uncertainty about how to approach, HIV and AIDS prevention with young peoples. For example, there continues to be widespread concern that sex education will encourage young people to become prematurely sexually active. As a result, many sex education programmes have concentrated solely upon abstinence. Well-designed programmes of sex education combining messages about safe sex as well as abstinence may delay sexual debut as well as increase preventive behaviours among those young people, who are already sexually active. Where they have been able to access appropriate knowledge, skills and means, young people have demonstrated a remarkable propensity to adopt safer behaviour.

The various projects discussed in this volume focus on community mobilization against HIV/AIDS throughout the world. The activities carried out in community projects are as diverse as the peoples and cultures that make up these communities. Some are entirely 'home-grown' and self-sufficient, while others have benefited from external advice and financing. Some are based in religious centres, others in medical institutions and still others in neighbouring meetings places. Many projects concentrate on public education, others on providing care and still others on prevention or other goals. One of the main roles of these projects is to frame effective and ethical policies and strategies for prevention and care and promote and support relevant research to develop new tools and approaches to HIV/AIDS. This role is best understood as being part of all these projects overall mission of leading and catalysing an expanded response to the epidemic to (a) improve prevention and care, (b) reduce people's vulnerability to HIV/AIDS; and alleviate the epidemic's devastating social and economic impact.

Once an initiative is discovered as doing any or all of the above well, the other 'core criteria' are used for best practice, relevance, efficiency, effectiveness, sustainability and ethical soundness.

The worldwide response of individuals and communities to the epidemic has been encouraging. With courage and compassion they have mobilized resources to care for and support those affected and to assist others in remaining uninfected. Striking has been the role of people living with HIV/AIDS who, within a short period of time, have given a human face to the grim statistics. Although only a small percentage of persons living with or affected by HIV/AIDS have come out in the open declaring their serostatus, those who have done so have been powerful catalysts. Their voice has been heard during the International Conferences on AIDS and STDs, providing insights into how to address problems, how to strive for positive living and how people can be empowered through the trauma and tragedy of the epidemic.

An environment characterised by high levels of denial, fear, and stigmatization has undermined the participation of those living with or affected by HIV/AIDS. Even when the political, legal and social environments are conducive the participation of those living with or affected by HIV and AIDS is seldom reflected in the formulation of policies and programmes. Reasons for this vary from country to country, a certain pattern emerges. First, there is an absence of appropriate mechanisms to ensure that the experiences, perceptions and capacities of those living with or affected by HIV and AIDS are expressed, valued, understood and taken into consideration in the development of policies and programmes. Second, even when an appropriate forum is provided, individuals living with or affected by HIV and AIDS often lack the skills necessary to engage institutions and governments in policy dialogue. Third, many individuals living with or affected by HIV and AIDS are not in gainful employment and are, therefore, too economically weak to engage in any serious discourse. Fourth, even when they are employed, the kinds of institutions they work for are unlikely to generate and initiate policy changes. The principle of greater involvement of people living with HIV/AIDS (GIPA) was critical to an appropriate, ethical and effective national response to the disease. This will strengthen the capacity and coordination of networks of people living with HIV/AIDS and community based organisations.

As the epidemic continues to ravage the developing world, it becomes evident that diverse strategies to confront the wide-ranging and complex social, cultural, environmental and economic contexts in which HIV continues to spread must be researched, tested evaluated, adapted and adopted. The majority of populations in developing countries have access to traditional health care and it is widely accepted that about 80 per cent of people in Africa rely on traditional medicine for many of their health care needs. Traditional healers are well known in the communities where they work for their expertise in treating many sexually transmitted diseases. There is a dearth of research actually testing the impact of involving traditional healers in HIV prevention efforts. This includes strengths and limitations of traditional medicines and healers with respect to collaboration with biomedicine and the continuing policy debate on the integration, cooperation, and collaboration of traditional medicine with national health care systems.

The future of any nation is directly linked to the future of its children — and by investing in children and in the families that sustain than, a nation is ultimately investing in its own development. Coping with the cumulative impact of over 17 millions AIDS deaths on orphans and other survivors on communities and on national development is an enormous challenge, especially in African countries with social and health services already reeling from lack of human and financial resources. Till now, approximately 15 million children younger than 15 years of age have lost either their mother or both parents to AIDS, with 95 per cent of these children living in sub-Saharan Africa. In spite of all hardships and stigma, these children also have a right to education, affection and cultural identity, as well as to services for the care of children. They have a right to be heard and to be protected from abuse, neglect, maltreatment and exploitation. They have the usual needs of children, including economic, social, educational, medical and psychosocial needs. The psychological effects are the least tangible and the most difficult for adults to address. Yet they impinge on all aspects of a growing child. The devastating wrought by HIV is very real, whether the impact is measured in terms of children's future prospects. Parents and organizations, religious leaders and counsellors are daily facing painful choices in relation to children to disclose the parental HIV status, to involve children in home care of the sick, to talk about the dying and death of a parent or sibling, to find ways and means of postponing orphanhood, and to secure the best future possible for each child, even in the midst of massive constraints. Such situations are regularly confronted worldwide and there is the need to address the tough questions related to the rights and needs of children affected by HIV/AIDS, with a focus on their psychosocial needs. The effect of listening and talking to these children affected by HIV/AIDS will be to make their perspective much better known to adults who are working with millions of vulnerable children throughout the world.

HIV infection rates among teenage girls are at times much higher than in teenage boys; the reason lies in girls' greater biological and social vulnerability. Compared with that of males, the female reproductive tract is more susceptible to infection with HIV and other STDs, particularly in younger girls. And girls often risk infection very early. Compounding the biological vulnerability of girls are complex and unhealthy societal expectations that mean girls and young women have less control over their lives and bodies than do their male counterparts.

Too many young girls find themselves at an early age in the sex business, usually for lack of other options for earning a living. Young girls are desirable because they are thought to be safe and uninfected with HIV but the risk of infection to them, and hence to their clients, is very high. There is a need for some responses to this problem, focusing on changing the attitude of girls and their parents in regard to prostitution and on providing a means for girls to avoid becoming sex workers through improved education and career opportunities. Such response takes into consideration regional and demographic differences in the nature and scope of the problem in the search for solutions.

States should ensure that government and the private sector develop codes of conduct regarding HIV/AIDS issues that translate human rights principles into codes of professional responsibility and practice, with accompanying mechanisms to implement and enforce these codes. In every country the workplace is one important front for preventing new HIV infections and promoting non-discrimination towards people with HIV/AIDS. This will serve several purposes. In countries where there have been no systematic activities around AIDS in the workplace it will be a guide on how to develop policy and build partnerships and will help carry forward the campaigns that have already started.

One

Home and Community Care for People with HIV/AIDS: Afro-Asian and Latin American Perspectives

Project Hope

Brazil has the fourth highest reported number of AIDS cases in the world, with 116389 cases of AIDS reported by the end of 1997. Over two-thirds of these cases have been reported in the industrialized south-eastern portion of the country. Nearly half of cases to date have been found among homosexual and bisexual men simultaneously the male-to-female ratio of AIDS cases has fallen from 9:1 in 1987 to the 3:1 at present.

In 1996, the Brazilian government passed a law to provide AIDS patients with free combination therapy and other medication, with poor and hospitalized patients given priority. This followed several lawsuits in which Brazilian courts ruled the government should pay for the treatment of people living with HIV/AIDS.

Project Hope—Brazil

In 1988, a nurse began to work on the problem of AIDS in Eastern Zone II of Brazil's largest city, Sao Paulo. A local bishop gave his support to her work and provided a small building in the working-class neighbourhood of Sao Miguel working as one of the project's centres.

Following a period of information-collection on the HIV/AIDS situation, the nurse made a large number of personal contacts in the area and brought together a group of volunteers. These volunteers were already well organized and making house visits of people living with HIV/AIDS and their families by the time the project was legally set up in 1991. Two new centres were formed in Guaianases and Vila Esperanca with the support of Brazil's National Programme on STD/AIDS, after a lapse of three years.

Project Hope was the first NGO in Sao Paulo to give home care. Their initiative was acknowledged as an important element in sensitizing government health authorities to the feasibility of home care, and changing the authorities original scepticism of this approach to AIDS care.

Objectives

The objective of Project Hope has been to improve the quality of life of people living with HIV/AIDS by:

(a) changing the behaviours and attitudes of people living with HIV/AIDS, and

(b) involving the community.

The project bases its home-care work on the following principles:

(a) the ideal environment and best therapy for a person infected with the virus is to be with his or family;

(b) families should be helped to accept and face up to the reality of living with HIV/AIDS; and

(c) infected individuals and their families should be helped to demand and fight for their rights as citizens.

Functioning in a Poor Urban Area

Sao Miguel covers an area of about 7.5 square kilometres with a population of approximately 1,03,000 persons. Most of the inhabitants are members of the working class, and many live in poverty. The epidemiological profile for the state of Sao Paulo may give a rough idea of patterns of HIV/AIDS in Sao Miguel. As of December 1997, the state of Sao Paulo reported 65350 cases of AIDS. Three-quarters of these cases are men. Sexual transmission accounts for just under half of all cases, while almost a third are the result of injecting drug use. Mother-to-child transmission accounted for just under 3 per cent of cases. Among the 28417 reported cases of sexual transmission, the official statistics attribute 39 per cent to homosexual exposure, 46 per cent to heterosexual exposure, and the remainder to bisexual exposure. Over 40,743,000 persons in the state of Sao Paulo have died of AIDS, till now.

Currently, Project Hope provides services to approximately 480 people who are living with HIV/AIDS. Of these, approximately 10 per cent seriously ill while 30 per cent are asymptomatic, with the rest showing some symptoms of the virus. There were 212 men, 189 women, and 68 children according to a recent count. In addition, the project was helping 94 orphans through its 'god parenting' programme.

Major Elements

Project Hope is structured around four programme areas:

(a) Health programmes, including support and orientation for people living with HIV/AIDS and their families, nursing care, occupational therapy, and mutual help groups for emotional and psychological support. Two professional nurses on staff provide care both at the project's centres or in patients' homes.

(b) Social programmes, alongwith a campaign for orphans.

(c) Educational programmes, including training of volunteers, production of educational material, and public debates aimed at specific groups such as students, young people and housewives.

(d) Mobilizing funds including fundraising from local donors and from national and international agencies.

Within these programmes, different activities can be further detailed as major elements of the project.

An average of 183 new cases are taken on by the project every year. Initial contact with the person living with HIV/AIDS is made in different manners most frequently through the initiative of the person or his or her family. Some introductions are arranged by the social services unit of the local hospital. The first home visit is generally aimed at collecting information. It is carried out by a nurse accompanied by a volunteer. The visit begins with learning about the background of the person with HIV/AIDS, and is followed by an assessment of his or her clinical condition. Finally, the social and economic situation of the person is discussed in order to make an evaluation of needs. Whether there are follow-up visits depends on the decision of the person with HIV/AIDS.

Every effort is made to establish a relationship of trust and friendship during the visits, and there is strict observance of the person's right to confidentiality. Between first visits and follow-ups, approximately 360 home visits are made every month. In approximately 90 per cent of the cases attended by Project Hope, the families undertake to look after the person living with HIV/AIDS.

An important job is carried out by paid staff who are known as 'multiplying agents'. These are young people (average age is 15 to 20) whose work is to promote awareness of HIV/AIDS and of the manners that individuals can prevent infection by or transmission of the virus. Examples include role-playing of how the condom use can be negotiated within a couple.

Role of Volunteers

Project Hope could not function without the voluntary contribution of time by different people. They include:

(a) 74 volunteers who work daily or weekly in the health programmes;
(b) 97 "godmothers" and "godfathers" who help with orphaned children; and
(c) 40-50 people who help from time to time with particular events such as fundraising bingos, raffles or bazaars.

The volunteers represent a cross-section of the Eastern Region's population. The youngest to date is 18 years old, while the oldest is over 70. Less than 5 per cent of volunteers have attended university, though 40 per cent have finished secondary school. The majority are women. A variety of religions are represented in the group. Many are persons who have received services from the project.

Volunteers are recruited in various ways, including campaigns on community radio, articles in print media, contacts with the neighbourhood association and word of mouth. Each candidate is interviewed to determine their personal history, why they got in touch with the project, and what their expectations are. At the same time, the interviewers describe the project and explain its objectives. If both sides are still interested, the volunteer enters an orientation period, learning in greater detail about Project

Hope's programmes and philosophy. The volunteer is free to choose a programme area to work in, based on this orientation. If his or her choice is to work in the health programme, the volunteer begins to accompany staff and more experienced volunteers on home visits. During these visits, the new volunteer acts only as an observer, and learns that everything divulged during the visit is confidential. This period of learning-by-experience is of two months duration. If all goes well, the volunteer receives formal training on:

(a) HIV and sexually transmitted diseases (STDs);
(b) medicines related to HIV/AIDS and STDs;
(c) the role of volunteers in home care; and
(d) the benefits of home care for people with HIV/AIDS.

Only then is the candidate considered a full-fledged volunteer who is authorized to do home visits alone.

Keeping Morale and Motivation High

Americo Nunes Neto is a long-time member of Project Hope. He says:

> "I've been HIV-positive for seven years now. I came into Project Hope as a client for their services in 1990. It was a good thing for me, as I really needed the support and also something to re-build my life around. After a while, I became a volunteer in the project and an activist in the struggle for the rights of people with HIV/AIDS. Today I'm vice-president of the project.

In my work of coordinating activities, I have to keep in mind the needs of the group. Our work can be very hard on people emotionally, so maintaining balance and harmony is extremely important in motivating our volunteers and staff. You can't just hope for that to happen, you need mechanisms for the organization to follow. We have a variety of these mechanisms.

One is simply good, consistent supervision. I know that sounds obvious, but you have to think about it to do it well, especially when everyone is so busy. Just telling people what to do and leaving them to it doesn't work - not just because you need to monitor the quality of what they do, but because they need the support and personal communication with someone knowledgeable. As well, our supervision of volunteers isn't just watching what they do; it includes updating them on what the project is doing, and ongoing training.

In formal terms, we schedule weekly meetings where we evaluate progress on individual cases and discuss what the client's needs are - and the needs of the volunteer, which as a coordinator I always have to keep thinking about. But we also do a lot of group reflection on issues that come up, especially concerns of the volunteers. Being included in decision-making and having your ideas listened to is a great motivator for a volunteer. I certainly was for me.

Another important point: even if you can't pay people for the work they do, you can be creative about compensating them in one way or another. Project Hope organizes things like games, group recreation, trips together - those are obvious, and people like them and they don't cost much. And they encourage friendships within the group, which is very important. We also can provide public transport passes so people can get around easily and cheaply on the city buses. Less obvious is therapeutic massage and psychological support. These are two services we offer to our clients, and we have professionals who do them, so it makes sense that volunteers should benefit from such supports as well if they need them.

Finally, we recognize people's limits. Everybody needs a rest sometime, and 'burnout' is a high risk in this kind of work. So we make sure people take a month's holiday from their volunteering duties every year."

Collaborations

An important component of the project is to find financial support for its programmes. This work is carried out in several ways, including promoting fundraising events with the local community, identifying and maintaining relationships with local donors, and contacts with supporting agencies both in Brazil and internationally.

Project Hope benefits from a great deal of community support, which is often expressed in contributions of materials or services. Fundraising or recreational events at times receive free food from local businesses, for instance. Local people with cars or trucks donate their time to do whatever driving is necessary, including driving patients to medical check-ups or treatment and delivering donated food and clothing to people unable to visit to the centres.

Project Hope has worked closely with the Brazilian Ministry of Health's National Programme for STDS/AIDS through an agreement that is subject to review on a yearly basis. The opening of the two new centres in Guaianases and Vila Esperanca was strongly supported by the Programme, which has maintained its financing for the centres' operations since their inception.

Donations and other support from outside Brazil have been very important to Project Hope over the years. The British agency CAFOD has supported some of the activities at the San Miguel centre for many years now, while CARITAS-Holland provides finances for Guaianases and Vila Esperanca. Besides the Austrian agency DKA funds part of education and prevention activities.

Project Hope participates with about 30 other NGOs in the Sao Paulo NGO Forum on AIDS. This association carries out state-level advocacy on behalf of people with AIDS. It deals with issues such as public health policy and prevention measures, hospital bed availability, and provision of medicines.

Project Hope holds weekly meetings of paid staff and volunteers to evaluate and follow up on individual cases. Activity reports are written daily and added to each patient's file, along with monthly reports written by agents, volunteers or staff coordinators. Summary information based on these files is provided to supporting agencies for evaluation and planning.

The single most important strength of Project Hope has been its ability to improve the quality of life of people living with HIV/AIDS. This is measured in terms of numbers of people visited, medical attention given, etc. There are other indicators that demonstrate success of different kind. An important indicator has been the project's ability to attract volunteers who do not have a direct 'stake' in HIV/AIDS. For example, besides the people living with the virus and their relatives, the project has attracted the involvement of a number of volunteers who are not seropositive and have no family members living with the virus. This solidarity indicate success in the project's participatory, community-based approach.

Project Hope's internal evaluations recognize different weaknesses. An important weakness is the lack of professional management training within the organization. Project Hope has also had difficulty in managing the relationship between paid and volunteer work, which has occasionally led to misunderstandings or conflict. On a broader level, the project shares the sense of many NGOs that encouraging true behaviour and attitudinal change among people living with HIV is a highly difficult goal to achieve.

Best Practice Criteria

- **Project Hope** is such an organization which has been successful in creating systems which are both effective and contribute to the organization's sustainability. These systems have allowed the project to create and maintain a team of volunteers and supporters in its local community. It has also been able to negotiate secure funding from external sources and generate linkages with both government and non-governmental institutions or groups working in the same field. These achievements demonstrate how Project Hope fulfils many of the best practice criteria.
- **Relevance:** Project Hope's activities align closely with goals of prevention, care and reduction of impact of HIV/AIDS. The project's institutional arrangements with the National AIDS Programme are an important guarantee that it will continue to remain relevant to national strategies while responding to the local conditions.
- **Effectiveness:** Project Hope's effectiveness in operational terms is indicated by the numbers of people visited and levels of service offered. The project takes on approximately 180 new clients each year and makes about 360 home visits per month. Its strategy of involving the community has clearly been successful, given that nearly 200 people participated on a voluntary basis. Project Hope acknowledges that it has been less effective in its other major objective of changing behaviours and attitudes of people living with HIV - a not infrequent finding in reviews or evaluations of community-based organisation.

- **Efficiency:** There are no indicators at present available on the efficiency of Project Hope's activities. However, the teaching strategy of "learning by observing" for home-visit volunteers seems to be highly cost-effective.
- **Sustainability:** Project Hope has existed since last 10 years indicating both that it responds to a need and that it has discovered ways to sustain itself. The organizers clearly recognize that sustainability is not only a question of securing financial resources but of concentrating to human issues such as morale, enthusiasm and communication. Having been successful in gaining relatively stable financial support from a different sources including local donors, Brazil's National AIDS Programme, and international donors, the project has placed a great deal of thought and energy in sustaining its volunteers who are such an important part of its programmes.
- For example, social activities such as dances and outings are used specifically to build morale and to recognize contributions by the volunteers in a non-monetary way. The limits of people's energy is recognized by the use of 'holidays' in order to prevent volunteer burnout and the provision of massage and other relaxation techniques. Regular meetings aid in communication between volunteers and between staff and volunteers by explicitly discussing volunteers' needs and perceptions. Finally, the project coordinators are highly aware that their responsibilities consist looking after the volunteers as people rather than as tools to provide services.

Sustainability has also been pursued through contacts with the local religious authorities, businesses and community members. These have led to a significant amount of in-kind services and goods such as driving services and the donation of food and clothing. The Catholic Church's support through provision of the project's first premises was crucial to getting Project Hope started.

- **Ethical soundness:** Project Hope has proved successful at involving people living with HIV in its work as volunteers and in its management as staff members. This is one of UNAIDS's main indicators of ethical soundness. Besides this, the project is socially inclusive, bringing together people from different walks of life within the community and serving clients, irrespective of their lifestyles. Project Hope emphasizes a holistic, active approach to HIV/AIDS that persuades seropositive people to live their lives as independently as possible.

Kitui, Kenya

The true number of HIV/AIDS cases in Kenya is not known. In 1997 it was estimated that nearly 2.1 million people were infected with HIV, of which some 200000 people had developed AIDS. The number of HIV cases is estimated to be rising at a rate of 7.5 per cent per year.

The HIV/AIDS epidemic in Kenya is likely to have a deep impact on the demography of the country. Demographic projections show that AIDS could potentially reverse gains made in increasing child survival and life expectancy.

According to one analysis, the number of orphans increased from the 1990 estimate of 25000 to roughly 600000 by the year 2000.

An analysis carried out on the socio-economic impact of HIV/AIDS in Kenya by Family Health International/AIDSTECH reveals that:

(a) By the year 2000, the cost of caring for people with AIDS could consume the MOH's entire recurrent budget unless appropriate alternative forms of health-care and health care financing are immediately promoted and adopted;

(b) On average, AIDS causes the loss of three-fifths of an infected person's productive life, or approximately 22 years;

(c) The total direct and indirect costs of AIDS to the country could reach 15 per cent GDP by the year.

Objectives

The objectives of the programme are:

- to reduce the incidence of HIV infection; and
- to enable people infected and affected by AIDS to live positively.

These goals are pursued by two means. The first is to provide counselling and holistic care to people infected by HIV/AIDS. The second is to cause behavioural change by increasing public awareness of both the impact of the epidemic and methods to prevent its spread.

The programme provides an important service to the local health system as it helps reduce the bed occupancy rate in the area's four hospitals. With home care offered as an effective alternative in a familiar environment; people living with HIV can be discharged as soon as they learn their sero-status and have been given counselling.

A Poor Rural Area

Kitui and Mwingi are two districts in eastern Kenya that constitute the diocese of Kitui. Together they cover an area of 29389 miles with a population of over 812000 people. Being industrially backward, most of the people depend on small-scale farming and livestock. Unfortunately, intermittent droughts result in frequent food scarcity and famine. Due to widespread poverty, there has been a marked migration of men between the ages of 16 and 50 years to the larger Kenyan cities in search of employment. Many return home during the Christmas and Easter holidays. Some women visit their husbands in town during these holidays or at the end of the month.

The population in the catchment area of Mwingi and Muthale Hospitals numbers about 102000 people, of which 46 per cent male and 54 per cent female. Of the estimated 43000 people in the sexually active age group (16-60 years), about 10 per cent are in primary school and 26 per cent are secondary school students. In the catchment area of Kitui Hospital, the population is 138000 and the sexually active age group contains 36800 people. Both catchment areas are situated on the lorry routes from Mombasa to Kitui and Nairobi to Garissa, with stop-off points in small towns along the way. The HIV/AIDS situation in the area is very serious. Some 40 per cent of beds in the area's four hospitals are occupied by people living with AIDS. Owing to poor nutrition, which is the result of frequent droughts in the area, resistance to infection is low, and people living with HIV present with many opportunistic diseases. Most cannot afford the treatment such diseases require.

It has been discovered that about 10 per cent of mothers are HIV-positive. The estimated number of HIV-positive adults (male and female) in the district was estimated at 30695. It is expected that this number will have grown to almost 33000 by the end of 1997.

Project's Major Elements

Pre-and Post-test Counselling

Some clients are referred for testing by doctors at the hospitals, while others simply arrive and ask to be tested. In both cases, counselling is given in all four hospitals both before and after tests are done. The home-care clinic provides the following standard services, the first three of which apply to all clients:

(a) introduction of people living with HIV to counsellors;
(b) ongoing counselling on living positively with HIV;
(c) clinical check-up;
(d) provision of drugs for opportunistic infections and STDs as required;
(e) preparation of people living with HIV for home visits and group therapy; and
(f) preparation of family members and friends for roles as care givers.

While some features of the counselling are general, some types of clients are handled in specific ways, according to their particular needs:

(a) TB patients who are referred for HIV tests are given pre-test counselling before they receive treatment with TB drugs.
(b) Children who may be infected with HIV are not tested until they are two years old. Their growth is monitored, and their mothers are taught how to maintain their children in good health.

(c) Elderly care givers who are taking care of orphans are given supportive counselling and are supplied with limited material support such as second-hand clothes and food.

Following the people living with HIV's discharge from hospital, a home visit is made by the counsellor. This visit serves to introduce the counsellor to these people's family and begin to develop trust with them. Again, home visits include some standard services:

(a) assessing home conditions and family needs;
(b) assessing physical, emotional, psychological, and physical condition of people living with HIV;
(c) supportive counselling for persons living with HIV and family members;
(d) identifying or meeting guardians
(e) providing simple curative medicines; and
(f) schedule next visit.

Several important issues are discussed in home visits. The person living with HIV is persuaded to identify a guardian from among close family members who will be responsible for the orphans. This guardian will also act as a contact person if the person living with HIV becomes ill and cannot visit the hospital. At these times, the guardian will go to the hospital to report on this person's condition to the counsellors. In addition, the guardian and other family members are given training in home care of people with HIV/AIDS. All information that comes up at these visits is kept confidential. Notes and other information are available to all counsellors and doctors associated with the project, but no one else.

Group counselling sessions or workshops for people living with HIV is an important way to assist people to come to terms with their condition. Typical activities at the sessions include:

(a) sharing experiences, both positive and negative;
(b) persuading people living with HIV to express their feelings and learn how to deal with them;
(c) assisting people living with HIV to discover their own strengths and talents; and
(d) discussing small-scale businesses and other income-generating activities.

Group counselling discussions have also been useful in identifying the need for workshops on health maintenance and ongoing education for personal growth.

The project attempts to provide members of the community with basic HIV/AIDS awareness, and to encourage the community to take responsibility for persons living with HIV and for orphans. For this, HIV education visits are occasionally made by counsellors to hospitals, schools, churches, workplaces, and public gatherings. Depending on the audience, the information is given in different forms, including Training of Trainers (TOT), seminars and workshops. The project also encourages competitions in drama, poetry, and songs on AIDS. Health education visits also target behaviour change in specific audiences. These have included youth groups, teachers, primary and secondary schools, men's and women's groups, traditional birth attendants, traditional healers, sex workers, and hotel and bar workers. It is established that such change is a gradual, ongoing process because there is still a stigma associated with the disease and some fear of programmes and personnel working in HIV/AIDS prevention.

Recruiting people living with HIV to act as volunteers is a recent and very important step of the programme. Denial and stigma still strongly prevail in Kenya, and this is an effective way to educate the community at large. To date, two persons living with HIV assisted by counsellors have made educational visits to locales away from where they live. In these visits, they have spoken of their sero-status and experiences. This activity is supported by group counselling which, in addition to helping people living with HIV come to terms with their condition, has encouraged them to see the need to assist in the education of the community. It is estimated that this activity will expand and develop in the near future.

The programme provides treatment and counselling to people who have sexually transmitted infections (STDs). This is an important service in this area, which has a high incidence of such infections.

A variety of services are given to people who are dying. These include helping them identify guardians for their children, and helping them write wills to ensure that their land and belongings are passed on to their children. Efforts are made to help people with AIDS spend their remaining days in familiar surroundings, and to die with dignity.

Encouragement

Some people living with HIV are helped to discover their existing talents and skills that might enable them to set up small businesses. Examples of products which might people living with HIV are taught to sell include second-hand clothes, utensils, and groceries. Skills that are taught include marketing and sales skills, book-keeping and simple accounts, stocktaking, and interpersonal customer relations.

Persons living with HIV/AIDS are provided with simple curative medicines, including anti-malarials, anti-diarrhoel, and anti-fungal drugs, multivitamins, and antibiotics.

Very needy clients are assisted with their food needs such as beans, maize, flour, eggs, and milk. This assistance is examined on the individual level in order not to encourage dependency. During the current famine conditions, seeds have been given to people living with HIV in each area.

Staff Training

All staff in the project are nurse/counsellors. Some are qualified as trainers of trainers, while others are trained as facilitators of groups, workshops, and seminars. Irrespective of their origin, all receive ongoing training in counselling and topics such as personal development, education for life, and behaviour change.

Staff are supported by central office as per requirement. However, all participate in meetings held every six months to plan, examine and implement the project's activities.

Confidentiality

Confidentiality is essential to the programme, since it is the only way to maintain trust in the relationships between counsellor and person living with HIV and between people living with HIV themselves. Confidentiality is emphasized to people living with HIV from the moment they participate in the programme. Candour between people living with HIV is essential to group counselling simultaneously since the practice of people living with HIV acknowledging their status at each group session is vital in their acceptance of their status. It is part of their education in self-awareness, and in acknowledging and accepting their feelings. In addition to spiritual care, these elements help people living with HIV in personal growth and overcoming stigma to a large extent.

Collaborations

The programme collaborates on an ongoing basis with Ministry of Health personnel. This collaboration started in 1993 with the secondment of two Diocesan nurse/counsellors to the government hospitals at Kitui and Mwingi. The ministry has financed some of the programme's World AIDS Day activities and the National AIDS programme has provided it with educational materials. Recently, all four hospitals have been accepted by the Ministry as Sexually Transmitted Infections centres, which will facilitate the programme in its work against HIV infection. The government hospitals supply to programme with some nursing materials such as gloves and disinfects, while others are bought by the programme. In addition, some free drugs are distributed to people living with HIV/AIDS in the government hospitals and the Mutomo Mission Hospital.

Monitoring and Evaluation

Group counselling sessions are conducted once every two weeks, and use self-evaluation. Monitoring of the programme's activities in home care clinics and hospitals is carried out on a monthly basis by supervisors. Every three months, programme personnel meet with Ministry of Health personnel. Evaluation and planning sessions for programme staff are held every six months.

Self-assessment by the programme indicates that staff are well trained and motivated, with the concrete benefit that minimal supervision of staff is needed. Provision of group counselling for staff is an additional source of strength for staff. Communication between the different groups in all four hospitals is good, as is collaboration with the Ministry of Health.

Our self-assessment is that two important elements in the programme itself need reinforcing:

(a) more effort is required in education aimed at changing attitudes and increasing acceptance of infected persons by families and the community; and

(b) there is not enough coordination between our programme and other NGOs, government departments, and the community. Regular meetings, even on a half-yearly basis, might assist ensure that all necessary activities are being given due coverage to avoid overlapping of efforts.

The main weaknesses seen to be directly associated with the increasing gravity of the epidemic and the lack of resources at hand to deal with it. For example, with 200 new orphans being discovered each month, the programme is unable to serve all orphans being left without caretakers. Similarly, there are not enough counsellors or material resources to meet the rising demand for counselling services, which are very time-consuming programmes. This results in increasing physical and emotional stress on counsellors. It has also generated a problem of confidentiality because it is impossible for only one counsellor to follow each person living with HIV, so information must be shared between counsellors. And it has made it difficult for counsellors to keep abreast of new practices in the field of HIV/AIDS.

The programme has resolved to fortify itself and improve its services in the following ways:

(a) increasing emphasis on mobilizing extended families to take care of orphans;

(b) running a workshop on behaviour change and education for life;

(c) continuing education for counsellors to keep up with HIV/AIDS developments worldwide; and

(c) increasing networking at local and national levels.

Role of NGOs/CBOs

Kenya AIDS NGO Consortium was set up in 1990 with more than 320 member organizations.

Important role played by NGOs and religious groups. Religious groups emphasize awareness and prevention activities. NGOs concentrate primarily on high-risk populations, emphasizing IEC, condom distribution and training for community-based workers.

Best Practice Criteria

The HIV/AIDS Programme exemplifies the types of action that can be undertaken to improve the quality of life for infected and affected persons.

The project illustrates UNAIDS best practice criteria in the following ways:

- **Relevance:** The programme is concentrated on two UNAIDS priorities: prevention and care. A wide variety of needs are provided for within this programme, from individual needs to care and counselling to community education.
- **Effectiveness:** From a top-down perspective, the programme takes a highly organized and professional approach to its activities, as could be expected when all staff are trained nurse/counsellors who are employed by a well-equipped mission hospital. Effectiveness also seems to be enhanced by a high degree of cooperation with the government health services, permitting collaboration between four hospitals in the area.

On the level of services, the programme has clearly taken into consideration diverse needs of specific groups of people living with HIV, and seems to have devised effective strategies for each. Different groups include PLWHAs with HIV-relevant medical conditions such as TB and STDs, seropositive or potentially seropositive infants, elderly care givers, and people who are in the terminal stages of AIDS.

Programme staff express concern that success in changing attitudes and behaviour in the greater community has so far been limited, particularly with regard to increasing acceptance of people living with HIV/AIDS. It appears likely that effectiveness in these areas of endeavour will remain limited unless greater resources become available for community education.

- **Efficiency:** There are currently no indicators available of the project's efficiency.

- **Ethical soundness:** The Kitui programme is operated by trained nursing staff with a strong grounding in their profession's ethics. Awareness of the need to safeguard confidentiality is solid, although the limited number of staff makes it necessary for counsellors to share information among themselves.
- **Sustainability:** The sustainability of the programme appears to be guaranteed by the support of both the mission and government hospitals, and the Ministry of Health. It is to be hoped that greater involvement with local community (i.e., less top-down approach to services) may become possible as more volunteers are recruited and the growing impact of the epidemic lessens the present stigma associated with it.

Ikhlas Community Centre-Drug User Programme in Malaysia

The first case of HIV in Malaysia was detected in 1986. Up to the end of 1996, the total cumulative number of HIV infections reported was 19019. Out of this number, 580 were AIDS cases. The major mode of transmission of HIV is through sharing of HIV-infected injection equipment among injecting drug users (IDU): this constitutes 77.4 per cent (or 14713 cases) of the total cumulative number of infections. Sexual transmission accounts for 5.9 per cent (or 1116 cases). (These figures probably contain a data collection bias since active HIV screening tests are conducted among injecting drug users incarcerated in the drug rehabilitation centres and prisons, whereas the number of people from other sectors of the population coming forward voluntarily for testing is still low). Of the total HIV infections reported, 83.4 per cent occur among those in the 20-49 years age group and 95.7 per cent of the infections are among males.

The national AIDS programme budget includes provision of drugs, including antiretrovirals. Public health officers, health clinics, and the rural health clinics are involved in provision of care for AIDs patients, along with district hospitals and general hospitals.

Ikhlas is a Malay word that means sincere. The Ikhlas community centre's drug user programme was started in 1991 by an NGO called Pink Triangle Malaysia. Operating in a drop-in centre and through outreach workers, it works with the intravenous drug user (IDU) population in a Chow Kit, a poor community of Malaysia's capital city, Kuala Lumpur. Chow Kit is bustling, traffic-congested area of Kuala Lumpur. Its ethnically mixed population is mainly comprised of working class Malays, Chinese, Indians, and a large migrant population of Indonesians. Chow Kit is a shopping and business centre, with a thriving retail and petty trade, but it is also a red-light district. Several of its side streets are lined with seedy brothels, and are safe haven to drug users. According to one estimate, there are about 8000 IDUs, sex workers, and transsexuals living and working in the area. An average of 1040 contacts with clients are made by programme staff and volunteers every month. Contacts include such activities as providing basic medical care and food, handing out and discussing information on HIV and harm reduction, and making referrals to other care and support services.

Objectives

The goal of Pink Triangle Malaysia in creating the drug user programme was to serve the IDU population of Chow Kit by:

(a) providing information on health, harm reduction, and HIV itself;
(b) providing care and support, including medication, nutrition, shelter, employment, and psycho-social support; and
(c) advocating for IDUs' needs and concerns.

Coverage

Pink Triangle was already an experienced organization in 1991, being the first NGO in Malaysia to work at the community-level on HIV and sexuality issues. It had started to work on behalf of a marginalized community - the gay community of Kuala Lumpur - in 1987, shortly after the first cases of AIDS were detected in the country. By the early 1990s it was well established, with its own HIV education and support programmes. One of the best known is Positive Living, a support and care project meant for people living with HIV.

At present, Pink Triangle has 18 staff and about 100 volunteers who participate in its HIV prevention and support programmes. One of the first services provided by Pink Triangle, and which is still being provided, is a telephone information and counselling service addressing issues of HIG and sexuality.

As their work evolved, members of Pink Triangle Malaysia were strongly aware of the fact that the gay community was not the only marginalized group of people who were especially vulnerable to HIV. They discovered groups such as injecting drug users, transsexuals and sex workers as particularly vulnerable. This was borne out by government data revealing the increasing number of HIV infections in Malaysia, particularly among IDUs.

As per official statistics, sharing of HIV-infected needles and syringes among injecting drug users constituted almost three-quarters of the total number of infections. In contrast, sexual transmission caused less than ten per cent. Little information was available about infection rates among transsexuals and sex workers, but Pink Triangle estimated that they too had high infection rates. Encouraged by their success among gay men, Pink Triangle Malaysia resolved to do something about the vulnerability of these other marginalized groups. The result was the drug user programme, based in an area of Kuala Lumpur known as Chow Kit.

Organisation

Pink Triangle Malaysia identified the importance of proceeding cautiously and systematically. Volunteers began by making contact with drug users and consulting them about their needs. Having learned a great deal from its own organization and continued operations since 1987, Pink Triangle Malaysia functioned on the following principles:

(a) trusting relationships had to be set up with the IDU community;
(b) the IDU community had to be consulted about what they wanted and needed;
(c) the immediate, basic needs of the IDU community had to be addressed before HIV education would take place;

(d) care and support services had to be given in safe spaces and be client-oriented (that is, concentrate on meeting the needs of the client);

(e) members of the IDU community could be motivated to take action to address their vulnerability to HIV/AIDS, and could involve actively in the project as per their own capacities;

(f) supportive relationships with other affected communities and concerned parties had to be set up and maintained.

These principles are applicable even today, more than five years after its birth. Before the first care and support work was undertaken, Pink Triangle applied the first three principles in order to understand their intended client group.

The IDU community is not an easy one to get to know. IDUs in Chow Kit set up close-knit peer groups or 'comradeship'. For example, one group that has stopped shooting drugs may exclude people who are still shooting drugs. However, prior to the start of the drug user programme, certain volunteers of Pink Triangle Malaysia had already set up contact and developed a good relationship with many members of the IDU community in the Chow Kit area. These contacts had been formed through the volunteers' work with the gay community there.

Through the initial contacts, an informal needs assessment was conducted among IDUs in Chow Kit. This was performed through outreach and discussion with the drug-using population in the area, who were consulted about the needs and concerns of the community. The informants were visited on their terms, in places where they felt most comfortable, including shooting galleries and meetings on the street. Key informants were selected at the time of outreach activities, based on their knowledge of the IDU community and on their contacts in Chow Kit. They included the so-called 'IDU doctors' who help other IDUs inject drugs for a fee, and who were identified as key agents of change. Demographic statistics was collected using a questionnaire. Later on, Ikhlas used the same principles to create project components especially for transsexuals and sex workers.

The informal needs assessment gave the Pink Triangle

volunteers a clear sense of what IDUs in a Chow Kit through as priorities for improving their lives. These priorities were extremely basic, emphasizing the extreme marginalization and vulnerability of the IDUs:

(a) basic medical care;
(b) shelter;
(c) food;
(d) jobs;
(e) children's welfare; and
(f) obtaining identification papers and birth certificates.

The Project — Major Elements

Guided by the information obtained in the needs assessment, Pink Triangle moved to set up the major elements of the drug user programme. They were, and remain the Ikhlas community (or "drop-in") centre, outreach services, and the ongoing motivation and involvement of the IDU community. The drop-in centre was conceived as a safe space in which many of the clients needs could be met efficiently but without intimidating them or making them feel unwelcome. It is situated on one of the side streets in Chow Kit, not far from the brothels and where the IDUs spend much of their time. It is located in one of a row of three-storey shop-houses. The building is rented from a landlord. Different programmes are carried out there, most of which reflect the original needs assessment.

Medical care and treatment is given by para medics, with referrals to hospitals/drug treatment centres given as needed. Counselling and psychological support are also available. As well as care and treatment, the drop-in centre has a strong education and prevention role to play. Information on harm reduction and on HIV and other STDs are available to everybody who want it. The centre also provides condoms and lubricant. Finally, the drop-in centre serves its clients with a variety of services not specifically related to HIV or STDs, but which respond to their stated needs and priorities:

(a) bathroom/toilet facilities are provided so that clients can maintain basic hygiene (bathe, wash clothes, etc.);
(b) food is served;
(c) referrals to job placements are done.

Drug programme workers do not only work in the drop-in centre, waiting for clients to come in to them. It has always been clear that the project must seek out and support clients in their everyday living and working environment. In addition to encouraging the participation of clients in the project's work, outreach is the most effective way to maintain first-hand understanding of people's needs and problems.

Outreach workers, both staff and volunteers, meet clients at home, in bars or on the streets—wherever the clients are most comfortable. The outreach workers also make visits to hospitals and to drug rehabilitation centres. Among the services provided by these workers are:

(a) transporting clients to hospitals;
(b) assisting with getting identification papers, birth certificates.

Motivation and participation of the clients was always a key element in the IKHLAS strategy, and has evolved as the project has gained acceptance in Chow Kit. The process started with the members of the IDU community who were involved in the initial needs assessment and early consultations. They not only contributed their knowledge but also became more aware of their vulnerability to HIV/AIDS. This provided some with the motivation to participate more actively, and the programme was ready with methods for them to do so. As time went on, IDUs who became aware the project were recruited as community health outreach workers. This recruitment included training in HIV education, harm reduction approaches and facilitation skills. The training was imported by HIV educators/trainers and health professionals from local hospitals.

There are many ways for clients to participate on a more basic level, and to take ownership of the project. For example, clients are persuaded to take responsibility for the nutrition programme and maintaining the cleanliness of the drop-in centre. Under supervision from the staff, they handle the shopping for food, do the cooking, and clean the bathroom/toilet facilities. This not only assists the project itself by making it more cost-effective, but is part of the process of 're-socialization' and self-esteem-building among the clients. An unexpected benefit from the interaction of clients with volunteers from hospitals, nursing schools, the corporate sector, and colleges in the programme is that it has stimulated some IDU clients to participate more actively in the programme. Apparently, the feeling of being accepted by people from the 'general community' is important to these clients for their re-socialization and self-esteem-building.

Collaborations

The programme is aware of the benefits its experience can offer to other groups, and the benefits that can be gained from the experience of others. Therefore, it has always made an effort to be open to volunteers from other affected marginalized communities who have a shared concern and identical vulnerability such as the transsexual, sex worker, and gay communities. Members of these are recruited and trained to do outreach work, and to offer support in the drug user programme. To date, six persons have been recruited in this way. One of them is a gay student who decided to give up his tertiary studies to work on the programme. Staff greatly appreciate his language and street skills, which have proven very useful for outreach work.

Cooperation — Social and Medical

The programme cooperates closely with all other organizations that can be of assistance to its clients. For example, clients are occasionally referred to drug treatment and rehabilitation centres, to other NGOs working with IDUs, to churches and to shelters. Such referrals go both ways, as many new clients come to the programme via referrals from these organizations. In addition, about 40 clients come to the Ikhlas drop-in centre everyday. Local hospitals regularly refer their IDU patients once they are able to leave institutional care. Many other NGOs working in the field of HIV/AIDS refer their clients and their affected families to the programme when they are satisfied that they could benefit from our services.

The drug user programme could not do the work it does without donations — in-kind and cash from various sources. Major donors include the European Commission (EC) and the Dutch agency HIVOS. Locally, great help has been received from:

(a) the Malaysian AIDS Council (MAC);
(b) theatre companies that have dedicated specific performances to the community centre. These have contributed not only finances but have given valuable publicity to their work.
(c) pharmaceutical and health-care companies that have contributed medicines and nursing materials (e.g., treatment drugs, gauze, bandages); and
(d) hotels and food manufacturing companies that have donated food to the nutrition service.

As well as gaining access to government services for clients and making its work popular the programme cultivates relationships with a variety of government agencies for reasons of advocacy. In particular, its objective is to create awareness and understanding of the needs and concerns of IDUs and to stimulate change at the policy-and decision-making level. This includes work with the National Anti-Narcotics Task Force, drug rehabilitation programmes, the police and prison authorities. In particular, staff have facilitated HIV education and counselling training sessions with personnel in prisons and drug rehabilitation centres. The project also maintains a close relationship with the Ministry of Health and hospital staff, from whom assistance of doctors to provide testing and counselling services at our drop-in centre is received.

Monitoring and Evaluation

The mechanisms employed for monitoring and evaluating the work are fourfold:

(a) seeking programme beneficiaries' feedback (stories);
(b) regular meetings for peer review and evaluation among clients, volunteers, and staff;
(c) monitoring referrals to and from other agencies; and
(d) obtaining feedback from affected families.

Main Strengths

These various evaluation methods indicate that the main strengths of the programme are as follows:

(a) In the project's six years of operation, it has been able to concentrate on what the clients want and need.

There are probably many reasons for this, but an especially important one is that the project is organised so that the ongoing participation and feedback of clients obliges staff and volunteers to keep this focus. Structurally, the programme is: community-based; situated within the area where its clients live, work and congregate; and largely run by IDUs/persons with HIV/AIDS for IDUs/persons with HIV/AIDS.

(b) This is associated to the previous point, but probably has more to do with recruiting. The concentration on immediate needs and the outreach component that meets clients in their own preferred places (homes, shooting galleries, street) provide clients with concrete evidence of concern.

(c) Nobody can relate to an IDU living with HIV/AIDS in the same way as someone who shares the same challenges and the same lifestyle. Providing a space and a structure in which people talk, share experiences and problems, and receive both relevant information and positive advice, is key to effective work at the individual level.

(d) *External relation:* Development of a good working relationship with governmental agencies and NGOs has paid off in different ways discussed earlier.

(e) *Fund-raising:* The programme has been able to create good support from Malaysia's corporate sector, both in cash and in kind.

Weaknesses identified by monitoring and evaluation mechanisms include the following:

(a) The work can be very intense emotionally. A high-risk, high-vulnerability population like IDUs presents special challenges. For example, the fact that clients and colleagues get sick and sometime die is very hard. The personal and legal problems encountered by clients inevitably affect the work of the project, and can get very complicated. The project's main way of dealing with such stress is to hold regular sessions among staff and volunteers for discussion of problems, ventilating and counselling.

(b) The programme has trouble getting interested and committed volunteers on an ongoing basis. One of its most effective tools for recruiting has been to recruit drug users and ex-drug users from the community.

(c) Better skills in management, administration, and so on are particularly necessary.

(d) Although the programme has been able to remain client-oriented, it at times encounters internal debate on how much effort and resources should be devoted to the collective needs of IDUs versus the individual needs of clients.

(e) Despite fund-raising success and good relations with outside agencies, the project occasionally experiences difficulty in getting access to adequate treatment facilities and drugs for our clients.

(f) Despite its efforts to maintain good relations with the police, the drop-in centre services are sometimes affected by police raids in the area. The project tries to deal with this problem through dialogue with the police at the decision-making level (i.e., not by trying to confront the police officers conducting the raid but by speaking with their superiors).

Threats and Opportunities

The project, like the population it serves, often finds itself in a position of vulnerability. It is most vulnerable to the withdrawal of government support. While it has achieved a strong profile in its field and can count on help from several professionals and influential people, the overall tolerance and support by government for its work is volatile. A change in the head of a government agency, or the government's need to respond to political or religious pressure can result in support being reduced or even withdrawn. While the project continues to build its profile and cultivate all the relationships it can with other agencies, this vulnerability is generally part of its environment and will continue to be so. Simultaneously, the time and effort spent building the programme's profile means that it at present has a highly visible platform from which to speak out. The project is well known to the media, who often give it sympathetic coverage. The project can speak both formally and informally with major players in the Government such as the Ministry of Health, Ministry of Home Affairs, and the Malaysian AIDS Council. So long as it maintains this profile and these good relations, and so long as it continues to participate and work on behalf of the real needs of IDUs and persons with HIV/AIDS, Ikhlas community centre drug user programme will continue to make its contribution to Malaysian society.

Other HIV/AIDS Agencies and NGOs

The Malaysian AIDS Council (MAC), an NGO umbrella association, was established in 1991 with monetary assistance from WHO. It groups 22 members, although only a few are AIDS-specific. The Council is supported in part with funds from the Ministry of Health. Council members generally focus on the most vulnerable groups in Malaysian society: women and youth, migrants, injecting drug users, gay men, and commercial sex workers.

Besides the National Council of Women Organisation promotes AIDS activities among its affiliate members.

Other NGOs active in HIV work are:

(a) Tenaganita, a women's group working primarily with migrant workers, in industry, and with sex workers in selected areas of Kuala Lumpur;
(b) PENGASIH which runs a halfway house for injecting drug users in Kuala Lumpur;
(c) Positive Living, another Pink Triangle Malaysia project for people with HIV/AIDS;
(d) The Malaysian Red Crescent Society, which runs a youth peer education project associated with HIV and reproductive health;
(e) The Federation of Family Planning Associations of Malaysia.
(f) Community AIDS Service Penang;
(g) National Council of Churches.

Best Practice Criteria

The IKHLAS Project strongly illustrates the community mobilization value of participation by persons living with HIV/

AIDS, and the resulting benefits in effectiveness and efficiency which are possible from being guided by such an ethical approach. In reality, the participation of infected persons from the injecting drug users community is probably necessary in order to reach this group, which is highly marginalized both socially and legally. The project illustrates best practice criteria in the following ways:

- **Relevance:** Since injecting drug use is the major form of transmission of HIV in Malaysia, the project's concentration on IDUs is extremely relevant to the national response to the epidemic. In terms of the proportion of activities, it is visible that two of the three project goals and a majority of activities are not devoted strictly to HIV/AIDS but to the more general needs of the target population. However, this in large part is a function of the marginalization of the injecting drug users, who do not seek or receive the same level of medical and social services as the rest of Malaysian society. It is possible that any other strategy than one that offers different services (not just HIV-associated ones) to this particular group would fail to engage their trust and participation and therefore not be effective at all.
- **Effectiveness:** There are no quantitative measures for the impact the project has had on IDUs in Chow Kit. However, the available evidence recommends that IKHLAS has been highly effective in gaining the trust of its target community (which is likely a function of its effectiveness in providing services this community wants or needs) and in attracting resources (food, medicines, services, funds) from the community at large. The project has also been effective in its advocacy activities through the favourable media profile it has been able to generate and the institutional links it has created with government and NGOs.
- **Efficiency:** The combination of a drop-in centre and outreach via staff and volunteers seems an efficient application of resources, particularly given the hard-to-reach characteristics of the target population. The cost-efficiency of the drop-in centre is maximized by application of client labour (under staff supervision) in cleaning,

cooking and shopping and by securing the services of medical staff on honorary basis.

- **Ethical Soundness:** IKHLAS's voluntary and participatory approach to HIV/AIDS is in accordance with current ethical standards in the field. The project's efforts to create a higher and more sympathetic profile for its clientele among the greater community, and to give them a channel for self-advocacy, supports basic human rights objectives.
- **Sustainability:** While recognizing the precarious nature of much its support, IKHLAS has made impressive strides in securing a variety of resources from a wide range of donors, institutions and individuals. This diversity of support has not only allowed the project to survive for more than six years but is probably the project's best guarantee of sustainability in the future.

Tateni Home Care Services: South Africa

The AIDS epidemic is well established in South Africa and continues to grow at varying rates in all nine provinces. In a November 1996 antenatal survey, 14.07 per cent of women attending public health service clinics were discovered to be infected with HIV. Over 10 per cent of all adults are estimated to be infected. If the estimates are accurate, this indicated just more than 2.2 million by the end of 1996. The majority of infections are the result of heterosexual transmission.

Analysis of reported AIDS cases is at present of limited value because of pervasive under-reporting. However, the present number of AIDS cases is estimated to be 43000 of whom 10000 are children born to infected mothers.

Levels of infection in Guateng Province, where Tateni Home Care Services is located, were 6 per cent in 1994, 12 per cent in 1995 and 20 per cent in 1996.

Mamelodi is a former black "township" of about 1.5 million people that lies west of South Africa's administrative capital city, Pretoria. The community consists approximately 250000 dwellings (including everything from proper houses to large boxes that people live in), with an average of six people per dwelling. A large proportion of the population is impoverished, and the incidence of HIV/AIDS is high.

Tateni Home Care Services identified a need for home-based care in 1995. Approximately 2000 dwellings were visited during the first year and identified about 1000 chronically ill persons, of whom 427 would benefit from home-based care. A consultant to the provincial department of health's Directorate for AIDS and Communicable Diseases, acted as an adviser to the group of developing home-based care policy and training materials. During the same year, the group started providing home-based care services.

In 1996 Tateni Home Care Services was asked by the department of health to join a team of key role players at the provincial, regional, and district/community levels. An integrated model of home-based care for the province was developed modelled partly on Tateni's work. Pilot projects based on the model are now being established in other locations in partnership with the provincial government.

Objectives

Tateni Home Care Services is a non-discriminatory, non-judgemental organization that aims to ensure that home-based care is provided in Mamelodi. The organization embraces the values of empathy, acceptance, hope, and the removal of discrimination against those infected or affected by HIV/AIDS. Its objectives consist:

(a) to provide counselling and support services to infected and affected persons;

(b) to implement home-based care that is affordable, accessible, equitable and efficient;

(c) to upgrade the collective capacity of the community to provide care and support;

(d) to enable and empower ancillary health careers to care for and cope with the chronically ill persons in their community; and

(e) to teach, advise, and provide guidance to the seropositive person and family members (or other significant persons in the patient's life) about relevant aspects of health care, infection, and health promotion.

The organization also bases its work on three important

principles. The first is the principle of decentralization, under which home-based care and support are decentralized from the provincial government to district and community level. Decentralization takes place through collaboration with other local health and social programmes. The second is the principle of partnership to include all stakeholders in policy development, strategic planning, and implementation of home-based care. Finally, the organization recognizes the principle of multisectoriality, which harnesses the knowledge and resources of a wide range of society in the response to HIV/AIDS.

Collaboration

In keeping with its primary principles, Tateni's activities complement existing health care services rather than duplicating or competing with them. The multisectoral approach means that, rather than working within the systems established by the Health Ministry (with its limited and often overburdened human resources of formal care givers and support personnel), Tateni adds new resources:

(a) the family and kinship network as primary care givers; and

(b) community resources as support services.

Tateni's approach recognizes the copying models of home-based care from industrialized countries, with their high levels of funding and extensive formal health systems, would lead to failure. First, doing so would set unattainable goals in an area with a large population and limited resources. Second, it would be inappropriate to the social and cultural context of the people of Mamelodi, whose African traditions emphasize complex family and community relationships of support, obligation, and consensus rather than formal, state-directed services.

However, collaboration with the formal health system is an important part of the approach. When essential, patients are referred to hospitals and other 24 hour institutions such as clinics for services like short-term admissions to control difficult symptoms, respite for primary care givers (that is, when the family needs a short break from looking after their seropositive member), or admission for more extensive treatment.

Major Elements

Tateni's home-based activities aim mainly at providing and enabling palliative care. However, HIV/AIDS prevention, education, and surveillance are also important parts of the work.

People with HIV and their families come to Tateni in a number of ways. Many come in search of services having heard about Tateni through word of mouth. Formal referrals are received from local clinics, general practitioners and the Pretoria Academic Hospital. Finally, Tateni receives clients through contacts with other local non-governmental organizations and CBOs community based organizations, notably those in the Mamelodi coalition of organizations working with Tateni (these include Women Against Abuse, Children's Day Care Centre, and various youth groups.)

Tateni's training activities are carried on at two levels. The first is training of community care workers. These are local people who typically live nearby the clients they will be assigned to work with once training is completed. The training is given by a professional nurse with help from a social worker. At present, the training is very basic and takes six months, but this is planned to be upgraded to twelve months in order to meet the standards of the National Policy for Health Workers.

The second level of training is carried out by the community care workers, with coordination and supervision by the professional staff. This training is directed towards:

(a) teaching persons living with HIV and their families how to provide effective home care. This consists discussing several aspects of HIV/AIDS itself, a holistic approach to wellness, and accessing the formal system as needed;

(b) teaching volunteers to provide services such as counselling and health promotion.

Partnerships

The model of home-based health care developed by Guateng province is based on devolution of decision-making responsibilities from the provincial level to the regional/district level. This creates a care interface between organizations at community level with health department officials who indeed have decision-making power, with the result that policy development, planning and monitoring activities are shared rather than shifted from one level to another. These planning and monitoring activities can thus be imbued with the core values of community mobilization since the lines of communication are not exclusively top-down. The arrangement also ensures that home-based care is delivered as per the health system's accepted standards of conduct and practice.

As discussed earlier, Tateni Home Care Services maintains an ongoing contact with local clinics, hospitals, and general practitioners. Referrals are made by all of these stakeholders both to and from Tateni. Clinic and hospital beds are used by Tateni clients both for purposes of treatment of patients and to provide respite to family care providers.

Financial support for Tateni Home-based Care Services comes entirely from local donors and the provincial government. There are at present no national or international sources of funding. The medicines and nursing materials dispensed by Tateni are only possible due to donors. In some cases, medicines may be supplied by a local clinic if the patient or a family member is able to go to the clinic and collect it.

Tateni maintains relations with several other community-based organizations and non-governmental organizations, including church groups, youth organizations, and women's groups. As discussed earlier, a number of these organizations are loosely grouped in the Mamelodi coalition.

Monitoring and Evaluation

At the end of its first year of operation in 1996, Tateni Home Care Services conducted a qualitative assessment of its work. A questionnaire was distributed to 500 participants, of whom 369 responded. In addition to showing overwhelming appreciation of the services provided, the results implied that most respondents preferred Tateni's home care and training to continue to take a general approach to health care activities rather than concentrate exclusively on HIV/AIDS.

Strengths and Weaknesses

Internally, staff feel that the basic strengths of Tateni are twofold: its success at encouraging community participation and its achievement of widespread feelings of community ownership. These are the reasons that Tateni has been able to reach and provide services to innumerable people in a relatively short time. These two strengths have given it enough credibility that the government services were willing to enter into a partnership with it.

The other noteworthy strength is the project's successful integration of government and community activities.

The organization notes two significant weaknesses:

(a) Resource mobilization is difficult, and the service is dependent on donors. Further partnerships and fund-raising will be essential if further progress is to be made; and

(b) although commitment from volunteers is high (some of which may be attributable to the newness of the organization); hours that can be volunteered are extremely limited. This is likely a problem in any impoverished community. The organization would like to add incentives such as travel costs, meals, and uniform to its budget as line items, but is unable to do so yet.

The Role of NGOs/CBOs in the National AIDS Programme

The work of Tateni Home-based Care Services takes place in a context of significant changes to South Africa's health system. A White Paper (in British parliamentary tradition, a White paper is a detailed discussion document presented to the legislature by the government, generally proposing significant changes to some aspect of government activity) for the Transformation of the Health System has been brought before the national legislature.

The document state that nongovernmental organizations should continue to play an important role in the delivery and management of services. It also proposed that community participation be guided by the following principles:

(a) All South Africans should be equipped with information conducive to caring for themselves or those in their community.

(b) People should be given the opportunity to actively take part in various aspects of the planning and provision of care counselling and support and preventive strategies.

(c) Civil society and the government sector will be involved mutually to check the transmission of HIV/AIDS.
(d) People living with HIV or AIDS will be involved in all prevention, control, and care strategies.
(e) The emphasis will be on sufficient capacity-building at all levels, including nongovernmental organizations to accelerate HIV/AIDS prevention and control measures.

In order to improve the effectiveness and ensure the implementation of the National AIDS Programme, government will develop partnerships with key NGO/CBO stakeholders and benefit from the collective experience of civil society. It also proposes the setting up of a committee to coordinate support for NGO/CBO programmes in HIV/AIDS prevention and control. Among others tasks, the committee will develop an NGO funding policy for the National AIDS Programme, process NGO applications for government funding, and evaluate progress by NGO/CBO organizations.

Best Practice Criteria

- **Tateni Home Care Services** exemplifies the community mobilization value of synergy, as achieved through shared planning and every day collaboration between community-based organizations, local institutions, and government. This synergy has made possible major benefits in both effectiveness (the impact on the target population) and efficiency (the use of available resources in the most effective way).
- **Relevance:** All of Tateni's proposed objectives are relevant to an enhanced response to HIV/AIDS. However, its goal of upgrading the collective capacity of the community to provide care and support is especially appropriate in an area where high HIV prevalences mean a large impact on the entire community. The creation of a CBO, even when the community has limited financial or physical resources to contribute, is also extremely appropriate given the provincial and federal government's adoption of

decentralization. Finally, the relevance of the project to actual needs in the community seems to have been ensured by the fact that the project began with a survey (in effect, a needs assessment) based on home visits to more than 2000 dwellings.

- **Effectiveness:** Tateni has only been providing services for two years, and formal measures of its effectiveness in terms of impacts are not yet available. Anecdotal evidence implies that the project's activities have lessened the lengths of some patients' hospital stays, which is an important benefit both to individuals and to the health care system.
- **Efficiency:** The project has adopted an efficient strategy of collaborating with clinics, general practitioners, and the local hospital ensures. This permits the project to avoid tasks already conducted by other organizations or institutions (particularly those better equipped for those tasks). A second efficient strategy is its two-level training activities. This allows formal, resource-intensive training of community care workers (selected from within the community) to be conducted simultaneously as less formal but much more widespread training of infected and affected persons. The project has also made a virtue of its lack of financial resources by being creative in acquiring or adapting premises (a vacant container used as a creche for parents receiving training) and equipment (a home-made training doll for demonstration of palliative care).
- **Ethical soundness:** Tateni's ethical standards are protected by its multiple interfaces with government, medical practitioners, and other community organizations (many of whom themselves participate in human rights activities such as reducing violence against women). This ensures that community values and wishes are not overwhelmed by the priorities of other levels of government or by the medical profession.
- **Sustainability:** Tateni's sustainability seems to be supported by the fact that the project is highly associated with needs as defined by the community. Linkages with

the formal health care system are another important element in its sustainability over time, particularly given the federal government's apparent support for the encouragement of community-based organizations in South African health care. However, the project acknowledges that it is highly dependent on outside donors for material resources, and that the poverty of the local community makes recruitment of volunteer labour extremely difficult.

Sanpatong Project: Thailand

By the end of the century, mortality due to AIDS could become the leading cause of death in Thailand. Two-thirds of the approximately 800000 persons at present living with HIV/AIDS reside in the northern part of the country. Rates of infection have historically been high among women who are or have been commercial sex workers, but recently the greatest rates of increase have been among women in stable relationships who have never been sex workers. HIV prevalence in the north among women attending antenatal clinics is between 4 and 8 per cent.

Based on current prevalence rates among pregnant mothers, by the year 2000 there were approximately 120000 AIDS orphans, and more than 60000 cases of infants with AIDS. Increasing AIDS-related mortality among infants and young children may reverse many of the gains made by effective national child health programmes, such as the Control of Diarrhoeal Diseases and Expanded Programme on Immunization.

The Sanpatong Home-based Care Project works in the Sanpatong area some 25 kilometres south of Chiang Mai city. A joint project of the Thai Red Cross Society health centre in Sanpatong and the district hospital, it at present works with approximately 600 people living with HIV/AIDS.

The project aims to make it possible for families to support and care for persons living with HIV/AIDS at home. The concept of home care is different in Southeast Asia than in Western countries, where it generally refers to home visits by doctors and nurses for purposes of treatment or monitoring. In contrast, people served by this project are taken into a hospital or clinic by their families when they need medical care. Services include training for family members, health care visits and referrals, provision of some basic necessities, meditation and spiritual instruction in the Buddhist tradition, and support activities, including a weekly club with visiting speakers and doctors.

Objectives

It is a convention in the Buddhist culture of Thailand for many generations of a family to live together, and to look after one another when one member is sick. The goal of the project is to reinforce this conventional value through home care training and other supports that will:

- allow primary health care for people living with HIV/AIDS to be provided at home;
- change negative attitudes of family members, friends and the community to HIV/AIDS; and
- promote self-care and self-reliance of families and individuals infected by HIV/AIDS.

As a secondary aim, it is hoped that this strategy of care will reduce costs both to individual families and to government health services.

A Holistic Approach

The Sanpatong area is one of the worst hit by the AIDS epidemic in Thailand. Since the late 1980s, the hospital system has been increasingly hard-pressed to provide care for all of those who needed it, with as many as 60 per cent of beds being occupied by persons with HIV/AIDS in recent years. The majority of these cases are of people in their most economically productive years. Families in which a member has HIV/AIDS face many devastating challenges, including:

(a) social stigma and discrimination;
(b) conflict between the desire to have children and the fear of infection;
(c) exorbitant emotional loss when family members die; and
(d) economic obstacles.

In 1992, a group made up of staff nurses from Sanpatong's

Red Cross health centre, volunteers from the faculty of medicine at Chiang Mai University, and Chiang Mai public health staff perceived an opportunity to create a new care project. Pooling its wide variety of practical and academic experience the group was able to agree on many fundamental ideas, the first of which was the importance of a holistic approach to care. As they witnessed it, a holistic approach should be one that provided bio-psycho-social support:

(a) *bio:* treatment of symptoms;
(b) *psycho:* helping to deal with stress and worry, solve problems, improve attitude; and
(c) *social:* improving ability to cope with, participate in, and be accepted by the community and greater society.

Their main idea was to help people living with HIV/AIDS be treated at home, a strategy that would reinforce all three parts of the holistic approach. Such a project, they knew, would necessitate education and skills training for many people: family members, volunteers from the community, and even village leaders. It would also require funding and resources to get started and to sustain itself. Simultaneously, the group, an NGO supported by several agencies recognised the significance of providing support for people who are HIV-positive but have not developed full-blown AIDS. In addition to meeting these people's needs for emotional support, the group's strategy consisted providing training on practical matters of self-care and self-reliance before the people get sick. Again, it was intended that this preparation would eventually reinforce all three parts of the holistic approach.

Major Elements

Since the project started, the group has pursued its holistic approach to care by creating a continuum of activities. These begin by dealing with the needs of individuals (health care, psychological reinforcement, etc.) and extend to community mobilization and income generating opportunities for people living with HIV. An essential ongoing activity is recruitment and training of volunteer medical personnel. The latter was assisted by the creation of a manual for these personnel. Recruitment of people living with HIV generally occurs either through word of mouth among community members or by doctors' referral. Besides this, the testing programme at the Sanpatong Hospital refers all persons detected HIV-positive to the project, usually to the HIV club that meets once a month.

At present, there are approximately 600 persons living with HIV served by the project, about 60 per cent female and 40 per cent male. The age range is from 25 to 45. About 60 per cent of people living with HIV are asymptomatic, with 20 per cent presenting some symptoms and 20 per cent having full-blown AIDS.

Modelled on the well-known Wednesday Friends Club in Bangkok, the Thursday Club is a monthly lunch gathering and support group for men and women with HIV/AIDS. It regularly attracts 40-50 people to its lunches, which consists meditation, exercise and talks from several guests. Visiting speakers and presentations consisted actors from a visiting international musical show, a Tao Yoga master from Korea, the White Line dance group (an AIDS education performance troupe) and vegetarian cooking classes from a Buddhist meditation centre. A particular highlight, and evidence of support from the highest levels of Thai society, was a visit by one of the King's cooks to prepare a meal for the club. Medical attention is available at each meeting, and food and herbal medicines (including honey tablets) are also given. The lunches are also used as occasion for the home care team to monitor the health of club members. Finally, the club is the first stage in the project's strategy of educating people living with HIV/AIDS about self- and home-care before grave illness has reduced their mobility and normal functioning.

Training People Living with HIV and Family Members

The project conducts regular one- and two-day training sessions about home care each month, mostly in Chiang Mai City. Thirty group sessions, each comprising 30 participants, have been held each year since 1994 and have thus reached about 900 persons since their inception. The sessions are open to all members of the public, and follow a format that has been worked out over time:

(a) "icebreaker" exercise to reduce participants' initial nervousness;

(b) individual introductions so that people get to know each other; and
(c) group meditation.

The sessions then break into small training groups based on two methodologies: problem-based learning and focus group technique. These smaller groups also follow a set format:

(a) HIV/AIDS education: all members are persuaded to tell their story and express their feelings, fears, and questions about HIV/AIDS. This leads to discussion and provision of information about the epidemic, its symptoms and the remedies. A particular attention is on practical methods to live with HIV/AIDS in one's life, including the significance of regular exercise, proper nutrition, condom use, etc.
(b) practicalities of home care: subjects discussed and demonstrated include universal precautions, dressing wounds, taking medication correctly, changing bed sheets, use of bed pans, bed baths and sponging, and utensils needed.
(c) developing confidence: the final part of the session aims to help participants gain confidence in themselves and their capabilities. In particular, they are shown how to feel strong and capable of self-care.

In all cases, home visits are made by both volunteers and nursing staff so that people living with HIV and caretakers can be supervised and monitored.

Extension of Club and Training of Health Care Volunteers

Once members have received the home care training and have had time to get experience doing it at home, they are persuaded to establish an HIV club in their own village. There are at present six such clubs in outlying villages. Not only people living with HIV but a variety of other people have aided in organizing these clubs, including village headmen, health system personnel, health volunteers and Buddhist monks.

Health care volunteers are also recruited to receive orientation and the home-care training. Once these activities are completed, the volunteers receive medicine boxes to use in their home-care visits. The medicines are for preliminary care of conditions such as diarrhoea, fever, cough, skin diseases, headaches, and stomachaches.

The project facilitates being together small support groups of about 30 persons living near each other in sub-districts. These support groups assist people living with HIV to share their experiences and concerns with each other. In order to create a family feeling, sightseeing trips and overnight camping at resorts are arranged for these groups.

Spirituality has always been important in Thai life, and so spiritual care is a well-accepted and necessary part of the project's work. In particular, meditation is taught by local Buddhist monks as a means of assisting hard-hit people find tranquillity and the mental strength to continue alongwith teaching meditation techniques, the monks provide people with spiritual guidance on how to protect themselves from suffering and how to put life and death into perspective.

As well, the Brahma Kumaris World Spiritual University runs free workshops for people living with HIV on such topics as positive thinking, self-esteem and meditation. It also does workshops on vegetarian cooking.

This activity was initiated as a way of providing practical support to families looking after people living with HIV. School funding (i.e. children's fees to attend school) blankets, clothing, food and milk are provided to these families, using donated funds and foodstuffs. A donation of 600000 baht (equivalent to US$ 17000) from the Thai Red Cross Society enabled the project to provide these amenities for two years. Medicines donated by private companies are also distributed.

Its goal is to get whole villages to accept and participate in the care both of persons living with HIV and their families. In coordination with existing Red Cross activities in villages in the Sanpatong area, the project holds monthly sessions in local houses. The sessions aim to involve village leaders in ensuring care for relatives of the deceased, and to encourage neighbours to help each other. At present, sessions are held in houses, village halls and health centres and have involved 300 people living with HIV and their families. A significant factor in the success of this activity is preparatory visits before the date of the session. These preparatory visits are used to explain the project to village leaders and gain their support, and to encourage participation by neighbours.

The project has established a self-supporting cooperative store a joint venture between the Red Cross health care centre and the Sanpatong Hospital. The shop sells food and crafts manufactured by people living with HIV/AIDS, and also provides work for some such people as shop attendants.

In northern Thailand, HIV infection has often resulted in the illness of women who are wives and mothers. The poorer families who cannot afford hospital care, this places the entire stability of the family at risk. Care-giving responsibilities in these situations often fall to grandmothers particularly. Although Thai grandmothers have always had significant roles in the care and upbringing of children and the running of households, this unexpected burden in their later years is a heavy one. This is true if they have no previous knowledge of HIV/AIDS or of basic home care techniques such as universal precautions. Grandmothers are also faced with significant emotional stress from the illness of their children and HIV-infected grandchildren, and often from the social stigma surrounding such illness. The project has started a new activity aimed at improving the ability of grandparents to function as home care givers and providing support to them as they do so. The project has identified the special needs of the care-giving grandmother as:

(a) training in home care techniques;
(b) ongoing, regular support from the home-care team to assist her look after her sick child or grandchild;
(c) support from medical personnel to keep herself healthy;
(d) financial support from the social welfare ministry;
(e) emotional support from the social worker or counsellor to help her express grief or cope with stress; and
(f) support and acknowledgment from neighbours and community.

Collaborations

The project has always had a strong orientation towards partnerships and alliance-building, since its inception. It has included people from three distinct organizations: the Red Cross health centre, the Chiang Mai University faculty of medicine, and Sanpatong district hospital (Thai Ministry of Public Health). Links with the all three groups remain strong. People living with HIV who come directly to the attention of the project and are in need of medical intervention or testing are first referred to the Red Cross health centre. Tertiary cases are referred to the Sanpatong hospital. In most cases, the Red Cross follows up with a home visit, and a letter to the health centre with an update on the case. The local public health office has donated 2000 baht per month for the Thursday Club monthly meetings.

The Red Cross works very closely with the local health system. Proposals are made jointly by the health personnel working with villagers.

The most important donors of funds, materials and other resources for the project are:

(a) The Thai Red Cross Society AIDS programme which offers medications and nursing staff;

(b) pharmaceutical companies which donate medications, and some prominent members of the industry who have made donations of cash;

(c) Rotary Clubs: Rotarians have been very philanthropic to the project; and

(d) milk companies: donations of soya been milk make possible the distributed of milk to families containing a member living with HIV.

In addition, the project ha an ongoing relationship with the Brahma Kumaris World Spiritual University, which provides workshops for people living with HIV.

Monitoring and Evaluation

Monitoring of progress is conducted by the home-care team once a month at the lunch club. Feedback from people living with HIV is listened to seriously, and discussed by the group. Project staff have noticed that few families now ask early whether confidentiality will be maintained, as used to be the case. This indicates that as there is an increased feeling of openness among people living with HIV and less fear of stigmatization. An objective measure of success in many people living with HIV has been the outcome of substantial weight gain in people living with HIV after three months in the project. No formal evaluation has yet been made of the project. Some indication of project success (as well as of demand for the kinds of services provided) has been the speed with which our community care activities have witnessed expansion from zero to 20 houses in several villages. People living with HIV feedback emphasizes the following benefits:

(a) increased ability to enjoy their lives;
(b) increased quality of life; and
(c) increased feeling of being respected, loved, and appreciated.

A major challenge facing the programme is to maintain huge resources in the face of rising needs. Funding from the Red Cross AIDS Programme and the Rotary Club has not always been ample, and staff have sometimes contributed from their own savings when money has been needed.

Although the actual challenge posed by the high infection rates of HIV in the region is daunting, it is hoped that the project is actually gaining energy. An important element in this is the increasing help offered by pharmaceutical companies, NGOs, and other organizations. For example, the Rotary Club and the Business and Professional Women's Club of Chiang Mai recently found a volunteer to work with the project.

Best Practice Criteria

The Sanpatong Home based Care Project is an example of how an organization's emphasis on participation and involvement of families in caring for people living with HIV/AIDS can result in efficiency and effectiveness benefits both to individuals and to the public health system. The project demonstrated best practice criteria in the following ways:

- **Relevance:** The goals and operations of the project are totally relevant to the present stage of the epidemic in Thailand, where a large number of people in local communities are presenting symptoms of AIDS. The bio-psycho-social approach fits very well with the concept of expanded response (i.e., an approach beyond the traditional goals of public health, which tend to be rooted in a purely medical model). Besides this, the goal of reducing the impact on government health services is extremely appropriate in a high-prevalence area where hospital and clinics are hard-pressed by the epidemic. The project's emphasis on support for orphans is similarly relevant given the infection rates among adults of child bearing age, particularly women in a stable relationship, in the North of Thailand.

- **Effectiveness:** Measured in numbers of homes visited (600 between 1994 and mid-1997) or reached through home-care training sessions (900) and types of service offered, the project seems to be effective in pursuing its goals of permitting primary health care to be provided at home and promoting self-care and self-reliance. Quality of service us safeguarded by the participation of aims of the formal health system (Thai Red Cross, Chiang Mai public health staff, and faculty of medicine at Chiang Mai University). While there is no evidence yet available on the effectiveness of using spiritual resources (talks from Buddhist monks, retreats, meditation techniques) to achieve psychological and physiological benefits for people living with HIV, experience from other fields of medicine recommend that this strategy is a beneficial one.
- **Efficiency:** The project's efficiency seems to be relatively high, in that it allows innumerable people to receive valuable services of useful quality at a low monetary and administrative cost. This is achieved by training unpaid human resources (mostly, though not entirely, family members of the persons with HIV) to assume care responsibilities that would otherwise be carried out by salaried medical staff in overburdened hospitals and clinics - or not at all. Efficiency is also enhanced by the emphasis on providing training to seropositive individuals and their families before symptoms of AIDS are witnessed. The use

of the lunch club, a strategy pioneered in Thailand, is one which has already been proven efficient as a non-threatening, low-cost access point through which infected people can receive services and information.

- **Ethical soundness:** The project emphasizes an open, non-discriminatory approach to HIV/AIDS that nonetheless protects confidentiality. It also emphasizes involvement of persons living with HIV and their family in the project. The simultaneous involvement of qualified academic, government, and non-governmental medical personnel appears to provide a sufficient set of checks and balances to assure that accepted standards of medical ethics are observed.

  Looked at from the outside, there may be an ethical concern in the component that supports grandmothers as care providers. This concern arises from the limited energy and increasing frailty of these older women and the assumption that they, rather than grandfathers, will assume this role. However, this concern is mitigated by understanding that the project aims to give grandmothers better skills to carry out a role they willingly assume (both through tradition and links of personal affection) and some measure of assistance through home visits and support groups. It relieves grandmothers of the sole responsibility for care by training other family members.
- **Sustainability:** The project reports difficulty in securing reliable financial resources. It is not yet clear whether the personal commitment and dynamism of some of the founding personnel are essential for the continued effectiveness and even survival of the project.

Chirumhanzu Project: Zimbabwe

Zimbabwe is one of the countries most affected by the HIV epidemic. Almost 22 per cent of the adult population (or about 1.2 million people) are at present HIV-positive. At present, the number of persons who have reached the stage of AIDS has totalled 150000. Some 400 people die of AIDS and its related diseases each week. In parts of the country, between 50 and 70 per cent of pregnant women attending antenatal clinics have been found to be HIV-positive.

Only one voluntary counselling and testing centre at present exists in the country, seeing an average of 30 clients per month. Another centre is planned in Harare in the near future.

Chirumhanzu District is a farming area in the central Midlands province of Zimbabwe. The HIV epidemic has struck the area hard. At St Theresa's Hospital, just over half of the 253 in-patient deaths occurring in 1997 were because of AIDS, and the numbers are still on increase. The Chirumhanzu Home-based Care Project began in 1994. It grew out of an initiative of Hospital health workers, including senior nurses, Dominican sisters, and expatriate doctors. Concerned by the overcrowded hospital wards, they were also well aware of the wish of local AIDS patients to stay at home under the care of their families up till, and including, the time of their death. Since then, a variety of HIV/AIDS-related services have been created, including home care for over 200 persons living with HIV. The home-based care part of the project is provided basically by family members under the supervision of home-care volunteers. These volunteers are themselves supervised by the project coordinator and the professional nursing staff of the hospital.

Objectives

The project is based on two main objectives:

(a) to meet the HIV-affected peoples' needs as near to their homes and relatives as possible;

(b) to provide the necessary information, skills, care, materials, and support to everybody involved or interested.

From its inception, the project has taken a comprehensive approach to care consisting not only meeting medical needs but also social and emotional needs. It promotes HIV awareness and prevention, both among the general public and among target groups within the public such as sex workers, students, and STD patients.

The project strongly believes in, and builds on, African traditions of family support and mutual obligation, including consensus to designate a direct care giver within each family. As project coordinator. Home care must be supported because it meets patients' needs effectively and not because it reduces demand on the local hospital beds. A final principle is the participation of persons infected or affected by the virus in all aspects of the project. This principle is important because it increases the profile of persons living with HIV in the community and thus serves to lessen stigmatization.

Background

The population of Chirumhanzu District is approximately 70000 people, of whom almost half are under the age of 16. The population in dry, hilly area is quite poor. The economy is based on subsistence farming, mostly of maize, and is highly dependent on adequate rainfall from year to year. The epidemic attacked the district in the late 1980s. Between 150 and 200 people have tested positive each year at St. Theresa's Hospital. About half of all beds occupied, and of all in-patient death, are HIV- associated. Moreover, HIV/AIDS statistics at the hospital (admissions, in-patient deaths) are still at a time when the hospital is already over-crowded.

An in-depth analysis of these statistics reveals that of all admissions ending with the patient's death while in hospital, AIDS patients stay longer in hospital than non-AIDS patients: Of the non-AIDS patients, the average stay before death was 8.2 days, with half dying after 4 days. In contrast, AIDS patients stay on average 14.6 days before dying, half of them dying after 8 days. The project began on the initiative of hospital staff who, realizing that home care would be necessary to look after the growing number of AIDS patients, went out to churches and communities looking for people willing to be trained in this task. The staff began giving workshops for trainers of home care givers.

Major Elements

The project is organizationally separate from the hospital but collaborates fully with it in referrals and has space in the hospital wing built by the Dominican Sisters. A full-time nurse paid by the hospital works with the project, while the group's full-time coordinator is paid a small honorarium from project funds provided by the Swiss NGO Solidarmed. A smaller honorarium is also given to a volunteer who assists the nurse and coordinator. The project's comprehensive approach includes three main elements:

(a) home-based care for AIDS patients;
(b) support groups for HIV-positive people; and
(c) awareness and prevention for general public and target groups.

The first two are aimed at meeting the medical, social, and emotional needs of persons with HIV/AIDS. The third concentrates on encouraging local society to take greater responsibility in accepting and caring for its HIV-positive members. The home-based care element of the project begins with the identification of clients. This occurs mainly in hospital through the admissions process or as a result of HIV testing. If discovered as HIV-positive, the individual receives counselling sessions that consist of assessment of individual needs and wishes. This assessment helps identify appropriate follow-up procedures once the patient has been discharged from hospital.

When patients are ready to go home, a letter is provided from the hospital to the patient's nearest local clinic and to the care giver and relatives. This letter confirms that the patient has been discharged for home care. A volunteer, who has been trained as a community-based care giver, undertakes follow-up at home. Each client is visited every week. The reports written by the volunteer following the visit are used by the project coordinator at the hospital to decide whether a home visit by a qualified nurse is needed. Nursing materials and drugs used in the home care service are mostly provided by the ministry of health.

Many patients diagnosed with HIV are mobile and able to take care of themselves. These people receive self-care training in nutrition, hygiene, and techniques such as caring for HIV-associated skin problems. The patient also receives training in positive living - taking on a forward-looking, optimistic attitude to life. When a person needs a greater degree of care and has come to St Theresa's for in-patient treatment, her or his family is asked to send a member over the age of 12 to take home-care training while the patient is in hospital. This relative is generally chosen in the traditional way by decision of the entire family, and is generally a female member relative (wife, mother, daughter or cousin). About one in ten of the care-giver relatives are male (fathers, husbands or sons. If coming from far away, the relative is able to stay in a guest house managed by the hospital during the training. Like self-care patients, family care givers receive training in nutrition, hygiene, oral rehydration and control of simple infections.

Most of the project's volunteer home care givers are recruited through the District's church parish councils and other base-level religious organizations. Criteria which guide the councils in their recruitment of these volunteers consist compassion and willingness to offer spiritual support and care. Most of the volunteers are HIV-positive themselves, though an increasing number are relatives of infected persons. There are at present approximately 30 volunteers in Chirumhanzu. Basic training is given in workshops that are supplemented occasionally with refresher courses. The basic course teaches how to provide care and supervise the home care provided by family members. The supervision of these volunteers is the responsibility of the project administrator and a qualified nurse. Concerns about individual clients are normally included in the reports written by the volunteers after their weekly home visit, and these can be discussed immediately with the administrator depending on their urgency. Meetings of all volunteer care givers are held each month to address more general problems.

Some incentive is provided to volunteers in the form of monthly pocket money. Since the actual sum of Z$8 is only enough to buy a small item such as a bar of soap, most volunteers prefer to receive the year's pocket money in a lump sum. Besides this, refresher workshops and monthly meetings at St. Theresa's are used partly as a way of thanking and motivating volunteers by providing a good meal and a social gathering.

The project has also created a number of support groups in the district. There are currently six groups with 12 to 22 persons in each group that come together each week on Thursdays. The numbers depend largely on how voluminous the population is in each group's village area, since there is no bus service to villages and members must walk to the support group meetings. Members learn about the groups through referral by the hospital or through word of mouth, and membership is, entirely voluntary. One of the objectives of the support groups is to increase the economic self-reliance of members by teaching sewing (by hand and by machine) and gardening skills. People within some groups are also involved in raising chickens together. Where such productive activities are underway, the groups appoint a small committee to oversee the work and to organize monthly meetings of the participants.

The project's important tool for awareness and prevention has been its drama group. The group has created a skit which it uses to entertain their public while providing information on HIV/AIDS. The group generally accompanies the nurse and coordinator when they attend village meetings, and performs at these meetings. Recently, the project has started to organize public netball and football clubs in the area for the community's young people. Games between clubs are used as an occasion to give talks and to show a video about HIV/AIDS. At present, eight women who volunteer with the project have taken on responsibility for prevention work. These women visit popular meeting places where they teach about HIV and sexually transmitted diseases, hand out pamphlets on these subjects, and also distribute condoms.

Partnerships and Alliances

Since it inception, the project has been careful to work with traditional leaders in the area in order to gain people's confidence and to overcome stigma and ignorance about HIV and AIDS. The project's primary outreach to villages begins with an invitation to the village chiefs and their advisers to visit the hospital or a clinic and to meet with the project staff. A video on home care and HIV/AIDS is shown during this visit. This is generally followed by a visit from the staff to the village, during which a public meeting may be held. This public meeting may consist of a presentation about HIV/AIDS by the project's drama group and a talk by the project's nurse or coordinator.

The Chirumhanzu Home-based Care Project was initially set up to work mainly in the hospital's catchment area, where there are about 150 identified HIV-positive client at present. The project also works with five government clinics in the district, with regular visits by the project nurse and coordinator. The project informs the Provincial Medical Director about its programmes through its annual report. Recently, the government provided five bicycles for the project to help project members move around the area more quickly and easily. During 1994-95, the project received funds from UNICEF through the Zimbabwean government. Since 1996, overseas donations have come from the Swiss NGO SolidarMed, and from German parishes and private donors with the assistance of the Dominican Sisters. The project is not aware of any other health-related organizations at present working on HIV/AIDS in the immediate region. However, the coordinator has represented HIV/AIDS support groups from the Midlands at capacity-building workshops given by the Zimbabwe National Network for Persons Living with HIV/AIDS (ZNNP+).

Monitoring and Evaluation

Monitoring of the project is conducted in the following ways:

(a) monthly review of home-based care activities by the project coordinator, augmented by visits to clinics and homes;

(b) monthly meetings of the project members, which consist reports from all activities within the project, discussion of problems, short- and long-term planning, policy review; and

(c) annual reports, consisting accounts and a budget are prepared for donor organizations.

These monitoring activities are ample for administrative purposes, but the project does not have enough personnel with the necessary skills to conduct the monitoring it would prefer to do. For example, more time to consider patient reports and examine the issues brought up at monthly meetings would probably allow the project to make some valuable improvements to procedures and policy. As the decentralization process moves more programmes out to the clinics from the hospital, it is anticipated that there will be increased challenges to monitoring. In anticipation of this development, the project has created a standardized monitoring form to be utilised to monitor the activities of home-based care workers operating from these clinics. Except for an evaluation of financial accounting systems carried out by the government in 1994-95, no formal evaluation of the project has been carried out as yet.

The Chirumhanzu Home-based Care Project has now existed for almost three years. During this period it has achieved a high degree of continuity in services and a stable financial basis for its operations through its donors. The connection with St Theresa's Hospital has been a particular source of strength and continuity, particularly due to the availability of trained health professionals to the project when needed. A significant feature of the project is the fact that it is managed by local people. Most of the project members are either HIV-positive or are directly affected in some way by the virus, such as having had a family member who died of AIDS.

Although the project has stable finances due to its donors and support from health, professionals in the hospitals, this dependence on overseas donors and foreign medical staff is not an ideal state of affairs. The area being a poor one, there are few options for greater resource mobilization locally or nationally. The project has not been able to get a great deal of active participation or support from local chiefs or village health workers. Some of the local chiefs are of the opinion that they should receive payment for supporting the project, as do the health care workers whose regular salary is very low. The project does not have the financial resources to provide any such payment, and this lack of participation has partly resulted in less community participation in the project than the project feels is possible. Another reason for this weakness may be the fact that the project is too centralized in the hospital. The decentralization of some of its activities to clinics further away from the hospital will have positive results.

Conclusion

In the short term, decentralization to surrounding clinics is one of the major objectives for the project. In future, the project hopes to cooperate with other home-based care or HIV/AIDS organizations on a provincial level. Recently, the project has begun to help establish a similar project in the neighbouring district of Mvuma. Progress to date includes informing local chiefs and selection by the community of designated care givers. Most important, the project wishes to make it possible for everyone in the area to talk about HIV and AIDS. In particular, it aims to empower all persons living with AIDS to be open about their sero-status if they wish to talk about it.

Two

Enhancement of Participation of People Living with HIV/AIDS in Sub-Saharan Africa

Introduction

By mid-2000, the number of people living with HIV throughout the world had risen to 34.3. million. Of this more than two-thirds inhabited in sub-Saharan Africa. Approximately 14 million adults and children have already died of AIDS since the start of the epidemic in the late 1970s. During 1998, it is estimated that 11 individuals around the world became infected every minute. The global response of individuals and communities to the disease has been encouraging. With courage and compassion, they have mobilized resources to care for and support those affected and to help others in remaining uninfected. Striking has been the role of people living with HIV / AIDS (PWHA) who, within a short period of time, have given a human face to the grim statistics.

Although only a little percentage of persons affected by HIV / AIDS have come out in the open, declaring their serostatus, those who have done so have been powerful catalysts in the subcontinent. At the regional level, the voice of PWHA has been heard during the International Conferences on AIDS and STD in Africa (ICASA), held in Kampala in 1995, and in Abidjan in 1997. PWHA can give important insights into how to address problems, how to strive for positive living and how people can be empowered through the trauma and tragedy of the disease. In many sub-Saharan African nations' an environment characterized by high levels of denial, fear, and stigmatization has undermined the participation of those affected by HIV and AIDS. Even when the political, legal and social environments are conducive, the involvement of those living with HIV/AIDS is seldom reflected in the formulation of national policies and programmes.

Although the reasons for this vary from country to country, a certain pattern emerge.

(a) There is lack of appropriate mechanisms to ensure that the experiences, perceptions and capacities of those living with HIV/AIDS are expressed, valued, understood and taken into consideration in the development of policies and programmes.
(b) Even when an appropriate forum is provided, individuals living with HIV/AIDS often lack the skills necessary to engage institutions and governments in policy dialogue.
(c) Many individuals living with HIV/AIDS are not in gainful employment, and are thus too economically weak to engage in any serious discourse.
(d) Even when they are employed, the kinds of institutions they work for are unlikely to generate and initiate policy changes.

These issues were exposed in one of the major outcomes of the Paris AIDS Summit for Heads of State, held in December 1994, where governments from more than 50 countries called for increased support for PWHA. Participants resolved that the principle of greater participation of people living with HIV/AIDS (GIPA) was critical to an appropriate, ethical and effective national response to the disease. They agreed to support a greater participation of people living with HIV/AIDS through an initiative to strengthen the capacity and coordination of networks of people living with HIV/AIDS and community-based organizations.

The Initiative

The initiative was necessary for the following reasons:

(a) To provide the required social setting debate on issues related to HIV/AIDS with those who are affected,
(b) To allow for the expansion of the national response by involving individuals whose representation has not been fully recognized such as parents who are HIV-negative but have nursed an adult child who is HIV-

positive, or families wherein one of the partners is HIV-negative;

(c) To give human face and voice to the current statistics of HIV/AIDS;

(d) To facilitate the acceptance of the presence of HIV/AIDS in the community; and

(e) To improve the economic status of those living with HIV/AIDS.

Using a participatory approach to design the project, a consultative process was initiated early in 1995 and preliminary studies were carried out to examine the impact of employing HIV-infected individuals in the insurance sector. The outcome of this process was a project document UNV project to support people living with HIV and AIDS. The project was approved in September 1996 with funding from the Special Voluntary Fund (SVF) and UNDP. Two countries - Malawi and Zambia - were selected to implement a two-year pilot project whose important task was to test the use of the National United Nations Volunteer (NUNV) modality as a possible mechanism for encouraging the greater participation of individuals living with HIV and AIDS in the national response. The project was initiated during the mid-1997 and it is being implemented with technical and financial support from UNAIDS and the UNDP Regional Project on HIV and Development for sub-Saharan Africa, located in Pretoria, South Africa.

UNV Pilot Project

The objectives of the project are to deepen understanding of the nature of the HIV epidemic and to strengthen the national capacity to respond effectively, through the participation of people infected with the epidemic. Specific key objectives include:

(a) to ensure that the knowledge and expertise of people infected with the epidemic contribute to decision-making at all levels and in all relevant institutions, and that their needs and insights are projected in policy and programme development;

(b) to strengthen the capacity of networks and organizations of those living with HIV and AIDS for strategic planning and programme management;

(c) to encourage recognition of the potential role of volunteers and volunteerism in the national response to the HIV epidemic.

Strategies

To achieve these aims, the project is adopting the following key strategies:

(a) Placement of NUNVs in carefully selected local institutions — both public and private — that are involved in HIV and AIDS eradication, care and support activities.
(b) Capacity-building for NUNVs through training to increase their knowledge and skills base in areas such as policy analysis and development, project development, and project/business management.
(c) Capacity-building for members of the national network and of organizations or support groups of PWHA through training to increase their knowledge and skills base in areas such as policy analysis and development, project development, and project/business management.
(d) Setting up of a micro-grants facility to promote and support community-based initiatives that will arise from the work of the NUNVs, and to develop and strengthen organizations of PWHA and their networks.

Implementation, Monitoring and Evaluation

To ensure long-term sustainability, emphasis is being placed on ownership by host institutions, the Network of African People Living with HIV and AIDS (NAP+) and government. An important characteristic of the project is the elaborate process of consultation at every major step of its design, implementation and monitoring. To reflect the consultative process at an institutional level, a governance network at global and country level has been put in place. These mechanisms are necessary to confirm the participation of all major stakeholders in the development, implementation and monitoring of the project. The processes defined below reveal how the consultation has taken place on the ground.

Selection of Pilot Countries

It was considered important to test the feasibility of using the UNV mechanism to promote GIPA in countries with a mature epidemic and relatively mature response. A preliminary evaluation of documents and discussions resulted in a shortlist of four countries, agreed upon during a joint UNAIDS/UNDP/UNV meeting, which took place in Geneva. Thereafter, an assessment mission supported by UNAIDS was carried out in the four short-listed countries. A combination of key informant interviews and group discussions with potential stakeholders was the *modus operandi* for the assessment mission. Although there was variation between countries, in general the following potential stakeholders were consulted: national support groups and networks of PWHA; National AIDS Control Programmes; AIDS service organizations; nongovernmental organizations (NGOs); UN Theme Groups on HIV and AIDS; and donors. Each of these groups was given the opportunity to participate in the initiative. Two English-speaking countries were selected, based on pre-set criteria. Using the pre-set criteria, the meeting held in Geneva, agreed that the piloting would be done in Malawi and Zambia. With the country selection process completed, two Country Project Coordinators (CPC) were selected and placed in Lilongwe and Lusaka.

Country Project Coordinators: Their Functions

1. To arrange the day-to-day operation of the project in the country of assignment.
2. To help negotiations, selection and placement of the NUNVs in institutions/organizations.
3. To support training of the national UNVs (NUNVs) - both formal and on the job - and provision of other kinds of support for skills development.
4. To work with and coordinate all necessary activities among the responsible national bodies/mechanisms, UNDP, UNV, nongovernmental organizations (NGOs), community-based organizations (CBOs), and NAP+.
5. To ensure the access of NUNVs to appropriate peer support, counselling and supportive services.
6. To offer appropriate guidance and support to the UNVs.

7. To help developing policies and strategies associated with disclosure, confidentiality, and public profile of the NUNVs.
8. To appraise the output of the NUNVs and provide feedback and of the NUNVs and output appraisal of the NAP+.
9. To administer the small grants component of the project.
10. To carry out on-going evaluation and refinement of the pilot project and drawing-up / sharing of lessons.
11. To work in coordination with all parties participating in the project formulation, implementation, monitoring and evaluation.

The Project Initiation

In the spirit of consultation, the launching of the pilot, initiatives in the two countries involved planning workshops the aims and objectives of which are discussed below.

(a) to reach consensus and common understanding on the aims and principles of the pilot project;
(b) to discover mechanisms for project implementation, alongwith selection and recruitment criteria of the national UNVs, their placements within institutions such as CBOs, NGOs, and ministries, training needs and methodologies, and support and supervision;
(c) to discuss aspects of project monitoring and evaluation; and
(d) to agree on an action plan for the way forward.

The Malawi workshop was held in Lilongwe, 27-29 May 1997, and the Zambia one in Lusaka, 2-4 June 1997. Participants included members from support groups and national networks of PWHA, AIDS service organisations, NGOs, NGO umbrella organisations, government ministries and co-sponsors of UNAIDS, and resource persons from such organisations as the Faces Project from South Africa, the Philly Lutaaya Initiative from Uganda and NAP+. The results of both workshops were similar. A consensus was reached on the purpose and basic principles of the pilot project and on the selection criteria for NUNVs. Mechanisms were discovered for implementation, including placement within host institutions and supervision methods. Training needs were also discovered along with potential resources for training in and outside the country. Finally, participants at each workshop came up with a three-month action plan to be carried out by the UNV Project Manager, with the assistance of a Project Advisory Group (PAG).

Monitoring and Evaluation

The uniqueness of the design of this pilot initiative was the participatory development of a monitoring and evaluation framework. A technical mission visited both countries and worked with the project's main stakeholders to develop three major elements of the initiative:

(a) a monitoring and evaluation framework;
(b) a process that will enable those involved to identify and meet the training and support needs of the project; and
(c) a decision-making process for the use and monitoring of the project's micro-grants facility.

Using the process facilitation approach as outlined in the UNDP manual, the facilitators worked with key players to achieve the following:

(a) a monitoring and evaluation framework for each country;
(b) guidelines for the management and operations of the micro-grants facility;
(c) a document on training and support strategies alongwith checklists for follow-up activities.

Candidates for NUNV Posts: The Future Training Needs

To assist the selection of NUNVs, a joint UNAIDS/UNDP mission was carried out in Malawi and Zambia in 1998. This mission was a follow-up to a meeting of the International Technical Advisory Group (ITAG) held in Abidjan in 1997. The selection process used a workshop modality to provide 'safe spaces' for potential NUNVs and host institutions to show their expected roles and responsibilities within the project, to better assist their informed decisions about their involvement in the project and to define an objective framework for selection of the first group of volunteers to be selected by the project. Specific objectives of the workshops were for the participants to:

(a) share their understanding of the project mission and proposed strategy, as well as their roles and responsibilities;
(b) express their vision, hopes and fears regarding their roles and the concept of volunteerism;
(c) clarify myths and misinformation about the project;
(d) discuss and demonstrate the implications of being open about their serostatus (on self, family and community); and
(e) understand the minimum criteria for selection of the first group of volunteers and define areas where the other candidates could contribute to the project.

The terms of reference for the mission are detailed below:

(i) Sharing of experience with various staff and management within the host institution;
(ii) Individual discussions / counselling within the host institutions. These are the one-to-one sessions which volunteers have at the work place with staff;
(iii) Out-reach activities to share experiences and performing HIV/AIDS awareness activities outside the host institutions e.g. residential quarters, churches and at community events; and
(iv) Other activities, not related to sharing experience but carried out by the NUNVs as in the case of volunteers with additional responsibilities.

In both countries, the important outcomes were:

(a) a greater understanding of the project's vision, mission, and proposed strategies, of the roles and responsibilities of each partner, of the concept of 'coming out in the open', and of the selection criteria for NUNVs;
(b) a strengthened commitment to the objectives of the project; and
(c) the completion of the selection method for NUNVs and host institutions.

Identification of Training Needs

The fifth phase of the project's implementation consisted training for the NUNVs, their associates in host institutions and members of many support groups and networks of PWHA. Following the Self-reflection and Selection Workshops, the following training needs were discovered:

(a) broader understanding of the epidemic;
(b) public speaking and media approaches;
(c) communication skills alongwith interpersonal skills and team work;
(d) peer counselling skills;
(e) writing skills (such as reports, project proposals, record keeping);
(f) micro-project financing (including formulation, monitoring and evaluation); and
(g) setting up and sustaining support groups.

In response, successful HIV and Development Workshops and a Skills Training Workshop have been held in Zambia and Malawi in 1998. The Skills Training Workshop included sessions on the basic facts about HIV and AIDS, peer counselling, basic nursing care, nutritional care, advocacy for ethics and human rights, communication skills, group formation, report writing and record keeping, project proposal writing and stress management.

Implementing the Framework

The framework for monitoring and evaluation which was developed necessitates under operationalization. Terms of reference have since been developed, especially for the special studies, and both countries can implement the evaluation framework. To inculcate a systematic process of learning at global and country level, a joint UNAIDS/UNDP/UNV meeting was help in Bonn to go over the experiences gained during the 18 months of the pilot initiative design and implementation. The following were the significant issues that emerged in the implementation of the pilot initiative in Zambia and Malawi:

(a) Consensus-building around key concepts and operational modalities is critical to the success of the initiative.

(b) It is necessary to set up a shared understanding of HIV and development. The assumption that stakeholders have a working knowledge of the broader developmental range of HIV is not valid. During the consultative and planning workshops, few stakeholders were not even convinced of the seriousness of the HIV epidemic in their countries. In future, consultative and planning workshops should give all the project's stakeholders the opportunity to reach a shared understanding of the HIV epidemic and its consequences. This would assist discussions on selection criteria for the selection of NUNVs, and on the roles and responsibilities of host institutions and NUNVs. The use of tools such as the HIV and development workshop before the consultative and planning process would address this problem.

(c) The facilitators should challenge selection criteria proposed during these workshops which may stop potentially good candidates from being recruited as NUNVs on the basis of their literacy level or their ability to communicate in the official language (e.g. English). Such criteria have prevented good candidates.

Development of Monitoring and Evaluation Framework

The monitoring and evaluation frameworks were derived directly from the project document and are reflection of the project's goals and objectives. They were developed with the involvement of many stakeholders before the selection and placement of the NUNVs. The job descriptions of the NUNVs seldom demonstrates the monitoring and evaluation framework. None of the job descriptions outlined the major function of the volunteer as that of giving a human face and voice to the HIV and AIDS epidemic. Besides this, the effective use of the monitoring and evaluation framework has been hampered by the fact that in neither country was a baseline assessment conducted at the initiation of the project. The framework for each country does not include simple monitoring targets, indicators and tools, which now need to be developed.

Recruitment of Candidates

The Self-reflection and Selection Workshop, whose important aim was to give an opportunity to candidates to reflect on what it means to talk publicly about their HIV status and their personal experience, was quite stressful for participants. It was felt that this process was necessary because future NUNVs would be required to be fully 'open' about their own HIV status, or about how they and their family have been affected by HIV and AIDS. There had also been an assumption that there would be a strong feeling of 'togetherness' among the members of a particular support group. It was expected that the group would take pride in, and support the selection of one or two of its members and that the NUNVs would be treated as ambassadors of the group in whatever role they were placed. However, this did not prove to be the case and the problem of competition arose manifold.

Ways should be discovered to minimize the stress induced by the exercise. Possible methods include shortening the selection process, and emphasizing the fact that the recruitment of ten (or more) NUNVs is only one aspect of the strategy/ activities implemented by the project.

The Micro-grants Facility

It was set up to help achieve the project's objectives. Funding made available under the micro-grants facility can be accessed for the purpose of:

(a) promoting and supporting community-based initiatives that have arisen from the work of the NUNVs; or

(b) developing and strengthening PWHA organizations and their networks.

Eligible activities may fall into any of the following categories: community group and workplace debates; capacity-building activities for the volunteers' own support groups; networking; legal assistance; training for members of community-based groups and PWHA organizations (e.g. public speaking, communication skills, skills training, counselling, psychosocial support, home- and community-based care, programme development, monitoring and evaluation, proposal and report writing); income-generating activities (including for survivors); psychosocial support (e.g. counselling, care for support group members and their families).

Training

The HIV and development workshop became a very powerful tool for bridging the knowledge and attitudinal gaps discovered among many stakeholders of the projects. However, this workshop should have been conducted much earlier in the consultative process to provide an in-depth understanding of the epidemic as a foundation for all subsequent stages of the process. There is also a need to modify some of the content and exercises used in the workshop to improve their tone and make them more user-friendly. The skills training programme has now been developed into a draft curriculum. This draft will be further refined in the expansion of the project. It was decided that the curriculum should be packaged in two portions: the workshop portion and the 'on the job' support and supervision of the development of specific skills (e.g. peer counselling, communication and public speaking, report writing, and support group formation). Most of these skills require practice and close supervision if they are to be mastered.

Placement of Volunteers

The overall objective of placing volunteers with host institutions is to provide human face and voice to HIV and AIDS. This human face and voice can be demonstrated within the workplace, and through the services offered by the host institution to its target group(s). Importantly, the volunteer must not merely be seen as just an additional employee, but as one who adds value by virtue of his experience of living with HIV/AIDS.

However, 18 months after the inception of the project, it seems that some host institutions, despite all the consultation processes put in place, still consider the volunteers as just an additional pair of hands. It has been reported in some instances that some volunteers regard it as a violation of their human rights for the project to expect them to share their personal testimonies during their work. This is a delicate issue since it is true that no one has the right to require another person to disclose their serostatus if they do not wish to do so. The requirement to 'be open' was explicitly included in the selection criteria and a very elaborate process was set up to ensure that those who were recruited as volunteers understood that they would need to use their experience as PWHA in doing their work. This results in frustration and resentment among those who were not recruited among the first round of volunteers and may consider themselves better qualified due to their openness about their HIV status. The networks of PWHA, who are full partners of this pilot initiative, are in the best position of legitimately resolve this dilemma. Appropriate mechanisms should be put in place to give their representatives more influence in the recruitment process.

GIPA in South Africa: UN Support

In South Africa, more than three million people are currently infected with HIV, yet the epidemic remains almost silent and faceless. The levels of discrimination and social stigma are unacceptably high and people continue to live under a conspiracy of silence. The National AIDS Review of 1997 suggested that greater participation of PWHA was crucial for effective HIV eradication and management. On the basis of this, the National AIDS Plan identifies GIPA as one of the key components for managing the epidemic in South Africa. The need for capacity building to enable PWHA to fulfil this role efficiently has been discovered and training programmes, such as those included in GIPA, are crucial to address this.

In January 1997, the UNAIDS Inter-country Team, together with UNV South Africa, held a meeting with partners from the Department of Health and the National Association of People Living with HIV/AIDS (NAPWA) to discover the scope of developing a National UNV project identical to the pilot projects in Zambia and Malawi. It was agreed that, in order to get a better and deeper understanding of the issues around GIPA and to avoid replicating existing efforts, an accelerated assessment should be undertaken. Two independent consultants (one a PWHA) participated in the National AIDS Review. They also visited and interviewed representatives from several public and private sector organizations to assess the need for such a project and inform the design and modality of the project management. As a strategy for expanding the response, the consultants were required to actively discover the role and interest of private sector organizations to participate in such a project. The accelerated assessment revealed that while some progress has been made in the participation of PWHA, the epidemic remains largely latent. The environment is not conducive to people revealing their HIV status due to the fear of rejection. NGOs that work with PWHA find that their contributions are not sustained due to a high 'burn-out' factor. Workplace HIV/AIDS programmes have not always been effective as people do not see the epidemic a reality if they have never seen an infected person.

Following the three-month accelerated assessment, the UN convened a one-day planning/consultative meeting. The objective of the meeting was to flesh out issues relevant to roles and responsibilities of the project partners, criteria for selection and recruitment of GIPA Field Workers (GFWs), and operational and management factors.

Following the planning/consultative meeting, a project document was drafted for financing and approval. The aim of the project was then defined as being that of:

(a) mobilizing the private sector to put in place effective, non-discriminatory HIV/AIDS workplace programmes and policies; and
(b) strengthening existing national programmes that involve PWHA.

To fulfil this purpose, the project is placing people living openly and positively with HIV/AIDS in partner organizations to assist with work-based HIV/AIDS policies and programmes. A National project manager was recruited in March 1998 and a Steering Committee and Advisory Board were set up.

The essential criteria for the GFWs agreed to by the Advisory Board was the need and importance of all candidates to be HIV-positive and willing to be open about their status. Other requirements included having good organizational, verbal and non-verbal communication skills, willingness to be trained, minimum educational qualification of Standard 10 and ability to work as a member of a team. The advertisement for the recruitment of the GFWs was placed in two national newspapers and circulated widely to partners. Following the receipt of approximately 100 application forms, 20 candidates were called upon to an intensive two-day Selection Workshop.

The workshop was structured to find out whether the individuals fulfilled the requisite qualification, as well as to promote self-growth and personal development. A highly participatory and experiential methodology was selected instead of straight interviews, since a workshop gives more time for evaluating applicants' strengths and weaknesses. It also offers a better insight into how applicants handle themselves in different situations. The various activities were selected with the objective of being informative, educational and personally empowering. A total of 12 candidates were selected as GFWs. In addition to the selection process for GFWs, the workshop was attended by guest participants from Mozambique and Swaziland who used the opportunity to become sensitized to the GIPA principle and to get motivated to kick-start similar processes in their own countries.

Since the selection workshop, GFWs have been placed in partner organizations. These include government partner the Ministry of Health, private organizations (Eskom Electricity Commission, Super Group Pty Ltd., Imperial Transport Holdings, Sowetan Newspaper, Lonrho Platinum Mines and Transnet), and NGOs (Lifeline and A.M.E. Church).

A comprehensive training and development programme was formulated for the GFWs to perform their duties effectively and professionally. The objective is to ensure that, with support and persuasion, each GFW can develop his or her own potential, on a personal an professional level. The GFWs have so far received the following training: basic computer skills; personal empowerment and guidelines to living positively with HIV, modelled on the field of psycho-neuroimmunology; communication and presentation skills; HIV and development; and HIV/AIDS policy and programme development. Further training in counselling and advanced computer skills is planned to follow soon.

GFWs also participate in several HIV/AIDS projects aimed at raising visibility and championing the cause of issues at hand affecting PWHA in South Africa. They participated in the UNDP Human Development Report for South Africa, the Ster Kinekor movie project, Stepping Stones Gender and HIV/AIDS training,

UNV workshops, and activities with the South African Broadcasting Corporation (SABC). GFWs have also assisted with regional workshops organized by UNAIDS to help kick-start GIPA activities in the region.

The main challenge is to sustain the project by continuing to import on-going training as well as support for the GFWs to fulfil their expected roles. This depends largely on availability of funds. The South African Business Council is being set up and it is hoped that the links with the GIPA project will go from strength to strength. The training and development programme for 1999 included: on-going skills building; development of a support system for the GFWs; electronic connectivity; an advocacy programme; developing participatory monitoring tools; and extending international opportunities to the GFWs (e.g. the International Conference on AIDS and STD in Africa, ICASA, and the Global Network of People Living with HIV/AIDS and International Community of Women Living with HIV/AIDS (GNP+/ ICW+) Conference in Poland.

Partner Organization: Selection

The rapid assessment process was important as it determined the direction of the project. One of the difficult aspects of the process was the selection of partner organizations. In hindsight, more time should have been devoted to screening the suitability of the organizations identified and interviewed. At least four-out-of-six original organizations have been considered unprepared or unsuitable to host a GFW. The desire of expanding the response was not fully realized and the choice of organizations was very limited in scope. These setbacks have delayed the implementation and the placement process of the GFWs. More effort had to be spent finding new partner organizations - a process that is both very slow and labour-intensive.

A much more intensive reference check is probably necessary to ensure that the selected GFWs have acceptable records with the communities in which they have to work. This might have to be backed up with preparing the community for the GFW and for talking about HIV/AIDS openly. This should help prevent the sort of unnecessary hostilities experienced in the past.

It is important to determine strategies that can sustain the interest of the GFWs and provide a certain financial security simultaneously. On-going training and support are crucial for the GFWs to continue operating at the energy levels required.

An agreement was reached on a number of follow-up actions on future collaborative programmes. One of the follow-up actions was the possible expansion of the pilot project to other countries in Africa and to other regions. Participants agreed to expand the project, particularly to French-speaking African countries, using a similar approach and building on the lessons learnt.

Therefore, a new project was designed to further develop suitable approaches and mechanisms for enhancing the involvement of individuals living with HIV and AIDS in response to the HIV epidemic. The proposal outlines an approach based on two separate but related strategies. The first strategy aims at ensuring, through an appropriate volunteer modality, the meaningful representation of individuals living with HIV and AIDS in key organizations and institutions engaged in the response to the HIV epidemic at community, district and national levels. The other strategy aims to strengthen the capacity of organizations and networks to participate at all levels in the formulation and implementation of policies and programmes that will generate supportive ethical, legal and social climate for an expanded response to the epidemic.

The NUNV modality provides an appropriate delivery mechanism for GIPA. Through this expansion, the NUNV modality and any other appropriate volunteer modalities will be further examined - this time in countries that are characterized by a lower HIV prevalence and poorly functioning national organizations and networks of PWHA. These several volunteer modalities will be considered in terms of the following questions:

(a) As currently developed, can they provide the appropriate space for individuals living with HIV/AIDS to influence policy and programming in host institutions, and at national level?

(b) Are these different volunteer modalities an appropriate delivery mechanism for economically empowering individuals living with HIV/AIDS, and for strengthening their organizations and networks?

(c) Is the NUNV modality, or any other volunteer modality, a feasible delivery mechanism for promoting GIPA?

Activities to initiate the expansion in two French-speaking countries began in February-March 1999. UNAIDS and the UNDP HIV and Development Regional Project will participate in the implementation of this expansion, to an even greater extent than for the pilot phase in Malawi and Zambia. The formal 'project' approach of placing individuals living with HIV/AIDS is only one approach to GIPA. The projects at present implemented in Malawi, South Africa and Zambia should provide an opportunity to review different approaches for enhancing GIPA. To that end, a round table discussion was conducted during the XIth ICASA in Zambia to create space for the sharing of experiences and lessons learnt from the different approaches to enhancing GIPA, particularly in sub-Saharan Africa. It was also intended to provide a venue for testing the following prioritization issues:

(a) Given the current trends of the HIV epidemic, should GIPA be considered a key element in the national response to HIV in sub-Saharan Africa?

(b) Which mechanism is the most appropriate for promoting GIPA, given the different political, economic, cultural and social contexts?

UNAIDS has made the GIPA principles a part of its policy because it has now been shown that GIPA is a key strategy in the response at all levels. A technical consultation on GIPA has taken place and key areas for action have been discovered.

Three

AIDS and Traditional Medicine in Sub-Saharan Africa

HIV/AIDS is at present the number one overall cause of death in Africa, and has moved up to fourth place among all causes of death globally.

As the epidemic continues to ravage the developing world, it becomes increasingly evident that diverse strategies to encounter the wide-ranging and complex social, cultural, environmental and economic contexts in which HIV continues to spread must be researched, tested, evaluated, adapted and adopted. The populations in developing countries in general have access to traditional health care and it is widely accepted that about 80 per cent of people in Africa rely on traditional medicine for many of their health care needs. Traditional healers are well known in the communities where they work for their expertise in treating many sexually transmitted diseases. As a result, the World Health Organization (WHO) has advocated the inclusion of traditional healers in National AIDS activities since the early 1990s.

The aim of the present discussion was to give a brief update on AIDS and traditional medicine in Africa, and to evaluate initiatives that have attempted collaboration between traditional and biomedical practitioners for HIV prevention. There is, however, a lack of research actually testing the impact of involving traditional healers in HIV prevention efforts. Most reports — even evaluation reports — often state only achievements and findings. The evaluation first looked as widely possible at all interventions involving traditional healers in HIV/AIDS prevention and care in sub-Saharan Africa.

Supplementary standards were defined that are specific to traditional medicine/biomedicine collaborative projects. Statistics were collected through published and unpublished literature, through personal contacts, e-mail correspondence, circulation of a questionnaire and by attending the First International Conference on AIDS and Traditional Medicine in Dakar, Senegal, in March 1999. It has been noted that some other illnesses and conditions not classified as sexually transmitted in biomedical nosology may be locally regarded as such by traditional healers and their clients.

Since the start of the epidemic, approximately 34 million people living in sub-Saharan Africa have been infected with the virus. In 1998, 70 per cent of the people who became infected with HIV and four-fifths of all AIDS deaths were in sub-Saharan Africa. Besides this at least 95 per cent of all AIDS orphans have been African. In the present discussion AIDS orphans are the people who lost their mother or both their parents to AIDS when they were under the age of 15. AIDS was responsible for an estimated 2 million African deaths, leading to 5,500 funerals a day. And despite the scale of death, today there are more Africans living with HIV than ever before: 23.5 million adults and children. The majority of new infections continue to be concentrated in Eastern and Southern Africa, no country being exception. In Botswana, Namibia, Swaziland and Zimbabwe, present trends indicate that between 20 per cent and 26 per cent of people aged 15-49 are living with HIV/AIDS. Zimbabwe, for example, is very hard hit. In 23 of 25 surveillance sites, over 20 per cent of all the pregnant women were discovered infected. About one-third of these women are likely to pass the infection on to their babies. In Central African Republic, Cote d'Ivoire, Djibouti and Kenya, at least one in ten adults is HIV-infected. In Rwanda, the median existence among women attending antenatal clinics in major urban centres was about 28 per cent and, in Uganda, the prevalence has dropped in recent years to 15 per cent in the same population. West Africa is generally less affected by HIV than Southern or Eastern Africa.

Interventions to stem the spread of HIV/AIDS on a global footing are as varied as the contexts in which we find them at present. Not only is the HIV epidemic dynamic in terms of treatment options, prevention strategies and disease progression, but sexual behaviour, which remains the basic target of HIV prevention efforts worldwide, is broadly diverse and deeply embedded in social and cultural relationships, as well as environmental and economic processes. This makes prevention of HIV/AIDS very complex. Most preventive interventions have relied on giving correct information about HIV transmission and prevention and imparting practical skills to enable individuals to lessen their risk of HIV infection. More recently, sociocultural factors surrounding the individual have been considered in designing prevention interventions. Besides this, beyond the individual and his or her immediate social relationships, larger issues of structural and environmental determinants also play an important role in sexual behaviour and thus are addressed in intervention design and implementation.

Monitoring and evaluation of prevention programmes have demonstrated that prevention does work. In countries that have implemented quick, well-planned efforts with support from political and religious leaders, alongwith sex education in schools, treatment of STDs (sexually transmitted diseases), and widely promoted condom use, HIV prevalence has been kept consistently low and has even decreased in some countries in the last five years. Yet, cases of decreased HIV prevalence are still the exception and many developing countries are struggling to find innovative, cost-effective strategies that are relevant to their AIDS situation. In resource-constrained settings, one avenue that has still been rarely travelled is cooperation with the indigenous health system.

The Importance of Traditional Medicine

Traditional healers represent a wide range of practices, consisting herbalism and spiritualism, as well as individuals who call themselves diviners, priests and faith healers, among other terms. Although many of the initiatives reviewed here did not differentiate between this classification, the term 'traditional healer' used refers to either herbalists, spiritualists, or to those involved in both practices. African traditional healers reflect the great variety of cultures and belief systems on the continent, and possess equally heterogeneous experience, training and educational backgrounds. This diversity is further enhanced by their adaptations to the dramatic social changes that have affected much of the region since colonization, such as urbanization, population migration and displacement, and civil conflict. The cost of traditional medical care varies with the nature of treatment, the type and severity of ailment and the relative wealth of the client. Whenever African healers' knowledge, attitudes, beliefs and practices about STDs and AIDS have been identified, findings have exposed the stage of the disease, the amount of information traditional healers have been exposed to, and their pre-existing belief systems about health and disease in general, and STDs and AIDS in particular.

Many traditional healers have treated STDs for generations, but their explanations of STDs and AIDS vary considerably, across ethnic backgrounds pertaining the nature, causes and modes of transmission of these diseases. However, the concepts underlying these explanations seem remarkably similar across national and cultural boundaries. Perhaps the most striking example is the origin of STDs: healers in many sittings, whether rural or urban, often ascribe these to transgressions of taboos associated with birth, pregnancy, marriage and death. Simultaneously some of Africa's gravest diseases, including AIDS and other STDs, are often understood within a framework of contagion which could include invasion of the body by dangerous microorganisms, pollution or environmental dangers. In many countries, healers could name and describe several types of STDs (which do not always correspond to the biomedical definition of STDs), few of them treat AIDS an 'African' disease. Traditional beliefs about the prevention of STDs or HIV/AIDS follow the logic of transmission and causation, and consist limiting the number of sexual partners, wearing protective charms or tattoos, having, 'strong blood', using condoms to reduce the risk of 'pollution', or undergoing a 'traditional vaccination' consisting of introducing herbs in skin incisions. In numerous cases at present, condoms have been acceptable to traditional healers, especially when they fit into their belief system. For example, many African healers consider semen an important element to nourish a growing foetus and maintain the mother's health and beauty, but their concern for family and cultural survival can override this belief and allow them to promote condom use.

Health Policy and Traditional Medicine

With growing interest and increasing need for wide health care in the past the governing bodies of WHO have adopted a series of resolutions. Policies regarding collaboration with traditional medicine have noticed deviation since the late 1970s. As early as 1974, the WHO Regional Committee for Africa decided that the topic for the technical discussions at its upcoming twenty-sixth session would be "Traditional medicine and its role in the development of health services in Africa." Three years later, the World Health Assembly adopted a resolution promoting training and research associated with traditional medicine. In 1978, in Alma Ata, WHO and UNICEF adopted resolutions supporting the use of indigenous health practitioners in government-sponsored health programmes. Further resolutions were adopted, encouraging specific measures governing the practice of traditional medicine to be incorporated within national health legislation, adequate budgets to allow promotion of traditional medicine, the development of traditional medicine systems, effective launching of these programmes, and inventories of medicinal plants. In 1990, the WHO Traditional Medicine Programme and the WHO Global Programme on AIDS came together in Botswana to find ways to involve traditional health practitioners more actively in measures to prevent and control HIV infection and AIDS in African communities. In 1994, the WHO offered further observations and direction regarding traditional healers, suggesting that upgrading their skills made more sense than training new groups of health workers, such as village health workers. Since then, changing policies and a growing body of statistics concerning cooperation with traditional healers have fuelled an ongoing debate on the public health relevance of investing in efforts for partnership with traditional healers. In this debate, the following points are made in favour of collaboration:

(a) Traditional healers often outnumber doctors by 100 to 1 or more in most African nations. They provide a large accessible, available, affordable trained human resource pool.

(b) Traditional healers possess many effective treatments and treatment methods.

(c) Traditional healers provide client-oriented personalized health care that is culturally appropriate, holistic, and tailored to meet the needs and expectations of the patient. Traditional healers are culturally close to clients, which facilitates communication about disease and associated social issues. This is especially important in the case of STDs.

(d) Traditional healers often see their patients in the presence of other family members, which reflects the traditional healers' role in promoting social stability and family counselling.

(e) When traditional healers engage in harmful practices, there is a public health responsibility to try to change these practices, which is only possible with dialogue and cooperation. Research has demonstrated that traditional healers abstain from dangerous practices when educated about the risks.

(f) Traditional healers are generally respected health care providers and opinion leaders in their communities, and thus are treating large numbers of people living with HIV/AIDS. Healers have greater credibility than village health workers especially with respect to social and spiritual matters.

(g) Since traditional healers occupy an important role in African societies, they are not likely to disappear soon. They survived even strict colonial legislation forbidding their practice. Even with the rapid sociocultural changes occurring in many African societies, traditional healers continue to play a crucial role in addressing the variety of psychosocial problems that arise from conflicting expectations of changing societies.

(h) Numerous studies document traditional healers' enthusiasm for collaborating with biomedical health providers and show that their activities are sustainable as they generate their own source of income.

(i) Many biomedical health providers want such collaboration.

(j) Especially since the 1980s, healers have been organizing themselves into traditional healers' associations, which makes it easier to set up collaborative programmes.

(k) Efforts at collaboration appear to improve health delivery in many ways:

  (i) increased knowledge and skills of traditional healers

  (ii) increased confidence in their practice

  (iii) increased transparency towards the community within their work

  (iv) earlier referral to hospital or health centre.

The weaknesses of collaboration include:

(a) The training and licensing of healers is not institutionalized, making it difficult to reach and train them regularly in a standardized manner.

(b) Quality control of healers is difficult in the absence of officially recognized licensing procedures.

(c) There is no general monitoring of healers' activities or claims.

(d) Traditional healers lack detailed anatomical and physiological knowledge.

(e) Traditional healers may include in many harmful practices or cause delays in referral to biomedical facilities.

(f) Promotion and improvement of traditional methods may undermine efforts to increase access to biomedicine.

(g) The effects of combining traditional and biomedical treatments are not known and may be harmful.

(h) Official recognition of traditional medicine gives legitimacy to traditional healers when their treatments and methods are still largely untested.

(i) Opening up collaboration with traditional healers raises their expectations of greater recognition from government, which governments may not be able to give.

Despite the limitations, it makes sense to at least attempt

collaboration, given the vast health needs in developing countries and the several realistic and practical advantages. The following section discusses eight projects that have developed collaboration between biomedical and traditional health practitioners for HIV/AIDS prevention and care. In addition, Guinea is also discussed as a supplementary case, since the government has tried to integrate traditional healers into many different aspects of health care, though not specifically AIDS.

Collaboration between Traditional and Biomedical Health Care

The African continent, should be an obvious place for collaborations between traditional and biomedical health care. Despite the multitude of health challenges affecting the African people, very little action has been taken to actually work with healers since the WHO's recognition of the significance of traditional medicine to basic health care, and of the need to include healers in national health strategies and policies. Considerable prejudice remains ingrained among many biomedical health practitioners about the justification, validity and integrity of traditional medical practices and practitioners. This is due to the absence of regulatory bodies governing the practice of traditional medicine in most of Africa, making it easier for charlatans to infiltrate the profession and abuse its reputation.

Nevertheless, the WHO recommendations are based on the premise shared by many researchers, physicians and public health experts that, as a highly respected, widely distributed and highly consulted group of health practitioners, recognized traditional healers have the cultural knowledge and skills to make an impact on the prevention of disease (including HIV/AIDS), as well as on health promotion and care. The traditional healer is frequently consulted as a religious and spiritual guide, legal and political adviser, and marriage and family counsellor. STDs are among the most common reasons for visiting the traditional healers in many African countries where many people are of the opinion that, while biomedicine can effectively cure physical symptoms of 'modern' diseases, healers are expected to completely heal the body and spirit, and to cure diseases considered distinctly 'African' (i.e., believed to be due to forces beyond modern medicine's comprehension) many people in Africa believe that biomedical health practitioners cannot effectively and completely cure STDs. Finally, women, whose social, cultural and economic position in Africa makes them especially vulnerable to STDs and AIDS, often constitute the majority of traditional healers' clients.

Since the start of the AIDS epidemic, there has been a renewed interest in collaboration with traditional healers in the hope of finding new, more effective ways to fight and prevent this disease. Initially, a number of projects attempted to assess the value of traditional herbal remedies for the treatment of illnesses related to AIDS. Other studies were conducted on traditional healers' perceptions of STDs, HIV and AIDS. With these results, collaborative efforts have created programmes that trained traditional healers as educators and counsellors to disseminate HIV/AIDS information and prevention practices among their peers and communities. As a means of involving traditional healers further, some projects have encouraged healers to empower and provide emotional support to clients living with HIV and AIDS.

With the realization that traditional healers could become effective health workers for HIV prevention, given their traditional roles as educators and counsellors in their communities, a number of projects started training healers in HIV/AIDS as early as the late 1980s. Some initiatives have noted that 'training' healers implies a different approach than that used with conventional health workers, to whom knowledge tends to be imparted unidirectionally. With traditional healers, only a respectful attitude of open exchange of ideas and information can win confidence and cooperation.

Botswana

In Botswana, where the 1997 national serosurveillance statistics demonstrated an HIV prevalence of 38.5 per cent among pregnant women in urban areas, the government has had a policy of actively promoting cooperation between modern and traditional medicine. Activities of the Ministry of Health/National AIDS Programme for traditional healers consisted seminars on AIDS, and implementing the Botswana Dingaka AIDS Awareness and Training Project. The project took place between 1991 and 1993 with the objective of training traditional healers as trainers who would pass AIDS information on to other traditional healers in selected pilot areas, and promoting cooperation and collaboration between traditional and biomedical health services. The original training of trainers lasted two weeks and involved 12 healers in six districts of Botswana. Trained healers were then to travel together to other districts to train 40 other healers in each district. Once trained, newly trained healers were expected to train more healers, obtain condoms from health centres and distribute them to their clients and communities.

Four of the five workshops planned for the second-generation healers took place. However, funding was terminated after the first phase of the project, so neither group of healers was followed-up or formally evaluated for effectiveness of the training or for accomplishment of stated objectives within the duration of the project. However, an independent assessment of the Botswana Dingaka AIDS Awareness and Training Project, conducted in 1994, interviewed 32 traditional healers, 19 nurses and 20 medical doctors; 72 per cent of the traditional healers interviewed stated that they had changed something in their practice in relation to the new information on AIDS and 80 per cent said that after training, they recommended condoms to their patients, while 31 of the 32 stated that they referred patients to clinics or to the hospital. Interestingly, 17 of 19 nurses, interviewed claimed that they also referred patients to traditional healers, but only 7 per cent of the medical doctors reported doing the same.

In a second assessment in 1995, three of the 12 first-generation healers interviewed said they were able to disseminate information in their communities, had referred patients to the hospital when their treatments failed, and had no hesitation in distributing condoms or talking about sexual issues with clients. All three healers also claimed they had many STD patients, yet had not, so far, had a patient whom they believed had AIDS. When asked how they would manage a person with AIDS, they all said there was nothing they could do, since they didn't have a treatment for AIDS. They were not aware of the clinical case definition of AIDS, and were not referring their clients for HIV testing and counselling. They did not see themselves playing a role in home-based care for persons living with HIV/AIDS.

Central African Republic

A one-year project to increase traditional healers' capacity to deliver preventive messages, provide support to persons living with HIV/AIDS, and modify their own risk practices was started in 1995 in the Central African Republic, where HIV seroprevalence among adults was approximately 15 per cent in Bangui and 4 per cent in rural areas. Over two months, 103 healers in four locations received six days (36 hours) of STD/AIDS information and training on community education. At the end of training assessment, traditional healers' knowledge had significantly improved regarding:

(a) the role of STDs in increasing risk of HIV infection
(b) condoms as a safeguard against HIV
(c) the causes of genital discharge and ulcers
(d) STD complications
(e) the modes of HIV transmission and prevention.

Knowledge and attitudes regarding traditional healers' risk practices of transmitting HIV and towards condom use did not improve. Evidently the attitudes towards condom use may not have changed due to the conflict with the desire to have children. The objectives supporting persons living with HIV/AIDS and changing healers' practices were not measured in detail in the first analysis. However, of the traditional healers who reported seeing STD cases, 76 per cent reported integrating partner referral into their STD treatment.

Guinea

In 1979, the Ministry of Public Health and its Department of Traditional Medicine began to collaborate with traditional healers on primary health care in Guinea. In the 1990s, when the prevalence of HIV was still below 1.5 per cent among women in prenatal care, an initiative was aimed at identifying how traditional medicine could increase the effectiveness of the National AIDS Programme and answer the following questions:

(a) For what STDs are traditional healers consulted?
(b) How do traditional healers diagnose and treat STDs?

A survey implemented by the Department of Traditional Medicine and a research study completed by ORSTOM (Institut francais de recherche scientifique pour le developpement et cooperation) both indicated that gonorrhoea was the STD most frequently diagnosed by the traditional healers. The National AIDS Programme financed two training workshops for traditional healers with the objective of increasing knowledge about HIV/AIDS transmission and prevention, clinical manifestations of AIDS, and AIDS care. Further training could not continue due to lack of funding. The educational messages should be specifically designed to reinforce, and not to contradict, traditional concepts of disease and illness. The objectives were "to bring traditional healers as effective educators at the community level, to give quality treatment, and to refer in time for all conditions he/she cannot treat." In one district of the country, the AIDS office, in collaboration with healer associations, organized training sessions for healer association members. It was realized that healers could play a significant role in health education, promotion and distribution of condoms, treatment of opportunistic infections, early referral, and participation in research on AIDS and STDs. In addition, traditional healers are involved in other basic health care issues such as immunization, nutrition education and sanitation. The district also did significant research and documentation on plants used in STD and AIDS treatment by traditional healer.

Malawi

In the Chikwawa District of Malawi, which in 1996 had HIV seroprevalence of approximately 30.5 per cent among women in antenatal care clinics in major urban areas, a series of orientations and focus group discussions were held with groups of traditional healers. AIDS activities were initiated within an already established eye care programme with the following objectives:

(a) To better understand the practices and roles of healers in their communities;
(b) To promote greater communication between traditional healers and the 'formal' health sector;
(c) To educate traditional healers about HIV/AIDS and STD transmission and prevention;
(d) To encourage community-based HIV/AIDS prevention and care activities by traditional healers.

A baseline survey was conducted with 89 healer regarding their knowledge, attitudes, beliefs and practices surrounding AIDS. As a result a curriculum was developed for one-day workshops in 14 sites emphasizing community education and condom distribution. Healers were selected through 'recommendations from community leaders to participate in training sessions. A total of 352 healers were reached in the first of 2 training programmes. Six months after the first training, 61 healers were randomly selected for an evaluation of the training sessions. The evaluation found that 64 per cent of the healers had conducted AIDS educational sessions and 89 per cent had distributed condoms. Those conducting educational sessions were more likely to distribute condoms compared to those who were not involved in AIDS education. When traditional healers ran out of condoms, many did not seek out health centres to replenish their supply. Moreover, changing community and traditional healers' values about STDs is more challenging than changing those about AIDS. Though the aspect of collaboration was not formally evaluated, investigators suggest that more collaborative referral networks need to be encouraged.

Mozambique

In 1996, Mozambique had an official overall HIV prevalence of 5.8 per cent in major urban areas and 19.2 per cent outside of urban centres. As early as 1991, a three-year programme was initiated by the Ministry of Health's Department of Traditional Medicine with the objective of decreasing the spread of HIV by reducing the incidence of STDs through a collaborative effort with a local healer organization. Preliminary qualitative research on traditional healers' perceptions of STDs and AIDS revealed a strong belief that biomedical practitioners "do not understand the true cause of STDs." The survey also demonstrated that all traditional healers had heard of AIDS, had complete faith in their medicines, advised avoiding biomedicine for STDs, and believed a number of illnesses (but not AIDS) to be sexually transmitted. A training strategy was proposed whereby new concepts such as promoting condom use would be integrated into existing notions of protection, and traditional principles (such as discouraging sex outside marriage of promoting sexual abstinence during STD treatment) would be reinforced. Simultaneously old practices, such as traditional vaccination involving healer-to-patient or patient-to-patient blood contact, would be discouraged.

Based on this strategy, two one-week workshops were conducted for 30 healers in two provinces of the country, in 1991 and 1994. An assessment of the 1994 workshop included 70 per cent of the trained healers and eight patients of trained healers. The evaluation found that most traditional healers had learned about the sexual transmission of HIV, 75 per cent reported condom use as a way to avoid AIDS, and 81 per cent claimed to promote condoms with at least their STD patients. However, confusion remained as to the relationship between STDs, HIV and AIDS and about whether AIDS is curable.

South Africa

In South Africa, HIV seroprevalence has been rising rapidly in the past few years, reaching 15 per cent in 1997 among women in antenatal clinics in urban areas and 18 per cent in more rural antenatal clinics. Traditional medicine has remained an important component of health services, despite a high rate of modernization. A project was started in 1992 to train 27,000 traditional healers nationwide about AIDS in three successive cycles. The strategy was to train 30 healers as trainers, who would each train a second group of 30 healers, who would then repeat the cycle.

Eighteen of the trained traditional healers reported having trained 630 second-generation healers in different regions of the country seven months after the first training. A preliminary evaluation of this second generation focused on 70 trained healers selected from 10 geographically representative sites. Ninety per cent of them thought that the demonstration of correct condom use was the most useful aspect of the workshop. These healers had correctly retained basic information on gonorrhoea, HIV as an infectious agent, HIV symptoms, and modes of HIV transmission and prevention. Of 18 healers who said they had treated cases of AIDS, three mentioned giving advice and counselling to their clients without being prompted. When prompted, the other 15 described promoting positive attitudes about people with AIDS, or showing care and understanding as to the type of advice or counselling given, while eight mentioned advising on condom use. The assessment concluded that the first generation of trained traditional healers selected and trained their peers for the second cycle more effectively than the western-trained trainers of the first generation, as the traditional healers' selection was less politically directed and the training more culturally appropriate.

Uganda

HIV seroprevalence is at the peak in Uganda. In the early 1990s, two NGOs the Ministry of Health and the National AIDS Commission launched an initiative called Traditional and Modern Health Practitioners Together against AIDS (THETA). The objective was to develop a true collaboration between traditional healers and biomedical health providers in the area of treatment, care, support and prevention of STDs and AIDS. In 1992, the first THETA project attempted a collaborative clinical study to examine herbal treatments for HIV/AIDS symptoms for which few or no therapeutic options were available in the region. Healers were unwilling to discuss AIDS with their clients because they feared losing them with this terminal diagnosis. These challenges motivated a second project to empower traditional healers to provide STD/AIDS counselling and education. The project had a particular emphasis on the healers' women clients in Kampala, where the prevalence of HIV had levelled around 30 per cent in pregnant women at that time. HIV seroprevalence has since declined in Uganda - to a level of 14.7 per cent in antenatal clinics in major urban areas in 1997.

For this study, 48 Kampala healers were selected through home and clinic visits to answer a baseline questionnaire related to their knowledge, attitudes, beliefs and practices surrounding STDs and AIDS. Following this survey, 17 healers were recruited to participate in a 15-month 'training' programme including an average of three training days a month. The original training curriculum was developed in collaboration with The AIDS Support Organization (TASO) and with the input of both healers and community women. Content concentrated on STDs and AIDS, but also covered general topics such as cultural beliefs and practices, counselling, leadership, sexuality, gender, and legal issues.

Healers' overall performance was examined systematically using various indicators with each traditional healer, his/her clients and the community. Research methods included oral and written tests, regular visits to the healers' workplace, client follow-up interviews, and sessions in which a trainer observed a healer practising education or counselling. Each healer was found to have applied the training differently, some using their new skills for community education, others for counselling and/or initiating persons living with HIV/AIDS, youth or women's support groups. Community education by healers proved to be a very interactive process whereby traditional healers designed their own training materials, and developed and used unique approaches such as story-telling, personal testimonies from persons living with HIV/AIDS, music, dance, poetry and drama to convey their messages. A preliminary assessment was conducted one year after the end of the training programme, comparing three communities where healers had completed the THETA curriculum with one community where traditional healers had not been trained. The community members with trained healers demonstrated increased knowledge about HIV/AIDS and reported increased condom use (50 per cent versus 17 per cent where the traditional healer was not trained) and reduced risk behaviour.

Healers' counselling was examined by interviewing 180 women clients consulting for HIV symptoms, STDs, or 'love' problems, with nine trained healers and following them up three and six months later. The proportions of women who reported having both received counselling from their healer (45 to 72 per cent) and been tested for HIV (46 to 64 per cent) had risen significantly by the second follow-up. During counselling, women said healers discussed facts about AIDS, positive living, condom use, and had demonstrated and offered condoms. Condom knowledge, attitudes and use were found to significantly increase over time among these women, as did condom negotiation by women with their sex partners. However, at six months, eight out of 39 (21 per cent) women still said that one could tell someone had AIDS by "pale skin or eyes". Finally, three of the trained healers spontaneously initiated the formation of 'persons living with HIV/AIDS' support groups for their clients, some of whom achieved local renown for their educational songs, drama and dance on AIDS. Based on these results, the THETA initiative has been expanded to six rural districts of Uganda. A participatory examination of THETA conducted in 1997-98 demonstrated that:

(a) 125 healers were trained in the first five districts selected;
(b) 60 per cent of trained traditional healers reported distributing condoms;
(c) 80 per cent of trained traditional healers reported counselling patients;
(d) 82 per cent of trained traditional healers reported giving AIDS community education;
(e) cross-referral of patients increased, with 97 per cent of trained healers referring patients.

Other benefits of training included: better hygiene, initiation of record keeping, decreased fees, initiation of patient support groups and improved collaboration with biomedicine. THETA conducts, clinical activities and has initiated the creation of a resource centre for traditional medicine and AIDS. Clinical activities have included a study assessing herbal treatments of traditional healers for specific HIV-related symptoms, and training for traditional healers on primary clinical diagnosis. The resource centre contains a library with material on traditional medicine and AIDS, and has produced two videos and a newsletter that comes out three times a year. It also conducts a monthly speakers' bureau where topics relevant to traditional 'medicine and AIDS are discussed and debated among practitioners of traditional medicine and biomedicine, as well as patients of both systems.

United Republic of Tanzania

HIV seroprevalence reached 13.7 per cent in 1996 in antenatal clinics in urban centres in the United Republic of Tanzania. In 1989, the impact of HIV motivated collaboration between traditional and biomedical health workers in the Tanga region of north-eastern Tanzania. A spirit of mutual respect was established, and experiences were shared on care and prevention of HIV/

AIDS as well as other mostly infectious diseases. Due to the enthusiasm of both sides of the partnership, the collaboration spread to the rest of the region, influencing the formation of the Tanga AIDS Working Group (TAWG) in 1992. The important objective of the organization was to stop the spread of HIV and other STDs and to reduce the impact of the disease in the region. With the assistance of existing village health projects and sensitization meetings with local leaders and the community, TAWG has been collaborating with about 120 traditional healers in two districts of Muheza and Pangani. Training of traditional healers consisted primary information about STDs, HIV and AIDS, and information on AIDS counselling and care, condom promotion and community behaviour change. Traditional healers were trained in hygiene and sterile procedures for their equipment. Field supervision and monitoring followed training. The results reported by TAWG demonstrated that 60 traditional healers and 60 traditional birth attendants have been trained and have:

(a) conducted home visits to 237 persons living with HIV/AIDS
(b) made 1,600 referrals for HIV testing
(c) made 5,400 referrals of biomedical health workers to TAWG for counselling
(d) organized 1,241 educational sessions reaching more than 19290 people
(e) promoted and sold condoms.

TAWG makes the following recommendations:

(a) Sensitization of biomedical and traditional health practitioners, as well as community leadership, is essential for setting up mutual trust and understanding of roles and expectations among the key players.
(b) Specific training on STDs and AIDS for particular groups, such as biomedical and traditional practitioners, is essential not only in imparting badly needed information and skills associated with their practice, but also to improve their confidence.
(c) The existence of local medicines for treatment of opportunistic infections provides a basic ingredient in home-based care services provided by counsellors.

(d) Involvement of traditional healers in identifying community needs for AIDS education leads to culturally grounded messages that are relevant, culturally sensitive and have the best potential for influencing behaviour change.

Zambia

HIV prevalence in Zambia is now one of the highest in the world, and was approximated at around 26.5 per cent in Lusaka. In 1978, the Ministry of Health designed a workshop to train healers about AIDS, which 40 healers attended. It was evident that their knowledge about HIV transmission, and their attitudes about people living with HIV and AIDS improved after the workshop. However 43 per cent of traditional healers still were of the opinion that abortion could cause AIDS.

HIV prevention activities with traditional healers were not followed up until 1994 and a training programme for STD/AIDS was developed for traditional healers. This consisted of three-day workshops and emphasized follow-up through healers trained in community education. In 18 months, the project trained about 2000 traditional healers in primary information on STDs and HIV/AIDS and 120 in community education. The curriculum, adapted from the THETA Uganda project with Zambian traditional healers' input, included STD/AIDS transmission and prevention, HIV testing, and condom social marketing. Traditional healers trained in community education, together with health centre staff, led monthly follow-up meetings. Mid-term survey results demonstrated that trained traditional healers scored significantly better than non-trained traditional healers on 13 of 17 impact measures, including knowledge about HIV transmission and prevention, advice for persons living with HIV/AIDS, and condom use. At the time of the mid-term review, 250 trained healers reported selling condoms to patients and community members through a social marketing programme. Trained traditional healers were also more likely to have discussed with their clients HIV and STD prevention, HIV testing, condom use and caring for persons living with HIV/AIDS. Most traditional healers' patients interviewed established that their trained traditional healers had taught them primary facts about AIDS, but they demonstrated poor knowledge about how HIV is not spread, HIV testing, the difference between HIV and AIDS, and AIDS symptoms.

Conclusion

Although advocacy for traditional medicine and attempts to involve traditional healers in primary health care had been undertaken well before the advent of AIDS in several African countries, there are still some collaborative efforts between traditional healers and biomedical health providers for HIV/AIDS prevention or care in Africa. It has been confirmed that there continues to be great enthusiasm on the part of traditional healers to collaborate with their western-trained counterparts and learn from them about STDs and HIV/AIDS. Experiences across countries demonstrate that modern and traditional belief systems are not incompatible but complementary. And if we accept with Green that, "traditional healers (in Africa) are unlikely to leave their way of interpreting STDs and other diseases as a result of any education directly with the prevalent beliefs", then collaboration can generate understanding and respect for both cosmologies so that they become harmonizing, and the interpretations healers make of them are beneficial for their communities infected by HIV. Once a common language is setup, it is possible to design, plan, implement and examine a collaborative project, as long as traditional healers' opinions and concepts are included.

Many programmes examined here have used a strategy whereby a core group of traditional healers is trained as trainers for periods ranging from one day to 15 months. These traditional healers are then encouraged to educate communities and/or train their peers. Some projects have also supported traditional healers in developing educational materials, condom social marketing, or giving basic counselling. Counselling may be one of the most essential services traditional healers have traditionally offered to their communities; since the AIDS epidemic, counselling has been an integral component of both STD/AIDS prevention and care strategies promoted globally. Counselling offers a bridge between prevention and care projects. Yet, only some of the projects examined above have reported on the effect of training traditional healers in counselling skills for STDs and AIDS. And the information available in these reports is still too limited to compare the elements involved in the counselling components of the training.

Basic assessments of some projects have established that 'trained' traditional healers quickly assimilate the new knowledge and 'integrate' it into their practices and the messages they deliver to communities, misconceptions remain, after short-term training. Few projects have planned, or have had the means, to systematically follow up healers after their initial 'training'. Yet, it is significant to provide longterm support to healers because, traditional healers can encounter significant difficulties in dealing with the issues of condom use, care and support, and death and dying elicited by AIDS. How can healers give their clients a diagnosis of AIDS when it means possibly losing their business? How can a traditional healer - the traditional advocate of the clan's fertility—counsel an HIV- positive woman who wants to have a child? And how can a traditional healer turn away a sick patient who has become dependent on his or her care and support? The THETA Uganda initiative indicates that, healers who have been regularly supported after training have sustained and even increased their STD/AIDS programmes in the community longer and more intensively than those who only participated in training.

Critical evaluations would be vital not only to assess the effectiveness of these strategies but also to examine the determinants of their success, or failure. For example, many projects discovered that traditional healers did carry out the educational and counselling activities they were 'trained' for, but some documents the content of these activities and discover how they impact on traditional healers' clients and communities. Not one evaluation included measures of cost-effectiveness of the programme. Systematic, more in-depth and longer-term evaluations would also assist answer the question of sustainability of traditional healers' involvement in HIV/AIDS prevention and care.

Biomedicine and traditional African medicine are based on concepts, languages and cultural constructs that are too distant for a simple mixing to automatically achieve positive results. Even when traditional or modern health concepts are translated in an attempt to bridge the gap between the two medical worlds, the lack of solid evaluations, together with a still-pervading scepticism among biomedical health providers against 'unscientific' approaches, cause collaborations to enter a vicious circle whereby the lack of statistics justifies the lack of funding, and vice versa. Yet, despite these difficulties, the projects examined here highlight that traditional healers are capable of performing their biomedical counterparts in their new roles as AIDS educators and counsellors.

Evaluation

Very few projects on traditional medicine and AIDS reviewed in the present discussion have been assessed thoroughly for effectiveness. Effectiveness is an activity's complete success in producing desired results and reaching overall objectives. Thus, to identify a project's effectiveness, there is needs to know objectives and outcomes, as well as what changed during the time the activity was implemented and why the change occurred.

Some projects aimed simply to train healers and evaluated their effectiveness by the number of healers trained and the information understood by healers. Others aimed to train traditional healers to reach fellow-healers, or the community served by healers, with AIDS information. Other projects aimed to change the sexual practices of healers' clients or community members. An objective of many projects was to enhance collaboration between traditional healers and their biomedical counterparts. Measures of effectiveness in each of these case included numbers of healers or community members trained by trained healers, behaviour change among healers' clients and/or community members, and collaboration indicators such as referral between healers and biomedical health facilities or links built between healers and health structures.

A significant increase in knowledge among trained healers regarding symptoms of HIV disease, HIV transmission and prevention and whether or not AIDS was curable was noted. One project in South Africa reported an increase in positive attitude about AIDS.

Other effectiveness measures consisted detailing how much of the information trained healers passed on to fellow-healers or clients and community members. In Botswana, healers trained in a two-week 'peer education' programme not only recalled information they learned two years after training, but they claimed to be training fellow-healers and community members as well. In Mozambique, South Africa, and Uganda, evaluation demonstrated that traditional healers were counselling clients in HIV/AIDS prevention and care. In Malawi, Uganda and the United Republic of Tanzania, trained healers were reported to be giving dynamic AIDS education, some using drama, song, and dance and many developing their own training materials.

Traditional healers were reported to be active condom promoters and distributors. Even after one-day training sessions, healers in Malawi reported having open discussions about condoms, and female traditional healers reported distributing condoms as frequently as male traditional healers.

The objective of increasing collaboration between the two health systems can be difficult to measure and some statistics were available. Projects reported increasing patient referral from healer to health centres, and strong links with local hospitals. In Uganda, healers have participated in policy-making bodies such as the National Drug Authority.

Even though most projects showed signs of at least short-term effectiveness, few completed comprehensive evaluations of long-term impact on traditional healers and/or communities. For this reason, it is difficult to assess whether they meet the best practice criteria for effectiveness. To do so, future projects should use indicators and tools to address and evaluate the issues.

Ethical soundness is measured as per principles of appropriate and acceptable social and professional conduct. Important concepts to be considered as regards ethical soundness include: confidentiality, mutual respect, community and government participation, and informed consent.

Measures of ethical soundness adopted by many of the eight projects evaluated here included setting up of a climate of mutual respect between traditional healers and biomedical health practitioners, signing agreements or working closely with hospitals or the Ministry of Health, and ensuring confidentiality of patients. Most projects had some connection with the Ministry of Health, but only two of them reported that they informed traditional healers and their communities of the projects' results (i.e., provided feedback). The Malawi project specifically addressed issues related to the negative or positive images relayed in awareness messages. Some projects also paid special attention to tailoring their messages to fit the understanding of traditional healers, or to strengthening resources in disadvantaged communities.

Two issues of particular concern to traditional medicine projects are: (1) whether any patients experience harmful effects because of traditional methods or treatments; and (2) respect of the proprietary rights of traditional healers over their herbal preparations. Nobody reported any harmful effects of herbal remedies and only one project discussed the measures in place to protect healers' rights over their treatments.

Ethical soundness issues were not necessarily addressed as part of a systematic plan, but rather out of concern and respect for traditional healers, their clients and communities.

Interest in efficiency has grown in recent years with the realization that resources are meagre and need to be used in the most cost-effective manner. The basic meaning of efficiency is the ability to produce the desired results with a minimum expenditure of energy, time, or resources. There are many economic evaluation techniques associated with measuring cost-effectiveness, but they all assist knowing the costs involved in project implementation and concrete measures of effectiveness. Measurement of efficiency included:

(a) cost of training per healer and per client or community member reached;
(b) number of traditional healers' clients and community members reached by healer initiatives (community AIDS education, drama, counselling);
(c) number of persons living with HIV/AIDS reached during home-care visits;
(d) number of fellow healers trained by trained traditional healers;
(e) financial control;

(f) regularity of activity and financial reports.

In the three projects that reported on cost of training, the figures varied, but not significantly. In Zambia, training costs were US$35 per day per traditional healer, in Botswana US$22, and in Uganda US$20. Figure available demonstrate that healers are able to attract large numbers of people to their community AIDS events, which translates into very large numbers of people reached for education, once healers are trained. The Tanzania AIDS Working Group estimated that, in three years, some 27,000 community members were reached in educational sessions, 4,300 persons living with HIV/AIDS in home visits and 450,000 people in drama groups. THETA Uganda estimates that it reaches between 150,000 and 400,000 beneficiaries annually (thus between 450,000 and 1,200,000 in three years). In comparison, another AIDS educational strategy in Uganda - the AIDS education through Imams initiative - reveals that they have reached 100,000 home in five years-a similar level. The cost per beneficiary was only available for THETA Uganda, where it was estimated to be between US$0.24 and US$0.71 annually.

One analysis in Botswana estimated that 30 per cent of persons living with HIV/AIDS would be admitted to a hospital during of their illness. Each user would average one re-admission, with each stay averaging 8.2 days and costing US$42 each day. Without home- or healer-based care, hospital treatment would cost US$241 per person living with HIV/AIDS.

Indicators that efficiency issues were being addressed included the prevalence of reporting and control of finances and administration. At THETA Uganda, accounts are audited annually and activity and financial reports are produced quarterly. Financial administration is tightly controlled. More details on finances and administration were difficult to acquire for other projects.

In-depth cost-effectiveness analysis would therefore necessitate specific evaluations whereby projects would be visited. Some project leaders did not have the expertise, resources or time to prioritize cost-effectiveness analysis. Ideally, efficiency evaluation should be planned for, budgeted and supported by funders from the very initial phase of project design.

Sustainability can be seen as the ability of a programme to

carry on with a certain degree of autonomy and to continue being effective over the medium-to-long term. Sustainability was assessed by finding out whether the information and skills passed on to healers were taken into consideration, and whether these skills were used over time. For example, an assessment was made of whether healers were continuing to practise counselling, condom distribution, and community AIDS education, and whether they were still collaborating with biomedical health practitioners.

An attempt to ensure sustainability by building relations with health structures has been made so that traditional healers could continue to receive support for their educational activities - including condoms for distribution - after completion of the intervention. None of the projects reported paying healers' salaries, but they often reimbursed expenses such as transportation costs to reach training sites. Many projects assumed that even if project activities were to officially end, healers had gained sufficient information and skills to continue to use that information in their practices. It has been demonstrated that healers recalled information imparted in training and that they claimed to be still using it through counselling and by educating clients and communities, as well as referring patients to hospitals and clinics. The South African healers who were trained by fellow-healers realised that they were ready to train a third generation of healers, but some of them preferred to have the assistance of a project facilitator during training. Project design generally included information in their curricula, but often failed to recognize the importance of incorporating into training the necessary skill-building sessions that would enable traditional healers to educate fellow-healers.

The healers continued to give education sessions in their communities and even started formal training of fellow-healers on their own initiative. Though THETA is no longer training the same healers it trained earlier, it is available to act as a guarantor for traditional healers' fundraising, or to facilitate occasional workshops organized by healers.

Sustainability is one of the most challenging issues facing HIV prevention efforts in general, and traditional medicine collaborative projects are no exception. One major problem is the definition and importance of sustainability given by different funders. It has been extremely difficult to remain active or to follow up with participating traditional healers over the long term, even though traditional healers remain active independently. A more systematic and standardized approach to sustainability is desirable in order to design long-term projects and measure their impact over time.

It has been formally recognized that, for developing countries, it is imperative to include traditional healers in primary health care. As discussed earlier, since the early 1990s, the same has been agreed upon for AIDS, especially in sub-Saharan Africa, where ministries of health cannot pay for adequate helath care services. Besides the debilitating direct and indirect costs associated with AIDS in many countries make the prospect of cooperating with traditional healers all the more appealing. In general, the basic fact underlying this approach is that African healers are accessible, affordable, and culturally appropriate and acceptable, thereby fulfilling the major criteria for low-cost, effective health care service delivery in most sub-Saharan African settings. Thus, the relevance of the overall approach of working with healers will be taken as a given, instead, it is the relevance of specific strategies that will be assessed.

Relevance is about how closely a project is focused on the HIV/AIDS response in the context of the society in which it is implemented. Issues such as cultural and political factors are generally considered. The emphasis was placed on how appropriate the particular strategy was to the HIV/AIDS situation and how the objectives related to the prevalence of HIV, needs assessments and the priorities of the National AIDS Programme. For instance, countries with a mature epidemic should combine prevention with counselling and care.

In the projects reviewed objectives were defined following baseline research with traditional healer, carried out either through surveys or focus group discussions. In only a few projects was it mentioned that needs were assessed as per the larger political context - specifically with reference to the AIDS epidemiology - or the surrounding community needs. However, in almost all the countries in this review, the prevalence of HIV was already high when the projects were initiated. The differences in political will to work with traditional healers between countries can play a significant role in the overall success of this type of collaborative project.

THETA Uganda may be the only project that conducted needs assessment in communities surrounding the traditional healers. It was disclosed their objective were directly based on National AIDS Programme priorities. The Malawi project reported that its objectives changed as the AIDS situation did. In the Central African Republic, it was noted that the content of the training curriculum was relevant to all types of healers trained, as the magnitude of knowledge and attitude change was not related to traditional healers' characteristics.

Measures of relevance therefore varied widely in the different contexts of evaluation. Where the relevance of involving traditional healers in HIV/AIDS control efforts is no longer in question, it is essential that the objectives and strategies be appropriate for a given context. This will have a considerable impact on effectiveness.

Additional Criteria

In addition to the general criteria used to assess a wide variety of AIDS-related projects, the following are considerations which apply specifically to collaborative projects between traditional medicine and biomedicine.

Due to the lack of regulatory bodies for traditional healers in most countries, selection of 'genuine' or 'authentic' healers can be a challenge for most new projects. In general, the projects generally consulted community leaders, traditional healer associations and the ministries in charge of traditional healer activities for approval and for recommendations of genuine or authentic healers. Many project leaders commented on the extensive time needed to select genuine traditional healers who were truly interested in collaboration.

In Senegal, criteria for selection were initially based on healers' reputations. The selection was enhanced by the use of children, considered innocent and unbiased. They were asked to which healer in their community they would refer someone with an ailment. In South Africa, the project first contacted five traditional healers' associations to select healers for training. However, in the second round of training, it was discovered that the trained healers were much more effective at selecting genuine healers than the traditional healers' associations were. Other initiatives also noted that it was preferable to avoid traditional healers' associations, as the internal politics of these associations can sometimes interfere with selection, training, or other project objectives. Such was the case in Uganda, where the criteria for traditional healers' selection used by THETA are the following:

(a) being recognized as healers by the community and local authorities;
(b) having regular patient attendance;
(c) having a clinic or shrine to receive and treat patients;
(d) knowing how to prepare herbal remedies.

Discussion, interviews and listening to traditional healers' needs were the most common methods used for building trust with traditional healers, and it was agreed that doing this gradually, without rushing the traditional healers, was important.

In Uganda, explicit recognition of healers' rights to their treatment secrets was emphasized in order to help gain trust in setting up the initial collaborative clinical research on herbal treatments for opportunistic infections. In both the United Republic of Tanzania and Uganda, a series of workshops were held after initial contacts to share ideas between representatives of the two health care systems. Other initiatives used repeated visits to healers' home/clinics or focus group discussions as a way of establishing trust.

Training Methods

With regard to content of training, most initiatives have had little difficulty with issues around AIDS symptoms, HIV transmission and prevention, condom use, condom promotion and distribution. The areas that provided the biggest barriers were home care, death and dying, mother-to-child HIV transmission and, in the Central African Republic, condom use, which is linked to a high desire to have children.

Collaboration

Healers in Uganda and the United Republic of Tanzania have been given access to hospitals, which has motivated them greatly. One project leader in the United Republic of Tanzania suggested setting up a cooperative relationship with a hospital or clinic to facilitate collaboration. THETA Uganda leaders noted as well that developing a lasting collaboration between the two health systems involves much effort on both sides of the collaborative relationship. Collaborative project designs cannot emphasize only the efforts required by healers and assume that the biomedical health workers will follow without as much time and energy input. In Malawi, similar lessons were noted, and it was suggested that more collaborative referral networks need to be encouraged between traditional healers and the formal health sector. It may be that what is needed is simply a change of attitude within the biomedical health structures and among personnel. The key is a true dialogue. Finally, THETA has suggested that the type of collaboration they have created in Uganda could be extended nationwide if emphasis were placed on building strong links at the community level with local leaders, health authorities, government and nongovernmental key players. These links ensure sustainability, reduce programme costs and increase healer recognition in their own communities.

Project Implementation

Collaboration has yield valuable public benefits. As longer-term projects have revealed, it is often not until after training that trained healers devise innovative initiatives for HIV prevention. For example, in Mozambique, it was noted that some trained traditional healers shared the information they gained from one workshop with other healers in their traditional healers' association. This may be evidence that the training was valued enough that some healers expanded the training without asking for resources. It is therefore critical to plan and secure funding for long-term monitoring, evaluation and follow-up of collaborative projects.

Given the changing epidemic and the dynamic relationship between the two health sectors, this issue becomes even more crucial if we are to take advantage of, and learn from, this exploratory field.

Research and Development (R & D)

More systematic evaluation of collaborative projects is urgently needed, especially to find out determinants of success and/or failure. Since many of these projects are still in an experimental phase, the statistics could be used to improve existing endeavours and help develop new ones. A multiplicity of variables needs to be examines and it is only with systematic and repeated evaluations, using a variety of methods, that we can hope to answer some of the crucial questions we are faced with. There is a dearth of rigorous, long-term measures of effectiveness and sustainability. Of particular interest is the question of cost-effectiveness; not one of the projects reviewed here officially reported on the efficiency of training with respect to cost-effectiveness. Without cost-effectiveness data it is easier for funding agencies to deny the usefulness of such projects.

Research, not only into the methods that traditional healers practise and the impact of training projects, but also into the relationship between the traditional and biomedical health care systems, is crucial if we hope to answer questions about collaboration between the two systems. Interesting questions, such as how each health system influences the other, and how the relationship could be mutually beneficial, deserve an in-depth analysis in order to build a sustainable link between the two sectors.

With greater emphasis on home care, it is possible that traditional healers may act as a critical link in the continuum of care from hospital to home. Research into the healer approach to care is another neglected area of research that shows great potential. In particular, a deep examination of the counselling provided by traditional healers, and how they integrate biomedical concepts into their traditional belief system and methods of practice, is still untouched by research. But it is crucial to our understanding of the impact traditional healers could have in both care and prevention of STDs and HIV/AIDS.

In the continuing struggle to provide comprehensive health care to a wider population, research into the role of traditional healers may lead to the development of innovative new strategies. For example, since the mid-1990s traditional healers have played a significant role in the promotion of condoms in a few countries in Africa. It is thus possible for them to play a role in providing greater access to other health care options such as family planning. This area has been looked at in some countries for basic health care, but has not been expanded to other areas of health or assessed on a large scale. The objective of maximizing availability of drugs in poor countries makes research on herbal medicine especially important today.

The question of standardization and regulation of traditional medicine training and traditional healers' practice has been discussed with respect to creating national policies. Consensus has not yet been reached, but the issues are complex as recognition often depends on organization of traditional healers. There is a danger that regulation and standardization of traditional healers' practices will cause a huge loss within these practices. However, many traditional healers are still interested in recognition by the biomedical structure and welcome official policy changes to this end.

Collaborative projects have much to learn from each other. An improved system of communication among traditional healers, as well as within and between countries, would be useful. Regular meetings and networking would benefit not only the projects concerned but their beneficiaries as well.

Four

AIDS Information Centre (AIC): Uganda

Introduction

A wide range of HIV/AIDS education and awareness programmes in Uganda since 1986 have resulted in many Ugandans asking the question: Am I infected? and a growing demand for HIV testing. Before the start of AIC, there were few HIV testing services in Uganda and almost none with associated counselling programmes. Recently an enormous burden was placed on the national blood bank where many Ugandans interested in knowing their sero-status went to donate blood. The blood bank was not able to give supportive counselling, and donating blood for the purpose of learning one's sero-status was an expensive misuse of blood banking services. In response to the growing demand for testing, several organizations allianced themselves to discuss the need for anonymous and voluntary counselling and testing services in Uganda. These organizations included: the Ministry of Health's AIDS Control Programme, Nakasero Blood Bank, Uganda Virus Research Institute (UVRI), TASO, USAID, InterAid, World Learning, Inc., Uganda Red Cross, Makerere University Faculty of Social Science, and the World Health Organization (WHO). The outcome of these collaborative discussions was the opening of AIC, in February 1990, under the direction of the late Lydia Barugahare, a Ugandan nurse trained in the United Kingdom.

Offering Ugandans an HIV counselling and testing service distinct from the national blood bank had a large positive impact. From 1989 to 1995 the amount of blood given by volunteer donors at Nakasero increased by over 400 per cent while the rate of HIV found in donations fell from 14 to 2 per cent.

In the beginning AIC offered services in Kampala, the capital city, through a main office in a downtown office building and several satellite sites in the Kampala area. Clients received Voluntary Counselling and Testing (VCT) over the course of two visits, receiving test outcomes after two weeks. In its first 11 months operation, AIC provided VCT to more than 9000 clients. This well surpassed the target of 5000 clients expected in the first year and confirmed the strong interest in VCT, which has continued up to the present. In eight years, AIC has grown from a single office with four staff into a multifaceted centre with four branches employing more than 80 persons. Since 1990 AIC has served over 380000 clients. In 1997, AIC merged its Kampala operations and opened its new headquarters in Kisenyi, an impoverished neighbourhood near the largest public transportation hub and Kampala's largest outdoor market.

By 1993, district branches were opened in Jinja, the industrial belt of Uganda, Mbarara, the largest city in the western region, and Mbale, near the Kenya border. Demand rose sharply from 1990 to 1993, and fell slightly in 1994. Large client numbers early on were partly a result of the several satellite that AIC operated. Owing to high operational costs, satellite services were halted and the total numbers coming to AIC declined, stabilizing at about 40000 per annum. Demand has increased in 1998.

Satellite Services

To serve Ugandans living in peri-urban and rural areas, AIC started operating satellite sites in 1992. These sites were in various locations, including health centres, community centres and churches. AIC counsellors and phlebotomists travelled to these sites either once a week, bi-weekly or monthly. Blood samples were sent back to Kampala for testing with counsellors returning to the site, with test results, two to four weeks later. By 1995, 20 satellite sites were operating. Although this worked well in some areas, there were many problems with the approach. Some sites had low numbers of clients with high costs of transporting staff, leading to high expenses per person served. Overall, the problem with satellite sites was one of logistics. Blood samples were sent from a satellite site to an AIC Branch, to AIC Headquarters, then to the Blood Bank. HIV test results were then taken from the Blood Bank to Headquarters for data entry, to the AIC Branch, then back to the satellite site. Due to the complexity of the routing, it was not easy for a client to return to a satellite site only to find that their test results were not ready. Since few if any rural clients have telephones, it was not possible to notify these clients in advance. Thus, some clients took unnecessary long walks or expensive trips and were too discouraged to return a third time. This experience revealed that affordable VCT for rural clients necessitated a decentralized approach with counselling and testing done locally, with same-day results.

Increasing Availability of VCT

AIC worked with health officials in 16 districts to address the sustainability of VCT and the necessity for integrated services. The result was an AIC expansion strategy that consisted integration of VCT into prevailing health facilities, at the district level, and technical assistance and training for district personnel. Due to this AIC introduced a pilot protocol for testing with same-day results, as well as procurement and distribution of test kits, support supervision, monitoring and evaluation. The expansion strategy required that AIC reorganize itself to provide adequate capacity for managing both the main branch and indirect sites. Collaboration was sought with district medical and political authorities and Memoranda of Understanding were signed. The steps of expansion included: needs assessment, site selection, personnel training, establishing the VCT facilities (in district hospitals and health centres), assessment of performance and phase-out. By 1998, 35 VCT sites were operating at hospitals and health centres, and more than 5000 clients had received VCT.

Present Contribution

The important objective of AIC is to contribute to the national efforts to prevent further spread of HIV infection, to enhance the psychosocial adjustment of those already infected, and to promote the adoption of healthy lifestyles. AIC currently offers:

(a) voluntary and anonymous HIV counselling and testing,

(b) rapid syphilis testing and on-site treatment for those testing positive,
(c) syndromic diagnosis and management of other STDs,
(d) condom education and distribution,
(e) information about family planning and FP counselling and commodities,
(f) TB education and referral,
(g) psychosocial and medical services,
(h) food supplementation and peer support,
(i) special services for discordant couples, and
(j) the Philly Lutaaya Initiative, with HIV-positive clients "going public" to advocate for VCT and behavioural change.

AIC also offers various training services to other organizations and health care providers in districts where AIC does not have a branch. AIC trains health workers in HIV test counselling, integrated HIV/STD/family planning counselling, the use of rapid tests for quick results, and record keeping. AIC extends its monitoring and support supervision to non-AIC sites offering VCT, and supplies a limited number of test kits to selected sites. Community mobilization and referral in districts without AIC branches are supported through outreach activities such as the Philly Lutaaya Initiative. The collection and evaluation of statistics and a number of research projects, are an important part of AIC's activities. Hundreds of professional and international visitors visit AIC every year to learn about AIC services while AIC representatives make frequent presentations at international conferences.

Who Comes to AIC and Why?

Demographic characteristics and HIV rates in clients

Demography

In AIC's first year of operation, the gender distribution was skewed, with 66 per cent of clients being male. With time, the number of women increased and in 1997, 49 per cent of AIC Kampala clients were female. In sites outside Kampala the numbers remain slightly skewed, with females constituting 44 per cent clients in Mbale, 45 per cent in Jinja and 47 per cent in Mbarara.

Overall, 47 per cent clients are women. An eight-year trend at AIC demonstrates that women clients are more likely to be HIV-infected than male clients.

About half of AIC's clients are young people between the ages of 20 and 29 years. This trend has been consistent over time, and is identical at all AIC sites. Infection rates vary considerably by age with older clients being more vulnerable. In 1997, there was a consistent pattern that women were more vulnerable than men in all age groups.

AIC functions in the four main cities of Uganda, which probably contributes to the high rates of education among AIC clients. In 1997, 57 per cent of AIC clients had some secondary or post-secondary education; only 7 per cent reported no education. This distribution was similar in all sites. Clients with at least secondary education ranged from a high of 63 per cent in Mbale to a low of 46 per cent in Mbarara. The Mbarara branch served the highest percentage of clients with no education (12 per cent). Other sites ranged from 3 to 9 per cent for clients with no education. A consistent pattern witnessed among AIC clients has been that clients with little or no education are more vulnerable than those with more education.

About half of AIC clients are single, many of them coming for testing before marriage or before starting a sexual relationship with a new partner. Most single clients are also young. Single clients are much less likely to be vulnerable than other clients. Those who are divorced, separated or widowed have higher vulnerability rates than those who report that they are at present married. Clients served at health centres and hospitals are more likely to be sero-positive because they have often been referred by their doctors for confirmation of a clinical diagnosis of AIDS.

The Visitors

Clients come to AIC for a broad variety of reasons. Interest in VCT is often "social", with clients demonstrating interest in knowing their sero-status before getting married, embarking on a new relationship, or making plans for the future. Pre-marital testing has increased over time and no doubt narrates the increasing percentage of couples who come together. "Medical" reasons for

VCT, such as feeling ill or having symptoms of AIDS, are stated less frequently. Although rarely mentioned in AIC's early years, 5 per cent of AIC clients in 1997 mentioned pregnancy as a reason for requesting VCT. Some of these clients wanted to know their sero-status before becoming pregnant; others were already pregnant. Recent revelations that short-course zidovudine (AZT) treatment can reduce mother-to-child HIV transmission, and that such treatment may become available in Uganda on broader basis, have been well reported in Uganda's press and may explain the recent increase in mentioning pregnancy when requesting VCT. Infection rates among clients vary widely depending on the reason for requesting VCT. Those who come for pre-marital testing have the lowest rates, at 5 per cent for males and 7 per cent for females. Those who want to use HIV test results to help them plan for the future have a little higher rates, as do those who report than they are worried or fear they have been exposed.

AIC provides VCT to about 130 clients daily in four sites in Uganda. More than 50 per cent of AIC's clients are served at the main branch in Kampala. The original AIC protocol (1990-97) consisted two client visits. In the first visit, called "pretest counselling", clients received a general orientation to HIV/AIDS, HIV tests and their meaning, counselling designed to assist clients decide whether or not to be tested, and counselling about how to prevent HIV transmission. At the end of pre-test counselling, clients had their blood drawn and were asked to return in two weeks for test results. In the second visit, clients received "post-test counselling", learned their test results, received additional counselling and referral to other services such as the Post Test Club, TASO, and other AIDS support organizations.

On average, 25 per cent of clients failed to receive their test results, either by not returning for the second visit or by returning but being discouraged when results were not ready. As rapid testing became more accurate, AIC decided to carry out trials to find out whether the laboratory protocol and the counselling protocol could be changed such that clients could receive counselling and HIV results simultaneously on the same day. Trials in 1995 and 1996 demonstrated that same-day services were popular among clients, preferred by staff, and feasible to implement, even at rural sites. As a result, the rapid testing and same-day protocol was implemented in 1997.

At present, clients come at AIC and are directed to the reception area where they are met by a receptionist. Here they help fill-out the top section of an AIC Counselling and Testing Card with brief demographic information. Each client is given a code number and information is collected such that client privacy is insured while simultaneously impostors can be prevented from seeing client records at later dates. Information on Testing Cards helps counsellors acquaint themselves with clients and support AIC data analysis and research. When the top section of the Testing Card is complete, the receptionist gives the client the tear-off strip at the bottom bearing the client code number and asks the client to take a seat in the waiting room until a counsellor is ready. In the waiting room, HIV/AIDS education brochures are available for reading, health education posters decorate the walls, and several HIV/AIDS and other locally produced health education videos are shown. In Kampala, the busiest site, clients wait an average of 20 to 30 minutes before joining a counsellor. At other locations, clients wait only a few minutes. VCT clients participate in a four-step process:

(a) test decision and orientation,
(b) phlebotomy,
(c) prevention counselling, and
(d) test results counselling.

The process includes group and/or one-on-one sessions with a counsellor. If particular clients or couples prefer not to participate in group counselling, they can request all services on a one-on-one basis. The entire process takes two to three hours.

Special Challenges in VCT

AIC clients are either served as individuals or couples. Routine statistics collected from clients since 1992 demonstrates an increase in the proportion of clients being served as couples, from 9 per cent in 1992 to over 26 per cent in 1997. AIC believes this is a positive sign. Couples are one of the most important targets for VCT, and adoption of risk reduction behaviour is often enhanced when couples receive both test results and prevention counselling together. The critical evaluation of HIV infection rates in couples reveals many interesting patterns. Overall, clients who come as couples have much lower rates of HIV infection than those who come as individuals. Among couples who are already married, AIC statistics reveal that 18 per cent of married couples are discordant and 15 per cent of married couples are both HIV-infected. AIC counsellors find it difficult to explain discordant results to couples who had been having unprotected sex. Counsellors also find it difficult to explain HIV-negative results to couples who are indulged in high-risk behaviour outside their marriage. In an effort to answer these perplexing questions, AIC embarked on research to learn more about discordant couples and high-risk negative couples, and how best to serve them. The 12-month research project is studying issues related to variability in transmission rates. Findings will be available in late 1999.

Recent research from Thailand has discovered that a short course of AZT during the last three weeks of pregnancy and during labour and delivery can largely reduce the probability that a baby will become infected with HIV. These revelations have been reported in Uganda's print media and there is at present increasing interest among pregnant women to get tested and, if positive, try to get access to AZT treatment. UNAIDS and UNICEF are now developing pilot programmes in Uganda to make AZT treatment in pregnancy available. As this is likely to affect the demand for VCT among pregnant women, AIC counsellors are now being trained in issues related to VCT during pregnancy.

Uptill 1997, blood was drawn from AIC clients "on-site" and testing was done "off-site" at the Nakasero Blood Bank (NBB). Standard ELISA tests were used with confirmation of positive test results. The whole process of sending blood samples to the NBB central laboratory, testing, recording of results, and distribution of results from NBB to AIC's headquarters and then to AIC's four branches, took two weeks. After many trials with an alternative system using rapid HIV tests, a rapid testing and counselling approach was initiated in 1997 that made it possible to provide counselling and test results within one two-hour visit.

In 1997, AIC established simple laboratories at each of the four main branches. All HIV testing is at present done "on-site" at AIC's four main branches, although 5 per cent of samples are retested for quality control at NBB. Besides this, selected samples, such as those which are weakly reactive and those which are negative but the client reports known exposure to HIV, are re-tested at the Uganda Virus Research Institute. At the time of this study, the Capillus test (Cambridge Diagnostics) is AIC's screening test. Confirmatory testing of all positives is done with Serocard (Trinity Biotech). If Capillus and Serocard are discrepant, a Multispot Test (Sanofi Pasteur Diagnostics) is carried out.

Several problems have been witnessed with this algorithm and the test kits. First, the kits require refrigeration that is at times unavailable at rural hospitals and health centres. Second, the packaging of these tests as part of a "kit' with 40 or 50 tests means that sites with low volume may use such small numbers of the confirmatory test that the kit expires before all tests are used. This is especially a problem with the third test, or the "tie breaker", which is very seldom used at rural sites but comes in a package of 50. A single-use kit that could be preserved at room temperature would lessen waste to a large extent. Research before the introduction of same-day rapid HIV testing demonstrated that 85 per cent of clients preferred to receive same-day results. Counsellors easily adapted to the new procedure and service delivery was improved overall. Now, the testing of samples for both HIV and syphilis occurs while the client is receiving prevention counselling. More than 99 per cent of clients now receive their results and post-test counselling in the same day.

Based on AIC's experience, there are few disadvantages to same-day testing. Clients not expecting to get their test results on the same day may experience stress, but most clients come to AIC expecting same-day results. Those who come unprepared to receive test results are persuaded to come another day. Counsellors frequently experience more stress will same-day testing as there may not be time to consult with colleagues on difficult cases. Overall, the move to same-day testing has brought advantages. All clients now receive their results and funds for testing are not wasted on clients who do not return. The probability for engaging in unprotected sex, while waiting for test results has been eradicated and couples who come in for testing just days before their wedding can have their results immediately.

Risk Reduction

There are many questions raised globally about the management, cost, and effectiveness of HIV counselling and testing programmes. An article written by staff of the US Centers for Disease Control and Prevention and AIC. As per a review on broad range of ethical, social policy, technical and economic issues that cause an impact on this HIV prevention service, some of the obstacles to VCT in the developing world are:

(a) widespread fear of taking an HIV test;
(b) potential for increased violence, loss of security, discrimination and isolation due to sharing of information about HIV seroposivity;
(c) scarce economic resources and competing priorities;
(d) lack of access to drug therapies, and psychosocial and clinical care.

Although these obstacles are substantial, AIC experience demonstrates that VCT plays an important role in Uganda's comprehensive HIV prevention strategy, benefitting both HIV-negative and HIV-positive clients. In 1992-93, AIC conducted an evaluation of its services. As part of this evaluation 2505 clients were followed for six months after receiving test results. Statistics collected during pre-test counselling sessions and three and six months afterwards showed that:

(a) although only 10 per cent of HIV-positive clients reported consistent condom use before receiving test results, by six months after receiving test results condom use went up to 89 per cent with steady, and 100 per cent with non-steady partners. By six months, the percentage of HIV-positive clients reporting sex with non-steady partners fell from 6 to 0.2 per cent;
(b) HIV-negative male clients increased their consistent use of condoms with non-steady partners from 34 to 93 per cent and with steady partners from 16 to 38 per cent;
(c) HIV-negative female clients increased their consistent use of condoms with non-steady partners from 14 to 94 per cent and with steady partners from 15 to 34 per cent;
(d) six months after learning HIV test results, 69 per cent

of clients who had learned that they were HIV-positive were reported to be refraining from any sexual activity, compared to 45 per cent prior to learning test results. In contrast, those who learned they were HIV-negative had increased their rates of being sexually active from 55 to 67 per cent but only 4 per cent reported having "non-steady" or casual partners.

Family planning (FP) services started in 1993 at AIC headquarters and have been available at all AIC branches since 1995. FP education is given to everyone who comes for HIV testing. AIC's FP clinics have served 28846 clients and provided modern FP methods to approximately 9000 clients. Reproductive Health Volunteers provide FP information while clients are in the waiting room. Volunteers are members of the Post Test Club and have undergone two weeks of training in integrated FP/ST/TB and HIV education. Volunteers help identify clients with particular FP needs and refer them to the appropriate nurse or counsellor. All AIC counsellors have been trained in integrated service delivery. They educate and counsel clients, and distribute pills and condoms when needed. AIC counsellors who are also nurses provide a wider package of integrated services, including examination and provision of a number of other FP methods. AIC statistics reveals that condoms are the most popular FP method, while 28 per cent of FP clients are using "dual methods". Condoms and Depo-provera are the most popular dual method, with condoms being used for HIV/STD prevention.

Information and Counselling on STDs

All clients who visit AIC for HIV counselling and testing also receive information and counselling on other sexually transmitted diseases and infections. As of 1998 the same sample of blood that is tested for HIV is also tested for syphilis, using the RPR test. In 1997, women clients had much higher rates of HIV infection than men while rates of syphilis among men and women were almost the same. In 1997, most AIC Kampala clients (77 per cent) tested negative to both HIV and syphilis; 17 per cent were HIV-positive but were negative to syphilis, and only 2 per cent were positive to both tests.

All clients who test positive to syphilis are provided on-site, same-day treatment with penicillin (injection) and are persuaded to bring their partners in for treatment. Unfortunately, only half of syphilis-positive clients accepted this service in 1997. In 1998 more efforts were being made to ensure that all RPR-positive clients receive same-day treatment. Clients are also offered an examination to detect other STDs that are then treated with a syndromic management approach. In 1997, 30 per cent of Kampala clients served by the STD clinic had syphilis and 53 per cent had other STDs. Numbers served by the STD clinic have increased in 1998 since the introduction of a simple screening device that alerts counsellors when it is necessary to use a more aggressive approach in making a referral to the STD clinic.

Information on Tuberculosis

Counsellors have given clients basic information on TB and the risks of co-infection since 1993. HIV-positive clients, especially those with TB symptoms, are persuaded to go for testing and possible treatment to any national TB control programme site. Between 1993 and 1995, AIC was an important site for recruiting HIV-positive persons into a trial of TB preventive therapy. This was carried out at Mulago Hospital under the auspices of Makerere University and Case Western Reserve University. Approximately 1000 clients participated in the study aimed at preventing HIV-positive clients from developing active TB. In 1998, AIC developed a proposal to give on-site TB preventive therapy for HIV-positive clients who are TB infected but do not have active disease. AIC hopes to implement this programme on a pilot basis at the Kampala main branch, using Post Test Club members as volunteers to ensure full compliance with courses of preventive therapy.

Post Test Club

The Post Test Club offers ongoing support to all AIC clients irrespective of the results of their HIV test. PTC members enjoy each others' friendship and support as well as a variety of services including: counselling, HIV/AIDS education, medical services including family planning and management of STDs, food distribution and recreation. The Kampala branch has 2500 PTC representatives. About 150 representatives meet every Saturday. The Saturday morning programme is dominated by food distribution for HIV-positive representatives and their families, sponsored by International Care and Relief. Representatives also enjoy board games, use the library, seek counselling, collect free condoms, and visit the Medical Booth for basic medical care. On average 60 PTC members stay for the Saturday afternoon programme lead by the PTC Counsellor-in-Charge. Programmes include guided discussions, films, guest speakers, and drama group presentations. Similar services and programmes exist at AIC sponsored Post Test Clubs in Jinja, Mbarara and Mbale. Approximately 65 per cent of PTC members are HIV-positive. Studies demonstrate that, over time, PTC members adopt and sustain risk reduction strategies appropriate to their HIV status. Their use of condoms is generally high and the PTC has become an important base for community dissemination of HIV prevention information.

Access to the Community

Many Ugandans admit they are afraid to go for an HIV test. Community outreach through PTC members participating in the Drama Group, Peer Education, the Philly Lutaaya Initiative and condom social marketing has made it possible to educate communities about AIDS, protected sex and the role of AIC's counselling and testing facilities. By giving AIDS a human face, AIC's community mobilization effort assists people make decisions that protect their lives and the lives of their loved ones.

All four AIC branches have a drama group. The Kampala group has 25 members who meet twice a week to practice song, dance and drama. All groups perform in English and local languages, at primary and secondary schools, churches, as well as gatherings managed by community groups. Members volunteer their time and are paid for travel expenses. In 1997, AIC drama groups participated in more than 70 performances.

Post Test Club members educate family members and friends about HIV prevention. Some PTC members participate in a 4-day training course to become Peer Educators and condom distributors. Peer Educators submit monthly reports showing numbers of peers talked to, peers' choices of protected sex options, numbers of peers referred for testing, and numbers of condoms distributed. Since 1992, Peer Educators have reached 180000 people and distributed 1200000 condoms.

Social Marketing for Change (SOMARC), a USAID-funded programme sponsored by the Futures Group, trains PTC members at AIC branches to market protector condoms. Social Marketers sell protector condoms in communities, at market price, and are generally consulted for information on proper use. Since the inception of programme in 1993, PTC SOMARC Social Marketers have distributed more than 180000 condoms.

Staff Training

AIC imports training for all its counsellors, supervisors, laboratory technicians, data entrants, peer educators and reproductive health volunteers. It also collaborates with other organizations to train their clinicians in the technical skills necessary to offer integrated HIV counselling and testing, family planning and STD management. Counsellor training forms the bulk of AIC's training programme. The curriculum was developed with technical assistance from the US Centers for Disease Control and Prevention to meet the special circumstances of HIV counselling and testing in Uganda. Counsellor training is of six months duration, although actual time in formal training sessions is four weeks. Counsellor training has four phases. The first phase lasts two weeks and HIV/AIDS/FP/STD/TB basic facts, as well as communication and counselling skills are given coverage. This is followed by a four-day practical training, after which the trainee is supervised while at work for a duration of not less than six months. The last phase of training lasts one week and covers advanced counselling skills.

AIC has a staff development programme that provides support for outside training to certain cadres of employees, with emphasis on areas that improve staff performance. All AIC Branch Managers and Heads of Department, including the Director, are trained HIV/AIDS counsellors. This facilitates in planning and supervising VCT services. All staff, regardless of their job, are given orientation in primary counselling skills to improve their client interaction. AIC refresher courses, such as integrated service delivery and rapid testing counselling protocol, are provided half yearly and help counsellors renew their commitment and further VCT skills.

Monetary Support

AIC was set up in 1990 with an initial grant of US$90000 from USAID and ample technical assistance from US-based experts in VCT. Based on the first year of successful implementation, USAID offered an additional $4345000 between 1991 and 1995. These funds were channelled through a US private voluntary organization, World Learning, Inc (WLI). During the period of 1991-95, WLI provided technical assistance in financial accountability, project management, grant writing, and personnel management. Beginning in 1991, the US Centers for Disease Control and Prevention (CDC) started providing technical assistance in areas such as monitoring and evaluation, counselling, training, and assessment of rapid test kits. A long-term CDC technical advisor, resident in Uganda, also provided sufficient technical assistance. As a result of AIC's institutional maturity and strength, AIC successfully negotiated a direct grant of $3565000 from USAID in 1996. This is for the period 1996 to mid-1999. AIC also started receiving support from the United Kingdom to the time of UK pound sterling 615316 ($820000) granted to AIC for 1996 to 2000. Since its inception, AIC has received smaller grants from other organizations and donors, including Uganda's Ministry of Health, InterAid, DED, UNICEF, UNDP, UNFPA, Christian Children's Fund, the governments of Japan and the Netherlands, and UNAIDS.

Cost of VCT

AIC has studied the cost of providing VCT with technical assistance from CDC and Emory University. Between 1994 and 1996, the unit cost per client was about US$12. Of this $5.13 was paid to the Nakasero Blood Bank. This amount included not only the costs of test kits but also personnel (both laboratory technicians and phlebotomists), supplies, equipment, technical supervision, and overhead. Recent analysis demonstrated that the unit cost of providing VCT services at AIC in 1997 was $13.39, a meagre increase over the 1994 figure. Of this unit cost, $4.59 was the cost of testing, including not only test kits but laboratory personnel, supplies, equipment, and technical supervision. The cost of counsellor time was $1.02. Taking into account all costs associated with direct services, the variable cost per client was $5.46 and the fixed costs for the building, administration, supervision, and monitoring was $7.93. This compares favourably with costs recently reported for VCT Kenya ($27) and Tanzania ($29). The incremental costs of adding family planning services were $1.17 per client and for adding STD detection and treatment, $1.76. It should be noted that these incremental costs for family planning and sexually transmitted disease management do not include the costs of drugs or commodities, but are AIC's costs in providing extra personnel and space for these services.

Costs were also calculated for the 'indirect sites' such as health centres and hospitals where AIC assists. At these sites, similar classifications of costs were examined for 'variable costs per client' and an average amount of $5.32 was calculated, which includes counsellor time, test kits and technician time, and the cost of the monitoring and supervision offered by AIC. The start-up costs of training personnel for these sites averaged $5.19 per client served in the first year after training.

Cost Sharing

When AIC opened in 1990, services were free-of-charge. A cost-sharing experiment started in January 1994 to facilitate a programme that was proving to be expensive, even from the donor's viewpoint. It was agreed that client fees were also necessary as a way for clients to attach value to the service. Experimentation with cost sharing began in Kampala with Uganda Shillings 1000 (about US$1) charged per client. Up-country branches charged Uganda Shillings 500 and satellite outreach stations charged Uganda Shillings 300. Fees have been revised upwards almost once a year, following analysis of fees and service utilization. Over 80 per cent of clients are willing and able to pay fees. AIC has Free Days for certain groups such as women, youth or couples regularly. Free Days are broadly publicized and the centre in Kampala can expect hundreds of clients to arrive on such a day. Clients who arrive in response to a Free Days advertisement are given coupons and advised to come on a specific day. Experience reveals that almost all clients with coupons return for free service. Regular free days include: World AIDS Day, Valentine's Day, International Women's Day and International Youth Day. AIC persuades couples to visit by offering two-for-one days. AIC has a fee exemption policy for those determined unable to pay. Counsellors forward recommendations for exemption to their supervisor for approval. Only 1 per cent of clients are exempted from paying fees, and less than 20 per cent of clients do not pay because of free testing days. During the 1997-98 financial year, AIC collected Uganda Shillings 77180000 (about $70000) in user-fees. While user-fee revenue represents a modest contribution to entire programme revenues, they are an important psychological contribution. User-fees play many roles:

(a) they are a move in the direction of financial sustainability;
(b) they are an indicator of value of the service to the client, and
(c) they are a way of discouraging inappropriate utilization.

Conclusion

Eight years of experience at AIC has revealed some important lessons for groups interested in offering HIV counselling and testing services.

VCT should be part of a comprehensive HIV eradication programme. In climates where there is significant discrimination against persons with HIV infection, or where there are no supportive services, it may not be suitable to offer VCT. Anonymity and protection of privacy are critical to ensure public trust in, and demand for VCT. Anonymity is more than just using codes instead of names. Especially when first offering VCT to the public, persons going for testing need to feel that they will not be readily discovered or stigmatized for entering the VCT service site.

Integrated services for family planning, detection of and treatment for other STDs, and education and referral for TB diagnosis and treatment are feasible and well received by VCT clients. Generally, an integrated approach benefits clients and public health. Effective counselling necessitates a client-centred approach with good rapport between counsellor and client, based on trust. Counselling should include information sharing, risk reduction planning and demonstration of skills. Good counsellors need preliminary training in one of the helping professions (social work, teaching, nursing or medicine) intensive training in HIV/AIDS counselling, specific training in other spheres such as couple counselling, sexuality, and bereavement, and periodic refresher courses. HIV/AIDS counselling is stressful and management must anticipate and address the potential for burnout. Managers who are trained as counsellors can better understand and supervise counselling services, and inculcate team spirit.

Once VCT becomes accepted by the public, large number of clients are likely to request VCT for 'social' reason such as testing before marriage or before a new relationship, and planning for the future, rather than 'medical' reasons such as already having symptoms of HIV infection or AIDS. A huge demand for VCT for social reasons is likely to increase the percentage and number of clients who come as couples rather than as individuals. On-going support through a Post Test Club assists HIV-positive members cope with infection and helps both HIV-positive and HIV-negative members adopt and maintain effective prevention behaviour. PTC members can contribute to the entire HIV prevention through their roles as community educators and condom distributors. Involvement of persons with AIDS makes for the most effective communication strategies because community members identify themselves with persons with AIDS. Post Test Club members also help change social norms in support of HIV risk reduction.

It is feasible to adopt cost sharing, although it is difficult to introduce fees in a service that is originally free. Fees-for-service may discourage some VCT clients, so it is important to have exemption policies as well as free days, two-for-one days, or other price reductions to encourage clients. A computerized Management Information System is critical for regular monitoring and quality control. AIC's system enables management to carefully monitor the numbers of persons served and many characteristics of AIC clients.

Five

Children Affected by HIV/AIDS (Zimbabwe and the United Republic of Tanzania)

Introduction

The basic needs of a child are food, shelter, clothing, love, and security, a combination of the material and psychological needs. Children infected by HIV/AIDS have similar needs, except the fulfilment of these needs is potentially in jeopardy when a parent or carer becomes ill and ultimately dies. Meeting these needs is significant for the growth and ability of a child to succeed through life. Meeting the psychosocial needs of children is not only a privilege, but also a right of the child. Organizations in sub-Saharan Africa have started to address the rights and needs of children affected by HIV/AIDS; however, many of them deal solely with material aid, such as school fees and food supplies. Financial assistance is also required, as narrated by a HIV positive mother from Tanga, United Republic of Tanzania, "There is nothing as bad as a spouse dying and then not being able to pay school fees."

Experiencing the Illness and Death of a Parent

Experiencing the illness and death of a parent is different for everyone. Despite the resilience of children, the illness and death of a parent always affects them, even if they cannot express it verbally. It can generate innumerable lasting problems for the child and alter the child's interaction with family, schoolmates, and peers. In order to help children through their grief, the possible ways in which they may express their grief must be discovered.

When a parent has HIV and is ill for a protracted period of

time, several changes occur in the family that affect the child both emotionally and physically. Out of necessity, children at times assume adult roles, such as that of care provider for an ill or dying parent, and this can prohibit their access to education. Frequently the disease process is not explained to children and they are left to draw their own inferences. Group counselling and the empowerment of parents to discuss their status and situation with their children should begin early in order to prepare children psychologically for the eventual passing away of their parents. Children whose parents have died of AIDS, whether they are infected themselves or not, are often referred to as AIDS orphans. The use of this terminology tends to label and stigmatize. Besides this, it excludes children whose parent(s) are infected with HIV but are still alive, a very important and substantial population of children.

The present discussion refers to children as either orphans or children affected by HIV/AIDS. The term 'orphan' is used for children who have lost at least one parent to HIV/AIDS. A wider category of 'children affected by HIV/AIDS' is used to refer to all children, affected or infected. The discussion also is intended for people concerned about and working with families affected by HIV/AIDS, such as social welfare officers, medical and nursing practitioners, health care workers, government agencies, non-governmental organizations (NGOs), churches, clubs and youth groups.

It highlights the experiences of children affected by HIV/AIDS, primarily those under the age of 15, through the use of their stories, poems and drawings. The role that older teenagers are fulfilling as resources for the younger ones is also narrated. Through providing examples of successful interventions being undertaken by organizations in Zimbabwe and the United Republic of Tanzania, the discussion shares experiences of essential psychosocial support to children who are infected and affected by HIV/AIDS in order to stimulate new awareness of needs and to open new doors for action.

It concentrates on what can be done for the child of an infected parent before and after the parent dies, to enable the child to cope better with the situation. It advocates for parents living with HIV/AIDS to discuss their status and situation with their children and to live positively and stay healthy in order to postpone orphanhood. The discussion also narrates how networking between organizations enables them to collaborate in addressing several children's issues that they could not tackle alone. It identifies lessons learnt that can be drawn upon in triggering and strengthening comprehensive programmes to address the psychological and material needs of children infected and affected by HIV/AIDS.

Child Rights and HIV/AIDS

To limit the adverse effects of the HIV/AIDS it is essential to ensure the childrens rights. In 1990, the United Nations Convention on the Rights of the Child came into being. The fundamental principle of the Convention is in the best interests of the child. This principle is based upon the understanding that children have full and equal worth, and that their vulnerability necessitates special support in order to enable them to enjoy full human dignity. There are 41 articles dealing with the rights of a child. The rights most relevant to HIV infected and affected children are summarized below:

The right of the child to:

(a) Affection, love and understanding;
(b) Ample nutrition and medical care;
(c) Free primary education and the opportunity for secondary, general and vocational education;
(d) Full opportunity for play and recreation. A name and a nationality;
(e) Special care if handicapped;
(f) Be first to receive relief in times of disaster;
(g) Learn to be a useful member of society and to develop individual abilities;
(h) Be brought up in a spirit of peace and universal brotherhood;
(i) Enjoy these rights regardless of race, sex, religion, nationality or social origin.

Psychosocial support for children affected by HIV/AIDS is directly associated to the rights classified in the United

Nations Convention on the Rights of the Child. Children are especially vulnerable to maltreatment or exploitation and a child cannot be physically healthy without also being psychologically secure.

Organizations, parents, carers, teachers and other people working with children, should therefore give priority to children's rights and make decisions based on the best interests of the child. Therefore; in order to seriously respect, protect and fulfil children's rights, it is vital that their psychosocial needs are met.

HIV/AIDS and African Children

(a) The number of people living with HIV/AIDS worldwide is 36.1 million, of whom 25.3 million inhabit in sub-Saharan Africa.

(b) Current UNAIDS figures estimate that 21.8 million adults have died of AIDS since the beginning of the epidemic, throughout the world, leaving an enormous number of children as orphans.

(c) there are approximately 1.4 million children living with HIV/AIDS worldwide.

(d) 95 per cent of the world's orphans live in Africa.

(e) Africa is home to 70 per cent of the adults and 80 per cent of the children living with HIV worldwide.

(f) In the year 2000, 3.8 million adults and children became infected with HIV and 2.4 million people at advanced stages of infection died of AIDS-related illnesses.

(g) Before the advent of AIDS, approximately 2 per cent of all children in developing countries were orphans. By 1997, this proportion increased to approximately 7 per cent and has today reached 11 per cent some countries.

(h) There are 13.2 million children under the age of 15 whose mothers have died of HIV/AIDS since the advent of the epidemic.

The HIV/AIDS epidemic has had an enormous impact on the world, especially in sub-Saharan Africa. The increasing rate of HIV infection affects African children in innumerable ways and in nearly every sphere of their lives. The number of children living with HIV/AIDS continues to grow everyday, as children are born to HIV-infected mothers, contracting the virus from their mothers during pregnancy. Besides this, there are millions of orphans who have lost at least one parent to an AIDS-associated illness. Although the number of orphans is staggering, its effects are only just beginning. HIV/AIDS has seriously impacted upon children whose siblings, relatives or friends have HIV; children who are suffering from or have died of AIDS-associated diseases, such as tuberculosis; and children whose homes are stressed with additional related orphans. Girls are especially vulnerable to HIV/AIDS and the negative effects of the virus. They encounter the chances of both physical abuse and the exploitation of their labour. When a family cannot afford school fees or there is sick parent who needs caring for, it is the girl child who is generally the first to drop out of school or to be given additional responsibilities.

The Effects

Economic

(a) Savings are used for medication/treatment and children must work to supplement the family's income.
(b) Illness lessens the economic performance of the household.
(c) Economic constraints make it necessary to look for alternative income generating sources, for example through prostitution, street children, or early marriage.
(d) When both parents have died or are unable to care for their children, they are shifted into the homes of the extended family, often taxing the financial stability of those households.
(e) Inability to maintain or repair the home.
(f) Lower nutritional status in households with less income and many children.

Educational

(a) The presence of AIDS in the household, and the additional responsibilities and burden it brings on the family, may cause children to drop out of school.
(b) Because of unresolved psychological trauma, the school performance of children is negatively affected by HIV/AIDS.

(c) Traditional skills die with the parent before being taught to the children.

(d) Orphans face stigmatization by other children, including at school.

Social

(a) In some communities it is taboo to take non-related children into one's home, especially if the children are sick.

(b) Dying is not talked about to children so they often do not understand what is happening in the household until the parent actually dies.

(c) Many times when a will is written it is disregarded by greedy relatives who leave nothing for the orphaned children.

(d) Medical concerns with opportunistic infections, such as tuberculosis, to other family members.

(e) Children and elderly people become the head of household.

(f) Poor families are more affected by losing a family member and may become impoverished forever, moving from poverty to destitution.

Psychological

(a) This is the least visible effect because it is not tangibly seen.

(b) Emotional suffering appears in various forms for everyone (e.g., depression, aggression, drug abuse, insomnia, failure to thrive, malnutrition, etc.).

(c) Children with sick parents worry about the future, where they will go and who will take care of them.

(d) Loss of consistent nurture, which can lead to grave development problems, and loss of guidance, which makes it more, difficult for the child to reach maturity and to be integrated into society.

(e) Psychological damage can arise at any time after the event (months, days, and even years).

(f) Children may not understand the situation and therefore cannot express their grief effectively. Even if they want to express their feelings, there is often no one to listen.

HIV/AIDS and Children in Zimbabwe

Innumerable elements have contributed to the difficulties facing Zimbabwe today. These include the effects of the present political impasse, the declining value of the Zimbabwean dollar, rapid inflation, lack of investment, rising unemployment, escalating costs of living, the effects of frequent droughts and the emergence of HIV/AIDS. The present political, economic and HIV/AIDS situation in Zimbabwe presents innumerable challenges to individuals, families, communities, and especially children living with HIV/AIDS.

On an individual level, the income of HIV/AIDS-affected families dwindles, usually because the breadwinner is ill or the family's savings are spent on medical care. Children in these situations are often forced to drop out of school and to work. The situation is exacerbated when the prices of food and household goods increase. Inflation has gravely impacted upon the country's health care system, more specifically on the diagnosis of HIV infection and the care of HIV/AIDS patients. Even diagnosing opportunistic infections is too costly for the majority of the population. For example, while treatment for tuberculosis is free, it costs a minimum of Zim $800 (US$16) to reach a diagnosis before treatment can begin. This excludes the cost of transportation and other expenses.

The fuel crisis in Zimbabwe has impaired the ability of AIDS organizations to care for families in need. In Harare, Mashambanzou is one non-governmental organization (NGO) that provides food for HIV/AIDS-affected families. The scarcity of petrol restricts volunteers for Mashambanzou and around the country from regularly reaching families with counselling, food, and blankets. HIV/AIDS has placed an additional burden on the extended family system. This structure has provided security for children and families for generations. Traditionally in Zimbabwe, family elders would meet and assign a family member, usually the father's eldest brother, to care for an orphaned child and raise the child as part of his own family.

Recently the capacity of families to cope with additional children has become more and more strained. Relatives are starting to look at their familial responsibility towards related children as more of a monetary hazard. There are additional problems for orphaned children without relatives owing to the stigma attached to caring for non-related children. In this emergency, additional support from outside sources is required to assist these children to cope. Early marriage is regarded as an option for households absorbing extra children. A man may marry to obtain assistance in taking care of his dependants. A woman may marry to reduce the number of dependants in her family's household, as well as to obtain additional income through the bride price, i.e. money or goods given to the bride's family by that of the bridegroom. The death of a mother or father can leave unsettled debts which impact negatively on the future care and resources left for the remaining children. In grave cases, the family of a deceased woman may not permit her burial until the surviving husband and his family have settled the outstanding debts.

The large part of the population reside in the rural areas. There are approximately two million people living on large scale commercial farms in Zimbabwe at present, nearly 20 per cent of the population. They help to produce major items of the country's economy: tobacco, maize, cotton, sugar, groundnuts, horticultural produce and beef. One million children live on these farms. It has been discovered that the average number of orphans at each farm was 12, in contrast to 2 in 1994. The average age of orphans was 11 years and most of the children were not infected with HIV/AIDS. Children living on farms encounter many challenges that are unknown to children living in towns. The livelihood and accommodation of families living on commercial farms is tied to their fathers' employment, as workers do not own the land they reside on. Families affected by HIV/AIDS therefore face the prospect of losing their homes once their fathers or breadwinners pass away from HIV/AIDS, often resulting in young boys having to become the breadwinner to prevent this from occurring. The recent farm invasions have also affected the lives of children living on the farms, endangering their physical and psychological security. For example, there has been a reported increase in the instances of rape among young girls living on the farms, thus making young girls in these areas more susceptible to HIV infection.

HIV/AIDS: Rural Life in United Republic of Tanzania

There are many traditional cultural similarities between Zimbabwe and the United Republic of Tanzania, such as early marriage and the bride price. Moreover 70 per cent of Tanzanians live in rural areas and depend on subsistence farming. Living with HIV/AIDS in the rural areas is especially demanding for several reasons. Subsistence farming meets only the family's immediate needs, so when the breadwinner becomes ill, there are no food or financial resources on which to draw. The epidemic is gravest in Dar es Salaam and in the north-western part of the country, where there are a large number of refugees from neighbouring Rwanda, Burundi and the Democratic Republic of Congo.

AIDS education is part of the national school curriculum; however, there is little general knowledge about the virus, especially in isolated rural areas. Access to health care can be difficult due to the distance, the road infrastructure and the lack of vehicles for transportation. There is also the problem of finding available HIV tests and confirming an HIV-positive diagnosis, even within health care facilities. The United Republic of Tanzania is a traditional society where even in the language youth respect their elders. This can be illustrated by the Swahili word for greeting an older person, Shikamoo, which means, I am beneath you. This respect keeps order in society, but is a challenge to AIDS education. Breaking taboos, such as talking about sex or death with some-one who is older and therefore more knowledgeable, is difficult. Writing a will also goes against tradition, and upon the death of a husband, his family generally takes as much of his property as possible, often leaving the widow and children with nothing.

It is estimated that by the year 2010, there will be 4.2 million orphans in the United Republic of Tanzania. Before this time, the country's support systems need to be strengthened to be able to cope with the needs of these children and to promote HIV/AIDS awareness, especially in rural areas.

Disclose of Parents' HIV Status

Talking to children about HIV/AIDS may appear like a desirable thing to do, but parents must overcome many obstacles both individually and within society, before revelation becomes an option. Below are some of these barriers.

Traditional Taboos

AIDS is such as taboo subject that people will refer to it as "the disease", or anything else in addition to AIDS. Most children whose parent or parents have died of an AIDS-associated illness attribute death to such illnesses as tuberculosis, poisoning or diarrhoea. It is not clear whether children really believe their parents died of these illnesses, or whether they simply say so to protect the family from the possible embarrassment and stigma that HIV/AIDS carries. Traditional healers commonly credit AIDS-related illnesses to bewitchment, which can leave children with the fear that they too will be bewitched or that they caused it in some way. As traditional healers are often used as counsellors, they too need information on HIV/AIDS and on providing psychosocial support for children affected by the virus.

In societies where there is little openness about HIV/AIDS, parents discuss whether revealing their HIV status would help or hurt their children.

Telling the Child

The views of parents differ on whether or not to reveal their HIV status. Disclosure is primarily dependent on how secure the parent is about the HIV-positive status. If the parent is not yet comfortable with being HIV-positive, HIV/AIDS education will not be shared positively with the child and may make the child feel uncomfortable with the information. Revelation can also depend on the age of the child. Children around the age of seven are mature enough to understand the finality of death and they have heard about HIV/AIDS in the community or at school. At that age children do not understand the stigma associated with the virus because they do not understand the implications of sexual transmission. The maturity of children and how curious they are about the virus can also affect disclosure. Some parents say revelation is necessary because children with information can safeguard themselves from contracting the virus when caring for an infected parent. Because the carer has such intimate contact with the infected person, it is probable that opportunistic infections or even HIV itself can be passed to the carer if proper precautions are not taken. Others admit that knowing about HIV in the family just makes the child's life harder. Eventually, it remains the decision of the individual.

Whatever is decided about disclosure, an HIV-infected parent must concentrate on living positively with the virus rather than on dying. People with HIV can prolong their lives with a better diet and a positive attitude. By facing the virus positively, parents can stay healthy longer and keep their children from becoming orphans for as long as possible.

Both traditionally and emotionally, HIV-positive parents face great difficulties in revealing their status to their children. Each individual must decide whether talking about HIV/AIDS will help their children to deal with the future or contribute to their stigmatization and discrimination. Although there are a few resources that assist in revelation, they are generally not easily accessible.

Discussion About Death

Once children realize that a parent may die, the future becomes a major concern. "Where will I go?" and "Who will pay my school fees?" are general questions. When children are not given the opportunity to express their emotions about the situation, these feelings are left to fester and could have long term effects such as depression or nightmares.

Fighting the Silence

It is a common belief that because children are resilient, they are not in need of counselling about death. This can be shown by the idea of comforting the widow at the funeral and sending the children out to play. Children are persuaded to keep their emotions inside and may hear such warnings as, If you cry, you will end up like your mother!

In the Shona culture in Zimbabwe, children do not actively involve in rituals surrounding death, and they are generally kept away from the funeral and the grave, although changes have been noted in this custom. Traditionally, families who have moved away from the rural areas return to the village to bury a family member. When this happens, the remaining children are left behind in town. Adults also avoid talking about death to children because it is too painful for the adults. The child's grief can evoke memories and strong feelings in the adults that they are not ready to deal with. Adults argue that by avoiding discussing death they are in reality protecting the child. Many parents hope to minimize the impact of the loss by avoiding talking about it, a conspiracy of silence.

This "conspiracy of silence" does help parents control their emotions, but even though nothing is verbalized, the parent is still communicating with the child about sickness or death, only it is something negative. Children are like a sponge; they absorb everything (emotions, tensions and actions) but adults do not realize there is so much water inside. Children's roles and lifestyles change dramatically when AIDS enters the household. The children often become the carers for a sick parent or they have to take on additional duties in the household, such as working to replace the income of the sick breadwinner or to supplement the money essential for treatment.

Children can see these stressors and sense that there is something seriously wrong, but they may not understand what it is or its implications. This can make them feel anxious, guilty, depressed and misunderstood. They do not express these feelings because they do not want to upset the situation further or they may be afraid of being overwhelmed by their feelings and try to keep them under control by keeping them inside. They get the feeling that whatever the secret is, it is too horrible to be talked about. By discussing the situation, children's fears are alleviated and they will be able to cope better with the stress.

Last Words to Children

Talking to children about death in advance gives them time to get used to the idea and steadily loosen the bond of attachment. Children who had the opportunity to say good-bye and were given last words of advice greatly appreciated it when the parent is gone. Having the probability to say actual thought-out good-byes to people, places or a familiar family structure is very healing for a child. Wishes and blessings can be exchanged, preventing the children from blaming themselves and leaves less unfinished to complicate the grief process. The children whose parents had talked to them about dying appreciated being able to use the time to share information and advice. For example, the children had the opportunity to learn how to do household tasks and could ask the parent, When you die, how should I do this?

Memory Book

Originating in Uganda, the memory book is a journal of facts and memories for children who are encountering loss or separation from a parent, including divorce,' any terminal illness or adoption, and it is appropriate for any culture or background. If children are separated from their parents, memories and identity tend to vanish. The Memory Book is an attempt to keep the memories alive and enhances the child's sense of belonging. The parent or caregiver fills in information and personal stories in different headings.

It helps children to understand the past and move on to a more secure future. It is a photocopiable resource, which makes it affordable and easy to distribute to parents and carers. There are various ways of completing the memory book. The parent can complete it and then to through it with the child or the child can assist in its completion. An important aspect of the book is that the child has the opportunity to ask questions about its history and future. If the parent wishes, the book can include input from other family members, photographs and other memories to remind the children of life before the separation from their family.

The Memory Book is a tool to help the parent and the child to deal with the past, present and future of the child. As it is common for orphaned children to be moved into a different area, the book serves as a reminder of their roots so they do not lose their sense of belonging. Revealing the parents' HIV status is not the important objective of the book, but it permits the opportunity to talk about HIV and facilitates revelation to other family members. The book is also beneficial with regard to HIV prevention, because the children see and understand the ordeal the parent is going through and do not want to repeat it.

Counselling

During the period of illness, parents or other carers may be busy with their own grief and would need the help of outside counselling. The aim of counselling for children at this time permits them to express grief and repressed feelings by allowing them to break down. Counsellors can persuade the child to deal with the reality of the loss and the adjustment to environment without the deceased. The child can then begin adjusting and exploring the circumstances as an independent person. Anticipating a parent's death begins the process of grieving early, which makes it easier for the bonds of attachment to fade gradually over time. It prepares them for what lies ahead instead of taking them off guard, and can promote the awareness that although change is hard, the child can manage grief and loss - what has happened is not so awful that it cannot be talked about.

Family Counselling

Bereavement counselling generally refers to counselling for families after a loved one's death. However, counselling can also start during a long period of illness, in anticipation of death. Many times, it is the parents who are counselled about death and due to the age-old idea that children are resilient and taboos on taking to the children, they are left out of the picture. It is important, however, that children are included in the family counselling.

Counselling for Groups of Orphans

When children are in difficult circumstances, usually they feel worse about it when they feel alone in their experience. Another way to assist children's psychosocial needs is to set up a peer group where they can share similar experiences and support each other.

Effective Responses

It is realized that at present, the majority of programmes working with children affected by HIV/AIDS have not strategically integrated psychosocial support issues in their existing programmes. To bridge this gap, accelerated learning through sharing experiences and information is the easiest way for an organization to grow and meet the varying needs of people affected by HIV/AIDS, especially their psychosocial needs.

Psychosocial Support

Adults must listen to what children are saying. At first, children will usually identify material needs, such as food or clothing, as their greatest concern. However, when adults take the time to listen to their stories and poems and observe their drawings, children can reveal their personal experiences and feelings. This is the most effective way to determine their needs to enable others to effectively assist them in having a better life. Through listening, the following lessons were learned from programmes in Zimbabwe and the United Republic of Tanzania on psychosocial support for children affected by HIV/AIDS.

(a) Respecting the rights of children, such as the right to protection against exploitation and discrimination, is essential for the well-being and growth of a child.
(b) Psychosocial support is an important aspect of children's rights and must be included by organizations associated with children as part of their programming framework.
(c) Children play a vital role in the future, so they should participate in decisions that affect them. Participation is a fundamental principle of the Convention on the Rights of the Child.

Acknowledging the Changing Roles

(a) Providing for the needs of children affected by HIV/AIDS necessitate not only material support for immediate needs but also skills from which they may benefit in the future.
(b) Children are aware of economic difficulties and changes within the household and these issues must be discussed with them in order to prepare them.

Enabling Environment

(a) Stigmatization of HIV/AIDS can be broken down through education and discussion.
(b) Educating family members, teachers, peers and other community members on the needs of children affected by HIV/AIDS increases their understanding of the situation and lets them respond positively.

(c) Teachers must not write off children with behavioural problems as "problem children", but should try to understand the reasons behind their misbehaviour.
(d) When they are given the knowledge about the needs of children affected by HIV/AIDS and the opportunity to do something about it, teachers will usually respond sympathetically and generously to their students.
(e) By reaching out and trying to understand a child's situation a teacher or caregiver can give love and guidance that the child essentially needs.

Permit Kids to be Kids

(a) Playing and adventure-based learning gives an opportunity for children to enhance their physical and psychological well-being.
(b) Giving children the opportunity to discuss their feelings and experiences with other children permits them to realize that they are not alone and helps to build their self-confidence.
(c) Listening to what a child has to say is a low-cost way of reinforcing the child's importance in an uncertain situation.

Participation of Youth

(a) Orphans will work together to create the family that they are missing at home and deal with the stigmatization from other children.
(b) If they are given the opportunity, youth will make responsible choices to improve the situation of others, such as the members of VSI educating younger orphans and helping the elderly.
(c) Giving them the opportunity to handle money may not always be flawless, but will give them a starting point from which to work.

Communication with Children

(a) HIV-positive parents must realize that living positively with the virus, such as providing proper nutrition and having a healthy attitude, benefits their children to a large extent because it prolongs their lives and postpones orphanhood.

(b) Revealing an HIV status to a child can be based on many factors, such as the child's age or maturity, but inevitably it is the choice of the individual parent.

(c) Providing food and shelter for children means little if it is not accompanied by psychological support, such as communication and tolerance.

(d) Traditional healers play a major role in several African societies, teachers circulate information on HIV/AIDS and religious leaders influence beliefs of their followers. Because all of these people can influence the situation of a child affected by HIV/AIDS to a large extent, they should be included in HIV/AIDS education.

About Death

(a) Children may not be able to narrate their thoughts and feelings easily, but this does not mean the illness or death of a parent does not affect them.

(b) Avoiding talking to children about illness in the household may make it easier for the parent to handle, but can make children feel anxious, guilty and depressed, and can even lead to long-term emotional problems.

(c) Talking about death and dying can be a positive experience for both parents and children. It gives children the opportunity to say good-bye and begin the process of healing and gives parents the satisfaction that the child will be prepared to live without them.

(d) Parents may also require counselling to assist them in talking to their children about death.

(e) Using a supplement such as the Memory Book is a useful tool to facilitate discussion on the child's family history and preparing for the future.

Education and Counselling

(a) HIV/AIDS education as part of counselling can be an effective way of prevention.

(b) Counselling prepares children for what lies ahead and

encourages them to believe that they can manage through grief and loss.

(c) Whether it is individual or within a group, counselling permits bereaved children to express their feelings and deal with their anxiety.

(d) An important part of counselling is working within family and cultural norms.

Concluding Tips

(a) Programmes dealing with children and HIV/AIDS should develop a holistic, multidisciplinary approach by bringing in equilibrium the supply of material and psychosocial support.

(b) There is no right way of addressing children's needs. Because their psychosocial needs are so wide and involve so many issues, organizations must work collectively to provide comprehensive, complementary services.

(c) Assisting only orphans isolates other children, such as children with terminally ill parents or from impoverished families, who are both as financially and psychosocially in need as the orphaned children.

(d) Include all children in orphan projects so as not to create or continue stigmatization.

(e) Giving the community a role in support programmes can make the programme stronger and more sustainable.

(f) Through networking, AIDS organizations can learn from each other how to deal more efficiently with children's issues.

(g) Following-up in children's own communities is important to the continued growth and empowerment of the child.

Six

Girls' Vulnerability to HIV/AIDS: The Thai Perspective

Introduction

HIV infection rates among teenage girls are at times much higher than in teenage boys; the reason lies in girls' greater biological and social vulnerability. In contrast to males, the female reproductive tract is more susceptible to infection with HIV and other STDs, particularly in younger girls. And girl frequently risk infection very early. Compounding the biological vulnerability of girls are complex and unhealthy societal expectations that mean girls and young women have less control over their lives and bodies than do their male counterparts.

In Thailand, too many girls find themselves at an early age in the sex trade, usually for lack of other options for earning a living. Young girls are desirable because they are thought to be 'safe' and uninfected with HIV, but the risk of infection to them, and thence to their clients, is alarmingly high. The present discussion narrates some responses to that problem, concentrating on changing the attitudes of girls and their parents in regard to prostitution, and on providing a means for girls to avoid becoming sex workers through improved education and career opportunities. The approach discussed is also an example of an AIDS response that takes into consideration the regional and demographic differences in the nature and scope of the problem in the search for solutions.

Factors Responsible for Girls' Entry in Sex Trade

The factors that girls enter the sex trade in Thailand have received much attention; innumerable research studies have attempted to discover the causes of and propose solutions to this problem. The causes have been divided into those at the societal level and those at the family level. At the societal level, Thailand's accelerated economic development is cited as one major cause. When Thailand adopted an industrialized, export-led economy, one of the consequences was that agriculture - formerly the backbone of the Thai economy - was devalued. Farmers went increasingly into debt and many were forced to move from their land to find employment in urban areas, usually Bangkok or provincial urban centres. Those who remained in the rural areas attempted several alternative family survival strategies, such as sending their children to cities to earn the family income.

Thailand's national policy, with its emphasis on economic growth, led at simultaneously to a rise in materialism in Thai society. Parental desires for a better, more comfortable standard of living - often encouraged by mass media advertisements - led some parents to encourage their children into the sex trade as a means of attaining their material objectives. Children who did not accede to their parents' demands were regarded as ungrateful, since respect for one's parents and providing for their care are paramount socio-cultural norms in Thai society, persisting even under Thailand's fast social and economic changes. In some rural villages in northern Thailand, where prostitution has become an acceptable occupation, families who do not sell their daughters may be seen as foolish by other members of the community.

The main reason for girls entering the sex trade is to satisfy their parents' urgent need for money, in some cases not for more material goods but simply for the family's survival. Earnings from unskilled labour are much lower than those from sex business. Thus, many parents decide to sell their daughters and earn quick money to meet their immediate needs. Though girls do not desire to become sex workers, many are forced or tricked into it. These children generally have little or no education and often do not live with their parents. Another group at special risk are children who live with a stepfather or stepmother. With weaker family ties and often less family support, they have become targets for recruitment into sex business, through force or deception.

The expectation that they will support their parents in any way they can is placed on daughters much more than on sons in

Thai society. A daughter's duty is to earn a living for the family to repay her debt of gratitude to the parents, while a son's is to spend time as a monk. Thus, the economic burden of the family is placed on the daughter's shoulders rather than on the son's. There is no reported incidence of the selling of sons by their parents, whereas selling daughters is quite common in some areas.

Indeed, the reasons males become prostitutes are different from those for females. It has been found that 51 per cent male bar workers in Bangkok were introduced to the job by their friends and 36 per cent by reading job advertisements. For male sex workers choosing this job is mainly their own decision. Even though there are far fewer male sex workers than there are females, it was estimated that there are only 3 or 4 male sex worker for every 100 females; national policies for preventing and solving the problems of sex workers given focus to both sexes. But different strategies are needed to cope with the different problems facing male and female sex workers. The present discussion concentrates on strategies for keeping girls from becoming prostitutes.

Vulnerability to HIV/AIDS

The first case of AIDS in Thailand was detected in 1984. Early cases were found among male homosexuals; thereafter the disease spread rapidly among injecting drug users in 1987 and 1988, and then to sex workers and their clients. It has now reached to the general population. The sentinel sero-prevalence survey shows that HIV has increased among all groups since 1989. In that time, the HIV prevalence rate for sex workers has risen especially rapidly, from 3.5 per cent to 29 per cent in 1996. Among AIDS patients, heterosexual transmission is now the predominant mode of HIV transmission.

Although the rate of new infections has started to decline by the year 2000 there were nearly 1.3 million HIV-positive persons in Thailand. A high rate of HIV infection among sex workers means that it is not only the women involved in sex business themselves who are at high risk of infection, but also their clients and others with whom they come into sexual contact. The problem is grave in the northern part of Thailand, where the rate of HIV infection among sex workers is alarmingly high.

Besides this, the risk of young girls' contracting HIV/AIDS is more than that of adults, and especially for those girls entering the sex industry. Estimates of the number of children involved in prostitution range from 13,000 to 100,000 or more.

An estimation technique to discover potential risk of becoming a sex worker designated three levels of risk: no risk, low risk, and high risk. Factors considered were area of current residence, migration, co-residence and school attendance. Those children who live in rural areas, are non-migrants, are living with family members and are attending school are identified as the no risk group. Those children seen as the high risk group are migrant children who live in an urban area apart from their families and are not attending school. The middle category, the low risk group, are those who have some, but not all, of the four risk factors. Based on an approximation of these factors, 1.7 per cent of the female population aged 11 to 17 lies in the high risk group, 68 per cent in the low risk group, and 30.3 per cent in the no risk group. There were between 30,000 and 100,000 female child sex workers. Among the low risk group, not attending school is the major factor: almost two-thirds of this group are not in school. There is ample evidence that child prostitution exists in great enough numbers to make it a significant social problem, one that also places such children at high risk of contracting HIV/AIDS.

Child Prostitution: Prevention Strategies

In 1992, a national effort was initiated to prevent child prostitution and to assist those at risk of entering the sex business. At that time, the problem of child prostitution became a high priority for the government, with several strategies implemented, including prevention, suppression, assistance, rehabilitation and legal measures to prevent entry into the sex business by children under 18. Preventive measures were seen as best practice, in that they could substantially reduce the children's risk of exploitation or of contracting a fatal disease. Some of the major strategies were:

(a) All children should receive nine years of quality primary education. Those impoverished children with no opportunity for further education need access to education and vocational training.

(b) The quality of education must be improved to enable a child to think and uphold moral principles, and be able to choose a way of life with human dignity. The educational curriculum and vocational training must be relevant to the local environment and conditions, as well as to the demands of the labour market.

(c) Girls and boys must have the same access to both formal and non-formal education.

(d) Counselling and guidance services for solving family and youth problems and job selection must be provided in every school and to out-of-school children.

(e) Recreational and social services should be provided so that children and young people can spend their leisure time appropriately.

(f) Campaigns to raise awareness about child prostitution should be conducted to foster correct attitudes among parents, guardians, teachers and the general public.

(g) Coordination with neighbouring countries in campaigns and publication about prevention and feasible solutions to problems associated with the sex business should be encouraged.

(h) An inspection surveillance system should be established to prevent coercion or deception of children into becoming prostitutes.

In response to the national policy, many project have been implemented, of which education and vocational training are witnessed as among the best strategies to prevent young girls from entering the sex trade.

Sema Pattana Cheewit Project

The Sema Pattana Cheewit Project is the most widely implemented of the strategies for carrying out the child prostitute elimination policy. In 1993, the Ministry of Education (MOE) conducted a survey of Thai sex workers both in Thailand and abroad to seek information about their hometown, age, education, reasons for becoming a sex worker, the channels used to find employment abroad, and so forth. This information, along with statistics on villages with high HIV/AIDS rates as well as the number of students who passed Grade 6 but did not continue their education, were used as the basis for planning the intervention. Eight provinces in the North (Chiang Rai, Phavao, Lampang, Chiang Mai, Mae Hong Song, Prae, Lampoon and Nan) were selected as the target area, since they were the highest risk areas for girls entering the sex business. These provinces also had high HIV/AIDS rates, as well as a high percentage of girls (43 per cent) who postponed their education after passing Grade 6. After the target provinces were selected, the seminar was organised to determine the reasons of the problem by concentrating on the factors that encouraged girls to become sex workers. From the seminar, five main factors were discovered and later used as guidelines for selecting girls for involvement in the project.

(a) *Poverty.* Agricultural areas that are not suitable for cultivation lead families living in them into a circle of debt trap.

(b) *Materialistic attitudes.* There was competition among households to own a nice house and possess expensive material goods as signs of social prestige. Households who had their daughter(s) working in the sex business and sending back income to buy goods and build new houses were accepted and recognized as successful families.

(c) *Lack of education.* Survey statistics disclosed that many sex workers had very little education. More than 95 per cent of sex workers had only six years of education or less, while others had no education at all because of poor family economic background. Even though the government provided free education, the families still had to pay for food, books, travel costs and other expenses not covered by the government.

(d) *Agent persuasion.* Agents for brothels who seek out young good-looking girls have several techniques to persuade girls and their parents that sex business is desirable. They may use either direct or indirect methods, depending on the attitude of the particular family. For those families who are not willing to send their daughter(s) to work in the sex business, agents may initially promise to find the girls well paying jobs in restaurants or factories, but later force the girls into sex trade.

(e) *Family difficulties.* Girls who live with a single parent, with other relatives or step-parents or in families with economic or drug addiction problems are at high risk of becoming sex workers.

The Cabinet approved the implementation of the Sema Pattana Cheewit Project and offered 4,000 scholarships to day students at 2,400 baht per year (about US$ 61) and 500 scholarships for boarding school students at 9,000 (about US$ 230) annually.

Education Programme

The Sema Pattana Cheewit Project aims to provide an education for girls in difficult circumstances enabling them to develop in maturity knowledge, and experience so as to be able to safeguard themselves from being deceived and so as to have a means of finding a socially acceptable job. The project's targets are these:

(a) To prevent girls at high risk from entering sex business, at least 500 girls are provided scholarships for boarding school.

(b) To provide 4,000 scholarships for day students to continue their education in schools located in their communities.

(c) To prepare scholarships for students who pass Grades 9 and 12 so that they can attend vocational training.

(d) To set up 94 Sema Pattana Cheewit centres in 94 districts in eight northern provinces. These centres will give information and conduct campaigns to stop girls from becoming prostitutes.

(e) To set up a collaborative system for working with other concerned organizations.

The Sema pattana Cheewit Project has three distinct phases. Phase I was implemented from 1994 to 1996 in the eight targeted northern provinces. Phase II (1997-1999) expands the project to other northern provinces as well as to Bangkok and Phase III (2000-2002) will cover high risk areas in the Northeast and the

South of Thailand. Students participate in the Sema Pattana Cheewit Project in three ways: in boarding school, in day school and receiving vocational training. Primary school teachers select students who meet the following criteria for boarding school participation in the project:

1. girls who are currently in Grade 6, residents of the eight target provinces in the North, who do not and will not receive other scholarships, and
2. Whose families have one or more of these characteristics:
   (a) Father or mother is deceased, disabled or in prison and unable to take care of their children;
   (b) A broken family, where children have to live with either a stepfather or a stepmother or other relatives;
   (c) Family members or relatives are or have formerly been in the sex industry, or the community of residence has a number of persons in the sex business;
   (d) Father or mother is a drug addict;
   (e) Family is otherwise in a situation that places the child at high risk of becoming a prostitute.

The selection criteria for day students are the same as for boarding school students except that the family is felt to be in a situation where girls can safely live with them, and the family will permit their children to go to school if they receive monetary assistance. The selection process consists of three steps. First, primary school teachers select candidates as per the guidelines issued by the Ministry of Education. Thereafter, each school sends the list of students to the district education office for screening. The district office forms a committee to select the number of girls according to a quota provided by the provincial education office. The district office list will then be sent to the provincial education office for finalization.

After the final list of students from each province is completed, it is sent for approval. The MOE should take approximately 45 days for approval, after which scholarships are disbursed to each province. After receiving a scholarship, each student opens a saving account under her name and sends the account number to the district office. The provincial education office then transfers the scholarship funds to the girls' accounts. In order for a student to withdraw the money, at least two out of three persons (homeroom teacher, principal and student) must sign the withdrawal form. For boarding school scholarships, the money is transferred to the bank account of that particular school. The money covers the cost of three meals a day, tuition fees, books, school uniforms and other education-related expenses.

The process of implementing the programme starts in early February, when the Ministry of Education announces the number of scholarships to be provided to each province, and each province determines the allocation of scholarships to each district and notifies the districts of that allocation. The district education office instructs each school to select girls to participate in the project under the conditions and characteristics specified by the Ministry of Education. A committee in each school selects eligible girls and sends the prioritized list, including a waiting list, to the district education office. The district level committee considers the list of students from every school and priorities it as per need. If the number of girls selected by the schools is more than the number of scholarships offered, girls who are not in urgent need, that is, whose family environment does not put them at particular risk, are put on the waiting list. The final list is then sent to the provincial education office. A provincial level committee reviews and revises the list and declares the names of the girls who are to receive scholarships. The final list is then sent to the Ministry of Education for recording.

By mid-April, the district education office must inform the schools the girls will enter about the process of receiving their scholarships. For three weeks in April, girls who receive scholarships for boarding school attend an orientation and training workshop to prepare them for the life in boarding school. In mid-May, school begins. Girls open their bank accounts and send the account numbers to the district education office, which examines all of the account numbers and names of girls and sends them to the provincial education office. After the provincial office receives the funds from Ministry of Education, the money will be transferred to the account of each girl. The time between receipt of the account number and the transfer of the money is more than one month.

If students drop out or change schools, the school in which

the student was originally enrolled must inform the district and provincial education offices. Girls on the waiting list will then be selected as replacements. School transfers are possible only for day students.

Girls who do not want to study in the regular school system but who do want to train in specific areas are placed in suitable vocational training programmes. At present, three areas of training are offered.

(a) *Agriculture training.* Starting in 1995, an operational centre for agriculture accepted 106 students who had passed Grade 6 for vocational training as part of a rural development project. Students are also enrolled in an out-of-school programme, and will graduate with a Grade 9 certificate after receiving agriculture training over a period of 18 to 24 months. In 1996, the Ministry of Education assisted approximately 40,000 needy ninth grade students to continue their education to a higher level. The Ministry of Education subsidized tuition fees and provided free housing. Another 5,000 baht (about US$128) per student per year was provided for raising cattle and growing vegetables for the period of their study. Students could sell the training products for profit, to give them experience in making a living after graduation.

(b) *Nurses' training.* Mahidol University in Bangkok provides 40 seats annually for girls who have finished Grade 9 in the North to train as assistant nurses for one year. After training, these students work in Siriraj Hospital and Ramathibodi Hospital, Mahidol University, for minimum two years. They are then encouraged to go back to work in rural areas. The Ministry of Public Health also offered seats for 50 students who passed Grade 12 in 1995 to train in nursing colleges under the Ministry, and another 80 seats in 1996. After training, they worked in public health centres or hospitals.

(c) *Working while studying.* At the beginning of 1996, UNICEF, in collaboration with the Dusit Thani Hotel (one of the leading hotel chains in Thailand), participated with the Sema Pattana Cheewit Project to organize a training programme for 60 students who had graduated from Grade 9 at hotels in Phetchaburi and Chiang Rai Provinces. There are plans to expand the project to other hotels in the Dusit Thani Kempinsky group in Thailand and in Europe. During their two years of training, students study general subjects via non-formal education through Thailand's distance education system. Students receive a salary of 2,000 baht (about US$51) per month. Graduates of this project are then recruited as staff for hotels within the Dusit Thani group at a salary of 5,000-6,000 baht (about US$128-153) per month. It is planned that this project will be expanded to other companies.

Budget

The Thai government provides a budget to cover scholarships for girls in Grades 7 to 9. The amount spent for both day students and boarding students grew from about 21 million baht (about US$537,000) in 1994 to just over 41 million baht (about US$1,048,000) in 1997. Several private businesses donate money to be used as a revolving fund for students attending nursing school and for personal expenditures for boarding school students. The total amount donated by mid-1998 was 8 million baht (about US$204,600).

Project Evaluation

Girls who are at present being supported by the project admit that their scholarships are very important for their study. Most of the girls have a positive attitude towards education and report that they will continue their education whether they receive a scholarship or not. The money needed for their education could come from family support or from loans, or they may decide to work and be self-supporting. Receiving a project scholarship helps to lessen the family's monetary burden for education, thus reducing the amount of debt the families might have incurred. Teachers who have selected girls for this project noted that some girls had already been sold to an agent. The teachers had to convince the girls' parents or guardians to change their minds prior to offering the girls their scholarships. It is not too dramatic to suggest that this project may save the lives of many girls and provide them an opportunity for a decent future.

Selecting the right girls is the most important step, to ensure that scholarships will reach the neediest children. In order for every school to use the same criteria, the project set standard selection criteria for each teacher to follow. From interviews with teachers in nine schools in three provinces, it was witnessed that 90 per cent of the girls selected conformed to the set criteria. Statistics collected from 86 girls in these three provinces disclosed that the majority were selected because of poverty (63 per cent), because their parents did not live together (19 per cent) or because they did not live with either parent (14 per cent). Other reported reasons, such as that the girls had good grades or their parents knew teachers in school, accounted for fewer than 5 per cent of the girls chosen.

The Provincial Education Office holds final approval of girls eligible to receive scholarships. Every province has set up a provincial committee to make decisions based on the criteria and the quota allocated to the province. However, the provincial level makes only very small changes to the list submitted by the district education office. Thus, the district level plays a crucial decision-making role. Since they have all of the detailed information about each of the girls selected from each school, district education authorities can more suitably prioritize the list by selecting the neediest girls first, regardless of the quota for each school. Keeping the decision-making power at the district level is important; at the district level, officials have greater information and greater access to each school. If necessary, district officials can visit the girls' families to observe real conditions. Decisions can thus be based on more immediate and accurate information.

At the project's beginning, provincial authorities transferred scholarships to the district education office, which then paid each student by cheque made payable to the girl's name. Students then opened a bank account and deposited the money. This process, however, was very slow: it took several months for the girls to receive the money. In some districts, girls received the first semester scholarship at the start of the second semester, which meant they had to use their own money for educational expenses during the first semester. Due to this problem the disbursement process was changed, having new students open a bank account and transferring the money directly to each student account. This streamlines the payment process. The students feel that the current disbursement system is satisfactory. About one-quarter of the girls admit that they had problems in receiving their scholarships, while about three-quarters admitted that they were satisfied with the money allocation. Of 22 students who reported having problems, just over half said that the money provided is inadequate for one year of schooling, while the rest said that the money allocation was delayed. No student reported problems in withdrawing the money.

The project's monitoring and evaluation process is implemented at every level. The Ministry of Education conducts a national survey on an annual basis by sending questionnaires to every project province asking about dropout rates, implementation problems, and follow-up information on those girls who have passed Grade 9. Furthermore, the monitoring team visits each province to solve problems at the provincial level. Information collected is used to adjust and revise the project as needed. At the provincial level, officials responsible for this project visit district offices for follow-up and monitoring. Likewise, district officials visit schools in their districts to collect information and provide guidelines for implementation and for addressing problems that may arise. A reporting system set by the MOE helps the education office keep track of required information.

Impact

In the first three years of implementation, 1994 to 1996, 1,395 girls received scholarships for boarding school and 11,500 girls for day school. Statistics were collected by the Ministry of Education about what the students who passed Grade 9 did after finishing their education (for the first group of girls receiving scholarships in 1994). However, only statistics pertaining to boarding school girls are available. This information demonstrates that of 395 girls who passed Grade 9 in 1996, 320 (81 per cent) continued their education in some form, two students took short training courses, 47 girls (12 per cent) began working, and 4 (1 per cent) dropped out of school.

The high percentage of girls pursuing an education after completing Grade 9 indicates the measure of success of this project. Girls recruited to be in boarding schools are those who have problems in the family and whose risk of being sold to an agent is very high. Boarding schools, which are located in provinces different from the girls' hometowns, take the girls away from home and their abnormal family environment. From focus group discussions with girls who are at present holding scholarships in boarding schools, it seems that the girls want to study when they have a chance. The three-week orientation programme to prepare girls before entering boarding schools helps them to adjust to life in school. Three years in school is long enough to provide knowledge of the dangers of getting HIV from becoming a sex worker, as well as to provide other means of making a living.

This project is financed by the government. Since project initiation in 1994, every Thai government has made a commitment to allocate a budget for it. The private sector and UNICEF participate by providing monetary support for the training of students who want to work and study simultaneously. Moreover, the Ministry of Education, together with the State Lottery Office, used lottery proceeds to establish vocational training fund for girls who finish Grade 9. They set a target of 600 million baht (roughly US$15,340,000), and use the interest from this fund to support short-course vocational training for 10,000 students annually. This part of the project is therefore potentially self-sustaining through the use of national support mechanisms from both government and the private sector.

Conclusion

After four years of implementation, the project processes have been adjusted in several manners to make them more efficient. Some of the lessons learned from project implementation are summarized below:

The most important aspect of student selection is choosing the girls most in need to participate in the project. Teachers who have worked in their schools for ample time know the girls' family backgrounds and select the neediest or the girls who have problems at home. Yet for those teachers who are new to communities, or who may have little contact with them (such as teachers who commute to work and do not live in the communities), a mechanism should be developed whereby they can objectively evaluate the needs and educational desires of students. This could take the form of collecting family background profiles containing such information as family size, structure, income, migration history of family members, etc., for each child. Community members could be classified to assist schools in collecting information on each girl.

This information, in addition to the students' academic records, could be used to identify those girls who could best benefit from scholarships, for either school or vocational training according to the project's objectives. Selection should start before the school year ends so that there is ample time for teachers to screen and nominate girls. If the time allowed for selection is too short, the school may make an announcement that anyone who is interested can apply. As a result, the objective of helping particularly high risk girls may not be achieved.

The disbursement procedure of transferring money to each girl's bank account has been found to be the most appropriate method. It cuts out unnecessary steps and shortens the time between approval and transfer of the money. However, the financial system at the provincial level must be made flexible enough to facilitate and speed up the disbursement process.

It appears that the quality of statistics from the monitoring questionnaire may be problematic, since several schools did not understand questions and provided incorrect information. For example, concerning the number of girls who drop out, many schools reported no dropouts because they had immediately replaced girls who had dropped out with those on the waiting list. Their understanding was that "dropout" referred to an unfilled position rather than to a girl who had left school. As a result, a very low number of dropouts seems in the official statistics, which in turn leads to insufficient attention to the issue of dropouts, the reasons and the ramifications for the girls who leave school.

Statistics from nine schools in the three provinces disclosed that 11 girls had dropped out, of a total of 346 students (about 3 per cent). Even though the percentage of dropouts is very small (and questionable), this group of girls necessitates greater attention. Based on information from the girls' friends provided during a focus groups discussion on the reasons for their dropping out, the girls who left school did so voluntarily since they wanted to go to work. Their work of choice was in the entertainment business: massage parlours, restaurants, etc., which places them at risk of becoming sex workers. Little has been done to follow this group of girls and help them to find other career alternative in line with the Sema Pattana Cheewit Project's objectives.

Besides this, the curriculum offered in school should provide more alternatives. Girls from poorer families may be at a disadvantage in terms of their educational ability, and they may not do well in a rigid academic environment. Students admit that their friends who drop out do so because they were bored with studying and unable to follow classes. If the school offered alternative programmes - such as vocational training in school and especially opportunities to gain important life skills - these might motivate girls to stay in school. Since the schools have no strategy to cope with girls who want to quit, it falls to each individual teacher to solve the problem. Some teachers may take it seriously and try to convince a girl to stay, but others may ignore the problem and simply replace one who wants to leave with the next girl on the waiting list. It is thus significant to have clear strategy for dealing with this problem, including guidelines for teachers to follow.

The district education office should serve as a centre of information about the girls' current situation both during their study and after they finish. Follow-up information about what the girls do afterwards is important, since it serves as an indicator of project success or the need for improved planning and implementation. Information about the Education Loan Project or other available scholarships should be distributed to Sema Pattana Cheewit girls before they pass Grade 9, so that they can make plans to continue their education.

The Thai Women of Tomorrow (TWT) Project

The Thai Women of Tomorrow (TWT) Project was commenced in 1992 by researchers at the Faculty of Social Sciences, Chiang Mai University (CMU) in northern Thailand. After completing several studies related to the incidence of sex work, child prostitution and AIDS, their causes and effects, the researchers turned to finding practical solutions to these problems. Since it is crucial to prevent young girls at high risk from being pushed or pulled into the sex business, the TWT proposal was submitted to the Women's Economic and Leadership Development Programme (WELD) under monetary support from the Canadian International Development Agency (CIDA). The first approved project, entitled *Reduction of Child Prostitution by Raisina Consciousness and Attitudes among Children and Parents in Rural Society*, was commenced in 1993. This was the TWT's first phase aimed at testing an attitude change model. The project targeted rural primary school girls at risk of becoming sex workers in two districts (Mae Jai and June) in Phayao Province, an area with major HIV/AIDS and sex workers problems. The project's objectives were to change the attitudes of both girls and their parents against sex work and in favour of higher education and good occupations.

After the model was tested with satisfactory results, the project moved to Phase II, *Providing Educational and Occupational Opportunities through Public-Private Partnership*. This phase built a public-private partnership to provide opportunities for girls for continuing education and skills training. The partnerships provided scholarship funds, skills training and job opportunities for girls after they completed their training programmes. Two provinces, Phayao and Chiang Rai, were the target areas and it was planned to expand the project to cover every province in the North and Northeast if the programme proved successful. The project received funding from the United States Agency for International Development (USAID) as well as private donations.

The third phase of the TWT project began at the end of 1994 after support from USAID ended. For the project to be sustainable, three activities were initiated. The first activity aimed to build a relationship with the private sector and other nongovernmental organizations for long-term support in providing scholarships to the students. The second activity was designed to transfer the idea and methodology of the public-private partnership to teaching institutions and public organizations, to link both study curriculum and training with the private sector. The third activity concentrated on strengthening media production and counselling to change the attitudes of young women and their parents regarding sex business; this activity received monetary support from the Government of Japan under the Small Scale Grant Assistance programme (SSGA).

Since the Faculty of Social Sciences at CMU is an academic institution, the fourth phase of the project then aimed to reduce its implementation role to that of academic support and continue the attitude change campaign. The fourth phase gained support from the International Labour Organization (ILO) under the International Programme on the Elimination of Child Labour (IPEC). The Last phase of this project is to set up a resource and research centre against child prostitution and abuse in northern Thailand. The centre's functions are:

(a) Providing information about child prostitution and child abuse;

(b) Promoting and coordinating a network of governmental and nongovernmental organizations and private agencies;

(c) Creating and using effective local media to change attitudes regarding child prostitution and child abuse;

(d) Promoting and supporting existing education and training institutes to adopt a comprehensive intervention module for eliminating child prostitution and child abuse

(e) undertaking an evaluation of on-going interventions and building academic support for network members.

Details about each of the TWT project's phases are presented below potentially useful for adaptation and implementation elsewhere.

First Phase

To change attitudes of rural girls and their parents against sex work and in favour of higher education. Target population was primary school students in rural areas who were at risk of becoming sex worker in two districts of Phayao Province. The four primary activities undertaken in this phase were:

1. To survey attitudes of girls and their parents about sex business.
2. To produce a 3-part series vide tape and attitude change materials.
3. To produce an attitude change manual including pre- and post-tests for the video tape, technical information for focus groups, counselling and home visits.

4. To recruit three teacher volunteers per district to be trained to work with students and their parents to change attitudes.

Second Phase

In September 1993, CMU conducted a seminar on its pilot three-step programme to find out practical solutions for solving the prostitution problem in northern Thailand. The seminar's conclusion emphasized that a public-private partnership was the best way to seek cooperation from every sector of society to deal with the problem. Informal discussions with private sector representatives were conducted to formulate the nature of the collaboration. Several private enterprises demonstrated a serious interest in this activity by offering scholarships, skills training and job opportunities. The project was expanded to cover two provinces, Phayao and Chiang Rai, with the aim of extending both educational and career opportunities.

The extension of educational opportunities activity has two main objectives: (1) to provide girls in Grades 5 and 6 and their families information about the consequences of sex work and AIDS, and (2) to provide girls from poor families who are at high risk of being lured into prostitution scholarships to continue their education upto Grade 9. Scholarships of 3,000 baht (about US$77) per year per student for 100 girls in two provinces in the North were provided by individuals and organizations in 1994. In 1995, the number of scholarships remained at 100, but it was increased to 300 scholarships in 1996 and thereafter.

The implementation steps for the first objective consisted: selection of counselling teachers in each district, for a total of 18 counsellors in the programme; training these counsellors to utilise media kits, focus group methods, person-to-person counselling, group counselling, and home visits; providing media kits (which include TVs and instructive videos) to counsellors, teachers, etc.; presentations by counsellors, development officers and public health officers, using the media kits, to target groups; and monitoring and evaluating activities by the provincial and district administrative committees and CMU.

The education extension activity commenced with an initial

provision of scholarships, then establishment of a long-term scholarship fund. The initial stage included: (1) conducting a public relations campaign, (2) acknowledging donor companies and organizations and (3) creating links between students and donors. The long-term objective is to set up a Thai Women of Tomorrow Foundation at the national level to raise scholarship funds.

The provincial administrative committee is responsible for regulating, managing and distributing the scholarship funds. The district committee controls the selection of students and monitors the programme as per the policies set forth by the provincial committee. The CMU Faculty of Social Science disburses scholarship funds to provinces and acts as a cooperative agency between scholarship students and donors. The counselling teachers and school principals nominate students for the scholarships and monitor their educational progress.

This activity provides job training and placement. Four job training programmes are offered: (1) an assistant health worker career programme; (2) a modern fashion and design programme; (3) a secretarial and computer training programme and (4) an assistant jewellery cutter training programme. There is also a (5) special training skills programme for girls who are too young to enter the other four programmes.

The objective of Assistant Health Worker Career Programme is to provide an opportunity for girls graduating from Grade 9, and aged 16 or more, to become assistant health workers, employed permanently in hospitals and child or elderly care centres. The programme target is 200 young women per year in the priority provinces for training and placement in the health care field. Its implementation steps are the following:

(a) The provincial administrative committee, public health, labour and public welfare offices consider the plan, training programme, and implementation steps in detail.

(b) The district administrative committee selects young women interested in this career as per the criteria and regulations established by the provincial committee.

(c) The CMU Faculty of Social Sciences, together with provincial administrative offices and private organizations, recommend career training opportunities and research available jobs.

(d) The Provincial Public Health Office, Provincial Labour Office, Provincial Public Welfare Office, Faculty of Social Sciences and private organizations recruit young women for the training programmes.

(e) A pre-training orientation session is conducted for the young women who have been recruited.

(f) The training programme is of three to six months duration.

(g) After training is complete, private organizations help provide permanent employment.

The objective of Modern Fashion and Design Career Programme is to help Grade 6 students aged 16 and above pursue a career in modern fashion and design and to work permanently in factories. This programme trains 180 young women graduates annually. Its programme steps are as follows:

(a) Chiang Mai University, the provincial administrative committee and private sector organization examine the plan, training programme, place for training, internship, and job placement opportunities.

(b) The provincial and district committees, especially the Provincial Labour Office and Provincial Public Welfare Office, recruit young women as per the criteria and regulation established by the provincial administrative committee.

(c) The young women selected attend a pre-training orientation session to develop an understanding of what they can expect during training.

(d) During the three-month training period, the trainees receive free lodging, food, transportation and a modest allowance. The trainees are able to earn extra income if the trainers find them part-time jobs or an internship during the training programme.

(e) Young women who pass the training programme will be placed permanently in the fashion and design factories in Chiang Mai and Lampang Provinces and be paid at par with their skills but not less than the minimum legal wage.

Secretarial Career (Computer Training) programme has as its objective to provide girls who have finished Grade 9 (aged 16 and above) with an opportunity to become a secretary. Fifty young women completing Grade 9 are trained for 250 hours in computer and other modern office skills. They receive certificates and support in finding suitable jobs. The implementation steps are as follows:

(a) USAID, CMU Faculty of Social Sciences and private business jointly create the training plan, programme activities, programme site and training, as well as making provision for jobs after training.

(b) The provincial and district administrative committees select young women who are qualified in accordance with the set up criteria and regulations.

(c) The girls recruited go through an orientation programme to assist them understand the training and working conditions.

(d) After training, students are tested and receive certificates.

(e) All private and public agencies participating in the programme cooperate in providing internship and jobs for trainees.

Assistant Jewellery Cutter Training Programme provides young women who have completed Grade 9 with an opportunity to become assistant jewellery cutters employed permanently in gem and diamond cutting factories and companies. The target was set at 120 young women to train and place in permanent jobs with the Thai Gem and Jewellery Traders Association. The implementation steps include the following:

(a) The district administrative committee and members of the Representative Committee from IQS (Public) Co. Ltd. (Gemopolis) in Bangkok recruit young women who want to accept this career.

(b) The faculty of Social Sciences along with provincial administrative offices and private organizations, cooperate with the Thai Gem and Jewellery Traders Association to provide jobs.

(c) Pre-training orientation is provided for girls who are recruited.

(d) The training takes place over six months at the Gemopolis Company, situated on the outskirts of Bangkok.

(e) After the training, the Gemopolis Company employed the young women permanently.

Girls who are not eligible to apply for one of the four training programmes discussed earlier because of their age are at risk of being pressured by their parents to work. Moreover, girls who are recommended for scholarship to continue their education to Grade 7, or those who are recommended for training programmes, may also be under pressure during the period (approximately two to three months) before school starts or before the training programme begins. Agents use this time to approach the girls' parents and offer money for loans. The Special Training Skills Programme was formulated to give these girls a special training opportunity within the province for this crucial two-to-three-month duration to prevent agents from pressuring the girls and their parents. The programme is implemented as follows:

(a) Local teachers/counsellors determine emergency cases in which girls are witnessed to be at high risk of leaving immediately to enter the sex business.

(b) The teachers or counsellors contact by telephone the Faculty of Social Sciences. Together they devise an appropriate alternative plan of action in a comprehensive and timely manner.

(c) Money from the special skills training programme is used by the teachers/counsellors to implement an immediate response to the needs of a particular girl in one of several training programmes, in skills such as hairdressing, cooking, cloth/umbrella painting or wood carving.

Third Phase

The TWT was able to enhance its ongoing activities and extend its efforts over a broader area and target population in northern Thailand. In this phase, previous experience working with the attitude changing programmes and the success stories of girls who completed there training and found permanent jobs were incorporated into several packages of campaign materials.

Fourth Phase

Three districts in each of four provinces in the north of Thailand: Chiang Rai, Phayao, Lampang and Chaing Mai were selected for this phase. Two projects were implemented during this period:

(a) a campaign against child prostitution and in support of the creation of new career attitudes, and
(b) development of education standards and skills training for girls attending boarding school under the Sema Pattana Cheewit Project.

This project is a continuation of activity from second phase, which concentrated on a campaign to change the attitudes of girls and their parents about sex work. Face-to-face discussion, focus group sessions, and home visits were among the campaign tools used. Scholarships were also provided to girls who passed Grade 6 to continue their education for three more years. This activity was coordinated with the Sema Pattana Cheewit Project implemented by the Ministry of Education. Girls recruited by the TWT project were treated the same as girls who participated in the Sema Pattana Cheewit Project. The TWT project, though, concentrated more attention on girls who passed Grade 9, to persuade them to continue their education or provide short-course training and discover appropriate employments for those who completed training.

Boarding schools involved in the Sema Pattana Cheewit Project receive girls at high risk of becoming sex workers, so that girls will be away from home to prevent their parents from forcing them into the sex work. However, it seemed to be necessary to provide girls in Sema Pattana Cheewit who were unable to follow the standard school curricula with other options. Girls from poorer families often have a disavantage in terms of education ability, and may be unable to attend classes. Such girls would benefit if school had alternatives such as skills training that could be utilised to assist them find employments after passing Grade 9.

Researchers in TWT project, in collaboration with the Sema Pattana Cheewit Project, conducted research to help develop education standards and skills training for girls attending boarding schools. The project for development of educational standards and skills training for girls attending boarding school has four important objectives:

(a) To improve and develop education models and standards so that they satisfy the needs of girls and can be used by them to generate income after finishing their education;

(b) To examine these models in participating project schools and evaluate their efficiency and effectiveness;

(c) To utilize the models as a skills training approach for girls in school and ascertain that they are appropriate for meeting local needs;

(d) To enable girls in this target group to earn some income during their education period.

Research activities and skills training in schools have been undertaken to accomplish these objectives.

Project Evaluation

This project's main objectives are to change the attitudes of girls and parents in the northern part of Thailand regarding sex trade and to provide a means for the girls to avoid becoming sex worker through improved education and career opportunities. Before the AIDS epidemic, parents learned from the experiences of other families that selling daughters into sex trade was a way to improve their economic status and satisfy their material desires. Since such parents had very few other alternatives for earning a living, they felt that sending their daughters into the sex business was a viable solution. Not every girl who entered into sex work was in this situation, however. Many were deceived and promised good jobs in the city, as waitresses in restaurants or as housekeepers, but were later forced to work as sex workers. With the spread of AIDS and the realization that sex workers are the most vulnerable group to HIV infection, many concerned organizations began taking this problem seriously. The TWT project focusses on preventive strategies to address the AIDS problem by providing opportunities for girls to enhance their education.

It is a common concept in the Thai community that the longer a girl stays in school, the greater the probability that she will stay out of sex work. Statistics indicates that Grade 6 graduates are more likely to enter the sex industry than Grade 9 graduates. Education is viewed as one of the best strategies to deal with the sex business problem and hence reduce the vulnerability of girls.

The project stresses encouraging girls who pass Grade 6 to continue school for three more years. This group is too young to legally enter the labour force but they are open to being forced into the sex business. Moreover, clients of brothels often prefer young girls under the assumption that they are free of HIV/AIDS. Those children mostly come from families in debt trap. Brothel owners have networks of agents who seek out families with young daughters and entice them with offers of money, and parents encountering economic pressures and a lust for consumer goods come to view their daughters as commodities that can be traded. The girls obey their parents' as a token of gratitude and to help secure the household income. Once sold, the girls are trapped in the sex network and find it very difficult to escape. They are subject to abuse and face the danger of being infected with HIV. Thus, keeping those girls from being sold is a very important step.

This project was initiated in 1992, two years before the Sema Pattana Cheewit Project started. The CMU researchers were interested in finding solutions to the child prostitution problem in northern Thailand, where the rates of both prostitution and HIV are alarmingly high in the country. This initiative should be viewed as a pilot project and, with respect to convincing girls and their families to continue their education, it has been successful. It was therefore used by the government as a model in implementing the Sema Pattana Cheewit Project and expanding it to other parts of the country with similar problems.

The project uses teachers trained as counsellors to monitor and discuss with girls their future education and careers. Teachers are aware of the problems of each girl and they also meet with the girl's parents or guardians to discuss the situation and encourage them to continue the girl's education. Teachers in this case play a significant role in identifying the target group. Approximately 95 per cent of the girls selected to participate in the project are in the specified target group. Since the project concentrates on education, it collaborates directly with the Ministry of Education at both provincial and district levels, the Ministry of Labour and Social Welfare and the Ministry of the Interior. These concerned agencies address such issues as training, job seeking, and selecting appropriate participants. The project's budget relied mainly on support from international organizations. A diagram of the partnership structure is presented in Appendix B.

Another difficult yet critical part is to discover proper jobs for girls after they finish their training. A job that can generate income at a satisfactory level is an incentive for both girls and their families. At the beginning, business sector participation in the project consisted only of a small scale garment factory in the local area that offered training and jobs. The advantage of this type of industrial unit was that the girls were trained in the entire process of dress making; the disadvantage is that the jobs are not well paid. The unit paid the girls much less than the minimum wage because they were trainees. The director of the project then contacted other, larger units where wages were according to labour laws. The girls were more satisfied with their monthly incomes and could send some remittance back to their families.

Originally, the project supported accommodations, per diem and meals for the girls and the unit provided training materials and other training related expenses. When the budget was cut, project personnel changed their role from monetary supporter to that of middleman for industrial units who wanted trained labour. The project conducted campaigns in all of the industrial units in the region, stressing that the project could recruit qualified girls to be trained to work in the unit. The project director also went to meet with the management to seek their cooperation to offer training and jobs to the girls. At present, seven companies are participating.

Another barrier encountered related to the culture of northern girls: they have to take a long vacation during the annual Sonkran Festival, during the Thai New Year (in April). For people in northern Thailand, this holiday is the most important of the year and they must return home for it. The vacation may take as long as 10 days. As a result, factories, especially those that must produce orders on schedule, prefer to hire girls who are not from the North.

The TWT project has successfully and effectively met several of its aims and objectives. The project recruited volunteer teachers in six districts of Phayao and Chiang Rai Provinces, trained them and assigned them the responsibility of making attitude changes among girls at risk and their families. Effective packages of campaign media and methods were produced; for example, one set of video tapes contains interviews with anonymous girls who are actually working as sex workers to let them tell of their suffering, the nature of which is generally unknown to villagers. When the girls and their families learn about how the girls might be abused, their attitude towards sex industry changes. Focus group sessions and home visits were also carefully prepared by TWT stall and delivered to target groups by volunteer teachers. These methods were continued with at risk families to monitor, follow up and try to affect decisions about the girls' futures. As a result, a great number of girls decided to either continue schooling or join vocational training programmes. The project offered more than 1,000 scholarships to girls who passed Grade 6. This means that these girls will not enter the labour market for at least three more years. Another 425 girls participated in vocational training in four areas:

(a) One hundred and forty girls attended the Assistant Health Worker six-month training programme at the Thai-Canadian Academy of the Care West Company. After training, they were employed by Care West and some private hospitals in Bangkok, Chiang Mai and Chiang Rai with legal wages and benefits.

(b) Seventy-five girls were trained for 250 hours at the Computer Centre, Chiang Mai University. They were then placed in secretarial positions at several reputed companies with reasonable salaries and benefits.

(c) One hundred and fifty girls were trained for three months at the Wing Group in Sankanpang, Chiang Mai and Sahapatana Groups at Lamphun. They were then placed at several garment and Leather-making companies in Chiang Mai with legal wages and benefits.

(d) Sixty girls were trained in the Gemopolis and the General Diamond Companies, the leading jewellery cutting trades. They were then employed as skilled jewellery cutters in these companies in Bangkok. The career is very promising and the benefits are higher than the minimum legal wage.

The project has been implemented for five years. The implementation strategies have been modified as per the changing situation. Since the project began in an academic setting. It has been oriented towards research. The intention was to develop a model that could be shifted to other areas on a larger scale. The project might be self-sustaining if it fully develops its partnership with both public and private sectors. Chiang Mai University has served as coordinator and the focal point of implementation. If funding from international and domestic donors can be found, the project could share expenses for training and providing student scholarships. If funds are terminated, it must work more as facilitator, coordinator and organizer for companies to select girls for their training programmes.

Since this project is being operated by an academic organization, it has not been possible to expand it to cover the entire target population. As a result, after examining their model and learning important lessons from its implementation, the project's organizers have changed their role to that of resource and research centre against child prostitution and child abuse in northern Thailand. Following are the conclusions:

(a) The project's premise was that changing the attitudes of girls and parents is the most important element for success. If parents and girls still have positive attitude towards sex business, it is difficult to convince them about the value of education. Even if the project can compensate the family by giving the children scholarships, the children might leave school before they pass Grade 9. The project therefore put its efforts into attitude changing activities, with scholarships and short-course training as supporting activities for those who wanted to have alternative manners of earning money. This strategy is crucial for the success of the project. Once families have negative attitudes towards sex work they will try to find other ways and means to earn a living regardless of the existence of this project. It is recommended that communities should participate in the attitude changing activities. The project, in collaboration with NGOs, may train community volunteers in attitude changing strategies. Once the communities have this knowledge and absorb the opinion of the danger of letting girls become sex workers, it is possible that the objectives of the project will be accomplished.

This strategy is different from that of the Sema Pattana Cheewit Project, which puts more emphasis on the scholarships. If the effort and strategies developed by these two projects can be combined the prospect of lessening the number of girls who enter sex work will be better.

(b) The short-course training provided for girls in rural areas had to be designed as per the girls' abilities. The computer training programme may not be appropriate because it necessitates skills in English, one major weakness of students in rural areas. It is difficult for them to learn the material and after they complete training their skills at times are still not at par with those of other well-trained persons. The training programmes that are best suited to the girls in this area are gem cutting and the garment industry. They can learn fast and get a well paid job after the completion of their training. Matching the right training programme with the target population should be a priority.

(c) Choosing the companies to participate in the project is another important issue. If the girls who finish training are placed in companies that exploit them with low pay or excessive work hours, it will discourage girls from such work and encourage them to become sex workers, who earn much higher incomes. As a result, past practices may re-assert themselves, with sex trade again being witnessed as the most viable form of work for rural poor women. Selecting the right business partners and involving them in every step of the project, especially in the planning and implementation stages, can increase their awareness and understanding of the objectives of the project and may reduce the likelihood of exploitation.

Education Loan Fund Project

The Education Loan Project was approved in January 1996 to provide educational opportunities to students who cannot afford to continue their studies after passing Grade 9. Human resource development and equal access to education for everyone are the project's major objectives. Since compulsory education in Thailand is six years, education to a higher level is thought to be up to individuals and their families. But families with meagre incomes may decide to put their children into the labour market rather than sending them to school. As a result, they will be trapped in low paying jobs and unskilled work, unable to improve their standard of life. This project offers low-interest loans to students to continue their education as far as the university level. Those who are eligible for loans must meet the following conditions:

(a) They must be Thai nationals enrolled in a Thai educational institution, either in high school (regular or vocational), earning but not having completed a bachelor's degree or participating in out-of-school programmes.
(b) They must not have a full-time job during their course of education.
(c) Their family can have a total income of not more than 120,000 baht (about US$3068) per annum and the student must have a satisfactory educational record.
(d) They must be free of bankruptcy.
(e) They must not be sentenced to prison.

Students can request to borrow money to cover tuition fees, education-related expenditures and living expenses. The yearly expenditure for each educational level varies from 53,640 baht (US$1372) for high school or equivalent to 76,500 baht (US$1956) for a bachelor's degree. Contracts are made on annual basis. After the first-year loan is approved, students are guaranteed to receive subsequent loans until graduation, unless they have educational problems and are unable to complete their studies.

Students must start to return their loans two years after the completion of their education. The loan reimbursement includes both interest and principal on the loan, and is paid back on a progressive schedule. The loan should be completely paid off within 15 years (that is, 17 years after students complete their education). The interest rate is set at 1 per cent per year. The loan is terminated when all the money is returned or the borrower dies.

In March or April, a committee and working group are set up

at the provincial level to consider guidelines for the allocation of loans and the implementation process. Information is disseminated to every educational institution student and the general public about the loan project. In May, the educational institutions make announcements for students to submit their requests and then screen the request forms. The institutes classify all students who wish to receive a loan and calculate the total amount requested.

In June, the provincial committee conducts a meeting to review the cases where the money requested exceeds the money allocated to the province. The committee may allocated less money than requested by each individual to spread it out to cover more students. The educational institutions advise students who are to receive loans to prepare a contract with Krung Thai Bank. In July, schools report the number of students and total money requested to the provincial education office, which in turn reports to the Ministry of Education and the Krung Thai Bank.

In August and September, the Ministry of Finance verifies all of the contracts and Krung Thai Bank transfers monthly stipends to each student account. The provincial working group later follows up on project implementation.

The project budget for the first year of implementation (1996) was 3000 million baht (about US$76,720,000); 60 per cent of that amount went to the Ministry of Education, and 40 per cent to the Ministry of University Affairs. In 1997, the budget was targeted at 950 million baht (US$280 million).

Project Evaluation

This project's target population is students (boys and girls) who have completed Grade 9 and want to continue their studies either formally or informally. The process of selecting students is carried out by a committee at each institute, under guidelines issued by the Loan Committee at the central office. The project is to help poor families irrespective of the risk children may be in with regard to entering the sex work. However, Sema Pattana Cheewit students receive priority in receiving education loans if they apply. Thus, although this project does not address the AIDS problem directly, it is viewed as a supporting project, helping to realize the objectives of the Sema Pattana Cheewit and Thai Women of Tomorrow projects.

However, regarding the chances of girls under the Sema Pattana Cheewit Project in securing loans, the Educational Loan Project is not fully successful. During focus group discussions with these girls about why they did not apply for the loan, most said they did not receive information about it. Loan project announcements are made at the high school level. Students at lower educational levels receive such information only from television or radio. Students who qualify to apply for loans must already be enrolled in a high school or higher level educational institution, which means that those who pass Grade 9 are unable to apply until they are already enrolled in a higher level educational institution. This process is different from that of the Sema Pattana Cheewit Project, where students who receive a scholarship know the result before they pass Grade 6; thus they are certain that they will have sufficient funds to continue their studies. The Educational Loan Project's process thus reduces the probabilities for poor students, such as those in the Sema Pattana Cheewit Project, who want to continue their studies but do not have sufficient information or are in doubt about getting approval.

With this loan money, more than 131,000 students studied in schools under the Ministry of Education and more than 21,500 students under the Ministry of University Affairs in 1996. The number of students receiving loans under the MOE rose to more than 373,000 (up 185 per cent) in 1997 and more than 65,000 (up 205 per cent) for students under the Ministry of University Affairs.

The project has been implemented for only two years. Its sustainability depends on whether the government has an ample annual allocation budget. Moreover, it also depends on whether students who have complete their education and start to work will promptly pay back their loans, which repayments will be put in a revolving fund and allocated to new students. It is too early to tell the rate of default (i.e., failure to repay the loans) or its impact on project sustainability.

Conclusion

(a) During the first year of implementation students did not understand the objective of the loan project and feared being in debt, thus the total loan amount requested by students applying for loans was less than the amount of money allocated. So informing the target population of the availability of funds and the terms of the loans is the primary need. Moreover, each school should receive detailed information in order to answer any questions that students may have. The implementation process is rather complicated and details of contracts need to be accurate. Many schools did not understand the projects process, which resulted in unnecessary delays.

The students who received loans during the first year of implementation had to wait about a semester before their loan was sanctioned. During the second year, when the students understood and learned from other students who had already received loans, the number of students who applied doubled and implementation was faster. Information dissemination and detailed implementation guidelines are crucial. Nongovernmental organisations can act as information disseminators to target populations, especially to the group in greatest need; this might involve identifying target groups and providing necessary information such as the availability of funds, the application process, the contract and repayment processes, and so forth.

(b) It was noticed to be important to avoid words that might be barriers for some population groups to apply for loans. For example, the word "interests" is not accepted by Muslims, thus lessening the probability for that group of students to apply for loans. The project therefore changed the word to "fee", which was acceptable to the target population.

The students who received loans, reported that they can concentrate more on their studies because they do not have to worry about earning money to pay for their education. They also said that they feel more responsible about completing their studies in order to get a job and pay back their loans.

Seven

Thailand's 100 per cent Condom Programme

Thailand was the first Asian nation to recognize that it had a major HIV/AIDS problem, a problem so grave as to deserve priority on the national agenda. While sporadic testing among female sex workers, injecting drug users (IDUs) , and men having sex with men detected little HIV through the end of 1987, the accelerated expansion of HIV infections among IDUs in early 1988 spurred efforts to watch the epidemic systematically. By mid-1989, a national sentinel serosurveillance system had been set up. In the first round of testing in 14 provinces conducted in June 1989, high infection levels were noticed among brothel sex workers in the country's northern provinces. By June 1990, with the system expanded to include all 73 provinces, HIV prevalence among brothel-based sex workers had crossed from 3.1 per cent in June 1989 to 9.3 per cent nationally (provincial median) and was rising fast. By June 1991, it had gone to 15.2 per cent. Prevalence was also growing rapidly among young Thai men from 0.5 per cent in November 1989 to 3.0 per cent in November 1991. Studies of behaviour and HIV infection among these and other populations soon demonstrated that most new HIV infections in Thailand were due to commercial sex.

Promoting the Condom Use

Since the advent of this disease, many Thai public health workers and researchers were of the opinion that widespread sex work would come to dominate the Thai epidemic, a viewpoint strongly supported by the available statistics from the early 1990s. Thus, a new approach to promote condom use in commercial sex was being pioneered in Ratchaburi province: the 100 per cent

Condom Programme.

The programme addressed the observation that sex work establishments requiring condom use or sex workers insisting on condom use would often lose clients and money to those who did not. Because many clients did not want to use condoms, there were economic disincentives for establishment owners who promoted safer behaviour at their establishments: men could simply go to another establishment or to a sex worker who did not require condoms. Regional Communicable Disease Control officials in Ratchaburi realized that one solution to this basic economic problem was to require that all establishments and sex workers in the province use condoms in every sex act. This would assure owners and managers that they would not lose business by enforcing the policies requiring condom use, since clients could not go anywhere else to obtain risky sex. They initiated a collaborative effort among local authorities, public health officers, sex establishment owners, and sex workers to ensure that clients could not purchase sexual services without condom use in the province. When this programme was implemented, the rates of sexually transmitted diseases (STDs) declined quickly and significantly. Soon after, the efforts were expanded into the provinces around Ratchaburi (e.g., Samut Sakhon province) and in some other provinces in other parts of the country with identical positive results. During this early period the Faculty of Medicine at Khon Kaen University was also piloting similar approaches in Khon Kaen, as was the Thai Red Cross Society in Bangkok and Pattaya.

A National Level Programme

Despite these initiatives, economic disparities still existed across provincial borders. If a man could not buy unprotected sex in Ratchaburi, he could always go across the border to any neighbouring province and purchase it there. Armed with strong epidemiological and behavioural statistics which demonstrated the important role of sex work in the Thai epidemic and the success of these pilot efforts, a set of planned steps to make this programme national policy was undertaken. In 1991, this included presentations to a regional meeting of provincial governors and their staff in April, to high level administrators of the Ministry of

Public Health in June, and to the permanent secretaries of various government ministries in July. In August, the national AIDS Committee issued a resolution to implement the 100 per cent Condom Programme on a national scale. The resolution stated:

> "The governor, the provincial chief of police and the provincial health officer of each province will coordinate to enforce a condom-use-only policy that requires all sex workers to use condoms with every customer. All concerned ministries will issue guidelines that comply with this policy".

Several national efforts in the early 1990s under the auspices of the National Condom Promotion Campaign were undertaken concurrently with the 100 per cent Condom Programme. Condoms were added into the Medical Device Act which required quality assurance. To ensure high quality condoms, a working group was set up between the Ministry of Public Health and Ministry of Industry to revise existing condom quality control directives, implement quality checks, and ensure enforcement of the guidelines. Condom use was promoted through mass media, peer education, and outreach programmes aimed at specific groups throughout the country. The Ministry of Public Health began providing approximately 60 million condoms a year free of charge, primarily distributed to sex parlours. After the adoption of the resolution, the Prime Minister's Office and Ministry of the Interior organized presentations at national meetings of all provincial governors and all district officers and provincial and district chiefs of police. The Ministry of Public Health also organized meetings of all provincial chief medical officers to persuade the implementation of the programme as fast as possible and to provide reports back to the Ministry of Public Health on a regular basis. These meetings revealed the high level of national commitment to the programme and instructed the audience to implement the programme locally. By mid-1992, all provinces reported that the 100 per cent Condom Programme was in place.

A Different Programme

Initially, many people did not believe the programme succeed. For example, reporters from a Thai daily went to

Chiang Mai in 1991, shortly after the implementation of the programme there, seeking to purchase sex without a condom. To their surprise, they were unable to do so. Small studies have examined the ability to purchase sex without a condom, and have found that most sex workers are quite resistant to the idea. Numerous other studies, as well as questions asked to sex workers during the national sentinel serosurveillance, now routinely show that condom use in brothels and massage parlours exceeds 90 per cent. These revelations confirm that the 100 per cent Condom Programme, in combination with other prevention efforts, has been very effective at discouraging unprotected intercourse in sex parlours.

There are clear indications that these efforts have had an impact on HIV transmission at the national level. Nationwide monitoring of condom use in brothel based sex parlours and of levels of reported STDs among men has shown a strong relationship between the increase in condom use and the rapid decline in STDs. Statistics from studies demonstrated gradual rise in their use of condoms with sex workers, a decline in the number of visits to sex workers, and a decline in reported histories of STDs and in HIV prevalence. Studies witnessed a tenfold reduction in STD incidence and a fivefold reduction in HIV incidence among young Thai men between 1991 and 1993. Thus, all indications are that the 100 per cent Condom Programme has been significant contributor to large-scale reduction of HIV transmission throughout the country.

Critical Evaluation

Such anecdotal evidence, small studies, and even national figures do little to tell us about the essential components of the 100 per cent Condom Programme to evaluate the factors that have contributed to its success, or to find out the programme's limitations. To address these issues, UNAIDS and the Ministry of Public Health of the Royal Thai Government (MOPH) supported the Institute for Population and Social Research (IPSR) of Mahidol University to formulate and implement a detailed study in mid-1997 examining the effectiveness of the programme at the provincial level.

The IPSR research team developed a two-phase strategy to discover the effectiveness of the programme in the provinces. In the first phase, they analysed existing statistics and conducted indepth interviews with key provincial officials participating in the implementation of the programme. The team used the statistics collected in this phase to discover the most important programme components and to develop ways of defining and measuring 22 programme input in the provinces. Detailed questionnaires were then designed to evaluate these inputs in the provinces. The second phase of the project surveyed implementing officials, pharmacists, and sex parlour owners and managers to evaluate the programme inputs at the local level. This phase also used surveys with sex workers and young men (many of whom were clients of sex workers) to find out the programme's local impact on behaviour. These research efforts are described in greater detail in the reports prepared by the team.

The study had three major components, conducted in approximately one-third of all Thai provinces (24 out of 76 provinces, 6 within each of the country's 4 regions):

- A review of prevailing statistics to find out the extent and nature of sex work in each province and to validate observed declines in STDs at government clinics.
- A series of in-depth qualitative and quantitative interviews in each province with government personnel participating in the implementation of the programme, owners and managers of sex parlours and local pharmacists. These provided quantitative measurements of the programme's inputs.
- Detailed surveys of both sex workers (approximately 100 per province) and young males (approximately 200 per province) to measure the effects of the programme.

The remainder of this document reports on the findings of this study in three key areas: the implementation of the programme at the provincial level; the effectiveness of the programme in the provinces studied; and a contextual analysis of the known limitations of the programme as well as the factors contributing to successful implementation.

Presence of Biases

Although the 100 per cent condom programme attempts to reach all types of sex parlours, the study laid emphasis on direct sex parlours that should be kept in mind. Sex work sites in Thailand are often divided into direct and indirect set ups. In direct establishments, such as brothels or hotels, the services available are primarily sexual and often take place on site. In indirect establishments, such as bars, massage parlours, cafes, or restaurants, sexuals services are offered in the context of other services such as food, massage, or entertainment, and sex often, but not always, occurs off site. The sites for interviewing sex workers in this study were primarily direct for two reasons. First, sites were selected from Ministry of Public Health lists that are routinely kept in each province. These lists are maintained locally from a combination of reports from STD patients about where they contracted STD, reports from sex workers coming for STD exams, knowledge of other sites by local health officials and police, and historical information on where sexual services are available. In some provinces, they may overrepresent direct sites, which are easier to discover and where more sex, and consequently more STD transmission, occurs. Second, the study team frequently faced difficulties in interviewing sex workers at indirect sites. Either the owners would refuse access or the sex workers would maintain that they did not offer sexual services.

An additional bias relates to the selection of provinces. While the first half were selected randomly, in some provinces it was not possible to locate the required number of sex workers for interviews. Thus, some provinces - where there were low numbers of sex workers or where the MOPH had more limited access to sex workers - were excluded.

As a result, these biases suggest that the findings presented here apply more to the situation at direct sex work establishments in areas of Thailand where the study team had good access. The findings of this study say less about what is happening in indirect sites.

Programme Implementation

The primary idea of the 100 per cent Condom Programme is to classify the aid of provincial administrative and health authorities, governors, the police, sex workers, and the owners and managers of sex parlours to make it impossible for clients to purchase sexual services without using a condom. In addition, the programme must be implemented with a large coverage, at least in a cluster of provinces so that clients cannot 'escape' the programme even if they visit sex parlours in the nearby province. This simple-sounding idea, however, latents a somewhat more complex reality. Many components and the cooperation of multiple agencies and individuals are needed to implement the 100 per cent Condom Programme effectively.

Organisation

Although the guideline to implement the 100 per cent Condom Programme came from the highest levels of the Thai government, the actual management and implementation of the programme's components make use of both existing and recently added health structures at the regional and provincial levels. In most provinces it was implemented fundamentally with existing local staff and health structures. Management at these levels makes the programme more responsive to local needs and helps to increase the relevance of the strategies and activities to the local situation. While there are many features common to most or all provinces, the actual programme implementation details do vary somewhat from place to place. This report will concentrate primarily on those features and factors that are common to most or all of the provinces.

Programme Management

Responsibilities for programme management are classified between two levels: the Regional Offices of Communicable Disease Control (RCDCs) and Provincial Public Health Offices (PPHOs). Each of the twelve RCDCs in the country has wide public health responsibilities for five to seven provinces, with the 100 per cent Condom Programme being only one of the many public health efforts the offices supervise. Within each RCDC, three units have responsibilities associated with the 100 per cent Condom Programme besides their other public health duties:

(a) the Pharmacy Section, accountable to the storage of condoms supplied by the Ministry of Public Health;

(b) the Implementation Support Section, responsible for evaluation of needs for condoms and managing their distribution to the provinces;

(c) the STD and AIDS Centre, with responsibility for providing STD examinations and prevention programmes for sex workers.

RCDCs have two additional units with the following responsibilities:

(a) the Health Behaviour Development Unit, providing HIV/STD prevention and care training for sex workers and the general population;

(b) the Epidemiology Unit, which helps in monitoring the use of condoms in sex parlours.

In the PPHOs, the AIDS and STD Section is responsible for prevention programmes for sex workers and other general public, especially male clients; for monitoring and evaluating the programme; and for the direct distribution of condoms to establishments, sex workers, and other groups. These activities may involve regional, provincial, and district hospitals and district public health centres when their assistance is helpful and relevant.

While the RCDCs have larger responsibilities for supervising the programme at the regional level in the provinces they cover, they also often directly participate in activities. Although the PPHOs collaborate closely with the RCDCs in the programme, the former is accountable for most field activities in their own provinces. This means that the activities related to the 100 per cent Condom Programme in any given province are the sum total of the activities of the RCDCs and the PPHOs.

Essential Components

From the initial qualitative analyses, the research team discovered five essential components of the 100 per cent Condom Programme:

1. Campaigns to build programme support and create demand for condoms;
2. Availability and accessibility of quality condoms;
3. Appropriate staffing, management strategies, and evaluation;

4. Checkups and STD care for sex workers and STD clients;
5. Collaboration between health workers, governors, police, sex parlour owners/managers, and sex workers.

After analysing its qualitative and quantitative research findings, the IPSR study team identified several activities within these five major components.

Demand Creation for Condoms

An obvious requirement of the programme is to classify the cooperation of the owners and managers of the establishments - they control access to the sex workers for prevention programmes and STD services. Various methods were used to set up a basis for cooperation.

Three-quarters of the provinces reported meetings within the last year with the owners and managers of the establishments, with anywhere from 10 to 100 owners and managers in attendance. At these meetings, the local AIDS and STD situation was narrated, prevention was discussed, the support of the owners and managers was classified for condom promotion, and better relationships were developed between provincial health officers and the owners and managers. Contact with owners and managers was maintained regularly in arranging site visits for prevention programmes or STD checks among the sex workers. Finally, implicit threats of police action could be used on occasion to enlist cooperation. In about one-third of the province, the police assisted in inviting the owns and managers in for the meetings. In most provinces, this strategy was rarely used; the PPHOs felt that, in the long term, developing cooperative, collaborative relationships with the owners was more effective than coercion. However, the participation of the police helped to provide legitimacy to the programme in the eyes of brothel owners, even if police did not participate in implementation activities.

The other significant activity witnessed in virtually all provinces was regular visits by health workers to the establishments to discuss prevention alternatives with sex workers and to provide STD testing and treatment. In interviews with the owners and managers, over 90 per cent reported that health workers had come to the establishments to discuss health problems. These visits were frequent, with more than half of the owners/managers saying they occurred at least once a month. The visits concentrated primarily on the sex workers: only about a third of the establishments disclosed that health workers had talked to any establishment personnel other than sex workers about prevention issues. These regular visits to sex parlours by pro-active health workers clearly play an essential role in raising awareness, building demand for condom use, and keeping the concentration on the issues.

Because the implementation of the programme was locally managed, a variety of other activities to promote condom use were undertaken in some provinces, but not in others. These included training peer educators among the sex workers, supplying two free condoms in all hotel rooms, and setting up projects to improve the relationships between sex workers and establishment owners. Other activities included the use of financial incentives, such as providing STD services at reduced rates if no STDs were reported.

Procurement and Distribution

It is obvious that, if condoms are unavailable, they cannot be used when commercial sex occurs. Thus, considerable attention was paid to the logistics of condom procurement and distribution at both the RCDC and PPHO levels.

Condoms were supplied from the central Thai government by the Ministry of Public Health to each RCDC as per the RCDC's annual plan - that is, a supply sufficient for the demand anticipated for sex business in that region. The RCDCs would then redistribute them to the PPHOs upon request. Most provinces requesting condom supplies about once a month. This system functioned fairly well. Most PPHOs admitted no supply problems at all, although five reported only one instance of shortfall. This was primarily related to a shortage of size 52 mm condoms, which were in high demand, while size 49 mm was oversupplied.

Personnel at both the RCDC and PPHO levels were well educated about the necessities for condom storage to protect quality. When possible, RCDCs stored condoms in air-conditioned warehouses on shelves constricted above the floor to avoid humidity. Those with no air-conditioning would place them in warehouses away from the walls in raised low stacks. Similar steps were taken at the PPHOs, with careful attention to avoiding sunlight and humidity, providing good air circulation, and keeping the condoms raised above the floor. However, the primary measure to ensure quality was to match supply and distribution so that the condoms were not long in storage. Health staff referred to this as a "fresh in and fresh out" policy.

The primary distribution mechanism was to provide boxes of condoms to the sex workers when they came for STD check-ups, which were required or strongly encouraged in each province. A sex worker would be given a box of 100 condoms at a time and could ask for more if she needed them. In only one-eight of the provinces surveyed were the condoms actually delivered to the establishment owner rather than to the sex workers. When the sex workers were asked where they got condoms, three-quarters reported a government source, and about one-quarter said from pharmacies, but only 10 per cent reported getting them from the sex parlours (the total is greater than 100 per cent because they could report more than one source). A number of the RCDCs also distributed condoms to STD clinic visitors, the military, NGOs, private enterprises, or other populations and places where they felt they would be used effectively to prevent HIV transmission.

It was clear that staff at both the RCDC and PPHO level paid attention to quality issues with the condoms they were distributing. Almost all of the RCDCs and three-quarters of the PPHOs reported some problems, including condoms breakage or shortages of condoms of the proper size. Besides this, they reported complaints from the sex workers and clients about the unattractive packaging and lack of different flavours or colours of the government condoms. Although the organizations were clearly tracking these problems, the high number of quality issues reported reveals a need for expanded quality control.

Sufficient staff, appropriate management strategies, and regular monitoring and evaluation are necessary to the effectiveness on any programme. This is particularly true of the 100 per cent

Condom Programme, where the behaviours in question occur behind closed doors in sites that are not always easily located, and the use of condoms can be ascertained only indirectly, through self-reports or condom distributing figures. Meeting the needs of this programme necessitates active staff able to go into the field frequently, well-thought-out strategies for locating and managing sites that have ongoing transmission, and concrete means of ascertaining that the programme is having an impact. These needs were met through a number of strategies.

Thailand has had a strong government STD care and prevention effort, which has expanded to a large extent in recent years as the gravity of the AIDS epidemic became apparent. These activities operate through STD/AIDS clinics at the regional, provincial, and district levels. The staff already involved in these activities were supplemented by additional staff as needed to mount overall HIV/AIDS prevention activities and ensure good coverage in each province. As discussed earlier the 100 per cent Condom Programme responsibilities were integrated into the responsibilities of a number of different departments or units at the RCDC and PPHO level, rather than generating a new vertical programme. This assisted to contain costs, produce a sustainable programme, and provide sufficient staffing to support the required activities.

The AIDS and STDs Section in each PPHO regularly maintained listings of sex trade establishments in the province and updated these every six months. Updates were based upon reports from men presenting at government clinics with STDs (who were asked where they contracted the STD) or results of STD testing among sex workers either in clinics or at the establishments themselves. These reports were then used to direct prevention efforts to those sites where STDs were still occurring, since continued transmission suggested failure to use condoms.

The existing infrastructure for STD prevention and care meant that STDs could be used as an indicator of ongoing risk behaviour and failure to use condoms consistently. Thus, when provincial officials discovered sites with ongoing STD transmission, they would make the owners and managers aware of this fact, expand the treatment services offered or step up STD testing at those sites, and increase the number of visits to those sites to ensure compliance with the programme. Because the programme had been initiated with strong support from the national government and both the governors and police were actively involved from the start, these groups could provide the necessary authority to ensure that owners and managers cooperated. But, while the authority clearly existed to close down sex parlours, that power was not being used very frequently. No RCDCs and only one PPHO reported closing a site in the preceding year. Instead, most expressed reservations about calling the police in for closures; they felt either that they already had good cooperation from the owners and managers or that it would damage their relationships with them, making it more difficult to conduct prevention activities.

All but two of the RCDCs and five of the PPHOs had set targets for the programme in terms of expected levels of condom use. Most RCDCs and PPHOs set either 90 or 100 per cent targets, but a small number of PPHOs set targets as low as 70 per cent, perhaps projecting their own field experience. In the last year, 3 RCDCs and 15 PPHOs examined the programme. The most common indicators for evaluation were STD incidence, followed by HIV infection rate among sex workers, and number of condoms used. Even in provinces that did not conduct a formal evaluation, almost all were closely watching STD rates. Approximately half of all provinces looked at numbers of condoms distributed and/or HIV infection levels among sex workers, and nearly half used the proportion of condom use in sex work, a behavioural indicator.

Care for Sex Workers

STD check-ups and care played the most important role both in directing prevention activities to the sites of greatest need and in evaluating the success of the 100 per cent Condom Programme, as discussed earlier. Thus, it is not surprising that most RCDCs and PPHOs placed a high premium on STD-related activities.

In every province, either the RCDC or the PPHO maintained an STD clinic, and each of these clinics provided physical exams for sex workers as part of its services. Many RCDCs and PPHOs directed sex workers to obtain check-ups between two and four times per month. Having regular STD checks provided an incentive to the workers to protect from infection, while at the same time permitting the follow-up of problem sites with field visits and expanded prevention activities.

These services were well utilized by the sex workers. In the survey conducted as part of this project, 91 per cent of the sex workers admitted receiving regular STD check-ups, ranging from 95 per cent in the brothels to a low of 86 per cent in the restaurant sites. More than 90 per cent of those getting check-ups received them at least twice a month, and over 90 per cent received these services from government clinics or hospitals. Only in the massage parlours did approximately one-quarter receive their care from private clinics or hospitals rather than from government sources. This implies that massage parlours represent the upper end of the commercial sex trade in Thailand, and many of the women working there can afford private medical services. Every province also had mobile teams that visited sex parlours to provide HIV and STDs education and conduct condom promotion activities.

Public sector STD clinics were used in three ways to facilitate the programme:

1. They provided information to health officials on establishments with ongoing sexual risk;
2. They permitted provincial officials to examine if sexual transmission of STD and HIV were still in prevalence; and
3. They permitted indirect evaluation of the success of the programme.

Collaboration

Although sex work is illegal in Thailand, it remains part of the sexual culture, and regular public health services such as STD care are provided for sex workers. Thus, rather than using legal approaches to restrict sex work, which could not curtail demand and would only drive the industry underground and make prevention efforts more difficult. Thailand chose the more pragmatic and effective approach of working cooperatively with all those who influence the sex trade. Thus, the 100 per cent Condom Programme consists a number of different actors and agencies. These include the National AIDS Committee, provincial governors, the police, regional and provincial health workers, the owners of the sex parlours, the sex workers themselves, and the clients. Each has different, but essential, roles to play in the implementation of the programme, and close collaboration among them is the key to the programme.

Since securing the support of the governor ensures the cooperation of others, the programme devoted considerable effort to educating and enlisting the support of governors. These efforts were largely successful in many provinces. Almost 60 per cent reported excellent cooperation from the governor, with another third reporting moderate cooperation. In at least one province, the governor even discovered sex parlours himself to ensure that condoms were available in every room. In some cases, governors would write letters to noncooperative owners or managers, insisting on their participation. Only one province reported low levels of cooperation from the governor.

While it might be hoped that the owners and managers of the establishments would be motivated to take a central role in prevention efforts at their establishments, this was not witnessed to be the case in this study. Most establishments did not have extensive education programmes of their own, despite often high turnover in staff. Less than half had meetings where they would debate health matters with the workers. Although those who did hold such meetings said they used them to discuss condoms and STDs, these topics were probably not high on their priority list; almost two-thirds claimed they had never witnessed STDs in their establishments or only saw them about once a year. Among the sex workers, less than 2 per cent reported anybody associated with the establishment as a major source of information about the 100 per cent Common Programme. In terms of enforcing the programme, about four-fifths of the owners and managers said they would negate a client who wouldn't use a condom, but the other fifth said it was up to the sex worker. Moreover, only a fifth said they would take any punitive action against a sex worker who didn't use a condom.

It is established that among sex workers' most of their awareness and information about the Condom Promotion Campaign came from television or health care workers. Health workers and, in some places, NGO workers provided training to sex workers on condom use and negotiation skills. Similarly, most STD care for sex workers and a major part of care for clients was provided through government clinics or government on-site STD services. Health workers also took the primary responsibility for managing day-to-day programme activities, condom distribution, and evaluation of ongoing efforts. These were the part and parcel of the core activities of the programme.

Because the provincial governors took the programme seriously, police did so as well in most cases. No doubt, in the early days of the programme, enforcement actions were initiated against establishments in some provinces to seek the owners' cooperation. However, the role of the police was noticed to be much less visible. The programme input survey found that police assisted in organizing meetings of owners in about a third of the provinces. Thus, at present their fundamental role seems to be one of potential enforcement, although most provinces are increasingly operating on a cooperative rather than confrontational basis with owners and managers.

While all the activities of the programme definitely helped to create a supportive environment for condom use and improved STD care, much of the persuasion for using condoms still came from the sex workers. Sex workers admitted that about one-fifth of men put on a condom without request and another two-thirds would let the sex worker put it on without objection. But there remained a core of about 10 per cent of sex purchasers who had to be convinced to use condoms, although ultimately less than one per cent would totally refuse. This suggests to a clear need for ongoing training for new sex workers in negotiating condom use with resistant clients.

Approximately two-thirds of those visiting sex workers admitted that condom use was their own idea, while about a fifth attributed it to the sex workers. This implies that most men have had the importance of using condoms in commercial sex impressed upon them, primarily through mass media campaigns (television, radio, and newspapers). It is not everything that these media messages were part of the National AIDS education and condom promotion campaigns and were efforts mounted by government agencies (e.g., the Office of the Prime Minister or the Ministry of Public Health), NGOs, or other organizations. Only about 20 per cent of the men listed health worker as a substantial source of information. That is, most of their information and motivation to use condoms came from sources other than the 100 per cent Condom Programme. This highlights the importance of implementing campaigns to reach the clients through other avenues at the some time.

Evidently, the effective implementation of this programme necessitates strong political commitment and the cooperation and assistance of several individuals and agencies.

Programme Inputs

As discussed earlier, all five major components of the 100 per cent Condom Programme have been implemented in most provinces in general. Thus, the overall level of programme inputs is uniformly high across the provinces, with only limited variation. This in itself is a noticeable achievement. Similarly, the level of success as measured by self-reported condom use by both sex workers and clients is also quite high.

The original intention of the present discussion had been to examine in detail the impact of various programme inputs on effectiveness as measured by overall levels of condom use in commercial sex. However, the limited variations witnessed in both the inputs and the outputs (i.e., levels of condom use) made this a Herculean task. Due to this, it was not probable to determine the influence of components present in almost all provinces, such as campaigns to reach sex workers or extensive STD testing and treatment, that definitely were among the most critical contributors to the success of the programme. It must also be remembered that national AIDS awareness and condom promotion activities were ongoing and certainly contributed as well.

To measure the implications of those factors that did vary somewhat from province to province, the analysis was redesigned to look at the sex workers' use of condoms with their regular clients as the output variable. This form of condom use demonstrated the greatest variation between provinces and different types of establishments. Thus, the impact of programme inputs on condom use with regular clients could be ascertained for those inputs that varied from province to province.

The two factors witnessed to influence condom use with regular clients were:

(a) the extent of collaboration between the various actors within the province;
(b) whether the province was home to one of the Regional Offices of Communicable Disease Control.

Increased collaboration with the governor, police, and establishment owners was witnessed to increase the level of condom use with regular clients. Provinces that were home to the RCDCs were also found to have higher levels of condom use with regular clients. These revelations can be tentatively interpreted to mean that the improved programme efforts that result from better collaboration within the province, and the expanded entire programme effort likely to occur in a province where both an RCDC and a PPHO are operating, increase the programme's ability to convince sex workers to use condoms with their regular clients, while RCDCs are effective in providing technical support and follow up.

IPSR made a further analysis of the effect of the different inputs on condom use with regular clients at different types of establishments. This analysis revealed that different inputs were important at different types of establishments. In particular:

(a) Accessibility and availability of condoms were more important in brothels than in massage parlours and hotels. This is probably because brothel workers depend largely on government-supplied condoms, while massage parlour and hotel workers also obtain condoms through private sources such as drug stores.
(b) In restaurants, the quality of the management of the provincial programme and the provincial staffing levels were witnessed to be more important to an effective programme than in the brothels. This most likely is associated to the greater difficulty of reaching the indirect establishments in the provinces. Only with good and effective management can the programme hope to reach these more challenging sites. Moreover, more staffing

implies more capacity at the provincial level to reach the sites that were more difficult to access.

Thus, the specific needs of different types of sex establishments may vary and the programme must adapt to these needs to maximize effectiveness.

Conclusion

The following important lessons can be drawn from experiences with the 100 per cent Condom Programme in Thailand and its success in producing high rates of condom use in commercial sex.

(a) Political commitment at both the national and local levels is important to the success of this programme. The strong and high level national commitment by the Prime Minister, the Minister of Public Health and the Minister of the Interior increased programme participation by local government officers and offices, and they subsequently were able to engage the owners and managers of sex parlours in the programme. The adoption of a national policy regarding the 100 per cent Condom Programme, coupled with aggressive efforts to enlist the aid of provincial governors, set the framework for active programmes at the local level and for using prevalent health and police infrastructures to ensure participation by sex parlours throughout the provinces. The political commitment is also translated into a consistent supply of good quality condoms for distribution free of charge to sex parlours. This is a crucial feature of the 100 per cent Condom Programme.

(b) STD care and 100 per cent Condom Programme support one another in such a programme. The 100 per cent Condom Programme had a demonstrable effect on the incidence of STDs in almost every province in the country. At the same time, using existing sources of STD care to evaluate the 100 per cent Condom Programme provided positive feedback indicating that the efforts were making a difference. These synergistic interactions contributed to the expansion of both 100 per cent Condom Programme and STD care efforts in the provinces and helped to build support for the two programmes. They also served to maintain regular contact between sex workers and health workers, improving the relevance of prevention efforts. In future attempts to replicate this programme elsewhere, careful attention should be paid to using STD treatment sources as both an avenue for 100 per cent condom programme and a means of examining the impacts of those efforts.

(c) While some enforcement may be helpful in launching a 100 per cent Condom Programme, in the future cooperation is the more effective approach. Although, in the early stages of the programme, the governor's backing and police cooperation clearly moved some establishment owners to participate, it is interesting that most RCDCs and PPHOs believed in applying police pressure sparingly. Many expressed the concern that such pressure would either damage the relationships they had built with owners or create negative feelings that would impede future prevention efforts. Similarly, many PPHOs resisted police closings of establishments because they felt it made the sex workers less accessible for prevention.

(d) Measurable positive results can be achieved quickly with such a programme. During the pilot phases of this programme, individual provinces would typically start to witness declines in STD rates with three to four months of implementation. National rates fell considerably each year. In situations like Thailand's, where much of the HIV transmission is occurring through commercial sex, concerted efforts to reach sex workers and clients can return major benefits quickly and can significantly slow the epidemic.

(e) Close collaboration of all the actors is necessary to the programme's success. Because each major actor had a different role to play, the programme could not have been successful without their combined assistance. The governors and police helped to open the doors, the owners provided the access, the sex workers convinced the clients to use condoms, the clients recognized the need for condoms. This reveals that the most effective prevention efforts are those that involve multisectoral efforts.

(f) Sex work is quite varied and takes many forms; programmes must take this into consideration to design the most effective prevention efforts. The variations by types of establishment in condom use and the factors influencing it witnessed in this study are likely to be much more pronounced in the early stages of the programme and will become more apparent as efforts expand to more extensive coverage of indirect sites. If programme managers recognize this, watch for the difference, and adapt their programmes flexibly, they will be more effective.

(g) When possible, existing health and government infrastructures should be used to keep costs low and increase sustainability. The programme in its present form in Thailand is quite sustainable as it has been well integrated into existing health structures, with a division of responsibility to avoid overburdening any one unit. This has also reduced the need for extensive special budgeting for the PPHOs beyond the provision of free condoms.

(h) A 100 per cent condom programme necessitates complementary efforts to reach the clients. The young men received little of their AIDS information or knowledge of the 100 per cent Condom Programme from the programme staff or directly as part of this programme. Instead, they received AIDS information, learned their skills and developed norms of condom use in commercial sex through complementary mass media, workplace education, and other prevention programmes. Such simultaneous efforts are essential to the 100 per cent Condom Programme and should be considered part of the entire overall package. The revelations here indicate that future prevention efforts must also strongly promote condom use with non-commercial partners for both clients and sex workers.

(i) The programme needs to adapt to the shifting balance of direct and indirect sites in sex work. While condom use has increased greatly at indirect sites over the last several years, the increase has not been as dramatic as at direct sites. With increased condom use, the role of direct sites in HIV transmission has decreased to a large extent. This makes efforts to reach all of the indirect sites increasingly important. New and innovative approaches need to be designed and implemented to access the harder to reach indirect sites effectively, a major challenge given their more clandestine nature.

Eight

HIV Prevention: Innovative Approaches

Introduction

By end-1999, approximately 34.3 million adults and children were living with HIV/AIDS in the world and 18.8 million deaths were reported. Sub-Saharan Africa remains the centre of the epidemic, with about 25 million men, women and children infected with HIV/AIDS. In Asia, approximately 7 million people are infected, and rates are increasing in countries such as India and China. Parts of central and eastern Europe are also demonstrating an alarming increase in HIV infection rates. Since last two decades, much has been learned about HIV prevention. Some of this new knowledge comes from carefully evaluation studies, programme reviews, the documentation of prevailing good practices, meta-analysis and reviews and the observations of field workers, nongovernmental organizations (NGOs) and health promotion practitioners. All of these information sources have proved to be valuable in revealing the most appropriate and promising interventions. By providing different kinds of information such as indicating changes in the prevalence and incidence of infection; changes in reported behaviours; increases in related service utilization or condom sales; or improved HIV associated knowledge beliefs, attitudes and skills - each contributes to our understanding of what can 'work' in HIV prevention. The following five criteria are valuable when examining HIV prevention programmes:

(a) *Relevance*

— perception as relevant by target groups

— cultural and contextual relevance

(b) *Efficiency*
   — well-coordinated planning and implementation
   — reach
(c) *Impact*
   — impact on reported rates of STD and HIV
   — impact on HIV and AIDS-associated knowledge beliefs and attitudes
   — impact on protected sex practices and protected forms of drug use
(d) Sustainability
   — generalizability to other contexts
   — cost-effectiveness
(e) Ethical soundness

The success of any intervention will depend considerably on the appropriateness of what has been done. Every intervention occurs within a specific context, and local context as well as the stage of the epidemic must be taken into account when planning, designing and implementing HIV prevention activities. Interventions at multiple levels are always needed in order to persuade people to adopt and sustain protected sex and drug use practices, as well as to set up the enabling and supportive environments necessary for reducing vulnerability to HIV infection.

Methodology

The identification of a number of innovative and promising Interventions was achieved through consultations with various experts in the field of HIV/AIDS prevention at the international, regional and local levels, as well as through reviews of published literature. Information was sought from key individuals working in international agencies and charitable foundations, and when necessary, followed-up at the regional level. Information was also gathered from individuals within UNAIDS and cosponsoring agencies as well as at regional and national levels.

Contact was then made with individual projects via their manager or coordinator and descriptions of their ongoing work were elicited under a series of headings. These included:

(a) the location of the project, contact details and the funding agency;

(b) an overall description of the work of the project;
(c) a statement of project activities and outputs to date;
(d) information about evaluation and project outcomes;
(e) a description of any innovative aspects of the work;
(f) a statement of constraints/obstacles affecting local activities and the succession of the interventions.

The activities undertaken as part of this work should not be regarded as comprehensive. Rather, the aim is to discover key studies and investigations on HIV prevention interventions beyond information dissemination. Thus, this work provides a set of intervention examples for HIV prevention and highlights some of the key issues to consider when designing, implementing and evaluating HIV programmes.

HIV Prevention

When the first cases of AIDS were reported in the early 1980s, individuals and groups acted to alert people to this dangerous new epidemic and the steps that could be taken to protect against it. Even before HIV was isolated, protected sex and protected drug use guidelines had been developed based upon epidemiological evidence associated with patterns of transmission. However, providing people with information about how to protect against infection has proven to be insufficient. People require enabling environments that will reduce their susceptibility and vulnerability, and allow them to change their behaviour based on their knowledge gained through information provision.

At the national level, political commitment at all levels is essential for programme success. Multi-level interventions that seek to involve a variety of partners in co-ordinated action have been more successful than those that work in isolation. The coordinated economic, political and social efforts are required to reduce societal vulnerability alongside programmes and interventions operating at individual and community levels. The following elements are among those central for effective national HIV prevention efforts:

(a) general awareness-raising activities to provide information and counter negative reactions among the general public;

(b) focused persuasive action to meet the needs of specially vulnerable groups and communities, with constantly expanding coverage;
(c) multi-sectoral and multi-level partnerships to deliver programmes and services across a range of contexts;
(d) community participation in programme and intervention development, and building upon the will of groups and individuals to contribute to national HIV prevention efforts;
(e) greater integration between prevention and care to lessen costs and to reduce levels of discrimination and stigmatization;
(f) action to build societal resistance to HIV transmission and reduce the systematic vulnerability of particular individuals, groups and sections of society.

A further set of principles has been identified outlining the factors that need to be taken into consideration if community-based prevention activities are to be effective. These include:

(a) engaging the community through existing organizations, groups and structures for education and support;
(b) building partnership and confidence through communication, networking and collaboration;
(c) including people with HIV/AIDS at all stages of the process so as to enhance visibility and benefit from their skills and experiences;
(d) creating an accepting community environment in which HIV and AIDS are acknowledged to be everyone's concern.

Besides these principles, community-based approaches need to confirm that resources are directed towards community capacity-building to ensure sustainability.

The following factors are central to programme success when adequately operationalized.

(a) the provision of information in culturally appropriate ways about how HIV is and is not transmitted;
(b) the inclusion of activities that persuade people (both as individuals and communities) to appraise the risks that encounter them personally;

(c) the provision of training in skills for communication and sexual negotiation;

(d) the provision of enhanced access to resources such as condoms and affordable health services, alongwith those for the early detection and treatment of sexually transmitted diseases (STDs).

(e) the involvement of target groups at all stages of design, implementation and evaluation;

(d) the monitoring of programmes/projects at all stages of development and implementation.

Prevention approaches need to be tailored to the needs of particular groups. When working with young people, for example, it is important to:

(a) take into account the diversity of young people and their needs;

(b) persuade youth participation in project design and implementation;

(c) work in a climate of openness that recognizes and respects the realities that young people face;

(d) focus on young men's sexual health, as well as sexual health issues associated with young women;

(e) evaluating the positive aspects of sexual health;

(f) promote greater awareness of sexual and reproductive rights;

(g) provide opportunities to address issues of gender, social status and sexuality;

(h) undertake work with young men to think about their role in relation to both their sexual health and that of their partners;

(i) promote more awareness of the structural issues affecting the sexual and reproductive health of young people, alongwith the need for improved rights and protection for young people;

(j) improve access to basic education and timely sex and HIV associated education;

(k) provide access to voluntary counselling and testing services, including appropriate referrals;

(l) increase access to youth-friendly health services.

When working with women, it is important to:

(a) use a multifaceted approach that addresses economic and other needs;

(b) focus on improving communication between sexual partners which acknowledges the difficulties women face in talking and negotiating with men about sex;

(c) increase awareness of the importance of including men in work for the prevention of HIV among men, women and children;

(d) address the need for improved health services for women;

(e) acknowledge the importance of a gendered approach to HIV eradication work, which includes discussions of power relations between men and women;

(f) provide access to voluntary counselling and testing services, including appropriate referrals;

(g) acknowledge the support that women can give to each other through debates and the development of networks.

When working with people who inject drugs, it is important to:

(a) concentrate on harm reduction as well as rehabilitation;

(b) advocate to safeguard the rights of people who inject drugs;

(c) adopt a multi-pronged approach including needle and syringe exchange and the provision of drug treatment, alongwith detoxification, substitution pharmacotherapy, HIV/AIDS care and social network interventions;

(d) provide drop-in services, mobile services and outreach work;

(e) work to improve the sexual health and sexual practices of people;

(f) undertake HIV prevention programmes;

(g) build trust between people who inject drugs and health professionals through outreach work;

(h) provide good access to sterile injecting equipment and condoms;

(i) provide access to voluntary counselling and testing services, along with appropriate referrals;
(j) establish high levels of knowledge about HIV infection and modes of transmission among people.

When working with men who have sex with men, it is important to:

(a) acknowledge the wider concerns of MSM in developing countries, including issues such as harassment, poverty and responsibilities towards family members;
(b) recognize the importance of raising public awareness about issues concerning MSM, countering prejudice and discrimination, and the promotion of human rights;
(c) provide training for professionals working with MSM, including health professionals, teachers and prison officers;
(d) address homophobia, including internalized homophobia;
(e) help MSM develop support networks;
(f) provide access to voluntary counselling and testing services, along with appropriate referrals;
(g) acknowledge the diversity of MSM in developing and developed countries.

When working with sex workers, it is important to:

(a) acknowledge the broader concerns and priorities of sex workers;
(b) address the prejudice and stigmatization that sex workers face;
(c) acknowledge the importance of helping to empower sex workers;
(d) provide improved and more accessible health services for the diagnosis and treatment of STDs;
(e) seek the cooperation and support of gatekeepers in the sex trade, including brothel owners and bar owners as well as employers of potential clients of sex workers;
(f) legitimize the role of sex workers as educators, providing them with the respect of their peers;

(g) acknowledge the importance of providing sex workers with financial incentives for peer-led work;

(h) work, where possible, with men as well as women through a concentration on clients and, in some cases, boyfriends.

Useful Approaches

There are, therefore, a number of different ways of creating knowledge about HIV prevention methods and their effects. All rely to some extent upon observation and the amassing of information, but each differs according to the rigour with which statistics and information are collected and studied. The kinds of relatively casual observations that contribute to intuitions and gut reactions are different in kind from the more systematic approaches used in observation studies and objectives-based evaluations. These in turn differ from the approaches at times applicable in more formally conducted experimental and comparative evaluations. It is crucial to consider the strengths and limitations of several approaches when making judgements about what works, and what might prove to be a promising approach in HIV prevention. No one approach can answer all the questions we may have about appropriateness and effectiveness. Altogether, different kinds of evidence, methodology can be persuasive to discover the most useful approaches to adopt in particular circumstances and with particular groups.

Young People

Approximately half of all people who acquire HIV become infected in their mid-twenties. Thus, it is crucial that work be undertaken to help young people protect their sexual health. However, there has been a lot of uncertainty about how to approach HIV and AIDS prevention with young people. For example, there continues to be widespread concern that sex education will encourage young people to become prematurely sexually active. As a result, many sex education programmes have concentrated solely upon abstinence. Several studies have demonstrated, however, that well-designed programmes of sex education, combining messages about protected sex as well as abstinence, may delay sexual debut, as well as increase preventive behaviours among those young people who are already sexually active. Where they have been able to access appropriate knowledge, skills and means, young people have demonstrated a remarkable propensity to adopt safer behaviour.

The experiences of young people vary as per social and cultural context, gender, socioeconomic status and sexuality. In order to be successful, HIV prevention programmes need to abandon stereotyped images of young people and take full consideration of their diversity while recognizing that all young people need accurate information. However, it is important to know that young people, especially girls in developing countries, do not always have the freedom to make their own choices about sexual behaviour. They may, for example, be vulnerable to forced or coercive sex, and may sell or exchange sex fire economic survival, or to gain the protection of adults. Young people in developing countries at times have immediate needs for shelter, food and clothes which take priority over the threat of an epidemic like AIDS which may or may not kill them in years to come.

It is important that programmes take into account these structural constraints, barriers and challenges for daily survival which young people encounter. In addition, it is critical that a dialogue begin with policy-makers to ascertain that the rights of young people are ensured, and that governments and international agencies work to address the specific needs of young people in especially vulnerable circumstances. It is also important to note that, while young people may be at special risk of HIV infection, they also present an opportunity for halting the epidemic, since their sexual and other habits may not yet be firmly established.

Recommendations

- Joint involvement of students and colleges administration in design and implementation of the school-based curriculum was found effective;
- Successful local campaign for young people's sexual health;
- Mass media linked to HIV/AIDS education in other settings can change social norms and attitudes, thus helping prevent HIV;

- A multi-faceted project incorporating shelter, food, health care, legal protection and HIV/AIDS education can improve the quality of life for young women involved in prostitution;
- Access to youth-friendly health services is an important part of HIV/AIDS prevention;
- Participation of young people in project development and implementation leads to beneficial outcomes;
- The anonymity of an AIDS Hotline can help people access information and counselling around the culturally taboo topics of sex and sexuality;
- Life skills approaches can enhance students, knowledge, attitudes and behaviours so as to lead to risk reduction;
- Life skills programmes may have beneficial effects for teachers as well;
- Three-part intervention increased reports of abstinence amongst Ugandan students;
- Outcomes attributable to the interactive nature of the intervention, not simply the provision of information;
- Combining together of intervention elements helped students process the information of a family member becoming HIV-positive in a way which led to positive behaviour change.

Women and Men

Approximately 55 per cent of all adults living with HIV/AIDS are women, with the difference between men and women being most pronounced in those under the age of 25. Not only have women been reported as having a heightened vulnerability to HIV infection, they also have an increased social vulnerability. Women have unequal access to education and economic resources. They wield less power than men in social and sexual relations. Entrenched stereotypes and differences in role expectations between the sexes also mean that women at times have less say in decisions about when and how intercourse takes place, including whether or not a condom will be used. Moreover, women are more likely than men to experience rape and sexual coercion, and are frequently forced to sell or exchange sex for their economic survival. In addition to their own increased risk of HIV infection, women also carry the lion's share of the social burden of the epidemic in terms of providing the care for relatives with AIDS. Women with HIV infection also at times encounter more social blame and stigma than men in the same position.

Women do not constitute a 'risk group' for HIV infection in the general sense of the term because women do not generally infect each other but instead acquire HIV mainly through their relationships with men. Research in different contexts demonstrates that women's attitudes towards sex and sexual behaviour differ to a large extent from those of men. Women report a preference for sexual relations based on mutual fidelity, intimacy and open communication. They have fewer sexual partners than men and a great many more women than men report having only one lifetime sexual partner. When women express a desire for protected sex, men are often obstructive. Perhaps not surprisingly, therefore, the major HIV risk for women is their regular sexual partner or husband. Dominant ideologies of masculinity, on the other hand, promote the display of sexual prowess, and encourage men to have multiple partners.

Many prevailing HIV prevention programmes fails to take ample account of the social vulnerability of women or the unequal power relations which make it difficult for women to influence decision-making in their sexual relationships. The major elements of many programmes - partner reduction, condom use and STD treatment - are not necessarily appropriate for women, who do not have multiple partners, cannot always influence the decision to use condoms, and may be asymptomatic for STDs. Indeed, open and honest verbal communication is one of the most difficult aspects of heterosexual relationships.

It is evident that existing ideologies of masculinity and femininity facilitate HIV transmission. There is also widespread agreement that the promotion of more equal gender roles is the key to preventing infection. It is crucial, therefore, not only to address stereotyped gender roles, but also to redress some of the stark structural inequalities between men and women, including the unequal distribution of economic resources and differentials in access to education and health provision. Women's empowerment, however, cannot be achieved by women alone but requires the support of men for its successful realization.

Recommendations

- Increase in knowledge about HIV and need to change sexual behaviours.
- Evaluation revealed high effectiveness in communicating accurate information credibility, and acceptance within the community.
- Issues of sexuality and HIV/AIDS more frequently discussed with staff.
- Staff more likely to recommend the use of condoms as a means of preventing HIV transmission.
- Innovative and multi-faceted approach to HIV/AIDS prevention.
- Participants showed increased use of condoms, fewer sexual partners, and increased ability to refuse unwanted sex.
- Reduction in incidence of alcohol misuse encouraged sharing of money in the home, and care for those who are sick.

People Who Inject Drugs

Approximately 6 to 10 million people throughout the world inject drugs. High rates of HIV infection among people who inject drugs have been found in countries as diverse as Brazil, Thailand, India and Myanmar. In many parts of the developing world, injecting drugs has become the most common risk behaviour coupled with HIV infection and HIV infection can spread very rapidly this way. For example, during 1985-87, HIV prevalence among people who injected drugs in Bangkok was one per cent. By the end of 1988, however, this figure had increased to around 40 per cent.

People who inject drugs risk HIV infection in two main ways first, through the sharing of syringes and other injecting equipment, and second, like other sexually active people, through unprotected sex with infected partners. Those designing HIV-associated programmes, aimed at people who inject drugs, encounter a number of challenges, not least the common fixed ideas about people who use drugs. Also, in many countries drug use is socially sanctioned, stigmatized and illegal. Not surprisingly, drug use in general, and injecting drug use in particular, is often latent. People who inject drugs are often marginalized, which means that they may find it difficult to access services and resources that might help them to protect their health. Some legal restrictions may serve as obstacles to HIV prevention, by prohibiting the open provision of sterile injecting equipment for example.

Evidence from Europe, North America and Australia suggests that people who inject drugs can make considerable changes to their behaviour to lessen the risk of HIV infection. It has been established that in developed countries participation in prevention programmes also leads to a reduction of risk behaviour among people who inject drugs. However, in developing countries there is highly variable access to appropriate information, education and services for people who inject drugs.

Recommendations

- At 18-month follow-up, 47 per cent of IDUs in intervention group reported reduction in needle and syringe sharing (cf. 35 per cent in controls).
- At 18-month follow-up, 30 per cent of IDUs reported always cleaning syringes (cf. 10 per cent in controls).
- In course of three years, reported 58 per cent reduction in heroin use and 30 per cent reduction in injection practices.
- At 9 month follow-up, reported decrease in high risk behaviour amongst the clients.
- Shortages of resources and organizational constraints have limited the effectiveness of the project.
- 25 per cent decrease in use of marijuana, heroin and speedball, six months after rehabilitation.
- Consistent behavioural change towards less risky behaviours.

Men Who have Sex with Men

In many developed nations, gay and other men who have sex with men were among the first to be affected by HIV, and continue to bear the brunt of the epidemic. In developing nations the situation is quite different. In many such nations heterosexual transmission constitute the vast majority of reported cases. However, it is not clear whether or not this is an accurate reflection of the real situation. In many developing nations, male-to-male sex is highly stigmatized, and in some it is legally prohibited. This can cause governments, political leaders and the general public to believe that homosexual transmission does not exist, when in fact it is simply latent.

As time has passed, a new willingness to 'lift the veil' on hitherto stigmatized and denied behaviours has come about. In sub-Saharan Africa, for example, where virtually no cases of homosexual transmission were primarily reported, there is now ample literature to suggest that same-sex contacts are far more common than previously thought. It is evident at present that across a variety of countries in both the developed and developing world men who have sex with men (MSM) are made more vulnerable to HIV infection due to the clandestine nature of their relationships, and the marginalization and discrimination they face. The challenge at present is to expand on the limited number of innovative programmes for men who have sex with men, and to address the structural factors that promote this discrimination and stigmatization.

Recommendations

- Raised profile of gay communities in a context where homosexuality remains illegal.
- Enhanced awareness of human rights.
- 85 per cent of participants reported improved knowledge of prevention practices and appropriate risk perception.
- 40 per cent increase in reported use of condoms, 30 per cent reduction in high-risk behaviour.
- Programme effectiveness attributed to the holistic nature of the intervention.
- Increased knowledge of HIV/AIDS prevention, and enhanced ability to communicate with sexual partners.
- Increased reported condom use and marked improvement in social atmosphere of prisons.
- Demonstrated clear value of friendship/social network approach.
- Holistic, non-clinical approach valued by clients.
- Increased knowledge and changes in attitudes towards homosexuality.
- Improved education and health service delivery for gay men.

Sex Workers and their Clients

Early in the epidemic, sex workers were recognized as a major group to involve in HIV-prevention work. However, sex workers have been difficult to fully participate in HIV prevention, since the illegality of prostitution in many countries means that women and men who exchange sex for money may not always be visible or accessible. Sex trade is also highly stigmatized in many societies and, in early reports about AIDS, the mass media often presented sex workers unhelpfully as 'conduits of infection' rather than as individuals who might be especially vulnerable and/or who have a major role to play in HIV prevention.

In developing countries, most female sex workers are characteristically poor, without formal education and relatively powerless. Often, individuals engage in sex industry to determine their own economic survival and, in many cases, that of their children and other family members. Rural to urban migration in many developing countries ensures both a large number of sex workers in cities and a ready clientele. A number of the clients of sex workers are men who have left their families behind to find employment in large cities. In some cultural contexts, sex before or outside of marriage regularly involves the exchange of money or goods. Importantly, existing HIV prevention programmes have rarely concentrated on the male client's of sex workers.

Sex workers are often highly mobile, making grassroots organization and HIV-preventive programming difficult. Additionally, while many sex workers do, or would wish to, use condoms, the largely illicit and sometimes illegal nature of sex work enhances vulnerability. In contexts where soliciting for clients is legal, carrying a large number of condoms may lead to arrest and fines. Similarly, the latent nature of sex trade may render sex workers vulnerable to rape and sexual coercion.

In prevention planning and programming it must be remembered that sex workers, like other groups, are far from homogeneous. They include women and men, those who identify as gay or bisexual, and young people, who may be relatively powerless and particularly vulnerable to exploitation and injecting drug users. There are a variety of contexts in which sex work takes place: for example, in brothels, bars, on the streets and through broker-mediated encounters.

Recommendations

- Reported increases in regular use of condoms.
- Increased use of counselling and testing services.
- Improved quality of life for sex workers.
- Increased awareness of civil and human rights.
- Reduced risk of HIV infection.
- Increased knowledge of prevention.
- Increased condom use, reduction in group rapes.
- Decreased levels of infection.
- Increased demand for condoms.
- Increased reported condom use.
- Fewer 'line-ups' and group rapes.
- Lowered levels of sexual harassment.

Nine

AIDS Prevention: Human Rights Approach

HIV/AIDS and Human Rights: UN Guidelines

States should ensure that government and the private sector develop codes of conduct regarding HIV/AIDS issues that translate human rights principles into codes of professional responsibility and practice, with accompanying mechanisms to implement and enforce these codes.

Introduction

In September 1997 the Council of the Southern African Development Community (SADC) unanimously approved a regional code on HIV/AIDS and employment popularly known as the Code. The objective of the Code is to create a regional standard on the best ways to manage AIDS in the employment setting. It aims to guide employers, employees and governments towards the most economically sustainable and humane methods to respond to HIV and AIDS in the workplace. The SADC is the first regional inter-governmental organization in the world to take such an initiative. The present discussion documents the Code and evaluates the factors why the SADC adopted it.

- To examine the state of the HIV/AIDS epidemic in Southern Africa and its impact on the workforce.
- To trace the process that was undertaken by SADC, trade unions, business organizations, governments and non-governmental organizations (NGOs) to promote the Code.
- To concentrate on the principles underlying the Code and explain why the issue of a uniform response to AIDS and employment is significant for Southern Africa and other developing countries.

- To look at some of the partnerships that were designed and strategies that were adopted in several countries during the process and to illustrate how lobbying and advocacy have drawn HIV/AIDS more fully to the attention of trade unions, business and government.
- To look at challenges for the effective implementation of the code and to present a number of methods in which employers, employees and governments can use the Code to introduce better activities around HIV and AIDS in the workplace.

In every country the workplace is a significant front for preventing new HIV infections and promoting non-discrimination towards people with HIV/AIDS. This 'Best Practice' will serve several purposes. In countries where there have been no systematic activities around AIDS in the workplace, it will be guide on how to develop policy and build partnerships. For countries in Southern Africa, it will help carry forward the campaigns that have already started.

The Southern African Development Community (SADC)

The Southern African Development Community (SADC) was established in 1992. At present, the SADC is an intergovernmental partnership of 14 countries - similar to the European Union (EU) or the Association of South East Asian Nations (ASEAN). It aims to integrate the countries of Southern Africa in a regional economic community that will be a building block towards an African economic community. The current SADC members are. Angola, Botswana, Democratic Republic of the Congo, Lesotho, Malawi, Mauritius, Mozambique, Namibia, Seychelles, South Africa, Swaziland, United Republic of Tanzania, Zambia, and Zimbabwe.

SADC has a permanent secretariat located in Gaborone, the capital of Botswana. The Secretariat coordinates its work through various sectors, which are located in different countries. The sectors are: Agriculture and Livestock Production; Natural Resources Research and Training; Culture and Information; Energy; Environment and Land Management; Finance and Investment; Food, Agriculture and Natural

Resources; Human Resources Development; Industry and Trade: Inland Fisheries, Forestry and Wildlife; Livestock Production and Animal Disease Control; Marine Fisheries and Resources; Mining Employment and Labour; South African Centre for Co-operation in Agricultural Research; Southern African Transport and Communications Commission; Tourism; Water. The SADC Employment and Labour Sector is located in Zambia. The Health Sector is based in South Africa.

SADC conducts an annual summit with heads of state or government. This is the ultimate policy-making institution of SADC. The Council of Ministers makes recommendations to the summit and ensures that policies are properly implemented.

When the Southern African Development Community was set up in 1992 HIV and AIDS was not considered to be an important issue by any of the governments of the Southern African nations. Sudden political developments had created the possibility for a united strategy against the region's twin evils, poverty and underdevelopment. Namibia had been independent since 1989 and in 1990 negotiations had started between the African National Congress and the National Party in South Africa to the ending of apartheid.

It was hoped that the strengthening of political and economic unity across the region would assist them to address these problems. Majority rule in South Africa would permit the most powerful economy in the region to be used to benefit all the people of South Africa but also to give a boost to development in its neighbouring countries. Thus SADC was intended to promote regional economic welfare, collective self-reliance and integration in the spirit of equity and partnership. Its important aims were economic well-being, the improvement of the standard and quality of life, freedom and social justice, and peace and security, for the peoples of Southern Africa. At the time of SADC's inception in 1992 cases of human immunodeficiency virus (HIV) infection had been detected in all Southern African Countries, but very few people were concerned that it could cross epidemic proportions. Unfortunately, however, the horrific social conditions under which most people lived also contributed to placing millions of people at risk of infection with HIV.

Conditions Responsible for Vulnerability

HIV does not discriminate between men and women, rich and poor, black or white. All people who are sexually active and who do not practise safe sex can be infected with HIV. However, the conditions under which some people live can put them at a greater risk than others. For example, people who are illiterate are more at risk since they cannot read printed messages about how to avoid infection with HIV. Women who are poor are more likely to sell sex than women who are rich and are more likely to be infected with HIV. This is called vulnerability. People in developing countries are highly vulnerable to HIV.

Southern Africa is one of the poorest regions of the world. The 14 member states of SADC have a population of 191 million people. In most countries the majority of people are illiterate and live below the poverty line. Millions live in rural areas at times without access to electricity, clean water or telephones.

There is large-scale migration of people between countries, and from rural areas of the cities. The constant moving and mixing of populations is related to employment or to the need to find employment to survive. Once people arrive at the cities they live in huge informal settlements or 'squatter camps' in conditions of deprivation that are identical to those in rural areas. Migrant labour is a feature of formal sector employment even at present. Approximately half of the workforce on South Africa's gold mines comes from the neighbouring countries of Lesotho, Botswana and Mozambique.

Ironically, peace across most of the subcontinent has also created additional vulnerability to HIV infection among many workers and their families. There has been an improvement in communications and trade. New roads such will soon make it possible for goods to be carried by truck from the west coast of Southern Africa (Windhoek in Namibia) to the east coast (Maputo in Mozambique). Poverty and high unemployment have created large informal production and trading sectors. Thousands of people from Zimbabwe, Malawi and Mozambique travel long distances by train and road to relatively prosperous countries like South Africa to sell woodcarvings, traditional cloths and African curios to tourists, or to try to find employment. In South Africa it has been approximated that there are between 500000 and 1.5 million undocumented or illegal immigrants. Large-scale legal and illegal (undocumented) migration makes it more difficult to combat HIV transmission and leads to vulnerability. Migrants who are in search of work or escaping political conflicts are often alone and far from their families. They are likely to sell sex or to pay for sex either for monetary gains or for pleasure. Illegal immigrants, who are afraid of being caught, are generally afraid to use health services. Victims of rape will not report to the police for fear of being deported. However, stricter measures to keep borders sealed will not serve the purpose because migration is driven by poverty. HIV prevention thus creates a further need for additional cooperation and common strategies on migration and regional development.

Most of the SADC region is at peace, but there are ongoing civil conflicts in Angola and the Democratic Republic of the Congo. These conflicts are creating large internal refugee populations and movements of people among countries. Refugees are vulnerable to HIV for the same reasons as migrants. In addition, they are often traumatized by war and violence. In such conditions, social norms break down. In refugee communities there is widespread rape and violence against women and children; there is almost no access to health services. Therefore, in the face of personal upheaval the risk of HIV infection seems to be a minor concern.

Many people in African societies still respect traditions and cultural practices that increase individual vulnerability to HIV. For example:

(a) the practice of mandatory wife inheritance by a brother if a woman's spouse dies;

(b) the 'cleansing' of virgins on reaching puberty through having forced sex with a disguised male;

(c) the minority status of women under conventional laws and low level of educational opportunity for the girl child.

All of the factors classified above create vulnerability to HIV infection. Some have no direct relationship with employment. But the implementation of creative employment strategies can address all of these problems. For example:

(a) workplace AIDS education can sensitively enhance

awareness about cultural practices that contribute to HIV;

(b) employers and employees can change workplace policies that necessitate workers to travel far from home without their families. In Zimbabwe a successful intervention programme was developed in the transport sector. In a joint effort between managers and workers through the National Employment Council for the transport industry, a peer education programme was developed and financed, to reach drivers and communities where long-haul drivers stopped en route.

Strategies like these assist to mitigate the worst impact of AIDS. The SADC Code on AIDS and Employment recognizes this. To tackle all these problems, some African leaders have become advocates of an 'African Renaissance'. They are of the opinion that it will be possible to extend development to the rest of the continent from countries such as South Africa, Botswana, Mozambique and Uganda where there is economic growth. Therefore, these countries will lead a renaissance' that will witness Africa emerge as a major economic, cultural and scientific centre in the 21st century. However, confronting the AIDS epidemic must be made a central part of economic regeneration..

HIV/AIDS Epidemic in Southern Africa: Present Trends

The AIDS epidemic is a major barrier to be encountered in Africa's aspirations for sustainable economic growth and development. By 1999, there were more people in Southern Africa infected with HIV than in Europe, North and South America combined. Approximately four million adults and children have died and in the times to come, many more will die. More than 10 million people in Southern Africa are infected with HIV.

Despite the shockingly high HIV prevalence in most Southern African countries the HIV/AIDS epidemic is still growing at an accelerated. In 1992, when SADC was launched, adult HIV prevalence across most of the region was under 5 per cent. By 1999, in cities and towns across the region, it averaged about 20 per cent.

(a) In 1997, in Francistown and Gaborone, the two largest cities in Botswana, HIV prevalence amongst women antenatal antendees was 42.9 and 34.0 per cent respectively.
(b) In 1995, in Harare, Zimbabwe's capital city, it was 37 per cent and 30 per cent in the second largest city, Bulawayo.
(c) In Namibia, by 1996, AIDS had become the largest cause of reported deaths, and national HIV prevalence was estimated to be 15.4 per cent.
(d) In 1996 in Blantyre, the largest city in Malawi, HIV prevalence at urban antenatal clinics was 34 per cent.
(e) In 1998 in three of the most industrialized provinces in South Africa (Gauteng, Kwa-Zulu Natal and Mpumalanga) adult HIV infection rates were more than 20 per cent.

Impact on Employees

The gravity of the economic impact of the epidemic is directly related to the fact that most of the infected persons are in the peak productive and reproductive age groups. AIDS kills those who grow the crops, work in the mines and factories, run the schools and hospitals and govern nations and countries. HIV is mainly infecting and affecting people of working age. Most infected people are aged between 16 and 35. Depending on the baseline mortality in a country and the extent of HIV infection, it has been approximated that as a result of AIDS, deaths of prime-age working adults will increase by a multiple of 2 to 10. UNAIDS and the World Health Organization (WHO) have opined that in an area where overall HIV prevalence is 8 per cent, HIV is the cause of four out of five deaths between the ages of 25 and 34. The implications of these realities for the workplace are serious. The consequences of AIDS for a country's economically active age group are evident from what follows:

(a) In the United Republic of Tanzania, it has been reflected that adult deaths will lessen the labour force by 20 per cent and the mean age of workers from 32 to 28 by 2010.

(b) In Botswana, Malawi, Zimbabwe and Zambia life expectancy has fallen dramatically. It is hoped that by 2010 in these and other countries life expectancy will have fallen by 20 per cent because of HIV/AIDS.

A decrease in life expectancy and an increase in adult and infant mortality will change the labour market scenario. This is not just something that might happen in the future. It is already happening. In various professions, regardless of sector and size, there are signs of an increase in illness and death amongst the workforce:

(a) In Southern Africa the mining industry employs approximately 750000 to 900000 people. Some mining companies estimate that up to 40 per cent of their employees have HIV. Although the numbers of reported AIDS cases in the mines are at present below 5 per cent of the workforce, this will rise in the years ahead. In South Africa some projections recommended that within 10 years up to 25000 mineworkers will die every year because of AIDS associated illnesses. AIDS will increase worker turnover by 3-6 per cent per annum.

(b) AIDS has created new direct costs for the mining industry. It also carries a voluminous social cost for the dependents of mineworkers who die and will no longer receive wage remittances. Six million people rely on mining for their bread. Deaths of the principal wage earner will result in increasing numbers of children having to work to compensate for parents who have died or who are too ill to work.

(c) In Botswana it is estimated at present that 33 per cent of employee deaths are due to AIDS. Between 1996 and 2004 the expected annual adult death rate because of AIDS will rise from 4 to 28 per one thousand (seven times).

These and other indicators of the impact of AIDS are drawn from medium-sized and large companies that have greater capacity to absorb the new costs and replace lost labour. In the formal sector HIV and AIDS will lead to declines in productivity due to lost time and absenteeism, increases in staff turnover, skills shortages and staff demoralization.

Impact on the Small and Informal Sector

Southern Africa also has a large micro or informal employment sector. Although this sector's share to traditional economic indicators such as Gross Domestic Product (GDP) is difficult to measure, this form of employment prevents millions of people from starving. This sector consists informal traders, peasant agriculturalists and women working in households.

Governments and formal sector employers cannot afford to be complacent about the impact of AIDS on the informal sector. In many countries industrial and economic policy attaches great importance to encouraging small and micro employment enterprises. Even in the most industrialized countries of the region, such as South Africa, small employment enterprises employ millions of people. In South Africa 37 per cent of private sector enterprises employ less than 50 people. They constitute 20 per cent of all those employed.

The small size of these 'employers' makes it much difficult to replace skilled and semi-skilled employees, for example motor mechanics, when they die or become too ill to work. Micro-enterprises will, thus, find it far more difficult to absorb the costs of increased absenteeism, staff-turnover and death.

Impact on Economy

Governments and employers must not conclude from suggestions that the net impact of AIDS on economic growth, particularly per capita Gross Domestic Product (GDP), might be small. Many traditional economic indicators do not give crystal clear image of the actual impact of AIDS on either employers or employees. For example, as the World Bank report explains, the deaths of a large number of people in the low-income brackets and smaller numbers of high earners could even result in an overall increase in per capita GDP. In fact, though, overall well-being will not have improved and the incomes of survivors will have been reduced.

HIV and AIDS have severe consequences for humans, and

social development. These factors will impact greatly on a country's ability to increase productivity and private and public investment. For example:

(a) Many employees will have children and spouses who are also infected.

(b) The death of one or both parents will mean that young people will be forced to go to work earlier, sacrificing their schooling.

(c) The sustainability of economic growth in countries like Botswana and South Africa will be endangered in a shrinking consumer market that could result from declines in population growth and the re-direction of consumer expenditure into caring for those who are ill.

(d) AIDS will dramatically affect the social environment in which all businesses operate, even if 'costs' can be contained. AIDS will have an impact on the morale of people in a similar way, for example, that rampant crime has visibly affected the morale of citizens in South Africa.

These facts are at present a part of the business environment in Southern Africa as well as in other developing regions of the world. They emphasize the importance of local, national and regional interventions that will assist to prevent the continued rapid spread of HIV. Employers, governments and trade unions must understand that a future beyond high AIDS-associated morbidity and mortality does exist, but only if they act decisively at present.

Ten

Necessity of a Regional Code

To facilitate regional economic integration and to standardize labour market policies and practices is one of the objectives of SADC. This necessitates a careful analysis of the effect that AIDS will have on the region's workforce and economies. Elements of such an analysis were discussed earlier. The present discussion looks at the process that was involved in the development of the Code. The SADC Employment and Labour Sector was initiated in 1995. Since its inception, it has set an example for other SADC sectors by operating in a way that has made it accessible to the opinions of trade unions, nongovernmental organizations and businesses. Commendably, it also recognized the importance of strategies to combat AIDS.

Its objectives are:

(a) To ensure that the Sector retains the tripartite relationship between labour, employers and government;

(b) To promote the formulation and integration of legal, economic and social policies and programmes which facilitate the generation of productive employment opportunities and income;

(c) To promote labour policies and measures which help free labour mobility, remove distortion in the labour markets, enhance industrial harmony and increase productivity;

(d) To provide a framework for regional cooperation in the sphere of employment and labour with the full participation and involvement of all the social partners;

(e) To promote a framework for regional cooperation in the collection and dissemination of labour market information;

(f) To standardize social security schemes;
(g) To harmonize regulations relating to health and safety standards at workplaces across the region;
(h) To promote the development of institutional capacities as well as vocational and technical skills across the region.

All of these objectives will be directly affected by HIV/AIDS and emphasize the importance of the Sector's activities in developing a Regional Code on AIDS and Employment.

In November 1994 the first proposal to develop a Southern African 'Code on AIDS and Employment' was made at a regional conference in Harare, the capital city of Zimbabwe. This conference brought together 70 participants from governments, non-governmental organizations (NGOs), employer and labour organizations across the region. It discovered a wide variety of issues relating to AIDS, economic policy and employment. In one of its resolutions the Conference noted the absence of policy guidelines about how to manage the effect and impact of HIV/AIDS on employment and economic development. The resolution warned that HIV will cost Southern African economies in terms of lost skills, lost production, a reduced tax base, increased social and health cost, reduction in household, company and national savings and incrcased consumption needs. The real costs of HIV/AIDS are poorly documented, not included in government budgets or estimates, or included as health costs despite their cross cutting economic/ employment impact and thus sectoralised to the health sector.

Delegates therefore proposed to exchange experiences and strategies for managing the impact of AIDS and concluded that a regional code on AIDS and employment would assist this and potentially serve two important functions:

(a) as a policy framework and guideline;
(b) as an entry point for a border review of regional issues associated with AIDS and employment and for a better exchange of information about the implications of AIDS on the labour market between SADC members.

A proposal for the drafting of a regional code was therefore made by the Secretary General of the Southern African Trade

Union Coordinating Committee (SATUCC) and it was agreed that Southern African countries [should] develop and legislate national codes of practice on AIDS and employment through a tripartite process with other affected communities involved.

Following the Regional Conference on AIDS and Employment the Southern African Labour Commission (the predecessor of the SADC Employment and Labour Sector) supported the recommendations. It proposed that national policies and programmes on HIV/AIDS and its implications on the workforce, productivity and the economy should be formulated through a process of tripartite consultations. In February 1995 the international Labour Organization (ILO) was asked to assist Southern African countries to formulate a process that would lead to the drafting of a regional code.

Drafting

In Zimbabwe in January 1996 the Organization of African Trade Union Unity (OATUU) and the ILO conducted joint workshop with tripartite representatives from the five Southern African countries that had earlier started to develop national employment codes - Botswana, Namibia, South Africa, Zambia and Zimbabwe. The objective was to amalgamate their experiences into a regional document. It was observed that the implications of the AIDS epidemic should not lead to despair, but rather should galvanize all social partners and sectors to optimum efforts for HIV risk prevention and plan for challenges ahead. The impact of AIDS will be lessened by collaborative planning and programming as well as promulgating supportive legislation. Support for a regional standard did not come automatically. Delegates debated the principles that necessitated to be included in a regional code and at the start, there was disagreement on various issues, as:

(a) whether pre-employment or pre-training HIV screening was justifiable;

(b) whether it was permissible to examine expatriate (foreign) workers for HIV. For example, although the National AIDS Plan in Botswana resists mandatory testing of local employees an exception is made for foreign people who are seeking to work in Botswana.

Some of these issues were referred back to national tripartite bodies for further discussion. Other issues were resolved at the workshop. On HIV testing, for example, it was agreed by everyone that pre-employment HIV testing is not acceptable, but representatives of business argued that in a few cases where an employee is being sent on a costly training course there may be some justification for HIV testing. Therefore, it was agreed that the Code should state that "in general there should be no compulsory testing for HIV." Overall however there was ample will to reach agreement and formulate a draft Code on which consensus was reached.

At the 'Mazvikadei Workshop' the SADC representative made a commitment that the Code would be officially tabled at the next meeting of the SADC Employment and Labour Sector, in May 1996. At this meeting, which was conducted in Lilongwe, Malawi, the Code was supported by officials from labour ministries across the region. Nonetheless, the SADC Ministers of Labour realised that there had not been enough discussion of the Code at a national level by business, trade unions and governments. The draft Code was thus referred back to the SADC member countries for further discussion. Meanwhile SADC undertook to conduct additional research to examine the impact that AIDS was going to have on employment in the region. The next discussion of the Code was scheduled for a year later.

Adoption of the Code

Between May 1996 and May 1997 advocacy for the Code continued. Lobbying was led by OATUU and by some NGOs. The first draft of the SADC Code was widely distributed through networks of AIDS service organizations, trade union federations and government bodies.

In December 1996 a Joint SADC/European Union Conference on Regional Approaches to the HIV/AIDS Epidemic was held in Lilongwe, Malawi. This conference examined impact that AIDS was likely to have on a range of issues, including employment, education, tourism and trade. It too resolved that a regional code on AIDS and employment was needed.

During 1996 national tripartite discussions on the Code took place in several SADC countries. When the Code was presented to the SADC Employment and Labour sector again in May 1997, it was agreed that there had now been ample consultation. The Code was then tabled at a meeting of Ministers of Labour from all the SADC countries (except Angola) that was held in Pretoria, South Africa, where it was overwhelmingly endorsed. It was forwarded to the SADC Summit in September 1997 for final ratification. At this meeting the Code was approved by Heads of Government as a new regional standard.

The SADC Code on AIDS and Employment is intended to influence labour policy practice in all fourteen of SADC's member countries. It is not a legally binding treaty or an instrument of law. However, the Code suggests that "SADC member states develop tripartite national codes.... that shall be projected in law." During 1998 two countries, Namibia and Zimbabwe, introduced a version of the Code into their labour legislation.

Namibia

In Namibia Guidelines for the Implementation of a National Code on HIV/AIDS and Employment were published in a Government Gazette in April 1998. In terms of the Namibian Labour Act the Code contains guidelines and instructions to be followed and adhered to by all employers and employees.

Zimbabwe

In Zimbabwe the national Code on AIDS and Employment was passed by parliament in 1998 as Labour Relations (HIV and AIDS) Regulations under the Labour Act. The code covers in a comprehensive manner: provisions for education of employees on HIV/AIDS; prohibition against HIV testing on recruitment; statements against discrimination on the basis of HIV status in promotion, transfer, job status, benefits or training; entitlement to sick or compassionate leave; provision of safe working environments where HIV exists; arid display of the Code in all workplaces.

To ensure that other countries follow the example of Zimbabwe and Namibia, SADC has been mandated to establish a mechanism to watch the Code's implementation and enforcement through national law.

The contribution that can be made to HIV/AIDS prevention at work and outside work by trade unions and employer organizations as recognized in national AIDS policies and plans. The workplace has a major role to play in society's efforts to check the AIDS epidemic. First, workplaces can be turned into 'adult class rooms' that teach millions of employees about HIV. In the present discussion, we look at the principles on which the Code is based and the recommendations it makes pertaining to workplace policy.

Decades of institutionalized racism and colonialism left most of the Southern African region underdeveloped and impoverished. At present, there are broad social and economic disparities within countries and between countries. For example, South Africa is considered a 'middle-income country'. In 1998, it was ranked 89th on the Human Development Index (HDI). However, within South Africa there remains abject poverty and inequality. Malawi (161st on the HDI) and Mozambique (166th on the HDI) are among the poorest countries in the world.

Political freedom for people in Southern Africa presented many new social and economic challenges in the 1980s and 1990s. The question of how to achieve sustainable social development became particularly important. It is here that the prerogatives of economic development and effective HIV prevention now coincide: managing the impact of the AIDS pandemic will be one of the greatest economic challenges Southern Africa will have to encounter.

Principles of the Code

Human Rights

- The Code is based on "the fundamental principles of human rights.... World Health Organization and International Labour Organization regional standards and Guidelines".
- In Southern Africa the reaction to AIDS in the workplace has repeated what has happened in many other parts of the world. Trade unions and NGOs have documented how the response of many employers (large and small) is to resort to acts of unfair discrimination.
- Some employers implement mandatory testing of job applicants for HIV. People with HIV are then denies work.

- Some companies terminate the services of workers with AIDS or only employ those who they think have a 'low risk' of being infected with HIV.
- Many company medical insurance schemes debar HIV from their medical benefits.
- Some industries have proposed a major restructuring of employee benefits to try and cut out the anticipated cost of HIV and AIDS.

Unfair discrimination is contrary to the principles of the Universal Declaration of Human Rights. Many of the practices discussed earlier latent people's rights to fair labour practices and equality of opportunity. They are in conflict with International Conventions and Treaties on Human Rights that most SADC governments have ratified and pledged to respect, protect, promote and fulfill. For example, employers who deny to train or employ people with HIV are acting in violation of the International Covenant on Economic, Social and Cultural Rights, which has been ratified by all the SADC member countries, except Botswana, Swaziland and South Africa. This is because their actions will be denying large numbers of people. The right to work, which consists the right of everyone to the opportunity to gain his living by work for which he may have a free choice or acceptance.

Unfair discrimination is also obviously against principles for the management of HIV and AIDS in the workplace that have been recommended by the International Labour Organization and World Health Organization. In 1988, a consensus statement issued by the ILO and WHO suggested that concern about the transmission of HIV/AIDS provides an opportunity to re-examine the workplace environment. It offers an opportunity to generate an atmosphere conducive to caring for and promoting the health of all workers. This may involve several issues and concerns, not only individual behaviour, but also address collective responsibility. It provides an opportunity to re-examine working relationships in a manner that promotes human rights and dignity, ensures freedom from discrimination and stigmatization, and improves working practices and procedures.

UN International Guidelines on HIV/AIDS and Human Rights

In recognition of the individual's human rights, health and economic effects of workplace discrimination the United Nations' International Guidelines on HIV/AIDS and Human Rights also consist several recommendations relating specifically to employment. In a Guideline on 'Anti-discrimination and Protective Laws' the United Nations proposes that laws regulations and collective agreements should be enacted so as to guarantee the following workplace rights:

(a) A national policy on HIV/AIDS in the workplace agreed upon in a tripartite body;
(b) Freedom from HIV screening for employment, promotion, training or benefits;
(c) Confidentiality regarding all medical information, alongwith HIV/AIDS status;
(d) Employment security for workers living with HIV until they are no longer able to work, including reasonable alternative working arrangements;
(e) Defined safe practices for first aid and adequately equipped first aid kits;
(f) Protection for social security and other benefits for workers living with HIV, including life insurance, pension, health insurance, dismissed and death benefits;
(g) Ample health care accessible in or near the workplace;
(h) Ample supplies of condoms available free to workers at the workplace;
(i) Workers' involvement in decision-making on workplace issues related to HIV/AIDS;
(j) Access to information and education programmes on HIV/AIDS, as well as to relevant counselling and appropriate referral;
(k) Protection from stigmatization and discrimination by colleagues, unions, employers and clients;
(l) Appropriate inclusion in workers' compensation legislation of the occupational transmission of HIV (e.g., needlestick injuries), addressing such matters as the long latency period of infection, testing, counselling and confidentiality.

When confronting AIDS it is important to learn from human rights violations of the recent past. If governments and employers stigmatize those who are infected and or affected they will perpetuate the social problems that have emerged as a result of racism. The negative consequences of discrimination against black people and discrimination against people with HIV/AIDS for economic growth and development are potentially very similar.

Sustainable development depends upon harnessing the skills and energies of as many people as possible. Racial discrimination worked opposite. I debarred large numbers of people from skilled employment, training and wealth. It left skills and purchasing power in the hands of a minority. Although there were temporary benefits for white people, keeping black people in low-skill, low-wage jobs eventually squeezed and distorted the consumer markets of Southern Africa. The result was economic crisis and political instability that undermined governments and employers alike. Unfair discrimination targeted at people with HIV has an identical effect. The effect of terminating or refusing to employ a person just because he or she has HIV is to deny that person the opportunity to earn a living and to spend their earnings on themselves and their families. This leads to the loss of dignity as well as several other globally accepted rights and opportunities including education, health and eventually life. Unfair discrimination entrenches the cycle of poverty. For example, denial to employ people with HIV or AIDS:

(a) increases the number of people who are unemployed and therefore dependent on those with jobs (already very high);
(b) decreases the number of economically productive people;
(c) wastes public resources that have been invested in the education and training of people before they were infected.

Unfair discrimination will decelerate the economic development of the region by increasing the dependency of people with HIV/AIDS and their families on the already meagre resources of their governments. One of the resolutions adopted at the Conference on AIDS and Employment noted that unfair discrimination by private employers does not extinct costs of AIDS disappear. If not borne by the private sector (employer, insurance, industry, etc.) they are shifted to the state or the household where the capacity to bear costs in lower and potentials for pooling the costs of risk between income group less.

These are the most important reasons why the framers of the Code set it within a framework of fundamental human rights. The Code does not generate new rights. It merely translates rights that SADC countries have already endorsed into the employment context. This is in keeping with the approach that had been developed in other countries, for example, the Ten Principles for the Workplace that have been framed by the National Leadership Coalition on AIDS in the United States.

Patient rights

The Code is based upon patient rights, medical and occupational health principles... and a human and compassionate attitude to individuals.

Unfair discrimination adds to the stigma around AIDS and in turns makes it more difficult to check the HIV epidemic. This contributes to larger numbers of people being infected with HIV, becoming ill and dying.

There is increasing recognition that public health at times provides an added and compelling justification for safeguarding human rights, despite the respect, protection and fulfillment which they merit in their own right. In the context of HIV/AIDS, an environment in which human rights are respected ensures that vulnerability to HIV/AIDS is lessened, those infected with and affected by HIV/AIDS live a life of dignity without discrimination and the personal and societal impact of HIV infection is alleviated.

In keeping with this, the International Guidelines propose that the human rights that should be protected at work include confidentiality, informed consent to testing, the duty to treat and the duty to ensure safe workplaces. These rights are all protected in the SADC Code.

Confidentiality: This ethical and human rights principle recognized that all people have rights to privacy about personal medical conditions. It applies fully to HIV infection and AIDS. In an employment setting it means that a person infected with HIV should have complete control over decisions about who, how and even if his or her colleagues are informed. Confidentiality must not be confused with secrecy. In a 'safe' workplace, where co-employees are educated about HIV and where unfair discrimination is prohibited people living with HIV are likely to want to be open about their infection.

Informed consent: This is an ethical principle deeply embedded in the medical profession. It means that when a patient is advised to undergo a medical operation he or she should fully understand the real and possible consequences of that operation. Applied to HIV testing it means that all people have a right to be fully informed about HIV and AIDS and to absorb how an HIV-positive result will affect their lives before agreeing to an HIV test. This can only be achieved through counselling.

The duty to ensure safe workplaces: HIV cannot be transmitted through casual contact between people at work. Therefore it is not justifiable to separate individuals with HIV from other employees. In workplaces where employees come into contact with blood or other bodily fluids, or where there are sometimes accidents that can lead to blood spills, universal precautions must be introduced and always practised. Employees should be taught to regard all blood as possibly HIV-infected.

Business Efficiency

The Code is based on "sound epidemiological statistics and prudent business practice.

Presently, conducting business in Southern Africa means operating in environment where HIV prevalence in the workforce and in the consumer market is approximately 20 per cent. This fact should influence business practice as much as other factors that distinguish industrialized countries from the developing world such as cultural and technological differences.

Unfortunately, emerging markets across the world are characterized by an accelerated incidence of HIV. At present, the AIDS epidemic is spreading equally fast in Asia and parts of Latin America. Therefore, businesses do not have the option or re-locating to other parts of the developing world to avoid HIV/AIDS.

Epidemiological principles inform us that in an area with a high or rapidly rising incidence of HIV infection it is not possible for a business (or any institution) to isolate itself from the AIDS epidemic. Unfair measures that seek to protect a company from AIDS do not work. Indeed, the experience of employers has been that measures that take away the rights of employees make the AIDS epidemic more expensive for the workplace for various reasons:

(a) They add direct costs. Identifying people at work - or applying for work - who have HIV requires compulsory testing, replacing skilled and unskilled labour and complex recruitment strategies. Denial to employ qualified and competent people because they have HIV may mean employing less suitable alternative candidates.

(b) They add indirect costs. These emerge from suspicion between employers and employees, and a demoralized, demotivated workforce.

(c) They may increase the prevalence of HIV. In the medium to long term they add to the burden of HIV/AIDS experienced by individual workplaces. For example, mandatory HIV testing of people joining the military services has not lowered the prevalence rate among soldiers. Compulsory testing does not lower the prevalence or incidence of HIV. The opinion that testing is a way to check HIV at the door of the factory or office is wrong. It undermines the real prevention messages of workplace education programmes.

(d) They prevent 'shared responsibility'. A unilateral response from employers paralyses the development of a common approach to AIDS by employers and employees. The Code is based on principles that recognize this. By combining strategies that are good for business, instil trust in employees and assist HIV prevention it aims to be as inclusive as possible.

Unfair discrimination makes people afraid to show interest in HIV prevention and therefore undermines workplace-based health education and HIV prevention. Workers who have HIV, or who are worried that they may be infected, are forced to latent their infection and their fears to protect their jobs. Unfair discrimination may reinforce people's opinions that AIDS is a punishment for 'immoral' behaviour and direct attention away from a realistic understanding of how HIV is transmitted.

Components of the Code

Based on the three principles explained earlier, the Code makes several specific recommendations about how to manage HIV/AIDS at work. It is important to note that the Code is not advocating 'special rights' for employees with HIV. In fact, it makes two important assertions:

(a) Employees with HIV should be treated the same as any other employee.

(b) Employees with HIV related illness, including AIDS, should be treated the same as any other employee with a life-threatening illness.

However, it explains that due to the gravity and impact of this unique illness special policies and measures are necessary. This is not a contradiction. Never before in modern history has an incurable virus affected so many people. Further, while there are many other illnesses in the developing world that cause illness and death none of them have gathered the same volume of stigma as AIDS. They do not primarily affect adults.

Education and Awareness

Key policy: The workplace is an excellent place to educate employers, employees and their families about how to prevent infection and live with HIV. Education, organized during working hours, is an investment that will benefit every workplace. If the promotion of health-seeking behaviour pertaining HIV is combined with other health issues (smoking, alcohol consumption, workplace safety, managing stress) it will result in increased productivity and morale. It is likely to instil trust and is the only way to reduce the long-term impact of HIV in the workplace.

Job Access and Job Status

Key policy: HIV, or the suspicion that a person may have HIV, should not be considered when employing, training or promoting an employee. Identifying employees with HIV does not immunize a workplace from the impact of AIDS.

Workplace Testing and Confidentiality

Key policy: Like any other health condition, infection with HIV is a private (confidential) matter. Employees or employers should not be forced to reveal their HIV infection to managers, medical officers or human resource personnel. Revelation is a matter of individual choice. Breaches of confidentiality will cause demoralization and disruption.

Privacy and confidentiality about HIV/AIDS will continue to be a major issue, which needs sensitive handling from all concerned. But what needs to be dealt with is a radical shift in norms and values, to a culture in which the question of how people get AIDS - the moral, ethical and cultural issues, must be superseded by the issues of how to support them, assist them to lead meaningful lives in the community, and how to prevent further spread of the disease.

Individual HIV testing is not associated with the day-to-day management of the workplace. However, education should explain the advantages of HIV testing if it is on a voluntary and confidential basis and is relevant to pre- and post-test counselling.

Managing Illness and Job Security

Key policy: Employees with HIV-associated illnesses should be treated as per to the rules that already govern sickness under company policy and in accordance with existing labour laws. Where it is possible, reasonable accommodation should be made for employees whose illness makes them unable to do jobs that become too stressful or strenuous, although this will depend on the size of the workplace concerned. It is justifiable to terminate employment as a result of incapacity, but it should be done fairly and without discrimination.

Occupational Benefits

Key policy: Greater illness and death will make it necessary to review and restructure many employee benefits (such as death and disability benefits, pensions and provident funds). This should be done openly and through negotiation. Benefits should not be restructured before there has been research to demonstrate the actual impact that AIDS will have on the viability of a benefit.

Once this has been done benefits should not be restructured in a manner that unfairly excludes employees with HIV, or drastically limits medical cover for HIV and AIDS.

Risk Management, First Aid and Compensation

Key policy: In the vast majority of workplaces there is not a risk of occupational infection. In working environments where there is a small risk (because employees come into contact with blood or other body fluids) the risk of accidental HIV infection can be eliminated by simple and cheap procedures. For example, teaching employees about infection control procedures 'universal precautions' and establishing and maintaining a properly stocked first aid box.

Protection against Victimization and Grievance Handling

Key policy: Fear of people with HIV - either among clients or co-workers - is caused by ignorance. Education leads to AIDS awareness, which takes away fear and create better relations at work. Disciplinary action is justified against employees who generate tear and hatred against co-workers with HIV, just as it is on the basis of sexual harassment or racial discrimination.

Information, Monitoring and Review

Key policy: HIV/AIDS is an evolving epidemic. Its impact on the economy of the region as well as on the individual workplace is still being analysed. All social partners should work together collect and share statistics. Policies, including the SADC Code, should be examine in the light of new statistics. Until this happens the success of the Code will depend on an ongoing campaign of advocacy, education and lobbying to encourage governments and employers at national level to integrate it into their national law and make it legally binding.

Now, the concentration has been on the role that was played by different organizations in Southern Africa to promote the SADC, Employment Code and the partnerships that emerged during its development. It focuses mainly on the experience of three SADC countries - Botswana, South Africa and Zimbabwe.

Botswana: The National Taskforce

In Botswana the process of developing a Code on AIDS and Employment led to a much broader cooperation between business organizations and the trade unions on issues of AIDS in the workplace than had existed before. Early in 1995 the Botswana Federation of Trade Unions (BFTU) framed an Employment Code with the assistance of the Organisation of African Trade Union Unity (OATUU). In November that year the BFTU hosted a tripartite workshop on economic and employment problems and HIV. This meeting was attended by several government representatives, trade unions and the Botswana Business Coalition on AIDS (BBCA). The meeting aimed to gather consensus on the need for an employment Code. It also led to a decision to set up a National Taskforce on HIV/AIDS at the Workplace.

Since 1996 the National Taskforce has carried out research and has supported many workplace programmes that have started to prepare employers and employees to deal with a number of challenges of HIV and AIDS. Among the Task Force's achievements so far are:

(a) An ill-health monitoring guideline which companies can utilize to carry out in-house impact assessments;
(b) A workplace action plan on HIV/AIDS, documenting resources and support for each activity;
(c) The setting up of bipartite health and social welfare committees in various companies.

Zimbabwe: The Intersectoral Committee

At the end of 1994 the National AIDS Control Programme (NACP) in Zimbabwe called together employers, trade unions and NGOs participating in workplace prevention programmes. This group consisted the Employers Council of Zimbabwe (EMCOZ), the Confederation of Zimbabwe Industries (CZI), government bodies, the Zimbabwe Congress of Trade Unions (ZCTU) and two nongovernmental organizations, SAFAIDS and the Matabeleland AIDS Council.

The group, which was initially called the 'Tripartite Plus', went through a number of brainstorming sessions on HIV/AIDS and employment. It was chaired by the NACP, but this role was later shifted to the Department of Labour. This approach resolved the issue of interministerial collaboration which, in many countries alongwith Zimbabwe is a persistent problem. The committee launched a policy formulation process:

(a) A consultation phase was planned to identify the issues, points of attention and resource persons.
(b) Consultative meetings were held in the two main industrial centres, Harare and Bulawayo.

These meetings permitted for an important categorization of issues into the following groups:

(a) those that could be made legally binding (if approved by the existing Tripartite) as Labour Regulations that would be gazetted as attachments to the existing Labour Relations Act;
(b) issues that were more of a policy nature, such as social security and occupational benefits, medical aid and general production and productivity issues.

The drafting phase involved holding various intensive meetings between the partners. This allowed for strong debate. It demonstrated considerably more consensus than was expected beforehand around key issues such as testing, occupational benefits and medical aid. The result was a draft set of policy recommendations. Thereafter a second round of consultative meetings in Harare and Bulawayo was organized to receive feedback on this draft. This collated further debate and permitted for amendments to the draft codes. This next draft was circulated broadly and in large numbers within the country as the *Draft Employment Code on HIV/AIDS - Volume 1 (Industrial Relations) and Volume 2 (Social Security and Production Strategies).* Individual members of the Intersectoral Committee then made formal and informal presentations to employer and employee bodies. These and other comments and submissions were used to finalize the draft code. This code was presented to the Labour Tripartite and approved after discussion and some variations. Thereafter, codification of the text in the appropriate language was undertaken through external expertise and submitted to the Attorney General's office.

In Zimbabwe several important lessons were learnt:

(a) A small motivated expert group of persons skilled in policy formulation and process thinking are required to take up the issue and to identify the probabilities for an open, consultative process. The informal networks of the members are essential for generating involvement in the debate. This includes having contracts with donor agencies to ensure access to appropriate funding.

(b) Taking the time for planning, consultation and discussion ensured wide acceptance of the opinion and permitted a wide range of views to be heard and incorporated. The distribution of the draft code is an essential part of this process.

(c) Formulation of an Employment Code necessitates patience, as it takes time for organizations to become involved. Bulk in the long term it is more likely to pay off rather than taking short cuts for quick limited results.

(d) Membership of the intersectoral committee: this expert group should include people with HIV/AIDS and representatives of NGOs that are experienced in running workplace programmes and are participating in information dissemination.

(e) Ideally, the government departments responsible for labour regulations and/or occupational health should be prepared to take a lead role.

(f) Enlisting wide participation of the parties concerned and affected by a proposed HIV/AIDS and Employment Code is a key to ensuring the necessary debate and focus for the formulation process. It is also essential for the achievement of consensus around critical issues.

(g) If possible, the drafting of a code should be linked to the existing structures such as the Labour Tripartite and Employment councils, as well as other existing umbrella bodies concerned, such as those for insurance and medical aid. Particular precaution should be taken to ensure the input of people living with HIV, human and patient rights bodies and the religious places.

South Africa: The Contribution of NGOs

In June 1993 the AIDS Consortium, a network of NGOs, AIDS service organizations (ASOs) and individuals based in

Johannesburg organized a conference on AIDS, human rights and employment. This Conference proposed that a 'Code of Conduct on AIDS and Employment' should be drafted and submitted to the government. It recommended that its principles be made legally binding on employers and employees. A committee that included human rights activists, business people and trade unionists was established and completed the first draft in August 1994. In 1995, the AIDS Consortium initiated a lobbying campaign to make the Code known. This campaign, which included seminars and workshops, targeted:

(a) Government: Meetings were held with senior government officials and politicians.

(b) ASOs and NGOs: The Code was made broadly available and through NGOs and ASOs copies found their way to hundreds of South African towns and cities.

(c) Trade unions: At the end of 1995 a young worker whose services were terminated from his factory because he had HIV addressed a conference of 500 delegates of the Congress of South African Trade Unions (COSATU) which has a membership of 1.5 million people. The Code was adopted by COSATU as its policy. The support of South Africa's biggest trade union federation added legitimacy to the Code. Thereafter many trade union members started to use the Code approach local workplaces with recommendations for workplace AIDS policies and prevention programmes.

As a result, the Code became a de facto guide for trade unionists and managers on acceptable policies and responses. Several major companies and trade unions simply adopted the Code as policy. In Gauteng, South Africa's most economically developed province, the Code became the official policy of the provincial government. This process helped to set up a wide sense of involvement with the Code.

Since 1996, the Code has continued to be used by employers and trade unions as a guideline to assist with the formulation of employment policy. Many of its recommendations have been incorporated into new employment laws, such as the Employment Equity Act and Medical Schemes Act (to be discussed later). It is also serving as a resource document for the drafting of a Code of Good Practice on Employment.

Analysis of the Process in Botswana, South Africa and Zimbabwe

Following are the differences in the approach taken in these three countries:

(a) In Zimbabwe the government played an important role initiating the process but the trade unions provided it an ongoing momentum.

(b) In Botswana the first draft of a Code was a trade union initiative but a national business organization used the Code as an opportunity to improve its HIV prevention programmes.

(c) In South Africa, NGOs took the lead in publicizing and promoting the Code, but they attempted to seek the support of government departments, trade unions and employer organizations.

Each response involved the combination of stakeholders who are needed for effective workplace HIV prevention. Each stakeholder brought different strengths to the discussions. The challenge for the implementers of the Code will be to continue to integrate these strengths.

The different approaches all led to the same end. Lobbying, research and negotiations around National Codes of Conduct contributed to the development of the SADC Code. By the time the regional Code was endorsed by the SADC Council in September 1997 the three campaigns mentioned above had guaranteed that the principles and objectives of such a Code were already well known by several governments, trade unions and the business community. Besides this, employment practice was influenced. The Code helped to make employees and trade unionists more aware of their rights. A broad consensus was reached on the principle that a policy framework for the response to issues of AIDS and the workplace must always take notice of the rights and needs of people with HIV or AIDS.

Importance of Trade Unions Participation

There are many advantages to trade union participation in campaigns on HIV/AIDS. Trade unions, is general have:

(a) Strong internal networks that can be used to carry information and messages about AIDS;
(b) A reservoir of potential peer educators amongst shop-stewards and other office-bearers;
(c) An interest in the health and safety of their members that makes them effective advocates of health promotion and disease prevention;
(d) Existing channels for discussion with employers and governments.

In Southern Africa the importance of the participation of trade unions is being proved in practice. A great deal of the initiative for the development of the SADC Code emerged from the Organisation of African Trade Union Unity's (OATUU) Health, Safety and Environment Programme. OATUU, which is located in Harare in Zimbabwe, worked in close cooperation with trade unions, businesses and NGOs and organized several workshops on AIDS and Employment.

One advantage of these workshops has been that there are many similarities between the codes that have been developed at national level and the Southern African Code. It also permitted experiences to be shared across countries.

Importance of Private Sector Participation

In South Africa the AIDS Law Project, an NGO, raised funds to publish the draft Employment Code in a national business daily. This brought it to the attention of business leaders. Many business houses arranged 'in-house' discussions on the Code, and the response was not supportive in the beginning. The opposition seemed to have been motivated by a desire to defend management's autonomy, particularly on matters that involve hiring and firing. The important issues that caused disagreement were the proposals to prohibit pre-employment HIV testing and the suggestion that there should be nondiscriminatory access to employee benefits. Thus, some groups drafted their own versions of an employment code/guideline. This reaction necessitated even greater lobbying on the part of NGOs and prompted research and the development of arguments (outlined earlier) to try and persuade business organizations that human rights and economic concerns can be accommodated. Two principles require mention here:

(a) It is important to identify spheres of agreement rather than disagreement. Often the gap between business and the community is a small one, but it gets exaggerated and eventually prolongs action on areas of agreement. This may be a barrier to the introduction of effective HIV prevention in the workplace, generating unnecessary conflicts that make collaboration with other social partners to limit the impact of HIV and AIDS more difficult.

(b) Some of the issues are complex and cannot be resolved by advocacy alone. For example, the question of the restructuring of employee benefits cannot be resolved without proper research into the impact of AIDS on the workplace. Such issues need to be discovered as early as possible so that plans for collaborative research can be set in motion.

The process of developing a Code on HIV/AIDS and Employment for Southern Africa was full of challenges and lessons for all the people and participant organizations. The outcome is a policy framework that has the support of the highest levels of government. But the greatest challenges is with the implementation and effective use of the Code by SADC member countries, trade unions, employers and governments. The drafting of national codes by several SADC member countries laid the foundation for a regional code. Now, the approval of the regional code by the SADC Council should be used:

- to proceed with the formal implementation of Employment Codes in countries where a 'draft' Code already exists, or has been legislated; and
- to initiate a process, similar to that undertaken by South Africa, Zimbabwe and Botswana, in countries where, till now, there have been no initiatives around AIDS and employment.

At a meeting of ministers and social partners of the employment and labour sector that was conducted in Swaziland in April 1999 reports were provided on the present status of the Code among SADC members.

In countries that are at war there are innumerable barriers to HIV prevention. However, unlike a decade ago, most of the region is at present at peace. AIDS has become the greatest threat to development, life and household security. At the SADC Employment and Labour sector meeting in April 1999 ministers and social partners urged member countries that had not formulated national policies and programmes on HIV/AIDS and employment and those that were not implementing the regional code to do so. However, trade unions, employers and NGOs should not wait or the Code's formal incorporation into legislation by their governments. There is a great deal that can be done now.

Role of Trade Unions and Employers

In South Africa less than 25 per cent of workplaces had implemented HIV or AIDS prevention programmes by 1999. This is also true in Botswana, Namibia and Zimbabwe. The SADC Code can be used by trade unionists and employers as a policy guideline for the initiation of HIV/AIDS prevention programmes.

Popularizing the Code

The Zimbabwean Labour Relations (HIV/AIDS) Regulations mention that every employer should provide education about HIV/AIDS during working hours. But in order to ensure that this takes place trade unions and employers will need to popularize the Code among their members. They will also need to conduct a survey of NGOs and other organizations that can be recruited to ensure that this proposal is carried out. Discussions can be organized around the Code within and between trade union federations and employer organizations. Thereafter it could:

(a) be presented for negotiations and adoption at industry level. For example, in South Africa the Southern African Clothing and Textile Workers Union (SACTW) has used the Code to develop a policy for its industry. This policy is being presented to the National Bargaining Council and after it is accepted will become a legal standard for all employers and employees in the industry;

(b) form the basis for a contract on joint responsibilities for HIV/AIDS prevention at factory level. For example, trade union members at a local engineering factory could use the Code to initiate negotiations with their managers over an AIDS prevention programme;

(c) be used as training tool for workers and managers on the shop floor on how to deal with issues of HIV/AIDS in the workplace.

Role of NGOs

Nongovernmental organizations employ hundreds of thousands of people in Southern Africa. They can set an example by adopting the Code as their own employment policy. They can also play a significant role by using the Code to make their own partners more aware of all the dimensions of the AIDS epidemic. For example, the Code can be used by organizations involved in development work, women's empowerment and children's rights. The South African National NGO Coalition has more than 1000 member organizations. At its annual conference in 1998 it adopted the SADC Code as its employment policy and resolved to lobby the government to make the Code legally binding on all employers.

Role of Government Departments and Members of Parliament

The decision of the SADC Heads of Government to unanimously adopt the Code gives it great political power. The Code's political authority can be used by government departments and National AIDS Control Programmes (NACPs) to introduce measures required for effective workplace programme. For example:

(a) The Code's recommendation that condom promotion should be a component of workplace programmes can be used by NACPs to approach employers and trade unions to discover ways for effective condom distribution in the workplace.

(b) The Code's proposals on nondiscrimination and safety at work can be used by ministries of labour and members of parliament to bring about changes in the law that would prohibit unfair discrimination and improve AIDS education and prevention in the workplace. For example, the South African Parliament has incorporated various parts of the SADC Code into new legislation. The Employment Equity Act, enacted in 1998, classifies 'HIV status' side by side with other constitutional bases where discrimination is considered to be automatically unfair. It also consists a clause that prohibits pre-employment HIV testing and states that testing of an employee to find out that employee's HIV status is prohibited unless such testing is determined to be justifiable by the Labour Court in terms of Section 50(4) of this Act. Besides this, the Medical Schemes Act of 1998 makes it unlawful for a medical insurance company to arbitrarily refuse a person membership of the scheme due to their state of health. Moreover, a new labour regulation has been approved by parliament that will make it mandatory for every workplace to have 'universal precautions' available in case of workplace accidents.

Objectives of Partnerships

The Intersectoral Committee in Zimbabwe and the National Taskforce on HIV/AIDS in the Workplace in Botswana are examples of partnerships that should be emulated by every SADC country. Partnerships on AIDS in the workplace should be formed to:

(a) initiate joint research into issues such as the impact of HIV and AIDS on employee benefits and to make commendations on how this impact can be managed;
(b) conduct surveys that will setup the real levels of awareness about HIV among employers and employees;
(c) implement and monitor pilot interventions and publicize examples of effective programmes.

As in other developing countries, especially in Asia, many of the challenges to society that AIDS generates are only just beginning to be encountered. Southern Africa has passed the 'hidden' or 'invisible' stage of the AIDS epidemic. Millions of people have HIV and there are hundreds of thousands of people with AIDS. The impact of AIDS on workplaces and homes is now obvious and yet stigma and fear mean that the majority of company responses are still characterized by silence. We must break the silence. Silence costs more to do nothing!

There are talks on "African Renaissance" in the present century. This Renaissance will depend on people to work, to create the nation's wealth and wealth for their own families and friends. It will also depend on politicians who recognize, enforce and take steps to realize the rights of all people to work, including people with HIV, AIDS or other disabilities. Implementing the SADC Code on HIV/AIDS and Employment will be central to the success of this dream.

SADC: The Code on HIV/AIDS and Employment

Human Immuno-deficiency Virus (HIV) infection and the Acquired Immune Deficiency Syndrome (AIDS) in the countries of the Southern African Development Community (SADC) (and worldwide) is a major health problem with employment, economic and human rights implications. As one response to this problem the SADC Employment and Labour Sector has set up this code on the industrial relations standards on HIV/AIDS, the "Code on AIDS and Employment". It should be noted that the provisions of this code applies only to workplaces and cannot and should not be construed as applying other areas of law such as national immigration laws, policies and associated administrative procedures.

Policy Principles

The same ethical principles that govern all health/medical conditions in the employment context apply equally to HIV/AIDS. However, the seriousness and impact of the HIV/AIDS epidemic and the potential for discrimination necessitate for a specific code on HIV/AIDS and employment. Simultaneously, given the increased risk of transmission of the disease under conditions of economic insecurity, nondiscriminatory approaches enable economic and public health management. The code will ensure nondiscrimination between individuals with HIV infection and those without and between HIV/AIDS and other comparable health-medical conditions. The regional nature and implications of the disease and the desire to harmonise national standards in dealing with HIV/AIDS motivate this regional code. This code aims to ensure that SADC member countries develop tripartite national codes on AIDS and Employment that will make projection in law. It presents guiding principles for and components of these national codes.

The code on AIDS and Employment is based on the primary principles of human rights and patients' rights, WHO/ILO and regional standards and guidelines, medical and occupational health ethical principles, sound epidemiological statistics, prudent business practice and a humane and compassionate attitude to individuals. The approach aim to achieve an equilibrium in protecting the rights of all parties, including those with and without HIV, employers, employees, state and others. This will include obtaining an equilibrium between rights and responsibilities, and between individual protection and cooperation between parties. Employees with HIV should be treated the same as any other employee. Employees with HIV-related illness, including AIDS, should be treated the same as any other employee with a life-threatening illness.

In its scope, the code should:

(a) cover all employees and prospective employees;
(b) cover all workplaces and contracts of employment;
(c) cover the specific policy components mentioned below, viz: job access, workplace testing, confidentiality, job placement, job status, job security, occupational benefits, training, risk reduction, first aid, workers' compensation, education and awareness, prevention programmes, managing illness, protection against victimisation, grievance handling, information, monitoring and review.

SADC member countries should ensure that interactions between them are consistent with the principles and policy components of this code and that they share and disseminate information to enable an effective and planned response to the epidemic. Policy development and implementation is a dynamic process so that the code on AIDS and employment should be:

(a) communicated to all concerned;

(b) routinely examined in the light of epidemiological and scientific information;

(c) monitored for its successful implementation and evaluated for its effectiveness.

Policy Components

Education, awareness and prevention programmes: Information, education and prevention programmes should be developed jointly by employers and employees and should be accessible to all at the workplace. Education on HIV/AIDS should where possible incorporate employee families. Essential components of prevention programmes are information provision, education, prevention and management of STDs, condom promotion and distribution and counselling on high risk behaviour. Workplace AIDS programmes should cooperate with and have access to resources of National AIDS Programmes.

Job Access: There should be no direct or indirect pre-employment test for HIV. Employees should be given the normal medical tests of present fitness for work and these tests should not include testing for HIV. Indirect screening methods such as questions in verbal or written form inquiring about previous HIV tests and/or questions related to the assessment of risk behaviour should not allowed.

Workplace testing and confidentiality: There should be no compulsory workplace testing for HIV. Voluntary testing for HIV on the request of the employee should be done by a suitably qualified person in a health facility with informed consent of the employee as per normal medical ethical rules and with pre- and post-test counselling.

Persons with HIV or AIDS should have the legal right to confidentiality about their seropositivity in any aspect of their employment. An employee is under no obligation to inform an employer of her/his HIV/AIDS status. Information regarding the HIV status of an employee should not be revealed to anybody without the employee's written consent. Confidentiality regarding all medical information of an employee or prospective employee should be maintained, unless revelation is legally required. This applies also to health professionals under contract to the employer, pension fund trustees and any other personnel who obtain such information in manners permitted by the law, ethics, the code or from the employee concerned.

Job Status: HIV status should not be a consideration in job status, promotion or transfer. Any changes in job status should be based on present criteria of equality of opportunity, merit and capacity to perform the work to a satisfactory standard.

HIV Testing and Training: There should be no compulsory HIV testing for training. HIV testing for training should be governed by the principle of nondiscrimination between individuals with HIV infection and those without and between HIV/AIDS and other comparable health/medical conditions.

Managing Illness and Job Security: No employee should be dismissed merely on the basis of HIV status, nor should HIV status influence retrenchment procedures. Employees with HIV related illness should have access to medical treatment and should be entitled, without discrimination, to agreed existing sick leave provisions. HIV infected employees should continue to work under normal conditions in their present employment for so long as they are medically fit to do so. When on medical grounds they cannot continue with normal employment, efforts should he made to offer them alternative employment without prejudice to their benefits. When the employee becomes too ill to perform their agreed functions the standard benefits and conditions and standard procedures for termination of service for comparable life-threatening conditions should apply without discrimination.

Occupational Benefits: Government, employers and employee representatives should ensure that occupational benefits are nondiscriminatory and sustainable and provide support to all employees including those with HIV infection. Such occupational benefit schemes should make efforts to protect the rights and benefits of the dependents of deceased and retired employees.

Information from benefit schemes on the medical status of an employee should be kept confidential and should not be used by the employer or any other party to affect any other aspect of the employment contract or relationship.

Medical schemes and health benefits linked to employment should be nondiscriminatory. Private and public health financing mechanisms should provide standard benefits to all employees irrespective of their HIV status.

Counselling and advisory services should be made available to inform all employees on their rights and benefits from medical aid, life insurance, pension and social security funds. This should include information on intended changes to the structure, benefits and premiums to these funds.

Risk Management, First Aid and Compensation: Where there may be an occupational risk of acquiring or transmitting HIV infection, suitable precautionary measures should be taken to lessen such risk, including clear and accurate information and training on the hazards and procedures for safe work. Employees who contract HIV infection during the course of their employment should follow standard compensation procedures and receive standard compensation benefits. Under conditions where people move for work, government and organisations should lift restrictions to enable them to move with their families and dependants. People who are in an occupation that necessitates routine travel in the course of their duties should be provided with the means to minimise the risk of infection including information, condoms and ample accommodation.

Protection Against Victimisation: Persons affected by or believed to be affected by HIV or AIDS should be protected from stigmatization and discrimination by co-workers, employers or clients. Information and education are necessary to maintain the environment of mutual understanding essential to ensure this protection. Where employers and employees agree that there has been adequate information and education and provisions for safe work, then disciplinary procedures should be initiated against persons who refuse to work with an employee with HIV/AIDS.

Grievance Handling: Standard grievance handling procedures in organisations in labour and civil law that apply to all workers should apply to HIV associated grievances. Personnel dealing with HIV associated grievances should maintain the confidentiality of the employee's medical information.

Information: Government should collect, compile and analyse statistics on HIV/AIDS, sexually transmitted diseases and tuberculosis and make it available in the public domain. SADC member countries should cooperate in making available national statistics for monitoring and planning an effective response to the regional health, human resource, economic and social impact of the AIDS epidemic.

Monitoring and Review: Responsibility for monitoring and review of the code and its implementation should lie with the parties to the tripartite at national and regional level and with the SADC Employment and Labour Sector.

The Namibian Code

This code applies to all employers in Namibia. Although the Namibian defence force is excluded from the general provisions of the Namibian Labour Act, it is bound by the Acts sections on non-discrimination. It is therefore believed that the Employment Code does apply to the NDF.

With the global marked increase in number of persons infected with the human immunodeficiency virus (HIV) and suffering from acquired immunodeficiency syndrome (AIDS) mainly in the economically active part of the population, the 20 to 50 years age group, the employers, employees and their organisations demonstrate a high level of anxiety pertaining to the impact of the pandemic on the work environment. From an initial response of denial, to a perception of AIDS as a medical problem, AIDS is continuously being recast as a development problem and an issue for all sectors. Loss of employment and individual income, loss of employees without sufficient availability of replacement, and a subsequent decline in production and national income can pose a deep and detrimental effect on the social and economic stability and the growth of a country. This is because of the fact that HIV/AIDS will affect economic growth and production through the illness and death of productive people and through the diversion of resources from savings (and eventually investment) to care.

Options and Responses: In response to the AIDS pandemic and its volatile and dynamic nature, the Ministry of Labour, in conjunction with the Ministry of Health and Social Services and with the wide tripartite consultation through the Labour Advisory Council, has formulated the National Code on HIV/AIDS and

Employment for HIV prevention and AIDS management. This code is proposed as an integral part of the government's commitment to address most of the key issues associated notably with the prevention of new infections, as well as to the provision of optimal care and support for the workforce. Workplace based activities that place HIV prevention and AIDS management in a sustained and comprehensive programme of health promotion have witnessed achievements in general health indicators. This implies a need for stronger public health approaches in the productive sectors.

Policy Principles: The same ethical principles that govern all health/medical conditions in the employment context should apply equally to HIV/AIDS. The gravity and impact of the HIV/AIDS epidemic and the potential for discrimination created the need for this "National Code on HIV/AIDS and Employment" to be based on the fundamental principles of human rights laid down in the Constitution of the Republic of Namibia, the provisions of the Labour Act (Act No. 6 of 1992), occupational health principles, sound epidemiological statistics, prudent business practice and a humane and compassionate attitude to individuals. This interdependency of SADC countries and people, nowhere more evident than in the transmission of HIV, demands equity and a shared approach to the challenges of HIV/AIDS. The Regional (SADC) nature and implications of the epidemic and the desire to harmonise national standards in dealing with HIV/AIDS motivate this Code.

Scope: Subject to the provisions of the Labour Act (Act No. 6 of 1992) this Code applies to:

(a) all employees and prospective employees;
(b) all workplace and contracts of employment;
(c) all human resources practices forming part of policy component of any organization.

Policy Development and Implementation: As policy development and implementation is a dynamic process, this Code shall be:

(a) communicated to all concerned;
(b) routinely examined in the light of new epidemiological and scientific information;
(c) wanted for its successful implementation and examined for its effectiveness in the workplace.

Policy Components: Information, education and prevention programmes should be developed jointly by employers and employees and should be accessible to all at the workplace. Education on HIV/AIDS should, where possible, incorporate employee families. Essential components of prevention programmes are information provision, education, prevention and management of sexually transmitted diseases (STDs), condom promotion and distribution and counselling on high risk behaviour. Workplace AIDS programmes should cooperate with and have access to resources of the National AIDS Programme.

Job Access: There should be neither direct nor indirect pre-employment testing for HIV. Employees should be given the normal medical tests of present fitness for work and these tests should not include testing for HIV.

Workplace Testing and Confidentiality: There should be no compulsory workplace testing for HIV. Voluntary testing for HIV on the request of the employee should be conducted by a suitably qualified person in a health facility with informed consent of the employee as per the normal medical ethical rules and with pre- and post-test, counselling. Persons with HIV/AIDS should have the legal right to confidentiality about their seropositivity in any aspect of their employment. An employee is under no obligation to inform an employer of her/his HIV/AIDS status. Information as to the HIV status of an employee should not be revealed without the employee's written consent. Confidentiality regarding all medical information of an employee or prospective employee should be protected, unless revelation is legally required. This applies also to health professionals under contract to the employer, pension fund trustees and any other personnel who obtain such information in the manners permitted by the law, ethics, the code or from the employee concerned.

Job Status: HIV status should not be a factor in job status, promotion or transfer. Any changes in job status should be based on prevalent criteria of equality of opportunity, merit and capacity to perform the work to a satisfactory standard.

HIV Testing and Training: In general, there should be no compulsory HIV testing for training. HIV testing for training should be governed by the principle of nondiscrimination between individuals with HIV infection and those without and between HIV/AIDS and other comparable health/medical conditions.

Managing Illness and Job Security: No employee should be dismissed merely on the ground of HIV status, nor should HIV status influence retrenchment procedures. Employees with HIV-related illness should have access to medical treatment and should be entitled, without discrimination, to agreed existing sick leave provisions. HIV-infected employees should continue to work under normal conditions in their present employment for as long as they are medically fit to do so. When on medical bases they cannot continue with normal employment, efforts should be made to offer them alternative employment without prejudice to their benefits. When an employee becomes too ill to perform his/her normal duties, standard procedures for termination of service for comparable life-threatening conditions should apply without discrimination.

Occupational Benefits: Government, employers and employee representatives should ensure that occupational benefits are nondiscriminatory and sustainable and provide support to all employees including those with HIV infection. Such occupational benefits plans should make efforts to protect the rights and benefits of the dependents of deceased and retired employees. Information from benefits plans on the seropositive status of an employee should be kept confidential and should not be used by the employer or any other party to affect any other aspect of the employment contract or relationship. Medical plans and health benefits linked to employment should be nondiscriminatory. Private and public health financing mechanisms should provide standard benefits to all employees irrespective of their HIV status. Counselling and advisory services should be made available to inform all employees of their rights and benefits from medical aid, life insurance, pension and social security funds. This should include information on proposed changes to the structure, benefits and premiums to these funds.

Risk Management, First Aid and Compensation: Where there may be an occupational risk of acquiring or transmitting HIV infection, appropriate precautionary measures should be taken to lessen such risk, including clear and accurate information and training on the hazards and procedures for safe work. Employees who contract HIV infection during the course of their employment should follow standard compensation procedures and receive standard compensation benefits. Under conditions where people move for work, government and organisations should lift restrictions to enable them to move with their families and dependents. People who are in an occupation that necessitates routine travel in the course of their duties, should be provided with the means to minimise the risk of infection including information, condoms and adequate accommodation.

Protection Against Victimisation: Persons affected by or believed to be affected by HIV or AIDS should be protected from stigmatization and discrimination by co-workers, employers or clients. Information and education are essential to maintain the environment of mutual understanding necessary to ensure this protection. Where employers and employees agree that there has been adequate information and education provisions for safe work, then disciplinary procedures should apply to persons who refuse to work with an employee with HIV/AIDS.

Grievance Handling: Standard grievance handling procedures in organisations, in labour and civil law, that apply to all workers should apply to HIV-related grievances. Personnel dealing with HIV-related grievances should protect the confidentiality of the employee's medical information.

Information: Government should collect, compile and examine statistics on HIV/AIDS, sexually transmitted diseases and make it available in the public domain. Stakeholders should cooperate in making available national statistics for monitoring and planning an effective response to the regional health, human resource, economic and social impact of the AIDS epidemic.

Monitoring and Review: Responsibility for monitoring and review of the Code and its implementation should lie with the parties to the tripartite Labour Advisory Council and with the Ministry of Labour.

The Zimbabwean Code (Statutory Instrument 202 of 1998)

This Code applies only to nongovernmental employers and employees.

Labour Relations (HIV and AIDS) Regulations, 1998

These regulations may be cited as the Labour Relations (HIV and AIDS) Regulations, 1998.

Interpretation: In these regulations:

(i) "AIDS" means acquired immuno-cleficiency syndrome and includes the AIDS-related complex;

(ii) "HIV" means human immuno-deficiency virus;

(iii) "testing", in relation to HIV, includes:

(a) any direct analysis of the blood or other body fluid of a person to find out the presence of HIV or antibodies to HIV; or

(b) any indirect method, other than the testing of blood or other body fluid, through which an inference is made as to the presence of HIV;

(iv) "related communicable disease" means any communicable disease whose transmission may be linked with HIV because of its transmission through body fluids or whose risk of clinical disease may be increased because of the presence of HIV;

(v) "medical practitioner" means a person registered as a medical practitioner in terms of the Medical, Dental and Allied Professions Act.

Education of Employees on HIV and AIDS: Every employer shall cause to be provided for the benefit of every person employed by him, and at such place and time during normal working hours as he may appoint, education and information relating to:

(a) the promotion of safe sex and risk-reducing measures pertaining to sexually transmitted diseases;

(b) the acquiring and transmission of HIV;

(c) the prevention of the transmission of HIV and AIDS; and

(d) counselling facilities for HIV and AIDS patients.

Education and information shall be provided in terms of sub-section (1) by persons who have proven sound knowledge and expertise in matters relating to HIV and AIDS, and who are able to communicate information with consistency and accuracy. The design of the education programmes shall be as per the guidelines approved by the relevant employer and employee organizations, in consultation with the Ministry of Health and Child Welfare and any other organization with expertise in HIV and AIDS-associated matters. The provision of the education referred to in sub-section (1) shall be at such intervals as the relevant employer and employee organizations may agree.

Medical Testing on Recruitment: No employer shall require, whether directly or indirectly, any person to undergo any form of testing for HIV as a pre-condition to the offer of employment. Sub-section (1) shall not prevent the medical testing of persons for fitness for work as a pre-condition to the offer of employment.

Testing of Employees for HIV and Confidentiality: It shall not be compulsory for any employee to undergo, directly or indirectly, any testing for HIV. No employer shall require any employee, and it shall not be compulsory for any employee, to disclose, in respect of any matter whatsoever in connection with his employment, his HIV status. No person shall, except with the written consent of the employee to whom the information relates, disclose any information associated with the seropositivity of any employee acquired by that person in the course of his duties unless the information is required to be revealed in terms of any other law.

Job Status and Training: No employer shall terminate the employment of an employee on the bases of that employee's HIV status alone. No employee shall be prejudiced in relation to:

(a) promotion;
(b) transfer;
(c) subject to any other law to the contrary, any training or other employee development programme; or
(d) status;

or in any other manner be discriminated against on the bases of his HIV status alone.

Eligibility for Employee Benefits: Subject to any other law to the contrary, the HIV status of an employee shall not affect his eligibility for any occupational or other benefit schemes provided for employees. Where in terms of any law the eligibility of a person for any occupational or other benefit scheme is conditional upon an HIV or AIDS test, the conditions attaching to HIV and AIDS shall be the same as those applicable in respect of comparable life-threatening illnesses. Where any HIV testing is necessary in terms of sub-section 2, the employer shall ensure that the employee undergoes appropriate pre- and post-HIV test counselling. Where an employee who opts not to undergo an HIV testing for the purposes of sub-section 2, no inferences concerning the HIV status of the employee may be drawn from such exercise by the employee of the option not to undergo the testing. Where an employee undergoes an HIV testing for the purposes of sub-section 2, the employer shall not, unless the occupational or other benefit plan concerned is operated by the employer, be entitled to information concerning the HIV status of the employee concerned.

Sick and Compassionate Leave: Any employee suffering from HIV or AIDS shall be subject to the same conditions relating to sick leave as those applicable to any offer employee in forms of the Act. Where a person is employed in an occupation or is required to provide services where there may be a risk of transmitting or acquiring HIV or AIDS, the employer shall provide appropriate training along with clear and accurate information and guidelines on minimising the hazards of the transmission of HIV and AIDS and associated communicable diseases. The working conditions and procedures pertaining to occupations referred to in sub-section 1 shall be designed to ensure optimal hygienic precautions to prevent the spread of HIV or AIDS and associated communicable diseases to employees and members of the public. Personal protective devices shall be issued, free of charge, by the employer to persons employed in occupations referred to in sub-section 1. The employer shall cause to be reviewed, for safety and efficacy, the use of any equipment, devices, procedures, including first-aid procedures used, or guidelines followed, in any occupation referred to in sub-section 1.

Copy of Regulations for Each Employee: An employer shall provide every employee with a copy of these regulations.

Offence and Penalty: Any person who contravenes any provision of these regulations shall be guilty of an offence and liable to a fine not exceeding five thousand dollars or to imprisonment for a period not exceeding six months or to both such fine and such imprisonment.

TABLE 1

SUMMARY OF DOCUMENTED EXAMPLES OF COLLABORATION IN SUB-SAHARAN AFRICA (1987-1999)

Country	*Project/ institution*	*Initiated/ supported by*	*Objectives*	*Methods*	*Achievements/findings*
Botswana	Seminars for traditional healers on AIDS, 1993	Ministry of Health	- Sensitization of traditional healers to AIDS - To coordinate activities of traditional healers with district health teams	No information	Seminars held sporadically with traditional healers on various diseases including AIDS
	Botswana Dingaka AIDS Awareness and Training Programme, 1991-1993	CIDA, WHO, Ministry of Health	- Providing a forum for exchange of information and experiences between traditional healers and biomedical health practitioners - Promoting cooperation and collaboration for health services - Creating awareness on AIDS among traditional healers - Training core trainers who will, in turn, pass on the information to other traditional healers in selected pilot areas	- 2-week TOT held with 12 traditional healers on AIDS from 6 districts of Botswana - Independent evaluation interviewed 32 traditional healers, 19 nurses and 20 medical doctors	- Trained traditional healers trained, on average, 45 other traditional healers per district in 2 years - 72% of traditional healers said they had changed something in their practice in relation to AIDS training - 80% said they recommend condoms - Educational video produced - Flip chart addressing practices of traditional healers produced

(Contd.)

(Contd.)

Country	Project/ institution	Initiated/ supported by	Objectives	Methods	Achievements/findings
Cameroon	KABP survey of traditional healers, 1990	NACP National traditional medicine programme	- To sensitize and introduce traditional healers to HIV/AIDS control	- National seminar on traditional medicine and AIDS to be conducted	No information
Central African Republic	Action to Define, Broaden, and Strengthen the Role of Traditional Practitioners (ADERT), 1995	Ministry of Health, University of Bangui, World AIDS Foundation, CDC, CIDA, University of Washington, USA	- To identify and reinforce aspects of traditional medicine believed to promote public health, while discouraging those that have negative health impacts - To enable traditional healers to deliver preventive messages, support persons living with HIV/AIDS and modify their own risk practices	- Focus groups to identify training topics and methods - Working group of traditional healers and Ministry of Health staff to develop curriculum. - 103 traditional healers at 4 locations (urban and rural) completed 6-day training - 96 traditional healers completed pre- and post-KABP questionnaires	Traditional healers' knowledge improved, except with regard to their own risk practices. Repetitive rather than single training model suggested
Ghana	Unit for traditional medicine established in Ministry of Health, 1990	WHO, Ministry of Health	- To involve traditional healers in primary health care	- Establishing a dialogue with traditional healers	Recommendations for involving traditional healers in management and treatment of AIDS
	Training manual for traditional healers	Save the Children	- To produce a document systematically train traditional healers in AIDS prevention and care	- Production of training manual	No information

(Contd.)

(Contd.)

Country	*Project/ institution*	*Initiated/ supported by*	*Objectives*	*Methods*	*Achievements/findings*
Guinea	Ministry of Health, traditional medicine unit. Integration of traditional healers into health activities, 1985	Ministry of Health	- To identify the factors within traditional medicine that can increase the effectiveness of the fight against AIDS in Guinea - To increase traditional healers' knowledge of modes of HIV transmission and prevention, clinical manifestations, care and support	- Survey of STDs known to traditional healers - Research on traditional treatments for fertility, AIDS, STDs - Baseline survey of traditional healers' knowledge of AIDS - 2 workshops organized for traditional healers - Each district has a physician in charge of traditional medicine	Traditional healers are registered with Ministry of Health. Research on 898 traditional healers since the beginning of the programme found that increasing numbers of traditional healers refer to health centres (using referral forms), hospitals and other traditional healers for diagnosis and treatment. Biomedical health providers also refer back. Traditional healers keep records on numbers of cases and treatment
Liberia	Anthropological Research on STDs, 1988	SOMARC/ USAID Johns Hopkins University, USA	- To learn how to promote condoms to limit the spread of HIV	- Focus group discussions with 53 participants - Conducted interviews with103 traditional healers	- Traditional healers advise against prostitutes. - Traditional healers should be taught STD diagnosis and referral because people believe in traditional medicine for STDs

(Contd.)

(Contd.)

Country	Project/ institution	Initiated/ supported by	Objectives	Methods	Achievements/findings
Malawi	Training on AIDS for traditional healers, 1992	International Eye Foundation, Malawi International Centre for Eye Health, UK	- To better understand the practices and roles of healers in their communities - To promote greater communication between traditional healers and the formal health care sector - To educate traditional healers about HIV/AIDS and STD transmission and prevention - To encourage community-based HIV/AIDS prevention and care by traditional healers	- Series of orientation and focus group discussion were held with traditional healers - An eye care programme formed the initial base of contact and collaboration between project staff and traditional healers - Baseline and follow-up (6 months post-training) were conducted with 89 traditional healers - One-day training sessions were held in 14 sites in one district (334 traditional healers)	- Increase in community education, condom distribution, and patient counselling activities 6 months post-training
Mozambique	Anthropological research and training on AIDS and STDs for traditional healers, 1991-1994	Ministry of Health, Swiss Cooperation	- To improve intersectoral cooperation in the prevention and treatment of STDs - To identify and reinforce aspects of traditional medicine believed to promote public health, while discouraging those believed to have negative health impacts	- Conducted interviews with 51 traditional healers specializing in STDs to develop training strategy - 5 focus group discussions were held, with 7 traditional healers per group - 2 one-week workshops in 2 provinces	- Developed culturally appropriate strategy for the NACP involving traditional healers for STDs - 30 traditional healers participated in workshop on STDs in 1991. In 1994, follow-up with 21 traditional healers; 8 clients were interviewed and showed increased knowledge on HIV transmission, condom use and promotion

(Contd.)

(Contd.)

Country	Project/ institution	Initiated/ supported by	Objectives	Methods	Achievements/findings
Namibia	Anthropological research on traditional medicine, 1995	PhD thesis fieldwork	- To analyse traditional healers' patients' health-seeking behaviour for illness in general	- Quantitative and qualitative methods	No information
Rwanda	AIDS research project (Project San Francisco), 1990	University of California, San Francisco, USA; Ministry of Health	- To analyse health-seeking behaviour of women patients with regard to AIDS and traditional medicine - To analyse knowledge, attitudes, practices surrounding AIDS and STDs	- Quantitative and qualitative methods including questionnaires, and in-depth interviews among 40 women involved in a prospective cohort study - 25 traditional healers interviewed on KABP on AIDS	- Majority of women used both biomedical and traditional systems and believed in greater effectiveness of traditional medicine for certain AIDS symptoms - All traditional healers had heard of AIDS, knew modes of transmission, signs and symptoms and that there was no treatment or vaccine
Senegal	Promotion of Traditional Medicine (PROMETRA), 1981	Centre for Experimentation of Traditional Medicine, Senegal Tulane School of Public Health, USA Morehouse School of Medicine, USA	- To promote traditional medicine	- 383 healers organized into an association called PROMETRA - Conducted training on diarrhoea and family planning, but not yet on AIDS - Needs assessment conducted prior to training	- 87% of interviewed patients were satisfied with traditional healers' services - 67% physicians interviewed stated they referred patients to traditional healers

(Contd.)

(Contd.)

Country	*Project/ institution*	*Initiated/ supported by*	*Objectives*	*Methods*	*Achievements/findings*
Sierra Leone	Counselling training for traditional healers, 1992	National STD/ AIDS Control Programme	- To train traditional healers in HIV/AIDS counselling	1-day training held with 150 traditional healers.	- 150 traditional healers trained in HIV/AIDS counselling - 80% of people with HIV/AIDS prefer traditional medicine treatment
South Africa	Training of trainers for healers, 1992	AIDSCAP, USA AIDSCOM, USA Ministry of Health, South Africa	- The initial goal was to determine the level of interest, knowledge, and skills of traditional healers in HIV prevention and whether they could serve as effective agents of behaviour change. - The ultimate goal was to engage traditional healers in combating HIV/AIDS in South Africa through training other healers and incorporating HIV/AIDS prevention into their practices.	- 1-year feasibility study - Preliminary 5-day workshop (Nov. 1992) 28 traditional healers 3 follow-up workshops (July 1993, Nov. 1993, July 1994)	- 630 traditional healers trained by 28 trained traditional healers on basic AIDS facts - 7-month follow-up:≥80% retained correct STD/AIDS information and practised counselling
	Pilot survey of traditional healers, 1992	Centre for Natural and Traditional Medicine, Washington, DC, USA	- To assess traditional healers' potential for AIDS prevention and care	No information	- Survey found traditional healers had high knowledge about AIDS, were treating symptoms of AIDS; and concluded that, "traditional healers are a force that cannot be ignored in the fight against HIV/AIDS".

(Contd.)

(Contd.)

Country	Project/ institution	Initiated/ supported by	Objectives	Methods	Achievements/findings
	Training programme for traditional healers in KwaZulu-Natal, 1994	AIDS Foundation of South Africa, National Traditional Healers' Association of South Africa	- To increase AIDS prevention, education and management in KwaZulu-Natal by providing training and resources to traditional healers - To help trained traditional healers become accepted by the biomedical system in KwaZulu-Natal	- Project emphasized strengthening resources in disadvantaged communities	- Traditional healers could identify signs and symptoms of AIDS after training - Traditional healers identified need for rural AIDS hospices and trained homecare personnel to care for persons living with HIV/AIDS - 75% traditional healers believed they could cure AIDS before training, none after
	Training of traditional healers in HIV prevention and collaboration, 1998	Government of South Africa	- To train traditional healers in every province of South Africa on AIDS prevention - To build collaboration between traditional and biomedical health systems	- 3-day workshop for traditional healers in every province of South Africa, using participatory methods	- Prevention training was successful, but collaboration was not. Recommends using traditional healers to train traditional healers because traditional healers respect their fellow-members.

(Contd.)

(Contd.)

Country	Project/ institution	Initiated/ supported by	Objectives	Methods	Achievements/findings
Uganda	Traditional and Modern Health Practitioners · Together against AIDS (THETA), 1992	Doctors without Borders, The AIDS Support Organization, NACP, Ministry of Health, Uganda AIDS Commission, Rockefeller Foundation	- To provide training for traditional healers in community counselling and HIV/AIDS education, basic clinical diagnosis and patient management - To provide a resource centre for information sharing on traditional medicine and AIDS - To advocate for traditional medicine among health professionals and other scientists in order to build a true collaboration	- Community mobilization, traditional healers training in AIDS education and counselling in 7 districts in Uganda, with 40 traditional healers per district since 1993 - Traditional healers' training in patient management with 30 traditional healers in Kampala in 1 year - Resource centre collects and disseminates information on traditional medicine and AIDS - Promoting collaboration between traditional medicine and biomedicine	- Increased counselling and AIDS education by trained traditional healers and increased knowledge and condom use among clients of trained traditional healers - Over 120 traditional healers trained and more than 96,000 persons benefited in 2 years - Collected a wide variety of materials on traditional medicine and AIDS - Produced 2 videos in Uganda and English for educational and informational use
	Community-based home care, 1993	CONCERN, Ireland Ministry of Health, Uganda	- To train volunteers to provide care and support to the sick using a primary care herbal kit developed by the project - To disseminate information on herbs and disease	- Workshops centred on skills and confidence-building in giving out herbal medicine	- Traditional healers trained 68 volunteers involved in home care and distributing herbs for common AIDS-related symptoms

(Contd.)

(Contd.)

Country	*Project/ institution*	*Initiated/ supported by*	*Objectives*	*Methods*	*Achievements/findings*
United Republic of Tanzania	Tanga AIDS Working Group (TAWG), 1990	Initiated by a physician and traditional healers Family Health International, Shaman Pharmaceutical Company, Evangelische Zentralstelle fur Entwicklungshilfe, GTZ	- Raise HIV/AIDS/STD awareness among traditional practitioners in 3 districts to safeguard both practitioners and clients from being infected during practices - Train traditional healers as community-based HIV/AIDS/STD educators and home-care providers for persons living with HIV/AIDS and their families - Promotion of community-based condom distribution	- Series of sensitization meetings between local govt., district PHC committees, village health committees, communities and traditional healers - 2 types of participatory approaches - ZOPP and LEPSA - were used to identify and train key people at the grassroots level - TAWG trained 120 traditional healers in 3 districts in 1994 - Health personnel at each health facility were trained to support the programme	- 160 traditional healers have been trained in HIV/AIDS and health information - Healers are involved in collaborative clinical work, AIDS education, counselling, home visits and village theatre groups - Training manual produced
Zaire	Workshops with traditional healers, 1989	CONNAISSIDA, Zaire Traditional Healers' Association	No information	- Action research using 2 experimental risk-reduction workshops with women in low-income area	- Demonstrated traditional healers' pragmatism and the role they can play in promoting behaviour change for safer sex practices

(Contd.)

(Contd.)

Country	*Project/ institution*	*Initiated/ supported by*	*Objectives*	*Methods*	*Achievements/findings*
Zambia	AIDS workshop, 1987	Traditional Practitioners' Association of Zambia, Ministry of Health	- To exchange ideas and experiences on AIDS and gain traditional healers' support in fighting its spread	- Dialogue between the Ministry of Health Education Unit and the secretariat of the Traditional Practitioners' Assn. of Zambia - Workshop held with 40 traditional healers	- 40 traditional healers attended - Knowledge increased, misconceptions still strong
	AIDS research, training and follow-up 1994-1996	Ministry of Health, USAID, More-house University School of Medicine, USA	- To educate traditional healers about HIV/AIDS and STD transmission, prevention and care - To enable traditional healers to educate their patients about these issues and motivate them to avoid high risk behaviour	- 25-40 prominent traditional healers selected to participate in 3-day workshops on AIDS between June 94 and Nov. 95 - Trained traditional healers attended monthly or alternate month follow-up meetings led by health centre staff	- 2000 traditional healers trained on AIDS facts and 120 traditional healers trained in community education - Knowledge increased, traditional healers started selling condoms through a social marketing programme
Zimbabwe	AIDS workshops, 1988	Zimbabwe National Traditional Healers Association (ZINATHA), Ministry of Health	No information	No information	- Workshops organized to train traditional healers in AIDS and counselling - Pamphlet in local language designed for traditional healers and AIDS

(Contd.)

Abbreviations:

AMREF	African Medical Research Foundation
BHP	Biomedical health practitioners
CDC	Centres for Disease Control and Prevention
CDD	Control of diarrhoeal diseases
CIDA	Canadian International Development Agency
KABP	Knowledge, attitudes, beliefs and practices
MOH	Ministry of Health
NACP	National AIDS Control Programme
PHC	Primary Health Care
SOMARC	Condom Social Marketing Programme
TH	Traditional healers
TM	Traditional medicine
TOT	Training of trainers
WHO	World Health Organization

TABLE 2

REVIEW OF EXAMPLES OF COLLABORATION ACCORDING TO UNAIDS BEST PRACTICE CRITERIA

*Project**	*Effectiveness*	*Ethical soundness*	*Efficiency*	*Sustainability*	*Relevance of approach*
Dingaka AIDS Awareness, **Botswana** 1991-1993	- Trained traditional healers passed on information to clients and fellow-traditional healers - 80% of traditional healers recommend condoms to patients - 31/32 refer patients - Nurses refer to traditional healers	- Programme worked with Ministry of Health	- Estimated cost US$22 per traditional healer trained per day - Traditional healers trained, on average, 45 other traditional healers per district	- Not sustainable as a project, but healers have continued to use the information they gained	- Objectives clearly stated, and relevant to the AIDS situation, but TOT and collaboration aspects of the project ambitious for time and resources allocated
Action to Define, Broaden, and Strengthen the Role of Traditional Practitioners (ADERT) **Central African Republic** 1994	- Significant improvement in traditional healers' knowledge on STD risk, condom use, and HIV transmission after training - 76% of traditional healers with STD cases report integrating partner referral into their STD care treatment.	- Programme worked with Ministry of Health - Specific attention to appropriateness of training topics and methods for traditional healers	- 103 traditional healers trained in 4 locations over 2 months - No cost-effectiveness measures	- No measures taken to ensure sustainability; activities ceased when funding stopped. - One healer interviewed in 1999 said he was eager to be involved in another project and he was still using the information gained	- Objectives clearly stated and relevant to needs assessed through baseline focus group discussion and working group of traditional healers and Ministry of Health staff - Magnitude of knowledge and attitude change was not related to traditional healers' characteristics, indicating that impact of training was uniform among practitioners. This implies that specific types of practitioners do not need targeting, and training content was relevant to all traditional healers in that setting and context

(Contd.)

(Contd.)

*Project**	*Effectiveness*	*Ethical soundness*	*Efficiency*	*Sustainability*	*Relevance of approach*
Training on AIDS for traditional healers **Malawi** 1992	- Increase in traditional healers' knowledge - 64% conducted AIDS education events - 89% distributed condoms - No evaluation of collaboration	- Collaboration with Malawi NACP - The purpose of the study was clearly explained to each traditional healer - Specific attention to positive images in educational messages	- In 6 months, 3000 community members reached in AIDS education	- Most healers within walking distance of training - Traditional healers encouraged to acquire condoms from health centre	- Goals and objectives clearly stated and relevant to needs assessed through baseline survey - Project changed significantly in response to changes in AIDS situation - Strategy did not include specific emphasis on biomedical health sector
Ministry of Health/traditional healers' association collaboration **Mozambique** 1991-1994	- 85% traditional healers able to describe HIV symptoms - 85% knew AIDS transmitted by sex - 81% traditional healers promoting condom use - traditional healers advise clients to avoid having many sex partners	- Programme started by Ministry of Health	- 47 traditional healers trained - No information on cost-effectiveness	- At least one follow-up workshop for traditional healers organized by the Provincial Health Dept within 10 months of the initial workshop - Traditional healers reported distributing condoms and cooperating in other areas with health department	- Objectives clearly stated and based on preliminary ethnomedical research, taking into consideration the national and local STD/AIDS programme priorities, as well as the political situation

(Contd.)

(Contd.)

*Project**	*Effectiveness*	*Ethical soundness*	*Efficiency*	*Sustainability*	*Relevance of approach*
Training of trainers **South Africa** 1992	- Traditional healers training other traditional healers, counselling clients, promoting condoms - Increased positive attitudes	- Collaboration with traditional healers' associations	- 1510 traditional healers trained, all but 28 by fellow-traditional healers in almost 1 year	- Second-generation traditional healers were prepared to train third-generation healers with minimal assistance	- Objectives clearly stated and based on feasibility of engaging traditional healers in the fight against AIDS
Traditional and Modern Health Practitioners Together against AIDS (THETA) **Uganda** 1992	- 200 traditional healers trained in 7 districts since 1993 - Traditional healers gained knowledge in HIV/AIDS and STD transmission, prevention and care - Traditional healers gained counselling, teaching, leadership and record-keeping skills - Trained traditional healers providing regular community AIDS education - Traditional healers distributing condoms - Traditional healers make increased referrals to biomedical health providers - THETA produces a newsletter, initiated a speakers' bureau, contains a library on traditional medicine and AIDS, and produced 2 videos - Conducted a study on the effectiveness of herbal treatment for opportunistic infections	- Research results are fed back to healers and community - Patient confidentiality is emphasized in training programmes - Agreement signed with Ministry of Health - Traditional healers have worked within the hospital for herbal study - Patients sign informed consent form - Mutual respect is emphasized from the beginning	- Admin. tightly controlled and reports produced quarterly - Costs per traditional healer client range between US$0.24 and US$0.71 - US$21/day per traditional healer trained - Estimated total number of beneficiaries range from 150,000 to 400,000 per year*	- Healers don't receive salaries - Strong links are built with community leaders in each district (i.e., local council, secretaries for women, etc.) for supporting continuing healer activities - Traditional healers involved in the training have formed their own associations that undertake various activities, including community AIDS education and drama, training of fellow-healers, and 'persons living with HIV/AIDS' support groups - THETA trained traditional healers involved in national policy bodies (National Drug Authority)	- Objectives clearly stated and based on baseline traditional healers' surveys and community baseline assessments - Objectives and implementation follow the National AIDS Programme strategy - Implementation of district activities is area-specific and based on feasibility assessments carried out in several possible sites before each new district is chosen

(Contd.)

(Contd.)

*Project**	*Effectiveness*	*Ethical soundness*	*Efficiency*	*Sustainability*	*Relevance of approach*
Tanga AIDS Working Group, (TAWG) **United Republic of Tanzania** 1990	- 120 traditional healers trained since 1994 - Drama group reached 55,000 people in 4 months - 1997 survey showed traditional healers had increased awareness of HIV/AIDS - Clients who were counselled reduced risky behaviour	- Mutual respect is a main TAWG principle - Counselled patients are given code numbers and confidentiality is assured - Ministry of Health authorised research; offices within hospital - Research results fedback to healers and NGO	- Traditional treatments are free for patients - In 3 years: 27000 community members reached in education sessions - 237 persons living with HIV/AIDS reached in 4,300 home-care visits	- As permanent members of the community, traditional healers will continue to practise their new research and counselling skills even if the NGO is not present - Healers don't receive salaries - NGO office is in the hospital; links between hospital and NGO are strong - 17 supervisors from the health facilities were trained to monitor and support traditional healers	- Objectives clearly stated and based on 7 years of experience working with traditional healers. - Linking prevention and care provides a culturally relevant approach for the Tanga region.
AIDS research, training and follow-up **Zambia** 1994-1996	- 250 traditional healers promoting and selling condoms - Traditional healers counselling on HIV and STD prevention, HIV testing and caring for persons living with HIV/AIDS at home	- Ministry of Health agreement - Project planned for feedback of results to province, district and local levels	- US$35/day per traditional healers trained	- Links built between traditional healers and local biomedical health practitioner and health facility	- Objectives clearly stated and based on preliminary assessments and national AIDS programme priorities.

*For ongoing projects, only starting date given.

TABLE 3
SPECIFIC CRITERIA/APPROACH FOR COLLABORATION

Country	*Criteria for selecting 'genuine' or 'authentic' healers*	*Approach used to build trust*	*Lessons learned*
Botswana	- Leaders from different traditional healers' associations in 6 districts selected 12 traditional healers for training	- Discussions and seminars with traditional healers	- Condom promotion easily integrated into traditional healers' practice - Home care difficult to integrate into traditional healers' practice - Follow-up necessary to sustain the intervention - Traditional healers see doctors as their counterparts - The legal status of traditional healers should be dealt with in order to improve organization of traditional healers and ultimately improve cooperation between health sectors - Biomedical health practitioners should be trained to acknowledge that patients share traditional and modern beliefs and values
Central African Republic	- The most influential traditional healers were selected by village leaders from a census list of traditional healers	- Central African Republic physician employed persistence, rapport building, and mobilizing skills to slowly gain trust - Traditional healers slowly found that collaborating with Ministry of Health would legitimize them in the eyes of the government	- Attitudes towards condom use did not change. Investigators linked this information to a high desire to have children - Authors found that design of curriculum adapted for training of traditional healers is useful for traditional healers' increase in knowledge; a one-time training cannot achieve a significant level of change in traditional healers' practice. Rather a repetitive model would be most effective for promoting cognitive, attitudinal and behavioural change.

(Contd.)

(Contd.)

Country	*Criteria for selecting 'genuine' or 'authentic' healers*	*Approach used to build trust*	*Lessons learned*
Malawi	- Older healers were reported to have more credibility with village leaders - Community leaders were consulted to gain approval and to recommend the most respected and most active traditional healers in their areas	- Focus group discussions were held with groups of traditional healers to build relationships between healers, Ministry of Health and project	- Traditional healers were open to condom promotion - Need for greater collaboration between health centre staff and traditional healers to maintain community-based education and condom distribution
Mozambique	- Traditional healers' association assisted in selection of traditional healers, seeking to provide balance by gender, age and district	- In-depth interviews and focus group discussions over 9-month period before training	- Much public health knowledge and practice is already found in beliefs and practices of traditional healers. Difficult to interview patients of traditional healers due to stigma of STDs. The use of indigenous disease names proved a great facilitator of communication as it was taken as a sign of respect
Senegal	- Selection based on healers' reputation, and pre-school children 4-6 years old were asked to identify traditional healers known for specific conditions	- Consent of local authorities - Series of contacts that lasted from several months to years - Healers provided names and addresses of other healers	- PROMETRA considers its work to be cultural research, medical practice, and views itself as an integral partner in dissemination of scientific information to a large community
AIDS Foundation, **South Africa**	- Traditional healers themselves selected traditional healers to be trained	- Traditional healers approached the AIDS Foundation of South Africa for training	- Traditional healers identified the need for rural AIDS hospices and trained home-care personnel - More work needs to be done to eliminate the tenuous and strained aspect of the relationship between traditional healers and biomedical practitioners

(Contd.)

(Contd.)

Country	*Criteria for selecting 'genuine' or 'authentic' healers*	*Approach used to build trust*	*Lessons learned*
Training of Trainers, **South Africa**	- 5 national traditional healers' associations selected traditional healers for first workshop based on gender and geographical balance - Trained traditional healers selected healers for future workshops	- In-depth interviews and focus group discussions over 1-year period	- Misconceptions about AIDS are easily dispelled - Second-generation traditional healers were as well, if not better, trained than first-generation healers due to better selection of trainees by traditional healers - Training on death and dying was not liked by traditional healers - It was advised to discontinue work with traditional healers' organizations to avoid political conflicts - Traditional healers wanted explicit condom demonstration - As traditional healers had access to intimate details of patients' physical emotional and spiritual lives, they experienced few problems influencing behaviour in sex and sexuality
Uganda	THETA selection criteria: - Being recognized as healers by their community and local authorities - Having regular patient attendance - Having a clinic or shrine to receive and treat patients - Knowing how to prepare herbal remedies - Questionnaire answered by each healer	- Emphasis on healers' right to ownership of their treatments - Initial contact through the Culture Officer of the Ministry of Gender and Community Development as well as through a TASO doctor and personal visits to traditional healer's clinic	- Research with traditional healers requires mutual respect and collaboration with biomedical health practitioner - Collaborative work requires time to build trust and continuous follow-up to monitor and evaluate a changing epidemic, and a dynamic relationship between the 2 health sectors - Traditional healers can come up with innovative ideas for AIDS prevention long after training is completed - This type of collaboration can extend nationwide if strong links are built at the community level with local leaders, government and non-governmental key players and health authorities.

(Contd.)

(Contd.)

Country	*Criteria for selecting 'genuine' or 'authentic' healers*	*Approach used to build trust*	*Lessons learned*
United Republic of Tanzania	- Two types of participatory approaches were used to identify key traditional healers and health personnel to participate in the training workshops	- Meetings were arranged between expatriate physician and traditional healers. Healers enjoyed being taken seriously and being treated like fellow professionals. Initial dialogues evolved into a series of workshops on patient care, treatment, education and cooperation between biomedical and traditional health practitioners	- Traditional healers should be respected as health professionals - Give traditional healers access to hospitals, clinics, and patients - Involve them in home care and training - Healers care about their patients and want to learn more - Traditional healers are keen students - Traditional healers love learning about research - Traditional healers enjoy mutual referral between them and hospital/clinics - Develop a cooperative and collaborative relationship between traditional healers and hospital/clinic
Zambia	- Traditional leaders assisted health centre staff in selection process. - Professional reputation within the community, willingness and ability to learn and communication skills	- Training was highly participatory - Health workers facilitating workshops underwent training in participatory methods - Effort was made to find terms that are more familiar to traditional healers' understanding of health and disease rather than using biomedical terminology	- Traditional healers came up with symbolic alternatives to high risk practices - After culturally appropriate exposure to explanations of public health, traditional healers can modify ritual practices

Index

E

F

G

H

I

ENCYCLOPAEDIA OF AIDS

ENCYCLOPAEDIA
OF
AIDS

(In 7 Volumes)

(Volume 6)

Editor

Dr. G.C. Satpathy

PUBLICATIONS

KALPAZ PUBLICATIONS

DELHI - 110052

ENCYCLOPAEDIA OF AIDS
(*Health, Reference*)

Rs. 7000 (Set)
Rs. 1000 (each volume)

ISBN: 81-7835-112-9 (Set)
ISBN: 81-7835-137-4 (Vol. 6)

Published in 2003 in India by
Kalpaz Publications
C-30, Satyawati Nagar
Delhi-110052
e-mail: kalpaz@hotmail.com

Laser Typeset at: Alphabet, Delhi
Printed at: Mehra Offset Press, Delhi

Contents

Preface

The later half of the twentieth century will be remembered in the history of medicine for two remarkable events, one good, that is the eradication of smallpox, and the other one bad, when the world was alerted to the first case AIDS in 1981, now running in a pandemic proportion. In a little over two decades it is estimated that over 36 million people are now infected with HIV/AIDS with 5.3 million being infected every year. India alone has about 4 million HIV/AIDS patients, the second highest number among all nations. Now it is well perceived as a serious threat to humanity, and the control of this epidemic lies not only in the hands of physicians alone but the entire society must involve to the task. No cure or vaccine is yet in sight. So the only mode of controlling it is prevention. The key to prevention lies in information, education and communication.

Twenty years of observation and study of the syndrome has generated profound interest among all branches of medicine, social activists, research workers, public health issues, health and sex education strategies, with innumerable clinical and pharmacological research being conducted on it all over the world. It is not possible to compile the whole saga of AIDS, which is unique in many ways and not yet fully understood. We have tried to accumulate as much information as possible in this seven-volume encyclopaedia, probably the first such attempt made ever. Since the process of acquiring information is never-ending, we hope to provide more and more information in future.

It has been a herculean task to compile the huge materials systematically, besides being an unique experience. In spite of the best efforts for accuracy and perfection, there may be shortcomings, which may be excused. It will be a success story for us if by this work the society to which the work is dedicated is benefited at large. The study does not end here. It shall be a continuous series in future with comprehensive details having a deep bearing on the subject.

Guwahati-23 **Dr. G.C. Satpathy**
Rathyatra-2002 **MD, IPM**

Acknowledgements

During the course of this research work, I happened to visit several academic fora which willingly afforded their support and facilitated my work. These are the Ministry of Health, Govt. of India, World Health Organisation, health departments of the States and academic institutions of higher learning. I have used the material from published works including scholarly journals and magazines to fill up the gaps in these volumes.

I have also taken academic support from several sources, which include universities, institutes, centres for higher learning, Acts passed in this direction, Statistical Year Book (UNESCO), voluntary organisations, legal luminaries, social activists, prison management, legal issues of AIDS, Legislation Enquiry Commission on HIV Law, Sri Lanka, Prevention of Brothels Act, Myanmar, Laws of HIV/AIDS in Pakistan, Documents in sub-Saharan, Africa, European Council Recommendations, UNESCO Courier, Philippines Overseas Employment Agency, Foreign Exchange Regulations Deptt., Central Bank of the Philippines, National Advisory Committee on AIDS in Singapore, Vietnamese National AIDS Committee, National Blood Transfusion Centre in Cambodia, Infectious Diseases Act, Thailand, AIDS Prevention Act in Korea, Labour Protection Law, Thailand, Social Security Act, Thailand, Homosexual Law Reform Act, 1986, Universities of Nairobi, Manitola (in Canada) and Washington, Institute of Systemic Therapy, Harare, Zimbabwe, The AIDS Service Organisation, Kampala, Uganda, Health Economics and HIV/ AIDS Research Division, University of Natal, Durban, School of

Public Health, University of Natal, South Africa Institute for Medical Research, Johannesburg, Centre for African Family Studies, Nairobi, Kenya, Malwai Institute of Management, Malwai.

I feel much grateful to these institutions and learned authors whose writings have proved useful in the texts of these seven volumes.

The publisher and myself feel much beholden to the panel of highly qualified and experienced advisers who are distinguished in their respective fields, for their valuable and timely guidelines, contributions and encouragement in making this work an epoch-making one.

I am grateful to several other research institutes and NGOs etc., scholars whose writings have been used in these volumes.

I am extremely grateful to my wife, son Anurag and daughter Anamika for their consistent encouragement to me during this stupendous research work.

Dr. G.C. Satpathy

Our Distinguished Panel of Advisers

1. Dr. A.K. Das, MD, MNAMS, Ph.D., FICA	Dean and Director-Prof. Dept. of Medicine, JIMPER, Pondicherry
2. Mr. D.K. Arya IPS (Retd.)	Former Director General, BSF
3. Dr. K.V. Dakhina Murty MD, DM, DNB, FISN	Prof. & Head, Deptt. of Nephrology, Nizam's Instt. of Medical Sciences, Panjagutta, Hyderabad
4. Maj. Gen. K.K. Ganguly	VSM (Retd.)
5. Col. M.K. Bhandari MD, FICA	Asso. Prof. of Medicine, Armed Forces Medical College, Pune
6. Dr. M.C. Dash	Vice Chancellor, Sambalpur University, P.O.: Jyoti Vihar, Orissa
7. Dr. N.C. Borah MD, DM	C.M.D. GNRC Hospitals Ltd. Dispur, Guwahati
8. Dr. P.C. Bhattacharya MD	Sr. Consultant, downtown hospital Dispur, Guwahati
9. Dr. S.B. Gupta MD	Physician and Cardiologist Central Railway Hospital, Mumbai

Introduction

As we leave the 20th century, there is still no cure in sight for one of the most frightening and devastating diseases the world has known.

HIV and AIDS continue to affect the lives of millions around the world. But they are not faceless millions. Almost all of us know a friend, family member or co-worker who has been affected. In our work as United Nations employee, we also see at first hand how the pandemic is ravaging the developing countries, particularly Africa and South Asia. Until a vaccine or a cure is found, our greatest weapon against HIV/AIDS is knowledge. The United Nations is committed to providing a supportive work place for its employees, regardless of their HIV status.

When the world looks back on the end of the 20th century, let us be remembered for our vigilance in combating one of the greatest killers in our life time. But let us also be remembered for our solidarity with all those who suffer from this terrible disease.

By the end of 1999, there were an estimated 34.3 million adults and children living with HIV/AIDS in the world and there had been some 18.8 million deaths. Sub-Saharan Africa remains the centre of the epidemic, with nearly 25 million men, women and children infected with HIV/AIDS.

Over the last two decades, much has been learnt about HIV prevention. Some of this new knowledge comes from carefully conducted evaluation studies, programme, reviews, the documentation of existing good practices (UNAIDS, 1999), meta-analysis and reviews and the observations of the field workers, non-governmental organisations (NGOs) and health promotion practitioner. All of these information sources have proved to be valuable in indicating the most appropriate and promising interventions.

Under the leadership of the Joint United Nations Programme on HIV/AIDS (UNAIDS) a new and more adaptable framework for HIV/AIDS communications has been developed. Unlike many earlier approaches this framework is based more on social and environmental context than on individual behaviour. UNAID'S basic assumption was that the logic and theory of HIV/AIDS strategies ought to evolve from within the meanings and values of the affected population. It responded to the increasing epidemic of HIV/AIDS by initiating a participatory research process to examine the global use communications for HIV/AIDS prevention, care and support. The primary aim was to examine the adequacy of existing communications theories and models for HIV/AIDS in Africa, Asia and Latin America and the Caribbean against a backdrop of contemporary communications uses in Western societies.

UNAIDS (1999) had reported that 90 per cent of the new cases of HIV are in Africa, Asia and Latin American and the Caribbean. Given the reality of the epidemics, information, education and communication on HIV/AIDS is still very important to reduce the spread of the disease and to strengthen efforts and programmes in care and support.

As HIV transmission is propelled by behavioural factors theories about how individuals change their behaviour have provided the foundation for most HIV prevention efforts worldwide.

Several studies have shown that economic factors have a strong influence on individual sexual behaviour, mostly through poverty and underemployment; Cross-nationally countries with the lowest standards of living are also the ones with the highest HIV incidence. Within both rich and poor countries, poverty is related to HIV and HIV intensifies poverty.

The proposed mechanisms for this relationship are : non-cohabitation between young married couples which can arise from critical economic situations forcing urban migration, seasonal work and truck driving, sex work, civil disturbances and war. Civil disturbance and war lead to displaced and refugee population and who not only lose their social and familial support systems but become highly vulnerable to HIV owing to intense social and economic strain in a alien culture. In such situations, HIV concerns take a very low priority in a risk hierarchy, and any previous or planned efforts for the control of HIV transmission are disrupted, if not destroyed.

Today, many of the interventions of HIV transmission, rather than using one of the behavioural theories in its entirety, have developed programmes based on one or many constructs often depending on the socio-cultural, political or economic situation and on the stage of the epidemic. Drawing on various models and modifying them to suit the population and context has been critical to implementation of prevention projects, especially in international settings, as nearly all theories were developed in the West. These trans-theoretical approaches are guided by critical constructs such as risk perception, social norms and sexual communication to form the basis of interventions worldwide.

Peer education is one approach to small-group HIV prevention usually aimed at individual behaviour. The peer health educator approach recruits leaders in communities at risk to be implementers of the education programme to their peers.

The peer educator approach has been used in as diverse populations. They performed differing tasks ranging from development and distribution of IEC materials including Video clips and pamphlets, as well as condoms discussion and distribution to conversations with peers on diverse topics such as empowerment, health and human rights and basic AIDS information.

Editor

One

Innovative Approaches to HIV Prevention

It has been estimated that, by the end of 1999, there were an estimated 34.3 million adults and children living with HIV/AIDS in the world and there had been some 18.8 million deaths. Sub-Saharan Africa is the centre of the epidemic, with nearly 25 million men, women and children infected with HIV/AIDS.

In Asia, around 7 million people are infected, and rates are on alarm increase in countries like India and China. Parts of Central and Eastern Europe are also witnessing rapid increase in HIV infection rates (UNAIDS, 2000). In the last two decades, much has been learned about HIV prevention. Some of this new knowledge comes from carefully conducted evaluation studies, programme reviews, the documentation of existing good practices (UNAIDS, 1999), meta-analyses and reviews (e.g., Gibney, DiClemente & Vermund, 1999), and the observations of field workers, non-governmental organizations (NGOs) and health promotion practitioners.

All of these information sources have proved to be valuable in indicating the most appropriate and promising interventions. By providing varied sorts of information - for instance, indicating changes in the prevalence and incidence of infection; changes in reported behaviours; increases in concerned service utilization or condom sales; or improved HIV-related knowledge, beliefs, attitudes and skills - each contributes to our understanding of what can 'work' in HIV prevention.

The following five criteria are specifically valuable when evaluating HIV prevention programmes:

(1) Relevance
- perception as relevant by target groups
- cultural and contextual relevance

(2) Efficiency
- Well coordinated planning and implementation
- reach

(3) Impact
- impact on reported rates of STD and HIV
- impact on HIV and AIDS-related knowledge, beliefs and attitudes
- impact on safer sex practices and safer forms of drug use

(4) Sustainability
- generalizability to other contexts
- cost-effectiveness

(5) Ethical soundness

It is potent to note, however, that the success of any intervention will largely depend on the appropriateness of what has been done. Every intervention occurs within a particular context, and local context as well as the stage of the epidemic must be taken into account when planning, designing and implementing HIV prevention programmes. It is also critical to remember that interventions at *multiple levels* are nearly always required in order to encourage people to adopt and sustain safe sex and drug use practices, and to establish the enabling and supportive environments required for reducing vulnerability to HIV infection.

Methodology

The identification of various innovative and promising interventions was achieved through consultations with a number of experts in the field of HIV/AIDS prevention at the international, regional and local levels, and through reviews of published literature. A parallel project supported by UNAIDS, and based within the East-West Center in Hawaii, has recently established an archive of HIV prevention studies. The objective of this report is to complement this and similar reviews. Information was sought from key individuals working in international agencies and charitable foundations at headquarters, and when required, followed-up at the regional level. Information was also accumulated from individuals within UNAIDS and co-sponsoring agencies at headquarters and at regional and national levels.

A standard *pro forma* was used to alert individuals to the nature of the project's work and to invite collaboration and participation. Copies of this *pro forma* were later sent by e-mail, fax or post to named individual contacts at intercountry and country level. This invited the nomination of local programmes, projects and activities to be considered for inclusion in this review.

Contact was then made with individual projects via their manager or coordinator and descriptions of their ongoing work were elicited under a series of heading. These comprised:

- the location of the project, contact details and the funding agency;
- an overall description of the work of the project;
- a statement of project activities and outputs to date;
- information about evaluation and project outcomes;
- a description of any innovative aspects of the work;
- a statement of constraints/obstacles affecting local activities and the success of the interventions.

The activities undertaken as part of this work should not be considered as comprehensive. Rather, the purpose is to identify key studies and investigations on HIV prevention interventions beyond information distribution. Thus, this work provides a set of intervention instances for HIV prevention and highlights some of the key issues to consider when designing, implementing and evaluating HIV programmes.

What Acts in HIV Prevention?

Over the last two decades, a great deal has been learned concerning effective interventions for HIV prevention. When the first cases of AIDS were reported in the early 1980s, individuals and groups acted to alarm people to this dangerous new disease and the steps that could be taken to protect against it. Even before HIV was isolated, safer sex and safer drug use guidelines had been developed based upon epidemiological evidence related to patterns of transmission. However, providing people with information about how to protect against infection has proven to be insufficient in and of itself. People require enabling environments that will reduce their susceptibility and vulnerability, and permit them to modify their behaviour based on their knowledge gained through information provision.

National Level

At the national level, political commitment at all levels has been shown to be inevitable for programme success. Multi-level interventions that want to involve a variety of partners in co-ordinated action have been shown to be more successful than those that work in isolation (UNAIDS, 1998a, 1998b, 1998c, 1999). Furthermore, coordinated economic, political and social effort are needed to reduce societal vulnerability alongside programmes and interventions operating at individual and community levels (UNAIDS, 1998d).

Global experience has shown the following elements to be among those central for effective national HIV prevention endeavours.

- general awareness-raising activities to give information and counter negative reactions among the population at large;
- focused persuasive action to meet the requirements of specially vulnerable groups and communities, with gradually expanding coverage;
- multi-sectoral and multi-level partnerships to deliver programmes and services across a range of contexts;
- community involvement in programme and intervention development, and building upon the will of groups and individuals to contribute to national HIV prevention endeavours.
- greater integration between prevention and care to minimize costs and to reduce levels of discrimination and stigmatization;
- action to build societal resistance to HIV transmission and reduce the systematic vulnerability of certain individuals, groups and sections of society.

Community Level

Following a recent review of successful community-based projects and activities (UNAIDS, 1999), a further set of principles has been recognised outlining some of the factors that require to be taken into account if community-based prevention activities are to be effective. These comprise:

- engaging the community through prevailing organizations, groups and structures for education and support;
- Making partnership and trust through communication, networking and collaboration;
- including people with HIV and AIDS at all stages of the process so as to enhance visibility and advantage from their skills and experiences;
- developing an accepting community environment in which HIV and AIDS are acknowledged to be everyone's concern.

Beyond these principles, community-based approaches require to make certain that resources are directed towards community capacity-building with a view to ensure sustainability.

Programme/Project Level

At the programme/project level, the following factors are important to programme success when properly operationalized.

- the provision of *information* in culturally proper ways about how HIV is and is not transmitted;
- the insertion of *activities* that encourage people (both as individuals and communities) to appraise the risks that face them personally;
- the provision of *training* in skills for communication and (where it is possible) sexual negotiation;
- the provision of enhanced *access* to resources such as condoms and appropriate and affordable health services, comprising those for the early detection and treatment of Sexually Transmitted Diseases (STDs).
- the *participation* of target groups at all stages of design, implementation and evaluation;
- the *monitoring* of programme/projects at every stages of development and implementation.

Group Level

Prevention approaches require to be tailored to the requirements of particular groups.

When working with *young people,* for instance, it is important to:

- take into consideration the *diversity* of young people and their needs;

- encourage youth *participation* in project design and implementation;
- work in a climate of *openness* that recognizes and respects the facts that young people face;
- focus on young men's *sexual* health, as well as sexual health issues concerning to young women.
- examine the *positive* aspects of sexual health;
- promote greater awareness of sexual and reproductive rights;
- give opportunities to address issues of *gender*, social status and sexuality;
- undertake work with *young men* to enable them to think about their role in terms of both their sexual health and that of their partners;
- promote greater awareness of the *structural issues* affecting the sexual and reproductive health of young people, comprising the need for improved rights and protection for young people;
- improve access to basic *education* and timely sex and HIV-related education;
- provide access to *voluntary counselling* and testing services, along with proper referrals;
- enhance access to youth-friendly health services.

When working with *women*, it is potent to:

- use a *multifaceted approach* that addresses economic and other requirements which may take priority over HIV/AIDS in the daily lives of women living in poverty in third world countries;
- focus on *improving communication* between sexual partners which acknowledges the problems women encounter in talking and negotiating with men about sex;
- increase awareness of the value of *including men* in work for the prevention of HIV among men, women and children;
- address the requirement for improved *health* services for women;
- accept the importance of a *gendered approach* to HIV prevention work, which includes discussions of power relations between men and women;

- provide access to *voluntary counselling* and testing services, along with adequate referrals;
- acknowledge the *support* that women can give to each other through open discussion and the development of networks.

When working with *people who inject drugs,* it is potent to:

- focus on *harm* reduction and rehabilitation;
- *advocate* to protect the rights of people who inject drugs;
- adopt a *multi-pronged approach* comprising needle and syringe exchange and the provision of drug treatment, comprising detoxification, substitution pharmaco-therapy, HIV/AIDS care and social network interventions;
- give *drop-in services,* mobile services and outreach work;
- work to improve the *sexual health* and sexual practices of people who inject drugs;
- undertake HIV prevention activities when *seroprevalence* is still low;
- develop *trust* between people who inject drugs and health workers through outreach work;
- provide good access to *sterile injecting equipment* and condoms;
- provide access to *voluntary counselling and testing services,* along with proper referrals;
- establish high levels of *knowledge* concerning HIV infection and modes of transmission among people who inject drugs.

When working with *men who have sex with men,* it is important to:

- *acknowledge the wider* concerns of MSM in developing countries, including issues such as harassment, poverty and responsibilities towards family members;
- identify the importance of *raising public* awareness about issues relating MSM, countering prejudice and discrimination, and the promotion of human rights;
- provide *training for professionals* working with MSM, comprising health workers, teachers and prison officers;
- *address homophobia,* comprising internalized homophobia;
- help MSM develop *support networks;*
- provide access to *voluntary counselling* and testing services, along with proper referrals;

- acknowledge the *diversity* of MSM third world and developed countries.

When working with *sex workers*, it is important to:

- *accept the wider concerns* and priorities of sex workers, which consists of social, legal and economic issues and concern for their families and children;
- address the prejudice and stigmatization that sex workers face;
- acknowledge the value of helping to *empower* sex workers;
- provide improved and more accessible *health services*, most particularly for the diagnosis and treatment of STDs;
- want the cooperation and *support of gatekeepers* in the sex industry, including brothel owners and bar owners as well as employers of potential clients of sex workers;
- legitimize the role of *sex workers* as educators, providing them related to their peers;
- acknowledge the value of providing sex workers with financial incentives for *peer-led* work,
- work, where feasible, with men as well as women through a *focus on clients* and, in few cases, *boyfriends*. This is important given the prevalent power relations between both men and women and clients and sex workers.

Sources of Evidence

There are clearly a number of various ways of generating knowledge about HIV prevention methods and their effects. All depend to some extent upon observation and the amassing of information but each differs according to the rigour with which data and information are accumulated and made sense of. The kinds of comparatively casual observations that contribute to intuitions and gut reactions are different in kind from the more systematic approaches used in observation studies and objectives-based evaluations. These in turn vary from the approaches often used in more formally conducted experimental and comparative evaluations. It is crucial to bear in mind the strengths and limitations of various kinds of approaches (and various kinds of proof) when making judgements about what works, and what might prove to be a promising approach, in HIV prevention.

By itself, no one approach can answer all the questions we may have about appropriateness and effectiveness. Taken together, various kinds of proof, and different kinds of methodology, can be persuasive in helping us identify the most useful approaches to adopt in certain circumstances and with particular groups.

The following sections provide case study instances in interventions conducted for the prevention of HIV/AIDS for the aforementioned most vulnerable groups, and describe promising HIV prevention interventions geared to addressing their particular needs.

What Works with Young People?

Near about half of all people who acquire HIV become infected before they turn 25. Thus, it is crucial that work be undertaken to help young people protect their sexual health. However, there has been a great deal of uncertainty about how to approach HIV and AIDS prevention with young people. For instance, there continues to be widespread concern that 'too much' sex education will encourage young people to become prematurely sexually active. Consequently, several sex education programmes have focused solely upon abstinence.

Various studies have shown, however, that well-designed programmes of sex education, combining messages about safer sex and abstinence, may delay sexual debut, as well as increase preventive behaviours among those young people who are already sexually active. Where they have been able to access proper knowledge, skills and means, young people have shown a remarkable propensity to adopt safer behaviour. The experiences of young people differ according to social and cultural context, gender, socio-economic status and sexuality. To be successful, HIV prevention programmes require to abandon stereotyped images of young people and take full account of their diversity while recognizing that all young people require accurate information.

However, it is important to be aware that young people, particularly girls in developing countries, do not always have the freedom to make their own choices about sexual behaviour. They may, for instance, be vulnerable to forced or coercive sex, and may sell or exchange sex to ensure their economic survival, or to gain the protection of adults. Young people in developing world often have immediate requirements for shelter, food and clothes which take priority over the threat of a disease which may or may not kill them in years to come.

It is important that programmes take into account these structural constraints, barriers and challenges for daily survival which young people face. Moreover, it is critical that a dialogue begin with policy-makers to make certain that the rights of young people are ensured, and that governments and international agencies work to address the particular needs of young people in especially vulnerable circumstances. It is also potent to remember that, while young people may be at special risk of HIV infection, they also present an opportunity for halting the epidemic, as their sexual and other habits may not yet be firmly established.

Youth Case Study 1

Setting	:	University
Country	:	Kenya
Intervention	:	Peer-led education
Sponsoring institution/ organization	:	Family Planning Private Sector (an NGO)

The **Kenyan** NGO, Family Planning Private Sector (FPPS) started a peer education project for sexual and reproductive health in assistance with staff and students in nine institutions of higher education. Students' representatives and Deans from all the institutions were brought together with a view to develop an outline curriculum. As a result, student leaders established 'AIDS Awareness Clubs' which became the chief coordinating bodies for activities. Peer educators organized a different kinds of activities, including condom distribution and the publication of newsletters. Qualitative evaluation carried out in five of the institutions by FPPS and Family Health International along with an external consultant during March-April 1997, revealed that around 19,000 students were reached through the programme, and the project substantially increased students' access to services as well as information. Among the most innovative aspects of the work was the way in which the project team got the support of the colleges' administration. In addition to, the initiative's success stemmed largely from the fact that young people themselves were involved in all aspects of project design and implementation.

Youth Case Study 2

Setting	:	Community: out-of-school youth
Country	:	Peru
Intervention	:	Advocacy, information dissemination, and youth empowerment
Sponsoring institution/ organization	:	Institute of Population Studies at Cayetano Heredia University

During 1995-1997, the Institute of Population Studies at Cayetano Heredia University in **Peru** designed, implemented and evaluated a community-based programme in youth and sexual and reproductive health in two neighbourhoods in Peru. Programme staff aimed first to mobilize community resources with a view to improve the quality and dissemination of information on related issues. Second, they aimed to develop more democratic models for sexual health promotion which respect the rights of young people. Third, they aimed to empower young people in identifying and knowing solutions to their own Sexual and Reproductive Health (SRH) problems. Besides, the project sought to motivate local municipalities, education and health sectors, youth groups and community-based organizations to direct more resources towards youth SRH services. In a preparatory phase, information on the perceptions and requirements of local young people was obtained. A survey of a representative sample of 800 young people was undertaken, along with focus group discussions, interviews with key members of the community and speedy assessment of health services within the area. An advisory committee including representatives from governmental, non-governmental, community and youth organizations was established. Later on, training programmes were designed and implemented with health workers, teachers and youth and school peer promoters. In addition to, a directory of reference services in youth health was compiled. The major output of the programme was the design and implementation of a campaign for improved sexual health among young people.

Qualitative and quantitative evaluation activities comprised the collection of data through activity records, individual and group interviews with key members of the community, post-workshop surveys and observations to asses the educational impact of SRH workshops. Besides, data were gathered on the functioning of the health services network and the referral system. Young people assessed the educational workshops positively since they were participatory, entertaining and centred on their own problems and perspectives. The young people were really committed to the programme strategy, as shown by their level of voluntary involvement as peer promoters. The level of involvement and help to the project from key people in the diverse working networks increased considerably. The evaluation concluded that the project strategy has high potential to impact on the SRH of young people, and to become established within the community.

Youth Case Study 3

Setting	:	Mass media
Country	:	Dominican Republic
Intervention	:	Communications campaign using radio, print and television
Sponsoring institution/ organization	:	Dominican Republic National HIV/AIDS Prevention Programme in collaboration with 20 government organizations and NGOs

In the period of 1994-1997, a media prevention campaign aimed at young people was developed via collaboration between the *Dominican Republic's* National HIV/STD Prevention Programme and twenty governmental and non-governmental organizations. Before the media campaign, extensive research, comprising a KABP survey, was carried out in order to establish a profile of the young people at whom the intervention was aimed. Proper messages about HIV/AIDS were then developed and sent through radio, television and print media in three phases. The first phase was designed to increase awareness. The second phase attempted to ensure consistency in messages from various sources, and included the production of a manual for teachers and youth workers. The third phase concentrated on making young people aware of how to protect themselves from HIV infection and providing information about where they could access services and support.

An evaluation conducted in 1996, which involved focus group discussions with young people, disclosed that the messages were perceived as well targeted, creative and imaginative. Young people reported that the messages had promoted discussion and helped them reflect on their behaviour. However, young people also reported that more work was required in order to encourage better communication between parents and children. The whole approach has now been replicated in Guatemala, and other countries in the region are also looking at how the method can be adapted for their own use.

Youth Case Study 4

Setting	:	Community: sexually exploited youth
Country	:	Nepal
Intervention	:	'Camps' or shelters
Sponsoring institution/ organization	:	Maiti Project

In *Nepal*, the Maiti Project has targeted young people subjected to sexual exploitation and abuse, including young women who are at risk of being sold into prostitution in India. The project has undertaken various range of activities, the focus of which is the establishment of camps in high-risk areas. Each of the camps functions as a shelter for approximately thirty girls who have been rescued from traffickers or who are in danger of being sold. The camps provide education and vocational training, and support and counselling. The project has worked closely with colleges, local pressure groups, village leaders, medical officers, lawyers and police. Evaluation suggests that the Maiti Project has prevented around 180 girls from being sold into brothels in India each year. Additionally, 105 people have been imprisoned as a result of the project's endeavours to expose child traffickers. In 1997 alone, 60 girls were repatriated from India and 75 per cent of these were subsequently reunited with their families. The project is most remarkable in its integrated approach to meeting the requirements of young people, and the ways in which it takes account of the complex social and economic circumstances of vulnerable young people.

Youth Case Study 5

Setting	:	Community
Country	:	Haiti
Intervention	:	Health services and training for young people, families and teachers
Sponsoring institution/ organization	:	Fondation pour la Sante Reproductive et I'Education Familiale (FOSREF)

In *Haiti,* the Fondation pour la Sante Reproductive et I'Education Familiale (FOSREF) has attempted to ensure the provision of reproductive health services directly designed for young people. Two big medical centres designed particularly for young people have been established. The project has also provided technical support to staff working in other clinical settings to enable them to cater more effectively to the requirements of young people. Other related project work has included the training of teachers and parents in order to expand the support network available to young people. Project staff have also played a central role in lobbying for national support for the creation of reproductive health services which properly respond to the needs of young people.

The participation of young people has been encouraged at every stage of development, management and implementation. Additionally, an extensive peer education programme with young people adopting the roles of trainers and health promoters was established. FOSREF staff carried out an evaluation in 1997 helped by an external consultant. By that time, more than 125,000 young people had been reached through the project. More than 4,000 had received training in family life and reproductive health, comprising 300 specializing in STD/HIV prevention. Two hundred schools, within the geographical area of the project, were incessantly visited by the peer educators. The training of peer educators was carried out by 18 youth specialist facilitators and assistant facilitators. More than 15,000 young people continuously attended the youth medical centres where they received a range of services including contraceptive counselling, prevention of STD/HIV, specialized HIV/AIDS counselling, antenatal care and support services. Besides this formal evaluation, two studies were carried by young people themselves to assess the appropriateness and acceptability of the services from the standpoint of the target group.

Youth Case Study 6

Setting	:	Community households
Country	:	Egypt
Intervention	:	Telephone hotline
Sponsoring institution/ organization	:	Ministry of Health and private sponsors

An AIDS hotline and counselling service evolved out of a trial telephone counselling service established during the early 1990s in *Egypt*. It was an effort to provide a channel for people to discuss issues surrounding sex and sexuality within a context where cultural taboos prohibit their open discussion in public. Even with limited advertising, people began to call, and an evident requirement for the service was identified.

In September 1996, after securing personnel and office space from the Ministry of Health (MoH), and funding from the Ford Foundation, the hotline was opened. Counsellors were appointed by the MoH and underwent an intensive 4-week training. The purpose of the project are to provide accurate information about HIV/AIDS to the general public, comprising young people, and to provide confidential and anonymous HIV/AIDS counselling services.

A team of expert counsellors answer all calls, and callers can choose whether to speak to a woman or a man. The hotline is advertised on bulletin boards, trains, metros, buses, and in Arabic newspapers. Supervisory monitoring of the calls is undertaken, to ensure the quality of the information and services provided. Evaluation has taken the form of monitoring the services and gathering basic demographic data on the callers using the service. Questions are asked to condition the level of education of each caller, how they learned about the hotline, whether or not they are married and from where they are calling. The volume of calls is monitored and daily statistics on the numbers of callers, their gender breakdown and the kinds of questions asked are recorded. Between September 1996 and May 1998, 18,628 calls were made, averaging around 1,000 per month. More than 50 per cent of callers are between the ages of 13 and 25 years, and 70 per cent are unmarried. Most callers have had a high school or university education, and less than 20 per cent are women. Although the project mainly focused on Greater Cairo, calls are also made from rural settings and from other countries where Arabic newspapers are read.

The number of calls made to the hotline has surpassed all expectations. The anonymity of the hotline seems to have provided a vital link to information and counselling services that would otherwise not be available. Through the hotline, people are able to discuss issues like sexuality, condom use, pre-marital sex and homosexuality, which are rarely addressed in public forums. At the time of its operation, this was the only HIV/AIDS Hotline run by a government service in the Middle East.

Youth Case Study 7

Setting	:	Schools
Country	:	Viet Nam
Intervention	:	Skills-based HIV/AIDS and STD prevention
Sponsoring institution/ organization	:	UNICEF and the Vietnam Ministry of Education and Training (MOET)

In *Vietnam*, a skills-based HIV/AIDS/STD prevention project was begun as a UNICEF-assisted HIV/AIDS prevention project of the Vietnam Ministry of Education and Training (MOET) in 1997.

The chief objective of the project was to work with schools to equip young people with information and skills needed for promoting healthy behaviour, and avoiding risky situations, especially concerned to HIV/AIDS.

The major focus was on student knowledge, attitudes and values and behaviours. An anticipated secondary result was a similar impact on teaching staff. The project trained teachers in skills-based health education for HIV/AIDS and other STD prevention, and supported them in practising the new approach in the classroom. Skills-based HIV/AIDS/STD-related lessons were developed for grades 1-12 and integrated into the prevailing curriculum. New teachers' guidebooks and student worksheets were developed by those trained. In the beginning implementation year, a total of 300 teachers implemented and 15,000 students studied life skills and HIV/AIDS prevention. Another 5,000 young people studied life skills and other topics with 140 Viet Nam Red Cross trainers supported by UNICEF.

Youth Case Study 8

Setting	: Schools
Country	: Uganda
Intervention	: School health education
Sponsoring institution/ organization	: Uganda AIDS Commission

A school health education programme in primary schools aiming AIDS prevention in the Soroti district of *Uganda* stressed improved access to information and other resources for healthy sexual behaviour decision-making; improved peer interaction related to information and decision-making related to HIV/AIDS, sexuality and health; and improved quality of performance of the existing school health education system. A cross-sectional sample of students, average age 14 years, in their final year of primary school was surveyed before and after 2 years of interventions. The percentage of students who said they had been sexually active fell from 42.9 per cent (123 out of 287) to 11.1 per cent (31 out of 280) in the intervention group, while no important change was recorded in a control group. The changes remained important when segregated by gender or rural and urban location. Students in the intervention group tended to speak to peers and teachers more often about sexual matters. Over the study period, these students became more likely to give as causes for abstaining from sex those associated with a rational decision-making model rather than a punishment model. A primary school health education programme which stresses social interaction methods can be effective in increasing sexual abstinence among school-going adolescents in Uganda. The programme does not have to be expensive and can be implemented with staff present in most of the districts in the region.

What Works With Women and Men?

It has been estimated the about 55 per cent of all adults suffering from HIV/AIDS are women, with the difference between men and women being most pronounced in those under the age of 25 (MAP, 2000). Not only have women been reported as having a heightened physiological susceptibility to HIV infection (International Center for Research on Women, 1999), they also have an increased social vulnerability. Women have not equal access to education and economic resources. They wield less power than men in social and sexual relations. Entrenched stereotypes and differences in role expectations between the sexes also mean that women generally have less say in decisions about when and how intercourse takes place, comprising whether or not a condom will be used. What is more, women are more likely than men to experience rape and sexual coercion, and are sometimes forced to sell or exchange sex for their economic survival.

In addition to their own increased risk of HIV infection, women also carry the lion's share of the social burden of the epidemic in terms of providing the care for relatives with AIDS. Women with HIV infection also generally experience more social blame and stigma than men in the same position. Gallois, Statham and Smith (1992) have argued that women do not constitute a 'risk group' for HIV infection in the usual sense of the term since women do not usually infect each other, but instead acquire HIV mainly through their relationships with men. Research in a variety of contexts exhibits that womens' attitudes towards sex and sexual behaviour differ considerably from those of men. Women report a preference for sexual relations based on mutual fidelity, intimacy and open communication. They have fewer sexual partners than men and a great many more women than men report having only one lifetime sexual partner. When women do express a desire for safer sex, men are often obstructive.

Perhaps not surprisingly, therefore, the major HIV risk for women is their regular sexual partner or husband. Dominant ideologies of masculinity on the other hand promote the display of sexual prowess, and encourage men to have multiple partners.

Various existing HIV prevention programmes fail to take proper account of the social vulnerability of women or the unequal power relations which make it difficult for women to influence decision-making in their sexual relationships. The basic elements of many programmes - partner reduction, condom use and STD treatment - are not necessarily proper for women, who do not have various partners, cannot always influence the decision to use condoms, and may be asymptomatic for STDs. Indeed, open and honest verbal communication is one of the most difficult aspects of heterosexual relationships.

There is now increasing recognition that prevailing ideologies of masculinity and femininity facilitate HIV transmission. There is also widespread agreement that the promotion of more equal gender roles is the key to preventing infection. It is crucial therefore not only to address stereotyped gender roles, but also to remove some of the stark structural inequalities between men and women, comprising the unequal distribution of economic resources and differentials in access to education and health provision. Women's empowerment, however, cannot be achieved by women alone but needs the support of men for its successful realization.

General Population Case Study 1

Setting	:	Community: women hawkers
Country	:	Namibia
Intervention	:	Prevention education
Sponsoring institution/ organization	:	Okatumbatumba Hawkers Association (a CBO)

The Okatumbatumba Hawkers Association was setup in 1989 in *Namibia* to support street sellers in their work. Initially, literacy and English courses were organized alongside training for effective negotiation with business establishments because these were the expressed requirements of its members. More recently, work has been extended to include HIV/AIDS, which the hawkers themselves raised concerns about. In October 1994, a training programme was started and a group of 16 women hawkers were trained in basic HIV prevention work. The overall view of the programme was to increase HIV/AIDS awareness and condom use among the community of Windhoek and neighbouring regions. An interactive, visual story-telling technique was the key learning tool used, and enabled people of all levels of literacy to participate in the programme. Prevention activities were carried out in *cuca* shops (informal/unlicensed drinking establishments), street markets, churches, local businesses and government agencies. Condoms and information leaflets were disseminated from these venues and the owners became informal information/support resources within their communities.

Trained hawkers from Windhoek later travelled to other regions where they trained their counterparts to provide local HIV prevention education in local languages. A training of trainers programme was later established in 7 of the 13 administrative regions of Namibia. This programme enabled the Hawkers Association to address the concerns of hawkers in other regions and to extend its business training, bulk purchasing and loan and savings programme to meet the requirements of hawkers who were reached through the AIDS awareness campaign.

In total, an estimated 11,000 people participated in education sessions. Follow-up visits have revealed a large demand from local communities for further education. Additionally, church leaders were very responsive to the initiative and expressed a wish to extend their role in terms of support to people living with HIV/AIDS. Evaluation has exposed an increase in knowledge about HIV and an increased awareness of the need to change sexual behaviours. Groups visited during evaluation talked about how they had communicated the information they had received to their children and families.

The effectiveness of face-to-face interaction was noted repeatedly. A further external evaluation of the work has been carried out by the regional directorate of the Ministry of Health, through observations of the intervention in the field. This disclosed a reported high degree of effectiveness in terms of communicating accurate information, credibility and acceptance within the community. The project's greatest innovation has been to build on the extensive social and interactive contact that street-sellers have everyday with their customers. The success of the project as a community-based initiative is important. It provides a clear illustration of how simply designed programmes can prove successful when proper strategies and acceptable and established channels are employed.

General Population Case Study 2

Setting	:	Family planning associations
Country	:	Jamaica, Honduras, Brazil
Intervention	:	Integrated prevention education and health service provision
Sponsoring institution/ organization	:	International Planned Parenthood Federation Western Hemisphere Region (IPPF/WHR)

In 1992, International Planned Parenthood Federation/ Western Hemisphere Region (IPPF/WHR) evolved a pilot project to integrate HIV/AIDS prevention into the programmes and services of Family Planning Associations (FPAs) in *Jamaica, Honduras* and *Brazil*. The outcome has been a shift of emphasis from the delivery of contraceptive services towards a more holistic approach that promotes sexual as well as reproductive health.

However, the aim of the programme was not just to 'add on' HIV/AIDS as an extra component, but rather to improve the overall quality of services by changing the manner in which they are provided, and effecting changes in interaction between clients and providers of these services. Initially, interviews were conducted with staff and clients, and observations were made at counselling sessions. As a consequence, staff were trained in basic information about HIV/AIDS and sexual health, counselling skills, communication skills, issues relating to gender and power, and the development of skills to train clients in more effective negotiation with their sexual partners. Special training according to professional needs was also provided - for instance STD management for physicians, and group facilitation skills for staff working with groups. Each FPA then adopted policies and practice to support the required changes in the provision of services.

Evaluation disclosed that work with clients had broadened from helping with contraception to more detailed discussion to risk behaviours, sexual relationships and power within relationships. Service providers changed the path in which they discussed family planning methods and now discussed each in relation to HIV/AIDS. Whereas before the intervention, staff at all three FPAs expressed resistance to condoms, they later not only discussed the role of condoms in relations to disease prevention but developed innovative ways of promoting their potential for enhancing sexual pleasure and destroying prejudices related to their use.

Moreover, whereas before there was a focus on the biological mechanics of preventing pregnancy, staff later discussed a wide range of sexual issues that were earlier considered taboo subjects. In response to this new approach, clients began to discuss with FPA staff previously sensitive subjects like homosexuality, anal or oral sex, extramarital affairs, impotence, premature ejaculation, sexual abuse and domestic violence.

General Population Case Study 3

Setting	:	Community
Country	:	Zambia
Intervention	:	Support and counselling services
Sponsoring institution/ organization	:	Society for Women and AIDS in Zambia (an NGO)

Established in 1989, the Society for Women and AIDS in *Zambia* (SWAAZ) represents an endeavour to respond to the various problems facing a society with a high prevalence and incidence of HIV/AIDS. The whole aim of this initiative was to strengthen the capacity of women, families and communities to respond to HIV/AIDS in Zambia. In Lusaka, SWAAZ is best known for the establishment of four family support homes in low-income communities rendering a wide range of services to women, young people, orphans, widows and people living with HIV/AIDS. Activities vary within each home, but include preschool and feeding programmes for orphans, women and youth clubs, small income-generating projects, like banking, knitting, sewing, gardening and carpentry, and community HIV prevention programmes. An evaluation was undertaken in late 1997 to access the impact of activities in Lusaka. The review team visited the four Family Support Homes in Bauleni, Chawama, Mtendere and Mandevu townships. In Bauleni, preschool provision and the programme for feeding orphans had a very positive impact, providing services to children which they would not otherwise have received. Other activities, comprising the income-generating projects, had not yet taken off. In Chawama, pre-school provision afforded opportunities for orphans to receive preschool education.

A Community Prevention Team (CPT) was using counselling as a method for controlling and preventing HIV/AIDS in the surrounding community. However, the review cleared that the Family Support Home at Chawama was not economically sustainable, being totally dependent on outside funding. At Mtendere, the preschool project was highly successful and economically self-sustaining. Additionally, a Youth Drama Club had been effective not only in its HIV prevention work but also in campaigning against poverty and raising awareness about mental health issues. The club generates income for itself and helps to subsidize the other activities of the support homes. In Mandevu, the pre-school project was the most successful and economically viable of all activities.

SWAAZ is respected for the innovative and multi-faceted nature of its interventions, addressing a wide range of economic and social requirements within communities affected by HIV/AIDS. Through close aid with other governmental and non-governmental organizations, SWAAZ has managed to sustain its work at times when this might not otherwise have been feasible.

General Population Case Study 4

Setting	:	Various organizations
Country	:	Uganda
Intervention	:	Participatory education and training
Sponsoring institution/ organization	:	ActionAID

The Stepping Stones (SS) project was designed to promote participatory education and training around the world. SS materials were originally designed for use in sub-Saharan Africa but have since been adapted and used in many other parts of the world. While focusing on the needs and special vulnerability of women, SS workshops also involve men. The aim is to help women and men explore their needs, analyse their sexual health problems and look at and practise different ways of behaving in relationships. The approach is highly participatory, using methods not requiring literacy. Workshop sessions are described in detail in a manual along with training guidelines. Sessions guide participants through building group trust, exploring issues to do with HIV and safer sex, analysing behaviour patterns, improving communication skills, and devising ways to change. Role-play, drama and drawing, along with other interactive methods, are used.

In 1997, the project completed a survey of people who had received training, with positive results. In 1998, a more in-depth review was carried out with four organizations and two communities in *Uganda* in which the SS approach had been implemented. A review team comprising representatives from international NGOs, local NGOs, health and education departments, and members of the Kabanga and Nabirumba villages where the training programme had been run, worked together to design the evaluation tools. Participatory meetings, using rapid appraisal techniques, were held with representatives of communities that had undergone training using SS, as well as those which had not received any training.

The participatory learning methods promoted by the project were highly valued, as was the good facilitation and the relevance of the content of the sessions. In terms of impact, the group receiving

SS demonstrated an increase in the use of condoms, fewer sexual partners, improved relationships with partners, children and friends and an increased ability to refuse unwanted sex. In addition, the project had a positive impact on other aspects of participants' life and reportedly reduced the incidence of alcohol misuse, encouraged the sharing of money in the home, and promoted more positive attitudes towards caring for those who are sick. Outcomes of the review have been used to further adapt the SS resource, and have been shared globally with those interested in participatory models of monitoring and evaluation.

The positive impacts brought about by the effective use of SS go beyond decreasing vulnerability to HIV infection and improving other aspects of women's lives. The programme challenges the notion that gender relationships within the household are not relevant to broader issues of development, and illustrates how personal issues impinge on the quality of life of individuals.

What Works With People Who Inject Drugs?

It has been estimated that between 6 and 10 million people across the world inject drugs. High rates of HIV infection among people who inject drugs have been found in countries as diverse as Brazil, Thailand, India and Myanmar. In various developing countries, injecting drugs has become the most common risk behaviour related to HIV infection and HIV infection can spread very rapidly this way. For instance, during 1985-1987 HIV prevalence among people who injected drugs in Bangkok was 1 per cent. By the end of 1988, however, this figure had rose to around 40 per cent. People who inject drugs risk HIV infection in two important ways: first, through the sharing of syringes and other injecting equipment; and second, like other sexually active people, through unprotected sex with infected partners.

Those designing HIV-related programmes, aimed at people who inject drugs, face a number of challenges, not least the common fixed ideas about people who use drugs. Also, in several countries drug use is socially sanctioned, stigmatized and illegal. Not surprisingly, drug use generally, and injecting drug use in particular, is often hidden. People who inject drugs are generally marginalized, which means that they may find it difficult to access services and resources that might help them to protect their health. Some legal restrictions may be barriers to HIV prevention, by prohibiting the open provision of sterile injecting equipment for instance.

Evidence from Europe, North America and Australia suggests that people who inject drugs can make considerable changes to their behaviour so as to subside the risk of HIV infection. There is clear proof that in developed countries participation in prevention programmes also leads to a reduction of risk behaviour among people who inject drugs. However, in developing world there is highly variable access to proper information, education and services for people who inject drugs.

IDU Case Study 1

Setting	:	Existing health and education service sites
Country	:	India
Intervention	:	Counselling and condom/bleach distribution
Sponsoring institution/ organization	:	SAHAI Trust (an NGO)

Outreach services for people who inject drugs were established in 1993 in Vepery and Royapuram, *India* by the SAHAI Trust, a non-governmental organization involved in prevention and treatment of drug use. A wide assessment of HIV risk behaviour among people who inject drugs was conducted in 1994 and identified an increase in many drug users injecting opiates as well as synthetic opioids such as buprenorphine. The research suggested that the sharing of syringes and needles and other injecting equipment was very common, as were high-risk sexual practices. Findings from this assessment provided the basis for the design of the outreach project. A team comprising ex-users and professional social workers provided education, counselling and support, as well as distributing condoms and bleach, to injecting drug users who were not reached through existing services or through traditional health education channels. Evaluation has comprised the collection of baseline data from 125 people who inject drugs and a follow-up assessment of 161 users eighteen months after the outreach intervention was introduced. Findings were compared with a control group of 87 drug users from locations where there were no outreach services.

The comparison at follow-up revealed that participants from the outreach locations had adopted important protective and risk-reduction behaviours. Nearly 47 per cent of participants reported decreased sharing of needles and syringes compared to only 35.5 per cent from control locations. Almost 30 per cent of users from outreach locations always cleaned syringes, compared to only 10.3 per cent of the control group. There was no considerable difference between the two groups related to reported sexual risk behaviour.

IDU Case Study 2

Setting	:	Community
Country	:	India
Intervention	:	Outreach and drop-in services including drug substitution
Sponsoring institution/ organization	:	SHARAN (an NGO)

SHARAN has carried on outreach work with people who inject drugs in the slum areas of New Delhi, *India*. The project began work in 1993 as a pilot drug substitution programme and, keeping in view its success, was funded in 1995 to introduce an expanded programme using sublingual buprenorphine tablets. A drop-in centre was established in a slum area (Nizammuddin), to serve the drug-using population from the poorest areas in Delhi.

The long-term objective of project was to produce significant reductions in levels of heroin and injecting drug use in New Delhi. It aimed to achieve this through providing accessible health and harm reduction services to people who inject drugs whilst simultaneously giving information on drug use and HIV/AIDS to their communities. The establishment of a drop-in centre providing medical care and a substitution programme has been complemented by the provision of outreach and community-based detoxification services. A specific staff-training programme has increased the capacity of the centre to address the needs of people who inject drugs. Substantial action, research, and the production and distribution of IEC materials are additional project outputs.

Initial baseline surveys were undertaken to inform the project design. Some original materials for awareness campaigns were created such as posters and street plays. Specialized training was provided to staff to develop counselling skills, and to give technical knowledge of drug use and HIV/AIDS. With the establishment of the drop-in centre, drug substitution treatment using sublingual buprenorphine, medical treatment comprising referrals to other services, and specialised care for tuberculosis, STD and HIV/AIDS management were introduced. In addition, the centre provides free needles, syringes and condoms. Outreach activities conducted by teams of peer educators include educational sessions on safer drug use and safer sex, referrals to relevant services, STD and tuberculosis treatment, and abscess management. Detoxification camps and home-based detoxification comprising the training of family and other community members) are further components of the project's work. These activities are supported through follow-up home visits to affected families, giving information and counselling.

An external mid-term evaluation of the programme was undertaken in August 1996 by two senior researchers from the Indian Council of Medical Research Unit on HIV/AIDS and Substance Abuse. Additionally, at the end of the first year, an evaluation of client responses was carried out by a private agency. Internal evaluations are also conducted to assess both the quality of life of clients (monthly) and the working of the programme (yearly). The mid-term external evaluation noted two major achievements. First, the programme has achieved a high degree of 'user-friendliness' and, as a consequence, the number of clients using the service has risen significantly. Second, the evaluation concluded that, as a trial of bupronorphine substitution, the programme had been very successful in proving its safety.

During the three years of its functioning, the project reached 1,611 clients, and 356 of these used the service on a regular basis (the centre had originally been contracted to service just 300 users). One hundred and fifty people who injected drugs had stopped injecting completely and 58 per cent had significantly reduced heroin use. There was a conspicuous reduction in the number of clients appearing with injecting-related abscesses, cellulitis, sinuses and thrombophlebitis coupled with an increased HIV/AIDS awareness. During its starting phase of operation, the project thus had a major positive impact on reducing the extent of heroin and injecting drug use in this area of New Delhi.

IDU Case Study 3

Setting	:	Community drop-in centres
Country	:	Ukraine
Intervention	:	Information provision and condom/needle supply
Sponsoring institution/ organization	:	Vera, Nadezhda, Lubov (a CBO)

In answer to the increasing number of people injecting drugs in the *Ukraine*, a project was begun in December 1996. Two stationary drop-in centres and one mobile outreach service were initially developed to provide free and anonymous services to people who inject drugs. Teams of three or four volunteer workers provided services, with each team including a volunteer who is medically trained, and a person who injects drugs. Services have comprised the supply of clean needles and syringes, condom distribution, information and counselling on HIV and production and distribution of leaflets. Services have been extended to comprise young men and women who sell sex.

Although the first impetus for the project came from the Southern Branch of the Ukranian AIDS Centre, in May 1997 the community organization Vera, Nadezhda, Lubov took over accountability for the implementation of the project. Records of attendance at centres together with daily project records, give important evaluation material. During the first four months of the centre's opening (up to April 1997), 4,889 visits from 1,216 people who inject drugs were recorded. It has been estimated that contacts with the outreach service crossed the total number of client contacts within the two drop-in centres. During the first six months of 1997, 114,000 syringes and 36,000 condoms were disseminated.

Between July and Mid-October 1997, about 3,000 injecting drug users were reported to have had contact with the service.

Pre- and post-intervention studies provide extra important evaluation data. The first survey (conducted in August 1996) involved 511 people who injected drugs and showed a high level of risk behaviours among respondents (58 per cent of whom were under 25 years old). Only 43 per cent reported using their own needles for injection, and condom use was reported as low as 16 per cent. In April 1997, a new sample of 200 people who injected drugs, recruited at drop-in centres and the outreach post, showed a much lower standard of both injecting and sexual risk behaviour.

This project has remained a community-based project and, in spite of major external difficulties, has managed to maintain a continuous service. It is run exclusively by volunteers who have other occupations as their means of income. The close involvement of people who inject drugs in programme design and implementation makes sure a high degree of acceptability. Project activities have had a positive impact on the reduction of risk behaviours. However, unfavourable political and organizational conditions have been a major constraint. This, coupled with a lack of basic resources comprising syringes and educational booklets and a dependence on volunteer involvement are limiting factors, together with severe financial shortages.

IDU Case Study 4

Setting	:	Prisons and community
Country	:	Mexico
Intervention	:	Harm reduction and rehabilitation
Sponsoring institution/ organization	:	Companeros A.C. (an NGO) with the support of the Pan American Health Organization and Mexican National AIDS Programme

Right since 1987, the non-governmental organization Companeros A.C. in Northern *Mexico* has been developing and evaluating prevention strategies among people who inject drugs.

In 1994, with funding from the Pan American Health Organization and with the support of Mexican National AIDS Programme, a strategy for the introduction of harm reduction was started based on Prochaska's model of 'stages of change'. This highlights the stages a drug user may go through before ceasing substance use.

The project promotes detoxification and rehabilitation alongside harm reduction

The overall objective of the work is to bring about changes in behaviour ranging from giving up the use of injected drugs, to gradual changes in behaviour, which reduce harm to those who continue injecting. Ex-injecting drug users are involved in outreach work. People who are at a perceived 'action' stage (a stage at which they have a strong intention to reduce harm or to stop using drugs) are identified by field workers and presented with a range of intervention options. Fieldwork is carried out in prisons as well as in the wider community, and people who inject drugs frequently come into contact with project workers. Information leaflets are produced and distributed by the field workers. Rehabilitation services given by the project incorporate complementary treatments like acupuncture and herbal medicine. Education and support is given to the families and partners of people who inject drugs.

Records detailing the type and extent of services provided to people using the project, together with follow-up surveys undertaken six months after a person enrols in the programme, provide the core of evaluation data. In addition, baseline data have been collected at the time of enrolment. These consist of demographic information and data on educational and social background and the age at which individuals began using drugs. By mid-1997, Companeros had delivered the following harm reduction services: community outreach services to 1,380 people who inject drugs; distribution of 55,373 harm reduction packets comprising condoms, bleach and education leaflets and 239 skills-building sessions with social networks of people injecting drugs, as well as 2,872 individual skill-building sessions. Between 1992 and September 1997, 928 heroin users enrolled in the rehabilitation programme.

Since the introduction in 1995 of a particular focus on young people (under 20 years), the percentage of young people making use of the harm minimization services has increased from 20 per cent to 32 per cent of the population group. Six months after completion of rehabilitation treatment, there was a 25 per cent decrease in the reported use of marijuana, heroin and speedball. Amongst those who continue using drugs, there has been change towards using drugs that are not injected. The extensive field and outreach work of the project, together with the stress on individual assessment and support, provides a personalized intervention approach. Recognising injecting drug users at stages when they are positively disposed to behavioural modification causes interventions to be better targeted.

IDU Case Study 5

Setting	:	Community
Country	:	Belarus
Intervention	:	Outreach and needle exchange
Sponsoring institution/ organization	:	Parents for the Future of their Children (an NGO) with the support of WHO and UNAIDS

Setup in mid- 1996 and funded by WHO and UNAIDS, a project was developed in *Belarus*. It was the outcome of an initiative from a group of Svetlogorsk residents who were concerned about the level of injecting drug use within their community, and the consequent risk of HIV infection from high-risk injecting and sexual behaviours. The group evolved into the NGO called 'Parents for the Future of their Children'. Svetlogorsk City authorities and the Republic AIDS Prevention Centre have also participated in the initiative. A needle exchange service is run at two exchange points. Disinfectant, condoms and brochures on safe behaviour and HIV/ AIDS prevention are also made available. Information materials for the families of people who inject drugs are produced and disseminated.

Volunteers provide outreach education services to 'difficult to reach' groups. Former injecting drug users voluntarily clear the area around the syringe exchange points. Since October 1997, a professional lawyer has offered free legal consultations to drug users. Anonymous diagnosis and treatment for STDs is undertaken at gynaecological centres by doctors who are specially trained and sensitive to the needs of people who inject drugs. Thirty peer educators have also been trained and a peer education project established.

Daily monitoring of services, together with behavioural, studies and a final project assessment undertaken in April 1998, form the core of evaluations of date. Additionally, and for the first time in the country, a method of sentinel surveillance using the blood residues in syringes was introduced. The syringe exchange points have consistently provided services to a minimum of 300 and a maximum of 700 people who inject drugs each month. The final assessment, conducted by a commission of international, regional and national experts, together with a second behavioural study, have identified a consistent behavioural change towards less risky practices among people who inject drugs coming into contact with the project. The primary behavioural study exhibited that 92 per cent of respondents had a high degree of risk of HIV infection. The secondary study showed this indicator to be subsided to 43 per cent. The number of representatives of the target group who did not use condoms likewise decreased from 71 per cent (pre-intgervention) to 30 per cent.

The quality and scope of the information and educational work were positively assessed. The fact that this project was launched at community level has given it a strong impetus and afforded it a high level of acceptance. Its focus on the close involvement of people who inject drugs in a range of project activities has rendered it highly accessible to members of the target group. The project has had an extra impact on promoting a positive attitude towards preventive interventions on the part of local authorities and the population of the city. There is a plan to reproduce the positive experience of the Svetlogorsk project in other regions of the country.

What Works With Men Who Have Sex With Men?

In various developed countries, gay and other men who have sex with men were among the first to be affected by HIV, and continue to bear the brunt of the epidemic. In developing world the situation is quite different. In many such countries heterosexual transmission accounts for the vast majority of reported cases. However, it is not explicit whether or not this is an accurate reflection of the real situation. In several developing countries, male-to-male sex is highly stigmatized, and in some it is legally prohibited. This can cause governments, political leaders and the public at large to believe that homosexual transmission does not exist, when in fact it is simply hidden (National Research Council, 1996). As time has passed, a new willingness to 'lift the veil' on hitherto stigmatized and refused behaviours has come about. In sub-Saharan Africa, for instance, where virtually no cases of homosexual transmission were initially reported, there is now a growing body of literature to suggest that same-sex contacts are far more common than earlier thought.

It is now explicit that across a variety of countries in both the developed and developing world men who have sex with men (MSM) are made more vulnerable to HIV infection following of the clandestine nature of their relationships, and the marginalization and discrimination they face. The challenge now is to expand on the limited number of innovative programmes for men who have sex with men, and to address the structural factors that encourage this discrimination and stigmatization.

MSM Case Study 1

Setting	:	Community
Country	:	Chile
Intervention	:	IEC campaign and training of health professionals
Sponsoring institution/ organization	:	The Lambda Centre (A CBO)

A project initiated in 1995 by the Lambda Centre, a gay association in Santiago, *Chile* in collaboration with other non-governmental organizations (NGOs) and some universities intended to address the high incidence of HIV infection amongst homosexually active men who then accounted for 82 per cent of all sexually transmitted HIV infections. Homosexual behaviour is a criminal offence in Chile and the political climate up until democratization in 1990 has made work with gay men difficult in

Chile. Nonetheless, a series of workshops with gay-identified men were held to encourage open discussion and encourage the development of social networks, alongside the training of health and other professionals on sexuality and discrimination issues. Posters were produced and disseminated, along with condoms and information on services. Work was carried out in terms of the defence of human rights and wider legal issues affecting gay men.

A strategy to develop a network of supportive individuals and institutions, comprising those within the public health system, was also developed. Over a five-year period, workshop content has been adapted and changed and tested out within different cultures and age groups in a variety of geographical locations. Attempts have been made to raise the profile of gay communities through their participation in public activities like World AIDS Day events, Gay Pride marches and candlelight memorials. A strategy to raise awareness within the public health system was employed to make care and support programmes more appropriate and accessible to MSM. This comprised the training of health workers on issues of sexuality and homosexuality. Other activities comprised the distribution of condoms, information leaflets and advice on where good-quality HIV counselling and testing services were available. Besides, work has been carried out in relation to the defence of human rights and wider legal issues affecting gay men.

Process evaluations were undertaken at each of the workshop sessions using an open-ended questionnaire format. The outcomes of this evaluation recognised a felt need among gay men for social forums where they can communicate openly on issues affecting them, and derive support for the difficulties they face. Evaluation data were also collected to assess the extent and scope of the work. Between 1995 and 1997, 172 activities were implemented with 1,576 people in seven Chilean cities. Groundwork has been laid for the development of a more systematic approach to HIV prevention for men who have sex with men, which can be consolidated upon and expanded in the future. The project has been specially innovative given the prevailing political climate, with gay organizations taking the lead in lobbying for changes in health care services, legal, civil and human rights and approaches towards homosexuality.

MSM Case Study 2

Setting	: Community
Country	: Jamaica
Intervention	: Counselling, education and outreach activities
Sponsoring institution/ organization	: Jamaica AIDS Support (an NGO)

A project was designed and implemented by *Jamaica* AIDS Support (JAS), a non-governmental volunteer-based support and education group for men who have sex with men (MSM). Widespread discrimination against MSM has made it difficult to implement HIV prevention work in Jamaica, and as men with HIV became unwell, very limited support has been available for them and their families. The main purpose of the outreach and risk reduction project was to increase JAS's capacity to support risk reduction among MSM in three discrete geographical areas. Comprising 80 volunteers, JAS met weekly and held educational outreach events and provided support to people living with HIV/ AIDS. Peer counselling was undertaken to promote self-esteem, a positive approach towards sexual health, and lasting behavioural change. Peer counsellors provided education to men who have sex with men and to their families, comprising 24-hour support for families of people living with AIDS.

Regular support group meetings have explored topics like safer sex, gay relationships, prostitution, education, homophobia and strengthening the gay community. Long-term counselling and support services for people living with HIV/AIDS have comprised telephone counselling and, importantly, the provision of home-based and hospice care at the 'Life' hospice established by JAS with financial support from their funders AIDSCAP. Monthly special events comprised parties, which featured safer sex skits and information booths. Condoms were distributed free of charge along with information leaflets and educational materials. Workshops were organised with drag performers to help them improve their ability to relay prevention messages through art.

Up until August 1998, a total of 106 support group meetings were organised nationally, and several more subgroups have met to discuss issues more intimately. A peer-counselling network has now been expanded from Kingston to two other cities, and four additional towns have been recognized for outreach activities. A total of 149 support groups of people living with AIDS have reached 737 attendees. Two KABP surveys were made in December 1995 and August 1996 and comparisons made. Eighty-five per cent of those surveyed in 1996 now reported knowledge of prevention practices and relevant perceptions of risk of HIV infection. A 40 per cent increase in the use of condoms and a 30 per cent reduction in self-reported high-risk behaviour was reported. The project is striking in its effort to provide wide-ranging support for MSM comprising those living with HIV/AIDS. The holistic nature of the prevention education workshops and the stress on counselling and peer support has been well received by MSM. The extension of the work from Kingston to other major towns and cities demonstrates the potential transferability of this style of work. The project has grown out of a self-help community initiative and this adds to its credibility among members of the target group.

MSM Case Study 3

Setting	:	Prisons
Country	:	Costa Rica
Intervention	:	Condom promotion and counselling
Sponsoring institution/ organization	:	ILPES (an NGO) with the support of the Costa Rican Ministry of Justice

The Instituto Latinoamericano de Prevencion y Educacion en Salud (ILPES) established a programme with men who have sex with men in *Costa Rican* prisons. In 1990, a study conducted among inmates of La Reforma Correctional Centre, the country's largest penitentiary, revealed a high proportion of HIV infection. No explicit policy on prison-based prevention measures had been formulated despite general recognition of the fact that sexual activity is common among inmates. Earlier there were no HIV awareness programmes directed towards the prison population, and access to HIV antibody tests was limited. In 1992, ILPES, in collaboration with the Ministry of Justice, initiated developing a Holistic AIDS Prevention Programme for inmates of Costa Rican correctional facilities. The central objective of this work has been to encourage changes in attitude towards HIV/AIDS on the part of inmates, but the approach also addressed the attitudes of correctional personnel. HIV prevention workshops were designed to explore and focus upon the several factors that contribute to or inhibit HIV prevention within prisons. To date, these have included work on power; AIDS and safe sex; anger management; sexuality, self-esteem; alcoholism and substance abuse; and holistic health.

Workshops use a participatory methodology in which all members take part on equal terms with one another, devising among themselves a system, of horizontal communication through such tools as games, exercises, role-play and meditation. Workshops have also been organised with prison personnel to increase awareness of HIV/AIDS related issues.

Evaluation, made during 1995, stressed on the outcomes of workshops for prison inmates. By this time, a total of 453 prisoners had participated in the programme and almost all the country's correctional facilities had taken part. A total of 188 individuals who took part in the programme during the first six months of 1995 were chosen to participate in the evaluation. A questionnaire was given to each of them before and after the experience, and changes in responses were systematically recorded. The percentage of inmates who proved knowledgeable about HIV/AIDS increased from 69 per cent before the intervention to 79 per cent post-intervention. Besides, the ability of respondents to communicate effectively with their sexual partners was reportedly increased by the workshops. There was a rise in the proportion of respondents who felt able to tell their partner what they liked from 56 per cent to 66 per cent, and a fall in the number of participants who stated that they never communicate with their partner about sexual preferences from 24 per cent to 12 per cent. In relations to condom use and attitudes towards condoms, the proportion of respondents who never used condoms decreased from 51 per cent to 36 per cent, and the number of respondents indicating that they found condoms enjoyable to use rose from 8 per cent to 19 per cent. The holistic workshops had an important effect on helping inmates feel better about themselves and as a consequence, a marked improvement in the social atmosphere in the prisons was observed. The uniqueness of conducting a project of this nature within state correctional services, mainly through a process of NGO/governmental collaboration should be noted.

MSM Case Study 4

Setting	:	Community
Country	:	Bangladesh
Intervention	:	Condom promotion and counselling
Sponsoring institution/ organization	:	The Bandhu Social Welfare Society (an NGO)

The Bandhu Social Welfare Society in Dhaka, *Bangladesh*, began its community-based work in October 1997. MSM are central to the project management and service provision. First ethnographic study, together with a risk and requirements assessment, was carried out in order to build a clearer profile of male-to-male sex networks. The programme was then designed on the ground of these findings. Primarily, the project is intended to develop and strengthen informal, friendship networks outside of the sexual environment. These are then used to address social concerns such as harassment and police victimization and other personal concerns that the men experience.

Outreach activities comprised an interactive approach to promoting condoms, encouraging discussion and sharing of experiences; the social marketing of condoms, ensuring referral; to sensitive and appropriate STD treatment services; and networking with women's sexual health agencies so as to build proper referrals for female partners. By providing opportunities for the men to explore other expressed interests like dance, fashion design, learning English and vernacular literacy skills, the project aims to enhance its acceptability and encourage longer-term attachment on the part of members of the target group. Since the project is still comparatively new, evaluation to date has largely involved monitoring of service provision and usage. Between October 1997 and January 1998, the Bandhu project received a total number of 960 visits (12 group meetings and 500 individual visits). Over 4,500 condoms were disseminated and 1,900 contacts established at public sex environments. Overall, there are conspicuous indications that a socializing/community building/friendship framework is more effective in this context than a more traditional peer education model.

Various aspects of the project's work have been important to its early success. The fact that the project is beneficiary-led is significant, affording it a high degree of acceptability and ensuring an ethical base for project activities. Similar projects employing this model of intervention have now been setup in Lucknow and in New Delhi. This demonstrates the project's transferability to other regional contexts. The holistic approach adopted, with the stress on developing extensive social and support networks, offers a non-clinical style of intervention and acknowledges the wider concerns of the target group. Outreach work, with its stress on friendship building rather than on condom distribution, is an approach that is well received by the target group. HIV/AIDS is still considered to be of relatively low significance, compared with other priority concerns of MSM including family, marriage, employment, income and harassment.

MSM Case Study 5

Setting	: Community
Country	: South Africa
Intervention	: Telephone service
Sponsoring institution/ organization	: Triangle Project (an NGO)

A project which has existed in different guises for the past 15 years, and which is now called the Triangle Project, works to meet the education and support needs of gay men in Cape Town, *South Africa*. The primary assumption of the project is that men are better prepared to protect themselves and partners in the context of HIV if they have a strong gay identity. To this end, the project works not only with gay men, but also efforts to address homophobia within the wider community, as well as to create safer and more accessible health and school environments and provide support and counselling services. A baseline requires analysis for gay men was carried out initially. Printed information was developed and distributed along with condoms and lubricants in bars and clubs. Outreach education on safer sex and empowerment was undertaken in the form of participatory workshops in bars, clubs and other gay venues. Counselling services were provided by telephone and face-to-face by a team of trained volunteers.

The project trains external groups such as teachers and nurses on issues related to homosexuality. More recently, training has been provided to counterpart agencies elsewhere in Southern Africa (such as GALZ in Zimbabwe). There is a strong focus on training volunteers with a view to expand the capacity of the organization to address the needs of gay men. The project is currently completing focus group research examining issues of sexual identity, self-esteem, health-seeking and risk-taking behaviours.

Between June 1997 and June 1998, 236,200 condoms were distributed at urban, township and cruising venues, along with 30,000 sachets of lubricant. Thirty-seven thousand leaflets on safer sex, alcohol and drug use, relationships, 'coming out', STDs and hepatitis B have been produced and distributed. A large variety of people have been given training on issues such as safer sex and attitudes towards homosexuality. Post-course workshop evaluations indicate enhanced knowledge and changed attitudes. Participants report valuing the non-didactic and non-prescriptive approach adopted during workshops. The project team is now in the process of developing and applying more systematic evaluation models. The project's focus on challenging negative attitudes to homosexuality has led to improvements in health service delivery and in education. Through nurturing a strong gay identity, the project has enhanced the accessibility of HIV prevention, education and support services to gay men in South Africa. However, government funding was curtailed by 90 per cent in 1997 when prevention of HIV within the heterosexual population was designated a priority.

What Works With Sex Workers and Their Clients?

Early in the epidemic, sex workers were identified as a key group to involve in HIV-prevention work. However, sex workers have been difficult to fully involve in HIV prevention, because the illegality of prostitution in many countries means that women and men who exchange sex for money may not always be visible or accessible. Sex work is also highly stigmatized in several societies and, in early reports about AIDS, the mass media often presented sex workers unhelpfully as 'conduits of infection' rather than as individuals who might be especially vulnerable and/or who have a key role to play in HIV prevention.

In developing world, most female sex workers are characteristically poor, without formal education and relatively powerless. Generally, individuals engage in sex work to determine their own economic survival and, in many cases, that of their children and other family members. Rural to urban migration in many developing countries ensures both a large number of sex workers in cities and a ready clientele. Many of the clients of sex workers are men who have left their families behind to seek work in large cities. In some cultural contexts, sex before or outside of marriage regularly involves the exchange of money or goods. Importantly, existing HIV preventing programmes have rarely focused on the male clients of sex workers.

Sex workers are generally highly mobile, making grassroots organization and HIV-preventive programming difficult. Additionally, while many sex workers do, or would intend to, use condoms, the largely illicit and sometimes illegal nature of sex work enhances vulnerability. In contexts where soliciting for clients is illegal, carrying a large number of condoms may lead to arrest and fines. Likewise, the hidden nature of sex work may render sex workers vulnerable to rape and sexual coercion.

In prevention planning and programming it must be kept in view that sex workers, like other groups, are far from homogeneous. They comprise women and men, those who identify as gay or bisexual, and young people, who may be comparatively powerless and particularly vulnerable to exploitation and injecting drug users. There are a variety of contexts in which sex work takes place: for instance, in brothels, bars, on the streets and through broker-mediated encounters.

Sex Workers Case Study 1

Setting	:	Community: male sex workers
Country	:	Morocco
Intervention	:	Peer education and outreach
Sponsoring institution/ organization	:	Association de Lutte contre le SIDA (an NGO)

The Association de Lutte contre le SIDA (ALCS) developed a project to focus on male sex workers in covert settings in Casablanca and Marrakesh in *Morocco*. The overall aim was to minimize the risks of STDs and HIV infection among male sex workers, their clients and their clients' partners. The project is also intended to meet the wider care and support needs of socially marginalized sex workers.

Between 1993 and 1994, observations and interviews were carried out with members of the target group in Casablanca and Marrakesh. In 1995, a structured behavioural survey was conducted with a sample of 172 men to give baseline data for the intervention. Peer outreach workers were then recruited and trained. The outreach workers began by making regular contacts at venues (around three times a week during 1995 in Casablanca) with male sex workers. They gave peer education and counselling, condoms, and referrals to local health services for STD diagnosis and treatment and HIV counselling and testing. A drop-in service was established along with a telephone hotline and discussion group. The project has begun to establish contacts in other cities where men are involved in sex work such as Tangier and Agadir.

In collaboration with WHO, an initial baseline evaluation was conducted in 1995 using questionnaires, interviews and a review of existing data. Behavioural change was measured by making comparisons with data collected earlier in 1993-1994. Extra process indicators provided data on the number of outreach contacts, the number and type of referrals, numbers of condoms distributed, etc. In relation to the acceptability of the project and the strategies employed, respondents had a positive attitude towards the outreach work and valued the opportunity to discuss issues concerned to sexual behaviour, health and HIV/AIDS. Ninety-three per cent of those surveyed preferred to access condoms though outreach workers rather than through more conventional sources. Increases in the numbers of men seeking voluntary counselling and testing were noted. Seventeen thousand individual contacts were made in a 10 months in 1995, reaching an estimated 530 persons (84 per cent of these engaged in sex work). Within a short period of time, reported regular use of condoms has increased. Detailed baseline research prior to the intervention, by interviewers who were related to the milieu of the target group, has confirmed the existence of situations of HIV/AIDS risk and vulnerability. The project has managed to set a precedent both within the country and the North African region in demonstrating the possibility of successful outreach HIV prevention work with marginalized and clandestine populations.

Sex Workers Case Study 2

Setting	:	Sex workers
Country	:	Venezuela
Intervention	:	Peer education
Sponsoring institution/ organization	:	Asociacion de Mujeres por el Bienestar y Asistencia Reciproca (an NGO)

A project implemented by the Asociacion de Mujeres por el Bienestar y Asistencia Reciproca (AMBAR) in Caracas, *Venezuela* intended to improve the quality of life of female sex workers through strategies which protect their health and at the same time guarantee their human and civil rights. In the beginning, a group of 40 sex workers were recruited to be trained as health promoters. Inclusion criteria used to identify potential health promoters comprised credibility and respect among their peers. After training, the women will be able to provide education on human rights, self-esteem, sexuality and reproductive health, prevention of STD/HIV and the effective use of condoms. Materials such as posters, leaflets and bulletins were distributed in establishments and public places frequented by sex workers. A manual and set of visual training materials have also been produced for use by peer health promoters when conducting talks and workshops. Outreach work is carried out both at working sites and at STD health services. Managers and the owners of clubs, hotels and bars where sex work takes place have participated in the project by assisting in the social marketing of condoms and the distribution of information. Weekly meetings have been held with health promoters to plan the peer education work, along with supervision and support sessions. Every Tuesday, free condoms have been distributed from AMBAR headquarters to sex workers who did partake in the promotion activities. Legal and psychological consultations have been made available alongside a programme to ensure that claims of violations of human rights brought forward by sex workers are channelled through organizations competent to deal with them effectively.

When the project began in 1995, 13,000 sex workers were registered with the Ministry of Health and Social Services. Later on, a register of 25,000 women using health and support services was established. Not a single case of HIV infection has been reported among those in contact with the project since 1995. Every Tuesday, a huge number of sex workers come to AMBAR headquarters to receive free condoms and to participate in educational activities. Police harassment has decreased as a result of the complaints processed by AMBAR. The social marketing of condoms has been a success, with sex workers assuming control of the market, and owners and managers selling condoms in their setup at affordable prices. Through successfully tackling human rights and health concerns, the project has gained a high degree of acceptance, verified by the extent of participation in the intervention. The project has achieved its goal of improving the quality of life of women involved in sex work and has considerably reduced the risk of HIV infection.

Sex Workers Case Study 3

Setting	: Community: sex workers
Country	: Cameroon
Intervention	: Peer outreach in urban areas
Sponsoring institution/ organization	: AIDSCAP

Between 1993 and 1996, AIDSCAP supported a project for sex workers and their clients in six urban areas of *Cameroon*. Trained peer educators worked in pairs to give weekly education sessions in bars, brothels, STD clinics, neighbourhoods and other sites where people were known to practise high-risk sexual behaviours. Moreover, educational sessions were held in prisons on request. Sex workers distributed condoms free of charge as a promotional activity and then sold condoms to peers and clients once demand had been established. A theatre group included sex workers performed interactive and humorous dramas at outreach venues where sex workers and their clients meet. Between 1993 and 1996, 200 peer educators and coordinators were trained and in turn conducted more than 5,000 education sessions in community and clinic-based settings. An estimated 5000,000 contacts were made through educational sessions comprising 52 workshops held at the central prison of Yaounde. Evaluation of the outcomes and impact of the activities has been conducted through baseline and follow-up KABP surveys collecting both quantitative and qualitative data. At baseline, information was elicited from 800 sex workers, 800 clients and 200 people being treated for STDs. Follow-up data were gathered from 818 sex workers and 661 clients.

The percentage of the target population able to recognise at least two means of HIV prevention rose from 40.2 per cent (sex workers) and 49.8 per cent (clients) at base line, to 85.6 per cent and 85.6 per cent respectively at follow-up. There was a decrease of 10-20 percentage points in the proportion of the target population reporting an STD in the three months immediately preceding the follow-up survey, coupled with an increase by 10 percentage points in the number having access to proper treatment for their last STD. The percentage of sex workers reporting having ever used a condom rose steadily from 28.3 per cent in 1988, to 88 per cent in 1996. Among clients, this percentage increased from 55.5 per cent in 1990, to 81 per cent 1996. Consistent condom use by sex workers with non-regular clients rose from 52 per cent in 1994, to 75 per cent in 1996.

A comprehensive assessment of the work already carried out during the preceding phase permitted this project to build on the strengths of an existing programme. As a result, project activities have been sustained over a substantial period of time, and the potential impact of the intervention has been maximized. Using drama as the chief means of HIV prevention communication has made it feasible to reach many people in an entertaining way within settings where they are most likely to engage in high-risk sexual behaviour. Sex workers have proved highly successful in the effective marketing of condoms. Indeed, the sale of condoms has become the chief source of income for some women who are now wholesalers.

Sex Workers Case Study 4

Setting	:	Community
Country	:	Papua New Guinea
Intervention	:	Outreach
Sponsoring institution/ organization	:	Papua New Guinea Institute of Medical Research

Research by the *Papua New Guinea* Institute of Medical Research in the early 1990s established that sex workers and their clients, mostly transport workers, were particularly vulnerable to HIV infection. In 1994, an ethnographical situation assessment was undertaken with transport workers and the women that sell them sex. Outreach work began even during the initial baseline surveys when informants were given potent information of HIV/AIDS, provided with condoms and shown how to use them. Training modules were developed and produced for sex workers and each of the target client groups. Workplace policy workshops were held with shipping firms, police, security firms and trucking firms with a view to secure their support.

Activities were designed to reduce the incidence of police 'line-ups' or group rape sessions to which sex workers in custody were subjected. Outreach work was undertaken with truck drivers at rest stops and through workplace training sessions, and with sailors and dock workers on wharves and aboard ships. A clinic providing confidential STD services for sex workers was established in Port Moresby. In Lae, sex workers could receive HIV testing and counselling at the project site, followed up, if necessary, with referral to local clinics for STD treatment. Theatre and music groups attached to the project also helped disseminate HIV/AIDS prevention messages. In addition to, a drop-in centre provided literacy and vocational training by the YWCA. A telephone Hotline provided counselling services for sex workers and clients. Formative research and ongoing monitoring have given some clear indicators of success to date. By mid- 1998, in Port Moresby 403 peer educators had completed their training. This corn 75 sex workers, 36 policemen, 16 policewomen, 14 wives of policemen, 20 security men, 163 sailors (from 24 ships), 65 dock workers and 14 hotel workers. In Lae, by March 1997 a total of 125 peer educators had been trained including sex workers, dock workers, sailors and truckers. Among sex workers, quantitative proof for increased condom use can be found in the progressive stages of baseline data denoting a rapid increase in condom use from the point at which the project was started.

Attempts to reduce the incidence of line-ups have been successful, with reported involvement by police officers in a line-up during the previous week being reduced from 10 per cent pre-intervention, to 4.2 per cent post-intervention. Additionally, the first successful prosecutions of police officers involved have occurred and the incidence of sexual harassment reported by sex workers has diminished. Demand for condoms has been steadily rising and in Port Moresby five condom depots have been set up on the wharves. During 1996-1997, between 1.5 and 2 million male condoms and 5,000 female condoms were distributed.

Extensive formative research on the real contexts of risk-taking in vulnerable groups has given guidance for the overall development of the project. The extent of involvement by a wide range of agencies is unique and was achieved by encouraging the highest level of participation in the project by a diverse range of concerned agencies, at every stage of its development. Addressing the human rights of sex workers has been of paramount significance.

Two

The Genesis of UNAIDS

The dire consequences of growing HIV/AIDS on societies has become clear by now, so there is a greater need for an intensive response. It was to strengthen the contribution of the United Nations system in the fight against AIDS by better coordination of its efforts and a stronger, more unified voice, that UNAIDS was established and began operations in January 1996 as the HIV/AIDS programme of six UN agencies. The partners in this pioneering effort at a joint response within the United Nations are the United Nations Children's Fund (UNICEF), the United Nations Development Programme (UNDP), the United Nations Educational, Scientific and Cultural Organization (UNESCO), the United Nations Population Fund (UNFPA), the World Health Organization (WHO) and the World Bank.

UNAIDS' mission, as the main advocate for global action on HIV/AIDS, is to lead, strengthen and support an expanded response aimed at preventing the transmission of HIV, providing care and support, reducing the vulnerability of individuals and communities to HIV/AIDS, and alleviating the impact of the epidemic.

Mother-to-Child Transmission (MTCT) of HIV

More than 4 million children below 15 years in age have become infected with HIV as the AIDS epidemic began, and more than 3 million of them have already died of AIDS. The huge majority of infected children get the virus from their mothers. Though Africa accounts for only 10 per cent of the world's population, to date around nine out of ten of all HIV-infected babies have been born in that region, largely as a result of high fertility rates combined with very high infection rates. In urban centres in southern Africa, for instance, rates of HIV infection of 20-30 per cent among pregnant women tested anonymously at antenatal clinics are common. Rates of 59 per cent and even 70 per cent have been recorded in different parts of Zimbabwe, and 43 per cent in Botswana. As there is a data from UNAIDS, there are very few places outside sub-Saharan Africa in which the existence of HIV infection among pregnant women has even reached 10 per cent, let alone the extremely high figures seen in this region. However, this is partly because the epidemic in other badly affected countries is younger and less advanced than in sub-Saharan Africa, so there is no room for complacency.

What are the Risks?

Following the lack of preventive measures, the risk of a baby acquiring the virus from an infected mother varies from 15 per cent to 25 per cent in industrialized countries, and from 25 per cent to 35 per cent in developing countries. The difference is mainly due to feeding practices: breastfeeding, now known to be a significant source of infection, is more common and generally practised for a longer period in developing countries than in the industrial world. Evidence suggests that the risk of Mother-to-Child Transmission (MTCT) is enhanced if the mother is newly infected with HIV, or is in an advanced stage of disease, or if the baby is highly exposed to her infected body fluids during birth.

During pregnancy child birth or breastfeeding the virus can be transmitted to the infant. It has recently been established that, among infected babies who are not breastfed, about one-third acquire the virus while still in the uterus and most commonly during the last three months of pregnancy. The other two-thirds become infected near the time of delivery. In populations where breastfeeding is the norm, however, infected breast milk may account for up to one-third of al! cases of MTCT.

Until very recently we knew of no way to minimize HIV-positive pregnant woman passing the virus on to her baby if she intended to give birth. But that is no longer the case. Scientific research has enhanced our understanding of this route of transmission considerably in recent years and offered a number of strategies for prevention.

The Breastfeeding Dilemma

Promotion of breastfeeding as the best feasible nutrition for infants has been the cornerstone of child health and survival strategies for the past 20 years, and has played a significant part in lowering infant mortality in many regions of the world. Therefore the evidence that has accrued over recent years that breast milk is an important source of HIV infection has caused real dilemmas for mothers, for the health personnel who advise and support them, and for policy-makers.

The cost of infant formula is often beyond the means of poor families in developing countries. Moreover, many lack easy access to the clean water and fuel needed to prepare replacement feeds safely. If used incorrectly - mixed with dirty unboiled water, for instance - a breast milk substitute can cause infections, malnutrition and death. But even if a mother has the means to feed her baby safely with a breast milk substitute, she may face other dilemmas. In cultures where breastfeeding is the norm, the very fact that she chooses not to breastfeed may draw attention to her HIV status and invite discrimination or even violence and abandonment by her family and community. For health care workers and policy-makers a further dilemma is how to make infant formula available to the small minority of women and babies who require it without undermining commitment to breastfeeding more generally, thus threatening the health and survival of many more children.

In August 1997, WHO, UNICEF and UNAIDS issued a joint Policy Statement on HIV and infant feeding. This takes account of the latest scientific proof of transmission via breast milk and promotes informed choice of infant feeding methods for HIV-positive mothers. The Policy Statement was followed in early 1998 by two complementary documents offering detailed guidelines for policy-makers and for health care workers on HIV and infant feeding. The guidelines stress that the provision of information and counselling on HIV and infant feeding should be part of an integrated package of care for all pregnant and lactating women. They stress too, that it is the individual mother's right ultimately to decide how she will feed her child, and she should be given adequate support for the course of action she chooses. Coercion, no matter what the circumstances or motives, is an abuse of her human rights.

What are the Options for Preventing MTCT?

The risk of MTCT of HIV can be minimized by mothers who know they are infected choosing an alternative to breastfeeding for their babies, reckoning on the two-to-one chance that the newborn infant is not already infected.

One study in Thailand showed, for instance, that this strategy alone reduced the rate of MTCT in a sample of 199 infected women to 18 per cent, compared with the "norm" for developing world of 25-35 per cent. But since 1994 there has been another strategy available for preventing MTCT, which includs is the use of the Antiretroviral (ARV) drug Zidovudine (ZDV, also known as AZT). The strategy was evolved by French and American scientists who found that when ZDV is given to HIV-positive women orally from the 14th week of pregnancy onwards and intravenously during labour, and to their infants for six weeks after birth, the risk of transmitting HIV from mother to child is minimized by over two-thirds if breastfeeding is strictly avoided. The strategy is now utilized routinely in the industrialized world. However, the regimen costs an average US$ 1,000 per mother/child pair and is complexed to administer, which means it is not suitable for widespread use in developing countries.

Early in 1998, trials in Thailand sponsored by the country's Ministry of Health and the US Centers for Disease Control and Prevention displayed that a shorter and simpler course of ARV drugs is able to cut MTCT by at least half if the baby is not breastfed. The treatment is provided to the mother only and consists of 300mg of ZDV taken by mouth twice daily from the 36th week of pregnancy and during labour. The cost of the drugs alone for each mother/child pair in the Thai trial was around US$ 50.

As part of these endeavours research is currently being conducted to test the effectiveness of an even shorter ARV regimen, using two drugs in combination. The PETRA study, as it is known, is supported by WHO and UNAIDS and started in 1995 in South Africa, Tanzania and Uganda.

So far, the success in minimizing MTCT using ARV drugs has only been demonstrated when breastfeeding is strictly avoided. No-one knows how effective the strategy might be if mothers do breastfeed their babies. It is critical that this issue be resolved as quickly as feasible since the majority of HIV-positive women who risk transmitting the virus to their infants come from cultures where breastfeeding is the norm, and where artificial feeding often presents great problems. Research is being carried out in a number of countries and results are due shortly. Preliminary results of this and other studies point to a limited efficacy in breastfed infants tested at six months of age.

From Research to General Practice

For ARV regimens to be introduced certain services have to be already in place. These include Voluntary Counselling and Testing (VCT) and good quality mother and child health services. All pregnant women must have ready access to antenatal and postnatal care and be able to give birth in a maternity ward or clinic with professional assistance, since skilled supervision of treatment is necessary. Other prerequisites are efficient systems of quality control, supply and distribution of drugs, and laboratory facilities with adequate capacity and skills. In reality, many countries are nowhere near able to meet these conditions. Some 40 per cent of the world's women lack access to adequate antenatal care. In sub-Saharan Africa, less than half of all births are attended by professional health staff, with proportions well below this being reported from individual African countries as well as from parts of Asia. Moreover, the proportion of people without access to health care at all ranges from over 40 per cent in some parts of Latin America and Asia to nearly 80 per cent in the poorest parts of Africa.

This represents a huge challenge for those committed to seeing that mothers and babies everywhere benefit from advances in science and technology. When results from the Thai study came in, UNAIDS, together with UNFPA, UNICEF and WHO, convened an international meeting in May 1998 to discuss how to promote the widescale adoption of strategies to reduce MTCT of HIV, and, crucially, what kind of support countries would need in order to set up programmes. Mechanisms are now being developed and put in place to mobilize resources, share information and lay the necessary foundations at national level. In addition, a number of documents discussing in detail the strategies for MTCT prevention have been prepared.

A package of measures developed by UNAIDS and its partners is being piloted in around 14 countries. The package comprises:

- measures to prevent HIV infection in women of child bearing age;
- measures for the prevention of unwanted pregnancies;
- VCT + ARV + replacement feeding.

Voluntary Counselling and Testing

The two most important interventions for the reduction of MTCT - avoidance of breastfeeding and antiretroviral programmes - require a woman to know whether or not she is HIV-infected. This means having access to Voluntary Counselling and Testing (VCT) facilities. Yet, at present, such facilities are scarce in developing countries where they are needed most. Ideally everyone should have access to VCT since advances in knowledge and understanding of HIV have greatly increased the benefits of knowing one's serostatus. People who know they are HIV-infected are likely to be motivated to look after their health, perhaps with behaviour and lifestyle changes, and to seek early medical attention for problems. They can make informed decisions about sexual practices and childbearing, including seeking abortion where this is desired and legal. Mothers can make informed decisions about infant feeding, and about seeking care for sick children without delay, and those whose test results are negative can be counselled about how to protect themselves, and their children, from infection. Furthermore, infected individuals can take steps to protect partners who may still be uninfected.

Since the primary purpose of VCT is to encourage informed decision-making and behaviour, it is very important that individuals have ready access to the relevant services. These include family planning services for those women or couples who wish to avoid or postpone pregnancy, or practice safe sex during pregnancy and lactation; abortion services, if legal, for those who choose to terminate a pregnancy; mother and child health and other health care and support services for HIV-positive people.

Experience to date in many countries shows great variation in willingness to make use of the VCT services that are available.

For example, a significant proportion of women who accept an HIV test during antenatal care fail to return for the results. The fear of stigma and discrimination if they test positive undoubtedly deters people - and has proved all too tragically realistic in a number of cases, where infected people have been rejected and even killed by their communities. However, this is only part of the picture and intensive research is being undertaken, especially in Africa, to identify the full range of factors that influence decisions to take an HIV test and what is needed to overcome resistance.

In 1997 UNAIDS issued a policy statement on HIV counselling and testing which endorses the value of this service as a critical part of an effective response to HIV/AIDS, and sets down the guiding principles. UNAIDS promotes the establishment of VCT services everywhere, offers technical assistance, and is currently supporting pilot projects in selected countries.

Odds Stacked Against Women

What is "gender"?

Whereas sex is biological, gender is socially defined. Gender is what it means to be male or female, and how that defines a person's opportunities, roles, responsibilities and relationships.

A person's gender is one of the most powerful factors of individual risk. Gender biases affect both sexes, and in a multitude of ways. In all its activities UNAIDS takes the broad definition of gender. However, our chief focus here is on the risks and vulnerability related to being female.

The factors that put girls and women at special risk from HIV are both biological and social. The risk of becoming infected with HIV during unprotected vaginal intercourse is two to four times higher for a woman than a man. Male-to-female transmission is more successful because, during vaginal intercourse, a woman has a bigger surface area of mucosa (the membranes lining the genital tract) exposed to her partners's sexual secretions than does a man. Furthermore, there is often a higher concentration of HIV in semen than in the sexual secretions of a woman. Age is also significant. The immature genital tract and scant vaginal secretions of young women put them at even greater risk than mature women as they provide less of a barrier to HIV. And there is evidence that the more fragile genital membranes and reduced vaginal secretions of postmenopausal women increase their vulnerability to HIV also.

Compounding women's biological vulnerability to HIV infection is a lot of cultural, legal and economic factors that put them at special risk. In many societies girls face discrimination from birth onwards. Typically they have less access to education, information and skills training than boys, which handicaps them for life. As adults they have limited opportunity for employment; generally no right to work or to own or inherit land and property in their own names; limited access, if any, to finance for their own business ventures; and generally limited access to health care services. The low status of women makes them socially sensitive to HIV, for all these discriminatory forces limit their opportunities to be informed about the functioning of their bodies, sexuality and health, and weaken their autonomy and power to protect themselves from infection.

In several cultures it is considered indecent for a woman to take the initiative in sexual encounters. Thus, they are inhibited from seeking out information on HIV or procuring condoms themselves. And several women dare not bring up the subject of safer sex even with a regular partner for fear of a violent reaction or even abandonment by a man on whom they are totally dependent for survival. While in several societies infidelity in women is strictly and often violently censured, they are often expected to tolerate infidelity in their menfolk even though, in the AIDS era, tolerance and silence may cost them their lives. A study from Pune, India, illustrates a situation common in very different societies. Of a sample of nearly 400 women attending the city's STI clinics, 93 per cent were married and 91 per cent had never had sex with anyone but their husbands. All of these women were infected with an STI and 13.6 per cent tested positive for HIV.

Given the high social value placed on female chastity and monogamy, it is a paradox that for millions of girls and women in the world sex is the "currency" with which they are anticipated to pay for all life's opportunities, from gaining admission to overcrowded classrooms to passing exams, securing employment or a market trading licence, or even crossing a border. In all these relationships women are relied on and subordinate to men, and therefore in a weak bargaining position in the sex act.

There are approximately 960 million illiterate adults in the world, of whom two-thirds are women. Women own only 1 per cent of the world's land and receive 10 per cent of its income.

—Source: UNFPA

If a woman is a reluctant partner, the risk of damage to the genital or anal mucosa is great, following the lack of lubrication and often rough handling by the male partner. The risk of infection with HIV is heightened too. Research confirms that non-consensual sex is a pervasive fact in girls' and women's lives. In a study in Papua New Guinea, for instance, half the young women questioned said they had been forced to have sex, often violently. A study in Malawi made very resemble findings, and in Nigeria one young woman in five questioned by researchers reported coercion. Cultural practices like female genital mutilation may also increase the risk of HIV transmission through trauma and tearing in the process of sexual intercourse. Currently, according to UNFPA, some 130 million women across the world are living with the consequences of this practice, and an estimated 2 million little girls are newly subjected to it each year.

Prostitution constitutes another situation in which women are unusually sensitive to HIV infection, yet for multitudes of women without skills or resources, it offers the best opportunity for making a living. Sex workers may have less knowledge about HIV and how to protect themselves. But even if well informed they may find it hard to stress on safe sexual practices for fear of violence, or fear that an unwilling client will take his business elsewhere. Furthermore, prostitution is illegal in various places and simply carrying condoms can be taken by police as testimony of sex work. Prostitution's illegal status often drives it into the shadows and makes it hard to approach vulnerable people with life-saving information and supplies. Among the most powerless and vulnerable people in the world are children and women forced into the sex trade by traffickers, for they have multiple sex partners and no autonomy whatsoever. As UNFPA says, an estimated 2 million girls aged 5-15 may be forced worldwide each year.

AIDS presents women with another dilemma in their sexual relationships. Safer sex - in particular the practice of condoms is incompatible with pregnancy, and those who wish a child and yet who believe they are at risk of contracting HIV therefore face painful choices. In some societies a woman's social status, and probably even survival, depends on bearing children, and where personal wish and social pressure coincide with very high levels of HIV infection, the choice for women is mainly cruel.

A Gender-Sensitive Response

Since its inception from 1996, UNAIDS has been committed to gender-sensitivity in all its policies and programmes, and to developing awareness of the paramount importance of this among all players in the field. UNAIDS believes that a gender-sensitive response must take into account the factors that increase women's risk and their vulnerability. Often this calls for fundamental social change, comprising the empowerment of women at the household, community and national levels. A key objective must be to engage men as partners in social transformation. Furthermore, gender and AIDS require to become mainstream concerns in the programmes of governments and non-governmental organizations in all the countries of the world.

Young People and HIV/AIDS

"The future of the HIV epidemic lies in the hands of young people. The behaviours they follow now and those they maintain throughout their sexual lives will condition the course of the epidemic for decades to come. Young people will continue to learn from one another, but their behaviour will base largely on the information, skills and services that the current generation of adults choose to equip their children with."

—AIDS Epidemic Update; December 1998

UNAIDS has estimated that every minute of every day, five young women and men are becoming newly infected with HIV. Worldwide, near about half of all new HIV infections today are in young people aged 10-25 years, and in the badly-affected countries the proportion is even greater, exceeding 60 per cent in some places. This grim statistic mentions the fact that, in advanced epidemics where there is a high prevalence of HIV in the general population, new infections become increasingly concentrated among young people since they run the risk of coming into contact with an HIV-positive partner almost as soon as they become sexually active. A study in Malawi, for instance, found that the annual rate of infection in teenage girls was six times higher than in women over 35 years.

In sub-Saharan Africa and Asia the virus is spread predominantly through heterosexual intercourse, whereas in Latin America the important route of transmission is sex between men, and in Eastern Europe it is needle-sharing between drug users. In places where the epidemic is heterosexually driven, young women are generally disproportionately affected, for reasons already discussed. Thus, studies sponsored by UNAIDS and its partners show that in western Kenya near about one girl in four between the ages of 15 and 19 years is living with HIV, compared with one in 25 boys in the same age group. In Zambia in this age period, 16 times as many girls as boys are infected. And in rural Uganda among 20-24 year olds, there are six young women who are HIV-positive for every infected young man.

Very alarming rates of teenage pregnancy and of STIs give an symbol of the extent of unprotected sexual activity among young people, and therefore of their vulnerability to HIV/AIDS. Demographic and health surveys conducted in sub-Saharan Africa between 1990 and 1996 show, for instance, that nearly 70 per cent of women in Uganda, Burkina Faso and Guinea were pregnant by the age of 19, and over half the women in Benin, Cameroon, Namibia, Tanzania and Zambia also became pregnant as teenagers. As far as STIs are concerned, the under 25 year olds account for around half of the 333 million new cases per year. Fortunately, several of these infections are easy to cure (for those young people with access to affordable youth-friendly health services), but left untreated they increase by as much as ten-fold the risk of acquiring HIV during intercourse.

Among young people, those who live on the margins of mainstream society are the most sensitive of all to HIV infection. They may be living on the streets, as orphans or fugitives from poverty-stricken or violent homes. They might be refugees or displaced people, young people growing up in urban slums, or young people segregated by prejudice and discrimination since they are homosexual in a society that refuses to accept or acknowledge homosexuality. Young people like these generally have limited access to education, services and supplies that might help them protect themselves, and their lifestyles, all too often, are loaded with risk. They may sell sex to survive, or use it to bargain for protection, a meal, a place to sleeps; or sex may give one of few opportunities for human warmth and intimacy. Violence, sexual abuse and exploitation are common experiences, and drug-taking is general part of the culture-a response to feelings of loneliness, boredom and despair.

Taking action to reduce the threat of HIV/AIDS to young people is more than a moral obligation. It is also completely necessary for halting the HIV epidemic. Experience to date illustrates that interventions for, and in partnership with, young people are among the most effective. Besides tapping into the energy and idealism of youth, such interventions advantage from the fact that young people are not yet set in their ways, and are often more willing than older generations to question social norms and change behaviour if important.

Towards a Safer World with Young People

A myriad of programmes have been set up around the world to protect the rights and meet the requirements of young people in the AIDS epidemic, and various lessons have been learned about what makes for success. It is very important, for instance, that young people be full and active partners, rather than passive recipients of programmes designed and run by adults. They should be involved at all stages of an HIV/AIDS programme, from the conceptualization and planning, to the running and monitoring of activities. This makes sure that it is truly relevant to their requirements while profiting at the same time from the energy and enthusiasm of youth, building their confidence and self-esteem, and promoting communication and mutual respect between the generations.

Building a safer world with young people means stressing on the individual to try to influence behaviour, as well as on the social context in which personal decisions are made and acted upon. It needs that young people be equipped with the knowledge, life skills and services they require to adopt healthy behaviour, resist unhealthy behaviour and protect themselves from diseases, comprising AIDS. And it needs at the same time that safe and supportive environments be created that are enabling and empowering. Such environments promote and protect human rights.

UNAIDS has always valued the rights and considered the needs of young people as a high priority. In 1998, UNAIDS, the Cosponsors and key partner organizations launched the World AIDS Day Campaign under the title "Force for Change: World AIDS Day Campaign with Young People". The intention of the 1998 campaign was to sustain the momentum of the 1997 campaign, whose basic theme was "Children Living in a World with AIDS", and to build on initiatives already taken. The 1999 campaign will build further on this foundation.

For the third regular year, the Inter-agency Working Groups on School AIDS Education and on Especially Vulnerable Young People will meet in 1999 to continue the recognition of effective policies and programmes. Furthermore, regional consultations will take place with young people, Cosponsors and youth organizations to develop further the elements of a global strategy on young people and HIV/AIDS. The background discussion paper on this topic was just welcomed by UNAIDS' Programme Coordinating Board (PCB) meeting, held in New Delhi in December 1998.

Three

AIDS and HIV Infection

United Nations
HIV/AIDS Personnel Policy
A. Information, Education and Other Preventive Health Measures

To enable the UN staff and their families to protect themselves from HIV infection and to cope with the presence of AIDS, should be provided with up to date and sufficient information.

(i) To this end, all UN bodies are encouraged to develop and implement an active staff education policy for HIV/AIDS using the handbook on AIDS for UN employees and their families produced by UNAIDS and recognising in the field local sources experienced in HIV/AIDS counselling, to give confidential follow-up.

The staff of the UN Medical Service should be fully involved in such staff education programmes. They should receive any extra professional education that may be required; and all substantial information material on HIV/AIDS, supplied and updated by UNAIDS, should be available through them at all duty stations.

(ii) All UN staff members and their families should be made aware of where safe blood may be obtained.

To complete this task, the WHO Blood Safety Unit, in cooperation with the UN Medical Service, should establish and regularly update a list of reliable and operational blood transfusion centres for circulation to UN headquarters, regional offices and duty stations. The UN Medical Service and local linked medical facilities should also make endeavours to make sure that blood transfusions are performed only when absolutely necessary.

(iii) UN Resident Coordinators must exercise their liability to adopt measures to reduce the frequency of motor vehicle accidents, not only because of their attendant high mortality and morbidity, but as they represent a particular risk for HIV infection in those localities lacking safe blood supplies. UN Resident Coordinators are, therefore, encouraged to consider the following devices for reinforcement or for general adoption if not already applied; and to circulate them to all personnel at the duty station together with instructions on the use of public transport:

- the fitting of and compulsory use of seat belts in all UN vehicles;
- adequate training in off-road use of 4-wheel drives;
- prohibition against the personal use of vehicles when an official driver is available;
- mandatory use of helmets for all riders of motorbikes;
- prohibition against substance abuse by vehicle drivers;
- organization of first-aid training sessions; and
- equipping UN vehicles with first-aid kits comprising macromolecular solutions (plasma expanders).

(iv) All UN staff members and their families should have access to disposable syringes and needles.

The UN Medical Service should make available disposable syringes and needles to staff on duty travel areas where there is no guarantee of the proper sterilization of such materials. They should be accompanied by a certificate in all UN official languages explaining the causes why they are being carried. Regional offices and other duty stations should stock disposable injection material for use by UN staff and their families. This stock required to be available at UN dispensaries, where such exist, or at the WHO duty station in the country.

(v) All UN staff members and their families should have access to condoms.

Condoms should be made available through the United Nations Population Fund (UNFPA) and/or WHO at those duty stations where there is not a reliable and regular supply of high quality condoms from the private sector. Access should be free, simple and discreet.

B. Voluntary Testing, Counselling and Confidentiality

Voluntary testing with pre-and post-counselling and assured confidentiality should be made available to all UN staff members and their families.

Adequate, proper and confidential facilities for voluntary and confirmatory testing and counselling should be provided locally to UN staff members and their families, with UN bodies acting in close collaboration with the UN Medical Service and WHO. Specific procedures must be developed by UN bodies to maintain confidentiality regarding to negative as well as positive results from an HIV test, including whether such a test has been taken. Only the person tested has the right to release information related to his/her HIV status.

C. Terms of Appointment and Service

Pre-recruitment and Employment Prospects

- The only medical criterion for recruitment is fitness to work.
- HIV infection does not, in itself, constitute a dearth of fitness of work.
- There will be no HIV screening of candidates for recruitment.
- AIDS will be treated as any other medical condition in considering medical division.
- HIV testing with the particular and informed consent of the candidate may be required if AIDS is clinically suspected.
- Nothing in the pre-employment examination should be considered as obliging any candidate to declare his or her HIV status.
- For any assignment in a country which needs HIV testing for residence, this requirement must appear in the vacancy notice.

Continuity of Employment

- HIV infection or AIDS should not be considered as a basis for termination of employment.
- If fitness to work is weakened by HIV-related illness, reasonable alternative working arrangements should be made.

- UN staff members with AIDS should enjoy health and social protection facilities in the same manner as other UN employees suffering from serious illness.
- HIV/AIDS screening, whether direct (HIV testing), indirect (assessment of risk behaviours) or asking questions about tests already taken, should not be needed.
- Confidentiality with respect to all medical information, including HIV/AIDS status, must be maintained.
- There should be no obligation on the part of the employee to inform the employer with regard to his or her HIV/AIDS status.
- Persons in the workplace affected by, or perceived to be affected by HIV/AIDS, must be protected from stigmatization and discrimination by co-workers, unions, employers or clients.
- HIV-infected employees and those with AIDS should not be discriminated against, comprising access to and receipt of advantages from statutory social security programmes and occupationally-related schemes.
- The administrative, personnel and financial essence of these principles under terms of appointment and service should be monitored and periodically reviewed.

D. Health Insurance Benefits Programmes

(i) Health insurance coverage should be available for all UN employees regardless of HIV status.
There should not be pre- or post-employment testing for HIV infection.

(ii) Health insurance premiums for UN employees should not be affected by HIV status.
No testing for HIV infection should be permitted regarding any health insurance scheme.

THE FACTS

What is AIDS?

AIDS implies for acquired immunodeficiency syndrome. It is a pattern of devastating infections caused by the human immunodeficiency virus, or HIV, which attacks and destroys particular white blood cells that are essential to the body's immune system.

When HIV infects a cell, it combines with that cell's genetic material and remain inactive for years. Most of the people infected with HIV are still healthy and can live for years with no symptoms or suffer only minor illnesses. They are infected with HIV, but they do not have AIDS.

After a good span of time, the virus becomes activated and then leads progressively to the serious infections and other conditions that characterize AIDS. Although there are treatments that can increase life span, AIDS is a fatal disease. Research continues on possible vaccines and, ultimately, a cure. For the moment, however, prevention of transmission may be the only method of control.

The Route of Infection in Adults

HIV targets two groups of white blood cells called CD4+ lymphocytes and monocytes/macrophages. Normally, CD4+ cells and macrophages aid recognize and destroy bacteria, viruses or other infectious agents that attack a cell and cause disease. In an HIV-infected person, the virus kill the CD4+ lymphocytes while the macrophages act as reservoirs, carrying HIV to a number of vital organs.

HIV attaches itself to the CD4+ lymphocyte and makes its way inside. This causes the cell to born more HIV but, in doing so, the cell is destroyed. As the body's CD4+ cells are depleted, the immune system got weak and is less able to fight off viral and bacterial infections. The infected person becomes susceptible to a wide range of "opportunistic" infections, like *Pneumocystis carinii* pneumonia, which rarely occurs in persons with normal immune systems. Tuberculosis (TB) poses a special threat to HIV-positive people, especially in areas of the world where both TB and HIV infection are increasing at higher rates. Millions of TB carriers who would otherwise have escaped active tuberculosis are now developing the disease since their immune systems are under attack from HIV. TB also progresses faster in HIV-infected persons, and is more possibly to be fatal if undiagnosed or untreated. TB is now the leading killer of HIV-infected Africans.

HIV-infected persons are also more susceptible to otherwise rare cancers like as Kaposi's sarcoma, a tumour of the blood vessels or the lymphatic vessels. HIV may also attack the brain, causing neurological and neuro-psychiatric problems.

In general, about 50 per cent of HIV-infected adults are probably to develop AIDS within 10 years after first becoming infected. The good news is that early treatment with improved drugs is considerably prolonging life for persons with AIDS.

The Route of Infection in Infants and Children

Most of the HIV-infected infants and children acquired the infection from their mothers before, during or shortly after birth, or during breastfeeding. Only a little proportion are infected through HIV-contaminated blood transfusions or injections. There are two patterns of disease progression in children infected from birth. About half these children progress rapidly to AIDS, while others remain symptom free for many years, as adults do. Studies illustrate that, in developed countries, approximately two-thirds of infected children are still alive at age 5 years. In developing world, the figure varies between 30 and 65 per cent.

How HIV is Transmitted?

To date, there are only four primary methods of transmission:

- sexual intercourse (anal and vaginal);
- contaminated blood and blood products, tissues and organs;
- contaminated needles, syringes and other piercing instruments; and
- mother-to-child transmission (MTCT).

Sexual Intercourse

HIV can be transmitted through unprotected sexual intercourse-that is, any penetrative sexual act in which a condom is not used. Anal and vaginal intercourse can transmit the virus from an HIV-infected man to a woman or to another man, or from an infected woman to a man.

The risk of becoming infected through unprotected sexual intercourse relies on four main factors: the possibility that the sex partner is infected, the type of sex act, the amount of virus present in the blood or sexual secretions (semen, vaginal or cervical secretions) of the infected partner, and the prevalence of other sexually transmitted diseases and/or genital lesions in either partner. Age may also be a determinent as young girls are physiologically more vulnerable.

The Probability of HIV Infection in the Partner

The prevalence of HIV infection among sexually active men and women varies according to geographical sphere or population subgroup, like heterosexuals, men who have sex with men (MSM), sex workers, or injecting drug users. Generally, the likelihood of becoming infected with HIV sexually is concerned to the number of sexual partners and unprotected sex acts you have. In other words, the more sexual partners you have, the greater your chance of becoming infected.

The Type of Sex Act

All unprotected acts of sexual penetration (anal, vaginal, oral) cause a risk of HIV transmission since they bring body fluids secreted during sex directly into contact with exposed mucous membranes (the lining of the rectum, the vagina, the urethra and the mouth).

- Men and women who engage in unprotected receptive anal intercourse with an HIV-infected partner involves the highest risk of becoming infected.
- The next highest risk is that associated with unprotected vaginal intercourse.
- Unprotected oral intercourse involves some risk as well, especially if there are mouth or throat injuries present such as bleeding gums, lesions, sores, abscessed teeth, throat infections, oral gonorrhoea or other STDs present.

This risk is minimized, although not entirely eliminated, by the proper use of condoms. Injury to the mucous membrane of the rectum, vagina or mouth may aid the virus enter the bloodstream. However, HIV can be transmitted even through unbroken mucous membrane.

Kissing has not been shown to transmit HIV, as saliva contains very little of the virus. Nevertheless, there is a possibility of theoretical risk of HIV transmission during deep or "wet" kissing (tongue kissing) if blood from gum or mouth sores is present in the saliva. There is no testimony that HIV has actually been transmitted this way.

Self-masturbation carries no risk of HIV transmission. There are yet no cases of transmission through mutual masturbation, either. However, masturbation of a partner involves a theoretical risk of HIV transmission if his or her sexual secretions come in contact with mucous membrane or broken skin.

The Amount of Virus Present in the Infected Partner

HIV-infected individuals become more infectious as they develop to HIV-related disease and AIDS. There is also an early one- to two-week period of infectiousness around the time of seroconversion-that is, when antibodies first develop.

The Presence of Other Sexually Transmitted Disease in Either Partner

There is a strong connection between sexually transmitted diseases (STDs) and the sexual transmission of HIV infection (3). The existence of an untreated STD-like gonorrhoea, chlamydial infection, syphilis, herpes or genital warts-can increase both the acquisition and transmission of HIV by a factor of up to 10. Thus, STD treatment is an important HIV prevention strategy in a general population.

Contaminated Blood or Blood Products, Tissues and Organs

Blood transfusions save millions of lives each year, but in places where a safe blood supply is not guaranteed, those receiving transfused blood have an increased risk of being infected with HIV.

In most of the industrialized countries, the risk of acquiring HIV infection from transfusions is very low. This is especially due to effective recruitment of regular, volunteer blood donors; improved donor testing systems; universal screening of blood and blood products with highly sensitive and particular tests for the antibody to HIV; and the appropriate use of blood.

In the developing countries, however, the risk is much higher. One estimate is that up to 5 per cent of HIV infections may be caused by transfusions in high-prevalence areas like sub-Saharan Africa. The lack of coordinated national blood transfusion systems, the lack of non-remunerated volunteer blood donors, lack of testing, and improper use of blood products compound the problem (4-6).

To prevent transmission by tissue and organ donation, comprising sperm for artificial insemination, the HIV-infection status of the donor should be carefully evaluated.

Contaminated Needles, Syringes or Other Piercing Instruments

HIV can be transmitted through the use of HIV-contaminated needles or other invasive instruments. The sharing of syringes and needles by injecting drug users is liable for the very rapid rise in HIV infection among these persons in several parts of the world.

A risk is also appended to non-medical procedures if the instruments used are not properly sterilized. Such procedures comprise ear- and body-piercing, tattooing, acupuncture, male and female circumcision, and traditional scarification. The actual risk depends on the local prevalence of HIV infection.

HIV transmission by means of injection equipment can also take place in health care settings where syringes, needles and their instruments, like dental equipment, are not properly sterilized, or through injury by needles and other sharps.

Mother-to-Child Transmission (MTCT)

Mother-to-Child Transmission (MTCT) is the very important source of HIV infection in young children. The virus may be transmitted during pregnancy, labour, delivery or after the child's birth during breastfeeding. Among infected infants who are not breastfed, most MTCT takes place around the time of delivery (just before or during labour and delivery). In populations where breastfeeding is the norm, breastfeeding may account for more than one-third of all cases of MTCT transmission (7,8).

Paediatric AIDS can be difficult to diagnose since some symptoms of HIV infection, such as diarrhoea, are also common in infants are children who are not infected. Therefore, these symptoms cannot be considered a reliable basis for diagnosis.

There are blood-based tests that permit early diagnosis of HIV infection in infants. These are used extensively in developed countries. However, these tests are rather expensive and are not readily available in developing world.

How HIV is Not Transmitted?

Family, friends and co-workers should not afraid of becoming infected with HIV through casual contact with an HIV-infected person at home, at work, or socially. These activities will not transmit the virus:

- shaking hands, hugging or kissing
- coughing or sneezing
- using a public phone
- visiting a hospital
- opening a door
- sharing food, eating or drinking utensils
- using drinking fountains
- using toilets or showers
- using public swimming pools
- getting a mosquito or insect bite.

AIDS and Work

For the huge majority of occupations, the workplace does not carry a risk of acquiring HIV. The exceptions include laboratory workers, health care workers, persons dealing with hospital waste products, emergency medical response personnel and any other occupation where there is a probability of exposure to blood. Their risk is very low, but real. Needle-stick injuries and other skin-piercing accidents and blood splashing into the eyes, these are the hazardous to which these persons may be exposed.

AIDS and Sports

There are no documented cases of HIV being transmitted during participation in a sports activity. The very low risk of transmission during sports participation would involve sports with direct body contact in which bleeding might be expected to occur.

It is theoretically feasible for the virus to be transmitted if an HIV-infected athlete had a bleeding wound or skin lesion with fluids that came in contact with another athlete's skin lesion, cut or exposed mucous membrane. Even in such an event, risk of transmission is very low. However, in sports involving direct body contact or combative sports where bleeding might occur, it is important to follow two simple procedures:

- cleanse any skin lesion with antiseptic and cover it securely; and
- if a bleeding injury occurs, interrupt participation until the bleeding has stopped and the wound has been both cleansed with antiseptic and securely covered.

PREVENTING HIV TRANSMISSION

PREVENTING SEXUAL TRANSMISSION OF HIV

Know Your Partner

Whether you are male or female-heterosexual, homosexual or bisexual—your risk of acquiring HIV infection is directly concerned to the likelihood that your partner is infected. Your risk is significantly higher if your partner has ever injected drugs, has unprotected sex with casual partners, or has a sexual history unknown to you.

Understand Which Sexual Acts Put You at Most Risk

All kinds of penetrative sexual intercourse (anal, vaginal, oral) with an HIV-infected man or woman bear a risk of transmission. Unprotected anal intercourse is one of the riskiest practices. This is fact even when a condom is used because of the increased likelihood that the condom will be damaged during this form of sex. Unprotected vaginal intercourse involves the next highest risk of infection. Oral sex also bears a small risk of transmission, particularly if there are mouth or throat injuries present like bleeding gums, lesions, sores, abscessed teeth, throat infections, or oral STDs present.

To protect yourself, always use a condom during penetrative sexual acts.

What You Need to Know About Condoms

Latex condoms lubricated with silicone or a water-based lubricant are recommended as a barrier method to minimize the risk of HIV transmission during anal, vaginal and oral intercourse. (If additional lubricant is desired, a water-based variety like K-Y Lubricating Jelly® should be used rather than an oil-based lubricant like Vaseline®, which can break down the latex). Latex condoms are only effective if they are used appropriately and do not break.

Natural membrane condoms, often made from sheep gut, are not recommended since they have tiny pores through which HIV could pass.

For very effectiveness, the condom must be put on the penis before it touches any part of the rectum, vagina or mouth. It should be put on when the penis is erect, taking care to leave a reservoir at the tip to contain the semen. Care should be taken during withdrawal of the penis (with the condom still in place) to avoid spillage.

Female condoms, like the REALITY® condom, are now available. The female condom is a soft relatively loose-fitting plastic pouch made of polyurethane (not latex) that lines the vagina. It has a semi-stiff plastic ring at each end. The inner ring is used to penetrate the device inside the vagina and hold it in place. The outer ring partly covers the labia area and holds the condom open.

Or, to be even safer, you can engage yourself in sexual practices that involve no penetration like caressing or massing any part of the body, masturbation (provided that sexual secretions do not come in contact with cuts or sores on the other partner's skin), and kissing that does not include heavy exchange of saliva and possibly blood. The safest course of all is abstinence.

Seek Medical Advice or Treatment for STDs

The presence of an untreated sexually transmitted disease-like gonorrhoea, chlamydial infection, syphilis, herpes or genital warts-can enhance both your acquisition and transmission of HIV by a factor of up to 10. If you suspect you have an STD, or have been exposed to one, it is necessary that you seek medical advice and treatment immediately.

Common symptoms comprise an unusual discharge from the vagina or penis, burning or pain during urination, and sores or blisters near the mouth or genitals. Other symptoms in women may comprise unusual bleeding (other than the menstrual cycle) and vaginal pain during intercourse.

Preventing Transmission of HIV via Blood and Blood Products

In industrial countries, the risk of transmission of HIV via blood and blood products is very rare for each unit of blood transfused.

It is also very rare to contract HIV in the health care setting. For instance, evidence from the USA hints that health care workers who accidentally puncture their skin with a needle contaminated with HIV have an estimated risk of less than five in a 1000 (0.5 per cent) of developing HIV infection.

Also, HIV is a fragile virus, meaning it is vulnerable to changes in temperature and other environmental factors, and has been shown not to be viable in dried blood for more than an hour. The concentration of virus particles of HIV per millilitre of blood is also very low in opposite to other viruses. In spite of the low level of occupational risk posed by HIV, safe work practices should be followed at all times by laboratory personnel and health workers. Don't be feared to ask your health care professional, clinic or hospital if they follow "universal precautions", or safety measures to stop the transmission of HIV in health care settings.

If you must travel to areas of the world where the safety of the blood supply is not guaranteed, you should follow these devices:

- before you start travel, identify sources of reliable medical help in your destination country;
- carry sterile disposable needles and syringes for your personal use (as part of the WHO medical kit);
- be aware of emergency medical evacuation procedures;
- minimize your risk of injury by following safety precautions such as using seatbelts and driving carefully; and
- if your are injured and lose blood, consider using a plasma substitute (crystalloids/colloids). If severe or acute blood loss has occurred, endeavours should be made to make sure that the blood has been screened for HIV and hepatitis B virus.

PREVENTING TRANSMISSION OF HIV VIA CONTAMINATED NEEDLES

Do not Share Needles or Syringes

Injecting drug use is one of the fastest growing routes of HIV infection in various parts of the world, primarily because needles, syringes and drug preparation equipment are repeatedly shared, enabling rapid spread of the virus.

Avoid Invasive, Skin-piercing Procedures

Ear- or body-piercing, tattoos, acupuncture or any procedure that needs invasive, skin-piercing instruments bear some risks of transmission. If you are considering any of these procedures, make it sure that all equipment is properly sterilized. Do not be feared to ask questions of the technician or health care personnel. HIV is easily destroyed by heat; instruments should be sterilized by steam or by dry heat. If this is not feasible, instruments should be disinfected by boiling.

Protecting Children

Parents should make sure that children should be well aware of the facts about HIV transmission and how they can protect themselves against infection. Specifically, children should:

- be aware that HIV is transmitted through blood;
- avoid any skin-piercing procedures or accidental injury from unsterilized needles and other sharp instruments;
- receive injections or other medical or dental treatment only when necessary and only with appropriately sterilized equipment;
- receive blood transfusions only when medically required and only with properly screened blood; and
- avoid the risk of traumatic injury necessitating blood transfusion.

Older children require information and encouragement that will help them avoid becoming infected through unprotected sexual intercourse or through sharing drug-injecting equipment.

Children also require to be reassured about the means in which HIV cannot be transmitted.

They should be encouraged to be sympathetic toward children and adults who are infected, and should not afraid of becoming infected through casual contact with these persons.

BEING TESTED

What the HIV Antibody Test Can Tell You

The standard tests to condition whether you are infected with HIV are based on detection of antibodies to HIV in the blood, not of the virus itself. Various types of antibody tests exist like the Enzyme-Linked Immuno-Sorbent Assay (ELISA) and simple rapid (S/R) tests. In recent years, tests have been developed that detect HIV antibodies in saliva and urine.

The first antibody test is called a screening test when a person gets it. If the screening test is negative, it means that no antibodies were found. The person tested is considered HIV-negative and confirmatory tests are not necessary. If the screening test is repeatedly positive, it must be confirmed. Confirmation can be done by using special tests, e.g. Western Blot or Line Immuno-Assays (LIA). It is also possible to confirm a positive result by using combinations of ELISA or S/R tests. Although the confirmation can be done on the same sample of blood, it is preferable to do the confirmation on a second blood sample with a view to avoid any errors.

HIV screening tests can sometimes give false-positive readings, particularly in populations where HIV is not present in high numbers, which is why confirmatory testing is always done on positive screening test results. This confirmation is needed to rule out false-positive screening results.

In regard to the accuracy of the antibody tests:

- It takes, on average, 25 days for an HIV test to show positive after a person becomes infected with HIV. This is a much shorter timeframe than before the introduction of very sensitive tests now used.
- If a person has been infected very recently, the test may show a negative result.
- When saliva and urine are tested, it takes longer for antibodies to become detectable.
- More than 99 per cent of infected persons will show positive after three months.

The HIV Antibody Test and Employment

In the great majority of occupations and occupational settings, work does not involve a risk of transmitting HIV between workers or from worker to client. The following recommendations have been put forward on AIDS and the workplace.

- Pre-employment HIV/AIDS testing as part of assessing fitness to work is not necessary and should NOT be required. This applies to both direct methods like HIV testing and indirect assessment of risk behaviours and questioning the applicant about HIV tests already taken. Pre-employment HIV/AIDS screening for insurance or other objectives raises serious concerns about discrimination, and merits close scrutiny.
- For persons currently employed, HIV/AIDS screening, whether direct or indirect, should NOT be needed.
- All medical information, including HIV/AIDS status, must be kept confidential.
- Employees should not be needed to inform the employer related to their HIV/AIDS status.
- Persons in the workplace who are HIV-infected (or perceived to be) must be protected from stigmatization and discrimination by co-workers, unions, employers and clients. Information and education are necessary to maintain a climate of mutual understanding important to ensure this protection.
- HIV-infected employees should not be discriminated against regarding their access to and receipt of advantages from statutory social security programmes and occupationally-related schemes.
- HIV infection alone does not limit fitness to work. If fitness to work is feebled by HIV-related illness, proper alternative working arrangements should be made.
- HIV infection is not a cause for termination of employment. As with several other illnesses, persons with HIV-related illnesses should be allowed to work for as long as they are medically fit for available, proper work.

While these measures are designed to protect your rights if you are HIV-infected, you also have a liability to adopt behaviour that does not put others in your workplace at risk of infection.

The HIV Antibody Test and Pregnancy

If you or your partner are worried about your HIV status, and you are thinking about having a baby, the HIV antibody test may help clarify your choices.

HIV testing should be available, with pre- and post-test counselling, on a voluntary, confidential ground. You and your sex partner should be counselled on the implications that positive test result will have for both of you, for the fetus and for the infant if pregnancy is considered.

An HIV-infected woman can transmit HIV to her infant. The most likely time for an HIV-infected pregnant woman to pass the virus on to her baby is either in the very early stages or in the developed stage of her infection. Thus, the risk of transmission is from low (if the HIV-infected woman has no signs and symptoms) to high (if she has AIDS). The transmission rate ranges from 12 per cent to over 30 per cent.

If you are pregnant and HIV-infected, you should be counselled on the alternatives of continuing or terminating your pregnancy (where abortion is legal) and about subsidizing mother-to-child transmission (MTCT) through treatment with zidovudine (Sometimes called ZDV or AZT) during your pregnancy.

Pregnancy does not seem to accelerate the progression of the clinical course of HIV infection.

LIVING WITH HIV AND AIDS

Coping with Confirmed HIV Infection

Learning that you are infected with HIV will change your life dramatically. You may realise a wide range of emotions-fear, loss, grief, depression, denial, anger, anxiety. No matter how reassuring the doctor, how effective drug therapies are now and will become, how minimal the physical impact of the infection, or how intellectually prepared you may be, your requirement for counselling and support will be great.

The psychological issues faced by most of the persons will HIV infection revolve around uncertainty. Your future hopes and expectations, your relationships and your career will all need some adjustment in order for you to cope with your illness and lead a happy, productive life.

The Impact on Your Health

The impact on your health is probably to depend on the stage of infection you have reached when you find out you are HIV-positive, the psychological support available to you, and your access to good medical care. Soon after becoming infected with the virus, some people experience a brief flu-like illness with fever, swollen lymph glands, skin rash or cough. You may then remain perfectly fit and healthy for several years despite being infected.

For approximately 50 per cent of infected persons, the time between becoming infected and the appearance of the opportunistic infections that characterize AIDS is more than 10 years.

Antiretroviral combination therapy, while expensive, has been shown to slow the onset of AIDS and long life expectancy. Your quality of life could also be improved by the preventive and therapeutic use of drugs that fight off common opportunistic infections and other diseases to which HIV-infected person are vulnerable, like tuberculosis. Active TB screening and contact tracing through sputum examination are also potent for families with an HIV-positive member.

Beside good medical care, psychological support-from family, friends and counselling-is critical. In various countries, there are support groups made up of persons living with HIV and AIDS. There are also several support groups and resources to be found on the Internet.

The Impact on Your Personal Relationships

Partners are probably to suffer the consequences of HIV infection and disease as much as the infected person, albeit indirectly. This is so even if partners know that they are not HIV-infected themselves. Their lives are probably to experience the same kind of pressures and upheavals, and they can realize similar feelings of uncertainty, grief, loss and anger.

Communication between the two partners and between partners and professional counsellors is important to develop understanding of the adjustments that will be needed. For instance, adjustments in sexual behaviour are necessary to stop further transmission of infection. Counselling can also address the physical and psychological changes and requirements that the partners will experience.

If you have HIV, you have an opportunity to make others more aware of the disease. By educating others, you may lessen the prejudice against persons with HIV or AIDS. However, consider carefully to whom you reveal your HIV status. Misunderstanding and discrimination do exist, and can affect you and the ones you love. Again, professional counselling can help with these issues.

Often, families are the important source of care and support for HIV-infected persons, and the type of care needed may change depending on the stage of the infection. Counselling for family members, both as individuals and as the family unit, can be very important, especially as the disease progresses.

The Impact on Your Work Life

How your work life is impacted will depend on how you realise physically and mentally, and at what stage your infection is discovered. Experience has shown that persons with HIV infection, with or without symptoms, should keep working as long as feasible. After the initial period of coming to terms with HIV infection, there usually comes a period of wanting to move on with life and work can be an important part of this transition. Although you are not obliged to inform your employer and colleagues of your HIV status, certain circumstances may make it necessary for your to do so. If your job calls for you to travel, for instance, you may need to go to countries where entry depends on a certificate that shows you are not HIV-infected. Additionally, you may require certain vaccinations.

Theoretically, you could become infected by the "live" but weakened pathogens in certain vaccines, particularly if your immune system has already been damaged by HIV. It is always very better to consult your physician to determine the risks involved with vaccines or if alternatives exist.

HIV AND YOUR INFANT'S HEALTH

Having a Baby

Pregnancy is something you and your partner will need to discuss very carefully with your physician and probably your counsellor if either or both of your are infected. It is very potent to receive medical care early in your pregnancy.

Your HIV treatment should not change very much from what it was before you became pregnant. If you decide not to discontinue your pregnancy, talk with your doctor about how you can prevent giving HIV to your baby. The chances of passing HIV to your baby before or during birth are about 15-25 per cent in developed countries and 25-45 per cent in developing world. Treatment with zidovudine (sometimes called ZDV or AZT) related to replacement feeding has been shown to greatly lower this risk.

Although you are pregnant, you should still use condoms every time you have sex to avoid contracting other diseases and to avoid spreading HIV. Even if your partner already suffering from HIV, he should still use condoms. After birth, your baby should be tested for HIV, even if you took ZDV and/or other drugs in the period of pregnancy. Talk with your doctor about your baby's special medical requirements and any medications he or she will require.

BREASTFEEDING

Breastfeeding is considered to be the best way to feed an infant. However, if a mother is HIV-infected, it may be preferable to replace breastmilk to minimize the risk of HIV transmission to the infant. The risk of replacement feeding should be less than the potential risk of HIV transmission through infected breastmilk, so that infant illness and death from other reasons do not increase. Otherwise, there is no benefit to replacement feeding. According to joint guidelines from UNAIDS, UNICEF and WHO, the following issues should be taken into account:

- replacement feeding requires to provide all the infant's nutritional requirements as completely as possible;
- breastmilk substitutes must be prepared and given hygienicially to avoid contamination with bacteria. This needs access to clean water and fuel;
- breastmilk alternatives must be affordable to families; and
- affordable family planning must be accessible, as women who do not breastfeed lose the child-spacing advantages that breastfeeding can provide.

Childhood Immunizations

Some parents may worry that their HIV-infected children might be adversely affected by routine childhood immunizations. In response, WHO and UNICEF have issued these guidelines. HIV-infected children should be immunized against diphtheria, tetanus and pertussis (with DTP); poliomyelitis (with OPV or IPV); and measles (with measles vaccine), as per standard schedules. Children with known or suspected HIV infection are at increased risk of severe measles, and these children should be given an extra dose of measles vaccine as soon after six months as feasible with the scheduled dose given at nine months as usual.

Parents of HIV-infected children are generally HIV-infected themselves and have a higher incidence of tuberculosis than the general population. Early protection against tuberculosis with BCG immunization is therefore recommended for HIV-infected children who are not symptomatic. Symptomatic HIV-infected children, however, should not be immunized with BCG or yellow fever vaccine.

A GLOBAL OVERVIEW OF THE EPIDEMIC

By the end of 1998, the number of people living with HIV is estimated to have grown to 33.4 million, according to estimates from UNAIDS and WHO. Most of these people do not have any knowledge that they are infected. The epidemic has not been overcome anywhere virtually every country in the world saw new infections in 1998 and the epidemic is frankly out of control in several places. More than 95 per cent of all HIV-infected people now live in the developing countries, which has experienced 95 per cent of all deaths to date from AIDS. These deaths are mainly among young adults who would normally be in their peak productive and reproductive years. The various repercussions of these deaths are reaching crisis level in some parts of the world. Whether measured against the yardstick of deteriorating child survival, crumbling life expectancy, overburdened health care systems, increasing orphanhood, or bottom-line losses to business, AIDS has never posed a bigger threat to development.

According to UNAIDS/WHO estimates, 11 men, women and children around the world were infected per minute during 1998-nearer to 6 million people in all. One-tenth of newly-infected people were under age 15, which brings the number of children now alive with HIV to 1.2 million. Most of them are thought to have acquired their infection from their mother before or during birth, or through breastfeeding.

Region	*Epidemic started*	*Adults and children living with HIV/AIDS*	*Adults and children newly infected with HIV in 1998*	*Adult preva-lence rate*[1]	*Percentage of HIV-positive adults who are women*	*Main mode(s) of transmis-sion for those living with HIV/AIDS*[2]
Sub-Saharan Africa	late '70s—early '80s	22.5 million	4.0 million	8.0%	50%	Hetero
North Africa and Middle East	late '80s	210,000	19,000	0.13%	20%	IDU, Hetero
South and South-east Asia	late'80s	6.7 million	1.2 million	0.69%	25%	Hetero
East Asia and Pacific	late '80s	560,000	200,000	0.068%	15%	IDU, Hetero, MSM
Latin America	late '70s—early '80s	1.4 million	160,000	0.57%	20%	MSM, IDU, Hetero
Caribbean	late '70s—early '80s	330,000	45,000	1.96%	35%	Hetero, MSM
Eastern Europe and Central Asia	early '90s	270,000	80,000	0.14%	20%	IDU, MSM
Western Europe	late '70s—early '80s	500,000	30,000	0.25%	20%	MSM, IDU
North America	late '70s—early '80s	890,000	44,000	0.56%	20%	MSM, IDU, Hetero
Australia and New Zealand	late '70s—early '80s	12,000	600	0.1%	5%	MSM IDU
Total		33.4 million	5.8 million	1.1%	43%	

1. The proportion of adults (15 to 49 years of age) living with HIV/AIDS in 1998, using 1997 population numbers.
2. MSM (sexual transmission among men who have sex with men), IDU (transmission through injecting drug use), Hetero (heterosexual transmission).

While mother-to-child transmission can be slow down by providing pregnant HIV-positive women with antiretroviral drugs and alternatives to breastmilk, the ultimate aim must be effective prevention for young women so that they can avoid becoming infected in the first place. Unfortunately, when it comes to HIV infection, women seem to be heading for an unwelcome equality with men. While they accounted for 41 per cent of infected adults worldwide in 1997, women now represent 43 per cent of all people over age 15 living with HIV and AIDS. There are no hints that this equalizing trend will reverse.

With the start of the epidemic around two decades ago, HIV has infected more than 47 million people. And though it is a slow-acting virus that can take a decade or more too cause severe illness and death, HIV has already cost the lives of nearly 14 million adults and children. An estimated 2.5 million of these deaths took place during 1998, more than ever before in a single year.

The UN Response to AIDS

Meeting the complicated long-term challenge of HIV/AIDS calls for an expanded response. Direct health interventions and action to influence AIDS prevention and care must be pursued and fastened, while innovative action must address the broader context of the epidemic, comprising its socio-economic causes and consequences.

The Joint United Nations Programme on HIV/AIDS (UNAIDS) was setup in January 1996 for this purpose. UNAIDS is a cosponsored programme that brings together the United Nations Children's Fund (UNICEF), the United Nations Development Programme (UNDP), the United Nations Population Fund (UNFPA), the United Nations International Drug Control Programme (UNDCP), the United Nations Educational, Scientific and Cultural Organization (UNESCO), the World Health Organization (WHO) and the World Bank in a common attempt against the epidemic.

The UNAIDS Cosponsors bring to this endeavour complementary mandates and multisectoral expertise, ranging from education and socio-economic development to women's reproductive health. They are committed to joint planning and action, giving UNAIDS a "cooperative advantage". Advantages include more effective advocacy, more effective of UN system resources through the sharing of costs, and greater coherence in United Nations support to national AIDS programmes.

Guiding Principles

- Strengthening of countries' capacity for long-term action ranging from prevention and care to impact alleviation.
- recognition and use of technically-sound policies, strategies and tools.
- Societal and structural changes to minimize the vulnerability of women, young people, migrants, drug users, sexual and ethnic minorities, and other population groups.
- Supportive social, political and legal environments that permit individuals to exercise their liability to protect themselves and others from HIV infection.
- Entitlement to all human rights without discrimination, comprising discrimination based on HIV infection status. These comprise the right to health, travel and privacy, the right to freedom from sexual violence and coercion, and the right to the information and means to prevent infection.
- Participation and partnership.
- National accountability to design, implement and coordinate the response to HIV/AIDS at the country level. The role of external partners, comprising UNAIDS, is to support and build on national action.
- Complementarity. Rather than undertaking itself what can be or is already being done by others, UNAIDS efforts to facilitate these efforts and to fill gaps in action and research.

Global and Local Impact

At the global level, UNAIDS is the AIDS programme of the seven Cosponsors and is liable for policy development and research, technical support, advocacy and coordination. At the same time, the seven cosponsoring organizations integrate HIV/AIDS-related issues and UNAIDS policies and strategies into their ongoing work. At the country level, UNAIDS can best be seen as the sum of AIDS-related activities undertaken by its Cosponsors with the backing of UNAIDS technical guidance and resources.

In countries where some or all of the Cosponsors are present, their representatives meet continuously in a special UN Theme Group to jointly plan, implement and evaluate AIDS-related activities. UN staff who are HIV-positive are encouraged to take participation in these Theme Groups for they lend both technical expertise and personal perspective to issues surrounding HIV infection. These staff also help educate their colleagues about the stigma and discrimination that infected individuals face in the workplace.

In addition, UNAIDS staff known as Country Programme Advisers are posted in selected countries to support the UN Theme Groups on HIV/AIDS, to strengthen cooperation with national partners and to provide technical support.

Important partners in national AIDS activities comprise governments (through both political leadership and the relevant ministries); community-based organizations; nongovernmental organizations (NGOs); the private sector; academic and research institutes; religious and other social and cultural institutions; and people living with HIV/AIDS.

The programme also supports research to evolve new tools and innovative approaches for slowing the spread of HIV and improving the quality of life of people living with HIV/AIDS. Instances are vaccine development, vaginal microbicides for women, methods of reducing mother-to-child transmission of HIV, and improved methods for preventing and treating the common opportunistic infections in HIV-infected individuals.

Four

Framework of Communication for HIV/AIDS

Introduction

A new and more adaptable framework with a view to HIV/AIDS communications has been developed under protagonist of the Joint United Nations programme on HIV/AIDS.

Unlike various earlier approaches, this framework is based more on social and environmental context than on individual behaviour. This framework was developed through a participatory process guided by both researchers and practitioners. Formulating this adaptable framework involved synthesizing experiences from the African, Asian, and Latin American and Caribbean regions and identifying and taking into consideration the various aspects of HIV/AIDS prevention, care, and support that need different approaches. Experiences from the United States and Europe were also comprised. UNAIDS' basic assumption was that the logic and theory of HIV/AIDS strategies should be evolved from within the meanings and values of the affected population.

To enable the synthesis of the new communications framework, UNAIDS sponsored five consultative workshops in collaboration with The Pennsylvania State University. They were organised in Geneva, Switzerland (November 1997); Abidjan, Cote d' Ivoire (December 1997); Washington, DC (February 1998); Bangkok, Thailand (July 1998); and Santo Domingo, Dominican Republic (January 1999). A number of other specialists and peers reviewed the reports, consensus, and recommendations of the workshops.

Executive Summary

The Joint United Nations Programme on HIV/AIDS (UNAIDS) responded to the increasing epidemic of HIV/AIDS by initiating a participatory research process conducted through five consultative workshops to examine the global use of communications for HIV/AIDS prevention, care and support. The main aim was to examine the adequacy of existing communications theories and models for HIV/AIDS in Africa, Asia, and Latin America and the Caribbean against a backdrop of contemporary communications use in Western societies. In the five consultative workshops (two global and three regional), 103 leading researchers and practitioners from various parts of the world were invited or consulted by UNAIDS in collaboration with the Pennsylvania State University (PennState).

The major finding was that five domains of context are virtually universal factors in communications for HIV/AIDS preventive health behaviour - *government policy, socio-economic status, culture, gender relations, and spirituality*. These interrelated domains formed the ground of a new framework that could be used as a flexible guide in the development of HIV/AIDS communications interventions. Individual health behaviour is recognized as a component of this set of domains, rather than the primary focus of health behaviour change.

Most HIV/AIDS communications programmes have been intended to achieving individual-based changes in sexual and social behaviour. While aspects of this approach are desirable and should be maintained, evidence from research and practice in different countries shows that existing approaches generally have major limitations; thus, a broader focus is required. Moreover, there is considerable inter-regional variation in the context of HIV/AIDS. Different of the theories, models, and frameworks currently in use in the regions do not adequately address the unique needs of HIV/AIDS communications. For instance, the cost effectiveness of interpersonal communication components of HIV/AIDS behavioural interventions in the regions has been underestimated.

The challenge of this new direction is to ensure a redirection of intervention programmes to recognize that individual behaviours are shaped and influenced by factors and domains within a broader contextual focus.

THE UNAIDS CONSULTATIVE WORKSHOPS

Methodology Process

Participatory research was utilized to plan and implement the development of the new framework. An important advantage of participatory research over traditional research methods is that it permits active involvement by those who will be the beneficiaries of the results of the research. The participant-beneficiaries are thus involved in defining the questions, establishing the parameters for the process, interpreting the result and directing the dissemination process. Consistent with the importance of participatory research, UNAIDS began this process by inviting comment and input from a broad range of leading researchers and practitioners from across the world. More than 80 per cent of the contributors and participants were from Africa, Asia, Latin America, and the Caribbean. Such broad consultation promotes flexibility for regional adaptation of the framework. Flexibility, in turn, promotes local ownership of the implementation process, since this last and vital step is realized at the local level - in the countries and communities.

There were five consultative workshops were organized altogether. Two of the workshops were of global nature, and three were regional, with one each in Africa, Asia, and Latin America and the Caribbean. In November 1997, fifteen leading researchers and practitioners in HIV/AIDS communications were invited to an inaugural consultative workshop at the UNAIDS headquarters in Geneva, Switzerland, to initiate reviewing the existing theories and models used to guide HIV/AIDS communications interventions. Under scrutiny was their adequacy both for universe and regional application - mainly in Africa, Asia, and Latin America and the Caribbean. Selected participants were invited to contribute papers on relevant subjects. *This first meeting concluded with unanimous agreement that is based on a review of the literature and of experiences in the field - most current theories and models did not provide a substantial foundation on which to develop communications interventions for HIV/AIDS in the regions.* It was agreed that further workshops should be held to seek input from researchers and practitioners in Africa, Asia, and Latin America and the Caribbean, with the ultimate objective of developing an adaptable framework.

In December 1997, the first regional workshop was organised in Abidjan, Cote d'Ivoire. This workshop took benefit of the wealth of experience among the participants at the concurrent International Conference on AIDS/STD in Africa. Two discussion groups on HIV/AIDS communications in Africa were held. One group discussion was conducted in English (nineteen participants) and the other in French (eighteen participants). Participants included practitioners and researchers involved in HIV/AIDS communications in Africa. Several of the participants were professionals engaged in HIV/AIDS prevention and care Information, Education, and Communication (IEC) and Behaviour Change Communication (BCC) interventions in various organizations and countries in Africa. The completion of this workshop echoed that of the inaugural consultative workshop in Geneva: *current theories and models did not sufficiently take into account the various situations among African countries and regions. It was unanimously agreed that a new framework that would comprise several identified issues and situation was an absolute necessity.*

In February 1998, a third consultative (and second global) workshop was held in Washington, DC, to review the input accumulated from the previous meetings. Since the conclusions reached at these meetings were so homogeneous, UNAIDS decided to hasten the development of a new strategy. To identify the requirements in Asia, Latin America, and the Caribbean, regional consultative workshops were organized in Bangkok, Thailand (July 6-8, 1998) and Santo Domingo, Dominican Republic (January 20-22, 1999).

Participants at these consultative workshops were selected on the ground of their expertise in communications and HIV/AIDS research and practice. UNAIDS was mainly interested in including those who had actually been involved in developing and implementing HIV/AIDS communications strategies in Africa, Asia and Latin America and Caribbean.

Participants discussed the approaches they had taken in their countries and regions, reviewed reports from previous meetings, and recommended step to be taken to develop a new approach or framework that would be more appropriate for their regions. Several participants provided examples from their countries and regions of successful communications programmes for HIV/AIDS. These instances confirmed that, in the future, HIV/AIDS prevention and care communications should ensure that measurable aims and outcomes are based on the experience of exemplar programs in each region and locality.

Goals

The ultimate goal for the participatory research workshops was to setup an improved framework and planning for HIV/AIDS communications in the African, Asian and Latin American and Caribbean regions. Initially, however, the goal was to generate ideas on how to develop a new framework and to gather input on the range of content the framework would be expected to support.

The sponsors and organizers realized that it was important for the contributors (and potential users) not only to evolve a new framework, but also to "buy into it" and commit to using it. Achieving a high level of participation by key organizations, therefore was a major process goal.

Objectives

These consultative workshops had three objectives:

(1) Review existing theories, models, frameworks, and planning for their potential effectiveness in communications programmes for HIV/AIDS prevention and care in Africa, Asia and Latin America and the Caribbean.

(2) Propose guideline for developing national and regional communications planning for HIV/AIDS.

(3) Advise on dissemination and implementation plans to activate more effective regional and national communications planning.

Commonly used communications theories and models were reviewed by researchers and practitioners and found to be limited in their applicability to HIV/AIDS prevention, care, and support. Several of these theories and models focus mainly on individual behaviour and make little or no allowance for the role or the social and environmental context of disease prevention interventions. This became increasingly clear as, during early discussions, the influence of factors of social and environmental context on the effectiveness of HIV/AIDS interventions in Africa, Asia, And Latin America and the Caribbean emerged.

Five

Sexual Behavioural Change for HIV

Introduction

The interventions to slow the spread of HIV across the world are as varied as the contents in which we find them. Not only is the HIV epidemic dynamic related to treatment options, prevention strategies and disease progression, but sexual behaviour, which remains the main target of AIDS prevention efforts worldwide, is widely diverse and deeply appended to individual desires, social and cultural relationships, and environmental and economic processes. This makes prevention of HIV, which could be an importantly simple task, enormously complex involving a multiplicity of dimensions.

Either implicitly or explicitly most of all the prevention interventions are based on theory. Most depend on the assumption that giving correct information about transmission and prevention will lead to behavioural change. Yet research has proved numerous times that education alone is not sufficient to induce behavioural change among most of the individuals. Thus, second-generation interventions were developed based on individual psychosocial and cognitive approaches that educate individuals in practical skills to minimize their risk for HIV infection. More recently, social researchers have come to percept that because complex health behaviours like sex take place in context, socio-cultural factors surrounding the individual must be considered in designing prevention interventions. Finally, beyond the individual and his or her immediate social relationships lie the larger issues of structural and environmental determinants that also play an important role in sexual behaviour.

The objective of this project was to associate outcomes of behavioural interventions around the world with the different models and theories of which they were based. There is however a lack of information on tests of the relevance of behavioural change models in differing contexts, particularly in non-industrialized countries and in regions at later stages of the epidemic. Most intervention reports, whether in peer-reviewed journals or conference abstracts, often do not clearly state the theoretical framework of the project. And in many cases, there was no clear intent to base interventions on behavioural change models as a great number of them have been propelled by the urgency to do anything to slow the epidemic, especially in resource-poor settings. The primary intention of this review was to look as broadly as possible at all interventions in order to recognize what has worked in the enormous variety of situations addressed. However, this would have implied analysing retroactively all prevention programmes to define their theoretical foundations, which was not possible within the scope, time and resources of this project.

This review thus focused primarily on the following types of reports:

- sexual behavioural change interventions for HIV clearly mentioning their theoretical approach
- studies testing theoretical models of behavioural change
- and reviews on impact of behavioural changes interventions.

Additional examples of developing world projects were used to balance the observations and conclusions drawn from the above sources with a view to compensate for the lack of tested models in these countries.

Most of the studies cited in this report comprise control or comparison situations and behavioural outcomes. Reports that included only knowledge and attitudes results were excluded. Also included were some interventions that used constructs from a kinds of theories attempting to incorporate social, environmental and cognitive elements, or used constructs alone without testing theories as a whole. Unfortunately, it was difficult to recognize interventions based both on a trans-theoretical approach and strong evaluation components.

Finally, this review was organized into four sections, comprising:

- a brief overview of theoretical models of behavioural change
- a review of basic approaches used to stem sexual transmission of HIV
- a summary of successful interventions targeting certain populations at risk
- and a discussion of remaining challenges.

Theories and Models of Behavioural Change

This chapter is divided into 4 sections that cover the most frequently used theories and models of behavioural change from different perspectives. It begins with theories that focus on the individual's psychological process, like attitudes and beliefs, then goes into theories emphasizing social relationships, and ends with structural factors in explaining human behaviour. This separation is artificial as there is essential overlap in categories. It might therefore be useful, as well, to see the theories as a continuum of models moving from the strictly individually centered to the macro-level of structural and environmentally focused.

(A) Focus on Individuals

As HIV transmission is propelled by behavioural factors, theories about how individuals change their behaviour have given the foundation for most HIV prevention efforts worldwide. These theories have been generally generated using cognitive-attitudinal and affective-motivational constructs. Near about all the psychosocial theories originated in the West but have been used for AIDS internationally with mixed outcomes. Only one of the psychosocial models discussed below, the *AIDS risk reduction model*, was developed especially for AIDS. Psychosocial models of behavioural risk can be classified into 3 major groups: those predicting risk behaviour, those predicting behavioural change and those predicting maintenance of safe behaviour.

Models of individual behavioural change often focus on stages that individuals pass through while trying to change behaviour. These theories and models generally do not consider the interaction of social, cultural and environmental issues as independent of individual factors. Although each theory is built on separate assumptions they all state that behavioural changes occur by changing potential risk-producing situations and social relationships, risk perceptions, attitudes, self-efficacy beliefs, intentions and result expectations. Central to HIV prevention interventions based on psychological-behavioural theory is the practice of targeted risk-reduction skills. These skills are often passed on to individuals in a process consisting of instruction, modeling, practice and feedback. The psychological theories and models that have been most instrumental in the design and development of HIV prevention interventions are briefly described below.

Health Belief Model

The Health belief model, developed in the 1950s, holds that health behaviour is a function of individual's socio-demographic characteristics, knowledge and attitudes. In conformity with this model, a person must hold the following beliefs with a view to be able to change behaviour:

(1) perceived susceptibility to a special health problem ("*am I at risk for HIV?*")
(2) perceived seriousness of the condition ("*how serious is AIDS; how hard would my life be if I got it?*")
(3) belief in effectiveness of the new behaviour ("*condoms are effective against HIV transmission*")
(4) cues to action ("*witnessing the death or illness of a close friend or relative because of AIDS*")
(5) perceived benefits of preventive action ("*if I start using condoms, I can avoid HIV infection*")
(6) barriers to taking action ("*I don't like using condoms*")

In this model, promoting action to change behaviour comprises changing individual personal beliefs. Individuals weigh the advantages against the perceived costs and barriers to change. For change to occur, advantages must outweigh costs. Regarding HIV, interventions often target perception of risk, beliefs in severity of AIDS ("*there is no cure*"), beliefs in effectiveness of condom use and benefits of condom use or delaying onset of sexual relations.

Social Cognitive (or learning) Theory

The premise of the Social Cognitive or Social Learning Theory (SCT) says that new behaviours are learned either by modeling the behaviour of others or by direct experience. Social learning theory focuses on the important roles played by vicarious, clandestine, and self-regulatory processes in psychological functioning and looks at human behaviour as a continuous interaction between cognitive, behavioural and environmental determinants. Central theories of the *social cognitive theory* are:

- self-efficacy - the belief in the ability to implement the important behaviour (*"I know I can insist on condom use with my partner"*)
- outcome expectancies - belief about outcomes such as the belief that using condoms correctly will prevent HIV infection.

Programmes built on SCT integrate information and attitudinal change to increase motivation and reinforcement of risk reduction skills and self-efficacy. Particularly, activities focus on the experience people have in talking to their partners about sex and condom use, the positive and negative beliefs about adopting condom use, and the types of environmental obstacles to risk-reduction. A meta analysis of HIV risk-reduction interventions that used SCT in controlled experimental trials found that 12 published interventions with mostly uninfected individuals all obtained positive changes in risk behaviour, with a medium effect size meeting or exceeding effects of other theory-based behavioural change interventions.

Theory of Reasoned Action

The *theory of reasoned action*, advanced in the mid-1960s by Fishbein and Ajzen, is based on the prescriptions that human beings are usually quite rational and make systematic use of the information available to them. People consider the implications of their actions in a given context at a given time before they decide to engage or not engage in a given behaviour, and that most actions of social relevance are under volitional control. *The theory of reasoned action* is conceptually synonym to the health belief model but adds the construct of behavioural intention as a determinant of health behaviour. Both theories lay emphasis on perceived susceptibility, perceived benefits and constraints to changing behaviour. The theory of reasoned action particularly focuses on the role of personal intention in conditioning whether a behaviour will occur. A person's intention is a function of 2 basic determinants:

(1) attitude (toward the behaviour), and
(2) 'subjective norms', i.e., social influence.

'Normative' beliefs play an important role in the theory, and generally focus on what an individual believes other people, especially influential people, would expect him/her to do.

For instance, for a person to start using condoms, his/her attitude might be "*having sex with condoms is just as good as having sex without condoms*" and subjective norms (or the normative belief) could be "*most of my peers are using condoms, they would anticipate me to do so as well*". Interventions using this theory to guide activities emphasis on attitudes about risk-reduction, response to social norms, and intentions to change risky behaviours.

Stage of Change Model

This model, developed early in the 1990s particularly for smoking cessation by Prochaska, DiClemente and colleagues, posits 6 stages that individuals or groups pass through when changing behaviour: pre-contemplation, contemplation, preparation, action, maintenance and relapse. Regarding condom use, the stages could be described as.

(1) has not considered using condoms (pre-contemplation)
(2) recognizes the requirement to use condoms (contemplation)
(3) thinking about using condoms in the next months (preparation)
(4) using condoms consistently for less than 6 months (action)
(5) using condoms consistently for 6 months or more (maintenance)
(6) slipping-up regarding to condom use (relapse)

In order for an intervention to be successful it must target the appropriate stage of the individual or group. For instance, awareness raising between stage one and two. Groups and individuals pass through all stages, but do not importantly move in a linear fashion. As with previous theories, *the stages of change model* stresses the importance of cognitive processes and uses Bandura's concept of self-efficacy. Movement between stages relies on cognitive-behavioural processes.

Among others, the CDC has used the *Stages of Change Model* in its AIDS Community Demonstration Projects for marginal populations in the US and in a research project intended to change women's sexual behaviour with their main partners.

AIDS Risk Reduction Model

The AIDS risk reduction model, developed in 1990 (Catania et al), uses constructs from the *health belief model, the social cognitive theory and the diffusion of innovation theory* (a social model described below), to ascribe the process individuals (or groups) pass through while changing behaviour with respect to HIV risk. The model recognizes 3 stages involved in reducing risk for HIV transmission, including:

(1) behaviour labelling
(2) commitment to change
(3) taking action.

In the first stage, knowledge about HIV transmission, perceived HIV susceptibility, and aversive emotions influence how people perceive AIDS. The commitment stage is shaped by four determinants perceptions of enjoyment, self-efficacy, social norms and aversive emotions. Again, in the last stage, aversive emotions, sexual communication, help-seeking behaviour and social factors affect peoples's decision-making process.

Programmes that *use the AIDS risk reduction model emphasize*:

- clients' risk assessment
- influencing the decision to lessen risk through perceptions of enjoyment or self-efficacy
- clients' help to enact the change (access to condoms, social support).

Conclusion

These psychosocial theories and constructs were very useful early in the epidemic to recognize individual behaviours associated with higher rates of HIV transmission. They continue to provide important guidance to interventions in formulating design and evaluation with diverse populations in a wide variety of settings. Theories also support in understanding study results. It is important, however, to pay special attention to these theories across cultures and genders as nearly all the individually based theories were developed in the West with little focus on the role of gender. Although several studies have proven the usefulness of these theories, it has become increasingly evident that alone they do not completely explain why some populations have higher HIV prevalence than others nor the complex interactions between contextual factors and individual behaviour.

(B) Social Theories and Models

Overemphasis on individual behavioural change with a focus on the cognitive level has undermined the total research capacity to understand the complexity of HIV transmission and control. Emphasize only on the individual psychological process ignores the interactive relationship of behaviour in its social, cultural, and economic dimension thereby missing the feasibility to fully understand crucial determinants of behaviour points out that, in several cases, motivations for sex are complicated, unclear and may not be thought through in advance.

Societal norms, religious criteria, and gender-power relations infuse meaning into behaviour, enabling positive or negative changes. A main difference between individual and social models is that the latter aiming at changes at the community level. Sociological theories assert that society is broken up into smaller sub-cultures and it is the members of one's immediate surroundings, the peer group that someone most identifies with, that has the most important influence on an individual's behaviour. According to this perspective, effective prevention efforts, particularly in vulnerable communities that do not have the larger societal support, will depend on the development of strategies that can enlist community mobilization to change the norms of this peer network to support positive changes in behaviour. A greater interest in the context surrounding individual behaviour led to increased numbers of interventions guided by the following theories and models.

Diffusion of Innovation Theory

The diffusion of innovation theory ascribes the process of how an idea is disseminated throughout a community. According to the theory, there are four important elements: the innovation, its communication, the social system and time. People's exposure to a new idea, which takes place within a social network or through the media, will condition the rate at which various people adopt a new behaviour. The theory posits that people are most likely to follow new behaviours based on favourable evaluations of the idea communicated to them by other members whom they respect. Kelly explains that when the diffusion theory is applied to HIV risk reduction, normative and risk behavioural changes can be began when enough key opinion leaders adopt and support behavioural changes, influence others to do the same and ultimately diffuse the new norm widely within peer networks. When beneficial prevention beliefs are instilled and widely held within one's immediate social network, individuals' behaviour is more likely to be consistent with the perceived social norms.

Interventions using this theory more investigate the best method to disperse messages within a community and who are the leaders able to act as role models to change community norms.

Social Influence or Social Inoculation Model

This educational model is based on the concept that young people engage in behaviours comprising early sexual activity partly because of general societal influences, but more specifically from their peers. The model suggests exposing young people to social pressures while teaching them to examine and develop skills to cope with these pressures. The model often relies on role models such as teenagers little older than programme participants to present factual information, identify pressures, role-play responses to pressures, teach assertiveness skills and discuss problem situations. Social influence model has been utilized to lessen smoking among young people as well.

Social Network Theory

The Social Network Theory looks as social behaviour not as an individual phenomenon but through relationships, and appreciates that HIV risk behaviour, unlike various other health behaviours, directly involves 2 people. With respect to sexual relationships, social networks stresses on both the impact of selective mixing, (i.e., how different people choose who they mix with), and the variations in partnership patterns (length of partnership and overlap). Although the intricacies of relations and communication within the couple, the smallest unit of the social network, is critical to the knowing about HIV transmission in this model, the scope and character of one's broader social network, those who serve as reference people, and who sanction behaviour, are basic to comprehending individual risk behaviour. In other words, social norms are best understood at the level of social networks.

One application of the Sexual Network Theory for HIV prevention is the concept of 'bridge populations' that form a connection between high and low prevalence groups. In Thailand, men who have both commercial and non-commercial sex partners form potent bridge population, which was an integral aspect of the spread of HIV in Thailand. Programmes using this theory to guide them would investigate:

- the composition of important social networks in a community
- the attitudes of the social networks towards safer sex
- whether the social network gives the important support to change behaviour
- whether particular people within the social network are at particularly high risk and may put many others at risk.

Although few network-based interventions have been tried, the concept has proved complementary to individual-based theories for the design of prevention programmes by emphasizing on the partnership as well as the larger social group. Analysis of network mixing gives the means to see efficiency of transmission and effective points of intervention.

Theory of Gender and Power

Unlike the psychosocial theories which are inevitably gender-blind, the theory of gender and power is a social structural theory addressing the wider social and environmental issues surrounding women, such as distribution of power and authority, affective influences, and gender-specific norms within heterosexual relationships. Using this theory to guide intervention development with women in heterosexual relationships can help investigate how a women's commitment to a relationship and lack of power can influence her risk reduction choices.

Programmes using the theory of gender and power would assess the impact of structurally determined gender differences on interpersonal sexual relationships (perceptions of socially prescribed gender relations).

Conclusion

Social theories and models see individual behaviours embedded in their social and cultural context. Instead of focusing on psychological processes as the basis for sexual behaviour, it tends to be social norms, relationships and gender imbalances that create the meaning and determinants of behaviour and behavioural change. These theories dictate that efforts to effect change at the community level will have the most significant impact on individuals who are contemplating changes and on those who have made changes but need support to sustain those changes. Social theories have been increasingly used with populations especially vulnerable to effects of partners and peers. These theories and models have been developed in the West and few examples have tested their relevance in developing countries.

(C) Structural and Environmental

Determinants of sexual behaviour can be seen as a function not only of individual and social but of structural and environmental factors as well. These factors include civil and organizational elements as well as policy and economic issues.

Theory for Individual and Social Change or Empowerment Model

This theory asserts that social change happens through dialogue to build up a critical perception of the social, cultural, political and economic forces that structure reality and by taking action against forces that are oppressive. In other words, empowerment should increase problem solving in a participatory fashion, and should enable participants to understand the personal, social, economic and political forces in their lives in order to take action to improve their situations. Werner (1997) states that, "*empowerment is the process by which disadvantaged people work together to take control of the factors that determine their health and their lives*". For this to happen he explains that feelings of powerlessness, which can come from lack of skills and confidence, have to be cast off. Although empowerment can only come from the group itself, enabling empowerment is possible by facilitating its determinants. The common struggle against gender or ethnic oppression, economic exploitation, political repression or foreign intervention is what builds necessary confidence.

A distinction is made between personal, organizational and community empowerment. Personal empowerment has to do with the psychological processes and is similar to self-efficacy and self esteem. Organizational empowerment encompasses both the processes that enable individuals to increase their control within the organization and the organization to influence policies and decisions in the community. An empowered community uses the skills and resources of individuals and organizations to meet respective needs.

Interventions using empowerment approaches must consider key concepts such as beliefs and practices that are linked to interpersonal, organizational and community change. Intervention activities can address issues at the community and organizational level such as central needs the community identifies, and any history community organizing among community members. The theory would prescribe including participants in the planning and implementation of activities.

Social Ecological Model for Health Promotion

In conformity with model, patterned behaviour is the result of interest and behaviour is viewed as being determined by the following:

(1) intrapersonal factors - characteristics of the individual like knowledge, attitudes, behaviour, self-concept skills

(2) interpersonal processes and primary groups formal and informal social network and social support systems, comprising the family, work group and friendships

(3) institutional factors - social institutions with organizational characteristics and formal and informal rules and regulations for operation
(4) community factors - relationships among organizations, institutions and informal networks within defined boundaries
(5) public policy - local, stage and national laws and policies.

Intervention strategies range from skills development at the intra-personal level to mass media and regulatory changes at other levels. The theory accepts the significance of the interplay between the individual and the environment, and considers multi-level influences on unhealthy behaviour. In this manner, the significance of the individual is de-emphasized in the process of behavioural change.

Socio-Economic Factors

Many studies have shown that economic determinants have a strong influence on individual sexual behaviour, mostly through poverty and underemployment. Cross-nationally, countries with the lowest standards of living are also the ones with the highest HIV incidence. Within both rich and poor countries, poverty is related to HIV, and HIV intensifies poverty.

The proposed mechanisms for this relationship are: non-cohabitation between young married couples which can arise from critical economic conditions forcing urban migration, seasonal work and truck driving, sex work, civil disturbances and war. Civil disturbance and war caused to displaced and refugee populations who not only lose their social and familial support systems but become highly vulnerable to HIV because of intense social and economic strain in a alien culture. In such conditions, HIV concerns take a very low priority in a risk hierarchy, and any previous or planned endeavours for the control of HIV transmission are disrupted, if not destroyed.

Conclusion

Community level theories, models or factors see human behaviour as a function not only of the individual or his or her immediate social relationships, but as depending on the community, organization and the political and economic environment as well. They are multidimensional with stress on linking the individual to the surrounding larger environmental systems. Interventions using this approach, thus, target organizations, communities and policy.

(D) Constructs Alone and Transtheoretical Models

Perception of Risk Construct

As behavioural interventions are designed to minimize higher risk behaviours, perception of risk is a construct in most individual psychosocial behavioural models and some interventions use the construct without applying any of the models in their entirety. Increasing perception of risk has been shown many times to increase HIV protective behaviour. Yet most behavioural models measure risk as individually conditioned which might not be relevant in many contexts. Not surprisingly, many women often perceive themselves at risk not because of their own behaviour, but due to the past or current, perceived or real behaviour of their sexual partner. Additionally, perception of risk as a predictor of future behavioural change has further complexities in circumstances where individuals report high perception of risk and high self-reported behavioural change. This condition may demonstrate limited realistic further behavioural change options, or feelings of fatalism.

Sexual Communication

Sexual communication has been noted in different situations to be predictive of condom use. Among incarcerated Latino adolescents with large numbers of sexual partners in the USA, it was reported that youth who communicated with their sex partners about each others' sexual history were importantly more likely to use condoms. In central Africa condom use was more likely if women reported discussion with their sexual partner about STDs or condoms. Sexual communication has also been reported as a source to self-efficacy among heterosexuals in Holland.

Key Approaches to Behavioural Change for HIV

Early in the AIDS epidemic, outcomes of population survey research alerted public health officials of the diversity of sexual behaviours and of the requirement to act quickly. The first interventions as well as the first applications of theories were propelled by the urgency to do anything to slow the major crisis at hand. Through popular public health channels, information was disseminated to populations at risk.

Today, a number of the interventions for the prevention of HIV transmission, rather than using one of the behavioural theories in its entirety, have developed programmes based on one or several constructs often depending on the socio-cultural, political, or economic situation and on the stage of the epidemic. Drawing on various models and modifying them to suit the population and context has been critical to implementation of prevention projects, particularly in international settings, as nearly all theories were developed in the West. These transtheoretical approaches are guided by critical constructs like risk perception, social norms and sexual communication to form the basis of interventions worldwide.

This section looks mainly at the most common approaches used to influence HIV risk reduction. Although these approaches are not consistently or directly derived from behavioural change theories or models, they draw on the different constructs mentioned above. The section is split between individual and community-level interventions, where the approach is mentioned and then specific examples of its use are reviewed.

(A) Approaches Aimed at Individual Level Behavioural Change

Information, Education and Communication

Mass and Small Group Education

As information was initially, for many, thought to be the key to behavioural change, HIV prevention programmes started with a focus on increasing awareness about the modes of transmission and prevention. Mass education for HIV prevention can take different forms but is often seen as a key component of a comprehensive AIDS prevention programme. Mass media, for instance, are directed to the general public and aim at teaching people essential facts, promoting healthy behaviour, quieting anxiety about casual transmission and preventing discrimination.

The description of the messages adopted by the information and education programmes of national AIDS control programmes of 38 different countries found that over 90 per cent emphasized on correcting misperceptions about AIDS. About 80 per cent provided information about personal risk assessment. In various countries, mass education provided the first step to national AIDS control programmes. Many mass education attempts successfully raised AIDS awareness by informing individuals of the risks of HIV infection, and in some cases education-based programmes were adequate to change high risk behaviours, increase condom sales, and reduce new HIV infections. The channels that national AIDS control programmes have used for mass education comprise targeted media, printed media and electronic media.

A review of 49 studies covering 18 countries to recognize empirical outcomes or evaluate impact of HIV-related mass-media campaigns in 1996 concluded that most campaigns with a view to "individual-level goals of knowledge, attitude or behavioural changes were generally successful at achieving these ends". However, behavioural end points of the projects reviewed were not mentioned. Additionally, as the author himself pointed out, large number of the project reports reviewed lacked methodological details; they were reported in conference abstracts. It is therefore not easy to conclude on the relative meaning of the term "successful", specially in relation to behavioural outcomes.

Small-group AIDS education is taking place across the world, advancing general knowledge of HIV in numerous communities. Small-group AIDS prevention programmes can be seen as having these important components.

- content
- context
- strategies.

Content comprises goals, objectives, and activities. The main content areas in most small-group intervention activities comprise: basic education about AIDS, sensitization to one's personal risks for HIV, instruction in individual actions that can minimize one's risk and exploring new ways to communication with sex partners. Entire interventions or research questions are erected on any one of these content areas.

The second component in small-group HIV prevention is the *context*. The various aspects of the intervention should be designed to fit the cultural, gender and developmental issues of participants. For instance, one investigator felt concerns of stigma and sexual identity were paramount to African American gay men and dedicated the whole session of this small-group intervention to focus on those issues.

The third component, *strategy*, is the process itself, where stress is placed on how the interventions are implemented between participants and group leader. Important elements to consider comprise how to foster trust, build group cohesiveness, promote motivation and mutual support among participants and between participants and the facilitator.

Although evaluations of small-group interventions have stressed on content and facilitation skills, all three components have been found to be critical to the success of this approach. The literature reports strong proof for the beneficial effects of small-group HIV prevention from randomized controlled trials of theory-based skills-building programmes. Many independent reviews of the literature as a whole found that small group HIV risk-reduction interventions result in meaningful changes in HIV risk behaviour.

Particularly in the USA, small-group AIDS prevention efforts have evolved since the starting of the epidemic from providing basic information in community groups and sensitizing people to personal risk sensitization. Later on, interventions began instructing people on condom use skills, eroticizing safer sex, and developing safer sex communication skills. Through interventions encompassing these elements, a number of people have reduced high-risk sexual behaviour, but not everyone is sensitive to small group behavioural interventions. For instance, small-group projects targeting heterosexual men for HIV prevention have not shown important intervention effects. Longer-term behavioural changes need ongoing support and modifications in the larger social environment within which these behaviours take place.

Peer Education

Peer education is one approach to small-group HIV prevention generally aimed at individual behaviour. The peer health educator approach recruits leaders in communities at risk to be implementers of the education programme to their peers. Selection of peer educators is a basic to the success of a programme and often includes:

- recognition by other members of the group
- being an opinion leader, thus well respected in the group
- willingness to be trained
- committed to the ends of the programme

Several interventions combine peer education with other approaches like the use of social networks, condom social marketing and outreach as these approaches can be complementary. Outreach work using peers has resulted in increased participation of targeted community members and increased diversity of participants.

The advantages of working with peers rather than with 'experts' from outside the social network are a lot depending upon the group at risk. Wingood noted that peer educators may be a more credible way of information for women, may communicate in a more understandable language, and may serve as positive role models. Other studies have revealed that when the group at risk is very different culturally from the majority, peers know the cultural risks and most proper and realistic risk-reduction strategies from experience.

The peer educator approach has been applied in as diverse populations as: dock workers in Nigeria, Arabian prisoners in Italy, street youth in Thailand, in—school youth in Armenia secondary school students in Argentina, taxi drivers in Cameroon low - and middle-class general population in Zambia, factory workers in Zimbabwe, sex workers in India, drug users in USA and traditional healers in South Africa, among many, many others.

In these various situations, peer educators performed differing tasks ranging from development and distribution of IEC materials comprising video clips and pamphlets, as well as condom discussion and distribution to conversations with peers on different topics such as empowerment, health and human rights, and basic AIDS information.

Surprisingly, all of the above studies, even though many were not randomly controlled, denoted positive results. But here again, many of these reports were conference abstracts lacking methodological details. In spite of, they show the astonishing diversity of populations and contexts with which peer education is being practised across the world.

Two studies analysed cost-effectiveness of peer education interventions among IDUs in the USA and factory workers in Zimbabwe. In Zimbabwe costs compared favourably to other HIV prevention programmes, and the US researchers concluded that the peer-driven intervention cost one thirtieth as much as the traditional (external) intervention.

As any other approach however, peer education has its limits. For instance, in Brazil, participants of a target group became health agents and lost their solidarity and support within the group, which is a main element to successful peer education. Another instance, comes from a convenience sample analysis of many peer education programmes in the USA that found a structural tendency for peer education programmes to employ low-income people and treat peer educators as the most marginal sector of the organizations's staff.

Testing and Counselling

In increasing numbers people in industrialized countries are receiving their HIV test outcomes as therapeutic options become available to more people. Research has shown various reasons developing nations should make Voluntary Testing and Counselling (VTC) accessible to their populations (UNAIDS, 1998).

Early identification of the virus enables referral for clinical care and psychosocial support. Ethically people have a right to know their serostatus with a view to protect themselves and others. And knowing their own serostatus and the options can motivate people to change higher risk behaviours. Additionally, De, Zoysa notes that HIV testing and counselling may have an important social impact through people knowing their serostatus sharing it with others and laying the groundwork for changes in social norms about HIV and AIDS. A positive HIV result has also encouraged some people to give personal evidences in community fora, a consequence that can have a powerful effect on individual attitudes, behaviours and social norms. In cultural contexts where fertility is highly valued, testing and counselling makes an important behavioural-change alternative to consistent condom use.

The theoretical foundation on which interventions providing testing and counselling are built principally includes the *stages of change model*. HIV testing and counselling may promote progression across the continuum of the stages of change. For instance, in rural south-western Uganda, a setting with high HIV prevalence, the majority of respondents in a research study reported that they had already made behavioural changes due to AIDS, but making further changes to protect themselves was contingent on knowing their HIV serostatus. It has thus been suggested that counselling promotes risk reduction through increasing perception of risk, self-efficacy and personal skills, and through reinforcing social norms or liability.

In 1991, in an extensive review of 50 testing and counselling studies in Africa, Australia, Europe and North America, Higgins *et al* found big risk reduction only among heterosexual couples with one infected partner. In other groups (homosexual men, injecting drug users, women) risk reduction was not very associated with counselling and testing.

An updated review of 35 studies conducted by Wolitski *et al.* in 1997 realised similar results to those of Higgins *et al* for some population groups. The clearest proof for positive behavioural effects of HIV VTC has been heterosexual sero-discordant couples where HIV counselling and testing was an important motivating factor to risk reduction. Studies of MSM have also indicated important risk reduction but it was not clearly related to their testing for HIV. Yet a UNAIDS report notes that among a sample of HIV-infected homosexual men in Norway the number of sex partners reduced from an average of 4.3 a year before to 1.6 after counselling and testing (UNAIDS, 1998). In HIV serodiscordant couples a consistent reduction in sexual risk practices followed HIV testing and counselling. Likewise, in most injecting drug users studies, counselling and testing proved to be beneficial in decreasing dangerous sexual practices. Across populations, individuals who learn they are HIV positive have been found to be more likely to change behaviour than those who learn they are HIV negative.

More recently a randomized controlled trial in 3 developing countries (Kenya, Tanzania and Trinidad and Tobago) displayed that couples receiving counselling and testing reduced unprotected intercourse among their spouses, mainly among serodiscordant and seropositive concordant couples. However, results mainly found that VTC produced important changes in reducing high-risk sexual practices with non-primary partners.

In the USA, a randomized controlled trial evaluating HIV post-test prevention counselling was made in 5 STD clinics comparing 3 arms: (1) HIV education comprising 2 sessions with brief HIV/STD messages, (2) HIV prevention counselling. 2 sessions intended to at increasing risk perception,)3) enhanced counselling, 4 sessions based on. theoretical constructs of behavioural change; self-efficacy and perceived norms, in a 12-month period. They got marked changes in condom use with both main and other partners across arms of the study. After 12 months, there were 19 per cent fewer new STD cases in the brief counselling group, and 22 per cent fewer in the increased counselling group, compared with the group that had received only educational messages. These findings help other studies showing benefits of client centered counselling combined with HIV test results.

Other, non-randomized studies in Rwanda, Uganda, Kenya and Zaire reported VTC to be a motivating factor mainly for couples to change behaviour. The AIDS Support Organization (TASO) provides counselling and support services to a number of clients with AIDS in urban and rural Uganda.

In an overall evaluation of TASO, it was marked that 90 per cent of all clients had revealed their HIV status to somebody following TASO services. On the countrary, a study in the Gambia showed no effect of individual post-test counselling on condom use among prostitutes who already had high rates of condom use before the intervention.

Wolitski sums up by noting that "*there is no question that HIV VTC can and does motivate behavioural change in some individuals*", but also that VTC alone does not always lead to changes and does not have the same effect in all populations and in different situations.

As with most other approaches, the stage of the epidemic and surrounding contextual factors will help to the outcome of the intervention. Moreover, the quality of the counselling provided is a key variable in predicting the impact of the intervention.

Conclusion

After years of experience with HIV prevention and different kinds of interventions aimed at individual behavioural change tested in different situations, certain characteristics of successful programmes point to key elements of approaches to behavioural change programmes. These elements comprise: increasing participants ability to communicate effectively about sex; helping participants increase their condom use skills; personalizing risk, achieving participants perception of risk avoidance as an accepted social norm, providing reinforcement and support for sustaining risk reduction. For individual level interventions to be successful, context particular information and skills are critical.

(B) Community-Level Interventions

Community-level approaches grew out of the realization that, in spite of the considerable risk reduction through individual-level behavioural change approaches, different approaches were required as well. Social epidemiology, pointing to differences in prevalence among many social categories within a given risk category in a community suggested intervening along these lines. The programmes in this section encompass the most widely publicized approaches to community level HIV prevention comprising interventions based on *social influence and social networks,* outreach programmes, school-based programmes, condom promotion and social marketing, community organizing and empowerment and policy level interventions. Each of these kinds of interventions either try to reduce individual vulnerability to or transmissibility of HIV, change community norms, limit dispersal of high seroprevalence networks or change community organizational structures making them less dangerous. Changing community cultures or community norms encourages motivation and reinforcement for individual HIV risk reduction. Several of the following programmes use ideas from the *theory of reasoned action* the *diffusion of innovations model* and the *theory of social influence* to mobilize peer pressure or to ostracize individuals who continue high-risk practices. Policy level changes like closing of bathhouses and enforcing condom use in brothels also account for important impact in community risk practices.

Social Influence and Social Network Interventions

Based on the *theories of social influence, diffusion of innovation, reasoned action and social cognitive theory,* these interventions use peers and social networks to send information. Social influence interventions recognizes key persons in communities who are capable of influencing others. The *social cognitive theory* posits that trusted role models are potent factor in the environment and the environment has a reciprocal relationship both with behaviour and the individual. In the *theory of reasoned action,* perceptions of social norms have a critical influence on behaviour. Social norms created by opinion leaders will ideally have a good effect on behaviour. Diffusion of innovation theory asserts that changing behaviour will more likely happen if the new behaviour is compatible with accepted social norms of particular social network, is simple to do, and has observable outcomes. One's social network can be a means of emotional and instrumental support and a reference that establishes social norms.

Research implemented using peer educators to influence social networks in gay communities showed important self-reported changes in safer sex practices after intervention. Encouraging results in changing social norms and safer sex behaviour have also been noted in a number of community-level social influence interventions in the USA. One programme implemented among men frequenting gay bars in three Southern cities started by identifying and recruiting opinion leaders. Project staff then trained leaders in risk-reduction, and the final stage involved opinion leaders in sending prevention messages to friends and other members of their social networks. In a later study using the same methods, researchers used a randomized experimental design with four test and four control cities and showed a reduction in population-level rates of risk behaviour after one year.

The empowerment project was like to the above studies but concentrated on young gay men in a midsize urban community in the USA, and included in the intervention package a publicity campaign and small-group sessions concentrating on individual behavioural change. In the test city, there was a 26 per cent reduction in unprotected anal intercourse compared to 3 per cent in the control city. A follow-up study examined the effectiveness of the various programme components (small groups, social events, and outreach) on post intervention sexual risk-taking. The small groups had large effect size, but reached significantly fewer men than social events and outreach. Although not as powerful, the social events and outreach were critical to the effectiveness of the programme as means of recruitment to the small groups and as a source of reaching men not interested in attending small groups. Authors concluded that the effectiveness of programme components were not independent; the synergy created by the whole programme makes the net effect of the intervention activities greater than the sum of its parts.

Sikkema *et al.* tested a comparable approach with women living in urban, low-income housing developments. The intervention comprised outreach, small groups and community activities to encourage social norms supportive of safer-sex and reduction of individual high-risk behaviour. Women who were identified as opinion leaders participated in a 4-session skills-building intervention centered on HIV prevention knowledge and behaviour. These women recruited other women who took participation in the same intervention and the cycle continued until about half the women in the housing development were reached. At the same time, social norm-changing events were being implemented. Outcomes of this randomized controlled trial found that condom use reported by women in the intervention site increased from 29 per cent at baseline to 41 per cent at 3-month follow-up.

The National AIDS Demonstration Research Projects effected in more than 60 sites in the USA to evaluate strategies among IDUs, combined research methodologies but stressed on the social networks of IDUs as the primary target group. The Indigenous Leader Outreach Intervention Model which combines medical epidemiology and community ethnography guided the project. Former IDUs were employed as outreach workers whose job was to recognize and access the social network, document the norms, values and situational factors relating to risk practices. Former IDUs were also liable for delivering the HIV prevention services. After a four-year intervention, incidence of HIV decreased from 8.4 to 2.4 per 100 person years. Sex risk practices decreased less dramatically than drug risk, but went from 71 per cent to 45 per cent. The same model was tested among sex workers in Indonesia with encouraging results.

Interpreting these outcomes for social influence interventions indicates that multi-component, individual and community level that combine cognitive-behavioural and norm-changing activities can result in positive changes for MSM and heterosexual women. In spite of the fact that all published reports mentioned here were based on interventions in the USA, since they are based on conversations with peers one could assume that they would be ideal for other populations (even non-literate) as well.

Outreach Interventions

Outreach interventions are conceptualized in a similar manner to social influence interventions in that they utilize individuals to pass on information within social networks, however the influential person may or may not be from the targeted community. The outreach worker enters the social system to encourage behavioural change as an individual change agent. Targeted communities are generally hard-to-reach groups such as drug users, sex partners of drug users, sex workers and isolated rural populations. The aims of outreach have often been harm reduction strategies like providing condoms to sex workers, but not necessarily addressing sex work itself.

Three large-scale research trials in the USA examined the effects of outreach delivered mainly to injecting drug users. The National AIDS Demonstration Research Projects targeted over 36,000 out-of treatment injecting drug users. Results denoted that sexual practices were much more difficult to change than sharing of drug using a equipment. The projects did show decrease in sex risk practices, but less dramatically than for drug risk practices.

A second step entitled the AIDS Evaluation of Street Outreach Projects supported by the CDC was taken in six US cities, and showed promising outcomes as well as being cost-effective. Again, this project found drug using behaviour easier to change than sexual behaviour. A third out-reach project (AIDS Community Demonstration Projects) was implemented in five US cities and had various target groups including. IDUs and their partners, MSM, female sex workers, street youth and men who have sex with men but do not recognize as gay. The health belief model, social cognitive theory, the theory of reasoned action and the transtheoretical stages of change model guided the outreach intervention. After the formative research, volunteer outreach workers implemented the intervention, by disseminating innovative, carefully designed materials and messages. The evaluation hinted that the communities moved across the continuum of stages of change due to the intervention. A dose-response effect was noted according to exposure to the intervention materials.

Interventions using outreach as a strategy have been carefully tested in the USA among diverse populations and have shown encouraging outcomes. This approach lends itself as well to hard-to-reach populations and has been used in various parts of the world though randomized controlled trials have not been reported outside the USA.

School-based Interventions

By the early 1990s, school-based programmes for HIV education existed in about three quarters of industrialized countries and 60 per cent of developing counters according to a survey of 38 countries. Besides interventions that simply give basic AIDS information in the classroom, multi-dimensional school-based programmes generally include classroom skills-building sessions, school-wide peer-led activities, and social norm changing programmes. Promotion of condom use was the theme most frequently followed in programmes for youth in and out of school. An extensive review of school-based interventions disclosed that no comprehensive school-based HIV-prevention interventions evaluated showed signs of promoting sexual acting out or fastening the onset of sexual intercourse (UNAIDS, 1997). It was found that effective interventions had a number of characteristics in common.

- proper information was provided about the risks involved in unprotected sex, enabling informed behavioural decision making
- programmes comprised skills building sessions increasing self-efficacy for safer-sex negotiating practices
- components were often based on social cognitive theory comprising modeling of safer behaviours
- activities were conducted in small groups or had a minimum of 14 hours of contact
- opportunities for youth to personalize information were given
- social pressures to engage in sex were addressed with strategies for resisting peer pressure
- reinforced supportive group norms and proper individual values for engaging in safer behaviour were stressed
- extensive training was given for teachers and/or peers who were to implement the training.

The element distinguishing school-based programmes from other interventions for youth was the supportive structural aspect played by schools and teachers, and the interaction between school, parents, students and community.

Condom Promotion and Social Marketing

It has now been proved numerous times that correct use of condoms is an effective method of preventing HIV transmission. Yet, countless research studies have recognized obstacles to their use in settings throughout the world, comprising inaccessibility and partner communication among other factors.

Most initial HIV prevention programmes included condom promotion and free distribution as part of a comprehensive HIV prevention package. Free distribution was inevitably aimed at introducing condoms where they were not previously available or distributing them to destitute populations at high risk such as sex workers and refugees. Although this approach accomplished its intended result of making condoms accessible without delay to large populations, the dearth of sustainability and reliability of free condom distribution programmes commanded the introduction of condom social marketing strategies mainly aimed at certain population.

Condom social marketing, which may well be the most developed of public health communication approaches, intends remove the barriers to condom use by using commercial marketing techniques like advertising and packaging to make the product accessible, affordable and attractive to all types of people. The theories underlying social marketing programmes derive from several different disciplines including operant conditioning and social cognitive theories as well as economic and marketing principles. Social marketing has been termed a 'strategic planning' approach based on the theoretical 'principal of exchange' which explains that people will only change their behaviour to something less pleasant (like condom use) if they perceive proper benefit (Kennedy, personal communication). Social marketing techniques highlight the significance of adapting the campaign to suit the characteristics of the population group being targeted. It dedicates sufficient time to formative research, which makes important asking the consumer always and often about his or her point of view. Modifying products needs a good understanding of the culture of the target group. Availing condoms at non-traditional outlets like as truck stops, bars, and hotels is integral to social marketing success. Flooding these non-traditional outlets with condoms aims not only to increase availability but also to increase social acceptability.

Consequences of these programmes have shown dramatic increases in condom sales in countries, such as Cote d'lvoire, Uganda and Malaysia where condoms were mainly unavailable before social marketing campaigns. After a 3-year peer-led condom promotion programme among sex workers in West Bengal, India, found that condom use rates rose from 3 per cent to 81 per cent, a social marketing campaign was launched. Six months into the project using peer education and community participation, free dissemination of condoms had decreased by 50 per cent and the same amount of condoms had been sold. Social marketing programmes have also been developed in Mexico, Dominican Republic, Canada, Brazil, Vietnam, Pakistan, Zambia, Botswana, Cameroon, South Africa and Haiti for HIV prevention. Evaluations have shown success in increasing condom use mainly among adolescents in Zambia and among married women in small urban areas in Pakistan.

Besides condom promotion, social marketing techniques have also been effective for other HIV prevention strategies like promotion of testing and counselling for adolescents in the USA, and the recruitment of research participants in Puerto Rico.

Community Organizing, Empowerment and Participatory Action Research

Empowerment approaches are built on the premise that positive public health impact is fostered by knowing the relationship between social structure and health, and by recognizing that lasting change is a process that starts from within a community. Empowerment regarding HIV in the USA has its historical roots in public health and community psychology. From the field of education, Wallerstein defined empowerment as:

"Empowerment education, as developed from Paulo Freire's writings, includes people in group efforts to identify their problems, to critically assess social and historical roots to problems, to envision a healthier society, and to develop strategies to overcome hindrances in achieving their goals. Through community participation, people develop new beliefs in their ability to influence their personal and social spheres. An empowering health education attempt therefore involves much more than improving self-esteem, self -efficacy or other health behaviours that are independent from environmental or community change; the targets are individual, group and structural change. Empowerment embodies a broad process that encompasses prevention and other goals of community connectedness, self-development, improved quality of life, and social justice."

Beeker suggests a definition of an empowerment intervention like.

"A community empowerment intervention seeks to effect community-wide change in health-related behaviours by organizing communities to define their health problems, to identify the determinants of those problems and to engage in effective individual and collective action to change those determinants,".

Empowerment approaches assume that health behaviours are not completely under volitional control of individuals, thus are not completely isolated events, but embedded within social, cultural and economic surroundings.

The impact of society's defined gender roles on protective health behaviour of women highlights the value of empowerment approaches, especially for HIV-vulnerable women. Beeker mentions ideally what the components of an intervention based on community empowerment for women would look like. The intervention would address the cultural environment by identifying gender roles that define women as subordinate to men; the physical environment by comprising access to appropriate services and materials such as battered women's shelters and both male and female condoms; the structural environment like opportunities for women to change their economic status; and the policy/legal environment like businesses providing paid leave for community service and child care.

Community participation at all levels of implementation is an integral aspect of community empowerment approaches. Interventions include community organizing, and Participatory Action Research (PAR) into their programmes. A strength of PAR resides in the ability of participants in connection with committed and creative professionals to adapt methods and content to diverse contexts. The positive results of PAR arise from its collaborative trust-building capacity, with direct community input that responds to emerging changes in social, political and economic situations. These interventions want to support communities to be self-determining in their ability to integrate HIV programmes into existing community structures by assessing their own requirements and priorities, defining, implementing and evaluating their own work.

Empowerment approaches have been used for AIDS risk reduction through various different strategies and in countless different settings and contexts. The literature mentions empowerment interventions directed at women, young gay men, youth, people with HIV and AIDS as well as many other communities at risk.

An intervention using PAR among lesbian women highlighted the power of community ownership of the project and its community over time that provided a space for engagement and commitment where women focused on community mores, values, and social expectations about sexual relating, drug use and HIV. The feeling of solidarity with peer educators enabled women to reduce risk behaviours.

Empowerment can have far-reaching positive health and welfare benefits. Schuler et al. describes the impact of involving women in credit programmes on contraceptive use. She found that, in Bangladesh, rural programmes for women can play an important role in changing fertility norms and accelerating contraceptive use by strengthening women's economic positions and fostering women's empowerment.

Other empowerment interventions for sex workers include a project in Zambia, where women fish traders who often experience sexual exploitation have been supported in forming economic cooperatives as a way of protecting themselves against HIV. A second example is a programme in India where women have been taught how to collectively save sufficient savings to pay bonds binding them to sex work.

Importantly, Beeker reminds us that empowerment approaches do not strive to substitute for individual psychosocial interventions, but to 'widen the lens to include person-in-environment' approaches. She notes that there is increased commitment to community participation, but that there remains a difficulty surmountable gap between empowerment rhetoric and practice. For that gap to be bridged, one key element is progress in operationalizing new concepts and constructs, and testing hypothesized relationships between, for example, community participation and community capacity to effectively address health issues. Although tools for measurement of single and multi-level (from personal to community level) empowerment have been developed and tested, they have not yet been used on a wide scale.

Policy Level Interventions

Policy level interventions are 'enabling' approaches that attempt to remove structural barriers at a larger level. Many believe that AIDS interventions are moving from solely investigating individual approaches to multidimensional models of community mobilization, empowerment and structural policy level interventions.

The earliest and some of the most effective efforts of community level change for HIV have resulted from social action. ACTUP, formed in 1987 in New York, is responsible for many successful policy initiatives for people living with HIV and AIDS as well as advocating for everyone's responsibility to practise safer sex.

Another widely recognized policy level intervention is the 100 per cent Condom Programme in Thailand that mandated condom use in brothels and during other commercial sex encounters. Components of the programme included a requirement that sex workers use condoms with all clients, that condom use be monitored, that brothel owners and managers assist in promoting condom use with uncooperative clients and that there should be sanctions against brothel owners for non-compliance. The programme showed a dramatic increase in self-reported condom use during commercial sex acts (14 per cent to 90 per cent), a decline in reported STD attendees in government clinics, and a decline of HIV positive army conscripts. Success of the programme has been attributed to the fact that it was based on harm reduction in a population at very high risk. It did not try to eliminate the brothels but attempted to reduce HIV transmission within them, and it used national policy which ensured a broad and lasting effort.

Conclusion

HIV prevention at the community level is an integral component to check further spread of HIV. By working with communities, in opposite to individuals, one is stressing on changing policy, social structures, social norms and cultural practices that surround individual risk behaviours. Community level changes working at the level of changing subculture have strength to effect long-term maintenance of changed behaviours, by changing the environment surrounding individuals to support safer behaviours. At the same time, many of these approaches highlight the significance of participatory methods of include and empower individuals. It is important to note that many of the interventions mentioned above may have initially stressed on one level (such as policy, or empowering individuals), but as the programmes developed they generally comprise more target levels including changing local cultures and subcultures. Programmes discussed here have been the most widely publicized approaches to community level HIV prevention yet several more innovative projects exist worldwide.

Finally, development of methods for application and evaluation of community-level programmes has not been operationalized on a broad spectrum. Assessing effectiveness of these programmes introduces a number of challenging issues like measuring community level changes using the community as the level of analysis rather than the individual. In addition, identifying elements of the intervention to measure, thus defining new community level indicators and obtaining large enough sample sizes to identify significance add new challenges to community level evaluation. This makes design of such programmes and the ability to carry them out possibly more complicated than individual-based programmes.

Examples of the Impact of Theory-driven Interventions

Theoretic models that have proved useful in explaining and predicting changes in HIV-related sexual behaviour give guidance in the design and implementation of prevention programmes. Reviews of theory-driven interventions have noted that these interventions focus both intrapersonal and interpersonal factors, provide skills training, try to change social norms and are thus more effective at reducing risk behaviour among participants. This section summarizes positive outcomes of theory-based interventions by particular population groups, comprising women, men, and youth.

Although injecting drug users fit into any of the above categories, we have placed them in their own group as interventions target them mainly.

(A) Women

A review of 51 reports through 1997 on studies worldwide noted the absence of interventions identifying the mechanisms of preventive effects and theoretical frameworks upon which interventions are built. This review found differences in effectiveness between target populations and between different kinds of interventions. Interventions targeting sex workers were the most likely to find increased condom use, decreased incidence of STDs, and decrease in unprotected intercourse (9 out of 10 studies). Effectiveness for other groups at risk was more varied: 13 out of 18 studies of African-American or Latino descent women were effective, as were 3 out of 10 studies for IDUs, 1 out of 3 for partners of IDUs, 2 out of 3 for STD clinic patients, 4 out of 7 for US college students, and 6 out of 14 studies for mixed gender community groups.

Ickovics et al. detected seven types of interventions tried among women globally: small group, community-wide, media, HIV counselling and testing, individual counselling, classroom education and laboratory experiment. Community-wide (12 out of 14) and small group interventions (13 out of 19) were more likely to show important results. Interestingly, Ickovics' review noted that higher intensity (5 or more sessions) were less effective than low-intensity small-group programmes for women. Authors suggested this may reflect the more resistant population targeted. Various international programmes incorporated peer-led *diffusion of innovations* approaches and all reported statistically significant increases in condom use (6 studies out of 6). In conformity with this review, less effective interventions for women overall were individual counselling (0 out of 4) and HIV testing and counselling (3 out of 6) as primary prevention. Testing and counselling and individual counselling, however, have demonstrated effectiveness as secondary prevention with serodiscordant couples (Ickovics, 1998).

A review of randomized controlled trials in the USA conducted by Wingood and DiClemente found that all effective interventions for women had a number of identifiable characteristics. In opposite to the review by Ickovics, the four studies mentioned were guided by the *social cognitive* theory (a theory based on the individual, taking into consideration environmental and behavioural factors, which places a strong emphasis on self-efficacy) provided skills in condom use and sexual communication and stressed support for continued maintenance of safer sexual behaviour. In addition, all effective interventions were peer-led and addressed gender-related influences like gender-based power imbalances within the relationship.

Generally, successful skills training interventions for women consider cultural factors and effort to personalize messages. Targeting women in the USA, and adolescents in the USA and Holland with behavioural skills enhancement programmes have produced positive effects. Studies among women in the USA have generally consisted of four to five sessions and demonstrated positive outcomes with medium-sized effects. Condom use has risen up to double the rate at baseline. Specific components of behavioural skills enhancement that have been tested comprised of: risk education and sensitization, condom use and safer sex skills training, and sexual communication skills training. Kalichman notes that behavioural skills enhancement training has not been tested experimentally outside the USA, so it is unclear to what extent it would give advantage to women in other countries.

An intervention among women in a New York City housing project was based on the *diffusion of innovation theory* in association with community mobilization. Women were recruited, organized and trained to help develop role model stores for the project newsletters. These women were also expected to begin discussions with their peers regarding HIV prevention. Information was diffused rapidly and seemed to promote discussion and condom use among the housing project women. Reported condom use of female sex partners within the housing project for IDUs rose for 15 per cent to 45 per cent.

The theory of gender and power given a model for the design of a successful gender-appropriate social skills intervention for African American women in San Francisco. The intervention addressed how to successfully talk safer sex and improve partner norms favourable to consistent condom use in comparison to a control group that received like training in a delayed fashion. The results showed significantly greater consistent condom use, greater sexual self-control, greater sexual assertiveness, and increased partners' adoption of norms supporting consistent condom use in the intervention group.

The sages of *change model* was used to guide a 6-month

longitudinal study among women in drug treatment, housing shelters, and hospital clinics in the USA, and showed that women exposed to individual stage-tailored counselling were twice as likely to report consistent condom use with chief partner 'at last sex contact' as women receiving free on-site reproductive health counselling and services. The stage-based counselling also proved useful at preventing relapse from consistent use further along in the process of change.

One study assessed the AIDS Risk Reduction Model (ARRM) with HIV-positive, largely disadvantaged, women in the USA and found that 6 variables representing the four important constructs of the model were associated with consistent condom use. The strongest predictor of condom use was perceived self-efficacy in influencing the partners's sexual behaviour, yet no important relationship between condom use and general self-efficacy was detected. The two other partner related variables associated with condom use were his seronegativity and his not wanting more children. The respondents' reproductive intentions were not significantly associated with condom use. The three variables that were negatively concerned to condom use were: having a conflictual relationship with primary partner, believing that condoms reduce sexual pleasure; and the use of drugs of alcohol in the previous four weeks.

Regarding to the *health belief model*, among heterosexual adults in Holland barriers to condom use, such as reduced pleasure of sex, were predictive but cues to action were not concerned to condom use intentions. The perception that most others in the reference group would engage in condom use with new sexual partners was an important predictor of condom use intentions and stresses the importance of the social environment with respect to AIDS protective behaviour.

Again internationally, an intervention guided by the social cognitive theory and community health promotion implemented in North-eastern Thailand targeting village women was evaluated using surveys, focus group discussions and village meetings. Elicitation research identified the significance of including total villages in the intervention rather than women alone. The evaluation found that eight of the nine result goals were achieved with significant increases in married women taking the initiative in reducing the risk posed to them by the sexual activities of their husbands. Certain measures taken by women included negotiating condom use with their husbands, and telling their husbands, and telling their husbands not to visit prostitutes. Men surveyed, however, did not change their condom use behaviour.

Sex Workers

Among the various studies including sex workers, only two will be highlighted here. A year-long intervention targeting sex workers, brothel owners and clients in Thailand used different small group sessions with peer educators who were experienced women and were called 'superstars'. The 'model brothel' aspect of the programme worked with owners to enforce essential condom use by sex workers, and clients were educated to use condoms. Volunteers were trained to pose as clients to test sex workers' condom negotiation skills. Results said that sex workers increased their refusal of sex without a condom rate from 42 per cent before the intervention to 92 per cent following the programme. The authors found that this multifaceted approach specifically focusing in sex workers, and accepting the importance of working with clients and owners was critical to their success.

A second study that mentioned the theoretical background and its usefulness for sex workers noted the utility of *health belief model and social cognitive theory*. One study guided by these two models worked with four groups of female sex workers in Indonesia and found that both increases in knowledge and condom use were mainly related to the number of intervention sessions the women attended. Results reflected the various social context of sexual behaviour of the four groups of sex workers and indicated that the four groups of women had different levels of knowledge about AIDS, different socio-economic levels, different numbers of clients and different self-efficacy. Beliefs about the advantages of condoms were highly predictive of condom use in 3 of the 4 groups. In the group with lower knowledge about AIDS, perceived susceptibility to other STDs, rather than HIV, was concerned to condom use. Self-efficacy was highly predictive of condom use in 3 out of 4 of the groups of sex workers. In the fourth group self-efficacy was already high as this group of sex workers do not depend on pimps and contact clients independently. Authors highlight that sex work is a complex business the comprises multiple sub-populations and distinct settings. These diverse realities must be considered in intervention design and implementation.

Conclusion

Interventions targeting women have lagged behind those of men historically. Women were left out of prevention efforts early in the AIDS epidemic particularly in Europe and the US. Today, considering gender, relationship and contextual issues as central to decisions with regard to sexual behaviour were universally important for the success of the interventions discussed above. Thus using gender driven theory across cultures might prove useful as sexual encounters in some situations can be imposed and gender roles and cultural values and norms sometimes define, or at the least, influence sexual behaviour. One international review found that peer-led community interventions guided by the *diffusion of innovation theory* were more successful overall than individual level interventions. Skills training particularly in condom use and sexual communication, and perception of risk were important variables among women in US studies. As with other populations, interventions easied by peers were often more successful than those using a facilitator from outside the target group as peers can generally target more appropriate, context particular methods for risk reduction.

Only one study, guided by the AIDS risk reduction model, reviewed here looked specifically at HIV-infected women and found that factors concerned to her sexual partner were more influential than many personal variables. Interventions with female sex workers often used the health belief model and the social cognitive theory with important results in diverse settings worldwide. Successful programmes often percepted the importance of including brothel owners and clients in their activities, thus considering the wider environmental factors associated with the behavioural practices included. The sex workers study conducted in Indonesia highlighted the importance of considering diversity among what is often generically termed a 'sex worker' population. By utilizing a theory driven intervention, investigators were able to recognize critical differences in predictive constructs between different sex worker groups.

(B) Men

Men Having Sex with Men (MSM)

A recent review of interventions with gay men found that studies mainly fall into 3 types: individually based, small-group and community-level. At the individual level, the review noted one unique study that randomly assigned men to one of 3 groups: (1) standard group that analysed HIV-prevention posters, (2) self-justification group that was asked to recall, as vividly as feasible, an occasion where they had unsafe sex and then justify according to a pre-determined scale, and (3) control group received no intervention. After 2 months, the self-justification group was importantly less likely to report unsafe sex than the other 2 groups.

One randomized controlled HIV-prevention study in the USA applying the small-group approach, used a 12-week intervention with 3 booster sessions among 104 men randomized to either receive, (1) the HIV risk-reduction intervention or (2) a waiting list control group. The four important areas covered in the intervention were HIV risk education, behavioural skills training, sexual assertiveness training and lifestyle changes for relapse prevention. The intervention group showed important reductions in rates of unprotected anal intercourse and increased rates of condom use immediately after the intervention, but 40 per cent relapsed 16 months later. Similar intervention components were tested among ethnic minority men and were found effective in reducing numbers of partners and rates of unprotected intercourse, with the strongest effects among Chinese and Filipino-American men.

In a third study using group intervention approach among African American men, components comprised: (1) discussions on being Black and gay or bisexual, building social support, and large-group discussion of AIDS misperceptions among Black men, (2) enhancing positive feelings about safer sex, practice of condom application skills, developing strategies to use condoms, and (3) dealing with issues of partner resistance, analysing one's own hurdles to staying safer, problem-solving safer-sex options, role play exercises, maintenance of safer sex, and establishing social norms for safer sex. Participants were randomly assigned to either a single session, a triple session or a wait-list control group. Outcomes indicated that men in the triple-session intervention group significantly reduced unprotected anal intercourse after 12 months of follow-up.

Controlled studies with men who have sex with men (MSM) have indicated various characteristics that have enabled men to change behaviour and maintain safer sex:

- eroticizing safer sex materials
- brief training on establishing and maintaining safer sex relationships
- how to discuss safer sex
- training on how to reduce stress
- intensive group counselling

Behavioural skills-enhancement interventions targeting MSM in different cultural settings have consistently demonstrated increased condom use during anal intercourse, with the greatest changes occurring with non-primary partners.

The diffusion theory has been shown to be effective in changing sexual behaviour of men who have sex with men of various studies in the USA. The model was tested in 3 small southern cities and consequences indicated systematic reduction in the population's high-risk behaviour with 15 per cent to 29 per cent reductions from baseline levels. Kegeles et al. used the diffusion theory to design an intervention to address determinants of high risk sex in young gay men in the USA. The authors recognized natural channels of communication to highlight sexual risk behaviour among the concerns of young gay men and to find alcohol and drug-free alternative environments for them. While comparison communities made no important changes, intervention communities showed important changes in unprotected anal intercourse with primary and non-primary partners.

Heterosexual Men

Within like populations like STD clinic attendees, self-efficacy was used to predict risk decrease in two different studies in the USA. Unfortunately, there is a dearth of information on behavioural interventions tested among heterosexual men. Kalichman notes that the behavioural interventions that have been tested in randomized controlled trials have not been effective in decreasing high-risk sexual behaviour. In one randomized controlled trial conducted among inner-city African American men a cognitive-behavioural skills-building intervention was compared with an AIDS educational intervention. No significant differences between groups was noted for AIDS concerned knowledge, intention to use condoms or condom use. Yet, there were some important lessons learned from this study. Greater value should be placed on relevant issues for the specific population. In a population with multiple competing risk practices, a social service programme that can give AIDs education along with drug treatment and job services may be more effective. The other two issues raised by this study were: the format of small group discussions was not well received by all men in the study and that cognitive-behavioural skills training programmes for HIV risk reduction should not be assumed to fit all vulnerable populations. Main reasons suggested by Kalichman were that heterosexual men may dearth a sense of vulnerability for HIV as they were not identified as engaging in high-risk behaviours for HIV as portrayed early in the epidemic in the USA.

Conclusion

The first decade of interventions with MSM noted major risk reduction with behavioural theory driven interventions comprising recognizable characteristics such as eroticizing safer sex, and improving sexual communication. Kalichman noted that we should not be too optimistic as applying again results to a dynamic epidemic may not continue to give intended outcomes (Kalichman, 1998). Our responses should be evolving as fast as the epidemic changes. More recently innovative programmes have initiated aiming at the community level rather than the individual. Interventions based on the *diffusion of innovations* theory have displayed community level change with gay men in the USA.

Most studies highlight that safer sex is easier with one's non-primary partner than with one's primary partner.

Choi points out the limited utility in strictly individually-based theories for particular groups at risk such as Asian-Pacific Islander men who have strong cultural demands and community stigma against homosexuality. Without considering these powerful contextual influences on behaviour, interventions cannot expect important results. Peterson describes how issues of being an African American MSM were directly addressed in their intervention along with social support and condom skills. As with other population groups, the intervention must be tailored to suit its population group, that is the group itself should be able to express its requirements and priorities for the programme to be successful.

In spite of the impressive results with gay men in diverse settings, there are few positive findings with heterosexual men in the industrialized world. As this group was not seen as vulnerable early in the epidemic, interventions concentrated on MSM and IDU populations. STD patients, however have been targeted with mixed outcomes. Two studies in the USA, guided by the social cognitive theory found increased condom use and one in the UK found no effect on behaviour. In developing world, approaches like testing and counselling have proven successful at motivating behavioural change among heterosexual men. Particular population groups, such as farm workers in Zimbabwe were targeted with an intervention guided by the social-ecological model for health promotion.

(C) Youth

Globally, most young people have started sexual intercourse by the age of 18 or 19 and at least half by the age of 16 (UNAIDS, 1998). In the USA about half of all adolescents are estimated to be sexually active and this percentage increases to over 80 per cent in some minority groups. Young people between the ages of 15 and 24 make up the majority of new HIV infections. Most of them live in the developing countries, but industrialized countries also face severe problems. USAID has estimated that by the year 2010 there will be a total of 41 million orphans who have lost their mother or both parents because of HIV/AIDS worldwide (UNAIDS, 1998a).

Intervention research with young people demonstrates that the success of the approach depends heavily on the youth's level of sexual experience. Comprehensive sex education among youth that have never had sex has been effective in delaying onset of intercourse among high school students.

A detail international review of 110 outcome evaluations with youth found that effective programmes.

- focused on understanding social and/or media influences on sexual behaviour to be able to make strong group norms against unprotected sex
- listened to what young people think and believe to ensure acceptable and appropriate programmes
- comprised modeling and practice of communication or negotiation skills
- integrated pregnancy and STD prevention with HIV programmes
- focused mainly on disadvantaged youth, providing access to resources and/or services to address their basic requirements (health care, legal aid).

This review also suggested that, although a clear pattern and full understanding are lacking, *social learning theories* have a greater strength than other theoretical frameworks in changing youth behaviour. Other cross-sectional surveys found that *the theory of reasoned action and the health belief model as well as the social learning theory* can help know behaviour of young people. All successful, theory-based interventions have consisted of skills training besides information and motivational components for young people.

Howard and McCabe showed success of the *social influence theory* using slightly older teenagers in the US to identify peer and social pressures that encourage negative health behaviours, to present factual information, teach assertiveness and discuss problem situations. Evaluation outcomes of the programme that included 536 students from a low-income population in Atlanta showed that among students who had not had sexual intercourse, those who took participation in the programme were significantly more likely to continue to postpone sexual activity through the end of the ninth grade than were similar students who did not take participation. A second carefully implemented intervention guided by *social influence theory* among US middle school students resulted in null findings. The authors note improper community and family-level intervention. Feasible dilution of the messages and perhaps over saturation of students with the programmes's health messages by the 8th grade.

In addition one study assessing the use of the health belief model to predict condom use among university students in Nigeria found that the major *health belief model* variables, comprising perceived benefits of condom use, perceived obstacles to condom use and cues to action, together with AIDS knowledge and male gender, significantly predicted condom use.

Reitman *et al.* suggest that behavioural constructs require to target specific behaviours. Their study, guided by the *health belief model* and the *theory of reasoned action*, among African American adolescents found that addressing condom use, decrease of the number of partners, or the frequency of sexual intercourse all concerned to different risk reduction strategies. The adolescents' positive attitude toward condoms emerged as the single strongest correlate of actual condom use.

Although multiple-session interventions have shown effectiveness, one project targeting African American adolescents demonstrated that a single-session workshop concentrating on cognitive behavioural skills training produced important increases in HIV-related knowledge, reductions in risk promoting faiths and lower frequencies of high-risk sexual behaviours.

One of the few studies that tested theoretical constructs in a manner that could delineate mediators of change was a single-session intervention among US college students to promote STD prevention. Researchers used regression analyses to show that changes in perceived advantages of condom use, acceptance of sexuality, sexual control, attitudes toward condoms, and self-efficacy for condom use were linked to behavioural intentions to use condoms. The authors found that the mechanisms for change in their intervention were affective attitudes toward condoms and condom users, and self-efficacy for condom use.

Conclusion

Together, the outcomes of these studies suggest that constructs subsumed in behavioural theory have greatly enhanced our understanding of risk behaviour among youth in different settings and situations. The *social influences theory* was also useful in one study but a *second study* using the same theory showed null findings. Skills training, attitudes, norms and self-efficacy have all proved effective in predicting behavioural change among young people. In intervention research, these constructs have also been useful in mediating actual risk behaviours. Outcomes have shown that young people who have already initiated sexual relations must be treated very differently than those who have not, and that interventions have to as well target particular behaviours rather than risk reduction in general. Although we noted one study in Nigeria, most theory-based research and intervention has been done in the USA. Without further research, these results may be not easy to apply in settings outside the USA. Reitman correctly concludes that condom use is a behaviour that might be particularly sensitive to situational or contextual variations especially among different populations such as the youth.

(D) Injecting Drug Users

Drug addiction is a major risk factor for HIV infection in about 80 countries across the world. Behaviours associated with drug use that are risk factors for HIV transmission are sharing of drug injection equipment and unprotected sex with an infected partner. As this report is stressing on sexual transmission, the sharing of drug injection equipment will not be discussed.

In a recent review of 19 interventions primarily in the USA targeting Injecting Drug Users (IDU), authors concluded that interventions comprised of:

- individual counselling
- HIV testing and counselling
- group interventions
- street outreach
- social interventions (Gibson, 1998)

In controlled studies, greater impact on behaviour was shown through intense and sustained interventions compared with their comparison conditions. Additionally, participants in successful interventions seemed to be more stable and better motivated than their counterparts who were a more heterogeneous group at many stages of behavioural change. The latter finding suggests that future interventions should target subgroups according to risk. As substantial to dramatic behavioural change resulted from both test and comparison groups in many studies, authors found that participating in evaluation research may itself have been a valuable intervention and the impact of behavioural assessments was understood partially responsible for this finding. One recommendation of this review was to consider a social change approach to HIV prevention in IDUs with a view to influence social norms towards safer behaviour.

Globally, it has been noted that IDUs need specific information targeting both the individual needs of the IDUs and the social/cultural context of injecting drug use. The support of particular health and social services is critical, for if an IDU has been motivated by a prevention message to seek treatment or use condoms, the service must be more easily available than drugs. Among 16 countries surveyed in 1992, the success in reaching IDUs varied widely with France reaching less than 5 per cent of that population and Sweden and Australia reporting over 90 per cent of IDU population reached. The gaps recognized in IDU prevention programmes centre around not addressing the social construction of addiction including poverty and social inequities that are strong predictors of HIV infection. If programmes only stress on harm reduction without approaching the larger issues, success will remain limited.

Conclusions

In contrast to what was commonly thought about IDU populations, reviews have noted substantial risk reduction among drug users especially as a result of sustained interventions. Reports on drug users generally emphasize drug use risk rather than sexual risk, but those reports that consider both have noted that sexual risk reduction is much more difficult to achieve than drug use risk. However, a review in 1998 stated that nearly all studies that assessed sexual practices found significant reductions in the number of sexual partners reported by subjects and/or increased use of condoms. Numerous studies have identified drug and alcohol intoxication as associated with high risk sexual behaviour, thus highlighting the importance of understanding and addressing the social construction of drug use. The *stages of change model* has been useful at guiding interventions with drug users. As with all of the above population groups, IDUs as well are an extremely diverse community, that should be seen and addressed in its complexity. Thus, interventions should target subgroups and consider the social construction of addiction to be effective.

Challenges

(A) Design/Context Issues

Design

Interventions based on theory have a better chance of success and theory can make it easier to understand why an intervention was or was not successful. Despite their contributions to the understanding of the psychological processes individuals go through while attempting to change behaviour, the limitations of the psychological theories of behavioural change have been well described in the literature. Most of these models are based on behaviours that are under intentional and volitional control, ignoring the fact that sexual behaviour involves two people, is often impulsive and is influenced by sociocultural, contextual as well as personal and subconscious factors that may be difficult to influence. Numerous studies have identified alcohol and drug intoxication as influencing sexual behaviour highlighting the importance of understanding the social context around sexual behaviour.

In a comprehensive review of behavioural interventions for HIV/AIDS prevention, Oakley *et al*. found that the most popular type of intervention was giving information. The review looked at 68 separate outcome evaluations among young people and adults, and suggests that sound and effective interventions are most likely to be skills-based interventions provided by peers or clinical psychologists in community settings using interviews or role plays and targeting behaviour or combined behaviour and knowledge outcomes.

The range of study designs is important to note. Randomized controlled trials were not considered exclusively for this report, as these conditions are almost inevitably only found in the industrialized world. In order for this report to consider countries with the highest prevalence, the least amount of resources and some of the most innovative responses the criteria remained broad.

The range of outcome measures encountered in doing a review such as this one, makes 'success' difficult to define. Many interventions oriented by theory rely on reported changes in behaviour as their behavioural outcome measure. Some however were satisfied with 'intentions' to change as intentions often predict behaviour. Others use markers such as changes in rates of STD infection, or HIV infection. All of these outcomes were treated as valid in this report, but were noted for the reader to distinguish the differences.

One of the greatest limitations of interventions and studies assessing these interventions was short follow-up time. Lack of follow-up time can undermine an intervention by not allowing positive feedback, not waiting for possible changes in social and cultural norms, and not taking maintenance of behavioural change into consideration.

Targeting

There has been much discussion around the issue of targeting AIDS interventions. From an epidemiological perspective it has been argued that to have an impact on the sexual transmission of HIV, interventions need to reach those most at risk of acquiring or transmitting the infection especially early in the epidemic. In information and education campaigns, many suggest that messages are more effective when they can be directed toward a specific target population as the language and approach ought to fit specific needs and solutions appropriate for different communities. Recent simulation studies have also argued that targeting interventions to priority groups would be an efficient and effective approach for HIV prevention in developing countries. For example, when addressing specific groups such as youth, it has been shown that interventions must look at those who have initiated sex as a different group from those who have not, to be effective. The danger arises, when the epidemic spreads into the general population, targeting most at risk populations is no longer sufficient to reduce transmission. Another concern with regards to targeting to reduce transmission is how to define the target group, by occupation, age group, geography. Identifying populations at risk and targeting too quickly can miss important vulnerable groups, such as male sex workers in Asia. Targeting populations that are more vulnerable should not be seen as singling them out and therefore increasing stigma. Working with priority groups is still important at any stage of the epidemic, but should be combined with other activities to reach a broader population equally at risk.

Targeting according to risk of transmission is one aspect, but a second issue is how much of the limited resources to place on primary prevention and how much on secondary prevention. Some studies address specifically targeting prevention efforts at already infected individuals.

(B) Gender

A significant number of studies have shown that gender influences HIV risk behaviour. As Ulin (1992) notes when referring specifically to women who are poor and dependent on their male sexual partners, reducing the risk of HIV transmission often means changing the balance of power in the relationship and could mean failure in their roles as women which are inextricably linked to their fertility. Many women are torn between the value of motherhood and the risk of HIV for either them or their child. The fear of their partners's violence has also been shown to predict whether women use condoms. In Uganda, stark gender differences were shown in perceptions of risk, women being more likely to perceive risk than men. The sexual double standard that sanctions many partners for men while restricting female sexuality has engendered confusing HIV prevention messages, such as reducing numbers of partners where this may not be protective. Data globally affirm that, not only are many women monogamous already, but it is unsafe for them to assume they are safe in their monogamous situation. Especially in high prevalence communities rates of discordance among married couples can be between 15 per cent and 20 per cent. Amaro notes that there is a growing body of knowledge that HIV among women has to be seen within the larger context. She suggests strategies such as participatory education that stress longer-term goals assessing root causes of gender differences including disempowerment and poverty. Wingood suggests a transition that will use gender-specific theories for research and programme development for women and HIV.

The same arguments apply with regards to sex workers in particular. De Zalduando emphasizes that the women within the broad category of sex workers represent an exceedingly diverse group with varied life histories and conditions. Without considering the actual situations within which these women live and work, it is impossible to envisage the services or supports needed by this vast range of range people. She advocates the use of enthnographic methods to understand key norms, sexual situations and interactions from the women's point of view.

(C) Changing Epidemic

As the HIV epidemic and the responses to the HIV epidemic evolve, people's experience accumulates predicting the need to update theoretical models and response. Since the development of anti-retroviral therapies, some studies have assessed preventive behaviour in relation to attitudes regarding combination therapies. In Uganda, where the epidemic has matured relative to many communities in the world, the need to incorporate temporal dimensions into measurements of sexual behaviour and perceived risk is clear. The impact of an epidemic where over 50 per cent of the population in a community knows more than 30 people who have died of the disease is profound. Measuring perceived risk should delineate risk due to past and present behaviour as interventions must target these risks differently. In a more mature epidemic Bunnell suggests "a theoretical framework which recognizes that perceptions of risk and sexual behaviour are not always individually determined, that gender and context are critical determinants of individual control over behaviour, that fear plays different roles at different stages of an epidemic and that lay communities can understand and utilize risk information".

(D) Null Findings

Few studies report on null findings but those that do are critical to complement our understanding of the relationships between context, population group, approach, intervention and theoretical background. In some populations behavioural skills training has failed to produce significant differences compared to control conditions. For example, non-impact has been shown with inner city African American men and STD clinic patients in the USA. Other reports of null findings include a randomized controlled trial among STD patients in the UK. The intervention was guided by *the social cognitive theory* and results indicated little difference in self reported behavioural change. It is suggested that community as well as individual interventions should address the environment in which risk behaviours take place. Two interventions that showed little effect were among youth. One was a brief programme based on constructs from the SCT and the *theory of reasoned action*. Authors suggested a longer intervention that addresses the multiple problems of this group that was drawn from a detention center and STD clinic. The second was based on the *theory of social influence* among middle-school students. Authors noted that inadequate community and family-level interventions, possible dilution of messages and over saturation of students with health messages by the 8th grade may have been responsible for the lack of positive results.

Conclusions

Safer sexual behaviour remains the single most effective method of preventing HIV infection. Although tremendous challenges still plague public health and the social sciences globally regarding AIDS prevention, much has been learned as well. It has become clear that effective HIV risk reduction interventions extend beyond basic information giving and help: sensitize people to personal risk, improve couples sexual communication, increase individual's condom use skills, the perception of lower risk practices as an accepted social norm, and help people receive support and reinforcement for their efforts at changing (Kelly, 1995). These principles form the foundation of successful HIV prevention strategies, but differences in individual, social, cultural and economic conditions dictate different design and implementation of programmes. Even if the principles underlying programmes are the same, tailoring to specific groups in specific settings will make programmes look very different. Not only should programmes be modified to fit certain cultural settings, but within cultural groups individuals may be at very different stages of readiness to change and successful interventions should take individual differences into consideration as well.

Changes in behaviour, such as dramatic increase in condom use, in very diverse population groups have taken place and some conclusions can be drawn. As Ulin suggests, when interventions have enabled the participants themselves to take part in mobilizing and setting goals themselves, efforts have been highly successful. Highlights have included the normative changes gay men in many US cities and sex workers in Thailand have made within their communities.

Another important point stressed by this broad overview of approaches to behavioural change is the need to see different levels HIV prevention initiatives as complementary. Individual approaches have shown impact, but to stem transmission on a larger scale for longer term maintenance of changed behaviour, community and structural level programmes are a critical complement. These approaches, despite showing great potential, have not yet been operationalized on a large scale. At this stage programmes should emphasize trans-theoretical approaches that combine individual level constructs with community-level projects that focus on subcultural norm changing. Community organizing can have the powerful affect of imparting a unified sense of purpose and new beliefs in the possibility of change.

An important element highlighted by a review by Oakley and Darrow was that the quality of evaluations was highly variable and often inadequate, which makes it difficult to conclude generalizable lessons about what works where from the heterogeneous literature. On the positive side, it is now possible to report that prospective experimental studies and long term follow-up in many different settings are feasible.

Despite the many advances in the field and many changes in behaviour observed, populations at highest risk have not received their share of the attention and resources allocated to AIDS interventions globally. The countries with the highest prevalences of HIV are those with the least resources and strained medical and social support systems. These countries with rapidly changing epidemics do not have the means alone to develop randomized controlled trials to test behavioural interventions, yet they are the communities needing the interventions the most urgently. Most theory-driven intervention research has been conducted in industrialized countries with very different epidemics to those in developing countries. It is therefore critical to test models and approaches across cultural, economic and social situations.

Following the findings of the importance of social norms and sexual communication for various groups including youth, MSM and heterosexuals, authors recommend community level interventions aiming at strengthening the perception that others also practice safe sex. Gender and power imbalances were also noted in many studies pointing to the necessity to build gender constructs into theories, models and interventions.

Recommendations for interventions aimed at women include greater emphasis on gender-related influences of behaviour. Studies in the USA and in Africa emphasize that self-protection, especially for vulnerable women may be affected by abusive partners, economic factors, and norms within sexual relationships. These recommendations apply to many different situations. In both West and Central Africa it has been noted that the ability to discuss sex and contraception with sexual partners as well as the imbalance of gender relations have a potentially significant impact on the capacity to enact changes in sexual behaviour. As Bunnell states, sharp differences in perceptions of risk between males and females in Uganda reflect underlying differences in societal power- the case in multiple settings around the world. To address women's needs for HIV prevention especially in developing countries, the development of female-controlled methods needs greater emphasis as well as a wider approach to HIV prevention that considers the social position of women.

In an epidemic where changes are occurring rapidly at the level of the virus, treatment context and within populations at risk multi-dimensional interventions based on theories and models which address individual as well as contextual and sociocultural variables such as gender, class and ethnicity, and their influence on sexual behaviour are urgently needed.

References

Aggleton P. Global priorities for HIV/AIDS intervention research. International Journal of STD & AIDS 1996; 7 (suppl 2): 13-16.

Ajzen I, Fishbein M. Understanding attitudes and predicting social behavior. Prentice-Hall, Inc., Englewood Cliffs, New Jersey 07632, 1980.

Alary M, Vincelette J, Dufour A, Otis j, Remis RS, Masse B, Lavoie R, LeClerc R, Parent R, Turmel B. Omega Study Group, Omega Cohort. Determinants of changes in patterns of unprotected anal intercourse (UAI) among men having affective and sexual relations with men (MASM) in Montreal. 12th International Conference on AIDS. Geneva 1998 [14204].

Allen S, Tice J, van de Perre P, Serufilira A, Hudes E, Nsengumuremyi F, Bogaerts J, Lindan C, Hulley S. Effect of serotesting with counselling on condom use and seroconversion among HIV discordant couples in Africa. BMJ 1992, vol 304: 1605-9.

Allen S, Serufilira A, Bogaerts J, van de Perre P Nsengumuremyi F, Lindan C, Carael M, Wolf W, Coates T, Hulley S. Confidential HIV testing and condom promotion in Africa. Impact on HIV and gonorrhea rates. JAMA 1992, 268: 3338-3343.

Alwano-Edyegu, M, Gumisiriza E, Campbell C Moore M, Marum E, Kaleeba N. HIV counselling and testing: Resolved that government/public resources for HIV prevention in the developing world should not be directed toward the provision of HIV counselling and testing services. 11th International Conference on AIDS Vancouver 1996 [We. 15].

Amaro H. Love, sex and power: considering women's realities in HIV prevention. American psychologist 1995, 50 (6): 437-447.

Ankrah M. AIDS: Methodological problems in studying its prevention and spread. Soc. Sci. Med. 1989, 29 (3): 265-276.

Asamoah-Adu A, Weir S, Pappoe M, Kanlisi N, Neequaye A, Lamptey P. Evaluation of a targeted AIDS prevention intervention to increase condom use among prostitutes in Ghana. AIDS 1994, 8: 239-246.

Asiimwe - Okiror G, Opio A, Musinguzi J, Madraa E, Tembo G, Carael M. Change in sexual behaviour and decline in HIV infection among young pregnant women in urban Uganda. AIDS 1997, 11: 1757-1763.

Auerbach J, Wypijewska C, Brodil K. AIDS and Behavior: An Integrated Approach. National Academy Press, 1994; 2101 Constitution Ave. NW 20418.

Bandura A. Social learning theory. Prentice-Hall, Inc., Englewood Cliffs, New Jersey 07632, 1977.

Banerjee B, Jana S, Banerjee A, Mukherjee S. Social marketing of condoms at red-light areas (RLAs) through community participation and peer promotion. 12th International Conference on AIDS. Geneva 1998 [33426].

Barton T, Borrini-Feyerabend G, de Sherbinin A, Warren P. Our people, our resources. IUCN, Gland, Switzerland and Cambridge, UK.

Beeker C, Guenther-Grey C, Raj A. Community empowerment paradigm drift and the primary prevention of HIVAIDS. Soc Sci Med 1998, 46 (7): 831-842.

Bianco M, Bianco M, pagani L. Evaluation of an intervention in training adolescents as peer educators in Argentina. 12th International Conference on AIDS Geneva 1998 [33539].

Bootan A. Strong youth, strong barriers to HIV. 12th International Conference on AIDS Geneva 1998 [33561].

Branson B, Rnsom R, Peterman T, Zaidi A. Randomized controlled trial of intensive group counselling to reduce risk behaviors in high-risk STD clinic patients. 11th International Conference on AIDS. Vancouver 1996 [Mo.D.1 753].

Broadhead R, Heckathorn D, Madray H, Mills R, Hughes J. The impact results of a peer-driven intervention to combat HIV among drug injectors. 12th International Conference on AIDS Geneva 1998 [33335].

Bunnell, R. Promoting or paralyzing behavior change: understanding gender and high levels of perceived risk of HIV infection in Southwestern Uganda. 1996 Doctoral Thesis; Harvard School of Public Health, Boston, Massachusetts.

Buunk B, Bakker A, Siero F, Eijnden R, Yzer M. Predictors of AIDS-preventive behavioral intentions among adult heterosexuals at risk for HIV-infection: extending current models and measures. AIDS Education and Prevention 1998, 10 (2): 149-172.

Campbell C, Marum E, Alwano-Edyegu M, Dillon B, Moore M, Gumisiriza E. The role of HIV counselling and testing in the developing world. AIDS Education and Prevention 1997, 9 (Suppl 13): 92-104.

Carael M, Buve, A, Awusabbo-Asare, K. The making of HIV epidemics: what are the driving forces? AIDS 1997, 11 (suppl B): S23-S31.

Case P. Injection drug use, in AIDS in the World: A global report 1992. Edited by Mann, J, Tarantola D, Netter T. Harvard College: 406-420.

Catania J, Kegeles S, Coates I Towards an understanding of risk behavior: an AIDS Risk Reduction Model (ARRM). Health Education Quarterly 1990 17 (1): 53-72.

Chan R, Wong M, Lee J, Koh D, wong C. A behavioural intervention programme to increase condom use among sex workers in Singapore. 11th International Conference on AIDS Vancouver 1996 [Mo.D 1747].

Choi K, Yep G, Kumekawa E. HIV prevention among Asian and Pacific Islander American men who have sex with men: a critical review of theoretical models and directions of future research. AIDS Education and Prevention 1998, 10 (Suppl A) (1): 19-30.

Choi K, Lew S, Vittinghoff E, Catania J, Barrett D, Coates T. The efficacy of brief group counseling in HIV-reduction among homosexual Asian and Pacific Islander men. AIDS 1996, 10: 81-87.

Choi K, Coates T. Prevention of HIV infection. AIDS 1994, 8: 1371-1389.

Coates T, Sangiwa G, Balmer D, Gregorich S, Kamenga C. Voluntary HIV counselling and testing (VCT) reduces risk behavior in developing countries: Results from the voluntary counselling and testing study. 12th International Conference on AIDS. Geneva 1998 [133/33269].

Coates T, Sangiwa G, Balmer D, Furlonge C, Kamenga C, Gregorich S. Serodiscordant married couples undergoing couples counselling and testing reduce risk behavior with each other but not with extra-marital partners. 12th International Conference on AIDS. Geneva 1998 [33268].

Coates T, Chesney M, Folkman S, Hulley S, Haynes-Sanstad K, Lurie P, Marin B, Roos L, Bunnitt V, Du Wors R. Designing behavioural and social science to impact practice and policy in HIV prevention and care. International Journal of STD & AIDS 1996; 7 (Suppl. 2): 2-12.

Cohen M. Prevention in AIDS in the World: A global report 1992. Edited by Mann, J, Tarantola D, Netter T. Harvard College.

Connell R. Gender and Power. Stanford, CA; Stanford University Press; 1987.

De Zalduando B. Prostitution viewed cross-culturally: toward recontextualizing commercial sex work for improved AIDS Intervention research. Anthropologists at work on AIDS; American Anthropological Association Task Force on AIDS 1990.

De Zoysa 1, Sweat M, Denison J. Faithful but fearful: reducing HIV transmission in stable relationships. AIDS 1996, 10 (suppl A): S197-S203.

De Zoysa 1, Phillips K, Kamenga M, O'Reilly K, Sweat M, White R, Grinstead 0, Coates T. Role of HIV counselling and testing in changing risk behavior in developing countries. AIDS 1995, 9 (suppl A): S95-S101.

DiClemente R, Wingood G. A randomized controlled trial of an HIV sexual risk-reduction intervention for young African-American Women. JAMA 1995 vol 274 (16): 1271-1276.

Edem C, Harvey S. Use of health belief model to predict condom use among university students in Nigeria. In Progress in Preventing AIDS? Dogma, Dissent and Innovation. Global Perspectives 1998. Edited by Buchanan D, Cernada G. Baywood Publishing Company Inc. Amityville, NY.

Elkins D, Maticka-Tyndale E, Kuyyakonond T, Miller P, Haswell-Elkins M. Toward reducing the spread of HIV in Northeastern Thai villages: evaluation of a village-based intervention. AIDS Education and Prevention, 1997, 9 (1): 49-69.

Farmer, P. Inequalities as co-factors for HIV transmission and for poor AIDS outcomes. 11th International Conference on AIDS Vancouver 1996 [Tu. D. 581].

Fishbein M, Hohnson W. The AIDS community demonstration projects (ACDP): a successful multisite community-level behavioral intervention. 11th International Conference on AIDS Vancouver 1996 [Mo.D.580].

Fishbein M, Middlestadt S. Using the theory of reasoned action as a framework for understanding and changing AIDS related behaviors. In Wasserheit JN (ed) Primary Prevention of AIDS: Psychological Approaches 1989.

Ford K, Wirawan D, Fajans R Factors related to condom use among four groups of female sex workers in Bali, Indonesia. AIDS Education and Prevention 1998, 10 (1): 34-45.

Ford K, Wirawan D, Fajans P, Meliawan P, MacDonald K, Thorpe L. Behavioral interventions for reduction of sexually transmitted disease/ HIV transmission among female commercial sex workers and clients in Bali, Indonesia. AIDS 1996, 10: 213-222.

Ford K, Wirawan D, Fajans P, Thorpe L. AIDS knowledge, risk behaviors, and factors related to condom use among male commercial sex workers and male tourist clients in Bali, Indonesia. AIDS 1995, 9: 751-759.

Fox L, Bailey P, Clarke-Martinez K, Coello M, Ordonez F, Barahona F. Condom use among highrisk women in Honduras: evaluation of an AIDS prevention programme. AIDS Education and Prevention 1993, 5 (1): 1-10.

Friedman S, O'Reilly K. Sociocultural interventions at the community level. AIDS 1997, 11 (suppl A): S201-S208.

Futterman D, Jean-Louis S, Hoffman N, Chabon B. promoting HIV counselling and testing to adolescents: contributions of social marketing. 12th International Conference on AIDS Geneva 1998 [33434]

Galavotti C, Gielen A, Armstrong K, Cabral R, Fogarty L, Cohen A, Milstein B. The effect of a theory-based HIV prevention intervention on condom use with main partners in samples of US women. 12th International Conference on AIDS. Geneva 1998 [14274].

Giami A, Dowsett G. Social research on sexuality: contextual and interpersonal approaches. AIDS 1996, 10 (suppl A): S191-S196.

Gibson D, McCusker J Chesney. Effectiveness of psychosocial interventions in preventing HIV risk behaviour in injecting drug users. AIDS 1998, 12: 919-929.

Giffin F. Beyond empowerment: heterosexualities and the prevention of AIDS. Soc Sci Med 1998, 46 (2): 151-156.

Gillmore M. Morrison D, Richey C, Balassone M, Gutierrez L, Farris M. Effects of a skill-based intervention to encourage condom use among high risk heterosexually active adolescents. AIDS Education and Prevention 1997, 9 (suppl A): 22-43.

Godin G, Savard J, Kok G, Forin C, Foyer R. HIV Seropositive gay men: understanding adoption of safe sexual practices. AIDS Education and Prevention 1996, 8 (6): 529-545.

Gold R, Rosenthal D. Preventing unprotected anal intercourse in gay men: a comparison of two intervention techniques. International Journal of STD & AIDS 1995, 6: 89-94.

Gordon J. The indigenous leader outreach model reaching out to sex workers in Indonesia. Research for sex work 1998, June. Den Haag offset, The Netherlands: 4-5.

Greenberg, J in AIDS Education: Interventions in Multicultural settings. Edited by Schenker 1, SaberFriedman G, Sy F. 1996. Plenum Press, NY 233 Spring St. New York, NY 10013.

Gregson S, Zhuwau T, Anderson R, Chandiwana, S. Is there evidence for behaviour change in response to AIDS in rural Zimbabwe? . Soc Sci Med 1998, 46 (3): 321-330.

Guenther-Grey C, Noroian D, Fonseka J, Higgins D. Developing community networks to deliver HIV prevention interventions. Public Health Rep 1996, 111 Suppl 1: 41-9.

Heaney C, Israel B. Social networks and social support. In: Glantz, Lewis and Rimer 1997. Health behavior and health education: Theory, research and practice. San Francisco, Jossey-bass (second edition).

Heise L, Elias C. Transforming AIDS prevention to meet women's needs: a focus on developing countries. Soc Sci Med 1995, 40 (7): 931-943.

Henry K. HIV/AIDS Policy in Kenya: Part I - Building a national response to the epidemic. NCIH Global AIDS Newletter no. 50: 8-9.

Higgins D, Galavotti C, O'Reilly K, Schnell D, Moore M, Rugg D, Johnsom R. Evidence for the effects of HIV antibody counselling and testing on risk behaviors. JAMA 1991, 266 (17): 2419-2428.

Holtgrave D. Public health communication strategies for HIV prevention: past and emerging roles. AIDS 1997, 11 (suppl A): S183-S190.

Howard M, McCabe J. Helping teenagers postpone sexual involvement. Family Planning Perspectives 1990, 22 (1): 21-26.

Ickovics J, Yoshikawa H. Preventive interventions to reduce heterosexual HIV risk for women: current perspectives, future directions. AIDS 1998, 12 (suppl A): S197-S208.

Israel B, Checkoway B, Schulz A, Zimmerman. Health Education and community empowerment: conceptualizing and measuring perceptions of individual, organizational and community control. Health Educational Quarterly 1994. 21 (2): 149-170.

James N, Gillies P, Bignell C. Evaluation of a randomized controlled trial of HIV and sexually transmitted disease prevention in a genitourinary medicine clinic setting. AIDS 1998, 12: 1235-1242.

James N, Gillies P, Bignell C. A randomised controlled trial of an intervention to reduce risk behaviour among STD clinic attenders. 11th International Conference on AIDS Vancouver 1996 [Mo.D. 1752].

Jemmott JB, Jemmott LS, Fong GT Reductions in HIV risk-associated sexual behaviors among black male adolescents: effects of an AIDS prevention intervention [published erratum appears in Am J Public Health 1992 May; 82 (5): 684]. Am J Public Health 1992 Mar; 82 (3): 372-377].

Jemmott B, Jemmott LS, Hacker Cl. Predicting intentions to use condoms among African American adolescents: the theory of planned behavior as a model of HIV risk-associated behavior. Ethn Dis 1992, 2(4): 371-380.

Kagimu M. Marum E, Wabire-Mangen F, Nakanjo N, Walakira Y, Hogle J. Evaluation of the effectiveness of AIDS health education interventions in the Muslim community in Uganda. AIDS Education and Prevention 1998, 10 (3): 215-228.

Kalichman S. Preventing AIDS: a sourcebook for behavioral interventions. 1998 Lawrence Erlbaum Associates Inc. Publishers. 10 Industrial Ave. Mahwah, NJ 07430.

Kalichman S, Hospers H. Efficacy of behavioral-skills enhancement HIV risk-reduction interventions in community settings. AIDS 1997, 11 (suppl A): S191-S199.

Kalichman S, Rompa D, Coley B. Lack of positive outcomes from a cognitive-behavioral HIV and AIDS prevention intervention for inner-city men: lessons from a controlled pilot study. AIDS Education and Prevention 1997, 9 (4): 299-313.

Kamb M, Kassler W, Peterman T, Zenilman J, Bolan G, Rogers J, Rhodes F,. Costs of preventing HIV via counselling: results from a randomized controlled trial (Project Respect): 12th International Conference on AIDS Geneva 1998 [33263].

Kamb M, Douglas J, Rhodes F, Bolan G, Zenilman J, latesta M, Peterman T, Graziano S, Killean W ' Fishbein M. A Multi-Center, randomized controlled trial evaluating HIV prevention counselling (Project Respect): Preliminary results. 1 1th International Conference on AIDS Vancouver 1996 [Th.C.4380].

Kathuria R, Chirenda P, Sabatier R, Dube N. Peer education to reduce STI/HIV transmission in Lusaka, Zambia. 12th International Conference on AIDS Geneva 1998 [33524].

Katzenstein D, McFarland W, Mbizvo M, Latif A, Machekano R, Parsonnet J, Basssett, M. Peer education among factory workers in Zimbabwe; providing a sustainable HIV prevention intervention. 12th International Conference on AIDS Geneva 1998 [33514].

Kegeles S, Hart G. Recent HIV-prevention interventions for gay men: individual, small-group and community-based studies. AIDS 1998, 12 (suppl A): S209-S215.

Kegeles S, Hays R, Waldo C, Pollack L. The whole is greater than the sum of its parts: An analysis of the intervention components of an HIV prevention program for young gay men. 12th International Conference on AIDS Geneva 1998 [43283].

Kegeles S, Hays R, Coates T. The Mpowerment Project: a community-level HIV prevention intervention for young gay men. Am J Public Health 1996 Vol 86 (8): 1129-1136.

Kegeles S, Hays R, Pollack L, Coates I Community mobilization reduces HIV risk among young gay men: a two community study. 11th International Conference on AIDS Vancouver 1996 [Mo.D.581].

Kelly J, Murphy D, Sikkema K, McAuliffe T, Roffman R, Solomon L, Winett R, Kalichman S. Randomised, controlled, community-level HIV prevention intervention for sexual-risk behaviour among homosexual men in US cities. Lancet, 1997, 350 :1500-1505

Kelly J, Kalichman S, Rompa D. Outcomes of a Randomised, intervention trial to promote consistent HIV risk reduction behaviour change maintenance in an ethnically diverse cohort of gay and bisexual men. 11th International Conference on AIDS Vancouver 1996 [We.C. 3497].

Kelly J. Changing HIV risk behavior: practical strategies 1995. The Guilford Press, 72 Spring street, New York, NY 10012.

Kelly J, Lawrence J, Stevenson Y, Hauth A, Kalichman S, Diaz Y, Brasfield T, Koob J, Morgan M. Community AIDS/HIV risk reduction: the effects of endorsements by popular people in three cities. Am J Public Health 1992, vol 82 (11): 1483-1489.

Kelly J, Kalichman S, Kauth M, Kilgore H, Hood H, Campos P, Rao S, Brasfield T, St Lawrence J. Situational factors associated with AIDS risk behavior lapses and coping strategies used by gay men who successfully avoid lapses. Am J Public Health 1991, 81, 1335-1338.

King R, Homsy J. Involving traditional healers in AIDS education and counselling in sub-Saharan Africa: a review. AIDS 1997, 11 (suppl A): S217-S225.

King R, Estey J, Allen S, Kegeles S, Wolf W, Valentine C, Serufilira A. A family planning intervention to reduce vertical transmission of HIV in Rwanda. AIDS 1995, 9 (suppl): S45-S51.

Kirby D, Short L, Collins J, Rugg D, Kolbe L, Howard M, Miller B, Sonenstein F, Zabin L. SchoolBased programs to reduce sexual risk behaviors: a review of effectiveness. Public Health Reports 1994, 109, 3: 339-360.

Kline A, Vanlandingham M. HIV-infected women and sexual risk reduction: the relevance of existing models of behavior change. AIDS Education and Prevention 1994, 6 (5): 390-402.

Laver S, Van Den Borne B, Kok G. Using theory to design an intervention for HIV/AIDS prevention for farm workers in rural Zimbabwe. In Progress in

Preventing AIDS? Dogma, Dissent and Innovation. Global Perspectives 1988. Edited by Buchanan D, Cernada G. Baywood Publishing Company Inc. Amityville, NY.

Lawrence J, Jefferson K, Banks P, Cline T, Alleyne E, Brasfield T. Cognitive-Behavioral group intervention to assist substance-dependent adolescents in lowering HIV infection risk. AIDS Education and Prevention 1994, 6 (5): 425-435.

Leite G, Cesar F. The continuity of peer education in Brazil. Research for sex work 1998: 10.

Levine, WC, Higueras G, Revollo R, Vega J, Aliaga A, Tinajeros F, Garnica M, Lewis J, Ugarteche J, Kaune V, Estenssoro M, Wright-Deaguero 1, Pareja R, Negron E, Posner J, Ransom R, Melgar M , Kuritsky J. Rapid decline in sexually transmitted disease prevalence among brothel-based sex workers in La Paz Bolivia: The experience of Proyecto Contra SIDA, 1992-1995. 11th International Conference on AIDS Vancouver 1996 [M o. C. 441].

Levy S, Phillips K, Rasher S, Schaffer T. Measuring behavior change among clients of communitybased organizations delivering prevention interventions in a large, urban setting. 12th Intemational Conference on AIDS Geneva 1998 [14285].

Lurie P, Fernandes M, Hughes V, Arevalo E, Hudes E, Reingold A, Hearst N, Instituto Adolfo Lutz study Group. Socio-economic status and the risk of HIV-1, syphilis and hepatits B infection among sex workers in São Paulo State, Brazil. AIDS 1995, 9 (suppl. 1): S31-S37.

Lurie, P, Lowe, R, Hintzen P. The impact of international monetary fund and World Bank policies on HIV transmission in developing countries. 10th International Conference on AIDS Yokohama 1994 [PD0380].

Maskovsky J, Davis J, Harley A, Shull J. The contradictions of peer education as employment for poor people with HIV//AIDS. 12th International Conference on AIDS Geneva 1998 [33523].

McLeroy K, Bibeau D, Steckler A, Glanz K. An ecological perspective on health promotion programs. Health Ed Quarterly 1988, 15(4): 351-377.

Moberg D, Piper D. The healthy for life project: sexual risk behavior outcomes. AIDS Education and Prevention, 1998, 10 (2): 128-148.

Morris M. Sexual networks and HIV-AIDS 1997, 11 (suppl. A): S209-S216.

Moughutou P. Education of road haullers and taxi drivers of Kumba town on STD/AIDS prevention: pilot project. 12th International Conference on AIDS Geneva 1998 [33557].

Nemoto T, Aoki B, Huang K, Ching A. Drug use and HIV risk behaviors among Asians in San Francisco. 12th International Conference on AIDS Geneva 1998 [14222].

Newcomb M, Stacy A, Ames S. Implicit sexual cognition and activation in HIV risk: predictors of sexual and drug abuse behaviors. 12th International Conference on AIDS Geneva 1998 [24152].

Oakley A, Darrow W. Social, cultural and political aspects. AIDS 1998, 12 (suppl. A): S189-S190.

Oakley A, Fullerton D, Holland J. Behavioural interventions for HIV/AIDS prevention. AIDS 1995, 9: 479-486.

Ogundare D. Evaluation of a workplace pilot behavioural intervention project among dockworkers in the two sea-ports in Lagos, Nigeria. 12th International Conference on AIDS Geneva 1998 [14369].

Oldenburg B, Hardcastle D, Kok G. Diffusion of innovations. In: Glantz, Lewis and Rimer 1997. Health behavior and health education: Theory, research and practice. San Francisco, Jossey-bass (second edition).

O'Leary A. The NIMH multisite HIV prevention trial: Social cognitive mediators of behavioral intervention effects on HIV/STD risk. 12th International Conference on AIDS Geneva 1998 [14279].

O'Leary A, Goodhart F, Jemmott LS, BoccherLattimore D. Predictors of safer sex on the college campus: a social cognitive theory analysis. J Am Coll Health 1992, 40 (6): 254-263.

Opare B, Tirtoree L, Bayor S. Strategy to attitudinal change in CSW, Wa, Ghana. 10th International Conference on AIDS Yokohama 1994 [PD0455].

Opio,A, Musinguzi J, Asiimwe-Okiror G, Byabamazima C, Turyaguma, Madraa E. Sexual behavior change due to HIV/AIDS: Results from population based surveys conducted in five districts of Uganda. 11th International Conference on AIDS Vancouver 1996 [LBD 6069].

Otto-Salaj L, Kelly J, Hoffmann R, Stevenson L. Outcome of a cognitive-behavioral HIV prevention intervention tailored to the needs of seriously mentally ill adults. 12th International Conference on AIDS Geneva 1998 [14279].

Parker R. Empowerment, community mobilization and social change in the face of HIV/AIDS. AIDS 1996, 10 (suppl. 3): S27-S31.

Peersman G, Levy J. Focus and effectiveness of HIV-prevention efforts for young people. AIDS 1998, 12 (suppl. A): S191-S196.

Pickering H, Quigley M, Pepin J, Todd J, Wilkins A. The effects of post-test counselling on condom use among prostitutes in The Gambia. AIDS 1993, 7: 271-273.

Prochaska J, Redding c, Harlow L, Rossi J, Velicer W. The transtheoretical model of change an HIV prevention: a review. Health Ed Quarterly 1994 Vol. 21 A: 471-486.

Prochaska J, Di Clemente C. Stages of change in the modification of problem behaviors. Progress in Behavior Modification. Eds. Michel Hersen, Ridhard Eisler and Peter Miller P. Sycamore, IL; Sycamore Publishing Company, 1992: 28.

PSI. Annotated catalogue of recent social marketing research and evaluation 1998. PSI 1120 19th St NW Suite 600 Washington DC 20036.

Re M, Pagani L, Bianco M. Assessing workshops on sexuality with Argentinian youth. AIDS/STD health promotion exchange 1996, 3: 13-15.

Reitman D, St. Lawrence J, Jefferson K, Alleyne E, Brasfield T, Shirley A. Predictors of African American Adolescents condom use and HIV risk behavior. AIDS Education and Prevention, 1996, 8 (6): 499-515.

Remien R, Wagner G, Carballo-Dieguez A, Dolezal C. HAART, Attitudes, and risk behavior among serodiscordant male couples. 12th International Conference on AIDS Geneva 1998 [14136].

Robles R, Marrero C, Matos, T, Colon H, Finlinson H, Reyes J, Sahai H. Factors associated with changes in sex behaviour among drug users in Puerto Rico. AIDS Care 1998, 10 (3): 329-338.

Roffman R, Stephens R, Curtin L, Gordon J, Craver J, Stern M, Beadnell B, Downey L. Relapse prevention as an interventive model for HIV risk reduction in gay and bisexual men. AIDS Education and Prevention 1998, 10 (1): 1-18.

Rogers EM. Diffusion of Innovations. Third Edition. New York, NY. The Free Press; 1983.

Rotheram-Borus. Seropositive youth make positive changes. 12th International Conference on AIDS Geneva 1998 [32426].

Roy A. Behaviour change among sex workers and clients can be best brought about by peer educators. 12th International Conference on AIDS Geneva 1998 [33540].

Roy 1. Role of peer educators in social marketing of male condoms to flat based sex workers (women) and rickshaw pullers of central Calcutta. 12th International Conference on AIDS Geneva 1998 [33441].

Schuler S, Hashemi S. Credit programs, women's empowerment, and contraceptive use in rural Bangladesh. Studies in family planning, 1994, 25 (2): 65-76.

Seema S. Prevention and control of STD/HIV transmission through peer educators amongst CSW. 12th International Conference on AIDS Geneva 1998 [33552].

Sepulvede J, Fineberg H, Mann J. AIDS: prevention through education: a world view. New York, Oxford University Press 1992 200 Madison Ave. New York, NY 10016.

Serwadda D, Gray R, Wawer M, Stallings R, Sewankamba N, Kone-Lule J, Lainjo B, Kelly R. The social dynamics of HIV transmission as reflected through discordant couples in rural Uganda. AIDS 1995, 9: 745-750.

Stevens P, Hall J. Participatory action research for sustaining individual and community change: a model of HIV prevention education. AIDS Education and Prevention, 1998, 10 (5): 387-402.

Svenson G, Johnsson K, Hanson B. Increased consistent condom use among students in a prevention study based on community organisation and action and the use of peer educators. 11th International Conference on AIDS Vancouver 1996 [Mo.D.582].

Sweat, M, Denison J. Reducing HIV incidence in developing countries with structural and environmental interventions. AIDS 1995, 9 (suppl. A): S251-S257.

TASO Uganda: The inside story, participatory evaluation of HIVIAIDS counselling, medical and social services, 1993-1994. TASO, WHO.

Tawil O, Verster A, O'Reilly K. Enabling approaches for HIV/AIDS prevention: can we modify the environment and minimize the risk? AIDS 1995, 9: 1299-1306.

Ter-Hoyakimyan A. Sargsyan D, Topchyan S, Zohrabyan L, Ghoukasyan G. Peculiarities of antiAIDS program aimed at teenagers in Armenia. 12th International Conference on AIDS Geneva 1998 [33554].

Torres-Burgos N, Serrano-Garcia 1, Galarza M, Henandez R. Social marketing principles applied to the recruitment of research participants: the university of Puerto Rico experience. 12th International Conference on AIDS Geneva 1998 [33435].

Ulin P. African women and AIDS: negotiating behavioral change. Soc. Sci. Med. 1992, 34 (1): 6373.

UNAIDS. Epidemics and behaviours: a review of changes in sexual behaviour in Uganda in the early 1990s. UNAIDS Best Practice Collection. Geneva: UNAIDS; 1997

UNAIDS/WHO. Report on the global HIV/AIDS epidemic June 1998, Joint United Nations Programme on HIV/AIDS; World Health Organization 1998. UNAIDS/98.10 -WHO/EMC/VIR/98.2 - WHO/ASD/98.2.

Vacondio P, Guaraldi G, Siciliano S, De Donatis D. Prevention of HIV transmission among Arabian prisoners of northern Italy using peer education methods: a video clip and a calendar. 12th International Conference on AIDS Geneva 1998 [33560].

Valdiserri R. HIV counselling and testing: its evolving role in HIV prevention. AIDS Education and Prevention 1997, 9 (suppl B): 2-13.

Van der Straten A, King R, Grinstead O, Vittinghoff E, Serufilira A Allen S. Sexual coercion, physical violence and HIV infection among women in steady relationships in Kigali, Rwanda. AIDS and Behavior, vol 2 (1), 1998.

Van der Straten A, King R, Grinstead O, Serufilira A Allen S. Couple communication, sexual coercion and HIV risk reduction in Kigali, Rwanda. AIDS 1995, 9: 935-944.

Visrutaratna S, Lindan C, Sirhorachai A, Mandel J. 'Superstar' and 'model brothel': developing and evaluating a condom promotion program for sex establishments in Chiang Mai, Thailand. AIDS 1995, 9 (suppl 1): S69-S75.

Wallerstein N, Bernstein E. Empowerment education: Freire's ideas adapted to health education. Health Education Quarterly 1988, 15 (4): 379-394.

Walter H, Vaughan R. AIDS risk reduction among a multiethnic sample of urban high school students. JAMA 1993 Vol 270 (6): 725-730.

Werner D, Sanders D, Weston J, Babb S, Rodriguez B. Questioning the Solution: the politics of primary health care and child survival with an in-depth critique of oral rehydration therapy. Healthwrights 1997. 964 Hamilton Ave. Palo Alto CA 94301.

Wiebel W, Jimeniz A, Johnson W, Ouellet L, Jovanovic B, Lampinen T, Murray J, O'Brien M. Risk behavior and HIV seroincidence among out-of-treatment injection drug users: a four-year prospective study. Journal of acquired immune deficiency syndromes and human retrovirology 1996. 12:282-289.

Wingood G, DiClemente R. HIV sexual risk reduction interventions for women: a review. Am J Prev. Med. 1996; 12 (3): 209-217.

Wingood G, DiClemente R. The role of gender relations in HIV prevention research for women. Am J Public Health 1995, 85 (4): 592.

Wolffers 1. About peer education. Research for sex work 1998: 3.

Wolitski R, MacGowan R, Higgins D, Jorgensen C. The effects of HIV counselling and testing on risk-related practices and help-seeking behavior. AIDS Education and Prevention 1997, 9 (suppl B): 52-67.

World Bank. Confronting AIDS: public priorities in a global epidemic. Oxford University Press, 200 Madison Ave, New York, NY 10016; 1997.

Six

HIV Surveillance

Reporting and Surveillance

(1) Who will be needed to report, what clinical information, with what personal identifiers, to whom?

(2) How will the proposed system help to a more accurate characterization of the HIV/AIDS epidemic?

(3) What is known about the completeness of reporting for other notifiable conditions, comprising those that bear some stigma? How can such experience be used to anticipate the desires to cooperate on the part of those who will be required to report?

(4) Given the limits of all reporting systems (e.g. error rates, failures to report), how will data derived from the proposed reporting system be intermingled with those derived from other sources (e.g. blinded seroprevalence studies) to give the most proper epidemiological picture that is practicable within available resources?

Reporting and Public Health Functions

(1) How will reported cases be used to 'improve endeavours at planning for prevention of HIV infection, for the provision of care?

(2) How and with what frequency will aggregate data based on reporting be "fed back" to the local level, to care providers?

(3) Will reported cases serve as the ground for partner notification? If so, how will the names trigger partner notification? Is reporting for other notifiable conditions used for partner notification, with what degree of effectiveness, and at what cost?

(4) What can be expected about the potential negative consequences of adopting the proposed reporting system on the desires of those at risk to undergo HIV testing, counselling, treatment?

(5) Will such registries be integrated with other disease, like tuberculosis registries?

Names, Coded Identifiers, Anonymous Reports

(1) In what way are names essential to achieve the epidemiological or other public health goal of reporting?

(2) In what way would coded or anonymous reports compromise the obtainment of public health goals of reporting?

(3) If coded identifiers are to be used, how complicated will they be? What identifying elements will be incorporated? What level of training and support will be necessary for those needed to report in order to keep error rates to acceptable levels?

(4) Will the code be unique, allowing the elimination of duplicate counts, the completion of inadequate reports, and the linkage of AIDS-related records?

(5) What, if any, experience is there with the use of coded identifiers for other reported conditions and what do they suggest about probable error rates?

(6) If error rates can be anticipated, to what limit are they acceptable or unacceptable given the goals of the reporting system?

(7) If anonymous reports without unique identifiers are used, what level of duplicate reporting would be anticipated? What contribution can such reports make to surveillance?

Legal Regimes Protecting Registries Containing Names

(1) What implementable legal regimes exist or will be put in place to protect the confidentiality of HIV/AIDS registries?

(2) What restrictions will there be on revelation in criminal or civil proceedings from such registries?

(3) What penalties will exist for the illegal revelation of data contained in registries?

(4) What does the experience with other disease registries disclose about the capacity of the system to protect the confidentiality of identifiable information contained?

Cost of Reporting

(1) What are the anticipated extra costs to adopting the proposed reporting system? Who will bear these costs? How do those costs compare with other aspects of the AIDS control programme? What are the costs of failing to enforce the proposed reporting system? Has some, even very basic, endeavour at a cost profit analysis of the proposed reporting system been attempted?

(2) What is the anticipated burden on those who will be needed to complete reporting forms? What will be the costs of supporting, training, and monitoring of the system? Who will bear them?

(3) What registry-based costs can be anticipated (computers, staff, encryption, etc.)?

Consultation

(1) What process of consultation with communities at risk, their advocates, and care-givers has been undertaken in the process of designing, planning and preparing for the enforcement of the proposed system of reporting?

(2) To what limit has such consultation produced consensus?

(3) To the extent that consensus has not emerged, what are the anticipated costs of enforcing the system of reporting in the face of resistance?

Conclusions and Recommendations

Reporting of HIV/AIDS may make an important contribution to elaborate epidemic surveillance. But the inevitable limits of such data necessitate also the use of other surveillance strategies.

A reporting system should only be followed with a clear understanding of the functions to be served and of the social, political and infrastructure context within which it would function.

A reporting system should not be followed before the expected costs of the system are compared to the alternative use of resources in AIDS prevention and care.

Careful consideration of the experience of disease reporting in general, its extents and contributions to the public health, should inform decisions about extending notification needs to HIV/AIDS. A decision to use names in a reporting system should be made only if strict and implementable regimes of confidentiality will secure the registries to be developed.

A decision to use unique coded identifiers should only be taken after a careful evaluation is undertaken of the capacity of those needed to encode data and of the capacity of those receiving to process such data. Even encoded systems need the creation of regimes of strict confidentiality.

Given the fears of those at risk for HIV infection and the existence of social contexts within which individuals have been subjected to discrimination, stigmatization, and acts of violence, it is decisive to engage in consultations with those most affected by the epidemic before adopting a reporting system.

Partner Notification

Beyond the objective of epidemiological surveillance, HIV/AIDS reporting may serve to trigger public health interventions like partner notification.

Partner notification endeavours are based on the assumption that those who have or may have been exposed by known index patients should be informed so that they may seek testing, counselling and clinical intervention where it exists. Yet there is much confusion about the limit to which partner notification should viewed as entailing a breach of confidentiality (the disclosure without consent of the identity of the index patient to his or her contacts), and the degree to which such endeavours must, by definition, rely upon coercion. In the last, there is profound disagreement over whether breaches of confidentiality or recourse to coercion - to the extent that they characterize the partner notification process - are justifiable.

Much of the confusion stems from the wide range of distinct activities and concepts involved in partner notification. One range of interventions is connected to the tradition of contact investigation, a second to the "duty to warn."

Contact Investigation and Sexually Transmitted Diseases

In various nations, contact investigation has been integral to efforts to control and prevent sexually transmitted diseases. After the diagnosis of an STD, the index patient is urged to reveal the names and feasible locations of past sexual partners so that they may be tested and treated. Such attempts thus not only serve the interests of those who are contacted but also of the public health, because a treated case can no longer transmit disease. In the 1930s, the senior health official in the United States declared: "We can break the chain of infection promptly by treatment; we can find the source and the exposed contacts, get them under treatment, and prevent new chains of infection.[1]

In the United States, the tradition of contact investigation has been characterized by a formal voluntarism. No sanctions exist for the failure to disclose the names of post sexual contacts. Considerable moral pressure may, however, be applied to index patients to give the names of partners. In exchange for providing names, index patients are assured that their identity will never be disclosed to those who are contacted. Index case anonymity and cooperation thus lie at the heart of the system.

Although founded on privacy and cooperation, contact investigation in the context of the AIDS epidemic has been the centre of heated debate. Various industrialized nations were not interested to adopt partner notification in the epidemic's early years. In Canada, for instance, the National Advisory Committee on AIDS stated in 1984 that "contact tracing is not necessary nor is it appropriate; in fact it is discouraged.[2] In the United States, few, if any, health departments applied in AIDS contact tracing those procedures related to the response to STDs.

By the 1990s the situation had radically changed. On a formal level, the CDC in the United States made partner notification an important feature of AIDS prevention efforts. In 1997 in Canada, the Federal/Provincial/Territorial Advisory Committee on AIDS stated "partner notification can make a positive contribution to a successful HIV/AIDS public health and prevention programme. Partners of HIV/AIDS persons should be notified of HIV exposure if at all feasible.[3]

While questions have been raised about the cost-effectiveness of such intensive endeavours in the context of the HIV epidemic, the gradual acceptance of contact notification can be traced to the recognition that, in its classic form, such efforts do not entail coercion, and protect the privacy of the index patient. Thus, even in cases where partner notification would disclose the identity of the index case (for instance, where the sexual partner of the index case is monogamous), the principle of cooperation, of engaging the index patient as a willing participant in partner notification or in voluntary behaviour modification to remove risk to the partner, leaves the patient with ultimate control over his or her privacy.

Duty to Warn

Very different has been question of whether clinicians or public health officials have a duty to warn unsuspecting sexual or needle-sharing partners when it becomes explicit that the latter will not do so and will continue to engage in behaviour that may lead to the transmission of HIV. Here the classic clash between the right to privacy of the patient and the "right to know" of the endangered individual is posed. It is a clash that confronts clinicians who become aware that their patients may cause a threat to third parties.

In the United States, the issue was faced directly by the California Supreme Court in the Tarasoff case,[4] where the question was whether a clinician had on affirmative duty to warn the intended victim of his patient. In that case the court ruled that such a duty existed, and "the protective privilege comes to an end where the public peril begins." The American Psychiatric Association objected that by creating such a duty the law would effectively discourage potentially violent patients from discussing their strategies with doctors who might dissuade them from taking action. Thus, it was asserted that Tarasoff was counterproductive. This objection would surface again in the AIDS epidemic. Critics afraid that patients, worried that physicians would inform partners of their HIV status, would be driven underground, away from the counselling, testing and treatment necessary to maintain their personal health and to preserve the public health.

The Tarasoff approach served as a backdrop to discussions of the duties of clinicians treating patients with HIV. The American Medical Association has stated that as a matter of professional ethics doctors have a duty to breach confidentiality to warn the unsuspecting partners of people with HIV. Most states have adopted "privilege to disclose" policies that treat such disclosures as permissible but not obligatory. This position echoes that of the *International Guidelines* on *HIV/AIDS and Human Rights*: "Public health legislation should authorize, but not require, that health-care professionals decide, on the ground of each individual case and ethical considerations, whether to inform their patient's sexual partners of the HIV status of their patient." The guidelines set forth criteria to help clinicians make decisions about whether to inform partners against the desires of the index case. The index case must have received thorough counselling yet continue to place others at risk; the index case must decline to notify partners or allow their notification; there must exist a "real risk" of HIV transmission to partners; the index case must be notified before his or her partners are informed; and those conducting the notification must protect the identity of the index case to the extent feasible in practice; finally, both index case and partners must receive follow-up an support after notification.[5]

Third Party Notification to Non-Endangered Individuals

Virtually all discussion of third party notification has centred on duties of infected individuals or others to inform sexual or needle-sharing partners. Some discussion has also concentrated on duties of health care workers exposed to accidental needle sticks. Such discussions have sought to weigh the competing demands of confidentiality and the interest of third parties in knowing about serious threats to life and well-being. There has been small discussion of whether there is a duty to warn others - family members and neighbours, for instance. Since the first years of the epidemic it has been explicit that such close but non-intimate contact posed no reasonable risk of HIV transmission. In the absence of risk there could be no duty to disclose. AIDS and HIV were, after all, not like tuberculosis, where exposed family members and co-workers could be placed at risk.

Third party notification to non-endangered individuals is not uncommon in a number a countries. The absence of strict regimes of confidentiality combine with culture to develop on informal and widespread system whereby not only partners but also friends, neighbours and employers may be informed of an individual's HIV infection. Explained one NGO: In Thai society for instance doctors and health officials will share information with their personal friends and associates. Such willingness to share information is also evident in hospitals. Generally, physicians will reveal HIV test results to family members, sometimes before revealing them to patients and even without disclosing them to patients. Health officials, too, are open to the cultural inclination to share information. Two NGO representatives reported that, in a recent meeting with school superintendents, several produced lists of children with AIDS or children whose parents had AIDS living in their districts. Provincial health officials had provided these lists.

The case of India underscores the complications that arise when countries begin the fundamental tasks of grappling with the dilemma of whether and how to notify both intimate and non-endangered third parties before establishing strict regimes to protect the basic rights of those with HIV/AIDS, and policies clearly delineating the duties and obligations of health care providers to both the infected individual and the health of the public. The changing legal horizon makes this a specially critical moment in India, for both recent Supreme Court decisions and emerging legislation threaten to muddy rather than clarify these principles.

While there may be no duty to reveal to non-endangered third parties, and while such disclosure may pose grave risks to those who are infected, isolation and secrecy are hardly ideal conditions for those who need and may be desperately dependent on the assistance of others. Besides, in a society of small, intimate villages like in Thailand, where most of the people receive little effective therapy for HIV/AIDS and most have come to recognize its symptoms, the notion that individuals can expect to live anonymously may be unrealizable.

References

1. Parran T. Shadow on the Land. New York. Waverly Press, 1937.
2. Commission of Inquiry on the Blood System in Canada. Final Report. Volumes 1-3. Ottawa: Minister of Public Works and Government Services Canada, 1997. p. 576.
3. The Members of the Federal/Provincial/Territorial Committee on AIDS Working Group on Partner Notification. Guidelines for Practice for Partner Notification in HIV/AIDS. Ottawa: Health Canada, January 1997. p. 2.
4. HIV/AIDS and Human Rights: International Guidelines. op.cit. p. 13.
5. HIV/AIDS and Human Rights: International Guidelines. op.cit. p. 13.

Seven

Prevention of Mother-to-Child

Major Elements of the Programme

An Option for Mothers-to-be

All The hospitals across Thailand have been informed of this programme with the help of Thai Ministry. Additionally, the mass media have provided the public with information on this programme by the means of Newspapers, pamphlets, magazines, and radio and television broadcasts. All these tasks on public notification have succeeded with the assistance of the Thai Red Cross public relation and fund-raising committees.

The health care provider who takes an intensive care of an HIV-infected pregnant women can make request zidovudine directly from the Thai Red Cross. It is suggested that the health care provider should discuss the following issues, which seem as a checklist on the drug request form, with the woman and her spouse prior to requesting the medication:

- The risks of HIV transmission from her to her unborn child and the choices of intervention
- The advantage of zidovudine in the prevention of HIV transmission
- The adverse side effects of zidovudine
- The way of taking the medication and the woman's desires to receive and take this donated medication
- The risk of HIV transmission through breast feeding and the family's access to formula feeding
- The mode to determine the child's HIV status and the couple's desires to bring their child for testing and for medical follow-up.
- The couple's willingness to raise the child
- The decision on a surrogate guardian for the child once

the couple can no prolong take care of the child in the future.

- Adequate family planning after the current pregnancy

The health care provider should inquire about the family income and occupation so that the donated medication is properly offered only to those who truly cannot afford it. The physician should stress to the couple of the risk for HIV transmission through breast-feeding. The Thai Red Cross supports that breast-feeding by HIV-infected women be discouraged. Alternative feeding should be comprehensively discussed with the couple. More than one counselling session may be needed. At all, times, the health care provider must assure the couple that their discussion will be based on the elements of confidentiality and that the couple's decision will be respected.

A Mission to Save the Child's Life

After all the discussions have taken place and the woman has agreed to take zidovudine, the health care provider fills out the drug request form. The information needed in this form comprises the family demography, family income and occupation, the history of pregnancy, the counselling checklist as above, the hospital address to which the medication should be delivered and the health care provider's name and signature. This form makes sure that all the important information has been discussed with the patient and provided to the Thai Red Cross. However, no patient's names are recorded on this form. The drug request form is then sent to the Thai Red Cross preferably by facsimile. The process of approval generally takes no more than one week. Once the request is approved, the health care provider will be notified. Zidovudine is generally delivered within two weeks after notification. The first shipment will be sufficient for one patient to use for 3 months. Later on, follow-up forms are to be filled out so that the medication can be delivered regularly to complete the whole course of the prophylactic regimen.

The Zidovudine Regimen used in this Programme is as follows:

(1) During pregnancy, a woman begins taking zidovudine any time between 14 and 34 weeks' gestation. The

everyday dose is 200 milligrams of zidovudine (2 pills) in the morning and 300 milligrams (3 pills) in the evening until the woman goes into labour.

(2) During labour, a woman takes 300 milligram of zidovudine (3 pills) orally every 3 hours till the birth of children.

(3) After birth, the infant takes zidovudine syrup at the dose of 2 milligrams per kilogram body weight every 6 hours until the infant is 6 weeks old.

This regimen is somewhat different from the ACTG 076 regimen. In the ACTG 076 regimen, a woman would receive 100 milligrams of zidovudine five times everyday during pregnancy. In this programme, the dose of zidovudine is less frequent for better compliance. Additionally, zidovudine was given intravenously (given into a vein) during labour in the ACTG 076 study. However, giving medication intravenously can be quite complicated, particularly in some community hospitals in rural Thailand. Therefore, a decision was taken to give the medication orally every 3 hours instead. It was found that the zidovudine level in the body remains rather comparable regardless of whether the medication is administered orally or intravenously.

New Life for the Child

All infants who receive Zidovudine from the programme gets free of charge HIV testing by the Thai Red Cross. Upon the parent's permission, blood samples are obtained by a heel stick or finger stick technique. We recommend that blood samples be obtained at birth, at 6 weeks and at 6 months of age. Small drops of blood are placed on the provided filter paper and permit to air-dry. The samples are then mailed with the similar form to the Thai Red Cross in the envelope provided. At the Thai Red Cross Laboratory, the dried blood spot samples are analysed for HIV. The technique being used is called the polymerase chain reaction assay. In a nutshell, the HIV gene is amplified if it is present in the dried blood spot. The gene is later detected using a standard laboratory technique. This method has proved sensitive and specific for the diagnosis of HIV infection in infants.

Once the outcome is available, the health care provider will be notified so that the parent will be informed of the child's HIV infection status. The Thai Red Cross makes encouragement that all children born to HIV-infected mothers be tested for HIV antibody at least once at or after the age of 15-18 months to confirm the child's infection status. This recommendation is appended in the last form as a reminder.

Donation Campaigns

All zidovudine being used in this programme comes from public donations. The donation campaign is under the direct liability of the public relation and fundraising committees of the Thai Red Cross. These committees include volunteers from various walks of life from chief executive officers to entertainers and from royal family members to government officers. The donations are get through four different ways as follows:

(1) Direct Donation

This is the very important source of the programme's fund. The Thai Red Cross accepts donation year-round from individuals, groups or organizations. The mass media continuously publicize the need for donations. One can donate in person at the Red Cross offices, by sending a cheque or a money order, or by transferring funds to the programme's bank account. There are no limits on the amount of donation. Additionally the donation is tax-deductible.

(2) Donation Through the Thai Red Cross Annual Activities

With the attempt of the public relation and fundraising committees, the Thai Red Cross has various activities for the general public each year. The important activities or events for instance are the Annual Thai Red Cross Fair, the World AIDS Day activities, the National Mother's Day celebrations, and the Princess Soamsawali's birthday celebrations. On these particular occasions, other than the donation campaign, there are countless educational activities concerned to HIV/AIDS prevention and care. This contribute to a better understanding of HIV/AIDS within the Thai society.

(3) Donation Through the Red Cross Red Ribbon Sale

Every year on 26 February, in recognition of the day this programme was founded, the Thai Red Cross holds the Red Cross Red Ribbon Sale over Thailand. This event, which is dedicated to those who suffer from AIDS, wants to raise public awareness of this disease. Parts of the benefit are directed to the zidovudine donation programme.

(4) Donation Through Miscellaneous Activities

The public relation and fundraising committees have worked with a number of non-government organizations and the private sector to establish a number of fund-raising activities. These comprise charity concerts, dinners, fashion shows, golf tournaments. gallery exhibitions, and the sale of special cassettes or compact discs, and so on.

PARTNERSHIPS AND ALLIANCES

The Roles of The Royal Family

As its patron, Her Royal Highness Princess Soamsawali has taken an active role in guiding and overseeing the zidovudine donation programme. Her Royal Highness has reserved her time to participate in various events related to this programme, has chaired the programme's annual meeting and has continuously donated funds and infant formula for the programme. One main event is the Spiritual Candle Light Ceremony on the World AIDS Day, when Her Royal Highness specifically meets with patients, volunteers and those who work in the field of HIV. On Her Royal Highness's birthday, there are abundant activities with regard to HIV/AIDS throughout the country. As the result of her dedication, Her Royal Highness has been accepted both by Thai and by the international community, comprising UNAIDS and UNICEF, as the foremost figure in HIV prevention and education in Thailand.

Her Royal Highness Princess Soamsawali is not the only royal family member associated with the Thai Red Cross. Her Royal Highness Princess Maha Chakri Sirindhorn is the patron of the Thai Cross Society. Although Her Royal Highness may not have an active role in the zidovudine donation programme. Her Royal Highness oversees all activities of the Thai Red Cross Society, comprising those related to HIV/AIDS and has provided valuable imputs for the operation of the Thai Red Cross AIDS Research Center. Moreover, parts of this programme's fund have come directly from Her Royal Highness's donations.

Ministry of Public Health

The Thai Ministry of Public Health, particularly the Division of AIDS, has played a potent role by providing information on the programme to all hospitals throughout the country. The Ministry has helped streamline the process by which hospitals take participation in the programme, and it continues to monitor and evaluate each hospital's participation. Such intervention has helped significantly in the smooth operation of the programme at these hospitals. Additionally, the Ministry has contributed zidovudine to be used in the programme.

Public Support

The reason that explains the success of this programme is its 'community-to-community' nature. The donation from the community ultimately returns back to the community. Being Buddhists, Thai people have strong belief that it is religiously important to support charities. Preventing one child from this deadly disease is considered by Thai as one of the very favourable and charitable attainments. Therefore, the programme is very well received and fits very well in Thailand.

Monitoring and Evaluation

From February 1996 to August 1999, there had been almost 2,900 HIV-infected pregnant women receiving free zidovudine from this programme. They were from 81 hospitals in 40 provinces throughout Thailand. The analysis of the transmission rate was performed by the Thai Red Cross in August 1999. The analysis was limited to a subgroup of 719 mother-infant pairs among whom dried blood spot HIV tests were available on infants at or after 4 weeks of age. The mothers started zidovudine during pregnancy at 14-34 weeks gestation and continued till delivery, and the infants received zidovudine for 6 weeks after birth. The transmission rate in this group was 5.9 per cent, which is agreeable with the rates reported from developed countries where zidovudine ATCG 076 regimen was implemented. Therefore, the scientific strength of this programme exists as it is now proven that zidovudine remains effective in reducing mother-to-child transmission of HIV outside the setting of clinical research in the less-developed region of the world. The analysis also confirmed that zidovudine is effective in the population with predominant HIV subtype E infection (HIV subtype E is the most common subtype in Thailand whereas subtype B is the most common subtype in the western world). The ACTG 076 study was performed in the United States and France where HIV subtype B is predominant.

This programme has demonstrated that the community can work effectively together to overcome the obstacle of the high cost of zidovudine. Donation of medication has proved feasible and can be used as one of the strategic tools to prevent mother-to-child transmission of HIV in less-developed countries.

Lessons Learned

Because the HIV/AIDS epidemic continues in Thailand, the Thai Red Cross foresees the inevitability of maintaining the zidovudine donation programme. A number of plans, with some modification, have been laid out for the continuation of the programme.

A subgroup analysis showed that the transmission rate of women who received zidovudine less than or amount to 8 weeks before delivery was not statistically different from the transmission rate in those who got zidovudine more that 8 weeks before delivery. In answer to this finding, by late 1999 the Thai Red Cross advised that antepartum zidovudine for pregnant women in this programme should be began at 32 weeks' gestation and be continued till labour. This will help save the fund and the medication without compromising the effectiveness of the regimen, enabling the programme to give the medication to more women. The intrapartum and the neonatal components of this prophylactic regimen remain unchanged. From time to time assessments have taken place thereafter to assure that the transmission rate remains within an acceptable range.

Since the medical knowledge in the field of HIV evolves rapidly, the Thai Red Cross recognizes that this programme may require to be frequently updated to provide the greatest advantage to patients. A recent study from Uganda (HIVNET 012) compared the safety and efficacy of nevirapine with zidovudine in the decrease of mother-to-child transmission. Both medications were well tolerated with no different adverse events observed in both groups. The transmission rate was near about 50 per cent lower among those receiving nevirapine compared with those getting the short-courses zidovudine. This new information has led the Thai Red Cross to evolve a new intervention strategy. In the year 2000, nevirapine as described in HIVNET 012 study will be incorporated into the programme's regimen. Both zidovudine and nevirapine will be provided to all participating pregnant women and infants. Theoretically, using both medications together to tackle the virus may lead to a further reduction of transmission.

The zidovudine donation programme has proved possible and successful in the Thai setting. The further step that the Thai Red Cross plans is to communicate with hospitals that have not yet taken part in this programme. Moreover, the Thai Red Cross has recently been made a UNAIDS collaborating centre. This will expand the role of the organization in this region. The model of this programme can probably be used as a demonstration or a prototype for other countries in this region.

Despite its Clear Effectiveness, the Programme has Some Weakness as Follows:

- Although the health care providers are asked to return all follow-up forms, this is not essential in practice. Several patient forms were missing. This makes a retrospective assessment difficult.
- There is no straight information on patient's adherence to the medication and to the medical follows-up. Without complete and accurate information, it is not easy to evaluate all aspects of the programme.
- Given that the programme is not a research project. Some health care providers did not send the infant's dried blood spots for HIV testings. It is feasible that some infants may not have been carried out in for follow-up, some families may have relocated, and some infants may have been tested locally by their primary care physicians.
- Although the programme has been publicized for almost 4 years, some antenatal care facilities may not be aware of it. As a result, the pregnant women may not be appropriately counselled, the decision to participate may

not be properly reached and zidovudine prophylaxis may not be properly offered.

- Whereas the programme focuses on reducing the number of HIV-infected children, the future of the uninfected children is not addressed, specially the issue of orphaning. In addition, there are no set medical care plans for the infected parents. Multidisciplinary approaches are highly necessary to solve the problems of this magnitude.

Although no formal evaluations have taken place, the Thai Red Cross periodically organises a meeting with all participating hospitals. The discussions are generally concentrated on the problems that health care providers and the Thai Red Cross faced and how to solve them. This has led all parties to a better understanding and cooperation, which eventually benefits pregnant women and children.

Best Practice

Relevance

The programme's chief objective is to make zidovudine accessible for HIV-infected pregnant Thai women with help from the community. The spread of HIV/AIDS in Thailand is mainly by heterosexual transmission. The increasing number of HIV-infected women has led to a large number of children born with HIV. Without interventions, the country will have to face an important number of paediatric HIV cases. The medical care for these children will be precious and may well be a burden for the country. Therefore, every attempt must be made to reduce the number of those affected children. This programme concentrates on providing free zidovudine to prevent transmission of HIV from pregnant women to infants and it should be considered as one of the alternatives for these women. This initiative should be viewed as a pilot project. Regarding convincing the society that intervention strategies can be implemented even in the resource-poor setting, it has been successful.

Effectiveness and Efficiency

The programme is administered by the Thai Red Cross AIDS Research Center headed by the Thai Red Cross Society. Because this is not a research project. The administration structure is organised to be efficient while maintaining flexibility in operations. The programme has set some criteria in an attempt to ensure that zidovudine will be provided to those who are truly unable to afford the medication. This has met the donors' expectation that the funds or the medication they donate should go to those who really require it. It also ensures that the programme will not be abused.

The programme, with the assistance from the public relation and fund-raising committees of the Thai Red Cross, has invited participation from the public and private sectors in both publicizing this programme and supplying financial support. This sort of cooperation has continued to grow.

As was earlier mentioned, the effectiveness of this programme has been reflected in the low transmission rate of 5.9 per cent. The programme and its consequences were recently presented at the Second Conference on Global Strategies for the Prevention of HIV Transmission from Mothers to Infants in Canada.

Ethical Soundness

This programme is operated by the driving force of charity and humanity from the community. The medication that the Thai Red Cross purchases is used only for the programme. In addition to, no request has ever been rejected and we have faith that the medication is equally allocated to all. The existence of this programme has stimulated health care providers in Thailand to involve the discussion of HIV as a relevant health concern for every pregnant woman and to provide the voluntary counselling and testing services. The programme also sets the standard of care for HIV-infected pregnant women and has helped shape the direction and the ethics of the clinical research on mother-to-child transmission in this country and in the developing countries.

Sustainability

This programme has been operating for near about 4 years. Judging by the number of requests, the level of donation, and the amount of the medication allocated each year, it is evident that there is a continuing requirement for this programme. However, it requires to be kept up-to-date with the new medical and social information. We believe that as long as HIV/AIDS is a public health problem for Thailand, the community-to-community' programme of this kind must survive. It could be one of a few weapons that the society has to combat and control this deadly disease.

References

1. Brown T, Sittirai W. The impact of HIV on children in Thailand. United Kingdom: Save the Children Fund: Bangkok, June 1995, Report No 16.
2. Weniger BG, Limpakarnjanarat K, Ungchusak, et al. The Epidemiology of HIV infection and AIDS in Thailand, AIDS 1991: 5(suppl 2): s71-s85.
3. Poonchareon W. Dilokwitayarat L. Current situations and trends of HIV infection in Thailand. The 7th National Seminar on AIDS. Bangkok. April 21-23, 1999.
4. Bunnell RE, Yanpaisarn S. Kilmarx PH. et al. HIV - 1 seroprevalance among childbearing women in northern Thailand: monitoring a rapidly evolving epidemic. AIDS 1999; 13: 509-515.
5. Khongphatthanayothin M, Rongkavilit C, Sirivichayakul S, et al. Thai Red Cross zidovudine donation campaign to prevent vertical transmission of HIV: results of the modified ACTG 076 regimen. The 2nd Conference on Global Strategies for the prevention of HIV Transmission from Mothers to Infants. Monteral. September 1-6, 1999 [abstract 100].
6. Annual Report. Thai Red Cross Zidovudine Donation Program: Bangkok, September 1997.
7. Annual Report. Thai Red Cross Zidovudine Donation Program. September 1998.

Eight

Female Sex Worker HIV Prevention Projects

Background

The three projects opted for case studies represent a range of situations, geographical locations, problems and solutions. Two of these, Sonagachi and SHAKTI, involve brothel-based sex workers in South Asia. The Transex project works with club or street-based sex workers in the Pacific nation of Papua New Guinea. SHAKTI comprises both brothel and street-based sex workers in Bangladesh. In each case, situations vary considerably. Sonagachi is a large, thickly populated red light district in the centre of Calcutta, housing 5,000 sex workers, of whom two-thirds are Indian and one-third hail from Bangladesh and Nepal. The project originates from the All India Institute of Hygiene and Tropical Medicine, funded by WHO in its earlier days and by the United Kingdom Department for International Development (DfID) more recently. Although it started when HIV prevalence was still rather low, prevalence has been increasing in West Bengal. In other regions of India, HIV prevalence has increased very rapidly. SHAKTI is the name of a project implemented by CARE, Bangladesh. It started at a brothel in Tangail, a medium-sized city in Bangladesh, and expanded to include street-based women in the capital city of Dhaka. DfID provided funding. The brothel at Tangail houses about 600 sex workers and the street-based intervention targets about 3000 workers. SHAKTI began when HIV was only sporadically found in returning migrants and some other groups of people in Bangladesh. As of 1998, HIV prevalence remained fairly low in Bangladesh, but appeared to be increasing slowly. The Transex project, enforced by the Papua New Guinea Institute of Medical Research, has two branches in the two big cities of Papua New

Guinea, Lae and Port Moresby. In both cities, the project works with independent, street-level sex workers. The project is mainly financed by AusAID and, to a smaller extent, had funding from UNAIDS for a single year. It is named Transex since it focuses on transport workers, i.e. sailors, truckers and dock workers, as well as police and security men, additionally the women who sell them sex. HIV prevalence was rising rapidly as the project started and continues to do so. The process by which these projects have been documented needs some mention. All projects were visited and documents reviewed. Taped interviews were conducted with some managers. Mid-term or final evaluations were carefully examined where available. Raw data were accessed for several projects and analysed. Sex workers from three projects were particularly helpful, as were outreach or field workers.

The first drafts of the case studies were examined by each project manager and then sent for review and comments to persons unconnected with the project in the same country and to persons outside each country. Each reviewer was a person closely involved with HIV prevention activities, comprising several known authors of published AIDS-related materials. After their comments were received, project managers were asked to respond, and then a full review of all materials took place in Geneva with UNAIDS representatives. As this process extended over a year, upto date information was sought from each project just before the completion of the last draft. Therefore, it is expected that this document is a fair and honest representation of the realities faced by the selected projects and their participants and that the reader will glean useful insights from the strengths and weaknesses these projects demonstrate.

Lessons in Best Practices in Sex Worker Interventions

The attempts made to document and analyse five female sex worker projects opted for the session at the conference in Manila in 1997 have resulted in three best practice case studies. Two have been set aside following inadequate documentation and lack of sound data to support claims of success. The other three illustrate different aspects of good practice and some not rather so good. There are lessons to be learned from all. In fact, it might be easier for most of us to see why some action fails than how an activity succeeds in bringing about change in complicated and difficult situations. This section will address several broad issues, illustrated by discussions of the case studies. Other more particular points will be listed below more precisely. The interested reader can refer to the full case studies for a more complete discussion.

The Individual vs. the Social

In nearly all settings, female sex workers are a stigmatized group of people. Their very existence challenges the standard family and reproduction-oriented sexual morality found in most of the societies. Yet they exist nearly everywhere, explicitly indicating that they fulfill a function for society. Hypocritically, most mainstream societies have relegated them to the margins, abused them, exploited them and restricted their rights as citizens. As women (in opposite to male sex workers), they are doubly powerless. With the advent of the HIV pandemic, they have been the first group in various nations to be targeted as vectors and seen as dangerous to the general population. They are seen as the source of infection and their clients as unwitting victims. Usually the sex trade or industry itself is left untouched. The contrasting perspective is that the sex worker is a person whose livelihood places her in a highly vulnerable situation for acquiring HIV. That livelihood, being illegal, is surrounded by layers of uncontrolled and therefore abusive persons. Sex worker projects must grapple with these variant perspectives, both in the society at large surrounding the sex worker and in the views of project personnel. Sometimes sex workers themselves are reluctant about their position in the epidemic, at times seeing themselves as actors, and at other times as victims. The strategies followed by HIV prevention projects for female sex workers reflect these perspectives and set the tone for the way in which the project is enforced.

Most of the projects appear to address high risk behaviour on the level of the individual, with persuasive methods, like advice, counselling, and peer education; enabling approaches that remove social constraints to safer sex (or conversely, put hindrances to unsafe sex in place) demonstrate greater success. These enabling approaches are exemplified by the projects documented here in various ways, which illustrate the way they function.

Formative Research

First, one must understand the structure of the sex industry, the position of women in it, who has power over them and who does not, and what the sex worker lacks to be able to live and work in a healthier setting.

Baseline quantitative survey research, while usually needed, is not able to supply the in-depth information required to design strategies for change. The Transex project was based on an optimal use of qualitative situational assessments and formative research. This made able the project to tailor the activities to local contexts and to be able to adjust to the realities in many sub-populations and cities. Sex workers themselves were involved in the project design and made their priorities explicit: they wanted help against police harassment.

The Sonagachi project conducted extensive surveys of sex workers, clients, boyfriends, and sex workers' children's requirements, gradually adding each piece of research, as issues become clearer. More qualitative information was collected somewhat informally, but was reflected frequently in the published documents on the project. SHAKTI conducted a formative survey, but it was not designed to uncover the power structure of the brothel. This information was collected in a less formal and less organized fashion, leaving project implementers somewhat confused about how to proceed. The force of events, however, in Bangladesh, moved the project advance.

Courage and Clarity of Commitment

But there is more. It also takes courage to face powerful political and social structures once these are delineated in the formative phase. The Sonagachi project is welcomed globally by sex worker organizations and AIDS activists alike for its integral involvement of sex workers. This could not have taken place without a palpable demonstration of courage and commitment shown by the project personnel. In this case, several community-based groups had been working in the Sonagachi area prior to the HIV intervention. They had themselves confronted the local gangs, a portion of the power structure, and had developed understanding of the social scene and the strength to stand up to it. As the HIV interventions started, they participated and helped intervention personnel to develop the strategy of empowerment that has been so successful. Gradually, women's groups, legal rights organizations, and even government agencies have joined the sex workers' endeavours to reform the social system around prostitution in Calcutta.

The Transex project in Papua New Guinea (PNG) operates in rather a different social setting. There are far fewer layers of control over the sex worker than found in the Indian sub-continent. The one salient power broker is the police force and the project took them on directly, addressing the highly vulnerable issues of group rape or line-ups. This has been one of the most potent aspects of the project, empowering the women through confronting police practices, sexual violence and issues of social marginalization. Gradually, the commitment of the project and its staff has become conspicuous to sex workers, who seem to be beginning to bond in a self-run organization. Both of these projects created a precedent by addressing social and sexual norms.

The SHAKTI project has endeavoured to bring about improved condom use without confronting the power structures and, in some ways, has been less successful than the other projects. Its original model of conflict resolution did not resolve the bigger conflicts surrounding the sex worker and hence, she has remained comparatively isolated in her attempts to induce safer sex in her trade, one that remains highly stigmatized in Bangladesh. Nonetheless, the participation of SHAKTI's sex workers, especially those who led in a fight against the closure of brothels in 1999, has been critical in bringing about a court decision mentioning prostitution as a legal way to make a living. While it is understood that all constraints in the social arena are not amenable to rapid change, the SHAKTI and Sonagachi projects demonstrate with clarity that even in highly repressive and abusive environments, the rights of sex workers can be addressed and sex workers themselves can be enabled to act.

Measuring Effectiveness

Unless a project creates sound ways of measuring its success, it is very difficult to defend its practices, even if they are subjectively thought to be successful. When screening various projects in the Asia-Pacific region, this issue loomed largest. Most projects are rather capable of maintaining process indicators, i.e. the number of condoms given out, the number of meetings held or peer educators trained. Measures of impact or effectiveness, however, are usually less well developed. In few cases, data are gathered which could be used to demonstrate impact, but there are no project personnel available with the skills to analyse and disseminate the results. In the case of SHAKTI, such a skilled person was available during the design phase and good indicators were established, but for a period in the project's life, those skills were not replaced. A similar skills gap occurred in the Transex project.

The types of indicators used must fit what the project is trying to accomplish and must accommodate all its greater effects. While all of the projects discussed aim at the control of HIV transmission, prevalence levels of HIV do not demonstrate impact very well. Incidence levels would be an improvement but need a cohort study, which becomes a major investment in research and is not feasible for most intervention projects. Levels of other STDs are considerably more useful in demonstrating improved sexual health, but are not particular to project components. It is not feasible to separate out the effect of improved recognition of symptoms, improved access to treatment, improved diagnosis and treatment, or improved condom use from such data. Further, some STDs, like chlamydia, are very often asymptomatic and not a good indicator in women. Results of STD surveys are very sensitive to modes of sample collection (e.g. how well a vaginal or cervical swab is taken), modes of laboratory testing (especially where cultures are needed, and modes of sampling. Unless well-trained persons are in place to carry out such surveys, they are repeatedly subject to failure, or at least, to questionable results.

In the case of Sonagachi, STD indicators produced a problem for several of the above-mentioned causes. Ultimately, the laboratory methods were improved. In the case of SHAKTI, laboratory methods were clearly well controlled, although some confusion resulted over the interpretation of negative controls on the PCR chlamydia results. Unfortunately, those with the clearest results, i.e. PCR-tested gonorrhoea and current syphilis (via VDRL at dilutions ≥ 1:8), showed no improvement over time. The Transex project was unable to develop its STD indicators at the starting of the project due to difficulties with availability of personnel as well as with the government. This work has begun but will need several years before an assessment of the impact of the project can take place. It is not likely that most sex worker projects will be able to utilize laboratory-based indicators and simpler modes of monitoring STD levels must be developed.

Self-reported condom use is always a difficult measure, though heavily depended upon by most projects. It is well recognized that women are under pressure by these projects to claim improved condom use and are highly likely to exaggerate. The major differences between mid-term survey outcomes and simultaneous monitoring outcomes for condom use at the Tangail brothel illustrates well the great pressure felt by sex workers when asked about their condom use by their own dedicated peer educators (as opposed to peer educators assigned to educate other cohorts of sex workers). SHAKTI attempted to address this question by collecting used condom covers, but this method did not appear to be appropriate.

Transex tried to diminish over reporting by ways of improved interview techniques, but had no other modes of verification. The use of condom is not a monitoring indicator and data on this aspect of outcome are only available through repeated surveys. Fortunately, the protracted period of first baseline data collection allowed a trend analysis, and the police component did have a follow-up survey. Its full evaluation was designed from the starting of the project to diminish bias by moving outreach workers from one city to the other to serve as interviewers in the follow-up survey.

While Sonagachi also simply asked women about their condom use in its earlier repeated surveys, more recently it has moved to asking how many condoms they are purchasing. This is a far better measures, assuming poor women will not buy what they do not plan to use, and is only possible when free condoms are not being disseminated. The very strong social marketing component of Sonagachi has enabled this to come about. Such a measure, however, does not accommodate the number of condoms supplied by clients or boyfriends, but, in the lack of targeted interventions for these groups, may well act as a proxy for all condoms available to Sonagachi's women. A similar attempt to selling condoms has occurred in the SHAKTI project and, in both cases, the sale of condoms by sex workers serves well to confirm the rising levels of condom use.

Monitoring is an on-going process. The majority of monitoring indicators for all projects concentrate on process or progress, not result. These are of value if project personnel are able to critically review their meaning and adjust activities accordingly. In all the projects discussed, time pressure and overworked personnel have been determinants working against the optimal use of monitoring indicators.

Monitoring growing levels of self-esteem or empowerment has been a weakness in all these projects, especially in a measurable form. Qualitative documentation does exist, e.g. anecdotes and newspaper articles. Only at Sonagachi has a quantifiable measure been developed, i.e. the number of sex worker meetings attended. This is feasible only because of the advanced nature of the intervention's approach to sex worker rights and self-directed activities, like training other sex workers elsewhere.

Strategies for Strength and Replication

All these projects have aimed at replication in other areas of their respective countries or regions. The West Bengal Sexual Health Project incorporates the Sonagachi experience directly and the Sonagachi sex workers' organization, the Durbar Mahila Samanwaya Committee, has given training to hundreds of sex workers elsewhere in West Bengal. Without the development of strong sex workers' organizations, each project has had to depend upon the interest of other NGOs. This has not been successful as yet in Papua New Guinea and is only partially successful in Bangladesh. However, in Bangladesh the strong collaboration of SHAKTI with government during its early phases was very effective in demonstrating the feasibility of targeted interventions for prostitutes in a highly conservative setting. Its strength grew as it linked with other legal and human rights agencies. In Sonagachi as in Papua New Guinea, the enforcing agency was a government affiliate. Nonetheless, other government sectors had to be convinced of the value of the project. Partnerships with NGOs were well developed in Sonagachi and have only recently developed in Papua New Guinea. In all cases, it is apparent that replicating the project must be done in a way that will allow local groups to adapt the overall plannings to their own situations and access the experience of the older project in the process. Planning for expansion or replication at the early stages of such a project is important for it permits the time for development of understanding and cooperative relationships with government agencies and NGOs.

Efficiency and Management

While levels of efficiency in such projects will never approximate to those in successful profit-making businesses, they can be tightened and improved. As per rule it is more efficient to address the top of a hierarchy that is in control of activities and behaviours of those lower down, as the Transex project did with the police, than to spend a great deal of time and money directly reaching the masses at the bottom.

Sonagachi also carried on repeated formal and informal advocacy meetings with senior government officials to win their cooperation. To a greater extent, this has paid off and allowed major international meetings of sex workers to take place in Calcutta. Large budgets are not always helpful. They can mislead inexperienced project managers into thinking there is ample room for mistakes to be made. Good budgetary control is needed and needs direct coordination with project strategies and particular activities. Even small budgets can thereby be well utilized.

AIDS prevention projects may attract NGOs and individuals who simply understand that there is funding available for this kind of work. When they percept the intensity of the problem, they may or may not be willing to commit themselves and a large part of their lives to working with stigmatized people. Leadership in sex worker projects needs honest commitment. It is not a job that suits everyone. The individuals who led the projects discussed were highly committed and personally involved. Their families became involved and their personal time was sacrificed. While this may lead to burnout, it may be necessary, at least at the starting of such projects. Others in such projects who are deeply committed also experience burnout and the project must build in methods to eliminate feelings of ineffectiveness, monotony, and grief. Persons living with HIV, whenever feasible, should be incorporated into project activities. This can help them and help everyone else remember why they are working so hard.

Specific Points

Peer education is one of a number of ways to convey information and persuade people to change their behaviour. Its great advantage is that peers can utilize their normal venues and modes of communication. If peer educators are separated from their colleagues with special privileges, the value of the approach may be lost.

- Addressing clients with particular programmes tailored to their requirements strengthens sex workers' abilities to negotiate condom use.
- Boyfriends, husbands and other non-commercial sexual partners repeatedly place sex workers at more risk than do their clients, especially after they have learned to persuade clients to use condoms. This aspect of the lives of sex workers requires specialized attention.
- Personnel well trained in current STD diagnostics and treatment must oversee the establishment and management of clinics for sex worker projects. Sex workers are people with other health problems as well and these also require attention.
- STD and other studies conducted with sex workers must be carried out with their full understanding and assure their right to refuse. Well-designed studies carried on properly are of value of sex workers too; poor studies waste their time and are seen as abusive. Results require to be fed back to the sex worker community in an appropriate fashion to make sure their understanding, and timely treatment must be given. Anything less is unethical and will destroy their confidence in the project and its messages.

- Project staff and sometimes sex workers too require training in human sexuality in order to be able to speak about sex with ease and convey clear messages.
- Lubrication, female condoms and promoting non-penetrative sex should be made part of the package of safer sex options.
- Documentation is more than periodic surveys and counting monitoring indicators. Writing and/or using tapes and film to document the history of a project is a worthwhile effort of its own and has potential value of several others.

Conclusions

The significance of designing and implementing successful targeted interventions for sex workers as part of HIV prevention and control cannot be over-emphasized. In almost every country, sex workers include a focal point of the epidemic, because, as women who provide sex for many men, infections can easily accumulate among them. They are the subject to discrimination, often violently intense, trafficking, legal persecution and societal ambivalence - as well as one of the first occupational groups to become very infected. From them, the infection passes back to their clients and into the general population of women, men and children. One of the clearest public health lessons originating from the HIV pandemic is that protecting the human rights of sex workers is one of the best ways to protect the rest of society from HIV.

Nine

AIDS and the Military

Facts and Figures

- Military personnel have a high risk of exposure to Sexually Transmitted Diseases (STDs), including HIV. In peacetime, STD infection rates among armed forces are generally 2 to 5 times higher than in comparable civilian populations. The difference can be even greater in times of conflict.
- Studies in the USA, the UK, and France show that soldiers from these countries have a much higher risk of HIV infection than equivalent age/sex groups in the civilian population. Recent figures from Zimbabwe and Cameroon show military HIV infection rates 3 to 4 times higher than in the civilian population.
- Although military personnel are highly susceptible to STD and HIV infections as a group, military service is also a unique opportunity in which HIV/AIDS prevention and education can be provided to a large "captive audience" in a disciplined, highly organized setting.
- Soldiers on deployment regularly have sexual contacts with sex workers (prostitutes) and the local population. For example, 45 per cent of Dutch navy and marines personnel on peacekeeping duty in Cambodia had sexual contact with sex workers or other members of the local population during a five-month tour. Often condoms are not used consistently.
- Like women everywhere, female military personnel are especially vulnerable. As well as being at higher risk of HIV for physiological reasons that all women share, they are often at a disadvantage in sexual negotiations, including negotiations for condom use.

- HIV is a threat not only to military personnel but also to their families and community. Military HIV programmes are most effective if there is close collaboration with civilian health authorities.
- Probably the single most important factor leading to high rates of HIV in the military is the practice of posting personnel far from their accustomed communities and families for varying periods of time. As well as freeing them from traditional social controls, it removes them from contact with spouses or regular sexual partners and thereby encourages growth of sex industries in the areas where they are posted.
- According to an international survey done in 1995-1996, HIV testing is carried out in some form by 93 per cent of reporting militaries. About 80 per cent of the military establishments that conduct pre-recruitment HIV screening reject candidates who test HIV-positive, and an equal percentage restrict HIV-positive personnel from combat, overseas deployment and piloting aircraft.
- UNAIDS believes that HIV-positive individuals in the military should be given every opportunity to do the tasks for which they have been trained and which they are still fit to perform. As well, armed forces should prepare to provide care and support for personnel and family members living with HIV and AIDS, including continuity of care as they return to civilian life.

Are Military and Civilian Populations Really that Different When it Comes to AIDS?

Military personnel are a population group at special risk of exposure to Sexually Transmitted Diseases (STDs), comprising HIV. In peace time, STD infection rates among armed forces are often 2 to 5 times higher than in civilian populations; in time of conflict the difference can be 50 times higher or more. Paradoxically - and fortunately - strong traditions of organization and discipline give the military considerable advantages if they move decisively against HIV/AIDS. Recently, relative studies of sexual behaviour in France, the UK and the USA showed that military personnel (both career and conscripted personnel) have a much higher risk of HIV infection than groups of equivalent age/sex in the civilian population. Armed forces in different parts of the world reflect the same phenomenon. A 1995 estimate of HIV in Zimbabwe, for example, places the infection rate for the armed forces at 3 to 4 times higher than the level in the civilian population.

What is there in the military environment that raises the risk of HIV infection?

- Military and peacekeeping service often comprises lengthy periods spent away from home, with the outcome that personnel are often looking for ways to relieve loneliness, emphasis and the building up of sexual tension.
- The military's professional methods ethos to excuse or even encourage risk-taking.
- Most personnel are in the age group at greatest risk for HIV infection - the sexually active 15-24-year age group.
- Personnel sent on peacekeeping missions generally have more money in their pockets than local people, giving them the financial means to buy sex.
- Military personnel and camps, comprising the installations of peacekeeping forces, attract sex workers and those who deal in illicit drugs.

Opportunities for Risky Behaviour

The number of sex partners that a person has is a potent factor in the risk of STD infection, especially HIV. The chances of encountering someone with prior exposure to HIV go higher as the number of sex partners goes up. The risk is especially high with partners who are "one-night stands" or sex workers when no condom is used. Military personnel on deployment often indulge in risky activities. For instance, a study of Dutch sailors and marines on peacekeeping duty in Cambodia found that 45 per cent reported having sexual contact with sex workers or other members of the local population during a five-month tour. Another study said that 10 per cent of US naval personnel and marines contracted a new STD during trips to South America, West Africa and the Mediterranean during 1989-1991. War itself provides for a particularly rich breeding ground for HIV infection. The mobilization of huge numbers of young men (already a high-risk group for STDs), the practice of intimidation through rape, and displacement of refugees (a highly vulnerable group) - all these factors increase the prevalence of virus. To make matters worse, war is often accompanied by the breakdown of health and educational infrastructures, crippling endeavours to subsides the spread of HIV during or following conflict.

The Risk-taking Ethos and other Attitudinal Factors

Military personnel are not only a special group because of objective factors like their relative youth, but also because of their attitudes. Some attitudes comprise both those purposefully inculcated by the armed forces in training and those which are learnt informally as part of military "culture" and strongly encouraged through peer pressure.

For example, willingness to accept risk is highly important in combat, but off the battlefield it may increase soldiers' desire to engage in needlessly risky behaviour (sex without a condom, purchased sex, etc.). A high value placed on aggressiveness may make soldiers prone to pursuing sex with several different partners as a type of "conquest". In the end, the sense of prestige that comes with being part of the uniformed armed forces, reinforced by bonding within units, may tempt soldiers to view civilians - especially women - as people over whom power can be exerted. This may increase the likelihood of soldiers engaging in anonymous, purchased or even coercive sex.

Separation from Accustomed Community

Probably the single potent factor leading to high rates of HIV in the military is the practice of posting personnel far from their accustomed community or their families for long periods of time. Aside from the emotional stress this places on individuals, the practice encourages use of commercial sex. As a result, local sex industries grow in response to demand from military bases and units. It is a prime challenge to military setup to re-think this traditional feature of operational practice in the light of health and social issues, both of which suggest the high value of finding ways to support strong family relationships and marriages. (Note that these issues must also be faced in relation to other people live long-distance truck drivers, migratory workers and labourers, prisoners and refugees.

Are There Especially Vulnerable Groups Within the Military?

Young, unattached men are a highly susceptible group both inside and outside the military. Typically, the young recruit on a weekend pass has both the time and motivation, especially under the influence of peer pressure, to indulge in high-risk behaviour. However, there are other groups within the military whose vulnerability should be addressed.

The increasing participation of women in the military in different parts of the world underlines the special vulnerability of women to STD and HIV transmission. Women are more likely to acquire any kind of STD from a single sexual exposure than men, and to have more asymptomatic STDs that are not easy to diagnose. Female military personnel are often at a disadvantage in sexual negotiations, comprising those for condom use. They are also subject to sex under duress and sometimes to outright rape.

The fact that in the military there are men who have sex with men is a vulnerable issue in various countries. Some sexual contacts occur between men who identify themselves as homosexual or bisexual. In few cases there is coerced sex (rape) among men. Finally, men who recognize themselves as heterosexual may experiment with male-to-male sexual activity (for instance, during periods of isolation from female companionship). Little research has been made on this, but recent studies suggest that such activity may be more widespread than generally assumed.

Impact can HIV/AIDS have on the Military?

Effects on Military Preparedness

Various countries are concerned that the armed forces' readiness can be compromised by HIV/AIDS. Commanders from some countries with high HIV prevalence concern about being able to "field" a full contingent for deployment on relatively short notice as the infection affects rising numbers of personnel. Even if new recruits can be found, readiness and smooth teamwork are compromised if absences are filled in by people who have not served together earlier. Preparedness is also affected as the skills and experience of highly trained individuals are lost because of AIDS and its opportunistic infections.

Impacts on Infected Individuals and Families

Apart from illness and death due to AIDS, the greatest impacts on armed force personnel who are known or even suspected to be HIV-positive may be on their career advancement and social lives, particularly in societies or workplaces where there are no measures to protect them from stigmatization. They will generally be discriminated against in different ways in both operational and social settings.

Opportunistic infections like tuberculosis or pneumonia or conditions like Kaposi sarcoma may not appear in a person with HIV for many years after the original infection. Onward transmission of the virus to spouses (and children), partners, sex workers, and other members of the community is therefore a serious risk, especially in those in the early stages of HIV infection before symptoms appear. The virus can be passed unknowingly between husband and wife, and to infants if a pregnant woman is infected.

Risk of Transmission to Civilian Populations

HIV/AIDS in the armed forces is a threat not only to military personnel and their families but also to the wider community. In several countries, a large proportion of the nation's young adults spends one or more years in the military either through conscription or high rates of volunteering. This implies that the number of people who return to civilian life is large both numerically and in its potential impact on all segments of society.

At risk from transmission by sexual intercourse are regular and casual sex partners and sex workers. As well, infected military personnel may also transmit the disease to the wider community through unscreend blood donations, sharing of infected needles, and to medical personnel who accidentally come into contact with their blood.

"Our study of the epidemiological data on HIV infection in French military personnel has shown us that tours of duty overseas multiply the risk of infection by a factor of 5. Despite our prevention efforts, some individuals remained impervious to the usual preventive messages, although there has been a considerable downturn in new infections in recent years. Nevertheless, the number of new (HIV) seropositive cases and of sexually transmitted diseases as a whole remains higher overseas than in mainland France, which implies that the preventive message targeted to overseas staff must be more insistent and more repetitive".

- General Jacques Abgrall, Deputy Director, Scientific and Technical Action, Central Directorate of French Army Health Services

CONCRETE ACTIONS SHOULD BE TAKEN

Seize the Opportunity for HIV Prevention

As mentioned earlier, large proportions of young adults in several countries spend one or more years in the military. While this may be seen as a potential threat to civil society in relation to HIV transmission after they leave the military, it must also be seen as a ubiquitious opportunity since, military service gives a disciplined, highly organized environment in which HIV/AIDS prevention and education can be provided to a large "captive audience".

In some ways, such attempts fit perfectly with the ethos of a profession that gives a high value on loyalty to comrades and the tradition of officers looking out for the well-being of those under their liability. From this perspective, HIV prevention and education are every bit as important to life and health as rescuing a wounded colleague on the battlefield or securing a position once taken.

While some armed forces have been slow to develop policies and implement HIV/AIDS programmes, others have moved with all the energy and decisiveness of which the military is capable when faced with a serious and clearly defined mission. Most of the programmes aim to change high-risk behaviours practised by a number of military personnel, while others effort to deal with the factors underlying the military's special vulnerability.

At the same time, the evolution of international power politics, advances in military technology and social changes within countries are pushing many armed forces to rethink their roles and missions. For example, relatively new missions such as peacekeeping, drug interdiction and disaster response all need soldiers to have skills and attitudes significantly different from previous generations of military personnel. All these contextual changes offer opportunities (as well as challenges) to armed forces' HIV/AIDS responses.

Approaches Addressing Risk Behaviour

Operational measures aimed at prevention have been instituted successfully in the armed forces of an increasing number of countries comprising Botswana, Chile, the Philippines, Thailand, Zambia and many NATO members. Among the measures taken are:

- Improved or expanded prevention education, comprising training of armed forces medical and nursing staff, and regular briefing of the troops themselves with specific HIV-related information.
- Condom education and distribution, an inevitable element in HIV prevention. Education must be clear and repeated to be effective.
- Expanded STD treatment, which, as has been demonstrated in civilian populations, has an important impact on HIV transmission rates when strongly promoted and made widely available.
- Provision of counselling and voluntary testing services, with regular encouragement to the personnel to take advantage of these services. (In several cases, troops headed for overseas deployment may be strongly advised to undergo HIV testing, or obliged to do so by the country to which they are deployed.)

Approaches Addressing Underlying Vulnerability Factors

Besides measures aimed at changing risk behaviour in the short term, armed forces are implementing or experimenting with activities that address the underlying factors that help to the high vulnerability of military personnel. These include:

- *Changes to posting practices*, including an emphasis on maintaining family life. Instances comprise shortening tours of duty away from home, and finding ways of helping soldiers to bring their families with them if long-term postings are unavoidable. Botswana, for example, has begun to shorten the length of time between visits home for troops stationed at remote border posts.

- *Changes to military culture.* The risk-taking methods will probably always be a necessary part of the military mind, but the increasing complexity of war will need soldiers to calculate risks better than earlier and take increasing initiative for neutralizing or reducing their risk. This fits in with the messages of HIV/AIDS campaigns, which stress understanding risks and taking personal responsibility for both one's own health and that of others.
- *Changes to military attitudes towards civilian populations.* With more missions bringing soldiers into contact with civilian populations, especially foreign populations, soldiers are learning new skills for dealing with people - especially people in crisis such as refugees, war-ravaged populations, and disaster victims. Concerns for human rights and the development of codes of conduct are taking on ever greater significance. However, these can only work effectively if military attitudes to civilians place greater value on protection, providing security, communication, compassion and understanding. These qualities will also contribute to improve the military response to HIV/AIDS, both within the armed forces and in their relations with civilian groups.

Partnerships with the Civilian Sector

All HIV/AIDS prevention and care endeavour must recognize the constant interaction between the military and civilian populations. The traditional separation of the military medical services from civilian input has been counterproductive in several countries. AIDS prevention and care programmes in the armed forces will be less effective than if there is more active help between the Ministry of Defence and the Ministry of Health or other civilian health authorities.

One approach is to have full participation by adequate

defence and military officials as members of the civilian National AIDS Programme and its committees charged with planning and management. A second is to have health-system officials participate directly in training, prevention education and care for the military.

Acceptance and Care of HIV-Positive Military Staff

Given the high rates of HIV infection in several military forces, an increasing priority is the creation of a non-stigmatizing and non-discriminatory environment within the military population for those who are HIV-positive. This must start with full confidentiality for HIV testing. As they pursue their careers, HIV-positive individuals should be given every opportunity to carry out the tasks for which they have been trained and which they are still fit to perform. In the end, armed forces should prepare to provide care and support for those who live with HIV and AIDS, comprising continuity of care for them and their families as they return to civilian life. This may comprise provision for home-care services and support of widows and orphans in places where civilian social services are not adequate.

"AIDS in the military, as well as in the national environment, is no longer an academic issue; it is a reality that has to be tackled with all the vigour and effort that is commensurate with its ramifications"

- *Major General Matshwenyego Fisher, Chief of Staff, Botswana Defence Force.*

Why don't They Just Make All Personnel Take an HIV Test?

Mandatory testing for the military was first established in the USA in 1985. By 1995, in conformity with a survey carried out by UNAIDS and the Civil-Military Alliance to Combat HIV and AIDS, HIV testing was conducted in some form by 93 per cent of reporting militaries (58 of 62 countries responding to the question).

Some 43 of the reporting countries stated that they impose essential HIV testing in some situations: pre-recruitment (25 countries); before foreign deployment (24 countries); before separation from active duty (12 countries), periodically (9 countries); and before a new assignment (8 countries). Rejection of candidates for recruitment based on a positive HIV test is the rule for 45 of 54 respondents, while 44 out of 56 impose restriction of duties for those who are known to be HIV-positive (for instance, banning them from combat or from piloting aircraft). In the last, 37 of 41 respondents exclude HIV-positive personnel from overseas deployment.

Pressure to Test

Military authorities in several parts of the world are under considerable pressure to institute or maintain essential HIV testing, whether before recruitment, prior to foreign deployment, or at regular intervals. At the same time, this policy has been criticized from various points of view. It is argued that mandatory testing is a violation of individual rights that cannot be justified by military-specific postulates; that testing is not cost-effective. It is also argued that a positive test in an asymptomatic individual does not bear on that person's right to work or "fitness for work". Another argument is that a strongly promoted and fully financed voluntary testing programme would be as effective as essential testing and possibly more so.

The role of the soldier is a special one, and the debate over voluntary testing must take this into consideration. Military policy-makers must consider not only the postulations of combat but also the fact that soldiers cannot question superiors' orders the way most civilians can.

UNAIDS believes that voluntary testing accompanied by counselling has a potent role within a comprehensive range of measures for HIV/AIDS prevention and support. It also believes that essential testing without informed consent is a violation of human rights, and there is no evidence that it achieves public health goals. With a view to justify mandatory testing (with its inevitable invasion of privacy and differential or discriminatory treatment), military forces should have to:

- demonstrate compelling aspects of the military workplace that make it different from other workplaces;
- show that HIV/AIDS is not being singled out for such treatment as compared with likewise diseases that raise comparable issues; and/or
- show that mandatory testing and its results (rejection,

limitation on deployment, dismissal) is the least restrictive means available and actually achieves the objectives being sought; i.e., that mandatory testing *achieves goals more effectively* than voluntary testing, counselling and prevention programmes.

"The first reaction of many organizations - not just the military - is to test in order to keep people who are HIV-positive from being recruited. But the fact is that most infections occur after people have been recruited. So testing isn't the answer to everything. In fact, it's doubtful that involuntary testing is the answer to anything".

—*Peter Piot, Executive Director, UNAIDS*

Ten

Prisons and AIDS

At a Glance

HIV rates are high in various prison societies. Other diseases are also often much more prevalent in prisons than outside, comprising hepatitis B, hepatitis C and tuberculosis.

Prisons are not closed-off worlds. Prisoners - and others, comprising prison staff and visitors - move in and out every day. Several prisoners are in for only short sentences, and some spend several periods there, returning to the outside world each time after their release.

All feasible steps should be taken to prevent HIV transmission in prisons - for the sake not only of staff and prisoners, but of society in general.

General factors in prisons which can facilitate HIV spread comprise: overcrowding; a general climate of violence, tension and fear; lack of information about HIV; and lack of adequate health facilities.

Certain factors responsible for the transmission of HIV in prison settings comprise: injecting of drugs with shared, unsterilized needles and syringes; unprotected penetrative sex between men, and tattooing with shared, unsterilized equipment.

Particular responses to the challenges of drug injecting and sex between men include:

- demand reduction and treatment for drug-dependent prisoners, comprising substitution or maintenance therapy, (e.g., with methadone)
- making full-strength liquid bleach available for sterilizing needles and syringes comprising those used for tattooing, together with instructions as to its proper use
- providing sterile needles on an exchange basis - one clean needle for a used one

- introducing peer education among injecting prisoners, using former prisoners and former injectors
- providing discreet and easy access to condoms
- providing education on the risks of HIV transmission to prisoners and prison staff alike.

General responses that could help minimize HIV transmission comprise:

- ensuring that all prisoners have their fundamental rights to health care observed, care which should be comparable to what they would get outside
- ending overcrowding;
- finding ways to lessen the climate of violence.

An important structural change that would facilitate several of the specific responses is to have health in prisons transferred under the control of public health authorities.

Isolation of prisoners on the grounds of their HIV status does not generally help subside transmission of the virus.

UNAIDS Best Practice Materials

The Joint United Nations Programme on HIV/AIDS (UNAIDS) is preparing materials on subjects of importance to HIV infection and AIDS, the causes and results of the epidemic, and best practices in AIDS prevention, care and support. *A Best Practice* Collection on any one subject typically comprises a short publication for journalists and community leaders (Point of View); a technical summary of the issues, challenges and solutions (Technical Update); case studies from around the world (*Best Practice Case* Studies); a set of presentation graphics; and a listing of key materials (reports, articles, books, audiovisuals, etc.) on the subject. These documents are updated as necessary.

Technical Updates and standpoint are being published in English, French, Russian and Spanish. Single copies of *Best Practice* publications are available free from UNAIDS Information Centres. To find the closest one, visit UNAIDS on the Internet (http://www.unaids.org), contact UNAIDS by email (unaids@unaids.org) or telephone (+41 22 791 4661), or write to the UNAIDS Information Centre, 20 Avenue Appia, 1211 Geneva 27, Switzerland.

Journalists seeking more information about a UNAIDS Point of View are invited to contact the UNAIDS Geneva Press Information Office (+41 22 791 4577 or 791 3387).

Background

In several prisons across the world there is a much higher prevalence of HIV than there is in society outside. There is usually also a much higher rate of some other diseases, like hepatitis B and C, syphilis and tuberculosis. Experiences have shown that there is a lot that can be done to check the spread of HIV, but for that to occur, those liable for the prison system must first identify certain risk factors and forms of behaviour in prisons.

Several of those who are HIV-positive in prison were already infected on the outside. Many come from parts of the population that carry a heavier than average burden of HIV infections. Additionally, many of those in prison are there because of drug use or trafficking, and they will try to continue drug use inside. Whether the authorities accept it or not - and however much they may try to repress it - drugs are introduced and consumed by prison inmates in various countries, and men commonly have sex with men in all-male prisons. Denying or ignoring these facts will not help solve the problem of the increasing spread of HIV - and both forms of behaviour are HIV transmission risks.

There has been a slow growth across the world of co-morbidity in prisons - that is, increasing numbers of prisoners with a combination of diseases like, typically, tuberculosis plus hepatitis C plus HIV. As in general populations, there has also been an increase in the incidence of multi-drug resistant tuberculosis.

Prisoners are generally in a highly vulnerable position — vulnerable to the power of prison authorities (as well as others in authority with whom they may come into contact, like the police), and vulnerable to the sexual and other demands of fellow prisoners, several of whom are violent by nature. Prisons are generally overcrowded, and operate in an ethos of punishment and of violence, and sometimes of systems of enslavement within prison hierarchies.

Prison officers are also open to infection with HIV. They risk infection, for example, by accidentally being pricked by a drug-injection needle while making routine searches of prisoners' beds and lockers. They can also be exposed to HIV through sexual contact with prisoners.

The high prevalence rates of HIV, tuberculosis and hepatitis in prisons should be of the greatest cause of concern to the community at large. The prison population, after all, is a fluid one, with people continuously moving in and out. Most prisoners are released into the community at some point, and some are imprisoned and released a number of times. For reasons of self-interest alone, if no other reason, the community and its leaders should react quickly and wisely to the problem of HIV in prisons.

There is much that can be done to reduce the increasingly spread of HIV in prisons, as several types of intervention around the world in the past decade have shown. As in other spheres of society where the spread of HIV is concerned, it is important, first of all, to end denial about what is going on - in this case, drug injecting and sexual contact. Then people should be given the important information, education and resources to avoid infection. In the case of prison populations one is starting at benefit here. The fact that prisoners are a "captive"" community generates an unusual opportunity for easy access to them, for the purposes of providing them with education and the important materials for HIV prevention.

THE CHALLENGES

The Phenomenon of Injecting

Drugs are commonplace in various prisons, since a number of prisoners come in with their drug habits already established, and they are generally successful in finding a way to continue drug use on the inside. Injecting is generally the preferred mode of consumption. Those who inject drugs almost always share needles and syringes, whereas a needle and syringe might be able to be smuggled into the prison, they cannot so easily be smuggled out again or thrown away. Sometimes, the equipment is even home-made, like needles from converted ball-point pens. In a normal prison setting, injecting equipment can rarely be sterilized properly; water on its own is not enough.

Sharing of injecting equipment is a very proper route of transmission for HIV - much more so than sexual contact. A recent survey in a women's prison in Lower Saxony in Germany exhibited that about a third of those sampled were injecting drug users. Of the women injecting, 4.9 per cent of them were HIV positive, as against 0.5 per cent for the non-injecting women. Much higher HIV rates among injectors in some other prison populations have been recorded.

(For those prisoners who are addicted, the availability of therapy comprising substitution or maintenance therapy) is generally non-existent or minimal. For those on treatment before entering prison, even continuation of the treatment may be refused.

Sex in Prisons

Sexual contact between men is common in male prisons around the world. Estimates differ considerably. A 1993 survey conducted in Rio de Janeiro, Brazil, suggested that 73 per cent of male prisoners had sex with other men in prison, while recent surveys in Zambia, Australia and Canada have come up with figures of between 6 per cent and 12 per cent. The sex may be consensual, but may also be forced, to a greater or lesser degree. Rape also exists. In some prisons rape is a "usual" event - sometimes as a kind of institutionalized initiation, where it can take the form of gang rape.

Several inmates are in prison for violent crimes. Some are mentally unstable. In the tense and claustrophobic atmosphere of prisons, with their own rules, hierarchies, alliances and enmities among the prisoners, attacks on prisoners - comprising sexual ones can easily occur.

The sex that takes place between men in prisons comprises anal sex; this may be more or less common, according to the particular place. Unprotected anal sex is a high-risk factor for transmission of HIV. The risk is even higher if lubrication is not used, and if the sex is forced, as in the case of rape. Condoms are not as per rule available in prisons.

In women's prisons where there are male prison staff, sex between men and women may also take place.

The Hindelbank Experiment: Access to Sterile Injection Equipment

A one-year experiment to provide sterile needles was launched at Hindelbank women's prison, in Switzerland, in June 1994. A year later, following the success of the project, it was decided to continue it.

The prison holds up to 100 women, in six wings, with most of the prisoners serving sentences for drug offences. In the project, dispensing machines were established in various accessible locations (showers, toilets, storage areas) to provide sterile needles. Prisoners were permitted to keep one (but no more than one) piece of injecting equipment, and only in a particularly designated cabinet.

The evaluation at the end of the first year of the project's operation exhibited that there had been no new cases of HIV or hepatitis in the prison and that the prisoners' health had improved. Furthermore, considerable decrease in needle sharing was observed, there was no evident increase in drug consumption, and needles had not been used as weapons.

Tattooing

Tattooing is common in prisons. Needles or tattoo guns for the purpose are repeatedly shared, creating a risk of HIV transmission. "Blood brother" initiation rites are also high-risk activities.

Lack of Information, and Testing Without Consent

There is little effort in most prison societies to educate prisoners about the risks of HIV. Testing for HIV among prison populations occurs in few countries, but frequently without informed consent being obtained.

Minimal Health Care

Health care for prisoners with HIV or AIDS is often non-existent or minimal, in comparison to what would be available outside.

Sometimes, the authorities realise that isolating prisoners with HIV or AIDS is the answer to stopping the spread of HIV in prisons.

A Denial of the Facts of Prison Life

Drugs of the sort that are injected recreationally are illegal in most of the countries. In some societies, for men to have sex with other men is illegal, or is criticised by sections of cultural or religious opinion. However, even in countries without inhibitions on sex between men in the community at large, such behaviour within prisons is repeatedly outlawed.

This strict illegality of various forms of behaviour in prison results in a denial that the activities take place and a great difficulty in even starting to discuss ways to overcome the problems.

The Responses

The legal and political authorities in some societies, and the mass of social, cultural and religious opinion, may be unable to bring themselves to accept particular forms of behaviour (whether in prison or outside), comprising sexual behaviour and drug injecting. But instead of pretending that the behaviour (and hence the spread of HIV) doesn't exist, it would be more productive for them to accept tacitly that the behaviour exists while tacitly permitting an adequate and effective response with a low visibility.

To make it easier for them to respond, the authorities might choose to consider some of their interventions against HIV in prisons as experimental. If successful (and some responses to date have really proved successful), the experimental period can be extended indefinitely.

Interventions for Injecting Drug Use

With the spread of HIV in various prisons fuelled by the sharing of injecting equipment, a strong response is called for. Banning drugs (in theory, this is the policy in just about every prison) has always failed. There are a kind of other feasible options, some of which are being tried. None are necessarily easy ones, and there are often problems - both practical and ethical - that require to be addressed.

- Provide demand-reduction measures and offer treatment for drug-dependent prisoners. It is potent to provide substitution therapy - e.g., with methadone -

for prisoners who wish to begin it or continue substitution started on the outside. Offering treatment to reduce demand or to help break addiction is another important measure.

- Provide full-strength liquid bleach for prisoners, together with instructions on how to sterilize needles and syringes. This has successfully been done in many prisons (comprising several in Europe and Australia, in some African countries and at least one Central American country) and trials are continuing in other prisons. Some people fear that the bleach could be misused, for attacks on prison staff or other prisoners or in suicide attempts. This has not occurred in any prison where bleach distribution has been tried.
- Provide free sterile needles and syringes, one an exchange ground (the prisoner receives a new needle for a used one). The first prison in the world to have a needle-exchange programme was Oberschongrun maximum security prison for men in Switzerland, in an unofficial scheme in 1993. This approach was then officially attempted and scientifically tested a year later in Hindelbank prison, also in Switzerland. It proven highly successful and the idea has since been launched in other prisons, comprising two in Germany. Under these schemes, the possession of drugs can still be considered illegal, but possession of a single needle is simply neglected and not treated as grounds for disciplinary action or for urine analysis.
- Enable peer education on HIV and drug-injecting to find place among prisoners who use drugs. This can also take the form of outreach work undertaken by former prisoners who are themselves injectors or former injectors. This response can help promote participation in drug cessation programmes among prisoners, or else - if they stress on continuing to inject - enable them to do so in a safe way, with the correct use of bleach or with needle and syringe exchange.

Protect Prisoners who have Sex in Prison

Provide condoms together with lubricant for prisoners in male prisons - either from dispensing machines, or, possibly better and more discreetly, in private from medical officers. This is now being done in more and more countries.

In women's prisons where there are male prison staff, both staff and prisoners should be given knowledge about the risks of unprotected heterosexual intercourse.

Reduce the Atmosphere of Violence

Find ways of preventing violent attacks on prisoners, comprising sexual abuse and rape. Condoms are not going to be of any use in this case. Prison staff should be trained to get rid of unnecessary force or brutality, and to respect the rights, dignity and well-being of prisoners.

End Overcrowding

Several prisons are hugely overcrowded. In the United States, for example, the prison population roughly doubled in the ten years up to 1995. The role that prison overcrowding plays in poor hygienic conditions, transmission of diseases and an increase of tensions, comprising sexual tensions, must be recognized.

Make Tattooing Safe

Much tattooing goes in prisons, often more than drug injecting, and repeatedly tattooing equipment is shared. It is important that liquid bleach should be supplied to sterilize equipment. Because tattooing is usually regarded by the authorities as an acknowledgeable activity (and many prison officers are themselves tattooed), there should be less opposition to the use of bleach for this objective. This in itself can provide a convenient means of introducing bleach to sterilize injecting equipment, particularly once it has been shown that the bleach is not used as a weapon. In any case, bleach is generally already present, unnoticed almost, in prisons, as an ordinary means of cleaning toilets and other areas.

Uphold the Human Right to Health Care

Basic human rights should be respected, comprising the right to health care. Prisoners have a right to the basic standard of health care that is available outside the prison. Informed consent should always be received before any testing for HIV takes place.

Supply Information

Education and information on HIV/AIDS should be supplied to all prison staff and prisoners.

No Isolation of Prisoners on Grounds of HIV Status

Isolating prisoners, or grouping prisoners in a special prison wing, if these are to be carried out, should be done without any reference to a prisoner's HIV status.

Put Prison Health Under the Control of Health Authorities

Experience in a range of prison systems has shown that health care in prisons can be delivered more properly by public health authorities than by prison management. This has the advantage, too, of strengthening the link between health comprising health education and counselling) in the community and health in prisons. Countries that have introduced this policy comprise Norway, which has operated it for some time, and France, which transferred control over prison health to its health ministry in 1994. Conditions in one of France's prisons, Les Baumettes in Marseilles, have reportedly improved significantly since the new policy was introduced.

Key Materials

World Health Organization (WHO) guidelines on HIV infection and AIDS in prisons. Geneva: 1993 (WHO/GPA/DIR/93.3). *10-page article written from public health perspective, proposes standards for prison authorities in efforts to prevent HIV transmission and provide care to those with HIV/AIDS in prisons.*

Joint United Nations Programme on HIV/AIDS (UNAIDS). HIV/AIDS in prisons. Statement to the fifty-second session of the United Nations Commission on Human Rights, Geneva, April 1996. Geneva: 1996. *2-page overview of basic human rights of prisoners with regard to AIDS, including access to education on HIV, access to health care and HIV prevention, and the right of security of person.*

Jurgens R. HIV/AIDS in prisons: final report. Montreal: Canadian HIV/AIDS Legal Network and Canadian AIDS Society. 1996 Sept. Comprehensive 150-page report *summarizing the history of HIV in prisons worldwide. Gives detailed analysis of practical, ethical and legal issues, particularly in the Canadian prison system.*

Kingma S.J., HIV/AIDS in prisons: emerging moral and legal dilemmas. Geneva: Joint United Nations Programme on HIV/AIDS (UNAIDS). Unpublished. Presented to the meeting of the Health in Prisons Network, Lisbon, 1996 Oct. 3-page speech advocating *HIV/AIDS prevention programmes in prisons. Gives overview of the legal and moral issues.*

AIDS & SOCIETY, International Research and Policy Bulletin Special Issue: AIDS in prisons. 6:3. 1995 Mar/Apr. 12-page issue. *Commentary on AIDS and criminal justice, short articles on global situation, China's approach to HIV control, AIDS education and New York police, updates on Canada, Scotland and Australia.*

Eleven

Brothel and Street-based Sex Workers in Bangladesh

BACKGROUND

Tangail Brothel

Bangladesh has had brothels for centuries that have steadily become part of the local culture. Some are residential, comparatively uncrowded, with small rooms rented to individual women. Others are crowded, with several small rooms housing three or more women together. Although not technically legal, brothel prostitution is regulated by the local authorities in Bangladesh. Sex work has been declared a blacklisted trade, and sex workers are highly denigrated by most members of society. Police exercise a degree of regulatory power, and for a fee varies from 5,000 to 15,000 taka (US$ 1 = 50 taka), place an affidavit with the court when a woman enters a brothel. This enables her to avoid arrest when working in the brothel. This system is supposed to make sure that only interested women who are at least 18 years old enter the brothels. The system is ambiguous and recognizes prostitution, but does not make it legal. At Tangail, the police, landowners, house owners and/or *bariwalli* (residential landladies), madams, *sardanis* (senior madams), and *mastans* or hoodlums related to local political parties, really run the establishment, which has a regulating body called the Shamaj. Although most of the women are "independent" operators, about 60 per cent of their income goes to the aforementioned authorities. A minority of newcomers, called *chhukris* (19 per cent), were completely under the control of senior sex workers or *sardanis*, and made to work for at least 6 months to pay them off, i.e., 100 per cent of their income was paid to their controllers.

At the time of the baseline survey, the average age of the women was 24 and 86 per cent were illiterate. Almost all (97 per cent) were Muslim and are engaged in the sex trade for an average of 7 years. Most (62 per cent) had long-term clients or lovers, whom they call *bhalobashai lokh* (literally, good home men), with whom they formed a marriage-like relationship. At the time the *lokh* are present, their women do not take clients. Some women have permanent relationships and give up taking clients altogether, but continue to live at the brothel. Some women are the children of sex workers and were raised in brothels, and in turn, several raise their own children at the brothel. Several send money to their mothers and other relatives. Tangail sex workers were not permitted to leave the brothel at will, and when out, could not wear any shoes or slippers; if they did, they would be fined by the police. This imposition on their rights was supposed to make sure they would not sell sex outside of the brothel. Their children were unable to register for school since they could not name their fathers.

Although violence has not been a big problem at Tangail, sex workers are heavily stigmatized by the surrounding community. Police exercise a greater control. Sex workers are made to pay extra money to the police if they take a client for the whole night. Consequently, some women have all-night clients. Most of the time at the brothel there is a very peaceful and sociable atmosphere, with open courtyards where women, children, lovers and friends gather. This isolated and controlled environment has afforded particular advantages for the SHAKTI project. However, it is not typical of all Bangladeshi brothels, is not stable, and it certainly is not an environment in which sex workers have sufficient control of their own lives and bodies. Pressure to earn for themselves, their families and their controllers, while facing eviction and forced rehabilitation at any time, makes safer sex a difficult objective to achieve. Their lives and livelihoods are literally at the mercy of political forces well beyond their control.

Street Sex Work in Dhaka

Street sex workers are the most visible of the various types of sex workers. In Dhaka, they are unique, found in most areas of the city, parks, railway stations, bus and truck stops, cinemas, markets and shrines. Several other sex workers operate in Dhaka as well, mostly out of hotels and residences that pose as normal family homes. It is well known that several university students, married women from middle-class families and others supplement their incomes through the sex trade. These women do not stand in public places, however, to get their clients, but instead have agents to bring clients to them or make appointments for them to go to particular sites. Public soliciting to sell sex is strictly against the law. Street-based sex workers include the lowest class of sex workers and, as such, are far more subject to violence perpetrated by clients, *mastans* and police. The police are often paid off to allow them their right to work, with sex and/or money. Territoriality is also evident, with some *mastans* or pimps fighting for particular spaces in which the women associated with them can work. Most street sex workers are independent, in the sense that they decide to work or not, as they require. A minority is bonded to a *dalal* or pimp, but a number of make use of local men on the streets, e.g., rickshaw pullers, hotel boys, guards, tea-shop owners, and others, to find them clients and then pay them with cash or sex for doing so. Additionally, some women have men who serve as their protectors; they may find them clients and, when required, help them avoid the police or stand as their husbands to want their release from police custody. Some sex workers even have "station husbands", special policemen who look after them in exchange for sex.

Street sex work must be seen as one of the more cheap street-based occupations in Dhaka, a crowded city of 10 million people. Male and transgender (*hijra*) sex workers also operate in several of the same contact venues as do the female sex workers. Generally, it seems the females have the greatest client numbers, *hijras* next, and males following. Besides thousands of paper pickers, beggars, sellers of flowers, tea, candies, fruits, or magazines, the streets are the home to many thousands of homeless individuals, both single adults and children and whole families. Some have plastic-covered "humpies' to sleep and cook in, others do not. Slums are packed with people and regulated by local politicians and their mastan gangs. From time to time, the police are instructed to clean up the streets and hundreds of women, sex workers and others, are arrested and placed in vagrancy homes, where their treatment is generally abusive. Less often, but more dramatically, instructions are given to the army to clean out slums, either by fire or bulldozer. When this happens, or when a severe flood drives thousands of people to Dhaka from hopeless rural areas, street sex work increases. Near about half of the people in Dhaka live on little over US$ 1 per day. The situation is very dynamic and unstable, creating an extremely challenging environment in which to carry out a sex worker HIV intervention.

Relevance

Many Bangladeshis consider their society to be sexually conservative. Probably for that reason, among others, most AIDS prevention messages have focused on the danger of going to prostitutes. The number of sex workers in brothels has variously been estimated as 10,000 to 100,000. The National Behavioural Surveillance of 1998, however, surveyed all brothels and found a total of only 6,584. Floating sex workers, male, female and transgender, are now thought to total up to 100,000 in the country as a whole. One survey has given a national estimate of 12,000 *hijras* with 2000 in Dhaka, most of whom also sell sex. Many early endeavours at research conducted with female sex workers demonstrated feeble knowledge of STDs and inadequate utilization of health services. These studies documented their social isolation and extreme marginalization. CARE is an organization devoted to working with the poorest and most marginalized members of society. Therefore, the project was seen as useful to both the requirements of poor, highly vulnerable women and the principles of CARE.

FORMATIVE STAGES

Brothel Baseline Studies

Tangail sex workers were distrustful when first approached by CARE, as other NGOs had come, promised different services, but were never seen again. CARE personnel, on the other hand, had never handled a sex worker project and were not certain and nervous in dealing with highly socially stigmatized women. After the starting phase of site selection during the first half of 1996, the project undertook, with the aid of external consultants, different types of formative research, comprising a qualitative assessment, a quantitative baseline study on behaviour and knowledge, and an STD survey. The total set-up phase covered one year, during which advocacy with those in the power structures and rapport building with the sex workers were able to proceed. A two-room set clinic, with nurse and physician, was established at the brothel on land donated by the Shamaj. Here STDs were treated, as were other sicknesses. Confidentiality was maintained on all records. Those who volunteered for the baseline STD survey were given a standardized clinical examination (n=296) and tested for HIV, syphilis, gonorrhoea and chlamydia. PCR techniques were available for gonorrhoea and chlamydia tests through collaborators in England, while the HIV and syphilis tests were undertaken at a government facility and later repeated at the national surveillance laboratories. For the purpose of blood sampling, the survey recruited 466 sex workers out of probable 593. The samples for HIV tests were unlinked to identifying information. Verbal consent was needed and cooperative sex workers helped secure the cooperation of others by showing them how the examination would be performed, utilizing a speculum and a medical school anatomical model. Women with symptoms were treated.

Important issues were revealed as a result of the formative research, some of which the project has been able to handle while others are unsolved. First, the levels of clinical signs of reproductive tract infections were high, with 63 per cent of the examined women having cervical discharge and 32 per cent having vaginal discharge. A further 2 per cent had ulcers, 6 per cent warts, and 26 per cent had lower abdominal pain. Laboratory tests confirmed somewhat lower rates, with 19 per cent positive by PCR for chlamydia, 20 per cent for gonorrhoea, and 18 per cent for a current syphilis infection (RPRD 1:8 and TPHA+). No woman had a positive HIV test. Tests were not conducted for other feasible causes of discharge or abdominal pain. The disparity between syndromic clinical diagnosis/treatment and the laboratory confirmatory tests revealed that the standard syndromic management strategy would only correctly recognize about half (45 per cent) of women with chlamydia or gonorrhoea as the others were asymptomatic. In addition, one-third would be overtreated since they would receive treatment for pathogens they did not have. Nonetheless, without proper treatment or screening strategies, the brothel clinic has had no alternate but to follow standard syndromic management guidelines. This issue is problematic for sex worker projects in most countries.

One aim of the project has been to reduce the time gap between when symptoms are recognized and when care is sought. Generally, the women did not desire to acknowledge current STD symptoms for fear of losing clients. At baseline, women with symptoms waited an average of 7 days before seeking treatment beyond their own home remedies. When they did want help, it was from paramedics, traditional healers, and medicine sellers, some of whom do not have safe injecting practices.

The project intends to improving levels of condom use. At baseline, only 3 per cent of women were using condoms for all instances of vaginal intercourse in the last 24 hours. Both oral sex and anal intercourse were reported as rare, but were perhaps under reported due to their shameful connotation. In the baseline survey, the women had an average of 3.5 clients per day; besides they had intercourse, on average, once a day with their lovers. Various barriers to increased condom use existed. First, the women saw condoms as a family planing device, and 45 per cent had already followed a mode of contraception. Others either sought a pregnancy or relied on menstrual regulation (legal in Bangladesh) or illegal induced abortion. At Tangail, 29.7 per cent of the women had never been pregnant and, to those who wanted children, infertility stood as problem. Second, 62 per cent of the women had lovers. While most of them did not live under the same roof with their private partners all the time, the position of the lover was like a husband and they saw no requirement to use condoms in their private relationships. Third, their clients did not like to use condoms. The sex workers feared that if they asked these men to use condoms, the clients would think that the sex workers were infected with a disease.

Street-based Sex Worker Baseline Studies

In late 1996 work started among street-based sex workers in Dhaka and by mid-1997, a baseline study was undertaken, with a capture-recapture component to estimate the population size. The capture-recapture method yielded an estimate of 4366 street-based female sex workers found within a two-week period. Many lived in slums (37 per cent) while others were homeless (30 per cent). Still others came into Dhaka to work from adjacent areas, often during the day only. More than half (60 per cent) were divorced or separated, while 21 per cent were currently married. Most of these women (80 per cent) had worked in other low-paying occupations, like in garment factories, as domestic servants in hotels or restaurants; 20 per cent had been in brothels. The average time they had spent in sex work was 3.5 years.

The STD study among these women disclosed much higher levels of prevalence than among those in the brothel. In a sample of 247 tested in the same way as the brothel sample, 48 per cent had chlamydia, 53 per cent gonorrhoea, and 31 per cent had current syphilis infections. None had HIV. Almost all (90 per cent) reported STD symptoms and on examination, 69 per cent had vaginal discharge, 62 per cent cervical discharge and 11 per cent had genital ulcers. In the previous three months only 54 per cent of those with symptoms wanted any treatment at all, mostly from medicine sellers. Most think that STDs were avoided by staying clean.

Some of the women were using condoms, mostly for prevention of pregnancy. They reported an average of 3.5 clients in the last 24 hours and only 14 per cent used condoms for more than half of all intercourse in the last 24 hours. Only 10 per cent had used condoms for all intercourse during the last 24 hours, but overall coverage was 18 per cent of all vaginal and anal sexual intercourse with any partner the previous day. Ten per cent of the women were pregnant while working.

IMPLEMENTATION

Working Strategies

The SHAKTI project has had four major working strategies. These are:

- to raise awareness
- to have repeated contact of high quality with sex workers
- to give the means of behaviour change (condoms and STD treatment)
- to create an enabling environment

This approach need mobilizing support from the power structures surrounding the brothel, i.e., the local administration, the police, local opinion leaders, clients that could be reached. The project design did not comprise training in negotiation of condom use, creative modes of safer sex or intensive work with client groups. It never anticipated the requirement for a strong advocacy component, and skills in this connection were not developed. As the project proceeded and events unfolded, new strategies were formed.

Peer Education

Peer education has been the main approach utilized by the project. This started in August 1996 in the brothel and in 1997 among the street women. After the mid-term review in 1998, the manner of handling peer education was changed in the direction of greater sex worker management of the project. During the first few years, about 50 peer educators were trained in the brothel, with 28 actively working (a ratio of 1 to 20 sex workers). They were each assigned zones in the brothel. A zone was made up of 10-14 apartments. Peer educators got 50 taka per day and worked a half-day, once per week. Their tasks were to visit the women in their assigned zones, discuss safe sex, HIV knowledge and STD treatment, and ask about condom use in the last 24 hours. They also collected the condom package covers. Rubbish bins for condom disposal were first placed in strategic locations, but later in each room. Used condoms in the bins were counted, but somewhat not regularly. These data were recorded with colour codes on a monitoring map, zone and room, wise by the peer educators. Then, the results were summarized on a monitoring board in the brothel. The process of peer education approached about 70 per cent of the women. The remaining 30 per cent were resistant. As these sex workers were not monitored, they were not comprised in the number who were using condoms at the first follow-up survey.

On the streets of Dhaka, drop-in centres were setup, a few at first, then more, and by the end of 1999 there were 8 drop-in centres at which women could rest, bathe and access STD treatment, as well as simple general health care. Peer educators were paid when they were at the brothel and assigned spots around the city at which about 35-40 sex workers could be reached per peer educator.

The trainers of peer educators, called field trainers, wore white laboratory coats and a badge around the brothel, while the peer educators themselves wore a badge and blue apron when working. This applied to the street-based peer educators as well and was copied from the Sonagachi project in Kolkata. The field trainers felt they needed these uniforms to distinguish themselves from sex workers, so that clients would not approach them for sex. While the peer educators have enjoyed the status these uniforms give them, the uniform marked them as somehow different and distinct from the other sex workers. The peer educators in both arms of the intervention were privileged with more attention, small amounts of cash and other rewards, such as lessons in literacy. A number of made repeated trips overseas and were often asked to represent the project at many AIDS meetings. Jealousy among the non-peer educator sex workers started to grow. The first step taken to address this was to drop the use of the blue uniform at the brothel. On the streets, the women were able to use the status symbolized by the uniform to protect themselves from police arrest and did not want to give it up. Gradually these markers have been removed and well-trained peer educators were elevated to outreach workers and given small daily payments, while a new cadre of volunteer, unpaid peer educators was developed.

By mid-1999, 55 outreach workers and 171 volunteer peer educators were working on the streets of Dhaka. These women approached about 3,200 sex workers on a regular basis for both group and individual discussions. Additionally, 6 *hijra* peer educators and 3 outreach workers were trained and through them at least 100 *hijras* are reached regularly. At the brothel, 21 outreach workers, 102 peer educators as well as 29 peer lover educators were trained and continue to work under the new scheme. The number of CARE staff at the brothel was drastically curtailed from 14 to 5 with the intention of decreasing reliance on CARE staff and increasing sex worker management of the project.

Health Care

The brothel clinic was staffed by a female doctor and two nurses, one male and one female. Although the doctor was committed to helping the sex workers, she had no specific training in STD management. In early 1999 she carried out short training with a clinic group in Dhaka and later in the year went abroad for a clinical training course.

The clinic is open 5 days a week in the morning from 9:00 to 13:00. The women were independent to bring their family members for any illness. STD drugs were given free, but drugs for other illnesses were bought elsewhere, with prescription given by the clinic. Immunizations were given to children by the government health service and special immunization campaign days were organized. Clients did not have access to the clinic, but the project opened the clinic in the evenings to the sex workers' lovers. Ultimately, technical support for clinic supervision was accessed through a partner clinical NGO. Sustainability of the brothel clinic is a greater concern for the sex workers. Through a workshop, the district health administration assured them that, if needed, they would assign a doctor to the brothel on a routine ground. Plans have been made to equip the sex workers with skills important to manage their own clinic, including an insurance scheme to cover costs.

Medicine sellers, whom the women generally consult, were given four training sessions on HIV and STD recognition and treatment, but need considerably more attention. They are known to give unnecessary intravenous injections of saline or other fluids.

In Dhaka, CARE's partner, the Marie Stopes Clinic Society, supplied services for the drop-in centres from the earliest days of the intervention. Problems arose repeatedly with regard to the way in which the clinic doctors treated the sex workers. Some covered their mouths when they addressed the women; others were curt and obviously not willing to touch them. The sex workers were very vulnerable to these slights and often complained. In addition, the clinic hoped to regain some of the cost of medicine, but it soon became explicit that many women were too poor to be able to pay the fees. Repeated meetings with the Marie Stopes directors gradually led to an intensive understanding of the needs of these women. The fee schedule was changed so that women now pay only 10 taka to gain a clinic membership card and all other treatment costs are free. As the street-based sex worker organization gained strength, it has been able to address the doctors more directly and this has helped improve doctor-patient interactions. Now several of the clinic activities are run by the sex workers themselves.

Empowerment: in the Brothel

The baseline survey recognized a number of concerns of the brothel sex workers and the project has endeavoured to address these. They were:

- economic stability and savings
- education, literacy
- medical services
- freedom of movement outside the brothel
- welfare of children
- social acceptance, including burial in Muslim cemeteries

Economic stability has not been addressed directly. Outreach workers are paid a small amount and have voluntarily chosen not to take clients for the few hours per day that they work as educators. For various reasons, in 1998 Tangail sex workers claimed that the number of clients had dropped. It was suspected that the high visibility SHAKTI brought the brothel, and the big number of visitors (nearly 200 in 1997) who desired to see the intervention, may have contributed to a decreased number of clients. Project management stopped all irrelevant visiting, and from mid- 1998 to mid- 1999 the brothel was visited only 17 times by outsiders.

Skills training in alternative modes of supplementing income started in February 1998. Various associated local NGOs began to provide training in embroidery and sewing to 20 women, with an intention to the sale of goods produced by the women. Such activities like sewing, however, cannot be expected to replace or even supplement a sex worker's income and most of the women are not very interested in this approach.

Several women had hired private tutors before coming to SHAKTI. Literacy and education are highly appreciated. Early in the project SHAKTI started a programme of literacy with the peer educators. Forty women attended but 12 dropped out. Literate peer educators started teaching literacy to 60 other sex workers, but the women lost interest following the inappropriate nature of the curriculum. A new curriculum was developed through consultation with 8 literate sex workers and several project staff, and now comprises issues like women's rights. A sub-contract was signed with a local NGO to run the education programme as of October 1999. Most importantly, literacy education was made available to all the sex workers and not just the peer educators.

The *sardanis, bariwallis,* and police exercise important control over the sex workers, especially over the *chhukris*. Independent sex workers are supposed to ask permission to leave the brothel and not to wear shoes or sandals. *Chhukris* are never permitted to leave until their period of indenture is completed. *Chhukris* are also not permitted to have lovers as such an attachment would diminish the number of clients they would be willing to take. Gradually, the peer educators (who are not *chhukris*) gained more freedom to wear shoes out of the brothel. In the early days of the project, continuous meetings were held with the gatekeepers of the brothel and efforts were made to encourage them to alter some of their practices. In a few instances, for instance on World AIDS Day, many women appeared in public wearing shoes.

The project started with a conflict resolution model (as opposed to one that focuses on the rights of sex workers) to convince those in the surrounding community, (e.g. religious and political leaders) that it was not encouraging illicit sex, only endeavouring to increase its safety. Numerous formal and informal meetings were held with these groups. This process was also monitored with indicators and a quarterly assessment. For the first few years, the project carefully avoided taking a strong stand in support of the sex workers. In 1996, sex workers were blocked by the local administration from taking participation in World AIDS Day activities. Protests were not lodged, but the next year, without confrontation, they simply seemed in the activities and nothing was said. Since considerable fear still exists that the police, local politicians or fundamentalist groups will close the brothel if the women offend local society, progress has been slow in transforming the social climate around the brothel.

After the mid-term review disclosed continuing disagreements about condom use among the women, meetings were organized at which the women were asked what they could agree upon. They all stated they wanted to wear shoes out of the brothel, but the *sardanis* did not like this. Although it changed the non-confrontational stance SHAKTI had taken previously, the women were advised to go out in groups of five with shoes but without make-up, to report what happened to the *sardanis*, and to wait a some days to see if the police came to threaten the *sardanis* or them. Within a few months, over 200 women had gone out of the brothel with shoes without any mishap and ultimately all have done so. Now they state they never percepted that the proscription against shoes was not a real law, but was only in their minds. Staff members had known there was no legal aspect to the taboo, but had never considered it wise to tell the women, lest they offend the local society.

In India and Bangladesh, children are a bigger issue in brothels. Women want their own or adopted children, partly to make sure an income when aged as well as to satisfy their own emotional needs for nurturing and attachment. Few sex workers have been able to educate their children by sending them away from the brothel, but most of them are unable to do this. SHAKTI has started coordination with another NGO to give a non-formal elementary school for brothel children. Currently about 45 children are enrolled. The partner NGO has purchased land on which it expects to build a training centre for the brothel children.

Various events have taken place in which selected peer educators have made public presentations about the project, both in Bangladesh and in other nations. A number of sex workers attended the Fourth International Asia-Pacific AIDS Conference in Manila in 1997 and the Twelfth World AIDS Conference in Geneva in 1998. Both sex workers and brothel keepers (owners and *sardanis*) participated the First National Sex Workers Conference of India in November, 1997 and the First Meeting of the Asia-Pacific Network of Sex Workers in March 1998. On other occasions, sex workers from Tangail have participated meetings with sex workers organizations in Kolkata, and Kolkata women have visited Tangail. Picnics, parties and other gatherings held by CARE for sex workers and CARE staff are other examples in which sex workers are given a small opportunity to percept less stigmatized. These are, however, inadequate to meet the requirements of all the women in the brothel and much larger structural changes to community attitudes and control will be needed before a sex worker in Bangladesh could feel equal to any other woman.

A small committee of sex workers, known as *Mukti Shangho* (Freedom Committee), was formed. The spirit of full participation, however, was compromised by the appointment of its leader by CARE personnel. Ultimately, it became clear that the committee was stagnant and unsupported by the sex workers. It was modified, renamed *Nari Mukti Shango* (Women's Freedom Committee), the sex workers elected the woman they wanted as leader and the organization initiated, the process of becoming formally registered as a social welfare organization. The committee collects 50 taka as a monthly subscription from its growing membership, gets 10 taka from each woman who registers at the clinic (donated by the partner NGO which supervises the clinic) and makes a small benefit on condom sales. Meetings are called regularly at which sex workers can take participation in making decisions about matters important to their lives. Leadership, however, continues to be problematic as the woman elected was later arrested and sent to jail. As the brothels of Bangladesh are nodes of political conflict and local politics can easily turn violent, growth of the self-run sex worker organization continues to be erratic. As of November 1999, membership stood at 230.

Empowerment: On the Streets of Dhaka

A lot of the problems of street-based sex workers were rather different from those of the brothel women. A number had no place to bathe, wash their clothes or even to sleep; others expressed that their greatest problem was police harassment. The obstacles to becoming skilled in practising safer sex included high levels of mobility, serious repeated legal problems, moving in and out of the trade, a large influx of new women, considerable levels of violence, as well as concerns for their children, health care, income stability and safety. Their social status is at least as low as the brothel women, if not lower, and their self-respect reflects their stigmatization. However, those who survive beyond some years on the streets are tough and smart. They are not threatened by *sardanis* and all-encompassing power structures, as several are in the brothels. These women took the lead and in early 1998 formed the first street sex worker organization, *Durjoy Nari Shangho* ("Undefeatable Women's Club"). They started to mobilize street workers, particularly in a local fight to re-open a previously closed brothel in Dhaka City. From the starting they saw their purpose as one of creating a collectivity strong enough to demand their rights. These comprise legal rights, burial rights, rights to shelter, education for their children, rights to safety from violence, mainly at the hands of the state, and the right to make a living. Gradually *Durjoy* formed 6 area committees with representation to a central one. They started registering their organization as a social welfare group. They opened a bank account into which they deposit the 50 taka collected as membership dues per month. They distributed food, water and medicine during Dhaka's severe flood of 1998, to sex workers and their families, as these women found it very difficult accessing relief goods at the regular sites. With the selling of condoms, the organization also get some earnings. By November 1999, membership had increased to 950 women. Sex workers manage several of the drop-in centres that can now provide space for some women to sleep, rest and bathe, as well as to undertake particular types of training. Both street and brothel sex workers have got some basic training in their legal rights, and many dozen street workers have got training in the martial arts as well.

A Turning Point

A crucial event occurred in July 1999 that galvanized street and brothel sex workers alike, and also shifted the stance of the SHAKTI project. A young sex worker named Jesmin at Tan Bazar brothel was beheaded by a fake client, an act easied by political forces that were working to close the brothel. The police and Social Welfare Department were taken into confidence to help close the brothel in the name of a rehabilitation programme. Violence and gross disregard of human rights ensued. This brothel and another nearby named Nimtoli, also likewise affected by these events, represented nearly 30 per cent of all brothel based sex workers in Bangladesh. Brothel sex workers throughout the nation were feared Women's rights groups and legal rights NGOs collected their forces to defend the brothels. Both *Durjoy and Nari Mukti Shangho* joined, leading the sex worker contingent, and staged a number of public demonstrations and made press releases. Within a short span of time, about 80 different human rights and women's organizations joined to start a group called Solidarity to stand with sex workers against the government. They met with the Prime Minister, but she would not alter the government's plans. She stated that she believed the only option for sex workers was rehabilitation, even though the women stated apparently that they did not want to be rehabilitated. The case went to court.

CARE's stance was simple and direct. It supported the sex workers in their fight for fundamental human rights, and started a stronger approach to working with government, UN agencies and other NGOs to bring this about. Besides various local groups, the International Network of Sex Work Projects, Amnesty and other international agencies were alerted to the major problems in Bangladesh and rallied support.

In March 2000, all who worked on advocacy and networking among the sex workers and other related groups experienced an astonishing victory. The High Court of Bangladesh made it clear that sex work was not illegal and that the women had a right to make a living. It further declared that state agencies liable for evicting women from the brothels had themselves acted illegally. The women were instructed that they could petition the lower courts to re-open their brothels. While it is not known how these events will impact on the future of the project, the court decision apparently gives a signal that human rights, and especially the constitutional right to work, will be protected for sex workers. This decision make strong the HIV prevention options for all concerned.

Condoms

Male condoms were purchased from a single source by the project and distributed free by peer educators. At the brothel, not all the women accepted condoms, reportedly since they did not like being asked how many clients they had the previous day and how many condoms were used. Those who did were supposed to receive as several as they requested. However, shortages and an effort to control scarce resources led to complaints by sex workers that they were not receiving the number they required. In mid-1998 the street based intervention only gave out 3 condoms per day to the women, i.e., the average number of clients reported during the baseline survey, and the brothel intervention gave out 4 per day. Problems had arisen when the condom dissiminator had a labour strike and no condoms were available. The government would not supply family planning condoms to these interventions at the amounts required. The future sustainability of the condom supply was in question.

Ultimately, condoms were available again from the chief source and by October 1998, three condom depots were set up in the brothel at which women could go freely to take as several as they wanted. This alleviated the pressure to ask questions and the 30 per cent of sex workers who had been resistant started taking condoms. Records were kept at the depots of how many condoms were taken, but this took the monitoring out of the hands of the peer educators. By December 1998, free condoms ceased to be available at the brothel. By a decision of the small sex worker-run organization, *Nari Mukti Shangho*, a system was established to purchase the same condoms at trade price from commercial depots in Tangail and sell them through the peer educators with a small advantage divided between the sales women and the organization. Meanwhile, government condoms started appearing at the shops around the brothel at prices lower than those bought by the sex worker organization. As they also were better lubricated, sex workers started purchasing them directly and to sell to others. Sales of condoms increased, but with the variety of feasible modes of access, it became more difficult to monitor.

Among the street sex workers, sales started and free condoms stopped being disseminated in February 1999. The street-based sex worker organization, *Durjoy*, was, by that time well organized and sales rose monthly, rising from 23,385 in February to 62,900 in August. A small benefit was made by the peer educators or outreach workers who sold the condoms and also by *Durjoy*. With this money, among other activities, they establish a trust fund for the poorest group of sex workers.

During 1998, female condoms were introduced to both groups of sex workers on a trial basis and found generally useful, especially among the street women. Because of their high cost and encouraging reports of safe re-use with washing, re-use with washing was also tried, but frightens of misuse prevented project managers from proceeding further with this alternate. Larger trials are planned after further research and training takes place. Additionally, a general demand for water-based lubrication has led to the development of a locally-produced product which is also under trial.

Clients, Non-clients and Lovers

Right from the beginning, little stress was placed in the SHAKTI project on the clients of sex workers. At the brothel these comprise traders and other businessmen, students, truckers, construction workers and others. In Tangail two AIDS information centres were established at a bus station and a court in the town of Tangail, but no targeted programmes for clients were developed. Working with the clients while they are in the brothel is difficult as they do not wish to be seen or recognized when entering the brothel. For this cause the brothel has several entrances. The brothel sub-culture is established for profit and the protection of clients and, although brothel keepers have stated they are worried about the loss to business that a rise in HIV would bring, concrete solutions to these issues have not emerged. Discussions with the brothel keepers, and selected other stakeholders, i.e., religious leaders and municipal personnel, have continued. To date, only awareness workshops have been organized with some client groups.

Street sex worker clients were enumerated in a study carried out in November-December 1998 by sex workers themselves. At 22 locations around Dhaka on one different day each week (during 7 successive weeks), thirty members of the *Durjoy Nari Shangho* interviewed five sex workers per day (every second one they met). Responses were recorded on a pictorial sheet. In total, for 923 sex workers, data were collected about 4,654 different clients. Rickshaw pullers were the most frequent, followed by a category called "service holders" which, in Bangladesh, means men who hold wage jobs, like government and private sector positions, and students. In this study, police were listed as clients but either paid nothing or very little, as they were generally simply given sex in exchange for protection. The study provided the project with information on types of clients, and other data, and gave the sex workers insight into the practice of research. It conspicuously demonstrated that illiterate women could undertake valuable research themselves, with minimal technical supervision.

The sex workers' prolonged lovers are important men in the brothel. Although some are abusive and exploitative, most of the women value their relationships with these men. Several of the lovers, pay the rent, buy them food and clothing, and help with their children. In February 1998, a study was conducted, showing that, among 233 of these men, 14 per cent were permanent residents of the brothel and 56 per cent visited for only one or two days at a time. About 30 per cent of women in the brothel had made claim they did not require to use condoms as they took no clients and remained faithful to their lovers, but project staff disputed this. The study, however, appears to corroborate this, with 28 per cent of the men stating their women took no clients. In the three months before the survey, 16 per cent of lovers reported having had sex with another sex worker in the same brothel and 16 per cent with a sex worker outside the brothel. Additionally, 60 per cent had wives. If it is true that about 30 per cent of sex workers were really taking no other clients than their long-term lovers, it is also right that these sex workers, and the others, were at risk from their lovers' multiple sex partners.

Street sex workers have long-term boyfriends or husbands too but they also are generally coerced into giving sex in exchange for protection. Pimps, guards, rickshaw pullers, police and *mastans*, among others, demand sex from these women. In conformity with the survey in October 1999, 36 per cent of women gave sex in exchange for protection (or some other favour) without pay the previous week, while 61 per cent had sex with their own private partners. Condom use differed accordingly, with 32 per cent of sexual acts covered among the casual or coercive partners and only 18 per cent covered with longer-term, private partners. Overall, 23 per cent of sex acts the previous week had been covered by condoms with men who were not paying clients.

Another survey among these women in 1998 disclosed that 13 per cent had at some time injected drugs, as had 24 per cent of their chief partners, far higher levels than among brothel women and their men. Moreover, these women more generally sold sex to men in groups, either for serial or simultaneous group sex, than did the brothel women. In most cases, group sex is riskier because the woman's capacity to control her safety is lessen and the men may be exposed to the semen of other men as well. In both 1998 and 1999, about one-quarter of the women sampled had hired themselves out to a group (averaging about 4 men) the previous week, and over half had done so the previous month.

Monitoring and Evaluation

During the first few years of SHAKTI, peer educators undertaken most of the monitoring of changes in knowledge, intent, trial and use of condoms. After the mid-term review, other modes of data collection were added. Biannual surveys carried out by independent interviewers were put in place, and, after condom sales started, the number of condoms sold was monitored. In mid-1998, new denoters on violence among street-based sex workers were developed. Data on the previous week's harassment were gathered at 444 group education sessions among 4,750 women in the drop-in centres between Sept 1998 and October 1999. Such an indicator could demonstrate a decrease (or increase) in violence over time and any impact the project might have on securing greater safety for sex workers through advocacy and better communication with street *mastans*.

The SHAKTI project has always made much endeavour to monitoring its own activities. Although at times changes were made that make comparisons difficult, overall the sampling and attention to accuracy, data management and analysis were proper to produce a clear picture of changing behaviour, major obstacles to greater success, and the impact of attempts to break those obstacles. One area in which monitoring was not fully appropriate was the changing composition of the target groups, a lesson for the future. Nonetheless, the attention to monitoring and research has made it possible to document the project very well, producing many presentations at international meetings and several useful publications.

Effectiveness

The peer educators gathered monitoring data that showed, after 14 months (as of October 1997), knowledge that STDs can be prevented through the use of condoms increased, as did intent, trial and reported condom use. Knowledge of the value of condoms increased from 36 per cent to 87 per cent. The intent to use condoms rose from 28 per cent to 64 per cent and the trial of a condom within the last 24 hours rose from 12 per cent to 59 per cent. Self-reported 'consistent' condom use increased from about 14 per cent to 28 per cent (consistency was interpreted as 50 per cent or more of all intercourse with clients during the previous 24 hours).

Surveys conducted in 1998 and 1999 separated questions about sex with clients and private partners more briefly than had been done earlier, using both the previous day and the previous week as recall periods. These showed a apparently rising trend in condom use.

Changes in composition of the brothel population continued over time. For many years the number of young women under 18 increased, until 1999, when a severe crackdown took place in a nearby brothel and panic spread. Towards the end of 1999, the government declared that all brothels would be closed and the women rehabilitated. While it may be doubtful that this objective will be accomplished, the combination of shifts in the resident population and reliance on syndromic management in a group of women with high STD prevalence, produced no important reduction in STD levels at the time of the mid-term evaluation in April 1998. The number of bonded sex workers (*chhukris*) continued to increase until 1999, as did the number of those under 18. A survey started in July 1999 was suspended for a month and finished in September because of trouble in the brothel. Violence at nearby brothels and at Tangail evoked police raids and some arrests. Outcomes of the survey showed that the number of bonded women had been decreased, young sex workers were fewer and, accordingly, the number of clients on the previous day was seriously diminished. Nonetheless, clients still liked the bonded young women. At that time, 52 per cent of independent sex workers had been without clients the previous day, while only 11 per cent of *chhukris* had no clients.

Among the Dhaka street sex workers, the baseline survey did not question use with non-paying partners in a conspicuous manner, but between 1998 and 1999 condom use with private and other non-paying partners improved. Outcomes of surveys over time demonstrate a clear improvement in use with all types of partners.

While the average age of those sampled remained about 22 to 23, the proportion under 18 decreased from 25 per cent to 14 per cent, and the average number of clients per week increased between 1997 and 1999 from 13 to 18. The sex workers reported several new women appearing on the streets during the 1998 floods and again after the Tan Bazar brothel was closed. No method of monitoring the changing composition of the street-based sex worker population ever evolved. The existence of current syphilis (TPHA+ and RPR=>8) did not shift between surveys in 1997 and 1998, with 32 per cent and 34 per cent respectively. It is not easy to understand if this was since the clinic work and condom use really failed to minimize the prevalence of syphilis or if the women accessing the clinics were regularly changing.

The first survey estimated about 4,300 street-based sex workers in Dhaka but continued estimates have not been made. The situation is very fluid, with a lot of women shifting from hotels to streets, or from city to city, and in and out of the trade. The actual number explicit at any one time appears to be highly influenced by police activity, but it is explicit that the women either find new venues or remain inactive for a while when police activity is high. Poverty, illiteracy, dearth of remunerative options and high rates of abandonment by husbands place a lot of women at risk of turning to the street sex trade for sustenance. Despite their many levels of vulnerability, street sex workers related to the SHAKTI project have demonstrated remarkable capacity to take control of their sexual health.

Efficiency

The excellent infrastructure of CARE, Bangladesh, CARE's largest mission, has certainly played a potent role in facilitating the operation of the project. Nonetheless, the project suffered in efficiency mainly due to the lack of experienced personnel at all standards and the continued need for training. SHAKTI was the first targeted intervention with a well-conceived behavioural change model particularly for sex workers in Bangladesh. Training of staff improved through the years with the addition of a newsletter, a journals club and increased access to reading materials translated into Bangla. Nonetheless, repeated disturbances developed by local politics and shifts in management were important factors that limited efficiency. Scaling up to cover all the nation's brothels through partnerships with other NGOs had been planned but dearth of funding, expertise, and, in the end, government's threats to close all brothels, have worked against this plan.

Ethical Soundness

Sound ethical procedures were put in place during the extended period of formative research. Confidentiality, non-coercive and informed consent processes and de-linking of HIV samples were used. All treatable infections diagnosed during STD surveys were treated. However, in the case of some STDs, outcomes were slow to approach the brothel due to sending the samples overseas for processing. Better collaboration with local laboratories has solved this problem.

Planning for the requirements of HIV-positive sex workers has also arisen as an issue that the project never explicitely considered in its early phases. A small support group for positive people has developed within the framework of the SHAKTI project, and plans to support its growth have been made.

Replicability and Sustainability

Throughout the life of the project, the AIDS programme of the Government of Bangladesh has been related to SHAKTI in numerous ways. The Tangail brothel and the street sex worker clinics have been comprised as sentinel sites in the National HIV Serosurveillance. Replicability through other NGOs will, however, need investment on the part of donors or government. Sustainability particularly of SHAKTI's sex worker interventions is considered achievable through the enhancement of skills among the sex workers themselves. Investment for the last year of the project is aimed at building capacity within the self-run organizations of sex workers for leadership, management, and monitoring. Continued help to these organizations will certainly be needed, but increasing numbers of functions have been taken over by sex workers.

Lessons Learnt

One of the most important lessons learnt in this project has been that, *even in a very conservative society, sex workers can be reached,* with a sexual health intervention in a non-judgmental way with prior inexperienced staff. *A step-by-step approach to behavioural change, with condoms sold by the sex workers themselves,* has worked to improve condom use. Monitoring of condom use and sales by the sex workers has contributed to their involvement in the result of the project. SHAKTI was a *well-planned project, informed by theory and epidemiology,* a factor which has helped hold it together through many changes of management and personnel. Considerable *investment in monitoring and documentation* has paid off a various ways for the project.

The fundamental approach of the SHAKTI project is explicitly replicable, with adjustments. There is now *a vision of sustainability through a sex worker-run project* that has evolved due to the endeavours of the sex workers themselves to band together for strength and safety. *Protecting the human rights of sex workers* has galvanized staff and sex workers alike and helped them to know the conditions required to ensure long-term HIV prevention. Their empowerment has become a principal aim of the project since it is explicit that sustainable operation of clinical services and an outreach programme will be best motivated by the women themselves. *Skills in advocacy* have emerged as a much required capacity when working with highly marginalized groups.

The dearth of evidence for a drop in STD prevalence illustrates the *requirement for regular monitoring of the changing composition of a dynamic target group* and the value of an indicator that will measure the frequency of contact with the intervention. It may also reflect the dearth of proper training for service providers and *the inadequacy of syndromic management alone* in a group with high levels of STDs. It surely also reflects the continued lower standard of condom use with regular partners, a serious issue requiring sensitive approaches and *better interactions with the men associated with these women.*

The problems faced by the SHAKTI project stress the *requirement for developing expertise among staff through continued training and practice.* As environmental, social and political situations are constantly changing, the project has had to be *flexible to survive.* Meeting the requirements of sex workers could not be accomplished by a single project, but has needed the *building of alliances with partners that have won victories for sex workers far beyond the immediate expectations of the project.*

Twelve

Red Light Area in Kolkata

Background

Calcutta, now renamed Kolkata, sometimes called 'the city of joy' is also a city of acute poverty, of Mother Theresa's domain, and the historical seat of the British Raj. It is a crowded and underserved city, struggling to clear itself up and modernize. It is also the conventional centre of Bengali culture and society, a culture that takes higher pride in its poetry, arts, music and political thought and action. The relentless oppression of women in India is powerful precisely since it is deeply integrated into class, caste and ethnic hierarchies. Resistance to class exploitation and social denigration has fuelled various movements in modern Bengali history. It is within this cultural and historical context that the Sonagachi project has grown. Adjacent to West Bengal are the states of Bihar and Uttar Pradesh in India and the nearby countries of Nepal and Bangladesh, all of which are substantially poor and disadvantaged, both ecologically and socially. From these areas hail a significant minority of Sonagachi's resident sex workers. Sonagachi is the derived pronunciation of a lane called Sanah Ghazi, named after dacoit or hoodlum, recast as a religious teacher.

The Sonagachi area was first recognized as a significant red light district of Kolkata when the British enacted the Indian Contagious Diseases Act in 1868. This was done in an attempt to control STDs reaching England via British soldiers serving in India. At that time, about 30,000 sex workers were estimated to work in the area. A survey carried out in the late 1800s noted three major reasons why women entered prostitution. These were seduction and abandonment, running away from the cruelty of husbands and in-laws, and becoming a family outcast due to personal efforts to break through the intense restrictions on the lives of young women. To this list today we must add poverty from birth, fake marriages and sale, situational poverty because of family losses, trickery and trafficking, abduction and sale. Additionally some family traditions of dancers and entertainers, e.g. Agrawalis, have gradually become family lines of sex workers.

The pattern of recruitment into the sex trade comprised cross-border movements and a significant number of young girls, approximately 15 per cent under the age of 15 at the time the project started entered in that way. The sex industry is controlled by police, politicians, local hoodlum gangs, brothel owners, madams and pimps. While few sex workers are independent, others, especially those newer to the trade, have madams and/or pimps. Some madam-controlled sex workers known as *chhukris* are totally bonded and each one is obliged to earn enough to pay off an advance given to her or, more generally, to the persons who 'sold' her into the trade. Another madam-controlled arrangement is called the *adhia* system, in which the sex worker turns over 50 per cent of her income to the madam. Pimps take 25 per cent of the sex worker's income and are organized in a hierarchical and regulated system headed by *mukia*, or political headmen. Rates of rooms got high. The sale of sex is legal in India if it takes place "within a room". Escaping arrest, freelance or 'flying' sex workers must also rent rooms at high hourly rates. The Prevention of Immoral Traffic Act, intended to regulating the flow of new women into the trade, in fact simply makes it easier for sex workers to be harassed, extorted, beaten, raped, and otherwise abused, when the Act is used to raid brothels on the pretext of removing younger women. The attitude of the surrounding society is often to despise and stigmatize sex workers on moral and social grounds.

Additionally, many sex workers have *babus*, men who begin as clients and then form longer-term relationships. While some of these men actually care for their women lovers and contribute to their expenses, several are abusive and exploitative. Nonetheless a lot of women require these companions for emotional and practical cause and are tied to these relationships.

The Sonagachi project area includes four main colonies of brothels, located comparatively close to each other, known as Sonagachi, Rambagan and Sethbagan, Jorabagan, and Rabindra Sarani. Collectively, this is the biggest red light area in Kolkata, with about 370 separate brothels housing about 4000 sex workers. The total number swells to about 5000 in September and October during the Hindu Puja season, a time of revelry and good earnings for sex workers. Additionally, on the crowded streets and tiny lanes below the multi-storey tenement brothel buildings, about 1500 flying sex workers operate. The whole neighbourhood is served by a number of small shops, itinerant traders, vegetable hawkers, youth clubs, wine shops, and medical clinics, some run by quacks. Prices at these establishments are much than in other neighbourhoods in Kolkata of same class. Hordes of people can be found at any time of day and night travelling on bicycles, scooters, rickshaws and on foot. It is a crowded, dirty, lively, and dangerous area where daily about 20,000 men come to drink and enjoy sex. Not only the sex workers, but their clients as well, are preyed upon by hoodlums. As in most such areas, the police either ignore or are involved in the ambient violence.

Each building has many brothels in it with 5 to 25 rooms. Sex workers fall into different categories according to their income, which is largely based on age and attractiveness. Higher-income women have pleasant rooms, sometimes with air conditioning, while the lower-income group may share a single room among up to five women, with beds separated by curtains. Ages range from 13 to 45 with incomes from Rs. 10 to 2,000 per night (Rs. 39=1US$). In spite of crowded quarters, the women live their lives in considerable isolation from each other and from the larger society. Madams and pimps impose rules that keep sex workers from visiting each other. Older sex workers, unless they become madams, are not able to secure a lot of clients and many work at housekeeping chores or baby sitting to make a living. Ultimately many become destitute.

Relevance

The AIDS epidemic in India is a rapidly growing one. As one of the world's most populated countries, its absolute numbers of HIV-infected and affected people are likely to become staggering in the next decade. With high proportions of very poor people and cultural patterns dictating very low status for women, Indian women are increasingly becoming the bearers of the HIV burden.

Sex workers represent those with the lowest status and the highest risk, among all women. The All India Institute of Hygiene and Public Health (AIIH&PH) has been known for its different health interventions and thus has been able to lead in the development of a broad-based support system for the project. This support mechanism is known as the conglomerate, and comprises NGOs, Community-Based Organizations (CBOs), and government institutions. At the time the project started, the prevalence of HIV was very low in West Bengal, providing an opportunity for a creative and flexible intervention.

Formative Stages

The initial baseline survey, carried on by personnel from the AIIH&PH with the help of an NGO that had been working in the area, the Society for Community Development, was undertaken from April to June 1992. The survey covered STD epidemiology, socio-demographics and behaviour. Flying sex workers were excluded. After the beginning count of 362 brothels housing 3,664 sex workers, the sampling methods were designed. Sex workers were grouped into those with charges higher than Rs. 100 per client (Category A), those with charges between Rs. 50 and Rs. 100 (Category B) and those with charges less than Rs. 50 (Category C). Sex workers were sampled randomly in proportion to the number in each category. Sixty-five brothels were randomly selected out of the feasible 362 and about 6-7 sex workers interviewed in each (with non-responder replacement), for a total sample size of 450 (12 per cent of the total). Additionally, 360 women from this sample were desire to undergo an STD examination undertaken at a two-room clinic set up in volunteer local club in the heart of the red light district. STD specialists from the Calcutta Medical College attended the clinic, and laboratory work was undertaken at the Bacteriology Department of the Calcutta School of Tropical Medicine.

In brief the social survey found that 85 per cent of the sex workers were between 15 and 29 years old. Most stated they entered the trade because of poverty (49.1 per cent), family disputes (21.6 per cent) or being misguided (15.6 per cent). Also, 85 per cent were illiterate and several were heavily dependent an alcohol, and 9.3 per cent were newcomers, having been in the trade for less than one year. In this sample 43 per cent of the women visited and worked in other areas of the city as well, staying there for few weeks or months before returning to Sonagachi. The majority had 3 to 4 clients per day for weekly incomes that varied between less than Rs. 300 to over Rs. 5,000. Several women (27 per cent) reported that men hired them in a group, a situation that seriously diminishes the woman's control. Around 40 per cent of the women had children, but the proportion with *babus* was not conditioned; 45 per cent of the women used some form of contraception but only 27 per cent did so consistently. Condoms were always practised by only 1.1 per cent and often used by another 1.6 per cent of women. At that time in 1992, 90.6 per cent of sex workers had never used condoms and only 31 per cent had heard of AIDS. More, 69 per cent, knew something about other STDs.

Endocervical smears detected 10.5 per cent positive for gonorrhoea, with 4.9 per cent confirmed by culture, although, for technical reasons, it later seemed that the methods used were insensitive and underestimated the true rate of gonorrhoea. *Trichomonas vaginalis* infection was detected in 11.1 per cent. Genital ulcers were seen in 6.2 per cent of the women. Serological testing for syphilis found 25.4 per cent positive by VDRL (dilution=> 1:8). The HIV positivity rate was 1.1 per cent.

Later in 1993 a client survey was conducted by 193 sex workers, as they had the easiest access to these men. Sex workers from each category of income were selected to conduct a precise questionnaire-based interview with one client each. As these women were mostly illiterate, they had to remember the questions and answers. Social workers visited them in the mornings and filled the form in with their support. Literate clients filled in their own questionnaires. The sample was biased towards men they knew, men who were spending the night, and fixed clients and, while useful, cannot be taken as representative of all clients. Those clients who entered and left the brothel quite quickly were under represented. Thirty-seven clients of sex workers of category A, the highest income group, were interviewed, as were 75 and 81 of categories B and C. respectively. Results disclosed an age range of 15 to over 40, with a tendency of younger clients to visit less expensive sex workers and more educated clients to visit the more precious women. The mean ages of clients by sex worker category were: A-42, B-39, and C-34. Of the clients, 87 per cent were literate and 44 per cent were businessmen. Others include wage-earners, professionals, drivers, students and police. The proportion of students (8.8 per cent) was as high as that of drivers (8.3 per cent). Slightly over half (52.3 per cent) visited the brothels once or twice a weekend and 9.3 per cent visited regularly. Most were alcohol drinkers and spent time entertaining themselves in wine bars. While vaginal intercourse was most common, 47 per cent also enjoyed oral sex. Anal sex was reported as rare, and 4 per cent paid to be masturbated.

Another survey of 200 *babus* was conducted, showing that 26 per cent were illiterate, but 9 per cent were graduates of universities. Likewise, 46 per cent had low incomes, less than Rs. 1,000 per month and 4 per cent had incomes over Rs. 2,500 per month. Although half had heard of AIDS, 73 per cent had never used condoms. Only 4.5 per cent reported using condoms continuously.

Additionally, in 1993 the project undertook another survey of sex workers to learn about their situations and aspirations regarding their children. Some 2,338 women were interviewed, 47 per cent of whom had children under 14 years old. Inspite of the considerable felt requirement for children, largely for emotional and social causes, pregnancy was a serious risk for these women, with 14 per cent stating they had deliberately terminated their pregnancies, several more than once. A total of 768 abortions had been experienced by 330 women, or an average of 2.3 abortions per woman. One woman had had 15 abortions and one live birth. An even major problem is the future of those born. About half were brought up in the brothel with little in the way of decent care. Some sex workers paid older sex workers to raise their children, but the most of kept their children with them, arranging makeshift creches when working. The others were brought up outside the brothel, either with family members or in orphanage homes, with 90 per cent of the financing supplied by the mother. Less than 5 per cent were raised in government or NGO-run homes. About half of the children had got some form of education, but drop-out rates from primary to secondary school were very high. None managed to go beyond secondary school. The mothers emphasised their requirement for hostel or boarding facilities with proper schooling and supportive environments for their children.

IMPLEMENTATION

Working Strategies

· The project started with a philosophy based on Reliance, Respect and Recognition, i.e. giving due respect to the women, depending on their knowledge and recognizing their profession. The project team members had to make it explicit to all that they would not disturb the prevailing power structure or seek to remove women from prostitution. Throughout the project's life, all those who influence the sex trade, even if in a negative way, have been drawn into its activities. At the same time, abuse by thugs, power brokers, unethical researchers, and others has been resisted by the sex workers and their supporters. The project itself has become a sentinel of resistance through organization and affiliation, to create a platform upon which sex workers could personally and collectively grow. Therefore, allies among government agencies, NGOs, CBOs, academic institutions, and many other organizations have been included in one way or another. Publicity in newspapers, dozens of public appearances, conferences, workshops, and visible campaigning have been practised to draw attention to the issues requiring reform. These issues are those most appropriate to the safety and well-being of sex workers, as defined by themselves. They comprise their rights as workers, the rights of their children, the safety of their neighbourhoods, their concern over the trafficking of children in the sex trade, and their legal and constitutional rights.

For project staff, misgivings had to be overcome. Some percepted endangered by being close to sex workers, and feared catching diseases. Others felt embarrassed having to deal so directly with sex. Hoodlums were a very real threat. Gradually, they eliminate their fears and have become true supporters of the women.

Police raids have been a greater problem in this project, keeping the sex workers insecure and feared. After every raid, staff believed that condom use declined and STDs rose among clinic attendees. Therefore, the AIIH&PH in cooperation with the Kolkata Police Department organised a training programme for police personnel. By April 1996, 180 police officers were sent for this training.

Health Care

A clinic, called the Health Service Centre, was setup in 1992 on the premises of a local youth club, Palatak, in the middle of the Sonagachi area. The Health Service Centre is staffed by one of two rotating STD specialist doctors and is open 6 days a week from 11:00 to 14:00 to sex workers and members of their families. Treatment is free and serum samples are gathered opportunistically for syphilis screening. Sex workers are encouraged by their peers to attend the clinic for screening even when asymptomatic. Follow-up on treatment is undertaken through the work of peer educators. On average, in 1998, 730 women came to the morning clinic per month. In 1993 another clinic was opened for evening sessions 5 days a week nearby in another club, particularly for clients. Demand has grown greatly and the clinic is now crowded; other clinic days are required.

Gradually, throughout the life of the project, because of the demand of sex workers, additional clinics of same kind have been opened. In 1994, one opened in Sethbagan and another outside the project area in Bowbazar, another red light district in Kolkata. These are operated, on behalf of the AIIH&PH, by the project with an NGO conglomerate. Between 1994 and 1998, 9 more clinics were started in red light districts in Kolkata particularly for sex workers and their families. As the many years have passed, the women have seen the value of good-quality health services and have noted the poorer quality and disrespectful treatment in other facilities in the city.

In 1995, the peer educators started a rapid assessment of the situation of sex workers in the rest of West Bengal. They found 254 red light districts and spots in all over the state. After prioritizing 30, they started organizing and, as of late 1999, 14 new projects had began. New clinics were constructed, peer education begun and condom sales carried out. This effort is financed by the project and managed by the DMSC.

Technical aspects of STD care, like resistance to antibiotics and verification of cure, remain to be handled. Aggressive screening and more referral and follow-up of *babus* and other clients are needed in the next phase of growth.

Peer Education

Peer educators were selected and trained, starting with an initial group of 12. By 1997 there were 65 trained peer educators who were paid the equal of US$1 per day. These women were given 6 weeks of training and utilized particularly designed flip charts, requiring little literacy, to explain the fundamentals of sexual health and safer sex to their peers. The Sonagachi area was divided into 11 zones that were covered by the 65 peer educators with 7 supervisors. From 10:00 until 13:00 every day, each group contacts 40 to 50 sex workers and 10 to 15 madams. They encourage the women to go for regular check-ups and seeking care when they have symptoms. Leaflets are given to those who are literate. Moreover video shows, slide presentations, small group meetings and ventriloquist performances have been used to approach larger groups of sex workers and clients.

They have also developed a performing group, Komol Gandhar, that comprises male and transgender sex workers, and perform at different cultural events. They perform plays about STD/HIV prevention and the issues surrounding prostitution. This dance/theatre troupe has become an important medium by which the sex workers can express themselves, forge a public identity and approach a large number of persons of all walks of life. It won first prize at a National Cultural Competition for Sex Workers, organized in Benares in mid-1997 and, in 1998, it performed at the Twelfth World AIDS Conference in Geneva.

After expanding to other brothels in Kolkata, the number of trained peer educators has increased 200 with a coverage of about 20,000 sex workers and babus. As the project has expanded, it has now increasingly become difficult to continue to pay all the peer educators required in order to maintain a ratio of one peer educator to 50 sex workers reached. Now the ratio is 1:160 with a view to deal with this problem, the project has developed an extra cadre of volunteers to help the peer educators approach women. Monitoring the quality of work of these volunteers represents a challenge in scaling-up, typical of most trainer-of-trainer like projects.

In 1998 the Positive Hotline was started and maintained by the sex workers in response to hearing about the sad situation of an HIV-positive woman who was not a sex worker. It has initiated with a single phone at one of the field offices and is staffed at night by the children of sex workers. This service to the larger community emerged from recognition of the requirement for counselling and support for HIV-positive people, whether sex workers or not. A core team has been developed of volunteers, a doctor, a nurse and a counsellor. Besides medical care, the service offers psycho-social and legal aid support and the team can be sent to the homes of HIV-positive people. As the number of HIV-positive people grows in India, the objective is to develop a model of community-based care for West Bengal.

Condoms

In the starting, the peer educators distributed free condoms and enquired about the extent of condom usage. Demand for the high-quality, imported condoms distributed by the project grew faster than the supply. During the first month of the project, 3592 condoms were distributed; by 1994, during the month of December, 79420 condoms were distributed. This rose to 110328 in December 1996. Following the budgetary constraints, the project was unable to meet demands.

In July 1995, the sex workers of Sonagachi formed a registered society called the Usha Multipurpose Cooperative Society Ltd., a consumers' cooperative which would support them save money and avoid the exorbitant interest charged on small loans by money lenders in the area. Registering as sex workers, instead of 'housewives', required a long struggle with authorities, but with a growing capacity for advocacy and publicity, DMSC was successful. Beginning with only 13 members, it now has over 1000 and regularly provides loans at low-interest rates to sex workers. Small investment schemes utilizing bank deposits have also been started. Its funds provide a creche for sex workers' children during working hours and it provides employment to older, out-of-work sex workers. In April 1997, it developed its first for profit business, the marketing of condoms. Bought in bulk, the condoms were sold to any group willing to buy. Recorded sales increased from a total of 213056 in 1997 to 443805 in 1998 and 730656 in 1999. The project still disseminate free condoms as well for newcomers to the brothel, to men who attend the STD clinics and to very poor sex workers.

In the meantime, condoms manufactured in India have improved and importing is no longer considered necessary. An activist-cum-sales arm of the Usha Cooperative, Besanti Sena, now markets condoms in 40 red light districts of West Bengal. With the profits made, they have purchased a piece of land outside of Kolkata at which they have been able to develop a training centre where they conduct most of their training. The older sex workers produce handicrafts there when particular market opportunities emerge.

Empowerment

Organization has been the basic to empowering the sex workers of Sonagachi. Several influences converged to encourage the sex workers of Sonagachi to organize themselves. First, an earlier organization of sex workers, called Mahila Sangha, was formed in the Sethbagan area in the 1970s, to fight against the incessant and violent extortion of money from sex workers by a local mafia. After gaining victory, they moved on to literacy and health programmes. Ultimately one of the leaders moved over to the Sonagachi project and led, the Sonagachi sex workers in their first appearance at the Kolkata Book Fair in 1992. Second, consecutive meetings of the peer educators began to knit them together and, to resolve conflicts, they formed an advisory Board and a committee to handle grievances. In 1993, the peer educators and supervisors held a candlelight procession against AIDS which made the headlines. Gradually step by step, new elements were added. The peers were given a green uniform jacket with a printed red cross on it and an identity card. With this they could realize like real health workers. Women started to take their clients into the clinic to have their STDs treated and were sought after for advice and information. It was found that, in the starting, women with children were the most enthusiastic about becoming peer educators as it gave them a more respectable status in the eyes of their children.

Running their own project and organizations needed that some of the women, at least, were literate. The women wanted a literacy project for themselves. One of the supervisors agreed to teach and they started, but soon it became clear that adult learners with special life experiences could do better if the literacy lessons grew from their own discourses. A new way of learning emerged which is participatory and has its own primer. A small newsletter with an attractive glossy format, *Namaskar*, was started, in which they can tell of their experiences. These are sold by the peer educators at fairs and meetings, specially the annual prestigious Kolkata Book Fair. Four editions have been produced so far. Additionally, daughters of sex workers were recruited to be teachers of literacy and there are 14 such teachers so far. This strategy has had the benefit of giving pride to the mothers and to the daughters, and helping them gain status in society. Indirectly, their new identities may make it easier to negotiate better positions regarding dowry and marriage at a later age.

DMSC started to develop cultural, sports and artistic activities for sex workers' children and, with the support of the project, placed at first 50, and now 100 children in mainstream boarding schools yearly. A creche now operates for brothel children and many other programmes sponsored by donors and operated by collaborating NGOs/CBOs.

In 1994, researchers, with the help of an NGO and police, accumulated blood samples from 50 Sonagachi women without their consent. This created panic in the area and the Institute registered its protest. Ultimately, the situation calmed down but left the women with determination to form an organization that could deal with local issues, like that one, which directly affected their lives.

In 1995, the DMSC Committee led a group of 1,000 sex workers to demonstrate against police raids in the Sonagachi area. They joined rallies against the eviction of sex workers in other parts of Kolkata and demonstrated against the unethical and illegal testing of an unqualified AIDS vaccine. They collected money to provide to the State for flood victims and, by 1996, started touring other parts of West Bengal to examine the situation of sex workers, which, in several cases, they found shocking. They visited sex worker projects in Bangladesh and Nepal. After some time, representatives of the Committee attended international meetings of sex workers meetings on the trafficking of children in the sex trade, and national and international congresses on AIDS. In late 1997, the Committee brought together thousands of sex workers, including males and transvestites, for the First National Conference of Sex Workers in Kolkata. They have taken on the role of the

Secretariat for the Asia/Pacific Sex Workers' Network. In March 1998, they organised another conference, the Follow-up Phase of the First National Conference of Sex Workers. This conference was attended by 2,000 sex workers from 48 red light areas across India. At this conference they were able to attain many of their objectives, particularly those related to networking. They now have a vision and a platform of objectives aimed at integrating themselves into a worker's world of rights and responsibilities. The Committee now has over 250 male and transgender members.

Three hundred sex workers have got legal training. As some wanted more than the short course originally given, another 60 had additional legal training.

One puzzling issue has been the presence of young sex workers in the brothel. This is both against the law, causing the police to make repeated raids, and a problem to older sex workers. The younger women have less capacity to press on safer sex, are biologically more sensitive to HIV infection and draw clients away from the older ones. The members of DMSC have taken the stand that they can regulate the entry of young women better into the brothels themselves than can the police or other agencies. They establish a system through which they could monitor new arrivals and counsel them before they actually enter the brothel trade. At first they were trying to send them back to their homes, but the majority simply declined to go having run away from abusive or difficult circumstances. With the assistance of the Social Welfare Department, they now have an arrangement whereby most the girls are sent to boarding schools sponsored by the Social Welfare Department. Over the years this process seems to have decreased the proportion of bonded sex workers, usually the youngest, entering the brothel, although indicators have not been recorded for this. With the objective of spreading this type of self-regulatory action, DMSC set up in 1999 three more Self-regulatory Boards at Sethbagan, Tollygunge and Rambagan in Kolkata. These boards are consisted of members from the state government, women's rights groups, other local people and sex workers. Members of DMSC frequently attend meetings and debates on trafficking, an issue of grave concern in the South Asian region.

Helping sex workers leave the sex trade has never been an

objective of the project but, essentially, growth in self-esteem and a sense of control over one's own life has led some women to opt to leave the trade. About one-third of the peer educators who have been active for at least several years have moved out of the brothel. They comeback daily to conduct their work; about 60 women have left sex work entirely. The low salaries they get from the project must be supplemented by other income and several of these women now sell saris and other small merchandise. In addition, the number of pimps and madams appears to be dropping. At Sonagachi, as elsewhere, the AIDS epidemic has led to the realization by several sex workers that they can avoid the repressive and unsafe conditions in illegal brothels by diversifying their work modes. A number of have moved into residential or hotel-based sex work, a situation having implications for future HIV prevention and evolving nature of the relations between the state and the sex trade.

Clients and Lovers

For clients, a clinic has been established with free treatment, free condoms and counselling, but no apparent mode of establishing client-targeted programmes has emerged. Police, youth groups and the general public have got several awareness programmes. Some clients have been reached at wine shops and through forms of 'edutainment' like ventriloquist shows. *Babus*, however, represent a special problem and, as fixed clients have got special attention. A meeting in the local Botanical Gardens was called in June 1997, attended by about 150 *babus*, which discussed the problems of the Sonagachi area and the role of *babus* in the establishment of safer sex norms. After this four meetings were held. Subsequently, a babu committee and a collective, known as Sathi Sangathan (Companion's Collective), were formed. The objective is to work with DMSC to fight against all kinds of harassment and violence against sex workers and their clients. One of their services has been to protect clients past the bands of *gundas*, or hoodlums that operate on the streets of Sonagachi.

Monitoring and Evaluation

The project accumulates data on several different monitoring indicators both at the clinics and through the peer educators. It also depends on periodic cross-sectional surveys for result on effectiveness, with one completed at the end of 1993, another in mid-year 1995 and the latest in 1999. The first external evaluation tookplace in 1996 and another in 1999. One potent recommendation made by these teams was that the project should develop different indicators. Instead of focusing narrowly on effectiveness in STD control, it should find a way to document the emerging strength and self-esteem of sex workers. By 1998 a number of new indicators were added. The attendance of clients at the project's clinics had been difficult to monitor as men sought treatment who may not have been clients. A referral card provided by the sex worker to the client (and later handed in at the clinic) now makes it feasible to monitor how many clinic attendees are clients referred by sex workers. The duration of self-recognized symptoms when the sex worker presents to the clinic is now recorded. Instead of continuing to ask how several sex acts were covered by condoms, the project now monitors how many condoms were sold, on the assumption that women will purchase what they will in actual use. Levels of empowerment and engagement in the community movement are now measured by asking how many times the sex worker manages to negotiate with landlords, police and other power brokers, and how many sex worker organization meetings or conferences she attends. Changing the indicators for monitoring the success of an evolving intervention is inevitable but must be done with care so that continuity with the past is minimally affected.

Effectiveness

At the end of 1993, 14 months after the intervention was implemented, the first follow-up survey was carried on. Sampling methods were necessarily the same as the baseline survey and 612 women were interviewed. Age distribution was resemble to the first survey and the literacy rate remained very low. The proportion of new sex workers (in the trade less than one year) was very higher (22.6 per cent) than at baseline (9.3 per cent). The median number of clients the previous day was 3. Group sex started to increase from 27.3 per cent at baseline to 48.7 per cent. The proportion of women reporting oral sex started to decrease from 74.4 per cent to 38.1 per cent. It is not unlikely that the questions were asked in varied ways in each survey, causing this puzzling result. The proportion of women reporting some knowledge of AIDS rose from 30.7 per cent to 85.8 per cent. The percentage of clients using condoms always or generally increased from 2.7 per cent at baseline to 69 per cent, a considerable increase. By 1998, this percentage rose to 90.3.

Although the methods utilized to detect gonorrhoea were too insensitive to identify all cases, these same methods were used for the baseline and first follow-up surveys. This showed a decrease in gonorrhoea from 13.2 per cent to 3.9 per cent. Neither HIV nor recent syphilis infections showed any significant change in prevalence.

In an effort to improve the survey methods, decisions were made for the second follow-up survey carried on in July-August 1995 to alter the sampling and STD detection techniques. This decision meant sacrificing some of the past data with a view to have improved measurement capacity in the future. However, the hoped-for improved random sampling methods did not work. True randomization is very difficult without recognizing the women in some way, especially because the sex workers were interviewed at the brothels and had to go voluntarily to the clinic for examination and testing. In fact, more went to the clinic than were randomly selected and it was hard to know who had really been interviewed. Additionally, although the laboratory methods to detect gonorrhoea were improved, laboratory capacity was not enhanced, and only 10 samples could be handled per day. In November 1995, when an external team of experts evaluated the project, it was recommended that in the future the laboratory work should be dealt by a commercial laboratory with greater capacity and that a reference laboratory be used for quality control.

Nonetheless, explicit evidence exists of a reduction in levels of recent syphilis and the presence of genital ulcers. Measures of current syphilis are higher for those who have more clients than others, are illiterate and have not taken part any meetings organized by sex workers.

Thirteen

Health Communication for HIV/AIDS

Introduction

An effective communication strategy is a critical component of the global endeavours in HIV/AIDS prevention and education. Such a strategy should be grounded in a sound theory such that the resulting framework is flexible enough for application in various regional and cultural contexts. Given the stress placed on HIV/AIDS prevention and care, mostly due to the absence of cure for or vaccination against the disease, employing effective communication strategies becomes pivotal in controlling the pandemic. Consequently, evaluating and redefining views to communicating proper messages to different populations and the public at large has become a critical aspect of HIV/AIDS prevention and care. Since HIV/AIDS was first reported, broad-ranging plannings based on social psychological theories and models of behaviour that are believed to be effective in guiding communication approaches to HIV/AIDS prevention and care have been introduced. These strategies range from a single universal approach to different integrated approach in understanding health behaviours. After more than a decade of battle with this pandemic, there are now serious questions raised with regard to the relevance of some of the most commonly used theories/models that guide communication strategies to prevent HIV/AIDS especially in Africa, Asia, Latin America, and the Caribbean as well as their diaspora. These questions focus not so much on the importance of the theories as such but on their adequacy, or lack thereof, in contexts different from those where they were initially developed and tested.

A critical point in this debate about proper health communication theories models is the recognition of culture as central to strategy implementation, and evaluation of health communication and health promotion programmes in general and HIV/AIDS prevention and care in special. In fact, designing a culturally relevant programme and communicating messages in small groups are two critical factors reported to influence positively the result of 37 community-based HIV/AIDS prevention programmes evaluated in the United States. It has long been known that very project implemented is guided by particular sets of assumptions, whether or not these assumptions are obvious to the interventionist, which are generally discernible as theories and models designed to facilitate the implementation of a given project in a population. Very often, however, these theories and models are not evaluated for their adequateness in project implementation.

Thus, much of communications research in HIV/AIDS tends to focus on theories "for" intervention rather than theories "of" interventions. Stated differently, commonly used communication strategies generally attempt to fit implementation processes into the rules of a dominant theory or model in social psychology rather than allowing the field experience to shape its own framework. Moreover, the role of cultural contexts in successful implementation of programmes often is omitted, even though evidence abounds that culture is an important feature in health behaviours and decisions particularly in the context of behaviours that may predispose people to HIV/AIDS. Consequently, it was essential that the integration of knowledge about the significance of communication strategies and the significance of culture in health behaviour became a critical component of HIV/AIDS prevention and care in the new millennium.

In this chapter, we discuss definitions and conceptions of commonly used theories/models in communicating HIV/AIDS messages and how these definitions/conceptions generally are offered through certain disciplinary and professional lenses that render adaptation in other contexts questionable at best. We examine strengths and weaknesses of commonly used social psychological theories as they relate to individual actions and behaviours with regard to HIV/AIDS prevention and education. We discuss also the role of culture in HIV/AIDS by addressing contextual aspects of culture rather than stressing only individual negative beliefs as is commonly the case. We argue that culture at the contextual level, rather than only individual beliefs, must be located at the center of all health HIV/AIDS prevention endeavours.

Theories and Models of Behaviour Change

Models of behaviour change typically utilized to guide health communication programmes are the same ones used to inform health promotion programmes. Some of the most potent theories and models include the Health Belief Model (HBM), the theory of reasoned action, social learning/cognitive theory, diffusion of innovation, and social marketing. The HBM was developed in the 1950s to predict individual response to, and use of, screening and other preventive health services. Accordingly, the response and use of disease prevention programmes will be predicated on an individual's perceived seriousness of the disease, severity of the disease, perceived advantage of services, and barriers to accessing such service:

In general, the HBM is a rational-cognitive model and assumes a "rational" decision-maker. Most adolescents, and several adults, do not seem to approach the AIDS issue from such a logical perspective, but seem rather capable of discounting risks and optimistically perceiving themselves as invulnerable to harm.

The theory of reasoned action predicts individual behaviour by examining attitudes, beliefs, behavioural intentions, and the observed expressed acts. In this linear progression from attitude to action, a given behaviour will be determined by an individual's intention. This theory also assumes that individuals are rational in their decision-making process, "a presumption that may not be totally relevant for AIDS-related behaviours that are heavily influenced by emotions". Besides, individuals evaluate information that may result in action within external constraints, which are mediated also by power relations in a society.

The social learning/cognitive theory demands that an individual behaviour is the result of the interaction among cognition, behaviour, environment, and physiology. The two primary domains widely used in HIV/AIDS programmes are modeling (imitation of the behaviour of a role model) and self-efficacy (one's perceived ability to adopt a recommended behaviour). Although this model is believed to be very useful in HIV/AIDS communication campaigns in the United States, there remains the question about its importance in cultures where individual decisions are the result of group norms whereby being individualistic is going against the grain. After all, the social learning/cognitive theory is an individual psychological model of behaviour change supports the need to focus on collective efficacy.

Diffusion of innovation focuses on the communication process by which a new idea or product becomes known and utilized by people in a given population. Two relevant principles of diffusion of innovation widely used in AIDS campaigns are generating awareness of HIV and using opinion leaders to influence attitudes and behaviours. "Diffusion of Innovation has been criticized for being too linear, for having a pro-innovation bias, and for widening the gaps between the `information haves' and `have-nots' in a social system. This gap has necessarily been observed in AIDS awareness and knowledge", given the positive correlation between knowledge of HIV and level of education. Despite its limitations, however, the use of opinion leaders in helping to shape culturally appropriate strategies is a component of diffusion of innovation that offers feasibilities in HIV/AIDS communications. This is particularly salient since the content (focusing on a community interpretation of disease meaning rather than an imposed germ theory), context (relationships and negotiation in families and communities), and language (codes of elasticity of usage were relevant) of communication will be a factor in the outcome of HIV/AIDS prevention and care. Soola says (1991) an "African communicator need not bother with the strictly technical aspects of information on AIDS (at least not for some 80 per cent of his audience), because of the non-beneficial effect of such information to a large majority of his audience". Indeed, Green (1999), based on his field work in Africa, has provided an African traditional healing theory of disease that is grounded in culturally defined codes and meaning.

Social marketing is an organized approach to encouraging acceptability of a social idea. Social marketing's four Ps-product, price, place, and promotion - have been applied extensively to HIV/AIDS prevention in condom promotion. A fifth P has recently been added to indicate positioning with regards recognition of competing campaigns on the same subject in the same location. Among the criticisms of social marketing in HIV/AIDS are ethical concerns, given that it sometimes utilizes manipulation, like fear, in promoting condom use. "Fear appeals stress the noxious consequences that will befall message recipients if they fail to adopt the recommendations of the source". Furthermore, it is believed also that social marketing employs a simple solution (such as condom distribution) to a complicated problem without addressing the social conditions that cause the spread of HIV. Social marketing targets individual behaviour only, "consequently reducing public health issues to individual-level problems and defining solutions within `information deficit' models". "How AIDS is discussed, how resources are allocated, who are defined as in the `risk groups,' and who makes the decisions about AIDS highlight the inseparable connection between AIDS and power in society". Regarding to the limitations of social marketing Smith's (1998) evaluation of social marketing denotes that product social marketing has been used widely and praised, whereas comparatively little effort has gone into behaviour social marketing (using social marketing to change and maintain behaviour change) and almost nothing has been done in the sphere of policy social marketing (using social marketing to influence policy to support HIV research and protection of persons living with HIV/AIDS).

The health belief model and other models and theories with identical principles were designed to address health prevention from an individual, linear, and rational perspective. Although these theories and models have proved effective in particular societies for addressing certain diseases, they appear to be inadequate for communicating HIV/AIDS prevention and care messages in Africa, Asia, Latin America, and the Caribbean. In fact the assumptions like individualism as opposed to collectivism) on which these theories and models are based are foreign to several non-Western cultures where these models/theories have been used to guide communication strategies for HIV/AIDS prevention and care. "We should not expect these models to be productive in explaining behaviour in social contexts where commonsense knowledge of the world takes a quite different form".

Theories and Models Applied to HIV/AIDS Prevention Programmes

Theories, models, or frameworks are designed to guide the implementation and evaluation of programmes along particular processes that are believed to yield an expected result. Even though practitioners in the field implement programmes without self-expressed pathways of models and theories, they are still guided by sets of assumptions that form the foundations on which the ideas, funding, and successful result evaluation of such projects are based. In evaluating the continuous reliance of health communication on social psychology, Lievrouw (1994) comments:

While there is no doubt that the social-psychological theory "classics" are appropriate to health communication and that they have been valuable exploratory tools, they nonetheless leave particular premises undisturbed. Chief among these is the presumption that communication in health is mostly a matter of interaction between institution message "sources", (e.g., medical research, professionals, government, foundations) and individual "receivers", (e.g., patients, their families, school children, employees).

Moreover, these theories and models of health behaviour change, such as social learning/cognitive theory and the hierarchy of effects, are based on individual psychology as opposed to family, group, or community locus of decisions. This application of individual and psychological models, in contexts where decision originates from group norms and processes, led to question claims made by researchers with regard to the program impact on behavioural outcomes from exposure to a radio drama on HIV/AIDS education in African countries.

Theories based on the individual, which may be effective and meaningful in a Western context, have lesser importance in self-effecting cultures of Asia, Africa, Latin America, and the Caribbean. In these regions, family and community are more potent to the construction of health and well-being than the individual, even though the individual is always identified as an important part of the cultural context. In these cultures, individuals are less likely also to express themselves and less likely to articulate their level of well-being from the standpoint of "ego" (the "I"). It is the state of well-being of family and community that regulates how individuals measure their state of health. Besides, theories and models based on measuring how the individual feels about himself or herself (e.g., "I feel good about myself") could never capture the health locus of control in various societies because such control rests somewhere outside the self. Within this self-effacing construct, individuals are not always habitual to expressing their attitudes and beliefs by utilizing extreme descriptors often found on social science survey instruments such as "strongly agree" or "strongly disagree". In fact, to do so within such a cultural context is considered disrespectful. Yet instruments designed to measure health behaviour, for example, self-efficacy, generally are presented on such a continuum of two extremes (strongly agree to strongly disagree) in cultures where such measures are not only irrelevant but could also be considered offensive. To capture the complexity of the context within which an individual is a part, one requires a framework that underscores the component of context that features culture as a central and organizing theme.

The professional and cultural partiality of the Westernized view to the understanding of self renders problematic findings from much social and behavioural science research in Africa, Asia, Latin American, and the Caribbean. For instance, one can appreciate differences between individual-centred versus family- and community-centered cultures by examining cultural differences in daily salutations. Greetings like, "How are you doing today?" may elicit a range of self-assured responses that captures how a Westerner actually feels on a given day—from "I'm well" to "Great" and "Wonderful". The same greeting among the Yorubas or Edos of Nigeria almost never elicits a state of being "Great" or "Wonderful" even if this is how the individual feels. Instead, a common, non-definite response is "O.K.," "Fine," or "We give thanks to the Almighty." Furthermore, such a response is consistent with cultural importance and meanings that promote and reward a tempered expression about one's well-being. The corpus of social psychology is based on the behaviours of people in Western cultures. According to Triandis (1994), culture is the man-made part of the environment; therefore, culture is a group's efforts to control its environment. Thus, the relationship between the individual and her or his environment is unidirectional with the individual always shaping the environment and never the reverse.

As a consequence, measures of skill acquisition and self-determination are based on the individual's perception of his or her ability to control his or her environment. Thus, controlling one's environment is a potent theme in Western conceptions of culture - a conception that eschews other cultural realities such as harmonizing with nature or adapting to one's environment or both. If controlling the environment is the raison d'etre of cultures, then the inability to control one's environment suggests retrogression, an obstacle to be overcome. Hence, "cultural barriers" (never cultural strength) become a common expression in this discourse.

Applied to health communication, limitations easily become self-evident. For instance, the cultural complexities of adhering to media messages about Sexually Transmitted Diseases (STDs) are seldom interrogated. The call for sexual negotiation at the point of initial contact between two people who are about to begin sexual relations contradicts most culturally sanctioned behaviour. Two people who are about to begin sexual relations typically avoid discussing their sexual past until they are more comfortable with each other at which point sexual intercourse commonly has occurred. In this case sexual behaviours precedes sexual knowledge, atleast in the context of relationship, which is generally the basis for most interventions on preventing HIV/AIDS. This reality of "behaviour first" renders the linear model of knowledge leading to attitude and behaviour counterintuitive in the context of relationships and culture.

Cultural Contexts and HIV/AIDS

Culture, generally appropriated as an exotic collective, is believed by many to exist only in Africa, Asia, and Latin America and in their descendants in the diaspora. According to Yoder

(1997), beliefs are used generally as a proxy for culture, such that beliefs and knowledge of illness become the focus of "culturally appropriate" messages and interventions. In fact, the term *belief* is often contrasted with knowledge such that "belief is used on denote ideas that are erroneous from the perspective of bio-medicine and that constitute obstacles to appropriate behaviour". Therefore, when "culture" and "belief" are coupled as in cultural belief, the resulting negative biomedical appropriation of the term becomes evident. As a result, culture is objectified and believed to be possessed by non-Western people, only identifiable through research. An instance, of this is found "in health education campaigns that seek information about local idioms of expression to better communicate health messages". As a consequence, it is reasoned that individual practices or behaviours found in these groups could be labeled cultural and often appropriated as a barrier. Thus, "barrier" often becomes the coupling metaphor with culture.

There are three vital themes that characterize perceptions about these notions of culture. First, culture is a *fossilized historical artifact*, which leads to such definitions as "culture is to a society what memory is to individual" (Kluckhohn, 1954). Second, culture is the observable aspect of individual behaviour that is understood better by locating behaviours (particularly those that are unfamiliar) within individual beliefs. Such beliefs are differentiated from knowledge since the Knowledge Attitude Practice Behaviour (KAPB) model places these domains in separate locations on a parallel continuum. In fact, belief and knowledge are thus constructed as a binarism and belief invariably becomes, a code for culture an obstacle that must be overcome. For instance, if you learned from your grandmother that chicken soup is good for your common cold, it is a "cultural belief". However, if you were to learn the same health information from a physician, it is "knowledge". A third theme is that culture is people's ability to *control/dominate* their environment. Thus, the onus of responsibility for adopting requisite behaviour rests in the individual. The assumption is that everyone desires to, and is capable of, changing their environment to suit their requirements. Each of these domains is an aspect of culture.

In the view of some scholars, culture is what society develops from in the process of development - a proxy for modernization. Modernization and culture are located often at two opposite ends of the spectrum. Given this impoverished notion of culture, "it appears urgent that we concentrate on studies of the distribution of meaning in social space, and on searching social sources of diversity and heterogeneity rather than focusing exclusively on cultural sharing, uniformity, and homogeneity".

Western cultures, to varying degrees, tend to view the self as a production of the individual, whereas various other cultures view the self as a production of the family, community, and other environmental influences for which we do not have, nor with, total control. Crawford believes "the heart of the cultural politics of AIDS is a contestation over the meaning of the self". A large part of this contestation includes the definition and construction of people with AIDS and those who have tested positive for HIV as "other". In its most basic sense, health is related to those who are not infected with HIV and illness with those who are infected with HIV. "The identity signified by HIV/AIDS comes to be seen as the other who is perceived not only as a physical danger, but as an equally threatening and dangerous identity".

The cultural politics of AIDS has caused the mobilization of several of these facets of culture with varying degrees of success. The mobilization of ethnographers to study these same risk groups has served a reductive function related to how culture is understood and conceptualized. "Despite their intention to break with the dominant public health models, most anthropologists are not really interested to distance themselves from the methodology and theorizing of what is perceived as 'real' science in public health". This problem is evident in the tendency to create epidemiological categories, thus reducing culture to recognitions of negative individual health practices in a subgroup of the population later generalized to be the definition of the larger group's culture.

In the literature dealing with cultural sensitivity, it is rare to see "strength" coupled with the concept of culture, although "cultural barrier" is commonly described as a reason for failure in public health and health promotion and communications programmes. For example, some health communication and health promotion programmes implemented in Africa have tended to undervalue the significance of oral communication as a genre. This practice is consistent with the academics' exaltation of written and visual modes of communication (slides and transparencies) as the only acceptable standard. For instance, traditional communication channels, which Ugboaja (1987) terms 'Oramedia', continue to maintain their potency in rural Africa.

We do believe and do support, as have others, that cultural sensitivity be central to health communication and health promotion theory and practice. This position is evident in cultural models such as PEN-3, a model practised in health promotion and disease prevention. In this model, cultural appropriateness in health promotion refers not only to the individual but also to the context that nurtures the individual and his or her family and community. This context is evaluated for attributes that are positive, existential, and negative. It is potent to promote the positive, recognize and affirm the existential, and contextualize the negative, such that opportunity costs and advantages for change are understood and appreciated. Regarding communication strategies for HIV prevention within the African context, for example, message segmentation is critical to reaching a population with a diverse mode of producing and acquiring information and knowledge:

In traditional societies, which most African societies are, the requirement for audience, message, and channel segmentation is important, considering the reach and influence of the various channels of communication and the absorptive capacity of the different segments of the population.

Conclusion

This examination of theories and models commonly used in health communication and promotion explicitly shows that HIV/AIDS communication often is based on the behaviour and decision-making process of so-called rational individuals who follow an established linear path from awareness to attitude to action. However, decisions about preventing HIV/AIDS are based on cultural norms that generally mediate individual decisions in ways that individuals may not always percept. Moreover, decisions about HIV/AIDS generally are based on emotion and thus may not follow any preestablished pattern of decision making advanced in most of the theories and models.

In an extensive review of the literature on theories and AIDS campaigns, Freimuth (1992) concluded that knowledge is not a sufficient condition for behaviour change. "Our analysis of survey data *rarely* [emphasis ours] found a close correspondence between changes in knowledge and changes in behaviour". Most theories offer approaches to initiating behaviour change but do not address maintainance of the new changed behaviour. Campaign planners need a greater understanding of their "target audience," which generally belongs to a culture and a social class different from theirs. Since the target population often is at a greater disadvantage related to the privileged location of professional researchers' income and level of education, the interventionist must be cautious about the imposition of foreign values on a group of people.

Cognizance must be paid also to the complementary forces of endogenous (within) and exogenous (outside) influences in setting the media agenda. Most theories used to inform campaign strategies do not comprise culture as a central concept. When they do, culture is treated as a "set of beliefs, values, and individual goals that pattern behaviour". Culture should become a pivotal domain in the new era of HIV/AIDS prevention and care. "Culture should be a central organizing concept in developing programmes of HIV education and assessing their outcomes". By culture we mean drawing from the potentiating feasibilities of a hybrid of traditional and modern culture. In the context of community development, Escobar (1995) argues that no longer should we focus on futile attempts at becoming modern by substituting the traditional but quite on a "hybrid modernity characterized by continuous attempts at renovation, by a multiplicity of groups taking the multitemporal heterogeneity peculiar to each sector and country". In Escobar's view, "traditional cultures" do not have to succumb to opinion of "development" and "modernity" but engage them in a constant relationship whereby the resulting hybrid communities can emerge with feasibilties for improving conditions of life whether it is HIV/AIDS prevention or community development.

With new challenges, such as a false sense of security generated by the prospect of a cure and hope for vaccine in the global endeavours to control HIV/AIDS, it becomes even more critical that we pay serious attention to contextual rather than individual theories and models that inform HIV prevention messages. Moreover, it is vital to understand the centrality of cultural contexts, rather than simply individual beliefs, in planning communication strategies. In the final analysis, media are a part of our culture and even more so in the definition and construction of what is considered to be media, which comprises folklore, storytelling, and the several nonstructural but established oral channels for transmission and confirmation of messages within communities. As we begin this new millennium, a new global communication strategy is timely. Such strategy should locate culture within a theoretical framework that will permit the flexibility for regional and national differences in communicating HIV/AIDS prevention and care messages.

References

Airhihenbuwa, C. (1995). *Health and culture: Beyond the Western paradigm*. Thousand Oaks, CA: Sage.

Airhihenbuwa, C.O., DiClemente, R.J., Wingood, G.M., Lowe, A. (1992). *HIV/AIDS education and prevention among African-Americans: A focus on culture*. AIDS Education and Prevention, 4(3), 267-276.

Bandura, A. (1986). *Social foundations of thought and action: A social cognitive theory*. Englewood Cliffs, NJ: Prentice-Hall.

Becker, M. H. (1974). The health belief model and personal health behaviour. *Health Education Monographs*. 2, 324-508.

Bibeau, G. (1997). At work in the fields of public Health: The abuse of rationality. *Medical Anthropology Quarterly*, 11(2), 246-255.

Bird, S E. (1996). CJ's revenge: Media, folklore, and the cultural construction of AIDS. *Critical Studies in Mass Communication*, 13, 44-58.

Crawford, R. (1994). The boundaries of the self and the unhealthy other: Reflections on health, culture, and AIDS. *Soc. Sci. Med.*, 38(10), 1347-1365.

Dearing, J. W., & Rogers, E. M. (1992). AIDs and the media agenda. In T. Edgar, M. A. Fitzpatrick, & V. S. Freimuth (Eds.), *AIDS: A communication perspective* (pp. 173-194), Hillsdale, NJ: Erlbaum.

Dillard, J. P., Plotnick, C. A., Godbold, L. C., Freimuth, V. S., & Edgar, T. (1996). The multiple affective outcomes of AIDS PSAs: Fear appeals do more than scare people. *Communication Research*. 23(1), 44-72.

Edgar, T., Fitzpatrick, M. A., & Freimuth, V. S. (Eds.). (1992). In *AIDS: communication perspective*. Hillsdale, NJ: Erlbaum.

Erwin. D.O., & Spatz. T.S. (1996). *An implementation guide for the witness project: A culturally sensitive, Community-based cancer education programme for African American women.* Linda Deloney (Ed.). Little Rock, AR: Arkansas Cancer Research Center, University of Arkansas Medical Sciences.

Escobar, A. (1995). *Encountering development: The making and unmaking of the third world Princeton,* NJ: Princeton University Press.

Freimuth, V.S. (1992). Theoretical foundations of AIDS media campaigns. In T. Edgar, M. A. Fitzpatrick, & V. S. Freimuth (Eds.), AIDS: *A communication perspective* (pp. 91-110). Hillsdale, NJ: Erlbaum.

Glanz, K., & Rimer, G.K. (1995). *Theory at a glance. A guide for health promotion practice.* Washington, DC: U.S. Department of Health and Human Services, PHS, NIH.

Good, B.J. (1994). *Medicine, rationality, and experience.* Cambridge: Cambridge University Press.

Green, E. C. (1999). *Indigenous theories of contagious disease.* Thousand Oaks, CA: AltaMira.

Green, L.W. & K Reuter, M.H., (1999). *Health promotion planning: An educational and ecological approach* (3rd ed.). Mountain view, CA: Mayfield.

Guttman, N. (1997a). Beyond strategic research: A value-centered approach to health communication interventions. *Communication Theory,* 7(2), 95-124.

Guttman, N. (1997b). Ethical dilemmas in health campaigns. *Health Communication,* 9(2), 155-190.

Jaccard, J., Turrisi, R., & Wan, C.K. (1990). Implications of behavioural decision theory and social marketing for designing social action programmes. In J. Edwards, R.S. Tindale, L. Health, E.J. Posavac (Eds.), *Social influence process and prevention* (pp. 103-142). New York: Plenum.

Janz, N.C., Zimmerman, M.A., Wren, P.A., Israel, B.A., Freudenberg, N., & Carter, R.J. (1996). Evaluation of 37 AIDS prevention projects: Successful approaches an barriers to programme effectiveness. *Health Education Quarterly,* 23(1), 80-97.

Kline, M.V. (1999). Planning health promotion and disease prevention programmes in multicultural populations. In R. M. Huff & M. V. Kline (Eds.), *Promoting health multicultural populations: A handbook for practitioners* (pp. 73-102). Thousand Oaks, CA: Sage. Kluckhohn, C. (1954). Culture and behaviour. In G. Lindzey (Ed.), *Handbook of social psychology* (vol. 2, pp. 921-976). Cambridge, MA: Addison-Wesley.

Lievrouw, L.A. (1994). Health communication research reconsidered: Reading the signs [A review essay]. *Journal of Communication,* 44(1), 91-99.

Lupton, D. (1994). *Medicine as culture. Illness, disease and the body in Western societies.* London: Sage.

Maibach, E., & Flora, J.A. (1993). Symbolic modeling and cognitive rehearsal: Using video to promote AIDS prevention self-efficacy. *Communication Research,* 20(4), 517-545.

McAllister, M.P. (1992). AIDS, medicalization, and the news media. In T. Edgar, M.A. Fitzpatrick, & V.S. Freimuth (Eds.), AIDS: *A communication perspective* (pp. 195-221). Hillsdale, NJ: Erlbaum.

Michal-Johnson, P., Bowen, S.P. (1992). The place of culture in HIV education. In T. Edgar, M.A. Fitzpatrick, & V.S. Freimuth (Eds.), AIDS: A communication perspective (pp. 147-172), Hillsdale, NJ: Erlbaum.

Paskett, E.D., Tatum, C.M., D'Agostino, R. Jr., Rushing, J., Velez, R., Michielutte, R., & Dignan, M. (1999). Community-based interventions to improve breast and cervical cancer screening: Results of the Forsyth County Cancer Screening (FaCaS) Project. *Cancer Epidemiology, Biomarkers & Prevention*, 8, 453-459.

Pelto. P.J., & Pelto, G.H. (1997). Studying knowledge, culture, and behaviour in applied medical anthropology. Medical Anthropology Quarterly, 11(2), 147-163.

Pliskin, K.L. (1997). Verbal intercourse and sexual communication: Impediments to STD prevention. *Medical Anthropology Quarterly*, 11(1), 89-109.

Rogers, E.M. (1983). *Diffusion of innovations* (3rd ed.). New York: Free Press.

Rogers, E.M. (1995). *Diffusion of innovations* (4th ed.). New York: Free Press.

Schoepf, B.G. (1991). Ethical, methodological and political issues of AIDS research in Central Africa. Soc. Sci. Med., 33(7), 747-763.

Seidel, G.(1993). The competing discourse of HIV/AIDS in Sub-Saharan Africa: Discourses of rights and empowerment vs discourses of control and exclusion. *Soc. Sci. Med.*, 36(3), 175-194.

Smith, W. (1998). Social marketing: Three approaches to HIV/AIDS prevention. Paper presented at the Fogarty Workshop on International HIV/AIDS Prevention Research Opportunities, San Francisco. April 18.

Soola, E.O. (1991). Communication and education as vaccine against the spread of Acquired Immune Deficiency Syndrome (AIDS) in Africa. *Africa Media Review*, 5(3), 33-40.

Sue, S. (1994). Instrumentation, measurement and evaluation strategies. Paper presented at the implications of cultural values, beliefs, and norms for health research: A methods conference. University of Milwaukee, Milwaukee. September 26-28.

Triandis, H.C. (1994). *Culture and social behaviour*. New York: McGraw-Hill.

Yoder, P.S. (1997). Negotiating relevance: Belief, knowledge, and practice in international health projects. *Medical Anthropology Quarterly*, 11(2), 131-146.

Yoder, P.S., Hornik, R., & Chirwa, B.C. (1996). Evaluating the programme effects of a radio drama about AIDS in Zambia. *Studies in Family Planning*, 27(4), 188-203.

Fourteen

Toward a New Communications Framework for HIV/AIDS

UNAIDS and the Future of Communications for HIV

Between 1997 and 1999, 103 researchers and practitioners were invited to take participation in two global (Geneva and Washington, DC) and three regional (Abidjan for Africa, Bangkok for Asia, and Santo Domingo for Latin America and the Caribbean) consultative meetings. A mixed group of practitioners and scholars in communication and behavioural sciences represented Africa, Asia, Latin America and the Caribbean as well as North America and Europe. Meetings were designed to review past and current approaches to HIV/AIDS communications and behaviour change and propose new directions that will accommodate a global and regional framework yet remain flexible enough for adaptation by countries and organizations. This effort involved synthesis of experiences from Latin America and the Caribbean, Africa, and Asia at consultative workshops through a participatory process, guided by inputs to experts on the methodology and outcomes. As indicated earlier, five domains were identified, by consensus as critical factors in the physical and social environment that influence health behaviours related to prevention, care, and support. These domains are crucial to effectiveness of HIV/AIDS communication programmes since they permeate and affect decision making in the context of HIV/AIDS. The discussions on regional issues also led to the identification of specific domains that have particular relevance to each region. For instance, in Latin America and the Caribbean the framework should emphasize advocacy as a crucial component, whereas in Africa community involvement was seen as fundamental.

Context as a Focus for a New Framework

The limitation of focusing on the individual at the exclusion of the context has long been a concern for leading research organizations. The Institute of Medicine (1994) in the United Sates raised this concern in its report on the future of preventive intervention research. Similarly, the Rockefeller Foundation sounded a call for a paradigm shift in its report on communication for social change (1999). Increasingly, researchers are questioning the serious methodological limitations in focusing on individuals to change their health behaviour without adequate attention to social and physical environmental factors that shape individual roles and expectations and thus their health behaviour. Thus, the identification of the five contextual domains is quite consistent with the call by institutions, scholars, and practitioners to develop a new direction for disease prevention.

Participants acknowledged that the individual is a crucial part of the context and that the new framework should recognize the role of the individual even though it is focusing on the context. To this extent, the new framework could draw on salient elements of existing theories and models. For example, the use of opinion leaders, a major component of diffusion of innovations, could be incorporated at the operational level by regions, countries, and communities as deemed appropriate. Such flexibility is a major feature of the new framework recognizing differences in cultures and locations. A discussion of the characteristics of each domain of the contextual framework follows.

The framework (UNAIDS/Penn State, 1999) is represented as a house whose structure varies in conformity with regions and countries. Every house has a foundation, a roof and a body designed to respond to the conditions in the environment — the context. In the new HIV/ADS communications framework, the five domains are represented in the foundation, the roof, and the body of the house depending on the goals, objectives, and strategies that will be employed in a given communications programme. For instance, communication programmes for condom availability and use by clients of commercial sex workers may locate the government at the roof in terms of policy to mandate 100 per cent availability and use of condoms. At the same time, gender can be located at the foundation to address the role and societal expectation of women in sexual negotiation while carefully examining the interrelatedness of other contextual domains - culture, SES, and religion. On the other hand, the reported inability to translate public awareness into positive health behaviour may necessitate locating the government at the roof. This will be crucial related to political interest to invest in varied strategies to focus on different population subgroups while locating culture at the foundation in terms of utilizing known aspects of learning processes within the culture to move families and communities from awareness to behaviour change. In this latter example, the role of gender, SES, and religion will be examined in determining proper strategy.

Finally, as one would expect in any house, there should be doors for entry and exit. In this framework, the double door will have the key issues and processes for implementing a strategy on one panel and the key steps and processes for evaluation on the other panel. The windows will offer opportunity for every region and country to address their certain conditions consistent with the stage of the epidemic in their context.

Government and Policy

Governmental policy and law play a critical role in programmes intended to controlling the spread of HIV/AIDS. Diop, in this volume, demonstrated how government action in Senegal has been a major factor in keeping the epidemic under control. Phoolcharoen (1998) reports how early government intervention at the policy level became a potent factor in the successful response of Thailand to the HIV/AIDS epidemic. The government quickly introduced legislation that supported Non-Governmental Organizations (NGOs) and community organizations' prevention endeavours. Similarly, Maadra and Ruranga-Rubaramira (1998) have pointed out that in Uganda "the openness of the government has created a conducive environment for interested agencies and organizations working in HIV/AIDS activities to work together". This attitude, coupled with political will on behalf of government officials, is highlighted as an important element in the Ugandan efforts to control the epidemic.

Government policy can either promote or hinder efforts at reaching the goals of HIV/AIDS communications programmes. Yet, as Deane says (1997) the reality is that public debate on HIV/AIDS issues remains, in many countries, too often poorly informed, sensationalist, and damaging to HIV/AIDS prevention. There are ethical, legal, and financial considerations that must be taken into consideration when discussing and planning communications programming to address these issues. Some of these challenges could be met by working through regional organizations such as Economic Community of West African States (ECOWAS), Southern African Development Community (SADC), Association of South East Asian Nations (ASEAN), Organization of American States (OAS), Caribbean Community and Common Market (CARICOM), and Central American Common Market (CACM), which can provide important channels for addressing some regional issues relating to HIV/AIDS. Some of the critical issues identified in this domain are as follows.

Agenda Setting

Role of government in setting the media agenda and how HIV/AIDS fits into it should be a part of the initial information gathering and analysis.

Image Management

Issues of tourism, migration, violence, and rape of women by military men require government support for adequate solution.

Collaboration

An important role of government is fostering inter-regional and intra-regional collaboration in HIV/AIDS programmes such as sharing lessons learned within and between regions and facilitating cross-border interventions.

SES

Economic status is an individual, group, and governmental factor in terms of adequate supply and consistent use of condoms as well as affordability of combination drug therapy in places where they are available. The contribution by Melkote, Muppidi, and Goswami in this volume discusses various studies and reports that have dealt with SES and various aspects related to AIDS in the developing world. Women with lower income and education report lower knowledge about HIV transmission and more misconceptions about AIDS. In fact, perception of risk was almost nonexistent among this impoverished population. Thus, socio-economic context is a crucial domain to be examined in communication strategies for HIV/AIDS. Furthermore, studies have shown that the commonly used criteria for SES (occupation, income, and education) do not reflect how the context differentiates between two individuals who share these characteristics. For example, two individuals earning the same salary may have different family obligations. For instance, a first-generation middle-class person tends to be financially responsible for more family members than a fourth-generation middle-class person. Higher education, income, and occupation may not equally leverage a woman's ability to negotiate the sexual behaviour of her partner. The following are key issues related to SES that must be considered in the framework.

Issues of Affordability

Affordability is a crucial indicator of SES, especially in clinical interventions such as combination drug therapy and technological interventions such as condoms. Many governments and most individuals cannot afford combination drug therapy even if it were available.

Compliance and Adherence

Even if the combination drug therapy is available, the potential difficulty with compliance and adherence makes preventive messages even more crucial. This is particularly salient for sustainability of behavioural outcome beyond the end of a planned intervention.

A Social and Developmental Problem

HIV/AIDS should be considered a developmental and a social problem. As a result the pandemic should be addressed within the context of other social and development problems in the regions relative to allocation and distribution of resources. Given that HIV/AIDS is a developmental problem, issues of accessibility of health care in general must be analyzed within a given context and the result incorporated into the planing of HIV/AIDS communications for media and interpersonal communications.

Culture

Culture refers to a collective consciousness of a people often shaped by a shared history, language, and psychology. As the contribution by Airhihenbuwa and Obregon in this volume indicates, culture is too often appropriated as a static and unchanging set of codes and meanings. Armed with a list of negative individual health beliefs and practices, the conclusion inevitably leads to blaming those beliefs and calling them cultural barriers. Western cultures, to varying degrees, tend to view the self as a production of the individual, whereas several other cultures view the self as a production of the family, community, and other environmental influences for which we do not have, or desire, total control. The following basic issues related to culture were considered in the framework.

Language Elasticity

This means differences in rules and codes of languages. Whereas some languages may be rigid and linear in their application, others are elastic and robust. A linear and rigid rule in cultural production (as in classical music) should not be implemented to an elastic and robust cultural production (as in jazz or calypso). By the same token, that a language is elastic does not suggest that such language dearth direction, nor does it imply that the rules are simple and easily understood.

Relationships within the Family and Community

This should be explored especially in the context of making decisions about adoption of preventive health behaviour and caring for the ill. The centrality of family and community rather than the individual in decision making must be taken into account. That is, the focus must be on group and family more than just on the individual. In fact, individual beliefs do not importantly explain the cultural context even though such beliefs may be a part of the culture. It is critical to understand who the caregivers are and their role in a culture. For instance, the use of home-based care in various cultures requires a systematic and regular information update to improve patient management and support.

Gender

Gender has been increasingly identified as one of the key dimensions in efforts aimed at transforming and improving the lives of huge numbers of people and around the world. Mendoza gives a comprehensive definition of gender:

Gender is what it means to be a male or a female and how that defines a person's opportunities, role, liabilities and relationships. Gender is a socio-cultural variable and refers to the roles, behaviour, and personal recognizes that the society or culture proscribes as proper for women and men. These attributes, opportunities, and relationships are socially constructed and learnt through socialization processes. Gender roles vary across determinants like race, culture, community, time, ethnicity, occupation, age, level of education. While sex is biological, gender is socially defined.

In HIV/AIDS communication gender plays a potent role in defining how programmes respond to the needs of both men and women. This implies creating supportive environments that would allow males and females to have proper means of protection against the disease as well as access to care and support when infected. For example, numerous HIV/AIDS prevention programmes have been carried out with a gender-based approach. However, a closer look suggests some basic problemmes that hinder women's equal chances of benefiting from these programmes. Mendoza (1997) argues that these programmes are concerned to gender roles in a society and include sexual norms that limit women's access to information by implying that they must be ignorant about sexual matters. Also, women's economic dependence on men, violence against women, and widespread acceptance of male promiscuity have worked against women's chances of protection against the disease. For example, in Zimbabwe, Kenya, South Africa, and Zaire, the enhancing financial insecurity that exists among a large number of female-headed households make transactional sex a "rational means of making ends meet".

Researchers and practitioners convened by UNAIDS agreed that besides suggestions made at recent international conferences on population and women issues, HIV/AIDS communication must take into consideration other dimensions. The following are key issues related to gender considered in the framework.

Male/Female Relationships

Attention should be paid to the roles and responsibilities of men and women, to sociocultural factors, and to how these factors affect their relationship. There must be recognition that in addressing gender, we are referring to not only women but also to men. It is critical to deem gender roles and the relations of power and negotiation within and between those roles.

Stereotyping

Communication materials should be formed to eliminate negative stereotypes of women and, on the contrary, used to promote positive images of women. Gender equity might be enhanced through reduction of negative stereotypes of men and women, which may influence ways and modes HIV is or has been spreading in the community.

Inclusiveness of Women in Planning

Needs assessment must have a gender analysis component. Gender issues should be taken into consideration not only at the beginning stage of planning a communication programme but also through implementation and evaluation of those programmes. In communication programmes for young people, be it formal or informal education, it is vital to take into account that both boys and girls are being targeted, as opposed to targeting a mass of young people only.

Spirituality

Spirituality is a much broader and a more inclusive concept than religion even though the two terms are often used interchangeably. According to Relv (1997).

Spirituality encompasses hope; faith; self-transcendence; a will or desire to live; the recognization of meaning, purpose and fulfilment in life; the recognition of mortality; a relationship with a "higher power," "higher being" or "ultimate," and the maintenance of interpersonal and intrapersonal relationships.

Proof from HIV/AIDS literature shows that there is a relation between spirituality and HIV/AIDS. This and the increasing urgency of the epidemic has encouraged the World Council of Churches' Executive Committee (1997) to issue a challenge to all churches to respond to the urgent call for actions resulting from the spread of HIV/AIDS worldwide. Spirituality encompasses faiths and value systems that range from organized religion to individual or collective values or both whose faith represent a guiding principle on which meanings are based. Spirituality is grounded in the belief that there is a supernatural being/force that regulates the interaction of living beings with their visible and non-visible environment. The scientific literature has given increased attention to the connection between spirituality and positive health behaviour. This link has always been known to exist among traditional healers whose healing modality is in part based on the belief in the power of supernatural forces to regulate human behaviour. The following are key issues related to spirituality to be considered in the framework.

Leadership Initiatives

Leaders of the different religious organizations have potent roles to play in HIV/AIDS prevention and care. At the very least, they can appeal to the moral conscience of their followers. Most importantly, they can provide a supportive environment for persons and families of persons living with HIV/AIDS.

Tolerance

One cannot assume that religion is a obstacle and that tenets are the same in all countries. For example, Senegal is 95 per cent

Muslim, and yet condom use seems to be readily accepted in the country, if the current high level of distribution and consumption serves as an indication.

Mind and Body

Traditional healers should be involved in planning of programmes where feasible.

Conclusion

The long-term solution to bridging clandestine and material inequity lies in structural reforms that change the manner in which resources are distributed in society. However, such transformations cannot be achieved in a short period of time. In the context of HIV/AIDS, short and medium-term solutions are required to alleviate the impact of AIDS along with long-term change strategies. The contextual domains present some challenges to be addressed since they do not lend themselves to linear intervention strategies directed to solving a problem without focusing on the causes. In fact, several of the relative success stories reported to date can be attributed to a focus on one or more of the five contextual domains identified. A focus on context not only addresses the physical and social environment, it also identifies the importance of bringing a project to scale rather than perpetuating pilot projects only that focus on individual behaviour. As the contributions in this volume show, countries are reporting success in their collective attempts to address HIV/AIDS through a focus on government policy (Diop), SES (Melkote, Muppidi & Goswami), culture (Airhihenbuwa & Obregon; Diop), gender (Esu-Williams; Melkote et al.) and spirituality (Diop). Peter Piot, executive director of UNAIDS, has called for social vaccines to aggressively control HIV/AIDS. These social vaccines comprise promoting continuation of mass education about HIV/AIDS prevention, 100 per cent condom policy, nondiscrimination against persons living with HIV/AIDS, and a protective environment for disclosure. Achieving these important aims will require collective efforts at different levels. The new UNAIDS framework offers an opportunity to meet these challenges.

References

Airhihenbuwa, C.O. (1999). Of culture and multiverse: renouncing "the universal truth" in health. *Journal of Health Education*, 30(3), 267-273.

Deane, J. (1997). *Surrendering the agenda: The future of HIV/AIDS communications*. Paper presented at the UNAIDS Consultation Meeting on Communications Programming, Geneva, Switzerland. November 7-11.

Fogarty Workshop on International HIV/AIDS Prevention Research Opportunities. (1998). University of California, San Francisco (UCSF) AIDS Research Institute, San Franciso, CA, April 17-20.

Gill, H., & Mohammed. S. (1994). Factors affecting control of AIDS in Nigeria. *International Conference on AIDS*, 10(2), 252 (abstract no. PC0371), August 7-12.

Gray, J. (1997). Spiritual pespective on social support in women with HIV infection: Pilot study. Image: *The Journal of Nursing Scholarship*, 29(1), 97.

Institute of Medicine. (1994). Reducing risks for mental disorders: Frontier for preventive intervention research. In P. J. Mrazek & R. J. Haggerty (Eds.); Washington, DC: National Academy Press.

Kelly, J.A. (1999). Community-level interventions are needed to prevent new HIV infections. American Journal of Public Health, 89(3), 299-301.

King, G. & Williams, D.R. (1995). Race and Health: A multidimensional approach to African-American health. In Amick, Levine, Tarlov, & Walsh (Eds.), *Society and Health*. Oxford: Oxford University Press.

Maadra, E., & Ruranga-Rubaramira, M. (1998). *Experience from Uganda, in UNAIDS: Partners in prevention: International case studies of effective health promotion practice in HIV/AIDS*. Geneva, Switzerland: UNAIDS.

Makinwa, B. (1997). *Communications programming and emerging challenges: Treatment drugs, vaccine trials, and rapidly changing science*. Paper presented at the UNAIDS Consultation Meeting on Communications Programming, Geneva, Switzerland. November 7-11.

McKinlay, J. B., & Marceau, L.D. (1999). A tale of 3 tails. *American Journal of Public Health*, 89(3), 295-301.

Mendoza, A.M. (1997). *Bridging information towards transformation: Can it work?* Paper presented at the UNAIDS Consultation Meeting on Communications Programming. Geneva, Switzerland. November 7-11.

Phoolcharoen, W. (1998). *Experience from Thailand*, in *UNAIDS: Partners in prevention: International case studies of effective health promotion practice in HIV/AIDS. Geneva, Switzerland:* UNAIDS.

Relv, M.V. (1997). Illuminating meaning and transforming issues of spirituality in HIV disease and AIDS: An application of Parse's theory of human becoming. *Holistic Nursing Practice*, 12(1), 1-8.

Rockefeller Foundation. (1999). *Communication for social change* [A position paper and conference report]. New York: Author.

Social Science Medicine (1993). Reassessing priorities: Identifying the determinants of HIV transmission [Editorial]. *Social Science Medicine*, 36(4), iii-viii.

Ugboajah, F. (1985). Oramedia in Africa. In Ugboaja (Ed.), *Mass Communication, Culture, and Society in West Africa*. New York: Hans Zell.

UNAIDS. (1999). *AIDS epidemic update*: December 1999 Geneva, Switzerland: UNAIDS/WHO.

UNAIDS/Penn State. (1999). Communications Framework for HIV/AIDS: A New Direction. *A UNAIDS/Penn State Project*. C.O. Airhihenbuwa, B. Makinwa, M. Firth, R. Obregon (Eds.). Geneva: UNAIDS.

World Bank. (1997). *Confronting AIDS: Public priorities in global epidemic*. New York: Oxford University Press.

World Council of Churches Executive Committee. (1997). *The impact of HIV/AIDS and the churches' response. Facing AIDS. The challenge, the Council's response. Geneva*: WCC Publications.

TABLE 1
OVERVIEW OF MOST FREQUENTLY USED THEORIES OF HUMAN BEHAVIOUR

Level	*Theory or Model*	*Behavioural Determinants*	*Examples of Programme Application*
Individual Level	**Health Belief Model**	Perceived susceptibility	Increase level of risk perception
		Perceived severity	Influence beliefs of severity
		Perceived benefits and barriers	Assess and influence beliefs about benefits/barriers of changing behaviour
		Cues to action	
	Theory of Reasoned Action*	Attitudes	Assess and influence attitudes
		Subjective norms	Assess and influence norms in the social group
		Behavioural intentions	Assess and influence behavioural intentions
	Social Cognitive Theory	Outcome expectancies	Sexual communication, need for social support to reinforce behaviour change
	Social Learning Theory	Self-efficacy	Modeling of safer behaviours
	Stages of Change	Precontemplative	Assess and influence outcome expectations and norms, perceived risk
		Contemplative	Assess and influence self-efficacy, intention
		Preparation	Assess and influence self-efficacy, intentions and outcome expectations
		Action	Assess and influence outcome expectations and norms
		Maintenance	Assess and influence norms, self-efficacy

(Contd.)

(Contd.)

Level	*Theory or Model*	*Behavioural Determinants*	*Examples of Programme Application*
	AIDS Risk Reduction Model	Labelling	Assess and influence risk perception, aversive emotions and knowledge
		Commitment	Assess and influence perceptions of enjoyment, self-efficacy and risk reduction
		Enactment and maintenance	Assess and influence communication, informal networking, formal help-seeking
Social and community level	**Diffusion of Innovation**	Change agent	Who are the influential people in the community
		Communication channels	Most effective means to spread information including community leaders
		Context	Assess type of social networks in community
	Social Influences	Context of social interactions	Equip young people with social skills including peer pressure resistance skills
		Social norms	Assess and influence social norms
		Social rewards and punishments	
	Social Network Theory	Social networks	Assess composition of social network
		Social support	Assess, build up social support

(Contd.)

Level	*Theory or Model*	*Behavioural Determinants*	*Examples of Programme Application*
	Theory of Gender and Power	Social sexual norms and power dynamics	Address social structure of gender relations
	Empowerment	Community organization Community building	Assess community priorities Assess key activities of the community and facilitate alliance building
	Social-Ecological Model for Health Promotion	Intra-personal (knowledge, attitudes, perception of risk) Social, organizational, cultural (social networks) Political factors (regulation)	Increase in knowledge, skills development, influence risk perception Community organizing, mass media Advocacy
	Socio-economic and Environmental Factors	Policy Resources; Living conditions Access to prevention	Advocacy; Community organizing Social services Increasing access to prevention (condoms)

* A more recent theory, theory of planned behaviour is an update of the theory of reasoned action. It was developed by one of the authors of the theory of reasoned action to account for behaviours that are subject to forces beyond the individual's control.

TABLE 2

MODELS AND THEORIES TESTED THROUGH RESEARCH OR REVIEWS

Author, Year	*Model/Theory/ Construct*	*Target group (n), country*	*Research Methodology*	*Results*
Edem, 1998	**Health belief model**	University students (395), Nigeria	Self-administered questionnaire distributed in classroom setting.	Three variables (condom benefit beliefs, cues to action, condom barrier beliefs) were significantly correlated to intentions to use condoms and past condom use.
Ford, 1995	**Health belief model**	Male sex workers (80) and clients (100), Indonesia	Individual survey interviews including questions on AIDS/ STD knowledge, sexual behaviour and psychosocial measures related to risk taking.	For tourists, factors related to condom use were condom beliefs, self-efficacy, susceptibility of STD infection, and STD knowledge. For sex workers factors related condom use were condom beliefs and self-efficacy.
Ford, 1998	**Health belief model + Social cognitive theory**	Indonesia - Female sex workers	Testing of 2 behaviour change models in 4 different groups of SW, in different socio-economic settings	'Results reflect social context of sexual behaviour'. Where knowledge of HIV is low, susceptibility to STDs and pregnancy related to condom use. Self-efficacy and belief that condoms can increase pleasure were related to condom use. In a more independent group self-efficacy not related, but susceptibility to HIV related to condom use. In higher priced group, condom use related to beliefs about AIDS prevention and pleasure as well as self-efficacy.

(Contd.)

Author, Year	*Model/Theory/ Construct*	*Target group (n), country*	*Research Methodology*	*Results*
Buunk, 1998	**Health belief model, Protection Motivation Theory, Anticipated regret, Social norms**	Heterosexual men and women at risk (711), Holland	Heterosexual adult females and males interviewed for predictors of intention to use condoms with new partners	A limited number of well described variables can explain variance in intention to use condoms: self efficacy, anticipated regret and descriptive social norms (belief that most others in the reference group would use condoms with new sexual partners)
Reitman, 1996	**Health belief model, Theory of reasoned action, Social cognitive theory**	African - American youth (312), USA	Interviews	Adolescent's positive attitude toward condoms was strongest correlate of condom use, and lower self-efficacy was most strongly related to high-risk sexual practices.
O'Leary, 1992	**Social cognitive theory**	College students, USA (923)	Survey on 4 college campuses	Stronger perceptions of self-efficacy to engage in safer behaviour, expecting fewer negative outcomes of condom use, and less frequency of sex in conjunction with alcohol or other drug use significantly predicted safer sexual behaviour.

(Contd.)

Author, Year	*Model/Theory/ Construct*	*Target group (n), country*	*Research Methodology*	*Results*
Nemoto, 1998	**Social cognitive theory Self-efficacy**	Asian community (254), USA	Interviews of Chinese, Filipino, and Vietnamese adults identified in needle exchange, jail, night clubs, and bars	Self-efficacy to practice safer sex was significantly associated with condom use in past 6 months. Cultural ideas such as shame and fatalism influenced condom use and self-efficacy.
Alary, 1998	**Theory of reasoned action, Theory of planned behaviour, Social learning theory**	Seronegative MSM (2000), Canada	Interviews and self-administered questionnaire every 6 months	Psychosocial variables associated with incident high risk sex were lower perceived behavioural control and perception of higher risk linked other sexual practices
Rotheram Borus, 1998	**Cognitive-behavioural**	Youth, USA	Review of cognitive-behavioural interventions for seropositive youth	Significant reductions in risk behavioural with cognitive-behavioural interventions.
Gregson, 1998	**Knowledge; Perception of risk**	Women (1294), Zimbabwe	Women of child-bearing age were interviewed	Effective behavioural change associated with greater knowledge, experience and personal risk perception, but obstructed by low female autonomy, marital status and economic status, alcohol consumption, labor migration.

(Contd.)

Author, Year	*Model/Theory/ Construct*	*Target group (n), country*	*Research Methodology*	*Results*
Newcomb, 1998	**Implicit cognition**	Men and women (579), USA	Participants completed a confidential questionnaire on a variety of health behaviours and predictors.	Memory association variable predicted unprotected sex, but poly-drug use was the strongest and most consistent predictor of the sexual behaviours.
PSI, 1998	**Condom social marketing***	Women and men (806), Zambia	Comparison of survey in 1990 with survey in 1996.	Findings suggest that condom marketing, promotion and distribution activities have been responsible for an increase in the use of condoms in Lusaka.
Levy, 1998	**Perceived self-efficacy, Perceived community norms Behavioural intention towards safer sex**	Prevention agencies for underserved populations (youth, IDU), USA	Evaluation survey.	Increase in the number of people who hang out with others who use condoms (community norms) Increase in number of people who used condoms the last time they had sex (behaviour) Increase in number of people who feel confident that they can tell their sex partners that they want to use a condom (self-efficacy)

(Contd.)

Author, Year	*Model/Theory/ Construct*	*Target group (n), country*	*Research Methodology*	*Results*
Godin, 1996	**Theory of planned behaviour**	Seropositive gay men (96), Canada	Cohort study, 6 month follow-up visits. Face to face interviews.	The best predictor of intention to use condoms (and of reported condom use) and of having sex without anal intercourse was perceived behavioural control.
Jemmott, 1992	**Theory of planned behaviour**	Adolescents (179), USA	Confidential self-administered questionnaire.	Attitudes and subjective norms predicted intentions to use condoms and perceived behavioural control significantly added to the correlation.
Lurie, 1995	**Socio-economic factors**	Sex workers (600), Brazil	Cross sectional study of prevalence of antibodies to HIV, syphilis, hepatitis B, behavioural factors and socio-economic factors.	Compared to those with a higher Socio-economic Status (SES), sex workers with a lower SES worked longer hours and had more clients. Sex workers with lower SES were more likely than those with higher SES to be infected with HIV, syphilis and hepatitis B.
Kline, 1994	**AIDS risk reduction model**	HIV-infected women (215), USA	HIV infected women from New Jersey medical and social service agencies interviewed.	Factors influencing condom use: • High perceived self-efficacy to influence partner • Partner HIV-negative • Partner doesn't want more children Negatively influencing condom use: • Conflicts with partner • Use of drugs and/or alcohol • Belief condoms reduce sexual pleasure

(Contd.)

Author, Year	*Model/Theory/ Construct*	*Target group (n), country*	*Research Methodology*	*Results*
Rickman, 1994	**Sexual communication**	Incarcerated Latino adolescents (2132), USA	Sexually active adolescents detained in Los Angeles county juvenile hall were interviewed regarding their sexual communication history and condom use.	High numbers of lifetime sexual partners, low rates of condom use. Respondents who communicated with their sex partners about each others' sexual history were significantly more likely to use condoms.

* Theories behind social marketing come from many different backgrounds including the commercial marketing, 4 Ps' (making the Product appealing, the Price acceptable, the Placement convenient, and the Promotion tailored to a particular audience), operant conditioning and social cognitive theories.

TABLE 3

INTERVENTIONS BASED ON MODELS AND THEORIES WITH VARIOUS TARGET GROUPS WORLDWIDE

Author, Year	*Target group (n), country*	*Model/Theory/ Construct*	*Research Methodology*	*Results*
Women				
Di Clemente, 1995	African American women (128), USA	**SCT and Theory of Gender and Power**	Community based intervention including 5, 2 hour group sessions led by peer educator focusing on gender and ethnic pride, knowledge, skills and norms	Increased consistent condom use, greater sexual communication and increased partners' adoption of norms supporting condom use.
King, 1995	Women (586), Rwanda	**Structural**	Participants were provided with family planning services and methods	Access to and information about hormonal contraceptives increased use and reduced attrition among both HIV+ and HIV- women in the study.
Elkins, 1997	Village women (600) and men (479), Thailand	**SCT and community health promotion**	Intervention was village-based including training, motivational audio-drama, posters and village meetings. Evaluation consisted of: KAP surveys, focus group discussions and village meetings.	Eight of the nine outcome goals were achieved with married women taking initiative in reducing risk posed to them by the sex activities of their husbands.

(Contd.)

(*Contd.*)

Author, Year	*Target group (n), country*	*Model/Theory/ Construct*	*Research Methodology*	*Results*
Galavotti, 1998	1289 at risk and 322 HIV-positive women USA	**Stages of change**	Behaviour change counselling intervention delivered by trained peer paraprofessional counsellors based on stage-tailored individual counselling sessions.	Women exposed twice as likely to report condom use with main partner at last sex and always use of condoms
Stevens, 1998	Lesbian and bisexual women (3665)	**PAR and Peer education**	Collective consciousness-raising qualitative field interviewing and individualized HIV-prevention education in an intense 2 year intervention	Outcomes suggest that the project supported changes to reduce risk, assisted participants in the realm of partner negotiations, and began to change community conventions about sexual expectations and practices.
Sex Workers				
Fox, 1993	Female sex workers (134), Honduras	**NS-information and accessibility of condoms**	SWs attending STD clinics given weekly talks and free condoms	Statistically significant increase in mean condom use from 64 per cent to 70 per cent of client contacts. Recommend targeting clients.
Asamoah-Adu, 1994	Female sex workers (107), Ghana	**peer education and condom promotion**	SW followed over 4 year study. Intervention included peer education and condom promotion.	Reported condom use increased dramatically in first 6 months. Relapse occurred after 3 years. Recommend targeting clients.

(Contd.)

Author, Year	Target group (n), country	Model/Theory/ Construct	Research Methodology	Results
Opare, 1994	Female sex workers (30), Ghana	**NS -audio-visual aids to influence attitudes and behaviours**	Education conducted through SW opinion leaders; video, discussion and condom demonstration conducted.	Condom use rose from 10 per cent to 100 per cent as sex workers identified very high perception of risk.
Visru-taratna, 1995	Female sex workers (500) brothel own-ers and clients, Thailand	**Perception of risk, condom negotiation, policy**	A year-long intervention. Small group sessions with SW and peer educators. Brothels required condom use through owners and education of clients. Specially trained volunteers posed as clients to test SW negotiation skills.	Sex workers increased their refusal of sex without a condom from 42 per cent to 92 per cent following the programme.
Williams, 1995	Female sex workers Nigeria	**NS - health education, condom promotion and STD services**	Health education using film, peer educators distribute educational materials, condom promotion with free distribution and later cost recovery and comprehensive, client oriented STD services.	Sex workers and clients knowledge about AIDS and STDs increased. Condom use among sex workers and clients increased between baseline and follow-up.

(Contd.)

Author, Year	*Target group (n), country*	*Model/Theory/ Construct*	*Research Methodology*	*Results*
Chan, 1996	Female sex workers, Singapore (128)	**Behavioural (sexual communication)**	Condom negotiation, support from peers and brothel owners and health staff.	Significant improvement in negotiation skill, in always refusing sex without a condom and significant decrease in gonorrhoea rates in intervention vs. control group
Ford, 1996	Female sex workers (300) and clients (300), Indonesia	**Health belief model and Social cognitive theory**	3 session series to: increase knowledge, perceived susceptibility and skills related to condom use and partner negotiation among SW. Increase knowledge among clients and pimps using outreach workers.	Knowledge and condom use increased significantly between baseline and followup for both SW (from 18-75%) and (29-62%) and clients of SW in both intervention sites.
Basu, 1998	Female sex workers India	**PAR- - though not stated explicitly**	Involving sex workers in research	Accurate sensitive data collected Rapport-building activity
Kelly, 1998	Female sex workers Viet Nam	**PAR - though not stated explicitly**	Involving sex workers in research	Regardless of method used, must involve participants in research

(Contd.)

Author, Year	*Target group (n), country*	*Model/Theory/ Construct*	*Research Methodology*	*Results*
Gordon, 1998	Female sex workers Indonesia (500)	**ILOM model**	Works on changing norms; sharing behavioural values	Mobilizes the community and changes culture
Youth				
Howard, 1990	Low income youth USA (536)	**Social influence**	5 classroom periods led by teenagers slightly older than participants presenting factual information, identifying pressures, role-playing responses to pressures, teaching assertiveness and discussing problem situations	By end of 8th grade students in the programme were five times less likely to have begun sex than similar students who were not in the programme. There was a stronger influence on girls than boys. The programme was not effective for students who had already initiated sex.
Jemmott, 1992	African American adolescents, (109), USA	**Social Cognitive Theory**	Intervention included a pre and a post-test + factual information, outcome expectancies about condom use and self-efficacy training.	Participation in the programme was associated with increased AIDS knowledge and intentions and self-efficacy to use condoms.

(Contd.)

Author, Year	*Target group (n), country*	*Model/Theory/ Construct*	*Research Methodology*	*Results*
Walter, 1993	Youth (72% Black or Hispanic) (1316), USA	**Health belief model, Social cognitive theory, and a model of Social influence**	School based, teacher delivered 6-session intervention.	Significant effects in intervention vs. control group in: knowledge, beliefs, self-efficacy, and risk behaviour scores (no. partners, consistency of condom use, high risk partners, diagnosis of other STD)
Re, 1996, 1998	Youth (389), Argentina	**NS - participatory methods**	Peer education workshops and community project	Peer educators were positive role models and were able to translate messages as 'peer gender specialists'; adolescents had low risk perception overall.
Gillmore, 1997	Youth in detention and at STD clinic (396), USA	**Social cognitive theory and Theory of reasoned action**	Testing of 3 behavioural interventions: • comic book • videotape • group skills training that emphasizes negotiating skills for condom use	Few differences among conditions; skill based intervention not sufficient to induce consistent condom use in heterosexually active high risk adolescents. Authors suggest longer intervention addressing multiple problems.

(Contd.)

Author, Year	*Target group (n), country*	*Model/Theory/ Construct*	*Research Methodology*	*Results*
Moberg, 1998	Youth (2483), USA	**Social influence**	Middle school students assigned to either of 3 conditions using blocked randomization: age appropriate, intensive and control	Null findings despite careful implementation of school-based component. Authors note, inadequate community and family-level interventions, possible dilution of message, and over saturation of students with health messages by 8th grade.
Kelly, 1992	MSM USA	**Diffusion theory**	Sequential stepwise lagged design, in 3 cities, opinion leaders were contracted to have conversations with peers to endorse actively and visibly the importance and acceptability of behavioural change as well as to convey strategies for change implementation.	Intervention produced systematic reductions of 15 per cent to 29 per cent from baseline in the population's high-risk behaviour with same pattern of effects sequentially replicated in all 3 cities.
Kegeles, 1996	Young MSM (300), USA	**Diffusion theory**	Implemented in 2 small communities with 1 control group, used natural channels of communication to create alcohol and drug-free alternatives and to place HIV risk among the concerns of young gay men.	Significant (27 per cent) reductions in proportions of young gay men engaging in unprotected anal intercourse with all men, but higher among secondary partners than boyfriends.

(Contd.)

Author, Year	*Target group (n), country*	*Model/Theory/ Construct*	*Research Methodology*	*Results*
Kelly, 1996	MSM (1/3 ethnic minority) (429), USA	**Cognitive-behavioural + maintenance**	Participants were randomly assigned to one of 4 1-day interventions: cognitive-behavioural risk reduction and relapse prevention, cognitive-behavioural risk reduction and personal relationships or the same 2 with 3 months of follow-up telephone and group boosters.	Greatest reduction and greatest maintenance of risk behaviour change among men in cognitive-behavioural group with discussion and problem-solving about personal relationship issues.
Infecting Drug Users				
Lawrence 1994	Drug-dependent youth (19), USA	**Cognitive-behavioural**	Substance dependent adolescents in residential treatment - received a 5 session HIV risk reduction intervention that provided HIV education, social competency skills and problem solving training.	Subjects showed increased knowledge about AIDS, better attitudes about prevention, greater internal and lower external locus of control scores, increased self-efficacy, and higher perception of vulnerability.
Wiebel, 1996	IDU (641), USA	**ILOM model**	Ex-addicts deliver HIV-prevention services targeting IDU social networks in community settings	Observed incidence of HIV infection decreased from 8.4 to 2.4 per 100 person years. Sex risk behaviour decreased but much less dramatically than drug risk behaviour.

(Contd.)

Author, Year	*Target group (n), country*	*Model/Theory/ Construct*	*Research Methodology*	*Results*
Fishbein, 1996	IDUs, female sex partners of IDU, SW, MSM who don't gay identify USA	**Stages of change**	Small media intervention materials were developed for each specific population focusing on key theoretical behaviour change variables as well as condoms.	Significant interactions indicating greater increases in intervention than comparison areas were found with respect to condom use with non-main partners, and similar but non-significant effect with respect to condom use with main partners.
Robles, 1998	Drug users (80% male) (1004), Puerto Rico	**Stages of change**	Enhanced intervention took place outside of office, included 8, 45 minute sessions using 'motivational interviewing' drawing on individual's perception of risk, motivation to change, continuous risk evaluation, negotiation and communication skills, Community and environmental resources were considered.	Use of condoms during vaginal sex increased from 26.4% to 36.9%. Significant predictors of condom use: HIV-positive, STD diagnosis, and participation in enhanced program. Effect stronger with non-primary partners.

(Contd.)

Author, Year	Target group (n), country	Model/Theory/ Construct	Research Methodology	Results
STD Clients				
James, 1996	STD patients (492), UK	**Social cognitive theory**	RCT - 3 groups (group A, group B, group C) • A - counselling intervention + leaflet + condoms • B - leaflet + condoms • C - no intervention	Group A were significantly more likely than group C to carry condoms, no difference between A and B or B and C. Intervention had no effect on self-reported behaviour.
Kamb, 1996, 1998	Heterosexual STD patients (4328), USA	**SCT+ Theory of reasoned action self-efficacy and perceived norms**	RCT - of 3 strategies: (1) educational messages, (2) brief counselling, (3) enhanced counselling (greater number of counselling sessions) with steps toward risk reduction beliefs, attitudes and behavioural intentions, skills training to increase self-efficacy	Decrease in rates of STDs in: brief counselling (19%), enhanced counselling (22%) vs. information only
O'Leary, 1998	STD and health agency patients, USA (3706)	**Social cognitive theory**	7 SCT interventions (1) randomized same-sex groups including information video with question and answer period, or (2) informational comparison condition.	Elements of SCT (self-efficacy, condom use skills, expectations of partner reaction) were significantly different between intervention and control group.

(Contd.)

Author, Year	Target group (n), country	Model/Theory/ Construct	Research Methodology	Results
STD Clients				
Wallerstein 1988	Hispanic, Native American, Anglo, USA	**Empowerment**	Visits to hospital and detention center, peer education strategies and training, social learning, resistance to peer pressure, life skills competencies and decision-making about alternative choices, analysis of media that influence consumption.	Statistically significant self reported perception of riskiness of drinking, driving and drug use
Kalichman, 1997	Inner-city African American heterosexual men (81)	**Theory of Reasoned Action**	RCT of a 4 session cognitive behavioural skills training intervention in comparison with an HIV education control condition.	Both interventions significantly increased AIDS-related knowledge, intentions to change HIV risk behaviours, and reduced unprotected vaginal intercourse. There were no significant differences between groups on any of the measures at post-intervention or follow-up assessments.
STD Clients				
Svenson, 1996	University students (37,000), Sweden	**Diffusion theory, community organization**	HIV-STD prevention approach based on community organization and action, target group empowerment and use of opinion leaders as peer educators	Consistent condom use with new sex partners was significantly higher among project-contacted students than controls, perceived safer sex social norms.

(Contd.)

Author, Year	*Target group (n), country*	*Model/Theory/ Construct*	*Research Methodology*	*Results*
Otto-Salaj, 1998	Seriously mentally ill patients (89 men and 103 women), USA	**Cognitive-behavioural (self-efficacy, personal risk assessment)**	Random assignment to one of 2, 7 session, skills building (assertiveness, negotiation to resist coercion to engage in high-risk behaviour and to initiate communication with partners about condom use or other safer sex practices), self-management of risk behaviours, reinforcement of safer behaviour	Compared to comparison group, participants in HIV risk-reduction intervention reported increases in both frequency and per cent of condom use in vaginal intercourse occasions, self-esteem, positive condom attitudes and risk reduction behavioural intentions. Risk reduction higher in females than males.
Hiebert, 1998	Canada	**Participatory action research**	Participants defining needs and figuring out how to meet those needs	Participants took control of project
Henry, 1998	Community leaders and governmental officials, Kenya	**Structural changes**	Government + religion + business; making changes at the policy level	Government's first comprehensive national policy on HIV/AIDS in 1997 through years of research, dialogue and consensus-building.

* = indicates year of publication; NS = theory not stated in the report; RCT = randomized control trial; SCT = social cognitive theory.

TABLE 4

SUMMARY OF THEORIES AND MODELS BY POPULATION GROUP

Population Group	*Theory/Model*	*Comments*
Heterosexual Women	**Social Cognitive Theory (SCT)**	Psychological theories such as SCT provided guidance to interventions (especially in the USA), suggesting skills training and strategies to modify perceived peer or partner normative beliefs about risk-taking. Skills training included talking with partners about sex and condom use and practicing condom use skills.
	Theory of Gender and Power	Among African American women in the USA, this model helped guide an intervention based on improving partner norms and increasing sexual communication skills.
	Diffusion of Innovations with Community Mobilization	This model was used effectively in among low income women in the USA
	Stages of Change	Stages of Change model was used to guide interventions in the USA. In the US study among women in drug treatment, investigators found stage tailored counselling more/effective than standard
	AIDS Risk Reduction Model	Authors noted that in this US-based study the strongest predictors of increasing condom use were partner-related variables
	Perception of Risk	This construct has been used in studies with women in Africa and predicted condom use especially in low HIV prevalence settings.

(Contd.)

(Contd.)

Population Group	Theory/Model	Comments
Sex Workers	**The HBM and SCT used together**	Different constructs were useful for different sub-populations, but self-efficacy and the benefits of condoms were predictive of reducing risk among many groups in Indonesia.
	ILOM	This model emphasizing changing cultural norms and mobilizing the community, was used in Indonesia.
	Diffusion of Innovations	This model was used effectively in community interventions with women internationally
Homosexual Men	**AIDS Risk Reduction Model**	This model was useful in guiding an intervention among African American men to address self-identity, social support, sexual communication and behavioural commitment.
	Diffusion Theory	The diffusion theory has been useful in guiding effective interventions with gay men in the USA in a few different studies.
	HBM, SCT and Theory of reasoned Action (TRA) combined	A combined behavioural model was used with Asian and Pacific Islander men in the USA and found greater than 50% reduction in unprotected anal intercourse in Chinese and Filipino men.
	TRA and SCT combined	Using constructs from both models, perceived behavioural control was most predictive for gay men in Montreal.

(Contd.)

(Contd.)

Population Group	*Theory/Model*	*Comments*
Heterosexual Men	**Social Cognitive Theory**	Elements such as self-efficacy, and condom use skills improved following an intervention.
	SCT and TRA combined	Self-efficacy and perceived norms were useful to predict decreases in STDs among men STD clinic attendees
Youth	**Social Cognitive Theory**	Interventions guided by SCT have increased self-efficacy and increased condom use in diverse youth populations in the USA
	Health Belief Model	Perceived benefits to condoms, perceived barriers and cues to action were predictive of condom use among university students in Nigeria
	HBM and TRA combined	Attitudes towards condoms - a strong predictor of condom use among African American adolescents
	Social Influence	This model has been particularly useful among youth in the USA who have not yet had sexual intercourse
	Stages of Change	An intervention guided by this model in Puerto Rico found increases in condom use among drug users
IDUs	**ILOM Model**	This outreach model has shown reductions in sex risk practices, but greater reductions in drug risk practices

Index

D

E

M

N

O

P

R

S

ENCYCLOPAEDIA OF AIDS

ENCYCLOPAEDIA
OF
AIDS

(In 7 Volumes)

(Volume 7)

Editor

Dr. G.C. Satpathy

PUBLICATIONS

KALPAZ PUBLICATIONS

DELHI - 110052

ENCYCLOPAEDIA OF AIDS
(*Health, Reference*)

Rs. 7000 (Set)
Rs. 1000 (each volume)

ISBN: 81-7835-112-9 (Set)
ISBN: 81-7835-138-2 (Vol. 7)

Published in 2003 in India by
Kalpaz Publications
C-30, Satyawati Nagar
Delhi-110052
e-mail: kalpaz@hotmail.com

Laser Typeset at: Alphabet, Delhi
Printed at: Mehra Offset Press, Delhi

Contents

Preface

The later half of the twentieth century will be remembered in the history of medicine for two remarkable events, one good, that is the eradication of smallpox, and the other one bad, when the world was alerted to the first case AIDS in 1981, now running in a pandemic proportion. In a little over two decades it is estimated that over 36 million people are now infected with HIV/AIDS with 5.3 million being infected every year. India alone has about 4 million HIV/AIDS patients, the second highest number among all nations. Now it is well perceived as a serious threat to humanity, and the control of this epidemic lies not only in the hands of physicians alone but the entire society must involve to the task. No cure or vaccine is yet in sight. So the only mode of controlling it is prevention. The key to prevention lies in information, education and communication.

Twenty years of observation and study of the syndrome has generated profound interest among all branches of medicine, social activists, research workers, public health issues, health and sex education strategies, with innumerable clinical and pharmacological research being conducted on it all over the world. It is not possible to compile the whole saga of AIDS, which is unique in many ways and not yet fully understood. We have tried to accumulate as much information as possible in this seven-volume encyclopaedia, probably the first such attempt made ever. Since the process of acquiring information is never-ending, we hope to provide more and more information in future.

It has been a herculean task to compile the huge materials systematically, besides being an unique experience. In spite of the best efforts for accuracy and perfection, there may be shortcomings, which may be excused. It will be a success story for us if by this work the society to which the work is dedicated is benefited at large. The study does not end here. It shall be a continuous series in future with comprehensive details having a deep bearing on the subject.

Guwahati-23
Rathyatra-2002

Dr. G.C. Satpathy
MD, IPM

Acknowledgements

During the course of this research work, I happened to visit several academic fora which willingly afforded their support and facilitated my work. These are the Ministry of Health, Govt. of India, World Health Organisation, health departments of the States and academic institutions of higher learning. I have used the material from published works including scholarly journals and magazines to fill up the gaps in these volumes.

I have also taken academic support from several sources, which include universities, institutes, centres for higher learning, Acts passed in this direction, Statistical Year Book (UNESCO), voluntary organisations, legal luminaries, social activists, prison management, legal issues of AIDS, Legislation Enquiry Commission on HIV Law, Sri Lanka, Prevention of Brothels Act, Myanmar, Laws of HIV/AIDS in Pakistan, Documents in sub-Saharan, Africa, European Council Recommendations, UNESCO Courier, Philippines Overseas Employment Agency, Foreign Exchange Regulations Deptt., Central Bank of the Philippines, National Advisory Committee on AIDS in Singapore, Vietnamese National AIDS Committee, National Blood Transfusion Centre in Cambodia, Infectious Diseases Act, Thailand, AIDS Prevention Act in Korea, Labour Protection Law, Thailand, Social Security Act, Thailand, Homosexual Law Reform Act, 1986, Universities of Nairobi, Manitola (in Canada) and Washington, Institute of Systemic Therapy, Harare, Zimbabwe, The AIDS Service Organisation, Kampala, Uganda, Health Economics and HIV/AIDS Research Division, University of Natal, Durban, School of

Public Health, University of Natal, South Africa Institute for Medical Research, Johannesburg, Centre for African Family Studies, Nairobi, Kenya, Malwai Institute of Management, Malwai.

I feel much grateful to these institutions and learned authors whose writings have proved useful in the texts of these seven volumes.

The publisher and myself feel much beholden to the panel of highly qualified and experienced advisers who are distinguished in their respective fields, for their valuable and timely guidelines, contributions and encouragement in making this work an epoch-making one.

. I am grateful to several other research institutes and NGOs etc., scholars whose writings have been used in these volumes.

I am extremely grateful to my wife, son Anurag and daughter Anamika for their consistent encouragement to me during this stupendous research work.

Dr. G.C. Satpathy

Our Distinguished Panel of Advisers

1. Dr. A.K. Das, MD, MNAMS, Ph.D., FICA	Dean and Director-Prof. Dept. of Medicine, JIMPER, Pondicherry
2. Mr. D.K. Arya IPS (Retd.)	Former Director General, BSF
3. Dr. K.V. Dakhina Murty MD, DM, DNB, FISN	Prof. & Head, Deptt. of Nephrology, Nizam's Instt. of Medical Sciences, Panjagutta, Hyderabad
4. Maj. Gen. K.K. Ganguly	VSM (Retd.)
5. Col. M.K. Bhandari MD, FICA	Asso. Prof. of Medicine, Armed Forces Medical College, Pune
6. Dr. M.C. Dash	Vice Chancellor, Sambalpur University, P.O.: Jyoti Vihar, Orissa
7. Dr. N.C. Borah MD, DM	C.M.D. GNRC Hospitals Ltd. Dispur, Guwahati
8. Dr. P.C. Bhattacharya MD	Sr. Consultant, downtown hospital Dispur, Guwahati
9. Dr. S.B. Gupta MD	Physician and Cardiologist Central Railway Hospital, Mumbai

Introduction

Encountering the vast devastating impact of HIV/AIDS on individual and community well-being and on development, life expectancy and childhood mortality; governments the world over have been reviewing the nature of their response to HIV/AIDS. Some have raised the issue of whether the principles of *confidentiality* and *informed consent* have hindered efforts to curtail the onward transmission of HIV. Particular concern has been expressed regarding the vulnerability of women to infection by husbands or partners who are not aware of their sero-status or refuse to disclose it or refuse to practise safer sex. This has led to calls to adopt policies such as named HIV case reporting, mandatory revelation of status and criminalising the deliberate transmission of HIV. The international consultation on these aspects have confirmed that the principles of confidentiality and informed consent are not barriers to effective prevention and care programmes. In fact, if employed appropriately, they are not only valid ethical principles but are also pragmatic mechanism by which to best protect both the non-infected and the infected. Rather it is HIV-associated *denial*, *stigma* and *discrimination* and the secrecy that results from these, that compose major impediments to an effective response to HIV/AIDS.

Although the epidemic is approximately two decades old and although HIV prevalence is very high in several communities, HIV/AIDS continues to be denied at the national, social and individual levels, to be lightly *stigmatised* and to cause grave *discrimination* based on HIV/AIDS status. There are many reasons for the stigma, denial, discrimination and secrecy that surround HIV/AIDS, and these will differ from one culture to another. However, in general, HIV/AIDS is a condition related to sex, blood, death, disease and behaviour which may be illegal—

commercial sex, homosexuality, injecting drugs. The fear and taboos related to these subjects lead to the denial, stigma and discrimination associated with HIV/AIDS, and breed the secrecy that hinder private and community discussion about the issues and behaviour involved. Denial causes individuals to refuse to acknowledge that they are threatened by a previously unknown virus which requires them to talk about, and to change, intimate behaviour, probably for the rest of their lives. Denial also causes communities and nations to refuse to acknowledge the HIV threat, and the fact that its causes and consequences will require them to deal with many difficult and controversial topics, e.g., the nature of cultural norms governing male and female sexuality, the social and economic status of women, sex trade, families separated by migration/work, inequalities in health care and education, injecting drug use. Stigma and discrimination and the fact that for many there is no available treatment, cause individuals to fear getting tested for HIV and to fear revealing it to health care professionals, for care, to families and communities, for support, and to sexual and drug-injecting partners, to prevent onward transmission of HIV.

The prevalence of denial, stigma, discrimination and secrecy imply that there is a clear and urgent need to 'open up' the epidemic. To achieve this, it is neither feasible nor desirable to force people; to get tested (and retested throughout their lives); to disclose their status, to change their behaviour. This would require the generation of a health 'police' state requiring vast amount of resources for testing and policing. It would also drive further underground the very kinds of behaviour that are already latent and need to be modified. However, it is feasible and desirable to open up the epidemic in ways that will reduce denial, stigma and discrimination, and will create are environment in which many more people have incentives to access prevention and care services, and are supported to change their behaviour for prevention purposes, to reveal their status to partners and families, and receive care, support and compassion. The offered guidance concerning how this might best be achieved by policies and programmes that encourage beneficial disclosure, ethical partner, counselling, and appropriate use of HIV case-reporting.

As UN system organisations, UNAIDS and WHO are committed to the promotion and protection of human rights, ethical principles and public health. The guidance provided here is based on the firm belief that human rights and ethical principles offer a framework by which the dignity and health of *both* those uninfected and those infected by HIV are protected. Moreover, adherence to human rights and ethical principles is essential to create an effective public health environment in which the most people are motivated to, and in fact do, change their behaviour, prevent their own infection or onward transmission, and receive care. Finally, individuals and communities can be, and should be, empowered to deal with the health challenges they encounter. In the context of HIV/AIDS, *beneficial disclosure* of HIV sero-status should be encouraged. This is disclosure that is voluntary, respects the autonomy and dignity of the affected individuals, maintains confidentiality as appropriate, leads to beneficial results for the individual, his/her sexual and drug-injecting partners, and family; leads to greater openness in the community about HIV/AIDS; and meets ethical imperatives so as to maximise good for both the uninfected and the infected.

In order to encourage beneficial disclosure, there should be created an environment in which more people are willing and able to get tested for HIV, and are empowered and encouraged to change their behaviour as per the results. This can be done by setting up more voluntary counselling and testing services, providing incentives to get tested in the form of greater access to community care and support, and examples of positive living; and removing disincentives to testing and disclosure by protecting people from stigma and discrimination. There already exist a number of community care and support programmes globally that are achieving these results. These should be replicated within and outside governmental programmes. Much more can be done by governments to encourage voluntary testing, counselling and beneficial disclosure by implementing public information and media campaigns that promote tolerance and compassion; enacting legislations and regulations and implementing legal and social support services that protest against discrimination; supporting community-based organisations associated with these activities;

and involving people living with HIV/AIDS in the formulation and implementation of HIV programmes and policies.

With regard to partner counselling (partner notification), ethical partner counselling should be encouraged which is based on the informed consent of the HIV-positive person, where possible. However, it also takes into consideration the serious probable consequences of *not* counselling partners—that is, HIV infection. Because refusal to counsel partners can lead to the onward spread of HIV, HIV counselling and partner counselling programmes should involve strong and professional efforts to encourage, persuade and support HIV-positive persons to notify and counsel partners. In some cases in which a properly counselled HIV-positive person refuses to counsel partners, the health care provider should be able to counsel partners, without the consent of the HIV-positive client, after there has been an ethical weighing of the potential harms involved, and appropriate steps have been taken. These steps consist of repeated efforts to persuade the HIV-positive client to counsel partners, informing the HIV positive client that partner counselling will occur, keeping his/her name confidential if possible; and ensuring social and legal support for the source client and other associated parties (spouses partners, family members) to protect them from any physical abuse, discrimination and stigma which may result from partner counselling. There is much that governments can do to create conditions to encourage ethical partner counselling. These include formulation of policies, laws and guidelines which protect confidentiality and informed consent, and outline clearly the limited circumstances under which partner counselling may take place without consult, training health care professionals and counsellors in ethical partner counselling, and increasing social and legal support for these who are involved in partner counselling. As regards appropriate use of HIV case-reporting, it has been suggested that HIV case-reporting, including named HIV case reporting (i.e. the reporting to public health authorities of each individual discovered as HIV positive) could provide accurate information on the spread of HIV, and allow effective actions to prevent further infections and ensure access to care services. However, in resource-poor settings, certain conditions result in the fact that HIV case-reporting does not provide accurate statistics for surveillance purposes and does not result in better prevention and care. These conditions are: little access to, or use of HIV-tests, reporting system which suffers from under-reporting, under-diagnosing and insufficient infrastructure to protect confidentiality; little or no access to anti-retrovirals; and limited resources which would be better utilised in increasing access to voluntary testing and care and improving prevention strategies. In countries where such conditions exist it is suggested that HIV case-reporting not be conducted.

Rather in assessing the use of HIV case-reporting and other surveillance strategies, countries should refer to the framework of second generation HIV surveillance, where a combination of both biological and behavioural surveillance tools is recommended. In general, such surveillance is cost-effective given the monetary and human resources available; refines, as well as reinforces, prevention and care strategies, maintains confidentiality, optimises access to available treatment options where this is practicable; and leads to regular and wide dissemination of information to the population in non-stigmatising ways that assist to open up the epidemic, decrease denial and increase commitment to encounter the epidemic. In underdeveloped countries, depending on the state of the epidemic and other factors, it is likely that HIV sentinel surveillance will be the most appropriate form of surveillance to employ.

One

HIV Voluntary Counselling and Testing: Evaluating Tools

Introduction

Voluntary Counselling and Testing (VCT) services have been considered important as an entry point for prevention and care interventions for HIV/AIDS recently. Access to VCT services, however, remains limited and demand is often low. VCT is not widely available and people are often afraid of knowing their serostatus in many high-prevalence countries because little care and support is available following testing, moreover the quality and benefits of VCT, in particular with regard to confidentiality, counselling and access to clinical and social support, vary to a large extent. Establishing VCT and ensuring a quality that will generate demand is thus a big challenge. Building in self-assessments, monitoring and regular evaluation is a significant tools to upgrade the quality of VCT. This chapter offers suggestions on monitoring and evaluation of the several aspects of planning and implementing VCT. It provides tools for the evaluation of VCT as part of a national programme, as well as VCT services at specific institutions, independent sites and services for special groups, consisting community-based non-governmental organisations (NGOs). It consists of monitoring and evaluation of VCT services related to the prevention of mother-to-child transmission of HIV (MTCT) and tuberculosis preventive therapy (TBPT). This chapter revises and adapts previous draft guidelines [1, 2, 3, 4] and incorporates relevant operational research outcomes.

Scope and Challenges

The scope and challenges of VCT have changed over the past decade. At the outset, VCT was primarily used to diagnose infection in symptomatic people to assist medical management, and testing was often accompanied by minimal counselling. It was also promoted, in a piecemeal way, as a component of HIV prevention. There were reports of obstacles to HIV testing due to the perceived stigma associated with a diagnosis, the lack of services and interventions available to those who tested seropositive[5] and adverse consequences, particularly for women, following testing[6]. The development of antiretroviral (ARV) treatment for people with HIV, less costly interventions to lessen the incidence of HIV-related infections, (such as tuberculosis preventive therapy[7, 8] and cotrimoxazole prophylaxis[9]) and comparatively cheap and feasible methods to prevent MTCT[10] have necessitated to promote VCT for people with asymptomatic disease more compelling. VCT services for young people are also being developed and services linked with family planning are becoming more widely available. The importance and cost-effectiveness of VCT in reducing HIV transmission are also at present recognised.[11] HIV testing methods have also become simpler and cheaper, making testing a more practicable choice in many developing countries.[12] The ease of HIV testing has also increased the role of the private sector in VCT in many developing as well as developed countries. The monitoring and evaluation of VCT services in the private sector brings additional challenges. VCT services have also been established for vulnerable groups such as commercial sex workers, prison populations, injecting drug users (IDUs) and refugees. These services need particularly careful monitoring to ensure such groups are not further marginalised and services are truly voluntary and confidential.

Reduced Incidence of Infection Contributes to Prevention

Studies evaluating VCT have concentrated on attempting to prove that VCT reduces incidence of HIV infection and thus contributes to prevention. This is because in planning and funding of VCT services it has been important to demonstrate that VCT 'works'. Studies on the virtue of VCT have largely focussed on the role of VCT in risk reduction and changing sexual behaviour.[13,14,15] Monitoring of VCT is dependent on reporting attendance, coverage and return rates. This chapter aims to provide guidelines to evaluate not only the implementation and effectiveness of VCT in HIV prevention, but also ways of assessing the acceptability and quality of services. It also focusses to assess the effectiveness of VCT in enabling people with HIV to better accept and cope with their infection and access appropriate services.

Cost Reduction

Besides reductions in the costs of HIV testing kits, VCT as a service will not be available in the times to come for the majority of people in high-prevalence developing countries, especially for those living outside the capital cities. Sometimes testing services will be offered intermittently when test kits are available. However, even where testing is not available, there are often well-developed counselling services for people with symptomatic HIV and their families, and services providing HIV prevention counselling (such as counselling about protected sex in family planning clinics). This chapter, although primarily focussed on evaluating VCT services, will also consist of counselling services where testing is not available, as in many settings this is a much more common choice.

Coercion to Test and Testing

As HIV testing becomes simpler to perform, it is widely available, often without counselling or without proper counselling or follow-up. Moreover, there are reports of coercion to test and testing which is not truly voluntary. Home testing and testing in the private sector pose serious challenges.

Counselling Sessions

A large number of people attending VCT, whether they test positive or negative, will attend one or, at the most, two post-test counselling sessions. It has been revealed that even when further counselling sessions are offered or referral to specialised counselling services is available, many people do not want further counselling, at least not in the immediate future.[16] Some people however, require ongoing counselling and some will attend for further counselling in the 1-5 years following VCT. This often coincides with a crisis or change in personal circumstances.

Following VCT, many people find other informal services or resources in the community to assist them with their emotional needs. Church groups, family members, friends and traditional medical workers at times offer emotional support. VCT services should therefore be flexible and either able to provide ongoing counselling or have close links with organisations providing this service. They should also be able to refer people to community organisations and spiritual/church groups when appropriate.

VCT Settings

Depending on demands and resources, VCT is being carried out in several settings in developing and developed countries.

1. Free-standing VCT settings
2. Hospital services
   (a) NGO within the hospital
   (b) integrated into general medical outpatient services in government hospitals
   (c) as part of specialist medical care, e.g., sexually transmitted infections (STI) clinic
   (d) dermatology clinic, chest clinic, antenatal and family planning services.
3. VCT as entry into the continuum of care/home-based care (consisting palliative care services).
4. Health centre - urban or rural.
5. Private sector (clinics and hospitals).
6. Workplace clinics.
7. Referral sites for legal requirements, pre-employment, pre-travel, pre-marital.
8. Youth health services and school health services.
9. Health services for vulnerable groups
   (a) commercial sex workers
   (b) prison populations
   (c) refugees
   (d) injecting drug users (IDUs)
   (e) men having sex with men (MSM)
   (f) children, orphans and street kids.
10. Self testing/home testing.
11. Attached to research project/pilot project
   (a) associated with antenatal services and interventions

(b) associated with tuberculosis (TB) services and TB preventive therapy

12. Blood transfusion services.

A number of models of VCT are available in many different settings in developing and developed countries. There is no single preferred model and the option of VCT service will depend on the needs of the community, HIV seroprevalence, maturity of the epidemic, attitudes towards HIV, political and community commitment to VCT, available monetary assistance and existing VCT resources.

VCT Evaluation Tools: Cautions, Difficulties and Limitations

This chapter includes a series of tools to evaluate VCT, in order to improve and develop services. The tools should be used with the cooperation and collaboration of counsellors, clients and service managers. They should be utilised in a flexible manner and should be adapted and modified as per the needs of the services. Some services may only require a single tool to evaluate a specific aspect of their service.

Utilisation of the Tools: Adaptation to Reflect Needs of the Service

These tools provide recommendations of content areas within counselling services to be evaluated. The tools are not intended to be prescriptive. It is desirable that managers of counselling services will assess and adapt the generic tools included in this discussion to project specific needs and local circumstances. Some of the sample questionnaires, which have been designed as comprehensive evaluation tools, are long and complicated to administer. Items which are less relevant to the VCT services under consideration may be reduced or discarded. The Appendix cites an example of how the tools could be modified when evaluating VCT services related to MTCT interventions. The tools are presented in a format so they can be photocopied if desired. These tools are also available via the UNAIDS website, and may be downloaded and adapted for local applications.

Selection of Tools

There are eight areas in VCT service development and provision for which monitoring and evaluation tools have been designed. Depending on needs and priorities of particular VCT services, only few of these eight areas will necessitate monitoring and evaluation. For example, when setting up VCT services, Tool 2 for VCT site evaluation: logistic considerations and coverage, can be used to help look at the suitability of sites. Tools 4.1, 4.2, 4.3 and 4.4 could be used in training or for periodic assessment of counsellors.

Monitoring and Evaluation: Participatory Nature

The tools are intended to be used by service providers enabling them to modify and improve practices and procedures in the services where they work. Providers need to have a sense of ownership of the monitoring and evaluation process so that it is clear that the tools are for their own use and benefit. The cooperation and collaboration of both providers and clients is desirable for the evaluation process. Before using the tools it is significant to explain their purpose to those participating in the evaluation. The results should be seen as a way of providing constructive feedback. Participants should be given an opportunity to discuss the assessment and provide additional comments and recommendations. It is hoped that the tools will be used repeatedly over time — for example, when assessing counselling quality and content — so that counsellors have the opportunity to respond to previous assessments and so that quality of counselling can be preserved. The counselling assessment is treated as a way of providing continous appraisal of, and feedback for, counsellors and could be built into training and supervision activities for counsellors.

Reporting and Feedback Mechanisms

Before considering using any of the tools, methods for statistics collection and analysis, reporting and feedback should be planned. Group discussion of the information needs for provisions of services is significant in this process. When evaluating individual counsellors/counselling sessions, immediate feedback following the counselling session (to the counsellor who is being evaluated) is suggested.

Client Consent and Preserving Client Confidentiality

Some of the tools require observation of counselling sessions by the assessor. In these circumstances it is important to explain to the client the purpose of the observation (which is to assist with training and development of the counsellor), reassure her/him that confidentiality will be preserved, and obtain her/his permission. If a client is unwilling or feels uncomfortable about having someone observe the counselling session, this must be given due consideration. When using Tool 7, a sample clients can be interviewed following a counselling session, or at a later stage. Clients should be advised at the earliest possible time, for example, when they make the appointment, that they may be asked to help with an assessment of the counselling service. If a client fails to attend this should be respected. If he or she wishes to be seen at a later time either at the centre or at home this should be managed. When this method was used during field-testing of this discussion in Zambia there were very few refusals and the majority of clients said that they had found the experience of speaking with the researcher useful. No adverse consequences were admitted.

Major Difficulties

Worries about acceptability of observation: In pilot settings where observational assessments have been used they have had a much higher acceptance by clients than was anticipated. Both clients and counsellors admit that the observations were much less intrusive than they feared, and several counsellors and clients said that they were unaware of the observer soon after the session began. Counsellors admitted once they had been reassured that the purpose of the observations was to assist them improve their counselling skills and that it was not a test, they felt more comfortable and could understand the advantages of the process. Some counsellors and counselling trainers explained that they thought clients would find it difficult to have an observer sitting in during a counselling session. They were worried that clients would be unable to discuss sensitive problems before a third person. However, in pilot studies it was observed that the majority of clients did not experience any difficulties with having an observer sitting in. A few clients said before the counselling session that they would prefer not to have an observer and this was respected. As with all the tools narrated it is important to explain their purpose (to the counsellor and/or the client), to ensure confidentiality and to permit them to defer or refuse to attend. In some countries counsellors have stated that it would not be acceptable to have counselling sessions observed by an assessor/counsellor. Alternative methods of assessing counselling sessions, which would be probable ways of overcoming this problem, include:

(a) *Audio recording of counselling sessions:* This has been successfully used in some settings and has been acceptable to both counsellor and client. Non-verbal communication cannot, however, be observed.

(b) *One-way mirrors:* Using a mirrored glass window through which a session can be observed by the supervisor has been used to assess counselling sessions. Although clients and counsellors may witness this less intrusive than having the observer in the same room it is an expensive choice. It is therefore unlikely to be practical to use extensively.

(c) *Dummy patients:* Dummy patients are volunteers trained to present to the counsellor with a particular problem. They can then report on the content and quality of the counselling sessions, but if the check-list tools are to be used they will have to fill these in after the counselling session. It is noteworthy that, if dummy patients are used, the counsellors are warned that this evaluation method has been chosen, otherwise counsellors may perceive a breach in trust between themselves and the supervisor.

(d) *Role-play sessions:* Role-play sessions can be very advantageous and have been used on a large scale in training of counsellors. Trainee counsellors or volunteers can present several case scenarios to the counsellor while the supervisor and other counsellors observe the role play. One VCT centre has used the four parts of Tool 4 (counselling evaluation) in training sessions for new counsellors where participants took it in turn to be clients.

(e) *Video recording of counselling sessions:* Video-recorded counselling sessions have been used in a few countries to assess counselling sessions. It is, however, appropriate only in very limited settings due to the problems with ensuring confidentiality and expense. If video recordings are used, the explicit consent of the client and counsellor must be given with the assurance that the counselling session will only be viewed by the counsellor and supervisor/assessor. Moreover, a fail-safe method of ensuring that the video recording be omitted following the assessment must be in place. Video recording of role-play sessions or dummy patients can, however, be advantageous and does not have problems with ensuring confidentiality.

Observation will bias the session: Having an observer sitting in a counselling session may change the dynamics of the counselling session and it could be considered that the counsellor will have an "improved performance" if he/she is being observed. However, the objective of the observations is to assist counsellors improve their counselling skills, rather than to test them. In field-testing counsellors admitted that although they initially felt nervous, the observed sessions were not different from "normal" ones to a large extent. Observers admitted that they found it easy to discover good aspects in the counselling sessions as well as the fields that could be improved.

Who should carry out the observation: The counselling observations can be carried out by:

A senior counsellor/supervising counsellor: The advantage of this is that there is no need to employ additional people. Logistic complications are minimised and it is easy to follow up an identified issues and provide continous assessment of trainees. Moreover, the counsellor may feel less frightened if he/she knows the person sitting in on the session.

However, there are some shortcomings. It could be construed that it is in the best interests of the supervisor to demonstrate that his/her counsellors are all competent, because this could be witnessed to reflect on his/her ability to train and supervise. However, it should be emphasized that the evaluation is not a pass/fail test of competence, but a way of upgrading performance and highlighting strengths and weaknesses in the service with an opinion to improving them. There is also the potential for personal dynamics to interfere in the evaluation of a counsellor by a supervisor, for example, if a counsellor likes or dislikes a particular counsellor.

Fellow/Counsellor: There are some advantages in using peer counsellors' observations. They can benefit from the experience of other counsellors and if this is a reciprocal practice it is likely to be unthreatening. The senior counsellor/supervisor must, however, have to take part in reviewing the process with the counsellors. This method has been used successfully in pilot-testing.

Independent Assessor: An independent assessor may offer a more objective assessment and can make comparative observations across sites. Providing and training an independent assessor may be expensive, especially if a service is to be evaluated as part of its regular programmes.

References

1. WHO draft report (Alfred Chingono). *Protocol for setting and monitoring locally acceptable standards of counselling in relation to HIV diagnosis,* 1994.
2. WHO draft report. *Guidelines for implementing HIV/AIDS counselling,* 1993.
3. NACO, India, draft report. *Counselling policy and related aspects: National AIDS prevention and control policy,* 1998.
4. Miller D, Casey K. *Thailand Department of Mental Health HIV/AIDS counselling: participant information and casework audit form,* 1998.
5. Baggaley R. *Fear of knowing: why 9 in 10 couples refused HIV tests in Lusaka Zambia,* Abstract number E.1266, 10th International Conference on AIDS and STDs in Africa, Abidjan, December 1997.
6. Temmerman M et al. The right not to know HIV-test results, *Lancet,* 1996, 345:696-7.
7. Mwingwa A, Hosp M, Godfrey-Faussett P. Twice weekly tuberculosis preventive therapy in HIV infection in Zambia, *AIDS,* 1998, 12:2447-2457.
8. WHO/UNAIDS. *Policy statement on preventive therapy against tuberculosis in people living with HIV,* document WHO/TB/98.255 UNAIDS/98.34, 1998.
9. Sassan-Morokro M et al. *Significant reduction in mortality attributed to cotrimoxazole prophylaxis among HIV-infected tuberculosis patients in Abidjan, Côte d'Ivoire.* Abstract 12461, presented at the 12th World AIDS Conference, Geneva, Switzerland, 1998.
10. Centers for Disease Control and Prevention. Administration of zidovudine during late pregnancy to prevent perinatal HIV transmission - Thailand 1996-1998, *MMWR,* 1998, 47:151-153.

11. Sweat M, Sangiwa G, Balmer D, *HIV counselling and testing in Tanzania and Kenya is cost-effective: Results for the voluntary counselling and testing study.* Abstract no. 33277, presented at the 12th World AIDS Conference, Geneva, Switzerland, 1998.
12. The importance of simple and rapid tests in HIV diagnostics: WHO recommendations. *Weekly Epidemiological Record,* October 1998, 73(42):321-328.
13. Coates T, Collins C. Preventing HIV infection. *Scientific American,* July 1998, pages 96-97.
14. Sangiwa G et al. *Voluntary HIV counselling and testing (VCT) reduces risk behaviour in developing countries: results from the multisite voluntary counselling and testing efficacy study.* Abstract 33269 presented at the 12th World AIDS Conference, Geneva, Switzerland, 1998.
15. Alien S, Serufilira A, Gruber V. Pregnancy and contraceptive use among urban Rwandan women after HIV counselling and testing, *Am J Public Health,* 1993, 83:705-710.

Two

Voluntary Counselling and Testing: Its Impact

Introduction

The various approaches to HIV prevention and care necessitate people to know their HIV status. The significance of voluntary counselling and testing (VCT) has brought about the broader promotion and development of VCT services. However, since the majority of countries where HIV has a major impact are also the poorest, the lack of resources has meant that VCT is often still not widely available in the highest-prevalence countries. For VCT services to be prioritized and for resources to be provided for their development, demonstrating the effectiveness of VCT is necessary. One of the difficulties in evaluating VCT's effectiveness is the technicality of the VCT process and the wide range of probable outcomes. The term VCT has also been used in many contexts to cover a broad spectrum of interventions. In this article it consists interventions that comprise a minimum of pre- and post-test counselling related to testing. However, it acknowledges that many VCT services offer ongoing/ supportive counselling. This chapter examines the different roles of VCT, considers the several outcomes of VCT that can be evaluated and discusses the limitations and difficulties related to VCT evaluation. Based on published and unpublished works, conference abstracts and case studies, this discussion focusses on information from developing countries. While some examples from developed countries are mentioned, this information is not comprehensive, hence review articles providing more complete information are described.

The Objectives

1. ***Prevention of HIV transmission***
   From positive-tested people to untested or negative partners
   From positive-tested mother to child
2. ***Prevention of HIV acquisition***
   By negative-tested people from positive or untested partners
3. ***Early and appropriate uptake of service***
   Positive-tested people
   (a) Medical care (consisting ARV therapy, treatment of OIs, prevention of OIs and HIV-related infections and screening for HIV-related infections and tumours)
   (b) Family planning (including counselling about reproductive choices)
   (c) Emotional care (including individual, couple and family support)
   (d) Counselling for positive living (ongoing counselling, nutrition, disclosure issues and discovery of safety network)
   (e) Social support
   (f) Improved coping and planning for the times to come
   (g) Legal assistance

   Negative-tested people
   (a) Emotional care
   (b) Family planning (including counselling about reproductive options)
   (c) Improved coping and planning for the times to come
4. **Societal benefits**
   (a) Normalisation of HIV
   (b) Challenging stigma
   (c) Promoting education
   (d) Supporting human rights
5. **Counselling for adherence**
   (a) Adherence to ARVs and preventive therapies
   (b) Coping with adverse impacts
   (c) Counselling about adherence in MTCT interventions.

Limitations

VCT services, which are available for many diverse groups of people in several settings, vary in their aims to a large extent.

This makes comparing VCT interventions difficult and sometimes misleading. The challenges of comparing interventions are summarised below.

The Challenges of Comparing the Interventions

Different Interventions

The content and quality of VCT services provided within and across countries vary considerably. It may thus be inappropriate to compare in-depth, long-term counselling services, where follow-up social and medical support is provided, for example, with routine VCT related to STI clinics, where such services are not at hand.

Factors Influencing Outcomes of VCT Interventions

(a) Theoretical articulation of counselling
(b) Content and quality of counselling
(c) Number of counselling sessions undertaken
(d) Individual, couple or group pre-test counselling
(e) HIV testing techniques employed in VCT sites (same-day simple/rapid testing versus ELISA)
(f) Related support services available to VCT sites
(g) Anonymous versus confidential versus mandatory testing and reporting of results
(h) Age/emotional maturity of clients
(i) Socio-economic issues (may affect access to treatment, prophylaxis)

Different Populations

Differences in impact and outcomes will be observed when assessing VCT interventions in different populations. In developed countries, many of the studies looking at VCT and sexual behaviour change have been conducted among injecting drug users (IDUs), homosexual men and attenders at sexually transmitted infection clinics. In sub-Saharan Africa, the majority of studies have been among the general population attending VCT centres, women attending antenatal clinics and among commercial sex workers. It is difficult to make comparisons between these groups as patterns and determinants of behaviour vary to a large extent.

Time Considerations

Timing of Evaluation

Many operational VCT projects are evaluated when they are set up, and research projects may establish VCT services to specifically look at their impact. This means that evaluations often take place before services have been fully developed or before communities have become accustomed to the intervention or realised its probable advantages. This is particularly significant in countries where VCT is a new service or where counselling has not previously been an element of medical care and support.

If the evaluation is repeated when services are well-established, different outcomes may be achieved. For example, when setting up the first VCT service in Lusaka, Zambia many people who attended during the first two years were symptomatic and thus the seropositivity rate of attenders was very high (more than 60 per cent). People, at this stage, attended for testing to confirm what they suspected or they were referred by health care professionals, friends or relatives who worried that they might have HIV. As the service developed and people became more aware of VCT's importance in HIV prevention, the seropositivity rate among attenders declined to less than 25 per cent. Many asymptomatic young people wished to know their HIV status and there was less stigma related to testing. Moreover, as accessible treatments became available people were less reluctant to be tested since they felt there was something that could be offered if they tested positive (Kara). In Uganda the population seeking VCT has also changed over time. In 1992, 66 per cent of clients were male. By 1997, more women were seeking VCT and the proportion of men had fallen to 51 per cent. Seropositivity rates of attenders also changed; in 1990, 35 per cent of female and 23 per cent of male attenders were seropositive. By 1998, seropositivity rates of attenders marked a decline to 26 per cent for females and 14 per cent for males.

The Epidemic: Maturity and Magnitude

The maturity of the epidemic may have a significant impact on outcomes. This is particularly true for uptake and return rates. In areas where the epidemic is new, ignorance, denial and stigma may be more closely related to HIV testing in comparison to the countries where the epidemic is more well-established. Countries where the epidemic is mature may also be experiencing a deep impact from HIV in terms of morbidity and mortality and other morbid symptoms such as rising numbers of orphans. These visual and practical consequences of HIV may be important in finding out how people perceive their own risk of infection, and thus their desire to undergo VCT. Countries where HIV-2 is the prominent infection may have high seroprevalence rates but low levels of morbidity, therefore fewer people will be encouraged to test for HIV since they witness less evidence of vulnerability in their community.

HIV Transmission: Its Prevention

HIV incidence/seroconversion. The most precise gauge of VCT's effectiveness in lessening HIV transmission is the *rate of new HIV infection* in people following VCT, in comparison to a control group who were tested but were unaware of their serostatus. However, due to ethical considerations and practical difficulties in performing such studies, approximations of seroconversion rates are used, or comparisons are made with other seroincidence/seroprevalence rates from other studies. An early, community-based study of patients with symptomatic HIV disease reported high rates of unprotected sexual intercourse and, consequently, high HIV transmission in incongruous couples following VCT (Hira, 1990[2]). People living in the same household as index patients with AIDS or symptomatic HIV disease in Lusaka, Zambia were clinically and serologically evaluated for HIV-1 infection. In the 150 households of male index cases, 92 (61.3 per cent) of their spouses were infected, compared with 57 (73.1 per cent) of the spouses of the 78 female index cases. Of the 52 discordantly infected couples followed for 1 year, 46 continued to have unprotected vaginal intercourse and 11 (21.2 per cent) of these seroconverted to HIV.

The study suggests that there is ongoing risk of HIV heterosexual transmission as infection advances in the infected partner. In this study, VCT failed to assist couples to adopt protected sex practices and prevent seroconversion. The study's objective was descriptive rather than to provide an intervention to prevent HIV transmission. It has been revealed that more effective counselling was a must. In a study from Kinshasa, Democratic Republic of the Congo (earlier known as Zaire), intensive couple counselling following testing was demonstrated to be effective in changing sexual behaviour in serodiscordant couples. The counselling resulted in a low rate of HIV seroconversion: 3.1 per cent per 100 person-years of observation in Congolese married couples with discordant HIV status who attended VCT. (Kamenga et al., 1991[3]). While this was an uncontrolled study, the low rate of seroconversion was identical to that documented in other prospective studies of married couples with serodiscordant results from the United States, who were counselled to use condoms (Goedert et al., 1987[4]). In a prospective study conducted in Rwanda, 60 serodiscordant couples were discovered, of whom 53 were followed up for an average of 2.2 years. During the follow-up, 2 of the 23 seronegative men and 6 of the 30 seronegative women seroconverted (seroconversion rates of 4 and 9 per 100 person-years). The rate was less than 50 per cent that approximated for similar women in serodiscordant couples where only the women had received VCT and the men were tested but unaware of their HIV status (Allen et al., 1992[5]).

A study of 1458 women, conducted by the same group, compared women who had been tested but whose partners were not aware of their status with women whose partners had also received VCT and were aware of their status. In the latter group, HIV seroconversion rates declines considerably (from 4.1 to 1.8 per 100 person-years $P<0.4$) (Allen et al., 1992[6]). In Pune, in Maharashtra State in India, the seroincidence rate in 1995 was approximated as 18 per cent per annum among patients who attend STI (sexually transmitted infection) clinics (Brookmeyer et al., 1995[7]). At the same site the impact of VCT in HIV prevention among those who tested negative was examined (Bentley et al., 1998[8]). Following VCT the risk of seroconversion was 6.1 per 100 person-years. Rates of seroconversion were examined in 144 heterosexual discordant couples recruited in California in the United States who were followed up for an average of 1.34 years (Padian et al., 1987[9]). Couples were generally counselled and tested in their own homes, and intensive follow-up counselling and support were available. Both condom use and sexual abstinence noted an increase over time. Most behaviour change was initiated between intake and first follow-up visit. No seroconversions were noted after 193 couple-years of follow-up. In this study, intensive couple counselling associated with social support seemed to be a very effective means to promote and sustain behaviour change among HIV-infected individuals and their heterosexual partners. It is noteworthy that the couples in this study were living in stable relationships, and in developed countries the gender inequilibrium in sexual negotiation may be less marked. In many high-prevalence countries women who are seropositive may find it difficult to ensure protected sex practices and prevent HIV transmission to uninfected partners.

Incidence of STIs

An appropriate proxy-indicator of adoption of protected sex practices (and hence a decline in HIV transmission) is incidence of STIs, following VCT. A study of Rwandan women recruited from antenatal and paediatric outpatient clinics revealed that VCT was associated with reduced rates of gonorrhoea (the prevalence of gonorrhoea noted a decline from 13 to 6 per cent $P<0.05$) among seropositive women following VCT. The greatest reduction in gonorrhoea was among those who admitted that they used condoms (16 to 4 per cent $P<0.05$) (Allen et al., 1992).

However, in the United States, a study from an STI clinic in Miami demonstrated a decrease in STI rates following VCT for those who tested seropositive, but a 103 per cent increase in rates of STI infection in those who tested seronegative. It was concluded that this may be partly due to the inadequate counselling received by those who tested seronegative (Otten et al., 1993[10]). Another study conducted among pair-matched seropositive and seronegative STI attenders in London (n = 218) demonstrated no significant association between serostatus and incidence of STI (George et al., 1998[11].)

Sexual Behaviour

The primary objective of VCT is preventive — to help people change their sexual behaviour so as to avoid transmitting HIV to sexual partners if seropositive, and to remain seronegative if negative. Thus, many studies that aim to assess the effectiveness of VCT have observed the changes in reported sexual behaviour following testing. There are, however, methodological problems related to these types of studies. Attempts at obtaining information on sexual behaviour must rely on self-reporting and there are some opportunities for checking information obtained against that from other sources.

Analytical Complexities and Interpretation of Statistics on Sexual Behaviour

Different Methods of Data Collection

There may be considerable inaccuracies and inconsistencies in collecting statistics about sexual behaviour. This can be compounded by different data-collection methods. Studies use innumerable data-collection techniques, including self-administered questionnaires, in-depth qualitative interviews, interview-administered questionnaires, telephone inteviews, summaries of clinical notes, postal surveys and methods using 'flash cards'. Different studies also report different sampling methods, length of follow-up, follow-up rates and processes, making comparisons between studies a challenge.

Cultural Differences

Attitudes about sexual behaviour differ amply and may influence reporting. In countries where discussing sexual issues is taboo, people may be reluctant to disclose intimate details or they may under-report sexual behaviour that is not 'approved of' or illegal (e.g., possible under-reporting of homosexuality in countries in sub-Saharan Africa, where it is criminalised). Other populations, which have strong cohesion and identity (such as homosexual men in San Francisco) may be less prohibited about discussing sexual practices. Interpretation of sexual terms may also vary between and within populations and may make interpretation of self-administered questionnaires complicated. For example, in Zambia at the time of in-depth interviews it was witnessed that some men considered themselves to be 'abstinent' if they were only having sex with their wife and other interviewees interpreted abstinence as not having sexual intercourse with anyone. Definitions of sexual practices may also vary with translation (which often occurs in studies where the participants are interviewed in their own language and the questionnaires are subsequently translated into English for analytical objectives).

Gender Differences

In most studies of reported sexual behaviour women report fewer sexual partners than men. In a national survey of sexual behaviour conducted in the United Kingdom the mean lifetime number of sexual partners was reported at 9.9 for men and 2 for women (Wellings et al., 1994[12]). Similar differences — a higher number of lifetime sexual partners reported by male than female students — were narrated in a survey among university students in Lusaka, Zambia and London, the United Kingdom (Baggaley et al., 1997[13]). These differences may be in part because of the social acceptability of men reporting multiple sexual partners, and male sex with commercial sex workers.

The ability to change sexual behaviour, as well as obstacles to these changes, may also vary considerably between countries and groups studied. For example, the use of condoms has been commonplace in many European countries for several decades and in developing countries, condoms are often unavailable and their use still very low. For example, until recently, condoms have often not been largely available in rural areas in sub-Saharan Africa. Even when they were distributed as part of a social marketing policy, condom use was still relatively low — 2.7 per cent of rural women and 6.9 per cent of rural men in Zambia said that they or their partner had used condoms (DHS, 1996[14]). This, in part, may be the outcome of economic and social issues as well as unfamiliarity with condoms. In some countries, religious or cultural beliefs preclude their widespread use or distribution.

Different Populations

Due to the wide range of groups studied it is difficult to make comparisons, or to perform meta-analyses of outcomes associated with sexual behaviour (Weinhardt et al., 1999[15]). It may be difficult or inappropriate to compare condom use among discordant gay couples from one place with discordant injecting drug users (IDU) heterosexual couples from another place.

Counselling can Lessen Risk Behaviour

Developing Countries

Studies demonstrating that sexual risk behaviour reduces significantly with counselling come from several developing countries. The recent multi-centre VCT efficacy trial was the first randomised trial of HIV counselling and testing from developing countries. It revealed that VCT resulted in greater behaviour change than health education alone. However, seropositive people were more likely than seronegative to demonstrate major changes in behaviour. However, some useful details are available in a scholarly write up.

Studies from Sub-Saharan Africa

Background Summary

(a) HIV transmission is widely because of heterosexual transmission. Although some groups, such as commercial sex workers, are more severely affected than others are, HIV affects the general population and is not just a issue that is limited to minority or vulnerable groups. The male-female ratio is approximately 1:1. Women have higher rates of infection in the younger age groups.

(b) The severest burden of HIV is in sub-Saharan Africa—more than 70 per cent of people living with HIV live in the region. Although the range of HIV seroprevalence in these countries is considerably large, many other countries are experiencing the widespread monetary and social impacts of HIV. These include the deaths of men and women between the ages of 20 and 40 — at a time when they are most economically productive — as well as a growing number of orphans. The average adult seroprevalence in sub-Saharan Africa is 8 per cent (range less than 0.5-35 per cent)[16].

(c) Counselling services prior to HIV were rare and the concept of 'formal' counselling was not known to most people. Often there were well-established systems for communicating and discussing health problems and issues associated with adolescent sexuality, commonly involving community elders or trusted family members as the educator. However, HIV has not often been adequately incorporated into these structures. Subsequently, HIV counselling services have been developed, though often in a piecemeal fashion or related to research projects. However, VCT services are now being expanded — often related to MTCT interventions.

Efficacy/Sexual Behaviour Change: Summary

(a) Studies among serodiscordant couples who are counselled and tested together demonstrate significant reductions in seroconversion following VCT.

(b) The majority of studies conducted among individual and couple attendees at VCT demonstrate that people can make some changes in sexual behaviour to reduce HIV transmission, but long-term changes are difficult without both partners being aware of their status.

(c) Although there are obstacles and difficulties for both men and women, most studies report that women, in particular, find it difficult to practice protected sex (or negotiate with their sexual partners to use protected sex methods) following VCT.

(d) Most studies in sub-Saharan Africa have been conducted when VCT services are initially established and longer-term analysis would be valuable.

Developed Countries

Studies Among Heterosexuals from Developed Countries

Background Summary

(a) There being increasing numbers of people with HIV who are infected with HIV by heterosexual transmission the largest numbers of cases are witnessed in people with 'risk factors'.

1. men who have sex with men
2. injecting drug users (IDUs)
3. people from Africa living in Europe.

(b) In Western Europe the adult seroprevalence rate is 0.25per cent and in the United States 0.56 per cent with less than 20 per cent of those infected being women[17].

(c) HIV prevalence remains relatively low among the general population and in many communities it is perceived as a problem of marginalised groups.

(d) The majority of the studies that have been conducted in developed countries have been among men who have sex with men (MSM) and injecting drug users (IDUs).

(e) VCT services are often available to the general population as well as for special groups in Europe and the United States. Uptake of VCT is generally low among the general population, though increasing numbers of women are being tested routinely for HIV at antenatal clinics.

(f) Services for persons living with HIV/AIDS (PLHAs) are generally well-developed with the majority of people being eligible for combination antiretroviral therapy.

Efficacy/Sexual Behaviour Change: Summary

(a) In general, the revelations are mixed, but many provided at least some evidence supporting the ability of VCT to encourage risk-reducing behaviour, however, some did not. The pattern of outcomes varied substantially across, and within, study populations and were often limited by methodological weaknesses.

(b) Counselling of serodiscordant couples has, however, been demonstrated to be very effective in eradicating HIV transmission.

(c) VCT in STI clinics and among students has only limited impact in changing sexual behaviour.

(d) Many of the studies occurred in settings with low seroprevalence. It has been established that people attending VCT may have already changed their behaviour prior to seeking testing, or did not perceive themselves to be at risk from HIV infection.

Pregnancy

Knowledge of HIV status can enable women to make informed decisions about whether or not to have children. Early in the epidemic there were no effective interventions to prevent mother-to-child transmission (MTCT) of HIV and women were sometimes motivated by health care professionals not to have children. Since the publication of the outcomes of the ACTG 076 trial in 1994 (Connor et al., 1994[18]) most seropositive women in developed countries are offered antiretrovirals (ARVs) to prevent MTCT and its rate is at present low. Before ARV interventions were available the incidence of pregnancy among women following VCT had been examined in three studies from the United States and two from Africa. The study of women and their husbands/partners in Rwanda (Allen et al., 1993)[19] demonstrated that VCT was related to increased use of condoms and reduced rates of gonorrhoea and HIV. However, pregnancy rates were identical for women testing seronegative and those women testing seropositive. There were also no differences witnessed in pregnancy rates in seropositive and seronegative women in Kenya (Kiragu et al., 1990[20]). The three studies from the United States also disclosed similar rates of pregnancy among women who knew they were seronegative and those who knew they were seropositive (Sunderland et al., 1988[21], Selwyn et al., 1989[22] and Cowan et al., 1990[23]).

Rates of termination of pregnancy were examined in one study that was also conducted before the recommendations to prevent MTCT were introduced (Sunderland et al., 1992[24]). Seropositive women were more likely to seek termination of pregnancy (TOP) than seronegative women. A study of female injecting drug users (IDUs) however, demonstrated no differences in the rates of termination of pregnancy (TOP) among seropositive and seronegative women (Pivnick et al., 1991[25]).

Since ARVs to prevent MTCT are at present widely available in developed countries, and are becoming increasingly available in some developing countries, counselling seropositive women about pregnancy has a different emphasis (to be discussed later in this text).

Voluntary Partner Notification and Partner Testing

One of VCT's important objectives is to lessen HIV transmission by motivating changes in sexual behaviour following testing. It is therefore important to be able to share HIV status with one's sexual partner in order to make appropriate changes in sexual behaviour.

Disclosure of HIV Test Result to Sexual Partner

It is difficult to make long-term changes in sexual behaviour without being able to share HIV test results with a sexual partner or partners. Disclosure to a sexual partner or partners can be witnessed as an important indicator of understanding and acceptance of HIV status. There are, however, societal issues that have a deep impact on rates of disclosure, particularly for women. The opinions of counsellors may also influence disclosure rates.

Disclosure after VCT

Most studies demonstrate that the majority of people share their HIV results with someone and disclosure rates increase over time as people adjust to their test result. Levels of disclosure to spouse/sexual partner/s are, however, generally lower. In studies from developing countries disclosure rates range from 24-79 per cent. Partner testing is lower (less than 1-75 per cent). Studies from developed countries also reveal that not all women are able to tell their partners that they have been tested.

Disclosure after VCT in Antenatal Settings

There is increasing emphasis on offering VCT to women attending antenatal clinics to enable them to take interventions to prevent MTCT. Thus, many studies are looking at disclosure to male partners in this context. Disclosure rates - and subsequent testing rates of sexual partners - vary considerably. It is often difficult for women in developing countries to reveal their HIV status with their partners/spouses and testing women alone (rather than as a couple) does not facilitate disclosure. Innovative ways of involving men in antenatal testing should be sought so that women are not blamed or isolated if they are identified to be seropositive. If men can be offered VCT they can take an informed and active role in decisions around the future, family planning and coping with MTCT interventions.

Couple Counselling

High rates of sero-discordancy among married couples have been revealed in many studies. Couple counselling prevents the problems of revelation to partners and has been a successful intervention where it has been promoted, although in some countries there are obstacles to attending.

Premarital VCT

Pre-marital testing is being promoted in some countries, especially by religious organisations. There are no statistics on the long-term outcomes of this strategy.

Disclosure and Domestic Violence

The fear of emotional and physical abuse as well as abandonment are main issues in low rates of disclosure among women, particularly from Asia and sub-Saharan Africa. Counsellor training could consist programmes that address violence awareness.

Counselling Clients about Disclosure

Often counselling clients about disclosure is just an instruction or suggestion to disclose and clients are not engaged in practical strategies of how to do this, i.e. problem-solving or role-playing. This may be an alleviating factor in the lower effectiveness of counselling interventions.

Partner Revelation from VCT Sites

Developing countries

A study from Lusaka, Zambia, demonstrated that while many people expressed worries about sharing HIV test outcomes, with time, the majority — both men and women — were able to disclose someone about their status. There was no major difference between those testing seropositive or seronegative. Some narrated that they had experienced difficulties following revelation. However, less than half of people with positive results were able to tell their sexual partners (Baggaley et al., 1997[26]). A very small percentage (less than 5 per cent) of partners subsequently came for counselling and testing. Inability to discuss HIV test outcomes with a sexual partner makes adopting safer sex practices more difficult. Many people who had not told their partner said that this was because they were ashamed of being seropositive or having gone for a test. Those who were seronegative said that even going for a test would make their partner suspicious. Some said that they feared blame, abandonment or abuse if their partner found out they were seropositive. Although both women and men expressed these opinions, women more commonly expressed them.

A prospective study of seropositive women in Rwanda established that after testing, 75 per cent said that they did not expect a supportive response from their partners when they told them about their status. However, when they were re-interviewed three years later, acceptance, understanding and sympathy were the general reactions of their partner after revelation. Nevertheless, 21 per cent had still not been able to tell their partner. Of the men, 48 per cent had tested for HIV following their partner's revelation of her seropositive status (Keogh et al., 1994[27]). Informing marital partners was found to be a major problem for most people with HIV in Zimbabwe. (Meursing et al., 1995[28, 29]). The major factors for non-disclosure were relatively good health and emotional status, denial of diagnosis, fear of rejection, limited knowledge of and belief in strategies to 'live positively with HIV', unacceptability of condoms and protected sex, and women's economic dependency and lack of power in sexual situations. However, with enhanced counselling 75 per cent were able to reveal to their partner/spouse.

Out of 3381 men who were enrolled in a factory, worker cohort 56 per cent returned for their HIV test result in Zimbabwe (Dube et al., 2000[30]). Although all men were motivated to bring their sexual partners for VCT, only 7 per cent did so. Twelve focus-group discussions (FGD) were carried on and several reasons were cited for this:

(a) They experienced difficulties with introducing the subject of VCT due to uncommunicative nature of their relationships.
(b) They feared that sero-discordant outcomes would lead to divorce.
(c) They feared that results would reveal their partners' or their own past, present or future infidelities.

(d) They thought that VCT was not a high priority relatively with other issues in their lives.
(e) Their wives were unable to attend the urban VCT site because they lived in rural areas.
(f) The men reported that the wives would assume they were negative if their husband was negative.
(g) The men reported a lack of interactive communication between their counsellors and themselves during pre-test counselling and they did not feel able to confide in them.

In Burkina-Faso, only 24 per cent of people who were seropositive and living in a stable relationship were able to tell their partner about their result. It has been established that in this mainly Muslim community non-disclosure may be justified in some situations, but acknowledge that it is a major barrier to HIV prevention (Badini et al., 1998[31]).

Developed Countries

A study from London also revealed differing patterns of disclosure. Although most people were able to share their HIV status with someone it was often difficult for seropositive people to share their HIV status with their sexual partner, especially if the partner was a casual or non-primary sexual partner (Miller et al., 1998[32]). Similar results were cited in a study of MSM from the United States (Huggins et al., 1991[33]). Following VCT, MSM were much more likely to tell regular partners than casual sexual partners.

Partner Revelation and Partner Testing Following Antenatal Testing

VCT services are being largely developed in MCH services in conjunction with MTCT interventions. In these settings women are generally tested alone, yet important decisions relating to their status should ideally be shared with their partner. In a small study from the Western Cape in South Africa less than half of seropositive women were able to reveal their HIV status to anyone and only a minority of these discussed it with their partner (Sigxaxhe, 2000[34]). In the MTCT programme in Botswana revelation to partners is also reported as being low and very few men are either tested together with their partners/wives or agree t test a little later (Mazhani et al., 2000[35].)

Information from 13 study sites offering VCT and MTCT interventions — from west (Abidjan, Bobo-Dioulasso), east (Addis Ababa, Nairobi, Mombassa, Dar Es Salaam) and southern Africa (Blantyre, Lusaka, Harare, Soweto, Durban) and 1 from Thailand — demonstrated low numbers of men agreeing to testing in most settings (Cartoux et al., 1998)[36].

In a study from Nairobi, Kenya, women provided VCT when they attended for antenatal care. Women were advised to tell their sexual partner their HIV status and to bring their partner for further counselling and testing, if desired (Temmerman M, et al., 1995[37]). However, of the 324 women who were identified to be seropositive only 66 (27.2 per cent) informed their test result to their partner and only 21 partners subsequently tested (5, or 23.8 per cent, were seronegative). Due to the adverse outcomes of partner disclosure that occurred during the study, the policy of partner notification was changed and women were counselled to make their own options about whether or not to involve their partner. Subsequently, only 109 out of 311 (35 per cent) of women with a seropositive result ever returned for their test result and only 9 (3 per cent) partners came for VCT. In Rwanda, of the 1 223 women screened for HIV at an antenatal clinic 70 per cent of the women who had post-test counselling said that they wished their partners to be tested for HIV. However, despite the persuasion of the counselling staff and the available infrastructure only 8 per cent of the partners were tested (Ladner et al., 1996[38]).

Results from a small qualitative study from the United States demonstrated following antenatal VCT, although all women had disclosed their HIV status to their partners, only 56 per cent of seropositive and 44 per cent of seronegative women knew their partner's HIV status (Lester P et al., 1995[39]).

Couple Counselling

Developing Countries

Many studies have demonstrated that a major proportion of couples in steady relationships have serodiscordant HIV test results:

(a) In a study from Zambia there were 52 discordantly infected couples from the sample of 245 (21 per cent) (Hira et al., 1990).

(b) In the multi-centre study (n = 589) 17 per cent serodiscordant (Coates et al., 2000).

(c) At AIC in Kampala, Uganda, of 1853 couples that attended together 7 per cent were serodiscordant (Baryarama et al., 1998[40]).

(d) A study from countryside Uganda showed that 7 per cent of couples were serodiscordant (Carpenter et al., 1999[41]). The risk of seroconversion, in this study, was discovered to be 105.5 per 1000 person-years for seronegative women married to seropositive men and 51.7 for seronegative men married to seropositive women.

This is crystal clear that married adults, particularly women with seropositive partners, are at very high risk of HIV infection. Married couples should be motivated to go for HIV counselling together enabling serodiscordant couples to be identified and counselled to help prevent transmission to the uninfected partner. Offering VCT to couples overcomes the problem of sharing test outcomes. Couple counselling and testing is aimed at enabling the couple to negotiate appropriate variations in sexual behaviour together. It also assists them plan together for their future and that of their dependants, with the support from their counsellor at both pre- and post-test. Couples seen together can be counselled to avoid blame and prepared, prior to testing, to coordinate the risk assessment and the reduction plans. The majority of studies of couple counselling among serodiscordant couples admit successful outcomes in terms of changing behaviour to prevent HIV transmission to negative partners.

Use of this model in Rwanda demonstrated that, relative to other VCT services, a far higher proportion of couples wanted to receive HIV counselling and testing together (Allen, 1993 see section 1). Moreover statistics from Rwanda have demonstrated that use of VCT services by cohabiting couples is effective in reducing HIV transmission within HIV discordant couples and diminishing the acquisition of new HIV infections in seronegative couples (Allen et al., 1992; Allen et al., 1993 see section 1). However, in other settings, often there has been large resistance to this approach (Baggaley et al., 1997[42]). Reasons for poor communication between partners are in part due to traditional beliefs about discussing sensitive subjects and roles of men and women within marriage. Teaching about HIV and gender awareness to young people may help future generations, but for women, in particular, who are at present in sexual relations, counselling and testing may fail to protect them from HIV infection from their spouses. In Uganda, although couple counselling was not popular when the services was established — in 1992 less than 9 per cent of attendees were couples — this services has become more popular, with 26 per cent of couple attendees in 1996 (UNAIDS, 1999[43]).

Couple counselling was shown to be effective in changing sexual behaviour in serodiscordant couples (Kamenga et al., 1991, see section 1a). Before VCT, less than 5 per cent of couples had ever used a condom. One month after VCT, 70.7 per cent of couples reported using condoms during all acts of sexual intercourse. At 18 months of follow-up, 77.4 per cent of the 140 couples still being followed reported continued use of condoms during all acts of sexual intercourse. Intensive counselling followed testing and this led to a low rate of HIV seroconversion - 3.1 per cent per 100 person-years of observation in Congolese married couples with discordant HIV status who attended VCT.

At AIDS Information Centre (AIC) in Uganda of 1 853 couples that attended together. 77 per cent said that they had never had sex but were intending to marry or start a sexual relationship; 92 per cent were both seronegative; 0.8 per cent were both seropositive and 7 per cent were serodiscordant (Baryarama et al., 1998[44]). Among the AIDS Information Centre (AIC) clients the probability of a seropositive man having sex with a new partner who was seronegative was 0.81, and among seropositive women 0.84. Thus, there is a high probability that people who are seropositive will develop sexual relationships with seronegative partners and, unknowingly, transmit HIV if VCT is not at hand.

Developed Countries

In a study from the United States, couple counselling was demonstrated to be highly effective in preventing HIV transmission. No seroconversions were reported after 193 couple-years of follow-up among discordant couples following VCT (Padian et al., 1993 see section 1). A study of 27 couples with a history of injecting drug user IDU from New York, however, showed that individuals who were aware of their HIV status for 6 months prior to the interview did not differ significantly in their type of sexual activity or their condom use from those unaware of their serostatus (Carballo-Dieguez et al., 1990[45]). There may, however, be different perceptions and priorities IDU couples that make changing sexual behaviour more difficult.

Premarital VCT

In many high-prevalence countries parents of young people and religious organisations are encouraging pre-marital testing. In Nigeria, Catholic community organisations are promoting pre-marital VCT (Ubane et al., 2000[46]). At AIC in Uganda, increasing numbers of people coming for VCT indicated that marriage plans was the reason they wish to be tested. In 1992, 6 per cent of those attending VCT did so due to pre-marital testing and this figure slumped to 35 per cent in 1998 (Turyagyen Da, 2000[47].)

Obstacles in Modifying Sexual Behaviour

Changing or modifying sexual behaviour is a complicated process, with individual, emotional, societal, practical and economic aspects. The expectation that VCT, one pre- and one post-test counselling session, will always result in protected sexual behaviour is often imaginary. Difficulties may be compounded if people are tested alone and feel unable to share their test outcome with their partner.

Communication Difficulties

It is often difficult for both men and women to discuss HIV testing in general and their own HIV status in particular due to cultural and social taboos surrounding discussion of sexual-issues (Baggaley et al., 1997, Machekano et al., 2000[48], Dube et al., 2000[49]). Without open discussion of HIV status it is difficult to make long-term modofocations in sexual behaviour to prevent HIV transmission. Interventions that provide young people with knowledge and communication skills will be significant for these difficulties to be overcome.

Gender Inequilibrium in Sexual Decision-making and Negotiation Obstacles for Women

Women are often unable to discuss protected sex with their husbands or sexual partners following VCT due to gender imbalances in sexual decision-making. This is a particular issue for commercial sex workers. A study from South Africa admitted that women need communication and negotiation skills so that they can discuss sexual and other problems with their partners (Karim et al., 1995)[50].

Difficulties in Modifying Sexual Behaviour

Many studies have demonstrated that women have less capacity than men do for making changes in their sexual behaviour:

Developed Countries

When seropositive women from San Francisco were questioned following antenatal VCT, although all admitted that they had informed their sexual partner of their positive HIV status, only 40 per cent said their partners used condoms. (Lester et al., 1995[51]). Reasons for not practising protected sex were refusal by partner, partner 'not liking them' or partner 'becoming too excited to wait to use condoms' and alcohol or drug use.

Developing Countries

A study from Rwanda disclosed that men control sexual decision-making (Straten et al., 1995[52]) and seropositive women were more likely to report coercive sex with their partner. If a woman was able to discuss her HIV status, or her husband had earlier been tested she was in a much better position to discuss or attempt negotiating for safer sex and condom use was higher. Involvement of the male partner is crucial for successful HIV risk reduction in couples. In Zimbabwe, women also admitted that it was difficult to make variations in sexual behaviour because of their lack of power in sexual situations (Meursing et al., 1995). Even if women were able to share their seropositive status with their sexual partners they were often unable to insist on (or even discuss) condom use. Men explained that they did not like condoms and they were not thought to be appropriate within marriage. In the multi-centre trial social obstacles were discovered that prevented women (both seropositive and seronegative) from being able to motivate male partners to use condoms (Sangiwa, 2000[53]). Women in Zambia narrated identical barriers (Chanda et al., 1994, Baggaley et al., 1998).

Desire to have Children

The need to have children may be witnessed as a greater priority than preventing HIV transmission. Thus, seropositive women may risk HIV transmission to a seronegative partner or seronegative women may risk acquiring HIV transmission from a seropositive partner (Allen et al., 1992).

Stigma

Uptake of VCT related to MTCT interventions can be inhibited because women fear that they will be discovered seropositive (and hence subject to stigma or discrimination) if they take antiretrovirals or do not breastfeed their infants (Botswana mid-term evaluation 2000). This was cited as a reason for registering a decline in VCT and MTCT interventions.

Economic Deprivation

In many high-prevalence countries abject poverty is the underlying cause of casual and commercial sex, with women and girls depending on money or gifts exchanged for sex (Chabala, 2000[54]). In many settings, while few couples receive VCT, they cannot always afford condoms, particularly if they are to be used for regular sexual partners. Many VCT centres do not provide free or subsidised qualitative condoms.

Checking HIV Transmission in Special Populations following VCT

Men Having Sex with Men (MSM)

The group that has been most widely studied in relation to sexual behaviour following VCT is MSM. These studies have been conducted largely in developed countries (North America, Australia and Europe). Reviews of VCT interventions among MSM are available (Higgins et al., 1991[55], Wolitski et al., 1997[56], Weinhardt et al., 1999[57]). Although unprotected sexual behaviour among MSM has decreased, it was witnessed to be declining prior to VCT being available. Since VCT has been available, some of the studies demonstrate that men have reduced risky behaviour but this is independent of testing. In those studies where VCT is associated with increased behaviour change, sexual behaviour change is more marked in people who are seropositive. Long-term studies have demonstrated that maintaining safer sex behaviour is difficult and many MSM are reported to resume risk behaviours with time (Kelly, 1998[58], Imrie, 1999[59]).

Studies among Men Having Sex with Men

Background Summary

(a) There has been a great variation in the sexual behaviour of MSM since the late 1980s. Much of this behaviour change was probably a result of the very high morbidity and mortality related to HIV in the gay community at the beginning of the epidemic in Europe and the United States. Many gay men witnessed friends die from HIV and it has been recommended that this direct experience resulted in behaviour change at an early stage. These changes were often noted before HIV testing became widely available.

(b) There is however, recent evidence that in some countries these changes in safer sexual behaviour among gay men are being eroded due to civility as life-prolonging ARV therapy is at present widely available. Having an 'undetectable viral load' is misconstrued as having a very low risk of HIV transmission and therefore not necessitating to practice safer sex.

Efficacy/ Sexual Behaviour Change: Summary

(a) Several studies demonstrated noteworthy decline in risk behaviour related to VCT, with seropositive men showing greater reduction in risk behaviour than seronegative men or men who are unaware of their HIV status. This may suggest that learning about being seropositive had a deep impact on changing behaviour and that seronegative men are still putting themselves at risk from infection.

(b) Although there are several studies that indicate that VCT is important in promoting safer sexual behaviour, many studies have inconclusive revelations and there is no consistent evidence to show that VCT is effective in promoting safer sexual behaviour among MSM.

Commercial Sex Workers

In many countries directing care and support to commercial sex workers (SWs) has been witnessed as an important approach in HIV prevention. An STI prevention programme in Kinshasa, the Democratic Republic of the Congo offering VCT, STI screening and treatment, group discussions about prevention and free condoms for HIV seronegative commercial sex workers succeeded in increasing condom use and lessening the incidence of HIV and other STIs (Laga et al., 1994[60]). In the Gambia, however, VCT for commercial sex workers did not result in an increase in condom use (Pickering et al., 1993[61]). Nevertheless, there was very high use of condoms before the intervention (89 per cent of women who subsequently tested seropositive reported using condoms before VCT and this leaves very little room for improvement. Moreover, the majority of HIV among commercial sex workers in the Gambia is because of HIV-2 and there was a low level of morbidity and mortality resulting from HIV in the Gambia at the time of the study. Thus, the effects of HIV infection may be perceived as being less harmful than in areas with high morbidity and mortality due to HIV-1.

A project from KwaZulu Natal in South Africa offered counselling and testing to commercial sex workers at truck stops (Morar et al., 2000[62]). Although uptake of testing was good, the majority of women did not want a positive result disclosed to them as behaviour change was very difficult for economic and social reasons. Following VCT, women also continued with unprotected sexual practices. This project demonstrates the difficulties and social and economic obstacles that must be overcome. It also reflects the limitations that may arise if commercial sex workers alone (and not their clients) are targeted for interventions.

Two studies among commercial sex workers from the United States report a rise in condom use and a decline in risky sexual behaviour following VCT (Corby et al., 1990[63], Cohen et al., 1988[64]). Projects offering peer counselling for commercial sex workers (without testing) have been demonstrated to be well-accepted and provide commercial sex workers information about safer sex and HIV prevention counselling (Cantillo, 1998[65]).

Studies among Commercial Sex Workers

Sex Worker: Summary

There have only been a small number of studies among commercial sex workers (SWs) in developing countries. Most of these studies have demonstrated that VCT can be acceptable and some result in significant variations in sexual behaviour to reduce transmission. However, in some settings economic and social pressures prevent SWs from practising safer sex. It may also be important to provide VCT and HIV education to clients if condom use is to be increased. In developed countries, such as Australia, innovative approaches have been developed to reach commercial sex workers, such as outreach buses and VCT related to IDU services for commercial SWs. In Russia and countries from the former Soviet Union, counselling services for commercial sex workers are beginning to be developed.

Although VCT (as well as other interventions, such as condom provision and screening and treatment of STIs) have been shown to be important and cost-effective interventions, there is still a great lack of provision of specially tailored services for commercial sex workers (Plummer et al., 1994[66]).

STI Clinic Visitors

In a study from the United States among STI attenders VCT was associated with a moderate decrease in STIs among people who tested positive, but the risk increased for people who tested negative. This recommends a need to improve post-test counselling in this setting, especially for people who test negative (Otten et al., 1993[67]). In another study from the United States STI attenders were randomised to either receive AIDS education alone or AIDS education plus VCT. At eight weeks follow-up the mean number of sexual partners noted a decline in both groups. However, compared with the AIDS education group, the VCT group questioned their most recent sexual partner more about HIV status, worried more about getting HIV and used condoms more often with their last sexual partner. VCT in this study was therefore shown to promote protected sex, at least in the short term (Wenger et al., 1991[68]).

Injecting Drug Users (IDUs)

In many countries IDUs play a significant part in HIV transmission. In the United States IDUs comprise one-fourth of the cumulative HIV cases. In New York alone there have been over 50000 cases of HIV among IDUs. Moreover, in the United States sex with an IDU constitutes 52 per cent of AIDS cases that are attributed to heterosexual contact. Of the paediatric AIDS cases, 55 per cent have been attributed to a mother who was exposed to HIV through her own injecting or that of her sexual partner (CDC HIV/AIDS surveillance, 1998). VCT can provide the opportunity for IDUs to know their HIV status and receive counselling about safe injecting practices and safer sex to prevent transmission to sexual partners. In Russia and the newly independent states of the former Soviet Union there has been a sharp rise in new cases of HIV infection — UNAIDS/WHO approximated that the number of infected people increased by a third in 1999 to 360 000. The majority of these were infected directly through IDUs or by having partners who were IDUs.

Studies Among Injecting Drug Users

Background Summary

* VCT services exist for many IDUs in Europe, Australia and the United States. Some IDUs are reluctant to attend them due to poor relationships with authorities and the police (with whom they may associate testing). Although services are being developed in the former Soviet Union and Russia their role in behaviour change has not as yet been fully examined.
* In most of the studies assessing the impact of VCT of safe-injecting behaviour and sexual behaviour, IDUs have been

recruited from drug programmes, some associated with methadone treatment and some with needle exchange.

* These studies often report major variations in behaviour. However, it is difficult to determine whether change occurs due to the treatment programmes or due to VCT.

Efficacy/Injecting Practices: Summary

In the majority of the studies there has been some reduction in risky injection practices (e.g., reduction in needle exchange) following VCT, although the effect of the associated treatment programmes may have a deep impact on this behaviour change.

Efficacy/Sexual Behaviour Change: Summary

In most of the studies there was a deep impact in sexual behaviour that could be directly attributed to the VCT component of the intervention/treatment programme. Changes such as increased condom use were generally more marked among IDUs who tested seropositive, than among IDUs who tested seronegative. Increased emphasis on providing safer sex counselling for IDUs who test seronegative is significant as they may be at continuing risk of HIV infection. In communities where VCT and needle programmes (NEPs) are available for IDUs there have been marked declines in the incidence among IDUs and the predicted rise in incidence has been pre-empted.

Prison Populations

HIV has been identified as a major issue in prisons because unsafe needle-exchange practices and unprotected anal intercourse are common (Macdonald et al., 1999[69], Dolan et al., 1999[70]). Mandatory testing of prisoners is necessitated in some countries and VCT is available in others (Wainstein et al., 1998[71]). It has not been examined whether VCT helps people in prison reduce HIV transmission or helps people to cope better or access services. In several countries preventing HIV in prisons is a very neglected area. Problems of confidentiality, lack of choice associated with coercive sex and lack of harm reduction and safe behaviour options need to be addressed. For the majority of people in custody there is no provision of condoms, clean needles (or access to bleach for cleaning needles), counselling and ongoing support for persons living with HIV/AIDS or adequate discharge counselling.

Truck Drivers

Long-distance truck drivers have been identified to be a vulnerable group at high risk from HIV transmission in sub-Saharan Africa (Wilson et al., 1994[72]). It has been demonstrated that truck drivers have higher HIV prevalence than the general population and in countries like Zimbabwe HIV prevalence is highest in trucking towns such as Masvingo and Rusape (MoH, Zimbabwe). HIV education and condom-promotion interventions have been implemented in several countries (Mwizarubi et al., 1994[73]). VCT has been offered as a component of these interventions in Kenya. VCT offered to truck drivers in Kenya resulted in a decline in sex worker contact, and a decline in the incidence of STIs (from 34 per 100 person-years to 10 per 100 person-years ($p = 0.001$). The percentage of men reporting extramarital sex decreased from 49 per cent to 36 per cent ($P < 0.001$) and the decline in sex worker contact went from 12 to 6 per cent ($p = 0.001$) but there was no change in reported condom use (Jackson et al., 1997[74]). This study provides motivating evidence that VCT programmes developed for individuals at high-risk of exposure can be successful in changing sexual behaviour resulting in a decreased incidence of STIs. In India it has been recognised that truckers are at moderately high risk of HIV infection and counselling services are being set up (Bamne, 2000[75]).

Blood Donors

Until recently VCT services have not been widely available in many sub-Saharan countries and many people who wish to know their HIV status attend blood donation sites. In Zimbabwe this was reported as being a major problem (Mvere et al., 1996[76]). In Zambia this tendency of people who wished to know their HIV status because they felt at risk from infection led to more than 38 of donation testing seropositive. This was not only expensive in terms of wasted units of blood, but also poses a transmission risk since 'high risk' donors may be in the window period. When a pre-test education programme was initiated explaining the rationale for blood donation and suggesting alternative venues for VCT for those who felt at risk, the prevalence rate declined to 8.6 per cent with a subsequent cost saving (Chama et al., 1993[77]). The objective of VCT related to blood donation is primarily to prevent those who are at high risk of HIV infection from donating blood. VCT services associated with blood banks may not be the appropriate sites for counselling individuals about coping with HIV infection and their own sexual behaviour. Referral to other VCT sites would often be more advantageous. However, in the United Sates VCT associated with blood donation may include person risk-reduction counselling. A study from New York among seropositive blood donors demonstrated a significant reduction in unsafe sex following testing (relative to their behaviour before testing), although 40 per cent still reported unsafe sexual behaviour at follow-up discussions (Cleary et al., 1991[78]).

Young People

Background

Young people aged 10 to 24 constitute more than one-half of all HIV infection occurring globally (excluding perinatal cases) (WHO/UNAIDS, 2000). Preventing HIV among young people is particularly urgent in sub-Saharan Africa where, in many countries, youth comprise more than 30 per cent of the population and general HIV prevalence rates exceed 10 per cent.

Several cultural, biological and environmental issues place young people, especially adolescents aged 10 to 19, at increased risk. For example, whether voluntarily or not, young people often begin their sexual lives at early ages. In Uganda, 30 per cent of women have had sexual intercourse by the age of 15 and 72 per cent by the age of 18 (DHS, 1995). In Kenya, the United Republic of Tanzania and Zambia, the average age of sexual initiation is reported to be 16 for females and 17 for males. Despite relatively high levels of knowledge among young people about HIV/STIs, a large proportion of them is involved in risky behaviours, with fewer than 10 per cent of the sexually active adolescent females from countries in sub-Saharan Africa reporting condom use (Zambia, DHS, 1996, the United Republic of Tanzania, DHS, 1996 & Kenya, DHS, 1998).

The immature genital tract of female adolescents makes them biologically more susceptible to the HIV virus, a risk compounded by innumerable social and environmental factors such as young girls engaging in sex with older men (Brookman, 1990[79], Weiss [80] et al., 1996). HIV prevalence rates among youth exposed the realities of these risks. Among pregnant adolescents 15 to 19 in sub-Saharan Africa HIV infection rates range from 4 per cent in Nairobi, Kenya to 32 per cent in Kampala, Uganda, with even higher percentages reported among pregnant women ages 20 to 24. Altogether, HIV rates are high among youth, HIV-infected females are disproportionately affected, with a ratio to infected males in excess of 4:1 in some populations (Munodawafa et al., 1996[81]).

VCT for Young People

While recent study results from sub-Saharan Africa disclose that high-quality VCT is an effective strategy for reducing HIV sexual risk behaviours among adults, little is known about VCT for youth, especially among adolescents ages 14 to 19. At present, though, experiences in several sub-Saharan countries reveal that youth actively seek and receive voluntary HIV counselling and testing, though many have expressed concerns about confidentiality, cost, access and lack of trust in their sexual partners.

Impact of VCT for Young People

There is very little information on the results following VCT for young people and whether they are able to change and sustain changes in sexual behaviour following VCT. Moreover, little is known about the experiences of seropositive young people and what impact a positive result has on their lives, who supports them and what their needs are.

There is very little information on VCT services and young people. In many high-prevalence areas, young people, especially young women, are at high risk from HIV infection yet they often have no access to VCT services. There have been many studies that acknowledge the special vulnerabilities of young people — and young women in particular — to HIV, but this has not been translated into increasing access to VCT services for them. Moreover, issues such as age of consent for VCT for young people, parental involvement in decisions to test, confidentiality and coercion to testing vary and need careful consideration in many settings.

Demand for VCT

In many developing countries VCT has not been available to young people. However, when young people are asked about whether they would like to be tested they often say they would like VCT to be more widely available and would like to be tested. In the pilot phase of a study of young couples in rural Western Kenya, 95 per cent of participants admitted that they would accept a free HIV test. If they had to pay for the service (a $ 4 fee), potential demand remained relatively high with 31-40 per cent saying they would pay for the test. The mean age of couples participating in this study is 22 (Damesyn et al., 1998[82]). In a study exploring knowledge and attitudes to HIV among university students in the United Kingdom and Zambia, 7 per cent of United Kingdom students (n = 217) and 10 per cent of Zambian students (n = 1240) had had an HIV test. A further 35 per cent of Zambian and 15 per cent of United Kingdom students expressed that they would like to be tested (Baggaley et al., 1997[83]). In a KAPB study from Rakai Province in Uganda 84 per cent of 865 young people questioned (18 to 25) said that they would like to see an HIV/AIDS counsellor in the future (Kelly et al., 1993[84]).

A participatory study from Uganda with adolescents (12 to 19) in Mpigi District, Uganda, revealed that the most frequently discussed topic initiated in peer group discussions was HIV transmission, followed by problems of sexuality and the initiation of sexual relationships (Bohmer et al., 1997[85]). Males (17 to 19) and females (14 to 16) demonstrated the greatest interest in HIV testing. However, many young people expressed concerns about issues of confidentiality, cost and location of services, as well as a lack of trust in their sexual partners to remain faithful after having the test. Very similar results were encountered in several focus group discussions and in-depth interviews conducted among young people from three provinces in Zambia (Baggaley et al., 1998[86]). There were 465 young people (m = 217, f = 248) ages 12 to 21 (mean age 17) who took part in the study. Young people proposed several theoretical reasons for HIV testing. Fifty-seven per cent of boys and 53 per cent of girls said that they would like to have the opportunity of going for an HIV test. However, the majority of them were not keen to have an HIV test currently, as they were worried that they would be positive (despite HIV prevalences being relatively low in this age group). Some young people said that they would consider having an HIV test in the future. The small number who had been tested thought it was better to know, even if the result was positive. There was a deep interest in pre-marital testing, which is promoted by several churches. Respondents witnessed this as an opportunity for a 'clean slate', although some said they would still be too afraid of the results to have a test, or felt there was nothing that could be done for them if they were identified to be positive. Some said that they would like pre-marital testing in order to prove their partner had been as careful as they had been, while others wanted to examine before exposing their marriage partner to risks they had taken themselves.

These studies project an abstract demand for VCT, which may not be immediately translated into actual demand, if VCT were made available, and emphasises the need for active promotion of the service and availability of support services for those who test seropositive.

Uptake of VCT

Young people do actively seek and receive VCT in many sub-Saharan countries such as Uganda and Kenya, even though the VCT services available have not been tailored specifically for young people (Nabwiso et al., 1993[87]). The AIDS information Centre (AIC) in Uganda has reported an increase in the numbers of youth seeking VCT, especially for pre-marital testing (Kakooza, 1992[88], Gumisriza et al., 1996[86]). About 15 per cent of AIC clients are between the ages of 15 to 19. By the end of 1995, 39 000 adolescents had visited the centre. Of these adolescents, 78 per cent were females and 40 per cent came to the centre with their sexual partners.

In Brazil uptake of VCT by young people (13 to 19 years) is reported to be increasing (Gomes et al., 2000[90]). In the United States 25 per cent of new HIV infections are in young people (13 to 21 years). To promote VCT in vulnerable young people in New York a social-marketing VCT programme aimed at young people has been developed (Flutterman et al., 2000[91]).

Impact of VCT

Very little is known about the impact of HIV testing on young people — whether it helps them make changes in the sexual behaviour; how young people who test seropositive cope; who they exchange their test result with; who provides emotional support and if they are able to access support services following VCT. A study from Nigeria narrated that the VCT service for young people increased uptake of condoms and decreased STIs but no detailed information was given (Ita, 1998[92]). A study from the United States revealed that VCT promoted a reduction in sexual partners among the majority of males but none of the females reported increasing safe sex practices (Flutterman et al., 1990[93]). Another study from the United States demonstrated that sexually active young people under 18 were less likely to visit VCT than their counterparts 18 to 44, although 50 per cent of new HIV infection in the United States is in men and women under 25 (CDC, 1998[94]). In order to study young people's attitudes and experiences to HIV testing, 73 high-risk (sexually active and economically or socially marginalised youth, living in urban areas with relatively high rates of HIV infection) were interviewed in depth (Kaiser family foundation, 1999[95]). Availability and acceptability of VCT services were found to be a major obstacle to attending VCT for these young people. Worries about confidentiality and fear that results would be shared with parent(s) without their consent also prevented young people from accessing VCT.

Care: Strengthening Access to Medical, Emotional and Social Support

VCT enables people with HIV to seek emotional, social and medical care, and in areas of limited resources permits services to be channelled appropriately. It also enables people who test seronegative to access suitable support and services.

Care Needs Following VCT

There are many supportive benefits of knowing one's HIV status, if seropositive. Studies have demonstrated that there are various major concerns following testing:

The major concerns for those who test seropositive are:

(a) Social support (alongwith material and financial support)
(b) Access to and provision of condoms
(c) Medical care (earlier access to appropriate medical care and preventive therapies)
(d) Emotional support and adjustment/coping (ongoing emotional support from counselling services, spiritual services, traditional medical services, partners, families and community)
(e) Sharing HIV status (with partner, family or close friend)
(f) Peer support (from peer-support groups, post-test clubs and advocacy)
(g) Future planning (making plans for their future and that of their dependents, alongwith making a will)
(h) Access to interventions to prevent MTCT (alongwith infant-feeding counselling, ARV interventions and special antenatal care)
(i) Family-planning services (consisting termination of pregnancy services where legal and safely available).

The major concerns for those who test seronegative are:

(a) Protected sex and staying negative
(b) Future fertility
(c) Exchanging result with partner
(d) Continuing risk of exposure (occupational, positive or untested sexual partner)
(e) Caring for relatives
(f) 'Worried well' (This refers to people who are at very low risk of HIV infection but worry much about being infected. This phenomenon is more common in low-prevalent countries where there has been a prominent HIV education campaign.)

Access to Medical Care

ARVs

In developed countries the development of highly active antiretroviral therapy (HAART) has had a moderate effect on the long-term survival of people with HIV. This has meant that there is great benefit for people with HIV to be aware of their seropositive status enabling them to start treatment earlier, thus avoiding HIV-related illnesses and prolonging their life. In Europe and the United States the death rate from HIV has fallen significantly over the past five years as a result of the availability of HAART (Carpenter et al., 2000[96]). Ongoing counselling has been demonstrated to be an important factor in ensuring adherence (Revsin et al., 1998[97], Greene et al., 2000[98]).

Preventive Therapies

Less costly interventions to reduce the incidence of HIV-related infections, such as tuberculosis preventive therapy (TBPT), have been shown to reduce the incidence of TB among people with HIV (Mwinga et al., 1998[99]), (WHO/UNAIDS[100]). Two studies from sub-Saharan Africa (Godfrey-Faussett et al., 1995[101], Aisu et al., 1995[102]) have revealed that VCT can be an appropriate site for screening and treating people who test seropositive for active TB, and providing TBPT to those without active TB. In Haiti, a community-based programme offering VCT and screening for TB was effective in diagnosing early TB and instigating prompt and effective treatment (Desormeaux et al., 1996[103]). In Zambia, a pilot project of integrated HIV and TB counselling for families is being promoted. Early results demonstrate that this is to be acceptable but longer-term follow-up is awaited (Ayles et al., 2000[104]). In Malawi, the Malawi AIDS counselling and resource organisation (MACRO) offers VCT at two sites. It also provides TB and STI screening and treatment and family planning. There is widespread demand for these services by people following VCT, even among people who visit VCT for primarily non-medical reasons (Phiri et al., 2000[105].) Other preventive therapies such as cotrimoxazole prophylaxis (Anglaret et al., 1999[106], Wiktor et al., 1999[107] Sassan-Morokro et al., 1998[108]) have also been shown to prevent morbidity in PLHA in some settings (seropositive TB patients in Cote d'Ivoire and Senegal). Cotrimoxazole is cheap, easy to administer and necessitates minimal monitoring. UNAIDS has suggested that it should be made more widely available to PLHA.

Family Planning Services

Referral for other services, such as contraception, can assist couples (both seropositive and seronegative) make informed decisions about family planning techniques and having children (Pugh et al., 1998[109]). In many high-prevalence countries the desire to have children is strong and there have been no major differences in the uptake of family planning services for seropositive and seronegative women. In Rakai, Uganda, 13 per cent of positive women and 12 per cent of negative women used female-governed family planning following VCT (Lutalo et al., 2000[110]).

Ongoing Medical Care

One of the most prominent services offered to people following VCT at Kara, Zambia, was the provision of basic, ongoing medical care for the treatment of HIV-related infections (Baggaley et al., 1998). Similar revelations were evident from The AIDS Support Organisation (TASO), Uganda, evaluation.

Complementary Medical Services

In many countries where ARVs are not available due to cost and lack of laboratory infrastructure persons PLHA may have symptomatic benefit from complementary/traditional medicines (Gouskov, 2000[111]). However, sometimes counsellors may have a role in challenging unrealistic faiths about complementary therapies or assisting clients in discussing the pros and cons regarding decisions about allocating limited family resources to these therapies.

Access to Ongoing Emotional/Psychological Care

Knowledge of HIV status can enable people to seek appropriate emotional support. Those who are seronegative will generally feel relief, but may have ongoing emotional difficulties, which need addressing. They may have a partner who is positive or who is untested and may therefore feel at continuing risk of HIV infection. Others may feel guilt at being negative, especially if a partner is infected or has died from HIV.

Developing Countries

People who test seropositive may experience a range of emotions from denial and anger to despair and suicidal ideation. These emotional responses are normal, but counselling can assist people cope with their emotional reactions and prevent grave or long-term intractable problems. Emotional problems were seen to be common in a study of 307 people who had attended VCT from six centres in Nairobi (Vollmer and Valadez, 1999[112]). Accessing emotional support has been shown to help people cope more comfortably with the psychological sequelae of testing seropositive.

A large number of people visiting VCT, whether they test positive or negative, will attend one or at the most, two post-test counselling sessions. In Zambia, although further counselling sessions or referrals to specialised counselling services were offered, many people admitted that they did not want to have further counselling, at least not in the near future. Only 10 per cent of seropositive people and 6 per cent of seronegative people had more than two post-test counselling sessions (Baggaley et al., 1998). Some people attended for further counselling in the one to five years following VCT. This often coincided with crisis or change in personal circumstances. When interviewed 6 to 18 months following VCT, many people admitted that they had found other informal services or resources in the community to help them with their emotional needs. Church groups, family members, friends and traditional medical professionals were cited as providing emotional support. In the multi-centre trial 86 per cent of people had only one pre-test and one post-test counselling session, although ongoing counselling was provided (Sangiwa, 2000). Those who tested seropositive were more likely to attend further counselling sessions.

Developed Countries

In lower prevalence countries, such as Romania, longer-term support may be needed for PLHA to help them cope, especially when the majority of people with HIV are from risk groups that are already marginalised (Buzducea et al., 2000[113]). Three studies among MSM (Hays et al., 1990[114], Catania et al., 1992[115], Peterson et al., 1995[116]) have demonstrated prominent that seronegative or untested men. However, people who were symptomatic were the most likely to seek help and it has been concluded that this may be a factor than knowledge of HIV status. However, VCT may enable MSM to receive services most fitting to their needs. A study of IDUs showed no difference in uptake of services between those who were seropositive and symptomatic, seropositive and asymptomatic and seronegative (Solomon et al., 1991[117]). This should not be regarded as an ineffective outcome as both positive and negative IDUs may be in need of emotional and medical support. VCT may mean that IDUs are able to seek health and psychological care services appropriate to their needs.

Spiritual Support

Ongoing emotional support can also be provided outside formal counselling services. Spiritual support for people with HIV has been shown to important in both developing and developed settings (Kaldjian et al., 1998[118]). In Thailand, Buddhist monks provide ongoing support for people with HIV and teach meditation to facilitate coping and relieve stress (Sittitrai et al., 1994 [119]).

Psychological Coping and Adjustment

One of the main advantages of counselling related to VCT is permitting people to accept and cope better with their HIV status. 'Coping' with HIV was defined by the TASO staff and clients to be *an acceptance of being HIV-positive and having a positive attitude towards making the most of each day.*

Summary VCT and Coping

Several studies have described enhanced coping following VCT:

(a) Acceptance of being HIV positive
(b) Alleviating anxiety and depressive reactions (Camara, 1991[120] Magura et al., 1990[121])
(c) Improving coping (Carvalho-Neto, 1991[122]; Mukisa, 1990[123]; TASO, 1995; Baggaley, 1998, Lie and Biswalo, 1996)

(d) Participation of family and friends in HIV care and support (Carvalho-Neto, 1991, TASO 1995)

(e) Bringing hope and relief (Zulu, 1990[124])

Coping mechanisms, following a seropositive test, reported in these studies include:

(a) Exchange of status with someone

(b) Sharing status with spouse or sexual partner

(c) Challenging beliefs about the meaning of an HIV diagnosis to facilitate adjustment

(d) Continuing to work or self care

(e) Enjoying social contacts and/or leisure programmes

In a study from an outpatient HIV counselling clinic in Zimbabwe, it was demonstrated that by providing 'enhanced counselling and support services' 75 per cent of PLHAs who were earlier fearful to undergoing VCT due to perceptions of stigma and rejection) wished to be tested (Meurising et al., 1995[125, 126] 1997[127] and 1999[128]). The counsellors were able to help people who tested positive to cope better by:

* Assisting in gaining of social support and acceptance from family, partners and employers by diffusing irrational fears, blame and anger.
* Facilitating discussions in marital and family relationships about 'shameful' sexual topics.
* Broaching difficult issues like planning for the future.
* Facilitating management of medical, practical and monetary problems.
* Encouraging disclosure within a supportive framework. With enhanced counselling 80 per cent of people were able to reveal their seropositive status to someone and 75 per cent were able to disclose it to their partner/spouse. In contrast, more than 50 per cent who refused counselling did not tell anyone else of their status, including those who were planning to marry or who were married. Importantly, none disclosing to family experienced total rejection.

Studies from the United Republic of Tanzania and Uganda have also demonstrated that counselling can enable people to gain social and emotional support and cope better (Lie and Biswalo,

1996[129]; Woudenberg, 1994; TASO, 1994 [130]. A study of HIV seropositive MSM showed that a specially tailored behavioural stress management intervention had a deep impact on decreasing anxiety and anger and alleviating stress (Antoni et al., 2000[131]). Seventy-three men were randomised to an intervention group or a waiting-list control group. Not only did the intervention group show significant psychological improvement over base line compared with the control group, but they had significantly less norepinephrine output and a higher CD3+CD8+ cell count at follow-up.

In Hong Kong, a study of 35 symptomatic, PLHA disclosed that group counselling/therapy and peer support enhanced mood, decreasing tension, anger and depression (Molassiotis et al., 2000[132]). Quality-of-life measures also improved with these interventions when compared with PLHA in a control group.

Sharing of HIV Test Result with Relatives and Friends

Sharing HIV status is not only important in enabling people to receive emotional support from relatives and friends and help in future decision-making, it also projects people's ability to understand and accept their HIV status. Rates of revelations to partners and family/friends vary considerably, but in many studies (particularly from developing countries) people have found it easier to discuss their HIV status with a close friend or family member than with their partner.

Advantages of Disclosure

Disclosure of one's HIV status increases both practical and emotional support for those who test seropositive (Holt et al., 1998[133]).

Developing Countries

People who tested seropositive from general VCT services in the United Republic of Tanzania shared their HIV test outcomes with a 'significant other' of the same sex. Those who were married or cohabiting did not choose their partner. The significant other was usually chosen among close family members, generally from the same generation as the patient (Lie and Biswalo, 1996[134]).

Similar findings were apparent from the Ugandan TASO/WHO evaluation (TASO/WHO, 1993-1994[135]). After counselling the majority of people (90.4 per cent) were able to disclose their HIV serostatus to close relatives. In that same evaluation, 85.3 per cent reported disclosing their HIV status to relatives other than household members and 67 per cent disclosed their status to household members. Only 36 per cent disclosed their status to spouses or regular sexual partners. This suggests that emotional support is sought over a wider family and community network. When the VCT service was first established in Zambia, people found it difficult to share results, especially immediately following testing (Kelly et al., 1994). A later evaluation from the same site demonstrated that most people were able to share their HIV status with someone (Baggaley et al., 1998). However, women in particular said it was shameful to have HIV and, if they were known to be seropositive, they worried they would be discriminated against, and were particularly reluctant to tell their partner.

In a study from Uganda, 22 families with 1 or more adult members with HIV were interviewed about their responses to HIV and stigma (McGrath et al., 1993[136]). Approximately 50 per cent of the PLHA interviewed said that they had not informed any of their family. They said that they feared their family would worry or would not understand. Some explained that they feared rejection if their families were aware of their positive status. Family members who were informed said that they were shocked or feared the loss of their relative with HIV. However, none rejected him/her or feared infection because of day-to-day contact.

Developed Countries

A small study from the United States revealed that when women from San Francisco were questioned following antenatal VCT many had not disclosed their HIV status to any friends (65 per cent) or family members (25 per cent). Many worried about being abandoned or rejected by loved ones if their seropositive status were known. They cited lack of public understanding about HIV infection as being a major issue and taboos about HIV infection, especially pertaining to women (Lester et al., 1995[137]). Despite not sharing their HIV status with family and friends, seropositive women said that they did receive good emotional support from them. A study from London also disclosed that people were more likely to share their test outcome when they had symptomatic HIV disease or needed treatment and that revelation enabled people to obtain additional support (Miller et al., 1998[138]).

Family Counselling

Where families can participate in counselling this can be more advantageous in helping the person with HIV be more accepted and supported by his/her family members (Lippmann et al.,1993[139]). A project from the Ukraine has demonstrated that by involving the families of people with HIV they were better able to accept and understand the problems of their HIV family member and to help that member cope following counselling (Pidlisna et al., 1998[140]). In Chaing Mai, Thailand, it has been proposed that post-test counselling should be conducted in a family setting to facilitate revelation and hence long-term support and normalisation. Preliminary enquiries have shown that this may be a feasible option (Srirak et al., 2000[141]).

Post-test Clubs/Support Groups

Peer support groups and post-test clubs have often been promoted in association with VCT, to help people cope following VCT by sharing experiences and providing mutual support. In some countries they have also permitted PLHA to form pressure groups to improve services and challenge politico-legal decisions. In Zambia, men were more likely to attend support groups than women (26 per cent seropositive men versus 3 per cent seropositive women). Some people who underwent VCT and tested negative also attended support groups—again men were more likely to attend than women (15 per cent men and 8 per cent women attended) (Baggaley et al., 1998[142]). Those who attended groups often did so in their own communities rather than in the support group associated with the VCT centre. Another study from Zambia has narrated the benefits of post-test clubs (PTC). Of the 810 people tested, 150 have joined PTCs. These provide peer support as well as outreach HIV education to the community (Katongo, 2000[143]).

Access to Social Support

An advantage of people aware of their HIV status is that it permits seropositive people and their families to benefit from social support services at an earlier stage. This may assist them to cope with their HIV infection and to have a better quality of life. In many developed countries there is broad range of social support services available for PLHA. In the United Kingdom people with HIV have statutory rights to certain services and there are a large number of NGOs that provide material and support services for people with HIV along with their families and dependants. It can therefore be an ample advantage to be familiar of one's status in order to be able to have access to these services at an early stage. Terrence Higgins Trust[144], a United Kingdom NGO, provides a wide scope of material and support services for people with HIV.

In middle-income countries with lower levels of HIV this is a more feasible option. For example, people with HIV in Russia have statutory rights to housing and other services (Russia Federal law, 1999[145]). In high-prevalence developing countries, although the needs for social support services are often much greater, resources are not frequently sufficient. Some developing countries have policies such as offering free or subsidised services to people with HIV, due to the overwhelming demand they may be difficult to implement. However, where VCT services have a close link to social support, these have been proved to be popular in many settings. In Uganda, TASO has been providing comprehensive support for HIV-infected and affected people since 1987. The participatory evaluation of the service revealed that there were many material needs of PLHA following testing. There are also innumerable examples of NGOs and religious/church groups offering support services for people with HIV. Problems of coverage and sustainability are common. In the Central African Republic, out of 2800 clients attending a VCT centre approximately 350 were seropositive. Of these, 80 per cent were referred for social support (Sehonou et al., 1999[146]). (Antenatal testing from sentinel survey sites in the country's capital Bangui disclosed a seroprevalence of 12-30 per cent).

Material Support to Persons Living with HIV/AIDS (PLHAs) and Their Families

Many of the countries that are most affected by HIV are also experiencing grave monetary hardship, and needs assessments often reveal that the most pressing requirement for PLHAs is material support. In Rwanda, seropositive women explained their most urgent needs as being food, housing and money (Keogh et al., 1994[147]). Linking material assistance to VCT services is controversial. Although it is popular among VCT service attendees and motivates the application of VCT services, if is often unsustainable and may lead to dependence and unmet expectations when supplies are short or donor support is limited (Williams and Kalinaki, 1999[148]).

At TASO a third of clients and family care-givers considered monetary assistance their major need. Although basic foodstuffs (e.g., rice, oil) are sometimes available, supplies have proved to be irregular and dependent on donations. When the VCT service was established in Lusaka, Zambia, seropositive clients were eligible for maize meal donated by the World Food Programme (WFP). This was a very popular service. The counsellors realised that they had something to offer people who tested seropositive. Widows with HIV, in particular, were often poor and supplies were welcome to help feed their children. However, this service was terminated when the WFP changed its policy, creating despondency among clients and counsellors. In the Kara study, the majority of people interviewed and not discussed 'Public Welfare' issues with their counsellor. This is understandable because, practically, there is very little available. The entire social welfare budget for Zambia for 1997 was US$ 634000 (total population approximately 9 million). The fund is targeted at unsupported women, the sick, elderly people and people with disabilities. In 1996, less than 150000 people had any contact with the social welfare services. Obtaining social welfare is cumbersome and involves assessment by the District Social Welfare Officer. This inevitably means travelling to the office and long waits for often no gains, as the criteria for qualifying for assistance are generally vague and arbitrary. Another study from Zambia also found that material needs (e.g., provision of basic food items and monetary assistance for school children) were a high priority for people who tested seropositive, but there were few resources at hand to meet these needs (Hamavhwa et at., 1998[149]).

Skills Training and Small Loans

Some people with HIV experience problems with employment due to:

(a) Irregular attendance as a result of intermittent ill-health.

(b) Employment-associated HIV testing. Some companies require employees to undergo HIV testing before they can take up a position or continue in employment.

(c) Discrimination or abuse by colleagues or employers.

(d) Women who lose their husbands as a result of HIV may also abandon their home and monetary security.

With a view to addressing these problems some VCT centres refer people who test seropositive to skills training workshops. Skills training for seropositive people following VCT has been running in Zambia since 1992. It is popular and provides a supportive climate for people coping with their HIV infection (Baggaley et al., 1995[150]). All the current trainers were originally trainees who entered the project following VCT, and some of the trainees have gone on to establish viable small businesses. TASO skills training has also been an integral part of services available for people following VCT. Although only 8.6 per cent of those attending TASO attended the day centre, 95.2 per cent said that they benefited from sharing experiences as well as from the emotional support of other PLHAs and 84.1 per cent said that they benefited from the skills training. The majority of day-centre attendees were women (81 per cent) and many were widows. In the TASO evaluation 60 per cent of those interviewed stressed the need for capital to initiate income-generating projects. When loans were made available, however, only 12 per cent repaid them.

In Kenya, women attending VCT related to a MTCT project were able to take part in income-generation projects and received help and information to improve the nutritional status of their children (Lukandwa et al., 1998[151]).

Support for Children of Persons Living with HIV/AIDS (PLHAs)

The TASO evaluation also identified school fee payment for needy children of PLHAs as a priority. Initially, TASO provided school fees for 35 per cent of children assessed as needing assistance. However, it was realised that this was only a short-term option as ongoing funding for this activity was not available. Other studies have shown the importance of providing counselling for children of PLHA and orphans to help them cope better and prepare for the death of their parent(s) (Krabbendam et al., 1998[152], Nanono Namatovu et al., 2000[153]).

Legal and Future Planning

Making Wills

If people with HIV are familiar of their status they can make plans for their future and that of their dependants. This may include making will and making decisions about the care of their dependants after they die. Property grabbing occurs in some countries in sub-Saharan Africa. It is the practice of relatives of the decreased seizing his or her property after death. This often results in women and orphans being left destitute following a death. Making a legally binding will may ensure that loved ones and dependants are provided for. In the TASO evaluation, making wills was discussed in 39 per cent of observed counselling sessions, with 51.3 per cent of people expressing willingness to make wills. However, only 16.8 per cent had made them and 22.3 per cent said there was no point in making a will as they had nothing to pass on. In Zambia, in an evaluation of 55 PLHAs, only 7 had written legal documents pertaining to their property (Ndawa et al., 1990[154]).

Planning for Dependants

In Zambia, 37 per cent of seropositive men and 35 per cent of seropositive women worried about the future of their dependants following their death. In the same study, 20 per cent of the men and 42 per cent of the women said that they had been able to make plans for their dependants' future following VCT. Other reports have revealed that as a result of counselling, HIV seropositive individuals have been able to make plans for their survivors (Ndawa, 1990[155]; Kaleeba et al., 1997[156], TASO 1994[157]).

Monetary Planning

In Zambia, 31 per cent of the men and 13 per cent of the women said they had made changes in their work life following VCT, in order to have better monetary options for the future. These changes included getting a second job, working overtime and saving.

Access to Interventions to Prevent Mother-to-Child Transmission: Specialist Antenatal Care and Family Planning Services

In developing countries inexpensive and plausible methods to significantly reduce mother-to-child transmission (MTCT) to HIV (CDC, 1998[158], Guay et al., 1999[159]), and advice on modifying infant feeding practices for seropositive women (Coutsoudis et al., 1999[160], Van de Perre, 1999[161]) are now available. These can reduce HIV transmission from mother-to-child to 10 per cent or less. For women and their children to benefit from these MTCT interventions it is significant for women to be offered VCT during the antenatal period. Counselling may also need to be ongoing after the initial post-test counselling session for seropositive mothers who take part in MTCT interventions, including modifying infant feeding practices (Chopra et al., 2000[162], Kibuuka et al., 2000[163]). VCT related to MTCT interventions should not be limited to ensuring uptake of and adherence to MTCT interventions. It is a much more effective intervention if counselling about HIV transmission to and from sexual partners is discussed and if men can be involved and agree to VCT as well. In a small study from Uganda, women attending VCT related to MTCT seronegative mothers preferred abstinence or condom use until their partners accepted VCT (Matovu et al., 2000[164]). The length of follow-up is at present short and it would be advantageous to know how long protected sex behaviour was maintained and what proportion of male partners accepted testing.

Access to HIV Transmission Prevention Services

Many people in high-prevalence countries or from among groups who are at higher risk from HIV infection imagine that they are already infected. This may prevent them protecting themselves from HIV infection. In Zambia, although the HIV prevalence rate among young men is low (less than 5 per cent in men under 19 years of age), many said that there was no point in adopting safer sex as it was likely that they were already infected (Baggaley, 1998[165]). Knowledge of HIV status can thus give people the ability to safeguard themselves from HIV infection and motivate access to HIV preventive services. A study from San Francisco revealed that people who tested seronegative but were at high risk of HIV infection were more likely to access HIV prevention services (Marx et al., 1998[166]).

Societal: Role of VCT

Eradicating the stigma related to HIV is the Herculean task to its prevention and care. It has been proposed that wider access to VCT and a larger number of people's greater awareness of their HIV status within a community are major elements in challenging stigma (Lambouray, 1998[167]). Countries where VCT is well-established, such as Uganda, have a less stigmatising attitude to HIV. However, for it to be effective in challenging stigma, HIV testing has to be a voluntary process related to counselling that assists people understand and accept their status (UNAIDS, 1999[168], UNAIDS, 2000[169]). For example, there are countries such as Russia, where HIV remains highly stigmatised, despite the fact that all women have routine testing as part of their antenatal care and a wide proportion of the population has been tested routinely for HIV. It has also been recommended that if VCT were offered routinely, and more people would accept VCT as a major component of medical care, it would promote 'normalisation' of HIV (De Cock et al., 1998[170], Godfrey-Faussett et al., 1998[171]). De Cock explains that the excessive caution around HIV testing has had the harmful impact of preventing people with HIV from accessing care. It also has contributed to the stigma and privacy related to testing. A study from Zambia contrasts the individual confidential approach to counselling with a more open, family-oriented one. It proposes that the latter generates more open and proactive responses at the community level (Goma et al., 1999[172]). There are, however, no studies that look specifically at the role of VCT in promoting openness in communities and this is an important area in which to prioritise future research.

Cost

Developing Countries

Cost-effectiveness analysis leaves out many of the latent benefits of VCT, particularly, in the fields of care and quality of life, which may be cost-saving. Results from the multi-centre trial have revealed that VCT can be a highly cost-effective intervention (Sweat et al., 1999[173], 2000[174]). Using a hypothetical cohort of 10 000 seeking VCT, they approximated that the intervention in Kenya and 985 in the United Republic of Tanzania. The cost per client for VCT was nearly US$ 29 in the United Republic of Tanzania, and US$ 27 in Kenya. In both these locations total costs were composed for 74 per cent for labour and infrastructure, 2 per cent for start-up, and 24 per cent for commodity expenses. The single largest cost was for counsellor salaries and benefits (36 per cent). The cost per HIV infection averted averaged US$ 346 in the United Republic of Tanzania and US$ 249 in Kenya. The cost per disability-adjusted life-year (DALY) saved was US$ 17.78 and US$ 12.7. VCT was witnessed as more cost-effective when targeted at seropositive people, couples and women. The most cost-effective intervention was VCT aimed at couples. If they increased the magnitude of couples attending VCT to 70 per cent this would reduce the cost per DALY to US$ 13.39 in the United Republic of Tanzania and US$ 10.71 in Kenya. VCT compares favourably to other interventions in cost per HIV infection averted in East Africa (e.g., US$ 251 per case of HIV averted for enhanced STI services in Mwanza. This intervention was approximated to cost US$ 10 per DALY saved (Gilson et al. 1997[175]). It can be inferred that the costs of VCT will fall as testing methods get inexpensive (Meda et al., 1999[176]) and innovative approaches to counselling may lessen costs. Moreover, if VCT is aimed at couples and at people of higher risk this will also increase cost-effectiveness.

The cost-effectiveness of blood-donor counselling has also been determined. There is no policy on donor notification and HIV counselling for blood donors in India. If existing staff and infrastructure are kept in consideration, the additional cost of providing these services to all blood donors would cost US$ 1.2 per donor (Dhiingra-Kumar, 1998[177]). This intervention would enhance blood safety by minimising blood wastage, reducing HIV seroprevalence in donated blood, promoting a health donor pool, besides facilitating life-style changes and behaviour modification in the donors.

Developed Countries

A cost-benefit analysis was performed on the CDC VCT, referral and partner notification service (Holtgrave et al., 1993[178]). Assuming that for every 100 people identified with HIV 20 new HIV infections are averted, the cost of the programme is US$188217600 and the monetary benefits of this expenditure are US$3781918000. The resultant benefit-cost ratio is 20.09. Sensitivity analysis demonstrated that the benefit-cost ratio is greater than 1 or for all considered cases, strongly recommending that publicly funded VCT, referral and partner notification services result in a net monetary gain to society. This analysis is highly dependent on the savings of treatment cost of the cases averted (TC) (lifetime TC for someone with HIV in the United States is approximated to be US$85000). In developing countries, although rates of seropositivity may be substantially higher, ARVs are not routinely available and treatment costs are much lower, this analysis may yield less cost-effective results. Another model from the United States also shows VCT (with or without partner notification) to be cost-effective in preventing HIV transmission (Varghese et al., 1999[179]). For 10000 people attending an STI clinic with a seroprevalence of 1.5 per cent, they estimated that VCT prevents 8 HIV infections and saves almost US$1000 000 (lifetime TC = US$175000). They estimate that the partner notification of the 113 people with HIV discovered by VCT prevents another 1.2 infections. The cost to the provider translates into a cost of US$32000 per case prevented by VCT and an additional US$28000 for partner notification. In demonstrating the cost-effectiveness of this programme, the high treatment cost is a major element.

A large multi-centre, randomised examination of VCT (brief or enhanced) versus HIV education estimates that brief counselling would result in prevention of new HIV cases at the cost of US$12098 per case prevented. Enhanced counselling may be a little more effective but much more costly (US$162795 per case averted) (Kamb et al., 1998[180]).

Cost Effectiveness Related to MTCT Interventions

Developing Countries

Several theories have been developed to examine the cost-effectiveness of MTCT interventions (costs included drug costs and VCT costs) in the prevention of paediatric HIV infection MTCT and the costs per HIV case averted and cost per DALY.

Developed Countries

Cost and Benefit to the Mother following VCT for MTCT

Antenatal testing is undertaken primarily to offer interventions to prevent MTCT. However, the diagnosis of HIV has implications for the mother herself. In many developed and some middle-income countries this diagnosis will permit her earlier access to ARV therapy for treatment of her own HIV disease and may prevent HIV transmission to a negative sexual partner. A theory has been developed that examines the health services costs and benefits for the woman of an earlier HIV diagnosis as a result of antenatal testing (Gibb et al., 1999[186]). They approximated that women were diagnosed a median of 20.4 months earlier as a result of antenatal VCT, with a cost of US$76887 per life-year gained.

Negative Results following VCT

Balanced against the advantages following VCT there are latent negative consequences of VCT for the individual and his or her family (Colebunders et al., 1993[187]). The putative disadvantages of VCT is that those who test seropositive may be discriminated against, suffer abuse or abandonment or may have grave emotional reactions to a seropositive result. However, while examining short- and long-term follow-up such negative outcomes are rare. Moreover, they can be minimised with ongoing counselling and support and sensitive discussion around revelation especially for women.

Abandonment and Abuse

Some studies from sub-Saharan Africa have reported high levels of abuse of seropositive women following VCT. However, these can be minimised when women have sensitive counselling about revelation and ongoing support following VCT.

Marital Break-up

In some studies marital break-up following VCT is reported as being high, especially for women in a sero-discordant relationship, leading to hardship for women, yet not always a negative outcome.

Discrimination

There are many anecdotal reports of people encountering discrimination following VCT in seeking employment, entry to religious orders, access to education, application for immigration and visas and access to health care. These negative consequences of testing seropositive should be challenged by advocacy and legislation and not be considered as a negative outcome of the VCT process.

Psychological Distress, Stress and Depression

Emotional distress upon learning that one has a seropositive HIV result is a rational response. However, for innumerable people, severe distress is short lived and can be eased by ongoing support from family members, friends and health professionals.

The stress following testing seropositive can be brought in equilibrium against the feelings of relief of those who test seronegative. Moreover, it has been demonstrated that untested people or people who are not aware of their HIV rest results (but feel at risk from HIV infection) are not free from this stress and uncertainty. Home HIV testing services may leave seropositive people particularly vulnerable since follow-up of clients is not ensured. Anticipating and meeting individuals psychological needs following HIV testing is thus important when developing a VCT service.

Abandonment and Abuse

Grave morbid symptoms for women following VCT has been reported in a study from Nairobi, Kenya (Temmerman et al., 1995)[188]. Seropositive women who received VCT in an antenatal setting reported high levels of negative outcomes. Of the 324 women who were diagnosed to be seropositive only 66 (27.2 per cent) communicated their test outcome to their partner and only

21 partners subsequently tested. Eleven seropositive women were chased away from their house or replaced by another wife, seven were beaten up and one committed suicide. Studies from Rwanda have also revealed the burden of physical and emotional violence, as well as the monetary difficulties that occur to women who test seropositive (Keogh et al., 1994[189], and Straten et al., 1995[190]).

In a study from the United Republic of Tanzania, 340 female clients were followed up for 3 months following VCT to evaluate the relationship between HIV serostatus, domestic violence and disclosure (Maman, 1999[191], Maman et al., 2000[192]). Both these who tested seropositive and seronegative encountered high levels of physical violence. In the study, 54 per cent of seropositive women and 32.3 per cent of seronegative women admitted that they had had at least one physically abusive partner *in their lifetime, before attending VCT*. Seropositive women were significantly more likely than seronegative women to report a physically violent story with their current partner in the last three months (31 per cent versus 16.2 per cent). It is not disclosed whether the violence following VCT was related to revelation of a positive status or a reflection of the higher level of violence encountered by women who subsequently were identified to be seropositive.

The multi-centre study (Gregorich et al., 1998[193]) found that the most commonly endorsed life events were, however, positive: strengthening of a sexual relationship (39 per cent more common among couples), increased emotional support from peers (29 per cent) and increased emotional support from families (23 per cent). Negative life events were also reported. Besides the break-up of sexual relationships (22 per cent), however, negative life events were uncommon (1-4 per cent overall). There were no significant differences between those who received VCT versus health information in reported levels of positive or negative life events. Although negative life events were uncommon in this study, they were significantly more likely to be encountered by people testing seropositive. Among those assigned to the VCT group at baseline seropositives were more likely than seronegatives to be estranged by peers (1 per cent versus 2 per cent $p = 0.01$), discriminated against by employees (1 per cent versus 2 per cent $p = 0.06$) and neglected by family (2 per cent versus 4 per cent $p = < 0.05$).

Seropositive women *enrolled as a couple* reported higher rates of physical abuse (18 per cent versus 5 per cent overall NS), and the break-up of a marriage (15 per cent versus 3 per cent overall NS). This emphasises the need for additional services for women in relationships who test seropositive.

Marital Break-up

A study of serodiscordant couples from Kinshasa demonstrated that at the time of testing 18 couples encountered acute psychological distress, such as threatened suicide, a husband's family chasing the woman from the house and allegations of infidelity. However, intensive home-based counselling by trained nurses resolved these difficulties in all but three couples, who later divorced (Kamenga et al., 1991[194]). In all three cases the woman was seropositive and the man seronegative. The counsellors enabled reconciliation in innumerable cases, but this involved providing high-quality, flexible and intensive counselling services for couples. In the multi-centre study high levels of marital break-up were reported (Gregorich et al., 1998). However, it was concluded that marital break-up should not be witnessed as a negative outcome, rather it may be a risk-reduction strategy. Simultaneously, women in sub-Saharan Africa whose husbands leave them may be blamed by their families and suffer, along with their children, monetary and material difficulties.

Discrimination

There are many anecdotal examples of discrimination following VCT, particularly for those testing seropositive.

Employment

Some countries have employment regulations that discriminate against people with HIV. This discrimination is at present being challenged. In South Africa the AIDS Law Project (ALP) acted on behalf of a job applicant who, during 1997, was denied employment by South African Airways as a cabin attendant because he was identified as living with HIV. In May 2000, the ALP successfully challenged the airline's policy of refusing to employ people solely because they test positive for HIV during pre-employment screening. However, in many other countries pre-employment HIV screening and discrimination continues to be practised even today.

Entry into Religious Orders

Many countries in sub-Saharan Africa emphasise on HIV-testing candidates before they enter religious orders, excluding those who test seropositive from training as priests or nuns (Baggaley, 1994[195]).

Insurance

Many insurance policies exclude people with HIV.

Education

HIV testing is required by some institutions before offering further education.

Foreign Travel and Immigration

Some countries require HIV testing prior to issue of a visa or entry permit.

Medical Treatment

Some people with HIV report discrimination from health professionals following VCT. A study from the United States revealed that when women from San Francisco were questioned following antenatal VCT they said that they had encountered higher levels of health care discrimination, personal isolation and negative psychological morbid symptoms than their seronegative counterparts (Lester et al., 1995[196]).

Psychological Distress, Stress, and Depression

Identifying that one is seropositive, as with other grave medical diagnosis, will almost inevitably cause shock and distress and have a severe impact on the individual and his or her family (Dautzenberg et al., 1992[197], Ankrah 1993[198], Lippman et al., 1993[199]). The objective of counselling is to assist the person understand, accept and cope with the diagnosis and prevent severe reactions such as suicide or long-term intractable depression.

Developing Countries

In Rwanda, a prospective study of seropositive women disclosed that although the majority reported good morale, chronic difficulties with sleep, performing daily routine and feelings of depression were reported by one-third of women (Keogh et al., 1994[200]). In Zambia, although many people who tested seropositive expressed sadness, anger or anxiety following testing this was comparatively short lived and no cases of attempted suicide occurred (Baggaley et al., 1998). Some people who had suspected that they were positive admitted that they felt at ease on receiving their result, since they were now able to understand symptoms and make schedules for treatment or for their dependants. People who tested seronegative expressed relief, but some also expressed guilt or sadness when partners or family members had tested positive.

In the multi-centre trial 81 people were interviewed in depth about their emotional feelings following VCT (Sangiwa, 2000[201]). Seronegative clients reported feelings of relief, decreased anxiety, improved hope and increased trust in themselves. Seropositive people reported better coping skills to deal with their circumstances, increased hope, disappearance of suicidal thoughts and help in decreasing isolation and normalising their situation. Among seropositive people, most distress was narrated as transient. However, some participants reported persistent feelings of sadness, desperation and a sense of loss as they felt they may have to give up having children and abstain from sex out of concern about infecting others.

Developed Countries

Men Having Sex with Men (MSM)

There have been several studies examining psychological outcomes following testing among MSM. Two studies show increases in stress and depression for those testing positive. Nevertheless, the long-term outcomes are not reported and the grave consequences (such as suicide) are not reported. In one study there was no difference in psychological outcomes between men who did not know their status and those who did. A study of homosexual men revealed that those who tested seropositive following VCT were more likely to suffer adverse consequences such as stress, depression and dissolution of their primary relationship than those who tested seronegative or those who refused testing (Coates et al., 1987[202]). Another study compared MSM who were aware of their HIV status with men who had been tested but refused to receive their test result (Doll et al., 1990[203]). Those who chose to learn their status were no more likely to report depression or anxiety following testing than those who opted not to know their status.

In a study of 22 seropositive MSM 22 seronegative MSM and 12 men who were tested (but did not want to know their HIV status), subjects who tested positive experienced an increase in anxiety, depression and AIDS anxiety. Subjects who tested negative experienced a decrease in these feelings after learning these outcomes (Huggins et al., 1991). People who did not learn their results experienced no change in these feelings. In a small study of injecting drug users (IDUs) attending a detoxification programme in Long Island, the United States, people testing seropositive demonstrated a wide range of emotional reactions to learning their results (Magura et al., 1990[204]). There were, however, no serious or damaging reactions. People with seronegative results were uniformly relieved. Almost all had informed someone of their status with unremarkable consequences.

Blood Donors

A study from New York of seropositive blood donors displayed that depressive symptoms scores for both men and women have substantially higher than scores typically found in representative population samples. More than 25 per cent of men and 33 per cent of women reported seeking psychological or psychiatric services in the first few weeks following notification of their positive result (Cleary et al., 1993[205]).

Home Testing

In the home sampling services, used extensively in the United States, seropositive people receive their test results over the phone (Branson, 1998[206]). From a sample of 865 seropositive people telephone counsellors explained that 7 per cent expressed shock or dismay at an unexpected positive result and 5 per cent hung up immediately and one client expressed suicidal thoughts (the phone counsellor ascertained he was with a friend who could give mental health support). Although 65 per cent of people accepted referral there is no information as to whether people took up the referral or the long-term psychological impact of this type of service.

Operational

Many VCT services are monitored by examining the statistics on demand and uptake of service, number of people being tested following counselling and rates for collecting HIV outcomes.

Uptake, Return, Rates and Acceptability

Uptake of services has often been considered as an important measure of VCT services 'success'. Uptake of VCT varies broadly within and between VCT service types, communities and countries.

MTCT Settings

Research Settings

Uptake and return rate of VCT related to MTCT interventions has been studied in detail. Thirteen studies from west (Abidjan, Bobo-Dioulasso), east (Addis Ababa, Dar Es Salaam, Mombassa, Nairobi) and Southern Africa (Blantyre, Durban, Harare, Lusaka, Soweto) and one from Thailand were included in a cross-sectional mailing survey about the acceptability of VCT and several MTCT interventions in antenatal clinics (Cartoux et al., 1998)[207]. All respondents represented research projects, rather than operational sites. The median overall acceptability was 65 per cent, ranging from 33-95 per cent. Where several studies were carried out in the same country, pregnant women had similar attitudes to HIV testing. The main reason for not wanting an HIV test was 'wanting to discuss with partner'. Five studies had overall acceptability rates of more than 70 per cent with high return rates. In the five studies where all information was available 1-4 per cent of *all women* offered VCT and 11-35 per cent of *all seropositive women,* were finally included in the MTCT intervention projects. These results were obtained from pilot research sites. It was concluded that fighting against HIV discrimination will be important to improve VCT acceptability and uptake.

A study from Zimbabwe offering VCT to women at delivery or post-partum had very poor uptake (Tavengwa et al., 2000[208]). This study offered vitamin A to mothers and/or babies in the 96 hours post-delivery and offered infant feeding counselling to women who tested seropositive. Of 1311 women who delivered 4 requested HIV tests at delivery and 118 (9 per cent) between 2 and 8 weeks post-partum. Even with free VCT and education and counselling on infant feeding most women opted not to learn their HIV status. This may project that the immediate/early post-partum period is not a practical time to offer VCT.

Operational Settings

It is likely that the uptake and return rates will be different in operational settings. There is limited information available, but preliminary outcomes from a large MTCT programme in Botswana display comparatively low uptake of VCT during the first eight months of operation (Mazhani et al., 2000[209]). This is because of fear of a seropositive result, lack of facilities where partners can receive counselling and testing, worry about partners' reactions and the lack of effective treatment available for infected women themselves. It should not be taken as a 'failing' of the project; it displays that women are able to make choices on testing without coercion from counsellors. Moreover, as the programme develops and the advantages of VCT related to MTCT interventions (for both mothers and children) are more widely known and understood it would be expected that uptake would increase. In Thailand VCT related to MTCT interventions provided by the antenatal clinic is routinely offered in some provinces. In a study exploring 24465 women attending 27 hospital antenatal clinics 99 per cent of women accepted VCT (Koetsawang et al., 2000[210]). Uptake of VCT in other operational settings varies largely in the UNICEF/UNAIDS MTCT pilot locations. Differences in testing plans, maturity of the epidemic, seroprevalence in the community and attitudes to and availability of VCT in the community are regarded to be important. It is also proposed that counsellors' attitudes towards testing at the sites may be a major factor in uptake.

Provisional results from the Khayelitsha Mother-to-Child

Pilot Project (funded by the provincial Government of the Western Cape in South Africa) display a high rate of acceptance of HIV testing (Sigxaxhe, 2000[211]). In Zimbabwe, 186 women attending an antenatal clinic in Chitungwisa were provided VCT as part of their antenatal care (Martin-Hetz et al., 2000[212]). Although most women endorsed the multiple advantages of VCT, uptake was low, with only 23 per cent women consenting to VCT. MTCT interventions have recently been introduced in antenatal clinic in Lusaka, as part of routine antenatal care. Prior to this a survey among antenatal attenders displayed that when VCT was offered to women at less than 28 weeks, 28 to 36 weeks and more than 36 weeks, 71 per cent, 62 per cent and 64 per cent respectively, of women said that they would agree to be tested (Chibwesha et al., 2000[213]). It is not known whether this proposed high uptake will be translated into action when the services are in operation.

VCT Centres

Uptake

Uptake of VCT in communities is dependent on societal issues as well as problem related to delivery of the service. There may also be proportionate differences in theoretical and actual uptake rates. For example, in Lusaka when students were asked if they wished to be tested for HIV there was a very high rate of interest. When the service was provided initially, uptake was very low. However, with time, there has been increasing demand for VCT in Lusaka (Baggaley et at., 1997[214]). Another study from Zambia evaluated the readiness to utilize VCT services offered to 4812 participants from countryside and urban sites. Although 37 per cent initially expressed willingness to use VCT services only 3.6 per cent in reality came for VCT (Rosensvard et al., 1998[215]).

Return Rates

The multi-site study from Nairobi and Dar Es Salaam randomised people to either receive VCT or health information. Of those assigned VCT 95 per cent were actually tested. Seventy-five per cent of those in the United Republic of Tanzania and 85 per cent of those in Kenya returned to collect their results (Balmer et al., 1998[216]). In the United Republic of Tanzania, those who were seropositive, or enrolled as couples were less likely to return for their test outcomes. When given access to unlimited counselling sessions most people opted to attend only two sessions, though those who tested seropositive had more counselling sessions. In the Central African Republic a tremendously high 98.5 per cent of a sample of 2800 clients returned for their HIV test result after one week (Sehonou et al., 1999[217]).

Couple Counselling

When couples can be tested together it has been displayed that this can be a very successful way of preventing HIV transmission in discordant couples. Uptake and acceptance of this option has been demonstrated to vary to a large extent. In Lusaka, where it was promoted as part of a VCT services, it was not popular and couples were very reluctant to be tested together (Baggaley et al., 1997).

In Rwanda, where couple counselling was offered as part of a research project looking at discordant couples, it was a popular selection. *No couple declined testing,* and none declined to authorise the investigators to divulge test results to a partner (King et al., 1993[218]). The remarkable difference in uptake of couple counselling in these two projects may represent a difference in the approaches of the counsellors and difference in the target populations. However, the uptake of VCT services by a community is dependent on innumerable factors, often beyond the control of the VCT service itself.

HIV Testing Techniques: Simple-rapid (S/R) Testing/Same-day Testing

If people are able to obtain their HIV test result within a few hours they are much more likely to receive their test result than if they have to wait one to two weeks. In the UNICEF/UNAIDS MTCT sites return rates were remarkably higher in sites using S/R testing than ELISA (discussed earlier). Other MTCT projects using S/Rs or changing to S/R testing have displayed high uptake rates:

(a) In Zambia, when S/R testing was offered in a pilot project at antenatal clinics, the overall acceptance was very high (81 per cent) (Bhat et al., 1998[219]). In the VCT services in Lusaka return rates were witnessed to be higher when S/R testing replaced ELISA (Kayawe, 2000[220]).

(b) In Rwanda, HIV rapid testing was offered to all women attending the antenatal clinic in the central hospital in Kigali. Of the 1223 women screened for HIV 68.7 per cent returned to collect their HIV test results. Women were more likely to return if they were seronegative (71.3 per cent) than if they were seropositive (63.9 per cent) (Ladner et al., 1996[221]).

(c) In Malawi, uptake of VCT had been low but increased fourfold when simple/rapid testing was available (Msowoya et al., 2000[222]). Moreover, 100 per cent of clients received their test results compared with 68 per cent when ELISA testing was used.

(d) In Kenya, same-day S/R testing has also been found to be acceptable but worries about confidentiality are still a concern (Arthur et al., 2000[223]).

(e) In Guatemala, introduction of S/R testing considerably increased return rates (Samayoa et al., 2000[224]).

(f) In Côte d'Ivoire, although S/R testing increased the proportion of women receiving an HIV test result during the antenatal period (compared with ELISA testing), there was, overall, very poor adherence to ARV interventions to prevent MTCT (Sibailly et al., 2000[225]). This reflects that while uptake rates of VCT can be improved using S/R testing unless women receive ample counselling to understand the advantages of testing it may not be translated into beneficial advantages for the mother and child.

Obstacles to the Uptake of VCT

Uptake of VCT services varies remarkably between settings and between countries. There are innumerable factors that may affect uptake rates or inhibit people from accessing services:

Method of Reporting/Confidentiality

VCT services have different methods of reporting HIV results, and this may have a deep impact on uptake of the service, especially where people are worried about confidentiality or belong to groups that are already unsupported or marginalised. Many VCT services offer a *confidential service* where the individual and his or her counsellor share the test result. Test results may be kept by the clinic or there may be a policy of reporting seropositive to a referral centre (named reporting). The logical basis for named reporting is that it is important for surveillance of HIV within communities/countries. Other VCT locations offer an *anonymous service*, where someone wanting a test can attend without giving his or her name.

A study from the United States weighed the impact of named reporting on the uptake of VCT services in publicly funded VCT programmes, where approximately 2.5 million people are tested for HIV each year (Nakashima et al., 1998[226]). It was feared that the introduction of named reporting to aid surveillance would cause some individuals to avoid testing. However, there was no severe impact on the use of testing facilities following the introduction of named reporting though in some states there was a statistically non-significant decline in testing among African Americans and IDUs.

Other studies recommend, however, that the introduction of anonymous testing increases testing in higher-risk populations, such as MSM and IDUs (Fehrs, et, al., 1988[227], Hoxworth et al., 1994[228], Hirano et al., 1994[229]). Other studies frcm the United States have also admitted that ending anonymous services results in a decline in testing of vulnerable populations (Hertz-Picciotto et al., 1996[230], Irwin et al., 1996[231]).

Stigma/Societal Issues/Current Trends

Stigma and discrimination may be important problems in the uptake of VCT in different communities. It has been postulated that political commitment to HIV prevention and care have resulted in less discrimination and, hence, increased demand for VCT in Uganda when compared to neighbouring countries. It has also been argued that, conversely, majority of the people who have been tested that is a major factor in promoting normalisation and reducing stigma and discrimination related to HIV. It has been displayed that a role model or valued member of the community declaring that he or she has been tested is important in reducing stigma and increasing the uptake of HIV testing. For example, when Magic Johnson declared that he had been tested and was seropositive there was a remarkable increase in people requesting VCT in the United States (CDC 1993[232]).

Availability of Treatment and ARVs

In countries where ARVs and other effective medical interventions (such as interventions to prevent MTCT) are available for people with HIV, there are considerable advantages to people with HIV being identified early. This has changed attitudes of health professionals as well as vulnerable people from HIV infection in developed countries to VCT, resulting in a greater uptake. In developing countries, the lack of ARVs and medical and social support services available for people with HIV is cited as a reason for the poor uptake of VCT (Baggaley et al., 1995)[233].

Simple-rapid (S/R) Testing/Same-day Testing

Many studies have demonstrated that if people are able to obtain their HIV test result within a few hours using simple/rapid technologies they are much more likely to receive their test result than if they have to wait one to two weeks. Thus, uptake rates of VCT can be improved using S/R testing. However, with S/R testing there is a probability that people may not have ample thinking time to make an informed and voluntary decision about testing.

Community Mobilisation and IEC

Unless VCT services are promoted as part of comprehensive HIV prevention, care and support uptake is likely to be poor. Provision of adequate IEC and community mobilisation is considered to be an important element in ensuring uptake of MTCT services related to MTCT interventions (UNICEF, 2000).

Poor Quality Services

In some countries VCT services are under-utilized because the services they offer are inadequate and do not meet client needs. A study from India revealed that some clients who had tested at hospital sites were found to be unaware of their HIV status and had not received any follow up (Abraham et al., 1998[234]). The services should match the needs of the target group, alongwith the medical and emotional needs, to maximise client uptake, participation and involvement. Poor quality of VCT services was also noted to be a considerable problem in a study from South Africa (Viljoen et al., 1998[235]). Only 85 per cent of people interviewed had given consent before being tested and only 48 per cent had had 'adequate' pre-test counselling. The lack of behavioural changes following the VCT services could be attributable to the poor standard of counselling observed.

In Kinshasa (Democratic Republic of Congo) counsellors noted that in clinical settings pre-test counselling was not often done. Consequently, results were often not relayed to the client. Medical staff themselves often had a non-cooperative attitude to VCT and were reluctant to give positive results to clients (Denolf et al., 2000[236]).

Client Satisfaction

Client satisfaction following VCT has been given due consideration in several studies. It is, nevertheless, difficult to promote objective measures of client satisfaction. In most studies levels of client satisfaction are reported as being high. This may be in part because clients do not want to upset their health providers, or feel that criticising a service would mar their future care. The following studies all used client exit interviews, either immediately following a counselling session or as part of a longer-term, follow-up study:

(a) A study from Myanmar (Kywe et al., 1996[237] and Thu, 1997[238]) considered the acceptability of VCT services. Statistics were collected on the content of counselling sessions and on client satisfaction of counselling. Of those people attending for VCT 90 per cent were 'satisfied with the counselling services they received'.

(b) In Zambia, of 377 people who had attended a VCT centre, 94 per cent had discussed safer sex with their counsellors and 89 per cent admitted that they had found the discussion helpful in making decisions. The majority said that they had found counselling an advantageous experience and that it had assisted them cope with their status. They also said that the links to support services were prominent (Kayawe et al., 1998[239]).

(c) The 'New Start' project in Zimbabwe has examined client satisfaction using exit interviews and discovered that 80 per cent were satisfied with the service (PSI, 1999[240]).

(d) In the multi-centre trial a sample of 81 clients were interviewed at 6 months following testing (Sangiwa, 2000[241]). Most were satisfied with the service and appreciated being made welcome, respected by the counsellors and provided with a level of continuity (seeing the same counsellor at pre- and post-test counselling). The service's privacy and the fact the counsellors told them the truth was also said to be important. Those who tested seropositive mentioned as significant the value of ongoing supportive counselling for coping with living with HIV and staying healthy.

(e) In Budapest, Hungary, in an evaluation of an anonymous VCT centre, 94 per cent of the 2000 respondents were satisfied with the services (Csepe et al., 1998 [242]).

(f) In Abidjan, Côte d'Ivoire interviews of counsellors disclosed that 99 per cent of clients appreciated VCT services (Doumatey et al., 2000[243]).

In a study conducted by the Kenya Association of Professional Counsellors 100 counselling sessions were examined through client exit interviews, counsellor self-assessment questionnaires and supervisor evaluation of audio taped sessions. The ratings by the three groups widely concurred and, in general, the sessions were deemed to be of high quality. Counsellors tended to under-rate their effectiveness, whereas clients and the supervisor ratings were very closely matched. This suggests that quality assurance in counselling could be carried out inexpensively and effectively using client exit interviews (Rachier et al., 2000[244]).

Counselling without Testing

In many settings HIV counselling is available without testing. This choice is inexpensive and does not necessitate a laboratory infrastructure and distribution system for test kits and has the potential to reach large numbers of people. In rural Uganda a community-based counselling service was set up to provide HIV counselling without testing (Mugula et al., 1995[245]). Attendance rose from 80 per month in 1993, to 400 per month in 1995. Counselling concentrated on safer sex advice and condoms were distributed by the project. Uptake of condoms also increased tremendously during this period. In other settings where HIV counselling is offered without testing this can led to client frustration since clients who following counselling are eager to be tested.

A study from the United States displayed that the type of counselling given was important in HIV prevention. The study considered the effect of 'brief and focused motivational/skills-building'. 'HIV risk-reduction counselling' versus 'educational counselling'. They discovered that condom use rose from 22-66 per cent (90 days after counselling) in the former group compared with 27-43 per cent in the latter group (Kalichman et al., 1998[246])

Other Behavioural Interventions

There have been several studies considering the efficacy of behavioural interventions without HIV testing to reduce HIV risk behaviour. Three studies have demonstrated beneficial outcomes of these interventions (measured as reductions in the incidence of sexually transmitted infections). The most successful behavioural intervention trial narrated is in ethnic minority women in the United States (Shain, 1999[247]). Six hundred and seventeen women with sexually transmitted infections were recruited and randomised to receive either group counselling (three weekly sessions of three to four hours) or a fifteen-minute health talk with a nurse. The women who received the group counselling had a 37 per cent reduction in sexually transmitted infections compared with the health education group over a 12-month period. A randomised controlled study from the United States demonstrated that brief group counselling reduced HIV-risk behaviour and resulted in better knowledge about HIV, stronger intentions to adopt safer sex and lower numbers of reported sexually transmitted infections among low-income women (Carey et al., 1998[248]).

In a study from the United States, 5758 seronegative people who attended an STI clinic were randomly allocated into 3 groups to examine the efficacy of counselling in promoting safer sex behaviour (Kamb et al., 1998 Project RESPECT[249]). The first group received in-depth 'enhanced' counselling, the second received 'brief' counselling and the third a brief didactic message that was typical of the normal care given by the clinics. In the first two groups receiving counselling a personalised risk-reduction plan was discussed. The participants were interviewed and examined at 6 and 12 months. Those who had received counselling (both enhanced and brief) had 30 per cent fewer sexually transmitted infections at 6 months and 20 per cent fewer sexually transmitted infections at 12 months than those who had received the information alone. Reported condom use was also consistently higher in the counselling groups. The study took place at five locations and the results were consistent over all locations. Some studies have demonstrated increased reported condom use but no significant differences in sexually transmitted infection rates:

A trial among high-risk clients from 37 clinics in the United States demonstrated that those who participated in a small group, 7-session HIV risk-reduction programme were more likely to use condoms consistently over a 12-month follow-up when compared with a control group. However, there was no remarkable difference in sexually transmitted infection rates (NIMH, 1998[250]). In a trial from a sexually transmitted disease clinic in London, men having with men either attended a seven-hour workshop or were given a twenty-minute session with a counsellor (Imrie et al., 1999[251]). Results revealed that while there was a small increase in condom use there was no reduction in sexually transmitted infections.

Testing without Counselling

Home Testing

Several different self-test kits have been promoted permitting people to self-test at home. Home collection kits are also available and these permit users to collect their own sample (blood or saliva) at home and send it to a collecting facility for testing. The client telephones the centre after one week for the test result. If the result is negative he or she will receive the result via a recorded message. If the test result is seropositive he or she will be 'counselled' over the telephone and referred for further follow-up if required. Although home-testing may improve accessibility and acceptability of HIV testing, it has been recommended to have limited HIV prevention advantages and may lead to undesired behaviour (Mertens et al.,

1994[252]). In the United States, 174316 people used home sample testing during the first year of its introduction and 97 per cent of these people phoned for their test results service. The percentage of those who were seropositive was 0.95 per cent. This is three times that approximated for the general population, and a similar rate to that found in VCT centres in the United States. A sample of 70620 seronegative and 865 seronegative people using this service has been examined (Branson, 1998[253]). Of all users 60 per cent (and 49 per cent who tested positive) had never tested before. Of those who tested seropositive, 65 per cent accepted referral for counselling, 23 per cent said that they already had some sort of follow-up and 5 per cent put the phone down immediately. Although there are no follow-up statistics on the people using this service it is used by people who are at risk from HIV infection and by many people who did not use other testing facilities.

While there are advantages to using home-collection and self-testing kits — they offer confidentiality and may provide a service for people who do not seek testing at VCT locations — they should be used with caution. Users must understand the need for a confirmatory test and about the window period. Regulations must be in place to ensure their quality and kits should have clear instructions and be easy to use. There are also worries that people using self-test kits have no pre-test counselling, or access to follow-up care and support, and that people may be coerced into testing (discussed earlier). There are still many reports of HIV testing being conducted in medical institutions without counselling. In a study from the Kenyatta hospital in Kenya, one-half of those tested did not receive any pre- or post-test counselling (Mwaura et al., 1998[254]). A study from Russia revealed that in 80 per cent of cases HIV testing was not accompanied by any pre- or post-test counselling (Nikitina, 1998[255]).

Peer Counselling

A study that introduced peer educators to communicate risk reduction among gay men consistently produced reductions in high-risk sexual behaviour (unsafe anal intercourse was reduced to 15-29 per cent of baseline levels) in the three intervention cities (Kelly et al., 1992[256]).

Conclusion

In this review of VCT outcomes, the majority of studies reveal benefits following VCT. However, many of the studies are narrative without control groups and have end points that rely on reported behavioural statistics (such as number of sexual partners or condom use) that are not supported with more objective results. In most of these studies there are, however, clear preliminary indicators that VCT is important in assisting people reduce risky behaviour, although societal and cultural pressures may sometimes override these. VCT is also shown to be important in enabling the person living with HIV/AIDS to access appropriate services, make decisions about future and family planning and benefit from interventions to prevent HIV-related infections and mother-to-child-transmission. VCT cannot prevent the person living with HIV/AIDS from the inevitable emotional stress when they learn about a seropositive result, but it can help people to understand, accept and cope. VCT services can also help those who test seronegative in future planning and in obtaining HIV preventive services to help them adopt and maintain protected sexual and injecting practices. There is, however, very little statistics on whether behaviour changes for both those test seropositive and seronegative can be maintained in the long term.

Changing sexual behaviour following VCT is governed by many factors and is easier if both partners can be counselled and tested together. Those studies that display the most consistent reduction in risky sexual behaviour are among couples who attended VCT together. A small number of studies report adverse consequences following VCT (such as violence, abandonment and dissolution of relationships) and many studies had anticipated that these would be difficulties. However, these were rare and could be minimised by counselling, particularly about disclosure.

Most of the studies that are more rigorously tailored and have more objective endpoints (such as seroconversion rates of sexually transmitted infection rates) are from developed countries and among MSM and IDUs. Although many of these studies demonstrate remarkable reductions in risky behaviour, the results are not consistent. Other societal and behavioural factors may be important in determining sexual and injecting behaviour in these groups and results cannot be generalised to heterosexuals from developing countries. When reviewing VCT studies it is difficult to make comparisons between the VCT interventions as these vary considerably between studies. In most studies the content and duration of the pre- and post-test counselling and the availability of ongoing counselling and support services were substantially narrated. Although several studies show that VCT is superior to health education and in-depth counselling superior to brief information-giving, it is not known what the key elements are in VCT that are most important in motivating long-term behaviour change.

Denial, stigma and lack of openness about HIV are considered as being major obstacles to HIV prevention and care in many high-prevalence countries. Although it is postulated that increased availability and uptake of VCT can overcome these obstacles there are no studies that have discovered this, and this field is in urgent need of investigation. Even though VCT does enable many people to change their behaviour not all are able to do so and not all VCT interventions are similarly successful in motivating behaviour change in different settings and among a wide range of populations. However, no single intervention (particularly HIV testing with a comparatively brief pre- and post-test counselling) should be expected to influence complex long-term behaviour in all people. VCT should be elastic and may need specific adaptation for specific groups of people. It should also be part of a more comprehensive programme that offers ongoing HIV prevention education and information, starting with HIV and sexual health education for youth before they become sexually active and reinforced at other contacts with health professionals. Innovative strategies are important to reach marginalised groups and groups who are not regularly in contact with formal health sector.

Important questions about the effective implementation of VCT remain unanswered.

These questions should be considered when designing VCT evaluations, particularly in developing countries that have the greatest burden of HIV.

(a) How can VCT services be improved to maximise the behavioural impact? Can VCT services be made less costly so that they can be implemented more widely in Third World countries?

(b) What are the long-term outcomes following VCT? How can VCT services be adapted to provide supportive care and HIV prevention for commercial sex workers and their clients and other marginalised groups?

(c) How can VCT services related to mother-to-child transmission projects include husbands/partners and will this improve uptake and influence sexual behaviour?

(d) Will the wider availability of VCT promote normalisation and reduce stigma in communities?

Studies from Developing Countries

Côte d'Ivoire

VCT services are available at several centres in Abidjan and in association with MTCT interventions at ANC clinics.

In an attempt to look at the effect of VCT on behaviour change, 208 seropositive people were interviewed from 7 different AIDS care centres there. Preliminary knowledge about HIV was good (Doumatey et al., 1998[257]). Reported sexual behaviour reported that many people were practising protected sex:

After testing seropositive

* 42 per cent used condoms always
* 28 per cent used condoms occasionally
* 26 per cent had abstained since receiving a seropositive result
* 50 per cent believed they were 'more responsible sexually'
* 12 per cent believed they may have infected their partner, even after testing
* 28 per cent had partners who were *not* tested

However, there was no pre-test behavioural statistics, so the impact of VCT on sexual behaviour could not be remarkably examined.

Democratic Republic of Congo (former Zaire)

Limited VCT services were available for antenatal women but were terminated due to political instabilities. (See studies from Kinshasa (Kamenga et al., 1991[258] and Ryder et al., 1991[259]). Also see study on sex workers (Laga et al., 1994[260]).

Ethiopia

A study of factory workers in Addis Ababa narrated their sexual behaviour prior to testing and knowledge about HIV transmission. Overall seropositivity among this group was 12 per cent. As yet there are no statistics on behaviour change following VCT (Sahlu et al., 1999[261]).

Kenya

VCT services are available at several NGO and government sites and in association with MTCT projects. In a study from Kenya women were provided VCT as part of their antenatal care. Women who tested positive and a comparison group of uninfected women were followed up for one year (Temmerman M, et al., 1990[262]). They had each received one session of post-test counselling where HIV, family planning and sexual behaviour were discussed. Family-planning use, condom use and pregnancy rates were identical in both groups. It was concluded that this single session of counselling was therefore ineffective in this setting, in influencing decisions on subsequent condom use of reproductive behaviour. However, it may be difficult for women to influence safer sex behaviour in their relationships since, in the majority of cases, their sexual partners did not know their HIV status. Moreover, in Kenya, as elsewhere, women often have difficulties in discussing HIV and sexual behaviour and insisting on condom use, especially with their long-term partner.

Rwanda

See under sections on seroincidence and couple counselling (Allen et al., 1992; 1993, Allen, Tice et al., 1992). See section on partner disclosure, (Ladner et al., 1995).

Uganda

Uganda has the most developed VCT services in sub-Saharan Africa. Since 1990 VCT has been available through the AIDS information centre (AIC) in Kampala, where more than 380000 people have been tested (UNAIDS, 1999[263]). Further VCT centres have subsequently been set up across Uganda (Magombe et al., 1998[264]). There are at present more than 20 satellite sites in operation.

The AIDS support organisation (TASO) is closely associated with AIC and offers ongoing counselling and a broad range of support services for people with HIV. There have been several studies aiming at the effectiveness of the VCT service and the ongoing support services provided by TASO and AIC. A study of 250 HIV consecutive positive and 250 HIV-negative people attending the AIC compared them with 200 consecutive clients who had earlier tested negative and were attending for a repeat test (Muller et al., 1992[265]). The majority of the people attending for repeat testing reported one sexual partner (67 per cent) or sexual abstinence (25 per cent). When compared with pre-test information from people attending the AIC for their first test, repeat testers were considerably less likely to report having casual sex (6 per cent versus 25 per cent). Repeat testers were also more likely to use condoms with casual sexual partners. Of the 200 repeat testers only 2 (1 per cent) had seroconverted. It is noteworthy, however, that the 'repeat testers' can differ from the 'first-time testers'.

An uncontrolled study of reported behaviour change at the AIC has displayed major changes in sexual behaviour following VCT (Moore et al. 1993[266]). Reported condom use increased from 10 to 89 per cent with steady partners, and from 28 to 100 per cent with non-steady partners of HIV seropositive clients. This study relied on reporting of sexual behaviour on a checklist questionnaire. A quantitative and qualitative analysis from the TASO counselling service demonstrates a good understanding of safer sex and a high level of safer sex behaviour following VCT (Kaleeba et al. 1997[267], and TASO, 1999[268]). When seropositive people in the TASO evaluation reported present sexual practices, 45 per cent (56 per cent females and 28 per cent males) said they were abstinent and 33 per cent (26 per cent females and 48 per cent males) said they used condoms. Of those who said they were using condoms 81.3 per cent said that they had done so after seeing the counsellors at TASO. Fifty-seven per cent of those who said that they had used from in their last sexual episode. The reported condom use was higher than that reported in the general population, where 10 per cent of people said that they had ever used condoms (Konde-Lule and Sebina 1993[269]). In the most recent evaluation of TASO 12120 records of clients attending between 1997-1999 were evaluated

(Mukasa-Monico et al, 2000[270]). Condom use increased from 23 to 41 per cent for women and 20 to 49 per cent for men following VCT. Further increases in condom use were witnessed in people who had further post-test counselling sessions. VCT in rural Uganda has also been examined. A small, uncontrolled study from rural Uganda reports condom use in 50 per cent of people following VCT (Kamaya, 1998[271]).

In a countryside community cohort from Rakai VCT was developed and provided free of charge (Lutalo et al 2000[272], Nyblade et al., 2000[273]). Behaviour change in the 20 months following VCT was evaluated in four groups: seropositive people who received VCT (n = 370); seronegative people who received VCT (n = 2304), seropositive (n = 562) and seronegative (n = 2860) who did not receive VCT. For all groups there was not a statistically major difference in *most* risk behaviours between those who had participated in VCT and those who had not. However, for both seropositive men and women who reported no condom use at the first survey, those who received VCT were more likely to report condom use at after 20 months relative to non-VCT recipients (23.5 per cent versus 12.8 per cent for men, 15.5 per cent versus 7.6 per cent for women p = 0.05 for both). Moreover, women who were seropositive and had received VCT had higher rates of condom use than seronegative women who received VCT (12.3 per cent versus 8.3 per cent). Among males condom use was moderately higher (but not significantly different) among seropositives than seronegatives following VCT (23.6 per cent versus 19.0 per cent). However, it may be more appropriate to compare both seropositive and seronegative with unaware controls as the objective of VCT is to promote condom use for all clients unless seronegative people are in a mutually faithful relationship with someone who had been tested negative.

Zambia

VCT services have been available in Lusaka since 1992, when Kara Counselling and Training Trust developed them in conjunction with support services for PLHA. Several studies from Kara have aimed at sexual behaviour, emotional and social outcomes and coping following testing. Other counselling projects have been developed related to hospitals or home-based care programmes (Jordan, 1995[274]). In 1999, a countrywide VCT service was initiated and is being introduced throughout Zambia (Ministry of Health interim report, 2000). Following successful pilot projects of VCT related to MTCT interventions, this service is also being expanded (see Chibwesha et al., Operational Aspects of VCT). Studies from the Kara Counselling service in Zambia have displayed some changes in sexual behaviour following VCT (Kelly et al., 1994[275], Baggaley et al., 1998[276, 277]). Following VCT both those testing seropositive and seronegative were more likely to use condoms and reduced their number of causal sexual partners, when compared with reported behaviour prior to testing. However, in other studies from Kara, some women expressed difficulties about using safer sex methods due to poor communication with their sexual partner/s (Chanda et al., 1994[278]). Also see under Seroincidence/Seroconversion (Hira, 1990).

Zimbabwe

VCT services in Zimbabwe were not broadly available until recently. Social marketing of VCT through The New Start project initiated in 1999, at present having nine operational VCT centres, with others planned (PSI 1999[279], Moses et al., 2000[280], Sangiwa et al., 2000[281]). An evaluation of these sites is currently taking place. These have been popular with both singles and couples. At present, 7000 people have attended the sites, 10 per cent being couples. There have been no statistics presented (till now) on the social and behavioural consequences of testing. VCT services in Bulwayo have been studied (see Meursing et al., 1993/1995/1999 on Access to Ongoing Emotional/Psychological Care).

The Multi-centre Trial: the United Republic of Tanzania, Kenya, Trinidad and Tobago

Recent results from the CAPS/AIDSCAP/WHO/UNAIDS multi-centre trial have given motivating results (Coates et al., 1998[283]; Sangiwa et al., 1998[284]; 2000[285]; Kamenga et al., 2000[286]; Balmer et al., 2000[287]; Furlonge et al., 2000[288], The VCT efficacy study group 2000[289]). This study was the first randomised trial of HIV counselling and testing from developing countries.

Participants were randomised for receive either health information or VCT. The study was tailored to compare the prevalence of self-reported, unprotected sexual intercourse at six months follow-up between the groups. Statistics on the social and psychological consequences of receiving VCT was also collected, and a cost-effective analysis performed. The results of the study (N = 3120, 1534 males and 1586 females) demonstrated that percentage of *individuals* reporting unprotected sexual intercourse with *non-primary* partners declined significantly, more for those receiving VCT than for those receiving health information (HI) only. (Males: 35 per cent reduction in VCT group versus 13 per cent in HI group; females; 39 per cent reduction in VCT group versus 17 per cent reduction in HI group).

Identical differences were observed in the number of unprotected cases with non-primary partners (males: 37 per cent in VCT group versus 12 per cent reduction in HI group; females; 42 per cent in VCT groups 12 per cent reduction in HI group); Among those assigned to VCT at baseline, those identified with HIV were more likely to change their sexual behaviour than those found as HIV negative. The rate of incident sexually transmitted infections among men assigned to VCT was 46 per cent was less than those assigned to HI only (3.5 per cent versus 1.9 per cent p = p 0.1), but rates among women were almost the same (6.2 per cent versus 5.6 per cent). Self-reports of unprotected sexual intercourse between baseline and first follow-up were strongly related to incidents sexually transmitted infections at the first follow-up. In *couples* (N = 586), 74 per cent were seroconcordant negative, 9 per cent seroconcordant positive, and 17 per cent were serodiscordant (6 per cent were M+ F- and 11 per cent were M- F+). At the first follow-up, both VCT and HI couples (in which one or both were seropositive) decreased significantly in the rate of unprotected sexual intercourse with their study enrolment partners compared with couples in which both were negative. Moreover, VCT couples were significantly more likely to report reduced unprotected sexual intercourse with their spouse than HI couples, but there was a slight change in reported sexual behaviour with secondary sexual partners.

This study, therefore, supports the efficacy of VCT in preventing HIV transmission in serodiscordant couples. Previous research in

Africa and the United States has also recommended that VCT is more effective for HIV risk reduction when both partners participate in the process together, share their test results and formulate risk reduction schedules based on their HIV test results.

India

The HIV incidence and prevalence is rapidly increasing in India. The predominant mode of transmission has been through heterosexual contact between female commercial sex workers and their clients. However, there is increasing seroprevalence among married monogamous women whose only risk factor was sexual contact with a husband who also has had a sexually transmitted infection. In north-east India the number of cases of HIV infection is increasing due to injecting drug users. By the end of 1999 there were 4 million people living with HIV in India. Efforts to provide VCT started in India in 1987. By 1992, there was a national training programme for counsellors. There are six regional VCT centres. However, private medical practitioners, some of whom do not offer adequate counselling or ensure informed consent prior to testing, conduct much of the HIV testing. Anonymous VCT services are also being promoted (Bhandari et al., 1998[290]). NGO services are popular and some report increased condom use following VCT (Kalyanasundaram, 1998[291]). In a study from Pune the role of VCT in HIV prevention among those who test negative was evaluated (Bentley et al., 1998[292]). There were 1628 seronegative heterosexual men recruited from a STI clinic. They were watched every three months for repeat VCT for twenty-four months. Counselling was concentrated on reinforcing messages of monogamy, condom use with sexual partners and provision of condoms. This ongoing counselling and testing was positively related to risk reduction behaviours. At six months men were 2.8 times - and at twenty-four months 4.7 times - more likely to consistently use condoms with commercial sex workers.

Thailand

In Thailand the first cases of HIV were detected in 1984 and 1985 among injecting drug users. The epidemic rapidly became more widespread with increasing seroprevalence witnessed among female sex workers, males attending STI clinics and women attending antenatal clinics. By 1993, 600000 to 800000 people were estimated to be infected. The Thai Red Cross quickly set up a network of VCT services. VCT services are also largely available in many government institutions (Guntamala et al., 1998[293]) and are now provided in some provinces related to mother-to-child-transmission interventions. In 1993, consecutive samples of 250 seropositive and seronegative patients were recruited to examine effectiveness of VCT in promoting behaviour change (Phanuphak et al., 1994[294]). Following VCT most clients expressed the intention to reduce HIV risk behaviour in response to a positive or negative HIV test result (more so if seropositive). This study relies on intention to reduce HIV risk behaviour and although the results are motivating they cannot be verified. A study from Bangkok compared self-reported behaviour of seropositive people who had received VCT with those from a matched sample of seropositive people who were unaware of their status (Muller et al., 1995[295]). Of the people who had received VCT 84 per cent reported that they had decreased their number of sexual partners since receiving it. They also reported more frequent condom use than did seropositive people who were unaware of their status.

Myanmar

There are approximated to be over 400000 cases of HIV infection in Myanmar. VCT services have been added to 28 pre-existing health services in townships across Myanmar (see Kywe et al., 1996[296] and Thu 1997[297] on the Operational Aspects of VCT).

Latin America and the Caribbean

VCT services have been promoted in many countries in Latin America and the Caribbean. In Chile the NGO FRENASIDA (Chilean Association to prevent AIDS) has operated a VCT centre in association with the government since 1991. The prevalence of HIV remains relatively low (in Santiago the approximated seroprevalence is 25.6 per 100000 Caceres et al., 1996[298] and UNAIDS 1999[299]). They report a relatively low uptake and low return for HIV testing but among those who do test almost 70 per cent report having changed their behaviour in some way, including increased frequency of condom use (Gonzalez et al., 1997[300]). In Brazil, at present all but two states there offer VCT services that are confidential and free of charge. Counselling services have been available since 1988, but the quality and uptake of these services varies considerably. Strategies to examine implementation of HIV prevention strategies by VCT locations have been developed (Passarelli et al., 2000[301]). During 1997, 10 public health services were visited. Although VCT counsellor were able to offer care and support for persons living with HIV/AIDS they were found not to be effective in helping persons living with HIV/AIDS to overcome their difficulties in adopting safer sex practices (Filgueiras et al., 2000[302]).

It is estimated that there are some 18000 people with HIV in Jamaica. The counselling and community outreach programme (CCO) has been promoted to offer psychosocial support for people with HIV.

Studies from Developed Countries

Students

A randomized-controlled examination of VCT versus HIV education alone was conducted among students (Wenger et al., 1992[303]). When interviewed at six months follow-up, the students in the VCT group had increased communication with sexual partners about the risk of HIV infection. However, no consistent differences among the groups in the number of sexual partners or the use of condoms were discovered at follow-up.

STI Clinic Attendees

In another study conducted by the same group in Los Angeles the effect of VCT versus AIDS education was looked at among consecutive attendees at a sexually transmitted infection clinic (Wenger et al., 1991[304]). At follow-up the mean number of sexual partners declined, but there was no significant difference between the groups. However, the VCT group questioned their most recent sexual partner(s) more about HIV ($p = 0.01$), 'worried more about getting AIDS' ($p = 0.03$), and tended to use condoms more often with their last sexual partner ($p = 0.05$). Of VCT subjects 40 per cent versus 20 per cent of the information group used condoms, avoided genital intercourse, or knew that their last sexual partner had a negative antibody test ($p = 0.005$).

Women Clinic Attendees

A study of women attending family planning and gynaecology outpatients revealed that being tested for HIV did not result in any major changes in condom use, self-reports of sexually transmitted infection or number of sexual partners in the four months following testing (Wilson et al., 1996[305]). Another study from the United States compared the effects of VCT on sexual behaviour among women attending four primary health care clinics (Icovics et al., 1994[306]). One hundred and fifty-two seronegative women and 78 women who had never been tested (matched for age and race) were questioned about their sexual behaviour at two weeks and three months after the VCT baseline. There were no major differences in the groups and no major changes in risk behaviour in either group. It was recommended that women who seek VCT may have already made changes in their sexual behaviour prior to requesting VCT.

VCT Sites

A study examining the free, anonymous, public VCT service at two sites in North Carolina, had disappointing results (Landis et al., 1992[307]). No major changes were discovered in high-risk sexual behaviour at follow-up.

Serodiscordant Couples

In these studies the prevalence of HIV was comparatively low. There were no people with seropositive results who took part in the intervention groups in studies by Wenger et al. In the study by Icovics et al., women were recruited from clinics in southern Connecticut, where there is little morbidity or mortality from HIV outside higher risk groups. Thus, while women are willing to undergo testing they do not perceive themselves to be at an alarming risk from HIV and therefore do not feel it is necessary to make changes in their sexual behaviour. This emphasizes the difficulties in making comparisons between studies from low-prevalence developed countries and much higher-prevalence developing countries.

Studies among MSM

Comparisons between Groups Before and After Testing Available

Some studies of sexual behaviour in MSM started before HIV testing was available, permitting comparisons of sexual behaviour before and after VCT was set up. A study from the United States followed a cohort of homosexual men from 1984, before HIV testing was available, until 1986 when HIV testing was available (Coates et al., 1987[308]). Men who were aware of their HIV status were significantly less likely to practise unsafe sex (12 per cent of seropositive men, 18 per cent of seronegative men and 27 per cent of untested men practised unsafe sex). All groups had, however, started to change their sexual behaviour before HIV testing became available. All reported significantly higher rates of unprotected sexual intercourse before HIV testing was available (48 per cent who later tested positive, 49 per cent who did not test and 41 per cent who later tested negative).

A study from the Netherlands also demonstrated that MSM had started to change their sexual behaviour prior to VCT being made available (van Griensven et al., 1989[309]). They also displayed that seropositive MSM were more likely to use condom during anal intercourse (with both steady and casual partners) than were seronegative and untested MSM.

Inconclusive Studies

Several studies recommended that although there were considerable reductions in risky sexual behaviour over time these were not clearly related to VCT. A study from Canada followed a cohort of homosexual men from 1984-1987 (Schechter et al., 1988[310]). Following VCT, the annual number of sexual partners declined for both those with seropositive and seronegative test results and there was a remarkable increase in condom use. More seronegatives than seropositives reported no condom used during anal intercourse with regular partners (45.7 per cent versus 23.4 per cent) and with casual partners (15.9 per cent versus 1.5 per cent). (There was, however, no control group of untested). A small group of people who had the largest number of casual sexual partners was also the most likely not to be using condoms with these partners. Although marked risk reduction was noted for MSM who were aware of their HIV status, some men continued to put themselves at an alarming risk. A study from Chicago disclosed that all MSM decreased risky sexual behaviour but there was no significant difference between men who were aware of their HIV status, and those who were not (Ostrow et al., 1989[311]).

A study from the United States compared MSE who were aware of their HIV status, with men who had been tested but declined to receive their test result (Doll et al., 1990[312]). Both groups had access to risk-reduction statistics. In both groups there was a notable decline in unsafe sexual behaviour, but these declines were independent of knowledge of HIV status and real serostatus. In a longitudinal study of 139 MSM from Boston, all groups (seropositive, seronegative and untested) demonstrated a decline in risky sexual behaviour, but there was no difference between the groups (Zapa et al., 1991[313]). Twenty-two seropositive MSM, twenty-two seronegative MSM and twelve men who were tested (but did not want to know their HIV status) were surveyed one week and six months after testing (Huggins et al., 1991[314]). All three groups altered their sexual behavior, with no major difference between the groups.

A study from four cities in the United Kingdom also showed no evidence for declining risky sexual behaviour following VCT (Dawson et al.,.1991[315]). In a study from 16 small cities in the United States there were mixed revelations (Roffman et al., 1995[316]). Although MSM who had undergone VCT reported more condom use and had more protected penetrative sexual episodes than untested MSM, they also had a considerably greater number of sexual partners. Therefore, overall untested and tested MSM reported a similar number of unprotected sexual episodes.

Decreases in Risky Sexual Behaviour, Related to VCT

Several early studies do, however, show significant decreases in risk behaviour related to VCT, with seropositive men showing greater reduction in risk behaviour than seronegative men or men who are unaware of their HIV status. It is recommended that learning about being seropositive had a deep impact on changing behaviour and showed that seronegative men were still putting themselves at risk from infection. In a study from Baltimore, United

States 1 001 MSM were provided VCT (Fox et al., 1987[317]). Of those, 670 elected to have VCT and 311 declined (the two groups had similar baseline characteristics). All were counselled about safer sex. In all groups unsafe sexual practices declined, although revelation of a seronegative test result led to a slight decline in these sexual activities. In Boston, MSM who tested seropositive were more likely to have protective sexual behaviour than seronegative or untested men (McCusker et al., 1988[318]).

Three cohort studies (Cohn et al., 1988[319], Zones et al., 1986[320], McKusick et al., 1990[321]) and three cross-sectional studies also demonstrated an association between VCT and reduction in risky sexual behaviour (Valdiserri et al., 1988[322], Frazer et al., 1988[323], Ross 1988[324]).

Long-term studies, however, have revealed that initial changes in sexual behaviour following VCT may be difficult to maintain. In a study from the United States, at two years 47 per cent of people and relapsed (not used protected sex practices) at least once (Abid et al., 1991[325]).

Studies among Injecting Drug Users IDUs

Significant Change in Injecting Practices Attributable to VCT

Some studies have found increases in safe injecting practices following VCT:

(a) In a study of 933 IDUs attending a detoxification centre in Milan (Nicolosi et al., 1991[326]) a preventive intervention based on VCT was associated with a significant reduction in sharing of syringes and unsafe injecting practices compared with risk behaviour in IDUs who had not received the intervention. The latter group showed no change—or even an increase, despite general information and HIV health education campaigns.

(b) In a small study of IDUs attending a detoxification programme in Long Island, United States both seropositives and seronegatives had reduced risk behaviour (Magura et al., 1990[327]). There was, however, no untested control group for comparison.

(c) In a study from New York City, seronegative IDUs attending a methadone maintenance treatment programme were less likely to use unsafe injecting than seropositive or untested IDUs (Magura et al., 1991[328]).

(d) In a study from 12 European countries, seronegative compared seropositive, seronegative IDUs and IDUs who had not received VCT (Desenclos et al., 1993[329]). Seronegative IDUs admitted higher rates of safe injecting than untested IDUs. Seropositive IDUs were also less likely to give their injecting equipment to other IDUs than to IDUs who had not received VCT.

(e) In a study of 5644 attendees at needle sharing programmes and detoxification centres in California, the factor most closely associated with not sharing syringes was having attended VCT (Watters et al., 1994[330]).

(f) Studies from Australia have shown advantages of needle-exchange programmes (NEPs), methadone replacement and VCT services, resulting in low HIV prevalence rates among IDUs. In Australia. However, it is difficult to attribute one intervention to this success (Drucker et al., 1998[331]).

(g) VCT and NEPs have expanded substantially in New York. The percentage of IDUs using NEPs has increased from 20-54 per cent and those using VCT from 51-81 per cent during 1990-1997 (Des Jarlais et al., 2000[332]). A meta-analysis of studies among over 11000 IDUs from New York during 1990-1997 has revealed that knowledge of HIV status and attendance at NEPs were associated with less risk behaviour. Using a NEP had an OR = 0.64 (p = less than 0.001) for sharing at last injection and knowledge of a seropositive status had an OR = 0.35 (p = less than 0.001) or unsafe sex with primary sexual partner. During this time the HIV incidence fell from 4.4 per 100 person-years to 0.8 per 100 person-years for those at risk. It was concluded that while there are manifold reasons in the process of declining HIV incidence among IDUs in New York there is a clear pattern of increased use of NEPs and VCT which were temporally related to a large reduction in HIV incidence.

No Significant Change in Injecting Practices Attributable to VCT

* In a study from New York (associated with a methadone maintenance programme) most people testing seronegative and seropositive curtailed injecting drugs. Those who continued to inject were more likely to use safe injecting practices, but there was no significant difference between those who were aware of their status and those who were not (Casadonte et al., 1990[333]).
* In a study from Washington, United States, 313 IDUs were randomly assigned to HIV education, HIV education plus VCT or a waiting list (Calsyn et al., 1992[334]). The sample as a whole decreases high-risk behaviour but there were no significant differences between the groups.
* In a study from Puerto Rico, VCT was provided to IDUs recruited from a street-selling area (Conlon et al 1996[335]). Of the 374 participants 88 per cent permitted to be tested and returned for their results and 73.5 per cent were followed up and interviewed six months later. Of the 176 IDUs who reported a seronegative test result prior to base line, 26 per cent subsequently diagnosed as seropositive. No significant difference was noted between seropositive and seronegative IDU risk behaviour.
* In a study from central Massachusetts, 4267 individuals were offered VCT at a multi-site programme including community clinics, drug treatment programmes and prisons. Half of those tested reported risk behaviour associated with IDU. A sample of 207 IDUs were followed up following VCT (McCusker et al., 1996[336]). Among those who continued to inject drugs there was a reduction in the percentage visiting shooting galleries following VCT but no other significant behaviour changes were reported.
* In a multi-centre study from the United States, 1174 seronegative IDUs who were in drug treatment programmes were asked about their injecting practices following VCT (Sabin et al., 2000[337]). VCT did not change risk behaviour in these programmes.
* In a study of male IDUs attending drug treatment centres in Northern Thailand there was no difference in changing

risk behaviours among those who had prior VCT and those who had not (Kawichai et al., 2000[338]). It was concluded that HIV prevention programmes, including VCT, have been extensively introduced over the past decade in Thailand and have reduced the incidence of HIV. A general trend in reducing risk behaviours in Thais might have been the cause for not observing significant change in IDUs following VCT.

* One study has evaluated whether VCT increases the probability of IDUs adhering to a drug treatment programme (MacGowan et al., 1996[339]). Knowledge of HIV status did not affect retention.

Significant Change in Sexual Behaviour Practices Attributable to VCT

The majority of studies show a reduction in risky sexual behaviour of IDUs following VCT.

* In a study from 12 European countries seropositive IDUs reported higher rates of condom use than seronegative and untested IDUs. (Desenclos et al., 1993).
* In a study from New York City, seropositive IDUs attending a methadone maintenance treatment programme were more probable to use condoms than seronegative or untested IDUs (Magura et al., 1991).
* A study from Bangkok and New York City showed that seropositive IDUs were more probable to practise protected sex than seronegative or untested IDUs (Vanichseni et al., 1992[340], 1993[341]).
* In a study from Puerto Rico, following VCT, seropositive IDUs were less likely to report being sexually active and more likely to use condoms, than untested or seronegative IDUs (Colon et al., 1996).
* A study from New York discovered that seronegative IDUs who had received VCT were more likely to always use condoms than seronegatives who had not received VCT (Friedman et al., 1994[342]). However, this difference was not witnessed among seropositive who received VCT than seropositive who were unaware of their status. The

researchers attributes the similarity in condom use between tested and untested seropositive IDUs to changes in condom use made by IDUs who suspected that they were HIV-infected and had thus made changes in their sexual behaviour based on this hypothesis.

These revelations recommend that community interventions aimed at providing VCT — and thus detecting seropositive IDUs, counselling them about their status and assisting them to reduce the risk of transmitting HIV — are effective in reducing the spread of HIV from IDUs to their sexual partner/s. In most studies, changes in behaviour to curtail sexual transmission of HIV are more remarkable among those who test seropositive than among those who test seronegative. It is crystal clear that seronegative IDUs may be continuing to put themselves at risk from sexual transmission of HIV (particularly if their sexual partner is also an IDU). Emphasis on providing counselling about prevention of sexual transmission of HIV for IDUs who test negative is significant.

References

1. UNAIDS (1999), *Knowledge is power: voluntary HIV counselling and testing in Uganda.* Geneva, (UNAIDS case study, Best Practice collection, UNAIDS/ 99.8E).
2. Hira S, Nkowane B (1990), Epidemiology of human immunodeficiency virus in families in Lusaka, Zambia. *Journal of AIDS,* 3:83-86.
3. Kamenga M et al. (1991), Evidence of marked sexual behaviour change associated with low HIV-1 seroconversion in 149 married couples with discordant HIV-1 serostatus: experience at an HIV counselling centre in Zaire. *AIDS,* 5:61-67.
4. Goedert J, Eyster M, Biggar R (1987), Heterosexual transmission of human immunodeficiency virus. *AIDS research and human retroviruses,* 4: 355-361.
5. Allen S et al. (1992), Effect of serotesting with counselling on condom use and seroconversion among HIV discordant couples in Africa. *British Medical Journal,* 304:1605-9.
6. Allen S et al. (1992), Confidential HIV testing and condom promotion in Africa: impact on HIV and gonorrhoea rates. *Journal of the American Medical Association,* 268 23:3338-3343.
7. Brookmeyer R et al. (1995), A new method for estimating current HIV incidence rates. *American Journal of Epidemiology,* 142:283-286.
8. Bentley M et al. (1 998), HIV testing and counselling among men attending STD clinic in Pune, India: changes in condom use and sexual behaviour over time. *AIDS,* 12:1869-1877.

9. Padian N, Marquis L, Francis D (1987), Male-to-female transmission of HIV. *Journal of the American Medical Association*, 258:758-790.
10. Otten M et al. (1993), Changes in sexually transmitted disease rates after HIV testing and post-test counselling, Miami, 1988-1989. *American Journal of Public Health*, 83:529-533.
11. George N, Green J, Murphy S (1998), Sexually transmitted disease rates before and after HIV testing. *International Journal of Sexually Transmitted Diseases and AIDS*, 9:291 -293.
12. Wellings K et al. (1984), *Sexual behaviour in Britain. The National Survey of Sexual Attitudes and Life Style.* London, Penguin Books.
13. Baggaley R et al. (1997), Knowledge and attitudes to HIV and AIDS and sexual practices among university students in Lusaka, Zambia and London, England: are they so different? *Journal of the Royal Society of Health*, 117:88-94.
14. Macro International, Inc. (1996), DHS and Central Statistic Office Ministry of Health Zambia Demographic and Health Survey 1996. Maryland, USA.
15. Weinhardt L et al. (1999), Effect of HIV counselling and testing on sexual risk behaviour: a meta-analytic review of published research 1985-1997. *American Journal of Public Health*, 89:9 1397-1405.
16. UNAIDS/WHO AIDS epidemic update, December 1999 (UNAIDS/99.53e-WHO/CDSCRS/EDC99.9-WHO/FCH/HIS/99.6).
17. UNAIDS/WHO AIDS epidemic update, December 1999 (UNAIDS/99.53e-WHO/CDSCRS/EDC99.9-WHO/FCH/HIS/99.6).
18. Connor E et al. (1994), Reduction of maternal-infant transmission of HIV type 1 with zidovudine treatment. *New England Journal of Medicine*, 331:18 1173-1180.
19. Allen S et al. (1993), Pregnancy and contraceptive use among urban Rwandan women after HIV counselling and testing. *American Journal of Public Health*, 83:705-710.
20. Kiragu D et al. (1990), Counselling of women with HIV infection: effect on contraceptive practice and pregnancy. Presented at the *6th International Conference on HIV/AIDS*, San Francisco, USA.
21. Sunderland A, Moroso G, Berthaud M (1988), Influence of HIV infection on pregnancy decisions. Presented at the *4th International Conference on HIV/AIDS*, Stockholm, Sweden, Abstract 1068.
22. Selwyn P, Shoenbaum E, Davenny K (1989), Prospective study of HIV and pregnancy outcomes in intravenous drug users. *Journal of the American Medical Association*, 261:1289-1294.
23. Cowan J et al. (1990), Reproductive health choices of women at risk from HIV infection. Presented at the *6th International Conference on HIV/AIDS*, San Francisco, USA, Abstract WCP117.
24. Sunderland A et al. (1992), The impact of HIV serostatus on reproductive decisions of women *Obstetrics and Gynaecology*, 79:1027-1031.
25. Pivnick A et al. (1991), Reproductive decisions among HIV-infected drug using women: the importance of mother-child co-residence. *Medical Anthropology Quarterly*, 5:153-169.
26. Baggaley R, Kelly M, Mulongo W (1997), To tell or not to tell: sharing HIV results with sexual partners. Presented at the *5th SANASO conference*, Mbabane, Swaziland, Oct. 1997, Abstract W322D.

27. Keogh P et al. (1994), The social impact of HIV infection on women in Kigali, Rwanda: a prospective study. *Social Science and Medicine,* 38:8 1047-53.
28. Meursing K, Sibindi F (1995), Condoms, family planning and living with HIV in Zimbabwe. *Reproductive Health Matters,* 5:56-62.
29. Meursing K, Sibindi F (1995), Living with HIV: help-seeking and preventive behaviour of seropositive people in Bulawayo, Zimbabwe, Abstract number TuD 662.
30. Dube S et al. (2000), HIV counselling and testing of couples in Harare: problems and prospects. Presented at the *13th International Conference on HIV/AIDS,* Durban, South Africa, Abstract D3773.
31. Badini D, Aprodec Y, Madina T (1998), What should a counsellor do if a volunteer refuses to share his/her HIV test result with his/her partner. Presented at the *12th International Conference on HIV/AIDS,* Geneva, Switzerland, Abstract 24325.
32. Miller R, Sabin C, Leask C (1998), To tell or not to tell: A review of HIV disclosure patterns at a London teaching hospital. Presented at the *12th International Conference on HIV/AIDS,* Geneva, Switzerland, Abstract 24329.
33. Huggins J et al. (1991), Affective behavioural responses of gay and bisexual men to HIV antibody testing. *Social Work,* 36:(1) 61-66.
34. Sixaxhe T (2000), Disclosure of HIV status among antenatal women in the Western Cape [MSc thesis] (submitted for publication).
35. Mazhani L et al. (2000), Report of mid-term review of the prevention on MTCT programme of Botswana, MoH/UNICEF, Botswana.
36. Cartoux M et al. (1998), Acceptability of voluntary counselling and testing (VCT) and interventions to reduce mother-to-child transmission of HIV. Presented at the *12th World AIDS Conference,* Geneva, Abstract No. 23310.
37. Temmerman M et al. (1995), The right not to know HIV-test results. *Lancet,* 345:696-697.
38. Ladner J et al. (1996), A cohort study of factors associated with failure to return for post-test counselling in pregnant women: Kigali, Rwanda 1992-1993. *AIDS,* 10:69-75.
39. Lester P et al. (1995), The consequences of a positive prenatal HIV antibody test for women. *Journal of AIDS and human retrovirology,* 10:(3) 341 -349.
40. Baryarama F, Kalule J, Marum E (1998), New relationships and HIV discordance rates among couples requesting HIV counselling and testing in Uganda. Presented at the *12th International Conference on HIV/AIDS,* Geneva, Switzerland, Abstract 23149.
41. Carpenter L et al. (1999), Rates of HIV-1 transmission within marriage in rural Uganda in relation to the HIV sero-status of the partners. *AIDS,* 13:10883-89.
42. Baggaley R (1997), Fear of knowing: why 9 in 10 couples refused HIV tests in Lusaka Zambia. Presented at the *10th International Conference on AIDS and STDs.* Abidjan, Africa, Abstract E.1266.
43. UNAIDS (1999), *Knowledge is power: voluntary HIV counselling and testing in Uganda.* Geneva, Switzerland (UNAIDS case study, Best Practice collection UNAIDS/99.8E).

44. Baryarama F, Kalule J, Marum E (1998), New relationships and HIV discordance rates among couples requesting HIV counselling and testing in Uganda. Presented at the *12th International Conference on HIV/AIDS*, Geneva, Switzerland, Abstract 23149.
45. Carballo-Dieguez A, Meyer-Bahlburg H, Ehrhardt A (1990), Persistent sexual risk behaviour among heterosexual IVDUs partners regardless of HIV antibody status. Presented at the *6th International Conference on AIDS*, San Francisco, California.
46. Ubane L, Faleyimu B-L, Ajayi P (2000), HIV testing, positivity and marriage counselling in a religious set up of a Nigerian community. Presented at the *13th International Conference on HIV/AIDS*, Durban, South Africa, Abstract D627.
47. Turyagyen Da J (2000), Planning for marriage and HIV counselling and testing in Uganda. Presented at the *13th International Conference on HIV/AIDS*, Durban, South Africa, Abstract D3736.
48. Machekano R, McFarland Bassett M (2000), Views and attitudes towards HIV voluntary counselling and testing among urban men: Harare, Zimbabwe. Presented at the *13th International Conference on HIV/AIDS*, Durban, South Africa, Abstract D3768.
49. Dube S et al. (2000), HIV counselling and testing of couples in Harare: problems and prospects. Presented at the *13th International Conference on HIV/AIDS*, Durban, South Africa, Abstract D3773.
50. Karim Q et al. (1995), Reducing the stigma of HIV infection among South African sex workers: socio-economic and gender barriers. *American Journal of Public Health*, 85:11, 1521-5.
51. Lester P et al. (1995), The consequences of a positive prenatal HIV antibody test for women. *Journal of AIDS and human retrovirology*, 10:3 341-349.
52. van der Straten A et al. (1995), Couple communication, sexual coercion and HIV risk reduction in Kigali, Rwanda. *AIDS* 9:8 935-44.
53. Sangiwa G et al. (2000), Client's perspective of the role of voluntary counselling and testing in HIV / AIDS prevention and care in Dar Es Salaam, the United Republic of Tanzania: The Voluntary counselling and testing efficacy study. *AIDS and behaviour* 4:1 35-48.
54. Chabala S (2000), The socio-economic realities that affect responses to HIV / AIDS in Kayama, Lusaka. Presented at the *13th International Conference on HIV/AIDS*, Durban, South Africa, Abstract D2617.
55. Higgins D et al. (1991), Evidence for the effects of HIV antibody counselling and testing on risk behaviours. *Journal of the American Medical Association*, 266:17, 2419-29.
56. Wolitski R et al. (1997), The effects of HIV counselling and testing on risk-related practices and help-seeking behaviour. *AIDS Education and Prevention*, 9:52-67 (supplement B).
57. Weinhardt L et al. (1999), Effect of HIV counselling and testing on sexual risk behaviour: a meta-analytic review of published research 1985-1997. *American Journal of Public Health*, 89:9 1397-405.
58. Kelly et al. (1998), Protease inhibitor combination therapies and perceptions of gay men regarding AIDS severity and the need to maintain safer sex. *AIDS*, 12:F91-95.

59. Imrie et al. (1999), HIV prevention and homosexual men: should we be optimistic about the new millennium? *Sexually transmitted infection*, 75:369-376.
60. Laga M et al. (1994), Condom promotion, sexually transmitted disease treatment and declining incidence of HIV-1 infection in female Zairian sex workers. *Lancet*, 344:8917, 246-8.
61. Pickering H et al. (1993), The effects of post-test counselling on condom use among prostitutes in the Gambia. *AIDS*, 7:271-273.
62. Morar N, Ramjee G (2000), Impact of voluntary counselling and testing among sex. Presented at the *13th International Conference on HIV/AIDS*, Durban, South Africa, Abstract C1030.
63. Corby N et al. (1990), Effect of condom-skills training and HIV testing on AIDS prevention behaviours in sex workers. Presented at the *6th International Conference on AIDS*, San Francisco, California.
64. Cohen J et al. (1998), Changes in risk behaviour for HIV infection and transmission in a prospective study of 240 sexually active women in San Francisco. Presented at the *4th International Conference on AIDS*, Stockholm, Sweden.
65. Cantillo C (1998), The role of peer counselling on HIV/AIDS education among prostituted women in Davao city. Presented at the *12th International Conference on HIV/AIDS*, Geneva, Switzerland, Abstract 24326.
66. Plummer F, Moses S (1994), Elements of targeted interventions.
Wilson D (1994), Provisional rapid assessment guidelines for prostitute interventions in sub-Saharan Africa. Plummer F, Ngugi E, Moses S (1994), The Pumwani experience: Evolution of a partnership in disease control. In: *Focusing interventions among vulnerable groups for HIV infection: experiences from Eastern and Southern Africa*, NARESA (No. 2).
67. Otten M et al. (1993), Changers in sexually transmitted disease rates after HIV testing and post-test counselling, Miami 1988 to 1989. *American Journal of Public Health*, 83:529-533.
68. Wenger N et al. (1991), Reduction of high-risk sexual behaviour among heterosexuals undergoing HIV antibody testing: a randomized control trial. *American Journal of Public Health*, 81:12, 1580-85.
69. MacDonald A et al. (1999), HIV prevalence at reception in Australian prisons 1991-1997. *Medical Journal of Australia*, 171:1 18-21.
70. Dolan K, Wodak A (1999), HIV transmission in a prison system in an Australian State. *Medical Journal of Australia* 171:1 14-17.
71. Wainstein C, Copie J, Rios E (1998), HIV counselling and testing for convicted people in Buenos Aires, Argentina. Presented at the *12th International Conference on HIV/AIDS*, Geneva, Switzerland, Abstract 43415.
72. Wilson D et al. (1994), Ethnographic and quantitative research to design a community intervention among long-distance truck drivers in Zimbabwe. In: *Focusing interventions among vulnerable groups for HIV infection: Experiences from Eastern and Southern Africa Network of AIDS researchers of Eastern and Southern Africa*, NARESA (No. 2).
73. Mwizarubi B, Mwaijonga C, Laukamm-Josten U (1994), HIV education and condom promotion for truck drivers, their assistants and sex partners in the United Republic of Tanzania. In: *Focusing interventions among vulnerable groups for HIV infection: Experiences from Eastern and Southern Africa Network of AIDS researchers of Eastern and Southern Africa*, NARESA (No. 2).

74. Jackson D et al. (1997), Decreased incidence of sexually transmitted disease among trucking company workers in Kenya: results of a behavioural risk-reduction programme. *AIDS*, 7:271-73.
75. Bamne A (2000), Reaching out to high-risk behaviour target groups viz., truckers entering Mumbai, India through innovative targeted intervention strategy and rendering clinical and counselling services. Presented at the *13th International Conference on HIV/AIDS*, Durban, South Africa, Abstract B1164.
76. Mvere D et al. (1996), Strong preference to "donate" among HIV-positive blood donors in Zimbabwe. *Lancet*, 347:902-3.
77. Chama D, Mkoma J, Mumba G (1993), The effect of donor recruitment policies in the provision of safe blood at UTH Lusaka. Paper presented at *VIIIth International Conference on AIDS/STDs in Africa*, Marakesh.
78. Cleary P et al. (1991), Behavioural changes after notification of HIV infection. *American Journal of Public Health*, 81:586-1590.
79. Brookman RR (1990), Adolescent sexual behavior. In: Holmes KK, Mardh PA, Sparling PF, et al. *Sexually Transmitted Diseases.* New York, McGraw-Hill, Inc. 77-84.
80. Weiss E, Whelan D, Gupta GR (1996), Vulnerability and opportunity. Adolescents and HIV/AIDS in the Developing World. *International Center for Research on Women (ICRW).* Washington, D.C.
81. Munodawafa D, Gwede C (1996), Patterns of HIV/AIDS in Zimbabwe: implications for health education. *AIDS Education and Prevention*, 8:1, 1-10.
82. Damesyn M et al. (1998), Locally sustainable administration of HIV counselling and testing to young couples in rural regions of Western Kenya. Presented at the *12th World AIDS Conference*, Geneva, Switzerland.
83. Baggaley R et al. (1997), Knowledge and attitudes to HIV and AIDS and sexual practices among university students in Lusaka, Zambia and London, England: are they so different? *Journal of the Royal Society of Health*, 117:88-94.
84. Kelly R et al. (1993), HIV prevention for adolescents in Rakai, Uganda. Presented at the *9th International Conference on AIDS*, Berlin, Germany, Abstract PO-D02-3440.
85. Bohmer L, Kirumira E (1997), *Final Report: Access to reproductive health services participatory research with Ugandan adolescents.* Pacific Institute for Women's Health, Los Angeles, California and The Child Health and Development Center, Makarere University, Kampala, Uganda.
86. Baggaley R, Sulwe J (1998), Young people talk about HIV Focus group discussions among young people in Lusaka, Mazabuka district, Southern Province and Mongu district, Eastern Province. *Final report UNICEF.* Lusaka, Zambia publications.
87. Nabwiso F et al. (1993), HIV counselling and testing (CT) in young Ugandans. Presented at the *9th International Conference on AIDS*, Berlin, Germany, Abstract PO-C25-3215.
88. Kakooza A (1992), Attitudes of young people to counselling services and HIV screening and testing. Presented at the *VIIIth International Conference on AIDS*, Amsterdam, the Netherlands (Abstract PoD 5325).

89. Gumisiriza E et al. (1996), Response of young people 15-19 to HIV counselling and testing in Uganda. *International Conference on AIDS*, Vancouver, Canada, Abstract Tu C333 XI.
90. Gomes M et al. (2000), Testing and counselling adolescents—Rio de Janeiro, Brazil. Presented at the *13th International Conference on HIV/AIDS*, Durban, South Africa, Abstract B5170.
91. Flutterman D, Guttmacher S, Rogers A (2000), Getting busy? Live with it. Get tested. Social marketing to promote HIV counselling and testing to youth: results from a six-city programme in the United States. Presented at the *13th International Conference on HIV/AIDS*, Durban, South Africa, Abstract B5390.
92. Ita M (1998), Counselling in reproductive health among young people in the Shitta community in Lagos State. Presented at the *12th International Conference on HIV/AIDS*, Geneva, Switzerland, Abstract 60857.
93. Flutterman D, Hein K, Kipke M (1990), HIV-positive adolescents: HIV testing experiences and changes in risk-related sexual and drug-use behaviour. Presented at the *6th International Conference on AIDS*, San Francisco, USA.
94. CDC (1998), Young people at risk. Epidemic shifts further towards young women and minorities, September.
95. Kaiser family foundation (1999), Hearing their voices. A qualitative research study on HIV testing and higher-risk teens, http://www.kff.org
96. Carpenter et al. (2000), (International AIDS society) Antiretroviral therapy in adults. *Journal of the American Medical Association*, 283:3 381-389.
97. Revsin N, Burgos M, Vilas A (1998), The importance of patient counselling and social support in anti-retroviral treatment effectiveness. Presented at the *12th International Conference on HIV/AIDS*, Geneva, Switzerland, Abstract 12454.
98. Greene D, VanDevanter N, Merzel C (2000), Counselling approach to adherence. Presented at the *13th International Conference on HIV/AIDS*, Durban, South Africa, Abstract D4588.
99. Mwingwa A, Hosp M, Godfrey-Faussett P (1998), Twice weekly tuberculosis preventive therapy in HIV infection in Zambia. *AIDS*, 12:2447-57.
100. WHO/UNAIDS (1998), Policy statement on preventive therapy against tuberculosis in people living with HIV, WHO/TB/98.255 UNAIDS/98.34.
101. Godfrey-Faussett P et al. (1995), An HIV testing centre as a recruitment site for tuberculosis preventive therapy in Africa. *Transactions of the Royal Society of Tropical Medicine*, 89:351-54.
102. Aisu T et al. (1995), Preventive chemotherapy for HIV-associated tuberculosis in Uganda: an operational assessment at a voluntary counselling and testing centre. *AIDS*, 9:267-73.
103. Desormeaux J et al. (1996), Widespread HIV counselling and testing linked to a community-based tuberculosis programme in a high risk population. *Bulletin of PAHO*, 30:1 1-8.
104. Ayles H, Chikwampu D, Mwale A (2000), Household counselling for HIV and TB. Presented at the *13th International Conference on HIV/AIDS*, Durban, South Africa, Abstract D3780.

105. Phiri P et al. (2000), Introducing clinical services at a voluntary counselling and testing centre in Malawi as part of the pro-test initiative. Presented at the *13th International Conference on HIV/AIDS,* Durban, South Africa, Abstract B5283.

106. Anglaret X, Chene G, Attia A (1999), Early chemoprohylaxis with trimethoprim- sulphamethoxazole for HIV-1 infected adults in Abidjan, Côte d'lvoire: a randomized controlled trial. *The Lancet,* 353:1463-1468.

107. Wiktor S et al. (1999), Efficacy of trimethoprim-sulphamethoxazole prophylaxis to decrease morbidity and mortality in HIV-1 infected patients with tuberculosis in Abidjan, Côte d'lvoire: a randomized controlled trial. *The Lancet,* 353:1469-75.

108. Sassan-Morokro M et al. (1998), Significant reduction in mortality attributed to cotrimoxazole prophylaxis among HIV-infected tuberculosis patients in Abidjan, Côte d'lvoire. Presented at the *12th International Conference on HIV/AIDS,* Geneva, Switzerland, Abstract 12461.

109. Pugh G, Narciso S (1998), Reproductive health counselling among PLHAs. Presented at the *12th International Conference on HIV/AIDS,* Geneva, Switzerland, Abstract 60711.

110. Lutalo T, Kidugavu M, Mawwer M (2000), Contraceptive use and HIV testing and counselling in rural Rakai district, SW Uganda. Presented at the *13th International Conference on HIV/AIDS,* Durban, South Africa, Abstract C246.

111. Gouskov D (2000), Establishment of an informational and promotional network with a multidisciplinary approach to HIV/AIDS focusing on natural and complimentary therapies, social support and counselling for HIV +diagnosed people in Ukraine: Tacis/LIEN project. Presented at the *13th International Conference on HIV/AIDS,* Durban, South Africa, Abstract E3927C246.

112. Vollmer N, Valadez J (1999), A psychological epidemiology of people seeking HIV/AIDS counselling in Kenya: an approach for improving counselling training. *AIDS,* 13:1557-67.

113. Buzducea D, Romica P, Carina J (2000), An attachment-based approach to counselling with clients affected by HIV/AIDS. Presented at the *13th International Conference on HIV/AIDS,* Durban, South Africa, Abstract D3741.

114. Hays R et al. (1990), Help-seeking for AIDS-related concerns: A comparison of gay men with various HIV diagnoses. *American Journal of Community Psychology,* 18:735-55.

115. Catania J et al. (1992), Coping with death anxiety: help-seeking and social support among gay men with various HIV diagnosises. *AIDS,* 6:999-1005.

116. Peterson J et al. (1995), Help-seeking for AIDS high-risk sexual behaviour among gay and bisexual African American men. *AIDS Education Prevention,* 7:2 2271-273.

117. Solomon L et al. (1991), Utilization of health services in a cohort of intravenous drug users with known HIV-1 serostatus. *American Journal of Public Health,* 81:1285-90.

118. Kaldjin L, Jekel J, Friedland G (1998), End-of-life decisions in HIV-positive patients: the role of spiritual beliefs. *AIDS,* 12:103-107.

119. Sittitrai W, Williams G (1994), Candles of Hope: The AIDS programme of the Thai Red Cross. ActionAid London, United Kingdom (Strategies of Hope series No. 9).
120. Camara et al. (1991), Changes in Psycho-therapeutical approaches applied to hospitalized AIDS patients, Brazil. Presented at the *Sixth International Conference on AIDS,* San Francisco, Abstract SB 399.
121. Magura S et al. (1990), Reactions of methadone patients to HIV antibody testing. *Advances in alcohol and substance abuse,* 8:97-111.
122. Carvalho-Neto LD et al. (1989), Effectiveness of preventive and educational aspects in a multidisciplinary study group with HIV-infected patients family members group, Brazil. *Second International Symposium on AIDS Information and Education,* Cameroon, Abstract 2.4-5.
123. Mukisa ER et al. (1990), The impact of caring for AIDS and HIV-infected people. *International Conference on AIDS in Africa,* Kinshasha, Abstract TPA 4.
124. Zulu R et al. (1990), How social aspects of counselling have brought relief and hope to HIV-infected and AIDS patients in their homes in Lusaka, Zambia. *International Conference on AIDS in Africa,* Kinshasha Abstract TPA 9.
125. Meursing K, Sibindi F (1995), Condoms, family planning and living with HIV in Zimbabwe. *Reproductive Health Matters,* 5:56-62.
126. Meursing K, Sibindi F (1995), Living with HIV: help-seeking and preventive behaviour of seropositive people in Bulawayo, Zimbabwe, Abstract TuD 662.
127. Meursing K (1997), *A world of silence. Living with HIV in Matabeleland, Zimbabwe.* Royal Tropical Institute, The Netherlands.
128. Meursing K, Sibindi F (2000), HIV counselling—a luxury or essential need? Emotional, social and information needs of patients diagnosed HIV-positive in Zimbabwe. *Health policy and planning,* 15:1.7 3-23.
129. Lie G, Biswalo P (1996), Positive patient's choice of a significant other to be informed about the HIV-test result: findings from an HIV/AIDS counselling programme in the regional hospitals of Arusha and Kilimanjaro, the United Republic of Tanzania. *AIDS, Care* 8:3 285-296.
130. TASO Uganda, the inside story: Participatory evaluation of the HIV/AIDS counselling, medical and social services 1993-1994 (WHO/GPA/TCO/HCS/95.1).
131. Antoni M et al. (2000), Cognitive-behavioural stress management intervention effects on anxiety, 24-hr urinary norepinephrine output and T-cytotoxic/suppressor cells over time among symptomatic HIV-infected gay men. *Journal of Consulting and Clinical Psychology,* 68:1 31-45.
132. Molassiotis A et al. (2000), The effect of cognitative-behavioural group therapy and peer support/counselling in decreasing distress and improving quality of life in Chinese symptomatic HIV patients. Presented at the *13th International Conference on HIV/AIDS,* Durban, South Africa, Abstract D4681.
133. Holt R et al. (1998), The role of disclosure in coping with HIV infection. *AIDS Care,* 10:1 49-60.
134. Lie G, Biswalo P (1996), Positive patient's choice of a significant other to be informed about the HIV-test result: findings from an HIV/AIDS counselling programme in the regional hospitals of Arusha and Kilimanjaro, the United Republic of Tanzania. *AIDS Care,* 8:3 285-296.

135. *TASO Uganda, the inside story: participatory evaluation of the HIV/AIDS counselling, medical and social services* (1993-1994) (WHO/GPA/TCO/HCS/95.1).
136. McGrath J et al. (1993), AIDS and the urban family: its impact in Kampala, Uganda. *AIDS Care,* 5:1 55-70.
137. Lester P et al. (1995), The consequences of a positive prenatal HIV antibody test for women, *Journal of AIDS and human retrovirology,* 10:3 341-349.
138. Miller R, Sabin C, Leask C (1998), To tell or not to tell: A review of HIV disclosure patterns at a London teaching hospital. Presented at the *12th International Conference on HIV/AIDS,* Geneva, Switzerland, Abstract 24329.
139. Lippmann S, James W, Frierson R (1993), AIDS and the family: implications for counselling *AIDS Care,* 5:1 71-79.
140. Pidlisna N, Lukyanova N (1998), Prevention of stresses in families of HIV infected patients. *12th World AIDS Conference,* Geneva, Abstract 33266.
141. Srirak N, Wichajarn M, Cheewawat W (2000), Feasibility of family-based HIV post-test counselling in a Thai community cohort. Presented at the *13th International Conference on HIV/AIDS,* Durban, South Africa, Abstract D3747.
142. Baggaley R et al. (1998), Kara coping study - interim report UNAIDS/WHO.
143. Katongo E (2000), Voluntary counselling and testing of HIV in Mufulira, Zambia. Presented at the *13th International Conference on HIV/AIDS,* Durban, South Africa Abstract D3738.
144. Terrence Higgins Trust Website: www.tht.org.uk.
145. Federal Law N 38-F3 of 30/03/95 (1995), Prevention of HIV transmission in Russian Federation. Approved by State Duma 24/02/95.
146. Sehonou J et al. (1999), Nongovernmental organization against AIDS in Africa: the Anonymous testing centre of Bangui for voluntary HIV counselling and testing in the Central African Republic. Presented at the *XIth International Conference on AIDS and STDs in Africa,* Lusaka, Zambia, Abstract 14DT4-2.
147. Keogh P et al. (1994), The social impact of HIV infection on women in Kigali, Rwanda: a prospective study. *Social Science and Medicine,* 38:8 1047-53.
148. Williams G, Kalinaki D (1999), The Kitovu Hospital Mobile Programme: Home care and orphan support in Ugandan rural communities affected by HIV/AIDS (draft report).
149. Hamavhwa C, Haworth A (1998), Critical realities of HIV/AIDS counselling in a developing country with high prevalence levels. Presented at the *12th World AIDS Conference,* Geneva, Abstract 33306.
150. Baggaley R et al. (1995), Skills Training for people with HIV (PWAs) in Lusaka, Zambia. *IXth International Conference on AIDS/STDs in Africa, December 1995.*
151. Lukandwa J et al. (1998), Counselling services for mothers attending a mother-child research clinic in Mulango hospital. Presented at the *12th International Conference on HIV/AIDS,* Geneva, Switzerland, Abstract 33308.
152. Krabbendam AA et al. (1998), The impact of counselling on HIV-infected women in Zimbabwe. *AIDS Care,* 10:1 S25-37.

153. Nanono Namatovu S, Matovu S, Sebikeje R (2000), Presented at the *13th International Conference on HIV/AIDS*, Durban, South Africa, Abstract D2533.
154. Ndawa G et al. (1990), Effectiveness of psychosocial counselling of HIV-infected clients in a referral clinic in Lusaka, Zambia. Presented at the *5th International Conference on AIDS in Africa*, Kinshasa, Abstract TPA 14.
155. Ndawa G et al. (1990), Effectiveness of psychosocial counselling of HIV-infected clients in a referral clinic in Lusaka, Zambia. Presented at the *International Conference on AIDS in Africa*, Kinshasha, Abstract TPA 14.
156. Kaleeba N et al. (1997), Participatory evaluation of counselling, medical and social services of The AIDS Support Organization (TASO) in Uganda. *AIDS Care*, 9:1 13-26.
157. *TASO Uganda, the inside story: participatory evaluation of the HIV/AIDS counselling, medical and social services* 1993-1994 (WHO/GPA/TCO/HCS/95.1).
158. Centres for Disease Control and Prevention (1998), Administration of zidovudine during late pregnancy to prevent perinatal HIV transmission - Thailand 1996-1998. *Morbidity and Mortality Weekly Record* 47:151-153.
159. Guay L et al. (1999), Intrapartum and neonatal single-dose nevirapine compared with zidovudine for prevention of mother-to-child transmission of HIV-1 in Kampala, Uganda: HIVNET 012 randomized trial. *Lancet*, 354:795-802.
160. Coutsoudis A et al. (1999), Influence of infant-feeding patterns on early mother-to-child transmission of HIV-1 in Durban, South Africa: a prospective cohort study. *Lancet*, 354:471-76.
161. Van de Perre P (1999), Breast-feeding transmission of HIV-1 how can it be prevented? *Journal of infectious disease*, 1 79:S405-409.
162. Chopra M, Schaay N, Piwoz (2000), What is the impact of an AZT programme on breast-feeding and infant care counselling and practices amongst health providers and HIV-infected women in Khayelitsha, South Africa. Presented at the *13th International Conference on HIV/AIDS*, Durban, South Africa, Abstract D203.
163. Kibuuka E, Lukandwa J, Matovu J (2000), The role of counselling in an antiretroviral drug trial study at Mulago hospital. Presented at the *13th International Conference on HIV/AIDS*, Durban, South Africa, Abstract D3763.
164. Matovu S, Ekideit H, Chimulwa T (2000), AIDS counselling as a strategy to prevent HIV vertical transmission. Presented at the *13th International Conference on HIV/AIDS*, Durban, South Africa, Abstract C5295.
165. Baggaley R, Sulwe J. (1998), Young people talk about HIV. UNICEF publications.
166. Marx R et al. (1998), HIV counselling and testing referrals given to high-risk negatives increase prevention service use. Presented at the *12th World AIDS Conference*, Geneva, Switzerland, Abstract 33273.
167. Lambouray JL (2000), HIV and Health Care Reform in Phayao, From Crisis to Opportunity. UNAIDS Best Practice publication (in press).
168. UNAIDS/WHO (1999), Technical consultation on notification and confidentiality and HIV/AIDS, Windhoek, Namibia. Meeting statement.
169. UNAIDS/WHO (2000), Reporting, partner notification and disclosure of HIV serostatus and/or AIDS. Public and human rights implications (in press UNAIDS/WHO).

170. De Cock K, Johnson A (1998), From exceptionalism to normalization: a reappraisal of attitudes and practice around HIV testing. *British Medical Journal,* 316 290-3.
171. Godfrey-Faussett P, Baggaley R (1998), Exceptionalism in HIV, challenges for Africa too. *British Medical Journal,* 316:1826-7.
172. Coma G (1999), Waller MK Denial of the HIV/AIDS epidemic in urban Zambia: Rethinking our approach to counselling. Presented at the *XIth International Conference on AIDS and STDs in Africa,* Lusaka, Zambia, Abstract 15ET1-4.
173. Sweat M, Sangiwa G, Balmer D (1998), HIV counselling and testing in Tanzania and Kenya is cost-effective: results for the voluntary counselling and testing study. Presented at the *12th World AIDS Conference,* Geneva, Switzerland, Abstract 33277.
174. Sweat M et al. (2000), Cost-effectiveness of voluntary HIV-1 counselling and testing in reducing sexual transmission of HIV-1 in the United Republic of Tanzania and Kenya. *Lancet* 356:113-21.
175. Gilson L, Mkanje R, Grosskurth H., Cost-effectiveness of improved treatment services for sexually transmitted diseases in preventing HIV-1 infection in Mwansa Region, the United Republic of Tanzania. *Lancet,* 1997, 350:1805-09.
176. Meda N, Gautier-Charpentier L, Soudre R (1999), Serological diagnosis of HIV in Burkina Faso through reliable, practical and less expensive strategies using commercial test kits. *WHO* Bull 77 731-39.
177. Dhiingra-Kumar N (1998), Cost-effective model for developing a blood donor counselling programme *12th World AIDS Conference,* Geneva, Abstract 33271.
178. Holtgrave D et al. (1993), HIV counselling, testing, referral and partner notification services. A cost-benefit analysis *Archives of Internal Medicine,* 1 53:1225-30.
179. Varghese B, Peterman T, Holtgrave D (1999), Cost-effectiveness of counselling and testing and partner notification: a decision analysis. *AIDS,* 14:1745-51.
180. Kamb ML et al. (1998), Cost of preventing HIV via counselling: results from a randomized trial (project RESPECT). Presented at the *XIIth International Conference on HIV/AIDS,* Geneva, Switzerland, Abstract 33263.
181. Marseille E, Kahn J, Mmiro F (1999), Cost-effectiveness of singe dose nevirapine regimen for mothers and babies to decrease vertical HIV-1 transmission in sub-Saharan Africa. *Lancet,* 354:803-809.
182. Mansergh G et al. (1996), Cost-effectiveness of short-course zidovudine to prevent perinatal HIV type 1 infection in a sub-Saharan African developing country setting. *Journal of the American Medical Association,* 276:2 139-145.
183. Mansergh G et al. (1998), Cost-effectiveness of zidovudine to prevent mother to child transmission of HIV infection in sub-Saharan Africa. *Journal of the American Medical Association,* 280:1 30-31.
184. Marseille E, Kahn J, Saba J (1998), Cost-effectiveness of antiretroviral drug therapy to reduce mother to child HIV transmission infection in sub-Saharan Africa. *AIDS,* 12:8 939-948.

185. Wilkinson D, Floyd K, Gilks C (1998) Antiretroviral drugs as a public health intervention for pregnant HIV-infected women in rural South Africa: an issue of cost-effectiveness and capacity. *AIDS*, 12:13 1675-82.
186. Gibb D et al. (1999), Costs and benefits to the mother of antenatal HIV testing: estimates from simulation modelling. *AIDS*, 13:1569-76.
187. Colebunders R, Ndumbe P (1993), Priorities for HIV testing in developing countries. *Lancet*, 342:601-602.
188. Temmerman M et al. (1995), The right not to know HIV-test results. *Lancet*, 345:696-697.
189. Keogh P et al. (1994), The social impact of HIV infection on women in Kigali, Rwanda: a prospective study. *Social Science and Medicine*, 38:8 1047-53.
190. van der Straten A et al. (1995), Couple communication, sexual coercion and HIV risk reduction in Kigali, Rwanda. *AIDS*, 9:8 935-44.
191. Maman S (1999), The intersection of HIV and violence: implications for HIV VCT in Dar Es Salaam, the United Republic of Tanzania. Presented at the *XIth International Conference on AIDS and STDs in Africa*, Lusaka, Zambia, Abstract 14DT2-2.
192. Maman S, Mbwambo J, Hogan M (2000), History of partner violence is common among women attending a voluntary counselling and testing clinic in Dar Es Salaam, the United Republic of Tanzania. Presented at the *13th International Conference on HIV/AIDS*, Durban, South Africa, Abstract C308.
193. Gregorich S et al. (1998), Being tested for HIV does not increase the incidence of negative life events in three developing countries: Results from the voluntary HIV counselling and testing study. Presented at the *XII International Conference on HIV/AIDS*, Geneva, Switzerland (Poster [24328]).
194. Kamenga M et al. (1991), Evidence of marked sexual behaviour change associated with low HIV-1 seroconversion in 149 married couples with discordant HIV-1 serostatus: experience at an HIV counselling centre in Zaire. *AIDS*, 5:61-67.
195. Baggaley R (1994), Compulsory HIV testing in religious orders. *AIDS Analysis Africa*, 5:10-11.
196. Lester P et al. (1995), The consequences of a positive prenatal HIV antibody test for women. *Journal of AIDS and human retrovirology*, 10:3 341-349.
197. Dautzenberg M et al. (1992), Coping behaviour of AIDS patients and caretakers in the United Republic of Tanzania. *International Conference on AIDS*, Amsterdam, the Netherlands, Abstract B224 VIII.
198. Ankrah M (1993) The impact of HIV/AIDS on the family and other significant relationships: the African clan revisited. *AIDS Care*, 5:5-22.
199. Lippman S, James W, Frierson R (1993), AIDS and the family: Implications for counselling. *AIDS Care*, 5:347-357.
200. Keogh P et al. (1994), The social impact of HIV infection on women in Kigali, Rwanda: a prospective study. *Social Science and Medicine*, 38:8 1047-53.
201. Sangiwa G et al. (2000), Client's perspective of the role of voluntary counselling and testing in HIV/AIDS prevention and care in Dar Es Salaam, the United Republic of Tanzania: the Voluntary counselling and testing efficacy study. *AIDS and behaviour*, 4:1 35-48.

202. Coates T, Morin S, McCusick L (1987), Behavioural consequences of AIDS antibody testing among gay men *Journal of the American Medical Association,* 258:1889.

203. Doll L et al. (1990), High-risk sexual behaviour and knowledge of HIV antibody status in the San Francisco city clinic chort. *Health Psychology,* 9:3 253-65.

204. Magura S et al. (1990), Reactions of methadone patients to HIV antibody testing. *Advances in alcohol and substance abuse,* 8:97-111.

205. Cleary P et al. (1993), Depressive symptoms in blood donors notified of HIV infection. *American Journal of Public Health,* 83:4 534-539.

206. Branson B (1998), Experience with home collection kits in the USA. *Journal of the American Medical Association,* 280:19 1699.

207. Cartoux M et al. (1998), Acceptability of voluntary counselling and testing (VCT) and interventions to reduce mother-to-child transmission of HIV. Presented at the *12th World AIDS Conference,* Geneva, Switzerland, Abstract 23310.

208. Tavengwa N, Ali F, Piwoz E (2000), The impact of counselling on infant feeding in the context of HIV on mothers' feeding knowledge, decisions and skills: Preliminary results from the ZVITAMBO Project (Harare, Zimbabwe). Presented at the *13th International Conference on HIV/AIDS,* Durban, South Africa, Abstract D5801.

209. Mazhani L et al. (2000), Report of mid-term review of the prevention on MTCT programme of Botswana (MoH/UNICEF Botswana).

210. Koetsawang S, Stewart R, Hewvuttiphan J (2000), Evaluation of counselling services in context of the perinatal HIV prevention trial in Thailand. Presented at the *13th International Conference on HIV/AIDS,* Durban, South Africa, Abstract D1478.

211. Sixaxhe T (2000), Disclosure of HIV status among antenatal women in the Western Cape [MSc thesis, submitted for publication].

212. Martin-Hetz S, Katzenstein D, Shetty A (2000), Predictors of acceptance of HIV testing and counselling by pregnant women in Zimbabwe. Presented at the *13th International Conference on HIV/AIDS,* Durban, South Africa, Abstract C5313.

213. Chibwesha C et al. (2000), Acceptability of HIV counselling and testing — Lusaka Zambia. Presented at the *13th International Conference on HIV/AIDS,* Durban, South Africa, Abstract C5449.

214. Baggaley R et al. (1997), Knowledge and attitudes to HIV and AIDS and sexual practices among university students in Lusaka, Zambia and London, England: are they so different? *Journal of the Royal Society of Health,* 117:2 88-94.

215. Rosenvard K et al. (1998), Readiness for HIV counselling and testing in a country with extremely high HIV prevalence levels. Presented at *XII International Conference on HIV/AIDS,* Geneva, Switzerland, Abstract 33261.

216. Balmer D et al. (1998), Counselling strategies: They work! Results form the voluntary counselling and testing (VCT) study. Presented at the *12th World AIDS Conference,* Geneva, Switzerland, Abstract 24312.

217. Sehonou J et al. (1999), Nongovernmental organization against AIDS in Africa: the anonymous testing centre of Bangui for voluntary HIV

counselling and testing in the Central African Republic. Presented at the *XIth International Conference on AIDS and STDs in Africa,* Lusaka, Zambia, Abstract 14DT4-2.

218. King R et al. (1993), Van de Perre Voluntary confidential HIV testing for couples in Kigali, Rwanda. *AIDS,* 7:10 1393-4.
219. Bhat G et al. (1998), Same-day HIV voluntary counselling and testing improves overall acceptability among prenatal women in Zambia. Presented at the *XII International Conference on HIV/AIDS,* Geneva, Switzerland, Abstract 33283.
220. Kayawe (2000), Kara counselling and testing service Lusaka, Zambia project report.
221. Ladner J et al. (1996), A cohort study of factors associated with failure to return for post-test counselling in pregnant women: Kigali, Rwanda 1992-1993. *AIDS,* 10:69-75.
222. Msowoya K, Marum E, Barnaba A (2000) Four-fold increase of voluntary HIV counselling and testing in Malawi with same day results counselling and confirmed, rapid finger-prick testing. Presented at the *13th International Conference on HIV/AIDS,* Durban, South Africa, Abstract LbPeA7012.
223. Arthur G, Mutemi R, Odhiambo J (2000), Voluntary counselling and testing: improved access for the poor through integrating same day services into primary health care clinics. Presented at the *13th International Conference on HIV/AIDS,* Durban, South Africa, Abstract C1028.
224. Samayoa B et al. (2000), Using a rapid test in counselling HIV test services in Guatemalan urban clinics. Presented at the *13th International Conference on HIV/AIDS,* Durban, South Africa, Abstract C4303.
225. Sibailly T et al. (2000), Impact of on-site HIV rapid testing with same day post-test counselling on acceptance of short-curse zidovudine for the prevention of mother-to-child transmission of HIV in Abidjan Côte d'lvoire. Presented at the *13th International Conference on HIV/AIDS,* Durban, South Africa, Abstract C549.
226. Nakashima A et al. (1998), Effect of HIV reporting by name on the use of publicly funded counselling and testing programmes. *Journal of the American Medical Association,* 280:16 1421-6.
227. Fehrs L, Fleming D, Foster L (1988), Trial of anonymous versus confidential HIV testing. *Lancet,* 2:379-382.
228. Hoxworth T et al. (1994), Anonymous HIV testing: does it attract clients who would not seek confidential testing? *Journal of AIDS public policy,* 9:182-189.
229. Hirano D et al., Englender S (1994), Hawkes H. Anonymous testing: the impact on demand in Arizona. *American Journal of Public Health,* 84:2 008-2010.
230. Heitz-Picciotto I, Lee L, Hoyo C (1996), HIV test-seeking before and after restriction of anonymous testing in North Carolina. *American Journal of Public Health,* 86:1446-1450.
231. Irwin K, Valdiserri R, Holmberg S (1996), The acceptability of voluntary HIV antibody testing in the United States; a decade of lessons learnt. *AIDS,* 10:1707-1717.

232. CDC (1993), Sexual risk behaviours of STD clinic patients before and after Earvin "Magic" Johnson's HIV-infection announcement. *Morbidity and Mortality Weekly Record,* 41:45-48.
233. Baggaley R et al. (1995), Barriers to HIV counselling and testing (VCT) in Chawama, Lusaka, Zambia. Presented at the *IXth International Conference on AIDS/STDs in Africa,* December.
234. Abraham J, Subrahmanian C (1998), 'Barriers towards the implementation/ utilization of HIV counselling services. Presented at the *12th International Conference on HIV/AIDS,* Geneva, Switzerland, Abstract 24339.
235. Viljoen J et al. (1998), Inadequate pre-and post-test counselling for HIV in two South African hospitals. Presented at the *12th International Conference on HIV/AIDS,* Geneva, Switzerland, Abstract 24340.
236. Denolf D, Nzila N, Tahiri M (2000), HIV testing without counselling and announcing the results. Presented at the *13th International Conference on HIV/AIDS,* Durban, South Africa, Abstract D3770.
237. Ktwe B et al. (1996), Feasibility of documenting the contents of HIV counselling sessions on Myanmar. Presented at the *XI International Conference on AIDS,* Vancouver, Canada, Abstract D5103.
238. Thu M (1997), AIDS central counselling team, Infectious Diseases Hospital, Yangoon, Myanmar Report on the Myanmar counselling feasibility study (unpublished data).
239. Kayawe I et al. (1998), Client's views on HIV counselling and testing - is it helpful? Presented at the *12th World AIDS Conference,* Geneva, Switzerland, Abstract 33265.
240. PSI (1999), New start VCT project background document.
241. Sangiwa G et al. (2000), Client's perspective of the role of voluntary counselling and testing in HIV/AIDS prevention and care in Dar Es Salaam, the United Republic of Tanzania: The Voluntary counselling and testing efficacy study. *AIDS and behaviour,* 4:1 35-48.
242. Csepe P, Simka J, Forrai (1998), Evaluation of anonymous HIV screening and counselling centre in Budapest, Hungary. Presented at the *12th International Conference on HIV/AIDS,* Geneva, Switzerland, Abstract 42150.
243. Doumatey L, Traore R, Adoko Y (2000), HIV counselling and testing: The experience of Abidjan Côte d'Ivoire. Presented at the *13th International Conference on HIV/AIDS,* Durban, South Africa, Abstract D3764.
244. Rachier C, Arthur G, Doyle V (2000), HIV/AIDS prevention and care (HAPAC) project: counselling services: how can they be quality assure? Presented at the *13th International Conference on HIV/AIDS,* Durban, South Africa, Abstract D3751.
245. Mugula F et al. (1995), A community-based counselling service as a potential outlet for condom distribution. Presented at the *9th International Conference on AIDS and STD in Africa,* Kampala, (paper WeD 834).
246. Kalichman S et al. (1998), Motivational enhancing and skills building risk reduction counselling interventions for women. Presented at the *12th World AIDS Conference,* Geneva, Abstract 33272.
247. Shain et. al. (1999), *New England Journal of Medicine,* 340:93-100.
248. Carey M et al. (1998), Reduced HIV risk among low-income women using motivational enhancement and behavioural skills training. Presented at

the *12th World AIDS Conference,* Geneva, Abstract 33274.

249. Kamb M et al. (1997), Efficacy of risk reduction counselling to prevent human immunodeficiency virus and sexually transmitted diseases: a randomized, controlled trial, *Journal of the American Medical Association,* 277:254-258.
250. The National Institute of Mental Health (NIMH) Multisite HIV prevention trial group (1998) The NIMA multisite HIV prevention trial: reducing HIV sexual risk behaviour. *Science,* 280:1889-1894.
251. Imrie J, Stephenson J, Cowan F (1999), A randomized controlled trial of brief small-group behavioural intervention workshop for 'high risk' gay men using an STD clinic presented at *the 13th meeting of the International Society for Sexually Transmitted Disease Research,* Denver, Colorado, USA.
252. Mertens T, Smith G, Van Praag E (1994), Home testing for HIV. *Lancet,* 343:1 293.
253. Branson B (1998), Experience with home collection kits in the USA. *Journal of the American Medical Association,* 280:19 1 699.
254. Mwaura J, Odhaiambo D, Maina N (1998), Pre- and post-test counselling in patients admitted to the Kenyatta National Hospital between May 1996 and July 1997. Presented at the *12th International Conference on HIV/AIDS,* Geneva, Switzerland, Abstract 42455.
255. Nikitina M (1998), Training of health workers in pre- and post-test counselling for HIV tests. Presented at the *12th International Conference on HIV/AIDS,* Geneva, Switzerland, Abstract 33319.
256. Kelly J et al. (1992), Community AIDS/HIV risk reduction: the effects of endorsements by popular people in three cities. *American Journal of Public Health,* 82:11 1483-11489.
257. Doumatey L et al. (1998), The impact of AIDS counselling in Africa: The experience of Abidjan Côte d'lvoire. Presented at the *12th World AIDS Conference,* Geneva, Abstract 24346.
258. Kamenga M et al. (1991), Evidence of marked sexual behaviour change associated with low HIV-1 seroconversion in 149 married couples with discordant HIV-1 serostatus: experience at an HIV counselling centre in Zaire. *AIDS,* 5:61-67.
259. Ryder R, Batter V, Nsuami M (1991), Fertility rates in 238 HIV-1 seropositive women in Zaire followed for 3 years post-partum. *AIDS,* 5:1521-27.
260. Laga M et al. (1994), Condom promotion, sexually transmitted disease treatment and declining incidence of HIV-1 infection in female Zairian sex workers. *Lancet,* 344:8917 246-8.
261. Sahlu T et al. (1999), Sexual behaviours, perception of risk of HIV infection, and factors associated with attending HIV post-test counselling in Ethiopia. *AIDS,* 13:10 1263-1272.
262. Temmerman M et al. (1990), Impact of single session post-partum counselling of HIV-infected women on their subsequent reproductive behaviour. *AIDS Care,* 247-252.
263. UNAIDS (1999), Knowledge is power: voluntary HIV counselling and testing in Uganda. UNAIDS case study. (Best Practice collection UNAIDS/ 99.8E).

264. Magombe J et al. (1998), Extension of HIV counselling and testing in rural sites: the Ugandan experience. Presented at the *12th International Conference on HIV/AIDS*, Geneva, Switzerland, Abstract 13427.
265. Muller O et al. (1992), HIV prevalence, attitudes and behaviour in clients of a confidential HIV testing and counselling centre of Uganda. *AIDS*, 6:869-874.
266. Moore M et al. (1993), Impact of HIV counselling and testing in Uganda. Presented at the *9th International Conference on AIDS*, Berlin, Germany, Abstract WS-C16-4.
267. Kaleeba N et al. (1997), Participatory evaluation of counselling, medical and social services of The AIDS Support Organization (TASO) in Uganda. *AIDS Care*, 9:1 13-26.
268. TASO Uganda, the inside story: participatory evaluation of the HIV/AIDS counselling, medical and social services (1993-1994) (WHO/GPA/TCO/HCS/95.1).
269. Konde-Lule J, Sebina A (1993), The impact of HIV in a rural Ugandan community. *East African Medical Journal*, 70:725-729.
270. Mukasa-Monico S, Bunnell R, Onyango H (2000), Impact of routine counselling on sexual behaviour of persons with HIV in Uganda. Presented at the *13th International Conference on HIV/AIDS*, Durban, South Africa, Abstract D4526.
271. Kamya M (1998), HIV/AIDS counselling in Butego community of Masaka district from 1993-1998. Presented at the *12th International Conference on HIV/AIDS*, Geneva, Switzerland Abstract 13419.
272. Lutalo T, Kidugavu M, Mawwer M (2000), Contraceptive use and HIV testing and counselling in rural Rakai district, SW Uganda. Presented at the *13th International Conference on HIV/AIDS*, Durban, South Africa, Abstract C246.
273. Nyblade L, Menken J, Wawe M (2000), HIV risk-behaviour change subsequent to participation in voluntary counselling and testing. Presented at the *13th International Conference on HIV/AIDS*, Durban, South Africa, Abstract D4731.
274. Jordan I-B, Haworth A (1995), The contribution of counselling in hospital and home-based care in a small town and surrounding rural area in Zambia. *Tropical Doctor*, 25:21-24.
275. Kelly M, Baggaley R (1994), Voluntary HIV counselling in Lusaka, Zambia. Who comes, why and does it help? Presented at the *Xth International Conference on AIDS*, Yokohama, Japan, Abstract 519B/D.
276. Baggaley R et al. (1998), HIV counselling and testing in Zambia: The Kara counselling experience (SAFAIDS 6(2) 1-9).
277. Baggaley R et al. (1998), Kara coping study - interim report (UNAIDS/WHO).
278. Chanda C, Baggaley R (1994), Does counselling help to empower women to negotiate for safer sex? Presented at the *Xth International Conference on AIDS*, Yokohama, Japan, Abstract 063D.
279. PSI (1999), New start VCT project background document.
280. Moses P, Sangiwa G, Ncube B (2000), New hope with "New Start": social

marketing of voluntary counselling and testing for HIV prevention. Presented at the *13th International Conference on HIV/AIDS*, Durban, South Africa, Abstract D3789.

281. Sangiwa G, Moses P, Ncube B (2000), "New Start" voluntary counselling and testing for HIV prevention in Zimbabwe: Effectiveness in reaching target populations. Presented at the *13th International Conference on HIV/AIDS*, Durban, South Africa, Abstract D3789.
282. Coates T, et al. (1998), Serodiscordant married couples undergoing couple counselling and testing reduce risk behaviour with each other but not with extra-marital partners. Presented at the *12th World AIDS Conference*, Geneva, Abstract 33268.
283. Coates T, et al. (1998), HIV risk reduction in individuals receiving voluntary HIV-+ counselling and testing in three developing countries and HIV risk reduction in couples receiving HIV counselling and testing in three developing countries (submitted for publication).
284. Sangiwa G et al. (1998), Voluntary HIV counselling and testing (VCT) reduces risk behaviour in developing countries: results from the multi-site voluntary counselling and testing efficacy study. Presented at the *12th International Conference on HIV/AIDS*, Geneva, Switzerland, Abstract 33269.
285. Sangiwa G et al. (2000), Client's perspective of the role of voluntary counselling and testing in HIV/AIDS prevention and care in Dar Es Salaam, the United Republic of Tanzania: The Voluntary counselling and testing efficacy study. *AIDS and behaviour*, 4:1 35-48.
286. Kamenga et al. (2000), The voluntary HIV-1 counselling and testing efficacy study: Design and Methods. *AIDS and behaviour*, 4:1 5- 15.
287. Balmer D et al. (2000), Characteristics of individuals and couples seeking HIV-1 prevention services in Nairobi, Kenya: the voluntary HIV-1 counselling and testing efficacy study. *AIDS and behaviour*, 4:1 15-23.
288. Furlong C et al. (2000), HIV risk factors in a population-based probability sample of North and Central Trinidad: The voluntary HIV-1 counselling and testing efficacy study. *AIDS and behaviour*, 4:1 49-62.
289. The VCT efficacy study group (2000), Efficacy of voluntary HIV-1 counselling and testing in individuals and couples in Kenya, the United Republic of Tanzania and Trinidad: a randomized trial. *Lancet*, 356:103-12.
290. Bhandari K, Gilada I (1998), Success of comprehensive HIV counselling and testing and care clinics in India. Presented at the *12th International Conference on HIV/AIDS*, Geneva, Switzerland, Abstract 12422.
291. Kalyanasundaram B (1998), Establishing counselling interventions within government STD clinics in Bangalore - an NGO's experience in the Indian context. Presented at the *12th International Conference on HIV/AIDS*, Geneva, Switzerland, Abstract 33260.
292. Bentley M et al. (1998), HIV testing and counselling among men attending STD clinic in Pune, India: changes in condom use and sexual behaviour over time. *AIDS*, 12:1 869-1 877.
293. Guntamala L, Chaiyawan G, Yachompoo C (1998), Anonymous counselling and testing clinics for HIV/AIDS in Thailand. Presented at the *12th International Conference on HIV/AIDS*, Geneva, Switzerland, Abstract 33290.

294. Phanuphak P et al. (1994), Knowledge attitudes and behaviour among HIV- positive and HIV-negative clients of a confidential HIV counselling and testing centre in Thailand. *AIDS,* 8:1315-1319.
295. Muller O et al. (1995), Sexual risk behaviour reduction associated with voluntary counselling and testing in HIV infected patients in Thailand. *AIDS Care,* 7:567-572.
296. Kywe B et al. (1996), Feasibility of documenting the contents of HIV counselling sessions on Myanmar. Presented at the *XI International Conference on AIDS,* Vancouver, Canada, Abstract D5103.
297. Thu M (1997), AIDS central counselling team, Infectious Diseases Hospital, Yangoon, Myanmar Report on the Myanmar counselling feasibility study (unpublished data).
298. Caceres C, Hearst N (1996), HIV/AIDS in Latin America and the Caribbean: an update. *AIDS* (suppl A) S34-S40.
299. UNAIDS (1999), AIDS epidemic update (UNAIDS/99.53E WHO/CDS/EDU/99.9 WHO/FCH/HIS/99.6).
300. Gonzalez M, Ministero de Salud, Fergadiott A (1997), Centre de deteccion y consejeria CONSIDA, Toro X., FRENASIDA, Santiago, Chile (unpublished document).
301. Passarelli C, Munhoz R, Mirim I (2000), Counselling and testing centres in Brazil: from care to prevention. Presented at the *13th International Conference on HIV/AIDS,* Durban, South Africa, Abstract D4479.
302. Filgueiras S, Munhoz R, Passarelli C (2000), Counselling on STDs and AIDS services: an evaluation. Presented at the *13th International Conference on HIV/AIDS,* Durban, South Africa, Abstract D1479.
303. Wenger N et al. (1992) Effect of HIV antibody testing and AIDS education on communication about HIV risk and sexual behaviour. A randomised, controlled trial in college students. *Annals of Internal Medicine,* 117:11 905-11.
304. Wenger N et al. (1991), Reduction of high-risk behaviour among heterosexuals undergoing HIV antibody testing: A randomized clinical trial. *American Journal of Public Health,* 81:1580-1585.
305. Wilson T et al. (1996), Testing for HIV and other sexually transmitted diseases: implications for risk behaviour in women. *Health Psychology,* 15:4252-60.
306. Icovics J et al. (1994), Limited effects of HIV counselling and testing on women. *Journal of the American Medical Association,* 272:443-448.
307. Lansis S, Earp J, Koch G (1992), Impact of HIV testing and counselling on subsequent sexual behaviour. *AIDS education and prevention,* 4:161-70.
308. Coates T, Morin S, McCusick L (1987), Behavioural consequences of AIDS antibody testing among gay men. *Journal of the American Medical Association,* 258.
309. van Griensven G et al. (1989), Effect of HIV antibody knowledge on high-risk sexual behaviour with steady and non-steady sexual partners among homosexual men. *American Journal of Epidemiology,* 129:3596-603.
310. Schechter M et al. (1989), Patterns of sexual behaviour and condom use in a cohort of homosexual men. *American Journal of Public Health,* 78:12 1535-1538.

311. Ostrow D, Joseph J, Kessler R (1989), Disclosure of HIV antibody status: behavioural and mental health correlates. *AIDS education and prevention*, 1:1-11.
312. Doll L et al. (1990), High-risk sexual behaviour and knowledge of HIV antibody status in the San Francisco city clinic Cohort. *Health Psychology*, 9:3253-65.
313. Zapa J et al. (1991), HIV antibody test result knowledge, risk, perceptions and behaviour among homosexually active men. *Patient Education and Counselling*, 18:9-17.
314. Huggins J et al. (1991), Affective behavioural responses of gay and bisexual men to HIV antibody testing. *Social Work*, 36:1 61-6.
315. Dawson J et al. (1991), The HIV test and sexual behaviour in a sample of homosexually active men. *Social Science and Medicine*, 32:683-688.
316. Roffman R et al. (1995), HIV antibody testing of gay men in smaller US cities. *AIDS Care*, 7:405-413.
317. Fox R et al. (1987), Effect of HIV antibody disclosure on subsequent sexual activity in homosexual men. *AIDS*, 1:4 241-6.
318. McCusker J et al. (1988), Effects of HIV antibody testing on knowledge on subsequent behaviours in a cohort of homosexually active men. *American Journal of Public Health*, 78:462-467.
319. Cohn D et al. (1998), Changes in HIV risk behaviour in a longitudinal cohort of homosexual and bisexual men. Presented at the *4th International Conference on HIV/AIDS*, Stockholm, Sweden.
320. Zones J, Beeson D, Echenberg D (1986), Personal and social consequences of AIDS antibody testing and notification in a cohort of homosexual and bisexual men. Presented at the *2nd International Conference on HIV/AIDS*, Paris, France.
321. McKusick L et al. (1990), Longitudinal predictors of reductions in unprotected anal intercourse among gay men in San Francisco: the AIDS behavioural research project. *American Journal of Public Health*, 80:978-983.
322. Valdiserri R, Lyter D, Leviton L (1988), Variables influencing condom use in a cohort of homosexual and bisexual men. *American Journal of Public Health*, 78:801-805.
323. Frazer I et al. (1988), Influence of HIV antibody testing on sexual behaviour in a high risk population from a low-risk city. *Medical Journal of Australia*, 149:365-368.
324. Ross M (1988), Relationship of combinations of AIDS counselling and testing and safer sex and condom use in homosexual men. *Community Health Studies*, 12:322-327.
325. Abid S et al. (1991), Relapse in sexual behaviour among homosexual men: a 2-year follow-up from Chicago MACS/CCS. *AIDS*, 5:757-760.
326. Nicolosi A et al. (1991), Positive modification of injecting behaviour among intravenous heroin users form Milan and Northern Italy 1987-89. *British Journal of Addiction*, 86:91-102.
327. Magura S, Shapiro J, Grossman J (1990), Reactions of methadone patients to HIV antibody testing. *Advances in alcohol and substance abuse*, 8:97-111.
328. Magura S, Siddiqi Q, Shapiro J (1991), Outcomes of AIDS prevention programme for methadone patients. *International Journal of Addiction*, 26:629-655.

329. Desenclos J, Papaevangelou G, Ancelle-Park R (1993), Knowledge of HIV serostatus and preventive behaviour among European injecting drug users. *AIDS,* 7:1371-1377.
330. Walters J et al. (1994), Syringe and needle exchange as HIV / AIDS prevention for injecting drug users. *Journal of the American Medical Association,* 271:115-120.
331. Drucker E et al. (1998), Measuring harm reduction: the effects of needle and syringe exchange programmes and methadone maintenance on the impact of HIV. *AIDS,* 12 A: S217-30.
332. Des Jarlais D, Perlis T, Friedman S. (2000), The roles of syringe exchange and HIV counselling and testing in the declining HIV epidemic among IDUs in New York City. Presented at the *13th International Conference on HIV/AIDS,* Durban, South Africa, Abstract D1124.
333. Casadonte P et al. (1990), Psychological and behavioural impact among intravenous drug users of learning HIV test results. *International Journal of Addiction,* 25:409-426.
334. Calsyn D et al. (1992), Ineffectiveness of AIDS education and HIV antibody testing in reducing high-risk behaviours among injecting drug users. *American Journal of Public Health,* 82:573-575.
335. Conlon H et al. (1996), Behavioural effect of receiving HIV test results among injecting drug users in Puerto Rico. *AIDS,* 10: 1163-1168.
336. McCusker J et al. (1996), Community wide HIV counselling and testing in central Massachusetts: who is retested and does their behaviour change? *Journal of Community Health,* 21:11-23.
337. Sabin K et al. (2000), Self-reported injection-related behavioural change among drug users after HIV counselling and testing in drug treatment centres 1994-1996. Presented at the *13th International Conference on HIV/AIDS,* Durban, South Africa, Abstract D5809.
338. Kawichai S et al. (2000), Impact of prior HIV counselling and testing on behaviour change among drug users in northern Thailand. Presented at the *13th International Conference on HIV/AIDS,* Durban, South Africa, Abstract C5383.
339. MacGowan R et al. (1996), Retention in methadone treatment programmes, Connecticut and Massachusetts 1990-1993. *Journal of Psychoactive Drugs,* 28:259-265.
340. Vanichseni S et al. (1992), HIV testing and sexual behaviour among intravenous drug users, Bangkok, Thailand. *Journal of AIDS,* 51119-1123.
341. Vanichseni S et al. (1993), Condom use with primary partners among injecting drug users in Bangkok, Thailand and New York City, USA. *AIDS,* 7:887-891.
342. Friedman S, Jose B, Neaigus A (1994), Consistent condom use in relationships between seropositive injecting drug users and sexual partners who do not use drugs. *AIDS,* 8:375-361.

Three

HIV Preventive Vaccine Research: Ethical Considerations

Introduction

This being the third decade of the AIDS epidemic, there still remains no effective HIV preventive vaccine. As the numbers of those infected by HIV and dying from AIDS are increasing alarmingly, the need for such a vaccine becomes ever more urgent. Various HIV candidate vaccines are at several stages of development. However, the successful development of effective HIV preventive vaccines is likely to necessitate that many different candidate vaccines be studied simultaneously in different populations globally. Subsequently it will require a large international cooperative effort drawing on partners from different health sectors, intergovernmental organizations, government, research institutions, industry, and affected populations. It will also necessitate that these partners be able and willing to address the difficult ethical concerns that came at fore during the development of HIV vaccines. In an effort to elucidate these ethical concerns, and to generate forums where they could be discussed in depth by those presently involved in, or considering, HIV vaccine develoment programmes, the UNAIDS Secretariat convened meetings in Geneva (twice), Brazil, Thailand, Uganda and Washington during 1997-1999. These meetings included lawyers, activists, social scientists, ethicists, vaccine scientists, epidemiologists, representatives of NGOs, people living with HIV/AIDS, and health care professionals. In the regional meetings, efforts were made to include people from a number of countries from that particular region. The entire process involved people from a total of 33 countries.[1] The objectives were to:

(a) identify and discuss ethical elements specific to development of HIV preventive vaccines;

(b) reach consensus when possible, and elucidate different positions, when not; and

(c) progress in ability to address these technicalities during pending or proposed HIV vaccine research.

In the present chapter, the important objective is to seek to offer guidance emanating from this process. This discussion does not purport to capture the extensive discussion, debate, consensus, and disagreement which arose at these meetings. Rather it reflects, from researcher's perspective, some of the critical elements that must be considered in HIV vaccine development programmes. Where these are considerably addressed, by other existing texts, there is no attempt to duplicate or replace these texts, which should be consulted extensively throughout HIV vaccine development programmes. Such texts include:

(a) the Nuremberg Code (1947);

(b) the Declaration of Helsinki, first adopted by the World Medical Association in 1964 and subsequently amended in 1975, 1983, 1989 and 1996;

(c) the Belmont Report - Ethical Principles and Guidelines for the Protection of Human Subjects of Research, issued in 1979 by the US National Commission for the Protection of Human Subjects of Biomedical and Behavioural Research;

(d) the International Ethical Guidelines for Biomedical Research Involving Human Subjects, issued by the Council for International Organizations of Medical Sciences (CIOMS) in 1993 (and developed in close cooperation with WHO);

(e) the World Health Organization's Good Clinical Practice (WHO GCP) Guideline (1995); and

(f) the International Conference on Harmonisation's Good Clinical Practice (ICH GCP) Guideline (1996).

It is hoped that this discussion will be of immense use to potential research participants, investigators, community members, government representatives, pharmaceutical companies, and ethical and scientific review committees participating in HIV preventive vaccine development. It suggests standards, as well as processes for arriving at standards, and can be used as a frame of reference from which to conduct further discussion at the international, national, and local levels.

Context

The HIV/AIDS pandemic is characterised by unique biological, social and geographical factors that, among others, affect the equilibrium of risks and advantages for individuals and communities who participate in HIV vaccine development programmes. These factors may necessitate that additional efforts are made to address the needs of participating individuals and communities, including their urgent need for a HIV vaccine, their need to have their rights protected and their welfare promoted in the context of HIV vaccine development programmes, and their need to be able to be full and equal participants. These factors include the following:

(a) The worldwide burden of disease and death associated with HIV is increasing at an alarming rate unmatched by any other pathogen. For many countries, it is already the leading cause of death. At present, available treatments are not ample because they do not lead to cure, but at best decelerate the progression of disease. The most effective treatment for decelerating HIV-related disease progression, antiretroviral medication, is complicated to administer, necessitates close medical monitoring, beyond reach of affected populations in monetary terms, and can cause significant adverse impacts. Due to this, antiretroviral medication is not readily available to the vast majority of people affected by HIV/AIDS. These are people living in developing countries and in marginalised communities in industrialised countries. There is, therefore, an ethical imperative to seek, as urgently as possible, a worldwide effective and accessible vaccine, to complement other prevention strategies. Moreover, this ethical imperative demands that HIV preventive vaccines be developed to address the situation of those people and populations most vulnerable to infection.

(b) Genetically distinct subtypes of HIV have been described, and different HIV subtypes are predominant in different regions and countries. Yet the relevance of these subtypes to potential vaccine-induced protection is not clearly understood. Thus, it is not known whether a vaccine targeted at one subtype will safeguard against infection from another subtype; and it is probable that a vaccine directed at a particular subtype will need to be tested in a population in which that subtype is prevalent. Therefore, developing a vaccine that is effective in the populations with the greatest incidence of HIV is likely to necessitate experimental vaccines be tested in those populations, even though these populations may for innumerable reasons be comparatively vulnerable to exploitation and harm in the context of HIV vaccine development. More and more efforts may need to be made to overcome this vulnerability.

(c) A few candidate vaccines may be conceived and manufactured in laboratories of one country (sponsor country or countries), generally in the industrialised world, and tested in human populations in another country (host country or countries), particularly in the developing world. (The term 'sponsor' has generally referred to the individual or institution who either owns the candidate necessary to conduct the vaccine development programme. Traditionally, the sponsor has been considered as a single corporate entity, such as a pharmaceutical company. In modern vaccine development programmes there are commonly multiple sponsors consisting of one or more corporations, one or more national governments and one or more international agencies.) The potential inequilibrium of such a situation demands particular attention to factors that will address the differing perspectives, interests and capabilities of sponsors and hosts with the objective of encouraging the urgent development of effective vaccines, in ethically acceptable manners, and their early distribution to populations most in need. Therefore, potential host countries and communities should be encouraged and given the capacity to make decisions for themselves pertaining to their participation in HIV vaccine development, based on their own health and human development priorities, in a context of at par collaboration with sponsors.

(d) HIV/AIDS is a condition that is both highly feared and

stigmatized. This is in large part because it is related to blood, death, sex, and activities which are generally not legally sanctioned, such as commercial sex, men having sex with men, and substance abuse. These are the problems which are difficult to address openly—at a societal and individual level. As a result, people affected by HIV/AIDS can experience stigma, discrimination, and even violence; and governments and communities continue to deny the existence and prevalence of HIV/AIDS. Moreover, vulnerability to HIV infection and to the impact of AIDS is greater where people are marginalized because of their social, economic and legal status. These factors increase the risk of social and psychological harm for people participating in HIV vaccine research. More and more efforts must be made to address these increased risks, and to ensure that the risks participants take are justified by the benefits they receive by their participation in the research. A key means by which to protect participants and the communities from which they come is to ensure that the community in which the research is conducted is meaningfully involved in the tailoring, implementation, and distribution of results of vaccine research, including the involvement of representatives from marginalized communities from which participants are drawn, where possible and appropriate.

Suggested Guidance

HIV vaccines development: Given the gravity of the HIV/AIDS pandemic in human, public health, social, and economic terms, sufficient capacity and incentives should be developed to foster the early and ethical development of effective vaccines, both from the viewpoint of countries where HIV vaccine trials may be held, and from the viewpoint of sponsors of HIV vaccine trials. Donor countries and relevant international organisations should join with these stakeholders to promote such vaccine development.

Given the global nature of the epedemic, the devastation being wreaked in some countries by it, the fact that vaccine(s) may be the best long-term solution by which to control the epidemic, especially in developing world, and the potentially universal advantages of effective HIV vaccines, there is an ethical imperative for worldwide support to the effort to develop these vaccines. This effort will necessitate intense international collaboration and coordination over time, including among countries with scientific expertise and resources, and among countries where candidate vaccines could be tested but whose infrastructure, resource base, and scientific and ethical capabilities could be insufficient at present. Though HIV vaccines should benefit all those in need, it is imperative that they benefit the vulnerable populations the most. Thus, HIV vaccine development should ensure that the vaccines are appropriate for use among such populations, among which it will be necessary to conduct trials; and, when developed, they should be made available and affordable to such populations. As HIV vaccine development programmes take time, are complex, and require infrastructure, resources and international collaboration:

(a) potential sponsor countries and host countries should immediately include HIV vaccine development in their regional and national AIDS prevention and control schedules;

(b) potential host countries should examine how they can and should participate in HIV vaccine development programmes either nationally or on a regional basis, including identifying resources, establishing partnerships, conducting national information campaigns, strengthening their scientific and ethical sectors, and including a vaccine research component to complement other prevention interventions;

(c) potential donors and international agencies should make early and sustained commitments to allocate ample funds to make a vaccine a reality, including funds to strengthen ethical and scientific capacity in countries where multiple trials will have to be conducted and to purchase and distribute future vaccines; and

(d) potential sponsors should set up partnerships with potential host countries, and begin discussions regarding community consultations, strengthening necessary scientific and ethical components, and eventual plans for equitable distribution of the advantages of research.

Vaccine Availability: Any HIV preventive vaccine displayed to be safe and effective, as well as other knowledge and advantages resulting from HIV vaccine research, should be made available as soon as possible to all participants in the trials in which it was tested, as well as to other vulnerable populations. Plans should be developed at the initial stages of HIV vaccine development to ensure such availability.

Although making a safe and effective vaccine reasonably available to the population where it was tested is a primary ethical requirement, it is feared that it could be a disincentive for industry to conduct studies in countries with large populations, or that it could account for an undue inducement for a resource poor country or community to 'cooperate.' Due to the gravity of the epidemic, it is imperative that sufficient incentives exist, both through monetary rewards in the marketplace and through public subsidies, to foster development of effective vaccines while also ensuring that vaccines are produced and distributed in a manner that really makes them available to the vulnerable populations.

As health and research communities plan HIV preventive vaccine research programmes, ample consideration should be given immediately to how a successful vaccine, and other benefits c resulting from the research, will be made readily and affordably available to the communities and countries where such a vaccine is tested, as well as to other communities and countries at high risk for HIV infection. This process of discussion and negotiation should commence as soon as possible and should be carried on through the course of the research.

At a minimum, the directly concerned parties should commence this discussion before the trials begins. This discussion should include representatives from relevant stakeholders in the host country, such as representatives from the executive branch, health ministry, local health authorities, and relevant scientific and ethical groups. It should also include representatives from the communities from which participants are drawn, people living with HIV/AIDS, and NGOs representing affected communities. The discussions should include subsidies, technology, royalities, decisions regarding payments, and intellectual property, as well as distribution costs, channels and modalities, including vaccination strategies, target populations and number of doses.

Moreover, the discussion concerning availability and distribution of an effective-HIV vaccine should engage international organizations, donor governments and bilateral agencies, representatives from widely affected communities, international and regional NGOs and the private sector. These should not only consider monetary assistance regarding making vaccines available, but should also assist to build the capacity of host governments and communities to negotiate for and implement distribution plans.

Capacity Building: Strategies should be implemented to build capacity in host countries and communities enabling them to practise meaningful self-determination in vaccine development, to ensure the scientific and ethical conduct of vaccine development, and to function as equal partners with sponsors and others in a collaborative process.

Potential host countries and communities have the right, and the responsibility, to take decisions regarding the nature of their involvement in HIV vaccine research. Yet disparities in economic wealth, scientific experience, and technical capacity among countries and communities can lead to undue influence over and possible exploitation of host countries and communities. The development of an HIV vaccine will necessitate international cooperative research, which should transcend, in an ethical manner, such disparities. Real or perceived disparities should be resolved in a way that ensures equality in decision-making and action. The desired relationship is one of collaboration among equals. Factors that may increase vulnerability to exploitation of host countries and communities may include, but are not limited to the following:

(a) level of the proposed community's economic capacity, such as is projected in the Human Development Index of the UNDP;
(b) community/cultural experience with, and/or understanding of, scientific research;
(c) local political awareness of the significance and process of vaccine research;

(d) local infrastructure, personnel, and technical capacity for providing HIV health care and treatment choices;
(e) ability of individuals in the community to provide informed consent, including the effect of class, gender, and other social factors on the potential for freely given consent;
(f) level of experience and capacity for carrying out ethical and scientific review; and
(g) local infrastructure, personnel, and technical capacity for carrying out the proposed research.

Strategies to overcome these disparities could consist:

(a) scientific exchange, and knowledge and skills transfer between sponsor countries and institutions, and host countries and communities;
(b) capacity-building activities in the science and ethics of vaccine development by relevant scientific institutions and international organizations;
(c) support to development of national and local ethical review capacity (to be discussed later in this chapter);
(d) support to affected communities and communities from which participants are drawn regarding information, education, and capacity and consensus-building on vaccine development; and
(e) early participation of affected communities in the design and implementation of vaccine development plans and protocols (to be discussed later in the present chapter).

Research Protocols and Study Populations: In order to conduct HIV vaccine research in an ethically acceptable manner, the research protocol should be scientifically appropriate, and the desired outcome of the proposed research should potentially benefit the population from which research participants are drawn.

In order to be ethical, clinical tests of vaccines should be based on scientifically valid research protocols, and the scientific questions posed should be rigorously formulated in a research protocol that is worthy of providing reliable responses. Valid scientific questions relevant to HIV vaccine development are those that seek:

(a) to obtain scientific information on the safety,

immunogenicity (ability to induce immune responses against HIV) and efficacy (degree of protection) of candidate vaccines;

(b) to find out immunological correlates or surrogates in order to discover the protective techniques and how they can be elicited;

(c) to compare different candidate vaccines; and

(d) to test whether vaccines effective in one population are effective in other populations.

Moreover, the selection of the research population should be based on the fact that its characteristics are relevant to the scientific issues raised; and the outcomes of the research will potentially benefit the selected population. In this context, the research protocol should:

* justify the selection of the research population from a scientific viewpoint;
* outline how the risks undertaken by the participants of that population are brought into equilibrium by the potential benefits to that population;
* address particular necessities of the proposed research population;
* display how the candidate vaccine being tested is expected to be advantageous to the population in which testing occurs; and
* set up safeguards for the protection of research participants from potential harm arising from the research.

These general principles will be further elaborated below.

Community Participation: To ensure the ethical and scientific quality of proposed research, its relevance to the affected community, and its acceptance by the affected community, community representatives should participate in an early and sustained manner in the design, development, implementation, and distribution of outcome of HIV vaccine research.

Participation of community representatives should not be witnessed as a single encounter, nor as unidirectional. The orientation of community participation should be one of partnership — towards mutual education and consensus-building pertaining to all aspects of the vaccine development programme.

There should be set up a continuing forum for communication and problem-solving on all dimensions of the vaccine development programme from first phase through third phase and beyond, to the distribution of a safe, effective, licensed vaccine. All participating parties should define the nature of this ongoing relationship. It should consist appropriate representation of the community on committees charged with the review, approval, and monitoring of the HIV vaccine research. Like investigators and sponsors, communities should assume appropriate responsibility for assuring the successful completion of the trial and of the programme.

Appropriate community representatives should be determined through a process of wider consultation. Members of the community who may contribute to a vaccine development process include representatives of the research population qualifying to serve as research participants, other members of the community who would be among the intended beneficiaries of the developed vaccine, relevant nongovernmental organizations, persons living with HIV/AIDS, community leaders, public health professionals, and those who provide health care and other services to people living with and affected by HIV. Participation of the community in the planning and implementation of a vaccine development strategy can offer the below-mentioned advantages:

(a) information regarding the health beliefs and understanding of the study population;
(b) input into the design of the protocol;
(c) input into an appropriate informed consent process;
(d) insight into the design of risk reduction interventions;
(e) effective methods for disseminating information about the trial and its results;
(f) information to the community-at-large on the proposed research;
(g) trust between the community and researchers;
(h) equity in choice of participants;
(i) equity in decisions regarding level of standard of care and treatment and its time period; and
(j) equity in plans for applying results and vaccine distribution.

Scientific and Ethical Evaluation: HIV preventive vaccine trials should only be conducted in countries and communities that have the capacity to conduct appropriate independent and competent scientific and ethical review.

Proposed HIV vaccine research protocols should be examined by scientific and ethical review committees that are situated in, and include membership from, the country and community where the research is proposed to be conducted. This process ensures that the proposed research is analysed from the scientific and ethical viewpoints by individuals who are familiar with the conditions prevailing in the potential research population. At present, some countries do not have the capacity to conduct independent, competent and meaningful scientific and ethical review. If the country's capacity for scientific and ethical review is inadequate, the sponsor should be responsible for ensuring that adequate structures are developed in the host country for scientific and ethical review prior to the commencement of the research. Care should be taken to minimize the potential for conflicts of interest, while providing assistance in capacity-building for scientific and ethical review. Capacity-building for scientific and ethical review may also be promoted in collaboration with international agencies, organizations within the host country, and other associated parties.

Vulnerable Populations: Where relevant, the research protocol should narrate the social dimensions of a proposed research population (country or community) that generate conditions for possible exploitation or increased vulnerability among potential research participants, as well as the steps that will be taken to overcome these and protect the dignity, safety, and welfare of the participants.

Some countries or communities, generally labelled as 'developing', have been perceived as inappropriate participants for a few phases of clinical research, due to a real or perceived increased level of vulnerability to exploitation or harm. The usefulness of the 'developing/developed' terminology for evaluating risk of harm and exploitation, however, is limited. It refers primarily to economic considerations, which are not the only relevant issues in HIV vaccine research. It also establishes two fixed categories, whereas in reality, countries and communities are distributed along a spectrum, characterized by innumerable different factors that affect risk. It is more useful to discover the *particular* dimensions of a social context that create conditions for exploitation or increased vulnerability for the pool of participants that has been selected. These aspects should be stated in the protocol, as should the measures that will be taken to overcome them. In some potential research populations (countries or communities), conditions affecting potential vulnerability or exploitation may be so severe that ensuring adequate safeguards is not possible. In such populations, HIV preventive vaccine research should not be carried out.

Some factors to be considered are those classified earlier in the article 'Capacity Building' which influence the disparity in real or perceived power as between sponsors and host countries, as well as the factors classified below that can also increase the nature and level of risk of harm to participants:

(a) governmental, institutional or social stigmatization or discrimination on the basis of HIV status;
(b) inadequate ability to protect HIV-associated human rights, and to prevent HIV-associated discrimination and stigma, alongwith those arising from participation in an HIV vaccine trial;
(c) social and legal marginalization of groups from which participants might be drawn, e.g., women, injecting drug users, men having sex with men, commercial sex workers, etc.;
(d) limited availability, accessibility and sustainability of health care and treatment options;
(e) limited ability of individuals or groups in the community to understand the research process;
(f) limited ability of individuals to understand the informed consent process;
(g) limited ability of individuals to be able to give freely their informed consent in the light of prevailing class, gender, and other social and legal factors; and
(h) lack of meaningful national/local scientific and ethical review.

Clinical Trial Phases: As phases I, II, and III in the clinical development of a preventive vaccine all have their own particular scientific requirements and specific ethical challenges, the option of study populations for each trial phase should be justified in advance in scientific and ethical terms in all cases, irrespective of where the study population is found. Generally, early clinical phases of HIV vaccine research should be carried out in communities that are less vulnerable to harm or exploitation, usually within the sponsor country. However, countries may choose, for valid scientific and public health considerations, to conduct any phase within their populations, if they are able to ensure sufficient scientific infrastructure and sufficient ethical safeguards.

Preliminary stages in a vaccine development programme entail research in laboratories and among animals. The transition from this pre-clinical phase to a phase I clinical trial, in which testing involves the administration of the candidate vaccine to human subjects to assess safety and immunogenicity, is a time when risks may not be yet well defined. Moreover, specific infrastructures are often required in order to ensure the safety and care of the research participants at these stages. For these reasons, the first administration of a candidate HIV vaccine in humans should generally be carried out in less vulnerable research populations, usually in the country of the sponsor.

There may be situations, however, where developing countries choose to conduct phases I/II and/or III (large-scale trials to examine efficacy) among their populations that are comparatively, vulnerable to risk and exploitation. For example, this could occur where an experimental HIV vaccine is directed primarily towards a viral strain that does not exist in the sponsor country but does exist in the potential host country. Conducting phase I/II trials in the country where the strain prevails may be the only way to discover whether safety and immunogenicity are acceptable in that particular population, prior to conducting a phase III trial. A country may also decide that, due to the high level of HIV risk to its population and the severity of HIV/AIDS already in country, it is willing to test a vaccine concept that is not being tested in another country. Such a decision may result in obvious benefits to the country in question if an effective vaccine is developed. It may also provide an important capacity-building experience, if phase I or phase II trials are carried out in a host country prior to a phase III trial being initiated there. Establishing a vaccine development programme that entails the conduct of some, most, or all of its clinical trial components in a country or community that is comparatively vulnerable to harm or exploitation is ethically justified if:

* the vaccine is anticipated to be effective against a strain of HIV that is an important public health problem in the country;
* the country and the community either have, or with assistance can develop or be provided with, adequate scientific and ethical capability and administrative and health infrastructure for the successful conduct of the proposed research;
* community members, policy makers, ethicists and investigators in the country have determined that;
* their residents will be adequately protected from harm or exploitation, and that the vaccine development programme is necessary for and responsive to the health needs and priorities in their country; and
* all other conditions for ethical justification as set forth in this document are satisfied.

In cases in which it is decided to conduct phase I or phase II trials first in a country other than the sponsor country, due consideration should be given to conducting them at the same time in the sponsor country where this is practical and ethical. Also, when the host country or community is not familiar with conducting biomedical research in human subjects, phase I/II trials that have been performed in the country of the sponsor should ordinarily be repeated in the community in which the phase III trials are to be conducted.

Potential Harms: The nature, magnitude, and probability of all potential harms resulting from participation in an HIV preventive vaccine trial should be specified in the research protocol as fully as can be reasonably done, as well as the modalities by which to address these, alongwith provision for the highest level of care to participants who experience adverse reactions to the vaccine, compensation for injury associated with the research, and referral to psychosocial and legal support, as necessary.

Participation in HIV preventive vaccine research may consist physiological, psychological and social risks. With regard to the physiological risks, the objective of an HIV preventive vaccine is to induce an immunological response in the human body to counteract the HIV virus if it enters the body, or to prevent it from entering at all. Vaccines at present being considered for human trials are not capable of causing infection, i.e. they do not include replicating HIV[2]. Several candidate HIV vaccines have been tested in laboratories, and some have been tested in human subjects. Not all of these candidate vaccines are the same, and not all candidate vaccines carry the same risks for harm. Thus far, however, major adverse biological effects have not been observed. Nevertheless, some of the more likely physiological risks of participating in vaccine research include the following:

(a) A person who has received a candidate vaccine and is then exposed to HIV may have a greater risk of developing established infection, or of progressing more rapidly once infected, than if the vaccine had not been administered. This potential harm has not been observed in trials uptil now.

(b) An HIV vaccine may require that several injections be given over months or years, resulting in pain, occasional skin reactions, and possibly other biological adverse episodes, such as fever and malaise.

(c) Injuries may be sustained due to research-associated activities during the course of the trial.

The potential for adverse reactions to the candidate vaccine, as well as possible injuries associated with HIV vaccine research, should be stated, as far as possible, in the research protocol and completely explained in the informed consent process. Both the protocol and the consent process should also narrate the nature of medical treatment to be provided for injuries, as well as compensation for harm incurred due to research-associated activities including the process by which it is decided whether an injury will be compensated. HIV infection acquired during participation in an HIV preventive vaccine trial should not be considered an injury subject to compensation unless it is directly attributable to the vaccine itself, or to direct contamination through research-associated activities. In addition to compensation for biological/medical injuries, appropriate consideration should be given to compensation for social or economic harms, e.g., job loss of employment as a result of testing positive following vaccine administration. With regard to psychosocial risks, participation in a complicated, lengthy trial involving intensely intimate matters, involving repeated HIV testing, and involving exposure to culturally different scientific and medical concepts may result in anxiety, stress, depression, as well as stress between partners in a relationship. Participation, if it becomes publicly known, may also cause stigma and discrimination against the participant if (s)he is perceived to be HIV-infected. Finally, some people may develop a positive HIV test after receiving a candidate HIV vaccine, even though they are not truly infected with HIV, i.e., a 'false positive' HIV test. This may result in the same negative social consequences that exist for those actually HIV-infected. The protocol should clearly state these, as well as ensure that the research occurs in communities where confidentiality can be maintained and where participants will have access to, and can be referred to, ongoing psychosocial services, including counselling, social support groups, and legal support. Consideration should also be given to establish an ombudsperson who can intervene with outside parties, if necessary and requested, on behalf of participants, as well as to providing documentation to participants that they can use to show that their 'false positive' is due to their participation in research.[3]

Advantages: The research protocol should outline the advantage that persons participating in HIV preventive vaccine trials should experience as a result of their participation. Care should be taken so that these are not presented in a way that unduly influences freedom of choice in participation.

A few of the activities associated with the conduct of HIV vaccine trials should benefit those who participate. At a minimum, participants should:

(a) have regular and supportive contact with health care

professionals and counsellors throughout the course of the trial;

(b) receive comprehensive information regarding HIV transmission and how it can be prevented;

(c) receive access to HIV prevention methods, including male and female condoms, and clean injecting equipment, where legal;

(d) have access to a pre-agreed care and treatment package for HIV/AIDS if they become HIV-infected while enrolled in the trial;

(e) receive compensation for time, travel and inconvenience for participation in the trials; and

(f) if the vaccine is effective, develop protective immunity to HIV.

Control Group: As long as there is no known effective HIV preventive vaccine, a placebo control arm should be considered ethically acceptable in a phase III HIV preventive vaccine trial. However, where it is ethically and scientifically acceptable, consideration should be given to the use in the control arm of a vaccine to prevent a relevant condition apart from HIV.

At present, vaccine with proven efficacy in preventing infection or disease from HIV does not exist. Therefore, the use of a placebo control arm is ethically acceptable in appropriately tailored protocols.

Participants in the control arm of a future phase III HIV preventive vaccine trial should receive an HIV vaccine known to be safe and effective when such is available, unless there are compelling scientific reasons which justify the use of a placebo. Compelling scientific reasons to use a placebo rather than a known effective HIV vaccine in the research population include the following:

(a) The effective HIV vaccine is not believed to be effective against the virus that is prevalent in the research population.

(b) There are convincing reasons to believe that the biological conditions that prevailed during the initial trial displaying efficacy were so different from the conditions in the proposed research population that the results of the initial trial cannot be directly applied to the research population under consideration.

In an effort to address the concern of lack of benefit to those randomly placed in a placebo control arm, apart from the benefits described in Advantages, it is recommended that the provision to these persons of another vaccine, such as for hepatitis B or tetanus, be considered. The appropriateness of such a step should be examined in terms of the scientific requirements of the trial, the health needs of the population of participants, and the equilibrium of benefits and risks to the active versus control arms of the trial.

Informed Consent: Independent and informed consent based on complete, accurate, and appropriately conveyed and understood information should be obtained from each individual while being screened for eligibility for participation in an HIV preventive vaccine trial, and before (s)he is actually enrolled in the trial. Efforts should be taken to ensure throughout the trial that participants continue to understand and to participate freely as the trial advances. Informed consent, with pre- and post-test counselling, should also be obtained for any testing for HIV status carried out before, during and after the research.

A process of consultation between community representatives, researchers, sponsor(s) and regulatory bodies should be used to tailor an effective informed consent strategy and process. Issues such as illiteracy, language and cultural obstacles, and diminished personal autonomy should be addressed in this consultative process. In some communities, special efforts may be required to achieve adequate understanding of 'cause and effect', 'contagion', 'placebo', 'double blind', and other concepts involved in the scientific design of the research.

HIV preventive vaccine trials necessitate informed consent at several stages. The first stage consists of screening candidates for eligibility for participation in the trial, which will involve, among other things, an evaluation of the individual's risk-taking behaviour and a test for HIV status. Informed consent should be obtained during this screening process after the candidate has received all material statistics regarding the screening procedures, as well as an outline of the vaccine trial in which he will be invited to enrol, if found eligible. Fully informed consent should also be given for the test for HIV status, which should also be accompanied by pre- and post-test counselling, and referral to clinical and social support services, if found positive.

The second stage at which informed consent is required occurs once a person is judged eligible for enrolment. That individual should then be given full information about the nature and length of participation in the trial, alongwith the risks and advantages posed by participation, so that (s)he is able to give informed consent to participate.

Once enrolled, efforts should then be made throughout the trial to obtain assurance that the participation continues to be on a basis of free consent and understanding of what is happening. Informed consent, with pre- and post-test counselling, should also be given for any repeated tests for HIV status. Throughout all stages of the trial and consent process, there should be assurance by the investigator that the information is understood before consent is given.

In some communities, it is conventional to require the authorization of a third party, such as a community elder, in order for investigators to enter the community to invite individual members to participate in research. Other circumstances which make individual informed consent difficult are those in which an individual requires approval of another person or group in order to make decisions, where there is coercion, and where there is a cultural tradition of sharing risks and responsibilities, e.g., a few cultures where men hold the prerogative in marital relationships, where there is parental control of women, and/or where there are strong influences by community and/or religion or hierarchy.

Such authorization or influence must not be used as an alternative for individual informed consent. Nor should trials be carried out where truly individual and free consent cannot be obtained. Authorization by a third party in place of individual informed consent is allowable only in the case of some minors who have not attained the legal age of consent to participate in a trial. In cases where it is proposed that minors will be enrolled as research participants, specific and full justification for their enrolment must be given, and their own consent must be obtained taking into considerations their evolving capacities.

In addition to the standard content of informed consent, prior to participation in an HIV vaccine trial, each prospective participant must be informed, using appropriate language and technique, of the below mentioned specific details:

(a) Prospective participants of phase II and III trials of HIV preventive vaccines should be informed that they have been selected as prospective participants because they are at comparatively high risk of HIV infection.

(b) Prospective participants for phase I, II and III trials should be informed that they will receive counselling and access to the means of risk reduction (in particular, male and female condoms, and clean injecting equipment, where legal) concerning how to lessen their risk of infection; and that in spite of these risk reduction efforts, a few of the participants may become infected, particularly in the case of phase III trials where several participants at high risk are participating.

(c) They should be informed that it is not known whether the experimental vaccine will prevent HIV infection or disease, and further, that a few of the participants will receive a placebo instead of the candidate HIV vaccine, when such is the case.

(d) They should be informed of the specific risks for physical harm, as well as for psychological and social harm, and of the types of treatment and compensation that are available for harm, and of services to which they may be referred should harm occur.

(e) All prospective participants of phase I, II or III trials should be informed of the nature and duration of care and treatment that is available, and how it can be accessed, if they become infected with HIV during the course of the trial.

Informed Consent: Special Measures: Special measures should be taken to protect persons who are, or may be, limited in their ability to provide informed consent bacause of their social or legal status. There are various categories of persons who are legally competent to consent to participate in a trial, and who have ample cognitive capacity to consent, but who may have limitations in their freedom to make independent options. Those who plan, review, and conduct vaccine trials should be alert to the problems presented by the participation of such persons, and either exclude such persons, if their vulnerability cannot be addressed, or take appropriate measures to ensure meaningful and independent ongoing informed consent, respect their rights, foster their well-being, and protect them from harm. The following are individuals or groups who should be given extra consideration with regard to their ability to provide informed consent in HIV preventive vaccine trials:

(a) Persons who are junior or subordinate members of hierarchical structures may be vulnerable to undue influence or coercion in that they may fear retaliation if they refuse cooperation with authorities. Such persons include members of the armed forces, students, government employees, prisoners, and refugees.

(b) Persons who engage in illegal or socially stigmatized activities are vulnerable to undue influence and threats presented by possible breaches of confidentiality and action by legal forces. Such persons include commercial sex workers, intravenous drug users, and men who have sex with men.

(c) Persons who are impoverished or dependent on welfare programmes are vulnerable to being unduly influenced by offers of what others may consider modest material or health inducements.

(d) Women living in cultures where their autonomy as individuals is not sufficiently recognized are vulnerable to influence and coercion from male partners, family, or community members.

Steps that might be taken to ensure that ongoing free and informed consent is given by participants from these groups include:

(a) appointment of an independent ombudsperson and/or group to monitor these factors;

(b) expansion of the responsibilities of the clinical trial monitor to include adherence to the informed consent and counselling process, or appointment of an independent counselling monitor;

(c) training of the counsellors on these factors; and

(d) group counselling and/or interaction with local NGOs representing the groups from which such participants are drawn.

Risk-reduction Interventions: Appropriate risk-reduction counselling and access to prevention methods should be offered to all vaccine trial participants, with new methods being added as they are discovered and validated.

Reducing the risk of HIV infection throughout the trial among participants is an essential ethical component of HIV preventive vaccine trials. All trial participants should receive comprehensive counselling concerning methods of decreasing the risk of transmission of HIV. This should include the primary principles of safe sexual practice and safe use of injection equipment, as well as education regarding general health and treatment of sexually transmitted infections (STIs). Investigators should offer trial participants appropriate access to condoms, sterile injecting equipment (where legal) and treatment for other STIs. All trial participants should also be counselled before enrolling in a clinical trial concerning the potential benefits and risks of post-exposure prophylaxis with antiretroviral medication, and how it can be accessed in the community.

The mechanism and frequency of counselling should be agreed upon by the community-host government-investigator-sponsor partnership, and should be based upon reliable information about the prevailing social and behavioural characteristics of the study population. Consideration should be given to providing counselling through an agency or organisation that is independent of the investigators in order to eradicate any real or perceived conflict of interest. Local capacity should be developed to employ such means in a culturally suitable and sustainable manner, guided by the best scientific statistics.

The provision of counselling to lessen the risk should be monitored to ensure quality and to minimize the potential conflict of interest between the risk-reduction objectives and the vaccine trial's scientific objectives. As new methods of prevention are discovered and validated, these must be added to the preventive methods being provided to trial participants.

Monitoring Informed Consent and Interventions: A plan for monitoring the initial and continuing adequacy of the informed consent process and risk-reduction interventions, including counselling and access to prevention techniques, should be agreed upon before the trial begins.

The value of informed consent depends primarily on the ongoing quality of the process by which it is carried out, and not solely on the structure and content of the informed consent document. The informed consent process should be tailored to empower participants to permit them to make appropriate decisions. Similarly, there are many ways in which risk reduction (counselling and access to means of prevention) can be carried out, with some methods being more effective than others in conveying the relevant information and in lessening the risk behaviour.

A method for monitoring the adequacy of these processes should be tailored and agreed upon by the community-host-government-investigator-sponsor partnership. Consideration should be given to the expansion of the responsibilities of the clinical trial monitor to include adherence to the informed consent and counselling process, and/or the appointment of an independent counselling monitor, as recommended in 'Informed Consent: Special Measures'. The appropriateness of such plans should be found out by the scientific and ethical review committees that are responsible for providing prior and continuing evaluation of the trial. This recommendation supplements the general guidelines for the monitoring of vaccine trials for safety and compliance with scientific and ethical standards and regulatory requirements.

Care and Treatment: Care and treatment for HIV/AIDS and its related complications should be provided to participants in HIV preventive vaccine trials, with the ideal being to provide the best proven therapy, and the minimum to provide the highest level of care attainable in the host country in light of the circumstances classified below. A comprehensive care package should be agreed upon through a host/community/sponsor debate which reaches consensus prior to commencement of a trial, taking into consideration the following:

(a) level of care and treatment available in the sponsor country
(b) highest level of care available in the host country
(c) highest level of treatment available in the host country, alongwith availability of antiretroviral therapy outside the research context in the host country
(d) availability of infrastructure to provide care and treatment in the context of research
(e) potential duration and sustainability of care and treatment for the trial participant.

Sponsors need to ensure care and treatment for participants who become HIV-infected during the course of the trial. At present, there is no global consensus regarding the level of care and treatment that should be offered. This was witnessed at the UNAIDS-sponsored regional workshops to discuss ethical issues in preventive HIV vaccine trials at which the following three different conclusions were reached. Care and treatment for those who become infected should be provided:

(a) at the level of that offered in the sponsor country, and should consist preventive risk behaviour counselling, general HIV care and treatment, post-exposure prophylaxis and antiretroviral therapy, as per the best scientific evidence for effectiveness available at the time of the trial; and should last at least for the duration for the trial, and longer, if so negotiated;
(b) at a level agreed upon by the host country, e.g., it might consist immunological monitoring, physician visits, prevention and treatment of opportunistic infections, and palliative care, but not necessarily antiretroviral therapy; and should be made reasonably available for the lifetime of the participants;
(c) at a level consistent with that available in the host country; there is no imperative to provide a level of care consistent with that in the sponsoring country, or with the highest available in the world.

Competing considerations that have led to disagreement about the standard of care and treatment consist:

(a) the need to achieve equity in care and treatment for all participants in HIV vaccine trials worldwide; in particular, to achieve equity between potential participants from sponsor 'countries and host countries;

(b) an ethical obligation of sponsors to provide care and treatment as per their resources;

(c) concern that a high level of care and treatment will account for undue incentives and inducements for countries and communities to participate;

(d) concern that governments might abdicate on their responsibility to provide care and treatment if sponsors fill this role;

(e) governments' will to be able to attract research into their countries in order to address the critical need of their populations for an HIV preventive vaccine;

(f) the right and responsibility of sovereign countries and communities to find out for themselves the equilibrium of risks and advantages they are willing to accept.

In the light of these competing concerns, it is recommended that:

(a) Consensus on the standard/level of care and treatment, its duration, and who will bear the costs should be reached before a decision to host HIV vaccine development.

(b) This consensus should emerge from an extensive dialogue involving the above-mentioned competing concerns among sponsors, and representatives from the potential host country and communities from which potential trial participants would be drawn, e.g., government officials, national scientific and ethical communities, affected populations, relevant NGOs, local religious and community leaders.

(c) Such a consensus should aim for achieving, as closely as possible, the ideal of provision of the best proven therapy for trial participants, taking in consideration the relevant conditions and concerns.

(d) Sponsors should seek, at a minimum, to ensure access to a level of care and treatment that approaches the best proven care and treatment that are achievable in the potential host country.

(e) Those participating in the planning of vaccine development programmes should seek to provide a comprehensive care and treatment package based, at a minimum, on standards of care developed by the community, but also taking into consideration the additional resources and higher standards brought by the sponsor into the research setting.

(f) Sponsors should contribute to the building up of both the research capacity and the health care delivery capacity of the community where the research is to be conducted, in such a manner that they become integrated into the infrastructure of the community.

Such a care and treatment package should include, but not be limited to, some or all of the following items, depending on the type of research, the setting, and the consensus reached by all interested parties before the trials begin:

(a) counselling
(b) preventive methods and means
(c) treatment for other sexually transmitted infections
(d) tuberculosis prevention and treatment
(e) prevention/treatment of opportunistic infections
(f) nutrition
(g) palliative care, alongwith pain control and spiritual care
(h) referral to social and community support
(i) family planning
(j) home-based care
(k) antiretroviral therapy.

Women: As women, including those who are potentially pregnant, pregnant, or breast-feeding, should be recipients of future HIV preventive vaccines, women should be included in clinical trials in order to verify safety, immunogenicity, and efficacy from their standpoint. During such research, women should receive ample information to make informed choices about risks to themselves, as well as to their fetus or breast-fed infant, where applicable.

Women, including pregnant women, potentially pregnant women and breast-feeding women, should be eligible for enrolment in HIV preventive vaccine trials, both as a matter of equity and because in many communities across the world women are at high risk of HIV infection. Therefore, the safety, immunogenicity, and efficacy of candidate vaccines should be established for women, and for their fetus and breast-fed child, where applicable. In these circumstances, the clinical trials should be tailored with the intent of setting up the effects of the candidate vaccine on the health of the woman and the fetus and/or breast-fed infant, where applicable.

Although the enrolment of pregnant, potentially pregnant, or breast-feeding women complicates the evaluation of risks and advantages, because both the woman and the fetus or infant could be benefited or harmed, such women should be viewed as autonomous decision-makers, capable of making an informed choice for themselves and for their fetus or child. As with all research participants, steps should be taken to ensure that pregnant or breast-feeding women who are enrolled in vaccine trials are capable of giving informed consent, as discussed earlier. Moreover, in order for (pregnant) women to be able to make an informed choice for their fetus/breast-fed infant, they should be duly informed about any potential for terato-genesis and other risks to the fetus, and/or the breast-fed infant. If there are risks associated with breast-feeding, they should be informed of the availability of nutritional substitutes and other supportive services.

Children: As children should be recipients of future HIV preventive vaccines, children should be included in clinical trials in order to verify safety, immunogenicity, and efficacy from their standpoint. Efforts should be taken to vaccine development programmes that address the particular ethical and legal considerations relevant for children, and protect their rights and welfare during participation.

Children[4], including infants and adolescents, should be eligible for enrolment in HIV preventive vaccine trials, both as a matter of equity and as a function of the fact that in many communities across the globe children are at high risk of HIV infection. Infants born to HIV-infected mothers are at risk of becoming infected during birth and during the post-partum period through breast-feeding. Many adolescents are also at high risk of infection because of sexual activity, lack of access to HIV prevention education and means, and engagement in injecting drug use.

Therefore, vaccine development programmes should account

the needs of children for an effective HIV vaccine; should identify the legal, ethical and health considerations relevant to their participation in vaccine research; and should enrol children in clinical trials tailored to set up safety, immunogencity, and efficacy for their age groups, once they can be so enrolled in terms of meeting the health needs and ethical considerations associated with their situation. Those designing vaccine development programmes that might include children should do so in consultation with groups dedicated to the protection and promotion of the rights and welfare of children, both at international and national levels.

Unless exceptions are authorized by constitutional legislation in the host country, consent to participate in an HIV vaccine trial must be secured from the parent or guardian of a child who is a minor before the enrolment of the child as a participant in a vaccine trial. The consent of one parent is usually sufficient, unless national legislation requires the consent of both. Every effort should be made to obtain consent to participate in the trial also from the child as per the evolving capacities of the child.

In some countries, individuals who are below the age of consent are authorized to receive, without the consent or awareness of their parents or guardians, such medical services as abortion, contraception, treatment for drug or alcohol abuse, treatment of sexually transmitted diseases, etc. In some of these countries, such minors are also authorized to consent to serve as participants in research in the same categories without the agreement or the awareness of their parents or guardians provided the research presents no more than 'minimal risk'. However, such authorization does not justify the enrolment of minors as participants in vaccine trials without the consent of their parents or guardians.

In some countries, some individuals who are below the general age of consent are regarded as 'emancipated' or 'mature' minors and are authorized to consent without the agreement or even the awareness of their parents or guardians. These may consist those who are married, parents, pregnant or living independently. When authorized by national legislation, minors in these categories may consent to participation in vaccine trials without the permission of their parents or guardians.

References

1. For a complete narration of the process and participants, see "Final Report, UNAIDS-Sponsored Regional Workshops to discuss Ethical Issues in Preventive HIV Vaccine Trials", available from UNAIDS. See also Guenter, Esparza, and Macklin: Ethical considerations in international HIV vaccine trials: summary of a consultative process conducted by the Joint United Nations Programme on HIV/AIDS (UNAIDS. *Journal of Medical Ethics* (February 2000), Vol. 26, No. 1: 37-43.
2. Some of the most effective viral vaccines are based on live-attenuated viruses and some investigators have proposed a similar theory for HIV vaccines. Any decision regarding testing a live-attenuated HIV vaccine in humans would have to be carefully examined in view of the significant safety concerns related to witty such a vaccine approach.
3. When a vaccine is tested, laboratory mechanisms should be available to differentiate HIV-positivity due to vaccination from that due to actual HIV infection.
4. As defined by the Convention on the Rights of the Child, Article "... a child means every human being below the age of eighteen years unless, under the law applicable to the child, majority is attained earlier."

Four

Carers for People with HIV/AIDS: Stress Management

Introduction

Latisa (name changed for the sake of confidentiality), manager of an AIDS care programme in Soweto, South Africa, tells a story that haunts her about her work in the township. She had gone to the home of a single mother with three boys aged 10, 7 and 5. The mother was terribly ill. She had sores all over her body that were oozing pus, recalls Latisa. The woman had nobody to care for her but the boys, and they were bathing their mother and trying to cope with everything themselves. The 10-year-old asked Latisa: 'how do I cook for my mother?' He was trying to do all that needed doing, but he didn't know how, When I left that home I was crying; couldn't keep my mind on the road ahead.

Gladys (name changed), a volunteer in a rural area of South Africa, says she was unprepared for all the social problems she finds in the homes she visits: 'I thought I was going to give health care, but then you find there's no food in the house, the whole family is hungry, there's no money coming in, and you feel you can do so little'. And in Uganda, Christine, a counsellor on the staff of an AIDS organisation who is herself HIV-positive, tells of her anxiety at being unable to reach her targets, as she is often too weak to handle the scooter she has been given to visit her clients. She feels guilty at having to lean on her colleagues, but cannot face the idea of retirement: "I have children to support—who will pay their school fees if I give up? And how will I manage without medical care?" she asks.

The strains on those caring for people with HIV infection and AIDS are enormous and wide ranging. And as the epidemic spreads and matures, overwhelming the capacity of the health and social services in many countries to cope, they are being borne increasingly by lay carers within families and communities. These people — pioneers of the home care movement, front-line workers in the efforts to curtail AIDS and to contain the damage it does to their societies—are a precious resource. The quality of care they provide and their ability to do so over a sustained period depend on the protection of their own well-being and morale.

The purpose of this report is to draw attention to the needs of carers and to what can be done to support them more effectively. It will concentrate on those participating in home and community-level care. And it will draw on the first-hand experience of individuals and AIDS organisations in Uganda, which was one of the earliest countries to be affected by AIDS and to respond with imagination, and South Africa, where the virus is spreading faster than almost anywhere else in this world. The report is intended for all those with an interest in the care of people with HIV/AIDS, but especially for those with direct responsibility for providing care or managing carers, for policy-making in this field, or for supporting AIDS, but especially for those with direct responsibility for providing care or managing carers, for policy-making in this field, or for supporting AIDS programmes.

Uganda and South Africa: Two Faces of the Epidemic

Ugandan Scenario

Some of the earliest cases of AIDS in Africa were discovered in 1982 in the fishing communities living along the shores of Lake Victoria in Uganda's Rakai District. Since then the virus has spread across the country, affecting rich and poor, urban and rural people alike. The most infections are transmitted through heterosexual intercourse. However, babies who have contracted the virus from their infected mothers before or during birth or through breast-feeding constitutes about one in five of all new infections.

At their peak in the early 1990s, HIV infection rates above 30 per cent regularly recorded at sentinel surveillance sites. These rates have been decreasing gradually over recent years — especially among women aged 15-19 years — and behavioural surveys suggest that youngsters are postponing their sexual debut, that people are having fewer sex partners and that they are using condoms more regularly. Still today approximately 13 per cent of the adult population is HIV-infected, with three times as many woman as men below the age of 25 being HIV-positive. As the epidemic matures, the burden of sickness is growing daily. Each year thousands of infected people develop AIDS, which is the number one cause of death among adults and the fourth most important cause of death among children under five years of age.

No family remains untouched by the epidemic. Everyone is caring for a sick relative, caring for the orphaned children of brothers, sisters, sons or daughters, or helping to support relatives who have lost their breadwinners and no longer have any money coming into the home. How to make ends meet—to pay the rent, keep children in school and food on the table, and find the money for drugs and treatment — is the main preoccupation of families, as AIDS rapidly impoverishes even comparatively well-off households and pushes those already encountering to survive over the edge into destitution.

Access to government health services in Uganda is extremely limited, with, 88 per cent of the population living more than 10 kilometres away from a health facility of any kind', and many clinics and health posts lacking trained personnel and short of the most basic medical supplies and drugs.

More than half of all hospital beds are occupied by AIDS patients, and many terminally ill people are turned away by chronically overstretched institutions. Therefore, a mass of organisations has emerged to fill the gaps in care and prevention. At present, some 1050 non-governmental and community-based organisations throughout the country are working in the AIDS field. They are the pioneers of home-based care for people with HIV and AIDS, which has recruited thousands of community-level volunteers and trained them to deliver a variety of services from primary preventive health care and first aid to practical advice and emotional support. The volunteers are supported by the staff of these organisations different professional skills, including especially counselling and nursing.

These organisations, backed by a government that has shown courage in acknowledging the nature and a volume of the epidemic encountering Uganda, have managed largely to overcome the despair and hopelessness that gripped communities early in the epidemic. When World Vision first went into Rakai in 1989, people knew so little about AIDS, except that it was a killer and they felt helpless in the face of it. 'When you visited houses you would find people had died; there were dead bodies and hopeless relatives not knowing what to do, full of fear and hurt and shame, weeping over the dead bodies. We would weep with them. Today people understand that a detection of HIV infection is not an automatic death sentence and that they can live for extended periods if they take care of themselves. With luck and positive thinking there is time to plan for the future. Whereas coffin-making was the growth industry some years ago, with carpentry workshops powdered with sawdust all along the road to Rakai, today brick-making has taken off too, since providing a secure house for their families, with brick walls and tin roof to replace the high maintenance mud and thatch, is a high priority for infected people. Everywhere, straw-topped brick kilns puffing like dragons send plumes of smoke rising among the banana palms in countryside plantations.

At present, the home-based care movement and all that it has achieved is threatened by weakened commitment from donors that has created panic for some of the most-valued enterprises, and threatened the morale of all organisations working in the field. This insecurity is just another reason of anxiety to people already carrying almost intolerable burdens. The staff and volunteers of AIDS organisations get no respite. Almost no one can shut the door on the problems and the pain of AIDS at the end of the working day, as most of the carers, like so many other Ugandans, go home to families bowed by disease, loss of loved ones and monetary problems of their own.

South African Scenario

Perhaps partly because of South Africa's isolation during the apartheid era, the AIDS epidemic was much slower to take off there than in other countries of the subcontinent. The first cases of AIDS came at fore among gay white men in 1983. It was not until the early 1990s that the virus gained momentum in the heterosexual community and began to spread like a bush fire. Today, South Africa has one of the fastest-growing HIV epidemics in the world, with approximately 1600 people becoming newly infected every day, and nearly 4 million believed to be infected by the end of 1998.

On the basis of results from anonymous testing at antenatal clinics, the South African Department of Health estimates that nationally around 23 per cent of pregnant women were HIV-positive by the end of 1998. But the spread of the virus is very uneven. KwaZulu/Natal—with its major sea ports, busy trucking routes, large population of migrant workers and history of social and political turmoil—has consistently displayed the highest prevalence of HIV. The rate for this province based on antenatal clinic statistics, was estimated to be around 32.5 per cent at the end of 1998, while HIV prevalence in the least-affected province, the Western Cape, was estimated to be around 5 per cent. Nearly everywhere else in the country, at least one adult in five was believed to be infected at the end of 1998.

To a great extent it is the secrecy surrounding AIDS that has permitted the virus to spread so rampantly. 'For two long we have closed our eyes as a nation, hoping the truth was not so real', said Thabo Mbeki, then deputy president, in an address to the nation in 1998. 'At times we did not know that we were burying people who had died from AIDS. At other times we knew, but chose to remain silent'.

More than a year has passed since Mbeki's speech, yet little has changed. So great are the stigma and fear surrounding AIDS present that in many places home care programmes are performing the work of treating and comforting terminally ill patients and their families without anyone ever mentioning the word AIDS. The case of Gugu Dlamini, a young Zulu woman who was beaten to death in her local *shebeen* (drinking house) by an angry mob after coming out in public as an HIV-positive person on World AIDS Day 1998, was reported globally. But it was not an exceptional incident: episodes of infected women, children and men being left to die in dark corners, abandoned by their families, or physically abused, are general, and make it hard to break the silence.

Nevertheless, more and more people in South Africa are finding the courage to speak out and show compassion for people with AIDS, as they themselves become infected or witness the suffering and death of people they love. Support groups of people with HIV and home-based care porogrammes are coming at fore in South Africa just as they have done elsewhere in Africa as the epidemic advances and reality can no longer be ignored.

'Carers' Defined

A revelation of HIV infection is always profoundly shocking. Feelings of fear, anger and despair, and thoughts of suicide, are general in the hours and weeks that follow. Where do people turn for comfort and guidance at such times? And who is most likely to care for them when they become too sick to look after themselves? This discussion concentrate at who the carers are, focusing predominantly on those outside the formal health services. The present discussion will look, too, at what motivates them to do this kind of work, how they are recruited and trained, and at the varieties of tasks they perform.

The different roles of caregivers are interchangeable and the demarcation lines between levels of care blurred. In areas badly affected by HIV and AIDS, many functioning as counsellors or nurses with non-governmental organisations, or a trained community volunteers, are also caring for someone at home who has AIDS. A few who work as professional or volunteer carers are themselves HIV-infected and registered as clients of AIDS organisations from which they receive care.

Family Carers

Lucy looked after her daughter-in-law and then her two sons when they were terminally ill with AIDS, and now she is helping to care for her little orphaned granddaughter who is HIV-infected. In the same city, 18-year-old Grace, one of a large family of children is caring for her mother who is bedridden and blinded by Kaposi's sarcoma that spread across her face within days of her noticing a small dark patch on her nose. Though no one in Uganda or South Africa has systematically listed who is doing the caring at family level, it is clear to those working in the field that the burden of care is borne predominantly by women and girls. A woman or girl child will find herself in the position of caregiver as a matter of course, of cultural expectation. And though many women are proud of their nurturing role and consider it natural, their subordinate status means there is likely to be little discussion within the family in assigning this responsibility, and little thought given to the personal sacrifices it will demand of females.

If a husband is ill, it is invariably the wife who looks after him, but if the wife is ill it's her children, or her sisters or mother who care for her, while the husband concentrates on earning money to support them all. Men are almost never the primary carers in the home. Men still are not coming along very well as carers. Many people in South Africa's townships today live in nuclear families far from their relatives. Often a mother will leave her home in a distant rural village to come and care for her daughter. Elderly mothers are finding themselves drawn into a role they just never imagined.

But AIDS is beginning to challenge traditional attitudes, and men, especially those who are infected themselves or who have worked with AIDS organisations and are knowledgeable and skilled, are increasingly willing to take on the physical care of sick partners and family members. "We have seen both extremes in the behaviour of men here in Soweto," says Mark Ottenweller, local director of Hope Worldwide. "Some have looked after sick partners or relatives magnificently, some have abandoned infected wives or thrown them out of the home." In KwaZulu/Natal, South Africa's worst-affected province, "it's not at all unusual to find men as primary cares," says Liz Towell, director of the Sinosizo Home-Based Care Programme, which has an extensive statistics on AIDS-affected families. "But most times they get tired of the job, or have to go back to work, so then they'll call their mothers from the farm. But that's only when things get bad—otherwise they just get on with it."

The least-acknowledged carers within the home are children. When one parent dies in a nuclear family there is often no one else but the children to look after the other parent who falls sick. This will be the case particularly in places where the intense stigma and shame of AIDS make people afraid of disclosing their infection. Many children are left to cope with terrifying conditions and witness the suffering of the person they most love and depend on in the world, without skills or knowledge and often without anyone ever having talked to them directly about what is happening. Nobody knows how many children in Uganda and South Africa are performing as primary carers, but it will become increasingly common as the epidemic matures simply because AIDS targets the parent generation. Anecdotal evidence from elsewhere in Africa suggests that it is often very young children, 8 to 11-year-olds, who are caring for sick parents, since older children tend to leave home to find work or seek survival on the streets as family poverty deepens.

Volunteer Carers

Volunteers are the backbone of community care programmes for people with HIV/AIDS. Some are what could be called 'informal' volunteers—friends or neighbours who step in to care for sick people they know, out of a sense of love or duty towards them. Or they are people, such as members of a church, who regularly commit some of their time to community service. But large numbers of people working for AIDS care programmes are 'formal' volunteers, recruited, trained and supervised by the organisations for which they work on an agreed basis. The organisations look for people who are:

(a) good listeners;
(b) non-judgemental and respectful of others;
(c) trustworthy and able to keep a secret;
(d) able to get on easily with people;
(e) sympathetic;
(f) self-confident; and
(g) committed.

Whereas most organisations stipulate that volunteers must be literate because they are required to keep records, Sinosizo, which works in some of the poorest and most disadvantaged rural communities in South Africa, has consciously developed a training programme and working practices that do not necessitate the ability to read and write. "We have Scribes' — at least one person in each group of volunteers who's literate and who sits down with the others and writes their reports for them," says Liz Towell. In her programme, information on home care — how to recognise conditions and what to do to prevent or treat them — is presented in simple drawings on cards that the volunteers keep for reference.

Motivating Elements

A sense of religious duty is the most frequently mentioned reason for taking on voluntary work, and seems to be what sustains people in the toughest times. While religious commitment is seen as a strength — and many care programmes are themselves church based — people with a desire to evangelize are not usually considered suitable as volunteers. Broad-mindedness, tolerance and acceptance of diversity are in particular important in caring for people with AIDS.

Simple compassion for others who are suffering is a common motivation for volunteering. 'In Africa there is a strong sense of community and a rich tradition of doing good work — reaching out to your neighbour or sick friend', says South African psychologist Pierre Brouard. Some people are motivated, too, by personal experience of AIDS in family or friends. They may have painful memories of the helplessness they noticed without knowledge or skills when AIDS came into their own lives, and what they learn as volunteers is both largely empowering and a source of pride. Alternatively, people who volunteer may simply want to join the effort to control a disease that is laying waste to their societies, and they cannot bear to sit by.

Large numbers of volunteers are HIV-positive themselves and have become involved in caring for others through joining support groups of people living with HIV /AIDS. The backbone of Hope Worldwide's care programme in South Africa is their support group members — people who have come together following a positive test for HIV, and part of whose strategy for survival and 'positive living' is to keep active, be useful and find purpose in life.

Self-interest is also usually part of the picture, even if it is not the main driving force for volunteering. Said Christopher, a volunteer in one of Uganda's worst-affected districts: 'I hope that when I get that problem myself someone will help me because I have helped them'. In his village there are some homesteads without graves marked with rough crosses among the coffee and cassava bushes. Many remember the days when people died, often with little dignity, in homes where no one knew what to do, and bodies were sometimes interred without ceremony by fearful and traumatised relatives.

Some people volunteer in the hope of promotion to paid employment with the organisation. Others are attracted by the incentives offered by volunteer programmes, such as preferential acccess to income-generating schemes and skills training, or perhaps food handouts. In Uganda, voluntary work in the community has, for a majority of people, been a stepping stone towards positions in local government. 'We motivate them to stand for local council elections because we feel political office will give them a wider platform to use the skills and knowledge they have learnt,' says a World Vision staff member responsible for supervising volunteers.

"I think people's motives for becoming caregivers are complex — we all do it for some reason of our own to start off with", says Pierre Brouard. "I guess I'm involved in this work because I lost a parent when I was very young. I am a gay man, so it has been very real for me, this disease. AIDS work helps me process all kinds of personal problems to do with mortality and spirituality, so there are very good selfish reasons why I do it. also feel a sense of responsibility a social bond, a concern for people who are victimised, because as a gay person I've experienced stigma and discrimination myself".

Purpose of Training

Volunteers are trained to provide innumerable services. The community volunteers with TASO and World Vision in Uganda are trained to counsel clients and their families, which essentially means listening to their concerns, giving comfort and information, and determining the options they have for dealing with various problems. They work closely with the local health services, acting as bonds between people in their homes and the clinic or hospital which may be many kilometres away. They collect drugs for bedridden patients, and will, if necessary, try to motivate a nurse or doctor to go out to treat a patient at home. Very often volunteers accompany people with AIDS to the health unit to assist them communicate with staff. Some are concerned that clinic staff may lack specialist knowledge about AIDS or skill in handling nervous and distressed patients.

Community volunteers with the South African programmes

offers much the same services. In both countries, overstretched staff in the health services are, generally speaking, grateful for the work volunteers do that lightens their own workload and augments their skills. In Uganda, for example, government health workers are deployed only to subcounty level, which means the most peripheral health teams each cover a population of about 30,000. Most programmes make a point of introducing volunteers to local clinics and setting up strong working relationships between them from the start. World Vision motivates mutual respect by involving local health personnel in their volunteer training programmes. Sinosizo's volunteers are members of the regional health forum, which gives them status and support. And Hope Worldwide worked with the health services, developing specialist skills in AIDS care, before they began their community programme.

Volunteers working with AIDS care programmes are trained to identify health problems, and to know which conditions they can treat themselves and how to do so, and which need referring to someone with greater skills, Sinosizo's volunteers in KwaZulu/Natal learn practical hands-on care, which means, for example, mouth care, how to perform a bed bath and how to prevent or treat pressure sores. Immediately following training they must display these skills with families in front of their supervisors to show that they are competent themselves and that they are able to pass the skills on successfully to the primary carers in the home. The aim is to empower families to do their own caring as far as practicable.

Some community volunteers are trained to supervise the treatment of tuberculosis. Some are given specialist skills in bereavement counselling. In Uganda, World Vision has added a component on communicating with children to their training curriculum, recognising the huge unmet needs of children, and the fact that more and more of them are being left with the responsibility of caring for sick relatives. Sinosizo, too, is promoting with the Psychology Department and Child and Family Centre at the University of Natal, a training package for its volunteers on the needs of children. And as the caseload of AIDS patients rises in this most heavily affected province, the programme is giving its keenest and most competent volunteers specialist skills such as terminal care and pain management.

Clarifying the relationship between the AIDS organisation and the volunteers, and what each can expect from the other, is crucially important for the success of a programme and the morale of everyone involved. This is generally addressed in training. Sinosizo starts its training course with a one-day seminar on the meaning of volunteering, which is an opportunity for those who are in fact looking for paid employment or are not truly committed to drop out before resources have been spent on them. Left Line, whose focus is on specialist counselling rather than home nursing skills, devotes a great deal of training time to "personal growth" in which trainees are helped to explore their own strengths, to deal with troubling issues in their own lives, discover their attitudes and build self-confidence.

A clear understanding of their own limitations, and what they are and are not expected to do, is crucial in volunteers, says Mark Ottenweller of Hope Worldwide. In his organisation, this issue is addressed in training, and thereafter there are generally regular discussions between volunteers and programme staff about what needs doing in their areas and how to allocate the workload. By and large, organisations choose to avoid drawing up formal contracts with volunteers because they want to motivate a sense of community ownership of the volunteer programme, rather than giving the impression that the volunteers are unpaid professionals of the organisation.

Functions of Volunteer Carers

The community-level volunteers who work with AIDS care programmes offer innumerable services, often combining both care and prevention. These include:

(a) emotional and spiritual support for people with HIV / AIDS, and their families wherever practicable;
(b) psychosocial counselling to assist clients resolve personal problems;
(c) practical advice about nutrition, hygiene, and preventive health care;
(d) primary nursing care to bedridden patients, and/or passing on such skills to primary carers within the home;
(e) help with domestic chores;

(f) liaison between the health and welfare services and patients in the community;
(g) supervision of tuberculosis treatment;
(h) peer counselling;
(i) community mobilisation against AIDS;
(j) public information and education; and
(k) condom distribution.

Additional Carers

Besides the support group members who are central to its home care programme, Hope Worldwide in Soweto uses the services of about 200 volunters linked to the Johannesberg-based Church of Christ. Everyone who offers time to the organisation is given primary information and education about HIV/AIDS. But a select group of about 150 volunteers who want to be more involved have been trained to do primary counselling so that they can give emotional support to people with AIDS in their homes or in hospital. The casual volunteers are called upon to do such things as prepare the ground for the vegetable gardens for support group members, or to mend the leaking roof of an AIDS-affected family living in a shack. A core group of specially committed church volunteers is used for the most demanding cases. If a family is nursing a terminally ill patient they will draw up a rota among themselves so that someone goes each day to assist with the household chores — cooking, cleaning, washing bedclothes and, of course, bathing the sick person.

Staff Carers

Most of the AIDS organisations visited have only a small complement of care workers — typically counsellors and nurses — on their staff. These employees may occasionally work diretly with clients and families, but their main prominent responsibility is to recruit, train and support volunteer carers in the comunity. TASO, however, employs several counsellors who are equally responsible for providing care themselves and for looking after teams of volunteers in the community. Besides the counsellors, the TASO centres each employ a number of health care workers who give medical care to clients. Very much the same things seem to encourage those applying for jobs with an AIDS care programme as those who volunteer their services. The most frequently stated motivations include:

(a) personal experience of AIDS that left painful memories of helplessness and catalysed a desire for knowledge and skills;
(b) personal experience that motivated a commitment to join the struggle against the epidemic;
(c) compassion for the sick and suffering; and
(d) a desire to serve others, often stated in terms of religious calling or duty.

Staff members may be recruited from amongst the volunteers working with a programme. But, since 1989, TASO has advertised for counsellors, looking for people with sympathy, resilience, patience and quick minds, preferably with a background in social science, education or health. An evaluation of the programme in 1998 recommended that it would be most cost-effective to recruit people with nursing qualifications a counsellors so that the same person could provide medical and psychosocial care.

TASO's training for its professional counsellors commences with a three-day exercise in self-reflection. 'This is our opportunity to examine a person thoroughly. We can observe their attitudes, beliefs and values, and help them change where essential', says training officer Hannington Nkayivu/Inappropriate traits include religious fundamentalism or bigotry, a tendency to be judgmental or moralistic, personal prejudices such as lack of respect for women or certain types of people, and inability to explain to children. "A counsellor must be prepared and able to treat everyone at par, whoever they are, and they must have respect for all ages and both genders," he says. After the initial exercise, the training course teaches the facts about HIV/AIDS, and promotes skills in counselling and general communication.

However, the curriculum is due for a change. 'TASO commenced counselling in a crisis', explains Sophia Mukasa Monico, TASO's director. "At that time nobody knew anything about HIV. But when a client comes to a counsellor today they know nearly everything about it, so what they want is not information but help with developing a coping strategy. We are finding the manners of addressing that". TASO also intends adding a module on 'communicating with children' to the training curriculum as counsellors and clients have become largely aware of the unmet needs of children.

At present, each of TASO's counsellors is assigned to a zone and is responsible for all the clients inhabiting that zone. They see their clients at the TASO Centre on clinic days, when they come for medical care as well. On non-clinic days the counsellors go on home visits to verify that people who have missed appointments at the Centre are all right, or they accompany nurses and medical assistants visiting bedridden clients as part of a home care team. Besides these duties, the counsellors are expected to mobilise comunities and establish several new volunteer programmes each year, as well as giving ongoing support to volunteer programmes already set up in their zones. Some counsellors are trained in aromatherapy, and offer this service to clients as well.

Most non-governmental organisations (NGOs) caring for people with HIV/AIDS work in close association with staff from government clinics. In South Africa, Hope Worldwide's support groups are based in local clinics, and rely on the nursing staff to provide medical care — at home if necessary and if resources permit — when they reach the limits of their own skills. Similar arrangements are common in other care programmes in Uganda and South Africa. However, government health professionals in these countries lack specialist knowledge and relationship skills in dealing with people with AIDS because these are not part of their training curriculum. In an effort to fill this space, TASO opertes AIDS Care Orienation Workshops for government health professionals to complement their basic training.

Traditional Healers

In her book about her family's struggle with AIDS[2]; Noerine Kaleeba, the founder of TASO, speaks of the frantic search for a local cure when her husband Chris became bedridden. She had the use of a car at the time, and she says: "If I heard that there was a healer in a particular part of Uganda I would drive there and come back with a bottle or jerrycan of preparation. I would go from place to place as people heard of effective healers and preparations. Relatives were bringing medicines by the jerrycan too, and soon there were medicines for wrapping, medicines for sniffing, medicines for drinking, and so on... Chris took all these remedies faithfully alongside the medicines he had been given (in the hospital)."

Traditional healers are the most widely used health practitioners throughout Africa, and the great majority of people with AIDS consult them at some time or another. Yet there has been litle official recognition of their importance within communities or commitment to informing and educating them about HIV and AIDS. "All along training has stopped where the road ends. At last this training is reaching beyond the road, where the real countryside people live," commented a traditional healer in South Africa, where the AIDS Foundation, in collaboration with traditional healers in KwaZulu/Natal, has promoted and recently commenced running workshops with them. Its objectives are to:

(a) increase the impact of AIDS prevention, education and management; and

(b) help trained traditional healers to be accepted within the mainstream health system.

In Uganda in the early 1990s, an expert in sexually transmitted infections based at Kampala's Mulago Hospital, and some colleagues, set up an organisation called Traditional and Modern Practitioners Together against AIDS (THETA), which has conducted research into the effectiveness of traditional herbal medicines and run training programmes. By the end of 1999, some 205 traditional healers from Kampala and several rural districts had been through the programme. In both countries training covers biological aspects of the disease, modes of HIV transmission, prevention, infection control and counselling issues, as well as addressing the relationship between the biomedical and traditional health services, and referral issues.

Despite these initiatives, traditional healers are, by and large, caring for people with HIV infection and AIDS without any support from non-governmental organisations or the statutory health services, and must cope with the stresses of the role and the problem of burnout in their own way.

Stress and Burnout

The Symptoms

Burnout not an "event" but a process in which everyday stresses and anxieties that are not addressed steadily undermine the carer's mental and physical health, so that eventually care-giving and personal relationships suffer. As a medical condition burnout has no clear definition, but as a psychological condition it has been well defined and is increasingly recognised by people in the caring professions. Managers and staff of the AIDS care programmes visited in Uganda and South Africa have discovered a few common features.

"Staff who are not coping will begin to be less punctual in coming to work or keeping appointments," says Tom Kityo, manager of one of TASO's centres in Kampala. The records they keep may demonstrate that they are regularly failing to meet their target or to see the clients assigned to them. Their reports may be handed in late and of poor quality. And they may become withdrawn from their colleagues and less interested in, and sensitive to, their clients.

Pierre Brouard, who works as a counsellor's counsellor in South Africa, says that chronic stress caused by the emotional burden of caring for people with HIV and AIDS typically manifests itself as either over-participation or under-participation on the part of the caregiver. "Over-participation is a kind of flooding response where you get so emotionally connected that you lose all perspective and burn out very quickly. Under-participation, on the other hand, is a withdrawn, unemotional, disconnected manner of working with people. Some of the counsellors get almost brutal, tough, because they get 'compassion fatigue'. I think both are very real dangers with an epidemic of this nature.

"Stress may also manifest itself in physical symptoms such as sleeplessness lethargy, feelings of restlessness and loss of concentration, and perhaps even shaking or tremors, and bowel disturbances", says Pierre Brouard. "Behavioural problems, such as irrationality, mood swings and depression, are frequent too".

Anne Finnegan, director of the Rustenburg branch of Life Line in South Africa, says that a counsellor may suddenly develop an antipathy for either telephone work or face-to-face counselling.

'Loss of trust with some aspect of the work generally tells us something is wrong — there is a problem the counsellor hasn't dealt with in their own life." Mark Ottenweller of Hope Worldwide comments that lack of initiative and enthusiasm, excessive fatigue, frustration, anger, quarrelsomeness and a tendency to complain are generally observed signs of stress, and things he has trained his supervisors to look out for and address before they cause illness.

The Signs

Stress among caregivers in the arena of HIV and AIDS manifests itself in a wide range of signs and symptoms, psychological, behavioural and physical. They include:

(a) loss of interest in and commitment to work;
(b) loss of punctuality and neglect of duties;
(c) feelings of inadequacy, helplessness and guilt;
(d) loss of trust and self-esteem;
(e) a tendency to withdraw — both from clients and from colleagues;
(f) loss of sensitivity in dealing with clients;
(g) loss of quality in performance of work;
(h) irritability;
(i) difficulty getting on with people;
(j) tearfulness;
(k) loss of concentration;
(l) sleeplessness;
(m) excessive fatigue;
(n) depression; and
(o) bowel disturbance.

Many of these feelings are not of themselves unhealthy, but they become so if they are neglected or suppressed and permitted to accumulate.

Talking of their personal experiences of stress, one counsellor in Uganda admitted that she regularly gets to the pitch where her 'brain feels so overloaded' that she cannot cope with another demand made on her, no matter how trivial. Another said that she found developing personal relationships outside her work very hard because she had so little emotional energy left. She would like to get married but did not feel the prospects were good. A counsellor working with HIV-positive mothers and babies commented: 'Some people take so much from you that you feel you are going backwards rather than forwards'. And a community health nurse in Soweto admitted that a year of working in a sexually transmitted diseases (STD) and AIDS clinic almost completely destroyed her interest in sex.

Though volunteer professionals may drop out of an AIDS care programme if stress becomes too great, the drop-out rate is not a good indicator of the levels of stress among staff members simply because, in poor countries, salaried employment is at a premium. Often there is an equilibrium to be struck between stress and monetary survival.

Many of the symptoms of stress discovered among people working for AIDS care programmes reflect exactly those experienced by primary carers looking after people with HIV and AIDS in their own homes and families. But, for those at home, such symptoms are less likely to be discovered and acknowledged, and they are more likely to be isolated with their problems, without easy access to anyone who can assist them find solutions or relief.

The Causes

Much of the stress encountered by cares is in the nature of the work itself—the fact that they are dealing with an incurable condition that kills largely young people and that causes terrible suffering. Moreover, it is a condition that stigmatizes not only infected individuals but very often uninfected people working in the field too. This is known as 'secondary stigma' and it can have a deep impact on the caregiver's status with family, friends and the public at large. But stress may also be caused by organisational factors—the way of care programme is tailored and managed.

Factors of Poverty

A survey by Hope Worldwide among its support group members revealed that food was their single most pressing need. This came as little surprise, for there is a great deal of evidence that monetary difficulties is one of the foremost causes of stress to carers. AIDS is often focussed among the very poor. But even those families who are not already on the margins of survival are swiftly reduced to poverty when the breadwinners are struck down by disease, or forced to give up paid employment or work in the family fields to care for a sick partner or relative.

Elizabeth lives in a neat, comfortable house in Soweto. There is TV and a modern, upholstered three-piece suite in the living room, a glass coffee table with books and a pot plant, and, outside, a neatly-tended garden. But Elizabeth's daughter Betty — a nursing assistant whose wages supported herself, her mother and her two teenage sons — is bedridden with AIDS and suddenly there is no money coming into the home. Elizabeth says there is no food in the house. The boys have stopped asking for bread when they come in from school because they know there is none. And when Betty needs drugs, Elizabeth must first go out to find washing or ironing to do in the neighbourhood, and use what she earns to take the minibus taxi to hospital, to buy the drugs and catch the taxi home.

Josephine, living in a tiny, sweltering shack made of corrugated iron sheets on the treeless plains of Hammanskraal to the north of Pretoria, has always been poor. But now, that she is too weak to find any work, the family is starving. Josephine, sitting at home in the shack she shares with seven others, is so hungry that she regularly loses her temper with her children. And given a bag of apples by the nurse from the home care team who comes to visit, she can hardly bear to share the fruit with her children.

For carers from outside, having to witness day in and day out the struggle of families to meet their most primary needs — for food, rent, medical care, clothes, kids' schooling — can be extremely stressful. 'The messages of TASO about living positively, eating well, looking after your health, can seem cruel when people are struggling to bring in any food to the home', says senior training officer, Hannington Nkayivu. "But in raining our counsellors we emphasise that they must recognise their limitations and make it very clear to their clients that they cannot do everything. Nevertheless, counsellors do feel the strain of expectations because the needs are so great." The director of a home-based care programme in South Africa asks: 'What good does it do to bring pain killers when you find that the caregiver in the household doesn't have the strength to roll the patient over because she is starving?'

The stress is often compounded by the fact that the carers themselves are in an identical circumstances. "It is hard to look after our own families when we are not earning even a cent for this work," said a volunteer in KwaZulu/Natal. 'We go to see hungry people and we are hungry too'. It is common for volunteer and staff carers alike to spend all day in the field visiting clients without anything to eat or drink, because AIDS care programmes on tight budgets rarely give allowances for refreshments. Besides demoralising hunger, volunteers frequently cite lack of money for transport to visit sick clients, or to fetch and pay for drugs, or buy paper and pens for record-keeping, or to fetch and pay for drugs, or buy paper and pens for record-keeping or rubber gloves for handling sick patients, as a major reason of stress because it undermines their ability to do their work and makes them feel inadequate. Sometimes their own families are resentful of the fact that they are working hard for no money. And, in a number of programmes, volunteers admit that partners have walked out on them, or that they themselves have had to leave home due to intense disapproval over their volunteer work.

Making ends meet is often a preoccupation for employees of care programmes, too. In Uganda, wages generally are so low that even professionally qualified people like doctors, nurses teachers and university professors have to do more than one job, or find other ways of supplementing their income, to earn ample to support their families.

Besides the preoccupation with personal hardship, the dependence of AIDS programmes on their donors is a constant background source of stress to many carers. Staff at all levels are often acutely aware of the insecurity of funding — and therefore of their own jobs — because they see organisations working in the same field flounder from time to time as donors change their focus or philosophies, or simply lose commitment.

And when a donor pulls out for whatever reason, a whole tapestry of activities, hopes and expectations unravels. Lucy Nsubuga is coordinator of an AIDS organisation staffed by HIV-positive people in Uganda that recently lost the support of its principal donor with very little warning. There is too little money to continue operating, yet Mrs Nsubuga cannot give up hope and dismiss her staff. 'They thought they were useful when they went out to the people, shared their life experience and counselled them. People identified with them. Now they are sitting at home', she says. 'Sometimes they can come to do proposal writing or to examine our training materials, but it is difficult when you don't know what is going to happen. And most of the time we are redundant, because most of our work is in going to the field with people with HIV/AIDS. Also it causes problems in the family. Husbands or wives ask: if you are not getting a salary, why are you going to work? What's the point? But if they stop coming, people will think they have resigned. So, they are puzzled and very much demoralised.'

AIDS care programmes are at the mercy, too, of government policy-makers who can change the rules for donating to non-governmental organisations. In Uganda, for example, food handouts have been the mainstay of many carer support programmes. News that the government was considering imposing tax on food aid from abroad led recently to the drying-up of free food supplies to one of the most widely respected home-based care programmes in Uganda, and the undermining of its activities and staff morale. Moreover, as of late 1999, NGOs were concerned that new rules being considered by the government would mean that donor funds could no longer be paid direct to individual organisations, but must be channelled through government structures.

More Work, Little Time

'There's so much to do and so little time to do it'. 'Time is very squeezed'. "If you are not careful, this job can take over your whole life." These comments from TASO staff in Uganda underline a root cause of stress in AIDS care programmes everywhere—overwork. The pressure to overwork may come from outside, when carers are set what they consider daunting targets by their managers or supervisors. A common feeling among professionals of care programmes is that pressure to achieve certain targets or population coverage comes primarily from donors, and failure to achieve them may cause the donors to withdraw support for the programme. Lack of control over the process of target-setting compounds the anxiety for carers.

Alternatively, pressure to overwork comes from inside—from individuals failing to recognise what is feasible and do-able in the face of overwhelming need, and pushing themselves beyond their own limits. Staff in several programmes admitted they regularly feel unable to take their annual leave because there is too much to be done. Though some programmes insist on staff taking the time off they are allowed, in others their sacrifice is gratefully acknowledged by their supervisors.

However, cutting back on vital rest and recreation time is not always a matter of personal option. In Uganda, TASO used to hold regular retreats for counsellors and health teams which were greatly appreciated as an acknowledgement of the complicables of their work as well as an opportunity to recharge batteries. But these have been curtailed for the time being as an unjustifiable expense. "It's a reality that outside donors are not really concerned with staff welfare matters—they are more interested in how many clients can be reached for the amount of money they give", commented a senior staff member.

A few carers say that the regular training courses they are offered by their programmes can be a double-edged sword. While they greatly appreciate the opportunities to upgrade their skills, it can mean they find themselves with additional tasks and responsibilities to fit into their working day. The job descriptions that staff members are given at the start of their contracts generally offer little protection. A counsellor with one programme commented, smiling: "Our job description is very open. It even states at the end of the prescribed duties: '... and any other tasks that may be necessary'!"

Volunteers too, feel the pressure of expectations from their communities. One of the most common requests from volunteers at meetings, said a supervisor from World Vision is how to manage their time effectively so that they don't become overwhelmed. "They tell us: 'People come and ask for my help even when I'm digging my fields.' Or `My neighbours knock on my door at any hour of the night'."

At the family level, caring for a sick person can leave little or no time for anything else — for paid work or food production, or for school if the carer is a child—and it is this that pushes families over the edge into destitution.

The Disclosure

"Our survey last year revealed that about half our support group members had disclosed their HIV status to their families, about half had not—that raises grave problems," said Mark Ottenwellet.

The isue of disclosure is especially problematic in South Africa because the stigma HIV and AIDS is still so strong that infected individuals risk serious discrimination or even physical harm if they disclose their serostatus. Moreover, there is a tendency to apportion blame: AIDS is known by many people as "the woman's disease" — a tendency encouraged by the fact that HIV infection rates found at antenatal clinics are used as prime indicators of the scale of the epidemic and are frequently quoted and the fact that most families only find out HIV is among them when a young woman becomes pregnant and goes for health care. But even in Uganda, where stigma is no longer so strong infected people still find it hard to tell family and friends that they are HIV positive. "You come out at your own risk," comments one young woman who works as a counsellor is Uganda. "It's not easy living with HIV. (Once you have disclosed your status) you are never treated the same again. You are always someone with the virus first and foremost."

The failure to disclose their status makes the task of caring for people with AIDS very difficult. A wife or husband caring for a sick partner, or a mother caring for a son or daughter who is wasting away before her eyes or persecuted by a secret he or she will not share, may suspect the problem is AIDS. But these family carers will be handicapped by uncertainty and inability to seek information and help openly. Or they may have no suspicion, and be left to care as best they can with a situation they do not understand. AIDS is an isolating disease anyway; secrecy makes it doubly so, and compounds feelings of helplessness and despair in primary carers.

For carers coming into the family from outside, the burdens or privacy are equally heavy. Unless a client has confided in a family member, the visiting caregiver cannot easily pass on knowledge or health care skills to anyone else and must carry responsibility alone. If I go to a house and find that no one knows, the person is all alone with the secret, I think to myself 'I'm too far away to help you,' and I worry too much about them," says Catherine, an AIDS care worker in Soweto. Jovah, a counsellor with TASO in Uganda, says: "If we get consent from the client, we prepare the family for what to expect and for the eventual end." But if the client has not told anyone, the home care team can do nothing to make death easier for the family.

Secrecy and widespread fear of revelation means that carers sometimes have to operate under false pretences. Either the word AIDS remains a strict taboo with patients and carers alike, as in a home-based care programme in the South African mining town of Carletonville where volunteers take over the care of terminally ill patients when the hospital can do no more for them. Between March and July 1998, the programme buried 40 people, most of them very young women, without anyone acknowledging openly the disease they were dealing with. In KwaZulu/Natal the Sinosizo programme, wishing to avoid being handicapped by the stigma of AIDS, has taken steps to be associated with others in need of home-based care as well, such as elderly people and cancer patients.

The issue of disclosing to children is particularly stress-laden for all concerned — sick parents, carers within the home and those coming in from outside. In neither South Africa nor Uganda is there a tradition of talking with children as equals and on an intimate basis. But carers have become increasingly aware of the suffering of children, who are too often hovering in the shadows of a sick room, seeing and hearing everything but never addressed directly. "We have this huge problem with children being excluded from the counselling all over the place. And some of them are so badly traumatized," says Liz Towell of Sinosizo. "Of course bereavement is part of life and they have to go through all that. But we've seen a lot of complicated grief, prolonged grief, and those are things that are not all right. Some of the children become mute with emotional trauma. We try to do the best we can, but it is not good enough."

Another particularly distressing aspect of secrecy for carers is when they find belatedly that one of their own colleagues has been living with HIV for a long time without telling anyone. The person begins to fall sick and the secret is disclosed. Typically colleagues react with feelings of hurt that he or she was not able to trust them, and feelings of sadness and inadequacy because they, whose special expertise is in giving comfort and suport, were not asked for help.

Commenting on why someone trained to care for people with AIDS, and therefore to be at ease with the disease, might be unable to disclose infection in themselves, psychologist Pierre Brouard said: "There's anxiety about disclosure because one of the things disclosure does is to take away a certain sense of control. 'I don't have control over who you subsequently tell, or how you see me. You may see me now as an ailing person, a dying person, a sick person.' And that perception change can be very difficult." A person who has become used to being a source of strength to others can find it extremely hard to reveal their own vulnerability. Moreover, they may have feelings of failure that they have been unable to practise in their own lives what they advise their clients.

Too Close for Comfort

In a country where almost no family is unaffected by AIDS, it is extremely difficult for carers to achieve professional detachment from their clients, or from the job itself. For most people it is not even possible to shut the door on AIDS at the end of the working day because they go home to care for relatives or friends, or children whose parents have died. The tendency to find themselves becoming over-involved is very real and the risks of stress and burnout as a consequence are high.

"When you work with a client you build up trust and closeness, and soon you begin to love them and they begin to love you. The relationship goes beyond the professional barriers", comments Hannington Nkayivu. "You get so close to a person, and then seeing them die in the end is very distressing." In Uganda, he explains setting professional barriers is specially difficult since the extended family system means that a person is rarely a stranger in a village or community. 'From your name people can see what clan you are from, and there is always someone to whom you are associated by clan'.

The pressure to become over-involved comes also from the intense neediness of infected people who tend to be isolated with their fears and suffering, without many people to turn to "Lay carers, especially, can feel easily manipulated by clients — that it is their job to take a patient to a clinic if they cannot get there themselves, or give them a bus fare if they have not got the money, or find a sandwich for a hungry person," says Pierre Brouard. "When you are faced with those real issues it is difficult to resist, to walk away from people."

Sometimes, the stress of over-involvement comes from the caregiver developing expectations of the client, and feeling a sense of personal failure or disappointment when advice is not heeded. For example, many carers admitted finding it difficult to cope with the news that an HIV-positive woman whom they had been counselling had become pregnant, putting the health of herself, her partner and her unborn baby at risk.

Carers interviewed recognised a number of other common stresses related to over-involvement. These include:

* inability to be there for their clients when they need them;
* inability to meet even the most pressing needs, such as the need for food or drink;
* feelings of inadequacy and sometimes guilt when they can do no more to help a person;
* feelings of loss and sadness at the death of a client; and
* lasting anxieties about the family members left behind, especially children.

For carers who are themselves HIV-positive, stress is a risk not only of getting too close to client but of personal recognition with a client's illness and impending death. Lucky Mazibuko is an HIV-positive man who writes a weekly column in a popular South African newspaper to try to dispel the silence and myths about AIDS. After seeing a man who was dying of AIDS, whose eyes looked huge in his emaciated frame, Mazibuko commented: "I could see myself in that man's battered body."

For the HIV-positive person, caring for someone else with the disease can be like looking into a mirror, says Catherine, a member of Hope Worldwide's suport groups in Soweto. "When I see other people with AIDS, I think to myself: am I going to be like that? It's so intimidating. At the family level, says TASO's director Sophia Mukasa-Monico, it is not uncommon for an infected wife or husband caring for a terminally ill partner to give up hope. "They say: after all, I'm going to go through the same thing, and who's going to look after me when my time comes?"

The Organisational Environment

A common cause of stress in the working environment, rather than in the work itself, is lack of communication between carers and their managers. Often, people say, the channels of communication are there, but they are not effective: their voices are either not heard or not heeded. Sometimes people feel they are given inadequate time to consider a policy issue before they have to comment, and decisions are made, simply because other business crowds it out until the deadline looms. Sometimes they give considered and strongly held views that are not represented in the decisions that are finally taken, and they are not given feedback or an explanation. A common feeling, in particular, in Uganda, is that carers lack any voice at the level of the donors, where they trust their work targets are being set without real understanding of what their work entails.

Volunteers working out in the community are particularly vulnerable to feelings of isolation and powerlessness in their work. A related issue is that of adequate training and preparation for the work carers are expected to do. "If your carers are not equipped to help people on many levels, you are sending them out into a minefield and they are going to get hurt', says Mark Otenweller. 'We concentrate on giving our people as broad a training and as much support as we can because they are our biggest resource'.

Counsellors working in centres rather than out in the field lack of adequate space to see clients in privacy as a source of stress. Administrative necessities, such as keeping records and writing reports, can also lead to stress if there is nowhere to which they can retreat to write them, or not enough time budgeted in their working schedule. Under such conditions, maintaining morale is an Herculean task.

Whether working in the community or in an institution, carers need to know there is someone they can turn to for guidance with a difficult case or just to confirm that they are doing things right, says Desiree, an AIDS counsellor with Life Line in South Africa. Carers also need to feel they have the authority to do what needs doing if they feel competent. Before joining Life Line, Desiree was working in a similar position at a hospital run by a mining house, but was extremely frustrated. 'At the hospital I always felt I wanted to learn and do more, and we were very much conrolled', she recalls. 'I think it is important to give a person responsibility for making their own decisions, and a chance to show initiative'.

The degree of authority and responsibility a carer is given depends to a great extent on their status within the organisation. This also affects the relative power they will have in decision-making and the priority given to their own needs. Herein lies a paradox. In both Uganda and South Africa, counsellors seem to be greatly respected by their clients and to have a high status within the community. Yet they are often comparatively powerless within the organisations for which they work.

"There are in fact many settings where the counsellor is valued but the actual counselling — in the sense of a professional set of skills that necessitate expertise and training—is undervalued in some way," says Pierre Brouard. "I think defining a clear area of competenc is a real difficulty with this work. It is almost as if there's a sense that `anybody can do it'— anybody who is in a relationship with a patient or client can do it. No way does it have the same status as doing a clinical examination." Lack of recognition and professional status are, he believes, root causes of why counsellors' own needs for care and support are too often given low priority within organisations.

Family Affairs: A Major Challenge

AIDS can have a severe impact on personal relationships and the equilibrium of power within families, which is a reason of stress to primary carers as well as to people offering assistance from outside the family. While the infected person is cast into a whirlpool of emotions and struggles to adjust to life with the virus, other family members are forced to encounter the implications of the diagnosis for themselves. Perhaps it means that a person has been unfaithful, in which case the other partner may feel anger, betrayal and fear that they too are infected. Perhaps parents are forced to recognise that a son or daughter in whom they invested great hopes is going to die without fulfilling them, and may be leaving grandchildren to be cared for as well. Or perhaps a child is encountered with the loss of one parent and fears that the other parent might be infected too.

Jackie, a mother of three children in Uganda who is HIV positive, remembers caring for her sick husband while coping with intense feelings of betrayal. "I just hoped at the time I found out we were both positive that he would be strong enough to receive my anger", she says. But he was already very weak and needed my help. So I did not have anybody to vent my anger on—I just had to be the simple wife and look after him. Sometimes I would look at him who was so vulnerable and realise that my anger would be a waste of time, it would be adding pain to the physical pain he was having. So I think I forgave him somehow. Jackie's feelings settled into deep depression after her husband died. For two years she was unable to return to the village to visit his grave.

Many carers state the difficulty, and sometimes personal pain, of looking after sick relatives who are moody, uncooperative and even hostile at finding themselves so vulnerable and dependent. But as a counsellor with TASO and an HIV-positive woman whose own health is deteriorating, Christine sees two faces of the same coin. "Being a patient can be hard", she comments. "I feel hurt sometimes when people show concern. You can be angry at being weak. And when you get very sick you can get disgusted with yourself and stop feeling there is any reason to care for yourself any more. I think it is important to help carers to understand the range of feelings of the patient, to advise them not to force care on a patient if they don't want it — especially when the end is coming. You must accept when the end is there."

Christine nursed her husband when he was terminally ill with AIDS and remembers him being in such pain that he wept. 'I didn't know a man could cry like that and I was shocked', she says. 'And I was fearful — I realized he was in pain and I didn't know what to do. He was rude to his mother because he saw her being unkind to me. And he was rude to all of us at the end, because he was fearful. When you are heading for death you are heading for the unknown, and it is intimidating'.

However, it is not always the sick person who is uncooperative and hostile. Latisa Mabe, coordinator of Hope Worldwide's programme in Soweto, says that relatives often believe a positive HIV test means imminent death, and they may withdraw from the infected person and neglect their needs until they have understood what it is they are in fact encountering. "I have been into homes where the husband just sat there and motioned to another room when we visited, saying: 'she is in there'. And you would find a very sick woman just waiting for us to come and help her, she says. Alternatively, families may become fatalistic. TASO's director, Sophia Mukasa Monico, says that the attitude that a sick relative is not capable of spending time and money on because they are going to die anyway is not uncommon.

Carers often require help and support in understanding and learning to deal with their own feelings as well as those of the sick person, expressed a World Vision staff member.

The Causes of Stress and Burnout

Some of the generally reported causes of stress and burnout among staff and volunteers working with AIDS care programmes are:

* monetary hardship;
* stigma related to HIV and AIDS;
* secrecy and fear of revelation among people with AIDS;
* oppressive workloads;
* over-involvement with people with AIDS and their families;
* personal recognition with the suffering of people with AIDS;
* fear of infection;
* the reality that AIDS is incurable;
* unmet needs of children;
* lack of space and confidentiality in work environment;
* lack of an effective voice in decisions that affect them and their work;

* too little autonomy or responsibility;
* lack of scope for initiative;
* inadequate support and supervision;
* inadequate training, skills and preparation for the work;
* lack of clarity about what the caregiver is expected to do;
* lack of referral mechanisms;
* lack of medication and health care materials;
* lack of recognition for their work; and
* lack of mutual respect or liking between caregiver and client.

Many items on this list are reasons of stress to carers at the family level also. Besides these, they might suffer from:

* isolation:
* the effect of HIV and AIDS on personal relationships and family dynamics;
* insecurity and fear for the future;
* difficulty in communicating with children; and
* difficulty in facing bereavement.

Managing Stress and Burnout: The Options

Personal Coping Techniques

Religious faith is a major source of comfort to several people in Uganda and South Africa. "I talk to God, pray or read my Bible," is often the first thing a caregiver will mention when asked how they cope personally with the stress of their work. But there are other widespread coping strategies that carers employ too. `I make a point of not talking about AIDS when I get home in the evening', said one lone mother who works for a care programme. Another reserves one day every week which she devotes entirely to her family. One South African remarked: "I always tell clients I'll do my best but that I can't do more than that. There are innumerable limitations out there that you have to find a way of not letting things get you down. Anyway, we know what it is to have needs and not get what we want — our background (in the apartheid period) has taught us not to have too high expectations'.

An elderly woman stated how, when nursing her two sons with AIDS, she learnt to anticipate stressful events and to plan ahead. She kept a suitcase full of fresh clothes and bed sheets in case her sons developed uncontrollable diarrhoea and there would be no time to search for things needed to keep them clean and maintain their dignity. A counsellor in Uganda explained that, if she is feeling overwhelmed, she will explain to a client politely that she cannot see them at that time and make another appointment. "If someone has grievance we sit down and talk it through then and there", said the supervisor of a care team in South Africa. "If necessary we say sorry to each other, if we've caused hurt or upset, then we start all over again. It's an African convention to talk things through — to determine problems in the *khotla* or the *indaba*'.

It is just these kind of strategies that Pierre Brouard tries to encourage in his training courses for counsellors. "I often say to trainees that the needs out there are like a hole in a bucket," he says "You can be pouring all your compassion and work into the bucket and it'll just go on pouring out. That is not to make them feel helpless or useless, but to make them have a certain sense of perspective — that if you stop pouring for 10 minutes it is not going to make a difference. A central message in our stress management sessions is that, to an extent, you have to take responsibility for yourselves. You cannot wait for someone else to come and say to you: stop and take a break.

Approaches to Deal with Stress

Though they share some common features, the programmes visited have a variety of approaches of dealing with stress and burnout among their staff and volunteer carers. This discussion will look at them in context, concentrating on those that are most imaginative and most likely to be applicable elsewhere.

The AIDS Support Organisation (TASO)

TASO gives high priority to the salaries of counsellors in drawing up its budget. At present they are paid about twice as much as government employees with commensurate academic qualifications. Counselling is one of the most demanding jobs a carer can do and, besides showing them that they are valued, TASO is keen to relieve counsellors of the stress of exploring for secondary sources is also a way of ensuring that people in whom

TASO has invested valuable time and effort in training are not easily lured away by other employers.

Income-generating programmes for its clients are also considered an important strategy for relieving the stress of families made poor by AIDS. But TASO has had mixed results. 'Our clients tend to be among the very poorest people in Uganda', explains Sophia Mukasa Monico. 'And when you give money to anyone who is very poor, the first thing they do is take care of their primary needs. You cannot think of generating income when you in fact do not have anything to start off with.'

After examining the situation, the organisation has decided to hive off this important activity to a separate organisation 'TASO 2', which can give it the undivided attention it needs. And it intends varying the paradigm from one in which making profit is the objective to one in which 'making a difference' — simply improving the standard of living within the home — is the important objective. This means, for example, that a family may be assisted through skills training and perhaps a grant to increase food production on their land so that they can eat twice instead of once a day. But training and loans will also be available to people wanting to commence small business enterprises. 'We intend working with groups so that they can assist each other and take collective responsibility for repaying the loans,' explains Sophia Mukasa Monico. 'We want to involve clients' family members too so that when a client dies the family's source of income would not collapse.'

For its staff carers TASO has instituted several measures to minimise stress and the risk of burnout. The organisation has promoted a culture of talking and sharing problems, in regular and frequent meetings between care teams and their supervisors, in workshops which bring management and staff together to discuss matters, and in inculcating the feeling that TASO is a 'family'. Respect for the principle of confidentiality between staff members as much as between staff and clients means that people can feel safe in admitting stress and seeking assistance, even if some do still find it hard to show vulnerability. During their preliminary training, counsellors are motivated to identify someone among their peers as a personal counsellor.

Members of staff who are sick continue to receive their salaries when they are unable to work, and will receive a further year's salary if they resign voluntarily due to ill health. TASO's director intends to introduce a policy whereby at least two children of a sick staff member are supported through school and even university. Another new idea for stress management is meditation. A teacher of meditation will shortly be joining TASO as a volunteer for six months, to observe the work of the carers and devise a programme of training them in meditation, which is hoped to become a routine part of the working day.

Mildmay International

The Mildmay Centre is located on a hillside on the outskirts of Kampala. Innumerable low brick buildings connected by covered walkways through bright gardens, Mildmay was opened in September 1998 as a referral centre to which severely ill patients can be sent by other institutions or programmes which can do no more to help them. It is a centre of excellence in palliative care, particularly the management of pain, which it offers on an outpatient basis. But, besides providing hands-on care, the Mildmay Centre's prominent function is as a resource for training others in the care of people with AIDS, offering advanced nursing and specialist skills, like pain management, that are rare but much expanding care, and to expanding the capacity to care effectively,' explains the director of clinical services, Dr Catherine Sozi. Both TASO and World Vision regularly take advantage of its training courses.

The Centre runs 'carers' workshops' every month at which its multidisciplinary team — representing medicine, nursing, child care, physiotherapy, occupational therapy, dietary advice, counselling and spiritual care — addresses every problem carers want to raise. 'We find that what most carers want is advice on how to deal with what they call 'difficult' patients — the patient who does not seem to appreciate what they are doing for them; the patient who is in distress and they do not know what to do; the patient with wounds; the patient who does not eat. And many are scared of dealing with the inevitable — which is facing end-of-life issues. So the workshops give them a forum', explains Dr. Sozi.

In association with the Ministry of Health, Mildmay has taken its "carers' workshops" to suburban and slum areas of Kampala, and has recently commenced running them in rural areas, too. Recognising the special and neglected needs of children, Mildmay runs separate workshops for different categories of people looking after children with HIV and AIDS — that is, one for health professionals, and one each for mothers and fathers. "We are planning to run workshops for schoolteachers, too," says Dr. Sozi. "They have told us: we have these children, they look so small, they are off sick the whole time and we do not know how to communicate with them".

Mildmay is at the forefront of teaching people how to communicate with children, both infected and affected. Christine, who has two young daughters, attended one of the Centre's "Positive Mothers" training courses and says it dramatically improved her relationship with her children, bringing them all very close. "I used to be rough with the children — ordering them to do this and that, and telling them to be quiet and stop asking questions. I did not want to tell them about my HIV status", she admits. "But I learnt at Mildmay that children need to know the truth, and that they need kindness and persuasion to talk. I learnt that they get depressed if they are left out, and that they get angry and resentful and then they are uncooperative because they are unhappy. In our training we were given the skills for communicating with our kids". Christine has, in turn, run workshops at her own TASO centre to pass on the skills she learnt at Mildmay.

To overcome the issue of stress among its own staff — who care for some of the most desperately ill AIDS patients, many of them children, at the end of their lives — Mildmay has engaged the services of an independent therapist from the institute of psychology at Makerere University to offer them individual counselling. She attends the centre once a fortnight. Mildmay's practice of working as an interdisciplinary team is itself an effective way of protecting staff from undue stress because it spreads the burden of care and responsibility.

Aware of the heavy demands of the Centre's work, Dr. Sozi believes in the value of taking time off and has set up a culture of respect for weekends and annual leave — no one is permitted to give up their free time lightly. Staff have their health and medical expenses covered, and these advantages are extended to up to four blood-related children, too.

World Vision

World Vision is well established in Uganda, carrying a wide range of developed programmes in 21 districts at present. The organisation commenced working with AIDS-affected communities in 1989 and, aware of the uniquely stressful nature of caring for people with HIV and AIDS, it has promoted a broad range of support techniques for carers at all levels. Primary carers are offered counselling, and primary training in health care. The organisation also makes them aware of the range of resources available and how to access them. And it offers them income-generating programmes to help them cope monetarily. Income-generation projects generally involve groups of people working together. "These have a value beyond simply helping people cope monetarily," explains Robinah Babirye. "Doing some activity as a group affords people the opportunity to talk and give each other mutual support. It can have a real impact on their emotions."

Support for its volunteers is given especially high priority by World Vision. To preserve their morale, the organisation tries to display its appreciation of their work as often as possible. It makes a point of acknowledging their presence and contribution and formally introducing them at every community gathering. It recognises, too, that volunteers' responsibilities often leave them little time for working their *shambas*, and that, as with primary carers, loss of food production and the encounters to feed their families cause great anxiety. World Vision therefore brought so that they could produce food more efficiently and with less effort. It provided an extra day's training at the end of their seminars, and was surprised at how ready people were to spend the extra time. At present World Vision has a system of "model farmers" whereby a few people, specially trained and using their own *shambas* as demonstration plots, act as a catalyst for training others in the community — especially families made poor by AIDS — who want to learn how to increase the output from their land.

Recognising the importance of knowledge and skills to self-respect, social status and confidence. World Vision devotes a large part of its budget to training programmes, alongwith refresher courses for volunteers and staff, and upgrading of skills. It also believes in flexibility and giving people as much scope for initiative as possible. "In World Vision, if you can defend your position and convince them of your viewpoint, you are permitted to do things your way," says Gladys Rukidi. "And if you need something from them, they will cooperate if they have the money to do so."

World Vision is aware of the risk of burnout in its staff, and regular retreats in which they are able to get away entirely from their normal work environment and spend time in structured Bible study and prayer, or simply relaxing and having fun, are one answer to this. The retreats inculcate a family spirit in which people can talk freely and share their problems—a spirit that is encouraged by the policy of using first names for everyone at all times, and no titles, says Robinah Babirye. Retreats are a tradition in TASO too, but, to the dismay of many counsellors, they have recently been suspended in some centres because they are considered an unjustifiable expense.

With HIV so widespread in Uganda, the probability of infection among staff members is high. To minimise anxiety about the cost of falling ill, World Vision has policy of reimbursing health care fees of up to 30 000 shillings (approx. US$ 21) a month for each staff member. "When it became clear that some sick people were needing more than this to cover their expenses and others were never using their allowances," said Robinah Babirye, "the staff had a meeting at which they agreed to pool the allowance. This way, there is more money for those who need it most".

Life Line

Life Line South Africa, inspired by a similar organisation in Australia, was set up in 1968 as a counselling service for people facing some kind of personal problem or crisis. As HIV infection has taken off in South Africa, Life Line's counsellors are finding themselves increasingly involved in helping people affected by the epidemic. At present, as well as doing telephone and face-to-face counselling, Life Line trains community volunteers who work in innumerable settings, such as clinics and schools. Their skills are broadly acclaimed, and Life Line is frequently called upon to train counsellors for other organisations, too.

Training commences with a "personal growth" course lasting 8-10 weeks. This is followed by an equally long course in communication skills and counselling, in which the issue of stress and how to cope with it is given special attention. "We impress upon counsellors the importance of looking after themselves, pointing out that if they permit themselves to get sick or burnt out they will be unable to help anyone," explains Anne Finnegan, director of one of Life Line's branches.

She narrates an exercise called 'Life is a Choice' used during training to bring home this truth. Working in groups of 7-10 people, trainees are asked to imagine themselves going on a special trip. They build a picture together of the destination and how they are travelling there, imagining themselves on a coach, a train, a boat or a plane. Then the facilitator informs the group that their chosen transport has crashed and all but three people have been killed. Each person in the group is asked to imagine he or she is one of the survivors and to argue their case before the others. Finally, everyone is asked to vote on who should survive and is given three pieces of paper to write down their individual options before reading them out to the group. "Only very rarely does someone vote for himself or herself with one of the three votes," comments Anne Finnegan. "Of course most people feel that it would be selfish to vote for themselves, and that selflessness and sacrifice are heavenly virtues. But in the discussion afterwards they are made aware of the fact that you have to be strong and healthy — and alive — to be able to help others," explains Finnegan. "Then we bring the focus back to HIV and ask.: how can you take care of another person if you do not take care of yourself?"

Once they are working in the field, the relationship with their supervisors is of prime importance in maintaining their health and morale, says Anne Finnegan. Counsellors working within Life Line are necessitated to fill in a debriefing form after every session with a client. The forms do not record the names of the clients, nor detailed narrations of their stories, since their primary purpose is to permit supervisors to monitor the counsellors' performance and state of mind. Counsellors are asked about their own emotional state at the end of a session, and where they felt they were most effective and most ineffective in their performance. "Entries such as 'I felt exhausted — this session was not in my diary' or 'I am unhappy about how fast time goes' are good indications of the strains of the job," comments Anne Finnegan. "We try to make sure counsellors do not get to the state of burnout. We look after each other at Life Line before we look after the community, because if we do not we cannot look after the community."

Hope Worldwide

"Rather than a single trauma that you have to work through, the traumas our people encounter are more like waves of the occean that keep rolling in to shore," comments Mark Ottenweller, the director of Hope Worldwide. "With the constant stresses on our counsellors, it is very important that we provide ongoing support and supervision so that they would not be agitated".

"The key to minimising stress and preventing burnout," says Ottenweller, "is to disperse the emotional burden". Hope ensures that no single caregiver is left sitting for long time with a sick or dying person by drawing in a large circle of people to do the caring. These may include members of the immediate family, the extended family, the support group or church volunteers. And in order to protect his staff from the deep impact of the epidemic as much as possible, Dr. Ottenweller makes sure there is variety in their duties so they do not get bored or too deeply involved in any one activity.

Another key to minimising stress on carers at all levels is to generate a widely supportive environment. This means networking, exploring and accessing local resources of all sorts, and creating mutually advantageous partnerships with others in the community. Hope's programme in Soweto is focussed on community health clinics, which provide accommodation for the support group activities, land for their vegetable gardens and medication, while Hope provides condoms, food, counselling and support to people with HIV/AIDS in the area served by the clinic. The organisation has enlisted support from local food retailers who donate food near the end of its shelf-life to the programme for its AIDS-affected families. And it has tapped into the volunteer network of one of the biggest local churches, whose members assist Hope's support groups in caring for sick individuals and families when the need arises.

Hope's staff also keep themselves uptodate with information regarding health, social welfare and legal matters. "When I visit a family at home," explains one of the coordinators, "I sit down with them and discuss all the resources available to them and give contact names and telephone numbers if possible. I talk to them about where to go with legal barriers like discrimination against an infected person, and what their rights are under welfare and human rights legislation. And I advise them on how to apply for the advantages they are entitled to."

Hope also helps organise income-generating projects for its support groups. Like TASO and others, it recognises that these are much needed but hard to set up successfully, so the organisation seeks expert advice, as necessary, on running small businesses and marketing. "Income generation takes patience and persistence to develop," says Mark Ottenweller. The vegetable gardens planted in the clinic grounds are supposed to bring in little income, but yields are unpredictable and they mostly just complement the diets of support group members.

The vegetable gardens are one answer to the need for food, which came top of the list in recent support group survey. "The surveys, carried out each year together with an evaluation of Hope's services, are important for monitoring the welfare and performance of carers," says Mark Ottenweller. "You have to have constant input from your clients, your community and your coordinators to sort out what your problems are and where people were experiencing difficulties."

Sinosizo

Sinosizo means "We Help" in the Zulu language. The home-based care programme commenced in the early 1990s under the auspices of the Catholic Archdiocese of Durban, but it is not church affiliated, "We have a spiritual dimension in that people are dying, people are intimidated, people are coming to terms with their own being, and so they need spiritual support, and that is clear," explains the director, Liz Towel. "But it does not have to be Catholic, or any denomination; it does not have to be church at all."

Sinosizo's primary objective is to strengthen the communities with which it works to care for their own people with AIDS. The function of its four staff members, who are all professional nurses with specialist skills in palliative care, is to train and supervise the teams of volunteers working at community level.

For volunteers to be effective they must have credibility, authority and status in the community. It is Sinosizo's policy, therefore, that none of its supervisors wear uniforms that might recognise them as professional nurses. Liz Towell explains: "If you put a nurse in a uniform in the community, the volunteer will have no status at all. Instantly! The family will say: `We want the nurse back'. So there is nothing to distinguish our supervisors as nurses. And when there are in the field with the volunteers they are not permitted to give hands-on care themselves — their job is to supervise."

The supervisor's job is also to introduce volunteers to staff at the local clinic and to promote good working relationships. "These are crucial to the success of home-based care for AIDS patients, but establishing mutual respect is not always easy — it can be fraught with suspicion, insecurities and turf rivalry. Here the supervisor's professional qualifications and rank are significant," says Liz Towell. Whereas a volunteer with little formal education might have great difficulty approaching or gaining the acceptance of health staff, the supervisor will automatically be recognised and respected at par. And having her support always in the background gives confidence to volunteers.

However, developing self-reliance in its volunteer teams is important to Sinosizo, since many of them work in remote areas beyond the reach of good roads and telephones, and the supervisors, are few. Volunteers generally work in pairs, when doing their home visits. This is primarily a matter of security: the townships and rural villages of KwaZulu/Natal have been rocked by sporadic political violence over recent years. But working in pairs also means that volunteers give each other moral support and share the emotional burden of care. In addition to promoting strong bonds with the team, the key to self-reliance and self-confidence, says Liz Towell, is to let things develop in their own time and to resist the pressure from donors to set inflexible timetables for the achievement of objectives. "If you rush volunteers, the programme will fail," she says. "If you let things happen in Africa Time, they will in reality work well."

Sinosizo's core donor, Caritas, has taken a deep interest in the programme and spent time with staff in the field. "They see every area we work in; they see the terrain that people are walking up and down; they see the level of education our volunteers have, they have a possibility to speak to whoever they want. So they leave with a crystal clear vision, and as a result it has made life so much easier for us, it in fact has."

Record-keeping is an important activity at Sinosizo, and literate volunteers who wish are given a two-day training course. Liz Towell has a record card for every patient, which she enters onto a computerised database and which includes details of dependants; support systems, if any; whether there are children at risk of being orphaned, the patient's monetary status who is looking after them as primary carer; as well as details of their medical condition. "At all times I can look and see exactly where the patients are, who is looking after them and how many patients each volunteer has, how many deaths they have encountered and how many orphaned children they have in their area," she says "For me it is a monitoring technique to make sure we are not overloading anybody emotionally. It also helps to have the data so that you can see where the growth areas are and where you might need to recruit more volunteers. You would not necessarily know if you did not have a database."

Constant Commitment to Good Schemes : Mentoring Programme for Counsellors

There are no records of the number of people involved in counselling in South Africa, nor of the drop-out rate, but there is tremendous anecdotal evidence that counselling is an unstable profession. Experience demonstrates that burnout and the decision to quit are often the result of lack of support once a trained counsellor gets out into the field. The HIV/AIDS Directorate in South Africa's Department of Health decided, therefore, to establish a mentoring programme.

Mentors, explained Thembela Kwitshana who devised the programme, are people with counselling skills and long experience themselves who look after counsellors working on the forefront. They are different from supervisors in that their responsibility is the welfare of the counsellors, not the quality or style of their work. "Supervisors often take on this role too, but there can be a conflict of interests, so that a counsellor may realise that her job will be on the line if she admits to the supervisor that she is struggling or has done something wrong, said Ms Kwitshana. "However with a mentor the counsellor should have absolute trust and know she can discuss any of their professional problems without feeling she is threatening her position." In addition, the job of a mentor is to be an advocate for counsellors' rights at every level, from the government to the organisations and institutions for which they work.

The programme was conceived in 1995, and the initial plan was to train people put forward by the provincial administrations, who would then employ them to support the counsellors in all organisations across the province. It was piloted successfully in KwaZulu/Natal, where four mentors were trained and subsequently provided support to a total of 900 counsellors across the province who came together regularly in small groups at a time, at local hospitals nearest to their places of work. They would spend some hours with the mentor, going over cases, discussing work-related issues and problems and perhaps having an expert give a talk on some relevant subject.

In KwaZulu/Natal the mentors were paid by the province but were seconded to the local non-governmental AIDS Training and Information Centres (ATICs), which had good contacts in the field. It was an inexpensive programme because of using hospital premises, said Ms Kwitshana. But it collapsed very suddenly when the budget for paying the mentors ran out after a year and their contracts were curtailed. It was a bitter blow to all who had invested so much hope and energy in the programme—and especially so since it was just about to be launched nationally.

"But I do not give up," commented Ms Kwitshana. "I try to understand why progress is slow, and see if there are ways round the barriers." Today she is working on the idea of bypassing local government and training mentors to work directly for a whole range of organisations. The new programme will offer training to people who are already working as nurses or counsellors or are in some other relevant profession, and who are therefore already receiving a salary from the hospital or NGO for which they work. She is aware of the danger that they might not have time to devote to another task, or to be able to keep up the commitment. But this is the best way at present of continuing with a programme which was already proved its worth, and Ms Kwitshana says she will address problems if and when they arise.

The Ark: Looking After South Africa's 'Shadow People'

The Ark is a barracks of a place standing among graceful but abandoned colonial buildings in Durban's old dockland area. Once a hostel of stevedores, it is now a shelter for destitute people and home to a thousand men, women and children at any time. These are South Africa's 'shadow people', says Alan, a resident who came to The Ark five years ago as an alcoholic who had lost his family, his friends and his job. "There are so many homeless people out there, it is unreal. But they are not seen. People walk past us and they do not care."

Two years ago The Ark opened a hospice for terminally ill AIDS patients, and today the 77 beds in seven small wards are mostly occupied. Care is given by residents of the Ark who have been rehabilitated and trained by Shirley Pretorius, who runs the shelter's general clinic. A pastor of the independent church that established The Ark in the early 1980s, she believes no one is beyond having something to give to society. And when AIDS began to manifest itself more and more strongly among the people who came in for shelter, Pastor Shirley, a registered nurse with specialist psychiatric qualifications, looked no further than the corridors and crowded dormitories of the hostel for people who could help her care them.

"In 1998 the hospitals were becoming overwhelmed with terminally ill patients. People with AIDS were being discharged;

many were too sick to get home, often to distant countryside: others were being rejected by their families, and they were ending up on the streets," Pastor Shirley explains. "We had a meeting at the The Ark and we decided this was a `gap' that needed filling. It goes against our Christian beliefs that anyone should have to die in the gutter without dignity. So it was given to me to establish the unit."

The Ark's clinic is at present a registered primary health care unit. Pastor Shirley has six people, trained by herself, to help her run the clinic and the hospice. "My six core members move from bay to bay in shifts throughout the day and night. In each bay I have a monitor, who lives with the patients and is there to give help where it is needed. The staff check every morning that everyone is bathed and dressed and cleaned. And if someone has an accident or a bed needs to be changed in between times, the monitor comes and calls the staff members on duty."

As well as primary health and nursing care, the clinic staff are trained in counselling of people with HIV and AIDS. Many patients have been rejected by their families, so reconciliation is one of the important objectives of counselling. "When somebody reaches the point of dying it gives them great peace of mind if they have been reconciled with their families", comments Pastor Shirley. "We have several people who are 'outside patients' — they just come in once or twice a week for medication and extra feeding. But they have gone home to their families when they thought they never would. Once the families have understood the problem, the reality that they are not going to attract AIDS from nursing, then they have wanted the patients home. And as a result they have been prepared to be trained. What generally happens is that the patient selects a family member who comes in, does two to three weeks' training, and then we send them home with the patient."

Recognising that many of her staff have struggled mightily with their own personal problems, Pastor Shirley spends a great deal of time with them looking at stress and how to manage it. "I find the more you involve people in the decision-making that is relevant to them, the more they feel they have got control of what they are doing and their lives," she says. "If a problem arises in sick bay — and we do get some very, very difficult patients — I will get the monitors and the staff for that particular bay and say: 'Right, what are the problems? We are going to brainstorm. Write down everything you can think of to solve those problems, and we will see if they are practical. And if they are, we will do them'. I find that because they feel they are in control of the situation, the stress level goes down."

Besides involving everyone concerned in the decisions about how the AIDS units are run, Pastor Shirley frequently starts the day with a short training session on stress management. "We deal with anger, we deal with shame, we deal with guilt. And we deal with 'getting tired of trying to measure up' ", she says. "This is a course I have put together, for people who are constantly feeling they have got to achieve someone else's standard because they do not feel good enough. We deal with all those types of things together."

Conclusion

Caring for the carers of people with AIDS is not only a humanitarian imperative, it is a social and economic necessity, for no country in Africa has yet seen the worst of the AIDS epidemic or experienced the full pressure on its health and social services. And no country can afford to squander the skills and commitment of the present day carers for they must be the carers of tomorrow, too, and the inspiration and role models for new generations of carers. As the earlier discussion has revealed, caring for carers necessitates action on several fronts. Managing stress and preventing burnout requires:

* Strengthening the capacity of the individual carer to cope with the duties and responsibilities of the role;
* ensuring that the working environment, practices and policies of care programmes offer a supportive climate to carers and are not causes of stress in themselves; and
* advocating for national policies and legislations that are sensitive to the needs of carers.

The present discussion is intended to make a projection of lessons and observations from the field that have wide relevance and that lend themselves to being adopted elsewhere.

The Inherently Stressful Work

A first requirement in supporting carers working in the field of AIDS is to acknowledge formally the fact that their work is inherently stressful, and that feelings of distress are legitimate reaction to their experiences, rather than signs of personal weakness or lack of professionalism. Bottled-up feelings lead almost inevitably to burnout, and carers need to feel confident and free to express doubts and distress and to seek timely help without fear of affecting their jobs or reputations. They will only do so if acceptance of the stressful nature of the epidemic is part of the culture of the organisation or institution for which they work.

Relief from the Burden

Carers at all levels need to be relieved of the burden of responsibility for things they cannot help. The message that 'bad things happen and it is not your fault' should be a litany of home-based care programmes. This is particularly important to child carers, since they are most vulnerable to feelings of guilt about suffering they cannot relieve.

Burnout, A Process and not an Event

Stress and burnout are complex phenomena with multiple causes and multiple manifestations. Thus no single, time-limited programme will ever be the solution. For AIDS programmes, managing stress among carers necessitates a broad-based, sensitive and continuous response, of which good support and supervision are desirable elements.

Stress Management Necessitates More Systematic Research

The management and mitigation of stress are difficult to get right unless one has a crystal clear picture of the problems. More systematic studies of stress among carers at all levels and in all settings are therefore needed, and more formal documentation of the different strategies used to cope with stress, how well they work, what they cost, and their effects of the quality of care as well as on the morale and commitment of carers. Moreover, opinions for carer support need to be exchanged between people working in this field, and the lessons of experience widely disseminated.

Knowledge: The Lasting Value

Knowledge is empowering — it gives people confidence, control and options in life, and it has lasting value. Thus training plays a central role in the management of stress and burnout among carers. Besides imparting the knowledge and skills needed to care for a person with HIV/AIDS, the training of carers should deal directly with the problems of stress and burnout. It should encourage self-reflection and self-knowledge and look at personal coping techniques. Another important issue is how to manage one's time effectively and how to recognise and accept one's own limitations. Ongoing training — both regular refresher courses as well as training in new skills — is important for maintaining confidence and morale. When planning refresher or advanced training courses, programmes should try, as far as possible, to fill the gaps in knowledge and skills that carers themselves recognise.

Importance of Valued Work

For the sake of their morale and self-confidence, carers at every level need to know that their work is recognised and valued. Words of praise or thanks are important, and some programmes understand this and make a habit of acknowledging and thanking people. Where volunteers are the first line of support to family carers, and perhaps doing much of the hands-on care themselves, they should be given the due recognition by their communities. Programmes should take great care to ensure that the staff members who train and supervise them, and who may be professionally qualified health professionals, do not undermine the authority or status of these front-line workers.

Volunteers are likely to have greater self-respect, more realistic expectations and deeper satisfaction from their work if they have a sense of ownership of their community programmes, rather than seeing themselves as unpaid employees at the bottom of the hierarchy of the organisations with which they are affiliated. The relationship between the volunteers and the organisation should be clarified at the time of recruitment and training. And because members of the public are not always clear about the status of volunteers and what they can expect from them, the message that they "are a part and parcel" of the community rather than of the NGO should be put across at every opportunity in public gatherings.

Relieving Poverty: A Top Priority

Income-generation schemes are much needed and much valued by AIDS-affected families and communities to relieve the stress of poverty. However, they are not easy to get right. Experience displays that necessity, commitment and enthusiasm are not sufficient to make small businesses successful: people need skills training as well as loans, and their enterprises need careful planning and management, and generally more attention to marketing, than is typically the case. Bringing in expertise to help with income-generation schemes is a sound idea.

Where food handouts are part of the strategy for relieving hunger, programmes should try to obtain supplies from sources as close to the community as possible, rather than from international food aid organisations. Not only will this involve less red tape, but local businesses are more likely to be reliable partners over the long term. Furthermore, their direct participation in the fight against AIDS will help to challenge denial and ignorance of the epidemic locally and to dispel stigma.

Dependable and Committed Donors

Because of the nature of their work — caring for people with incurable conditions and many needs — AIDS programmes have limited scope for self-reliance. Thus the preoccupation of donors with "sustainability" is a constant source of anxiety, and the pressure to demonstrate effectiveness too often means that staff welfare measures get pushed aside in the interests of population coverage.

To relieve the anxieties of dependence and insecurity, there needs to be greater constancy of support from donors. Moreover, donors cannot afford to concentrate narrowly on population coverage problems alone. Unless they look more sympathetically on issues of staff welfare, they will be falling into the classic trap of so many development aid donors in the past — that of purchasing vehicles for development projects but making no allowance for fuel or maintenance! There is much to be gained on both sides by donors visiting programmes on their own home territories, going into the field with carers and seeing for themselves what their work entails.

Stress Management: Not a Luxury

Stress management is not a luxury: burnout is a very real threat to people who spend their time with the sick, the dying and grieving, and watching the struggle of families to survive. Thus staff welfare should be a high priority for all AIDS programmes. Effective measures for managing stress include:

* setting realistic targets for work;
* regular time off that is respected;
* annual retreats for carers;
* health care provision and paid sick leave;
* team work and regular meetings to discuss issues and share problems;
* the appointment of a carers' counsellor; and
* an effective voice for carers in decisions that affect them.

Having good policies and mechanisms in place is only the first step, however, it is important to see that they do not get pushed aside by pressures of work and lack of money. Maintaining staff welfare requires constant commitment and the political will to see that it remains a priority. The value of having strong and sensitive managers, aware of their responsibility for the health and well-being of their staff, cannot be ruled out.

Emotional Burden

An effective way of minimising the stress of working in the AIDS field is to assign several people to the care of a client where appropriate, so that no one carer has to shoulder the responsibility or the emotional burden alone. This is difficult to manage, however, if a client is fearful of disclosure. Helping clients identify someone with whom they can safely share their diagnosis is an important part of counselling, and an important element in generating a coping family situation as well as in dispersing the burden of care. However, the dangers of being recognised as HIV positive are very real in some settings, and disclosure is an extremely sensitive issue that necessitates careful handling. Clients must never feel coerced into revealing their status.

Rather than sending in carers from outside, AIDS programmes should encourage and empower communities to do their own caring as much as possible. Not only does this trend help to disperse the burden of care, but it also helps to dispel stigma and prejudice by bringing home to people the reality of the epidemic — the fact that it is not just a problem for other people "out there", but is in their own midst, affecting friends and neighbours and perhaps their own relatives.

Battle against Prejudice, Discrimination and Stigma

A powerful lesson from experience is that the battle against prejudice and stigma is never conclusively won. The association of AIDS with grim suffering, death and behaviours that people everywhere find difficult to talk about, and to accept, means that the stigma of AIDS needs to be constantly challenged.

Clear Job Descriptions and Good Referral Mechanisms

Carers need a clear understanding of their duties and the limits of their responsibility for any client. They also need to know who or where they can refer clients to when their condition calls for greater expertise or they are unable to manage the situation alone. Good communication and referral mechanisms within AIDS care programmes are therefore essential. And programmes should aimd to strengthen their own foundations and generate a supportive environment for carers at every level through networking and partnerships with other organisations and individuals with something relevant to offer.

For carers at home, being made aware of the resources available locally and other sources of support is a great comfort.

Independent Evaluation

Independent evaluation of programmes at regular intervals is important for a number of reasons, not least because it gives everyone working for the programme a fresh perspective on their daily activities. By putting services, working practices and relationships under the spotlight, it can determine problem areas and suggest alternative ways of doing things that might not be obvious to the people involved. Several programmes spoke with enthusiasm about the exercise, saying that it permitted them to refocus their activities and to change things that were not working as well as they should. One director said that independent evaluation had given her programme a new lease of life — she and her colleagues seemed to be caught in a downward spiral of overwork and inadequate resources, and were on the point of giving up when the evaluation team analysed what they were doing and showed them how they could restore the equilibrium.

Evaluation of Legislations and Policies

Government policies and laws can create a supportive environment for the care of people with HIV / AIDS, or they can be obstructive. Of particular significance are laws and policies regarding:

* HIV testing;
* access to drugs;
* the prevention of mother-to-child transmission;
* the human rights of people with HIV infection, and AIDS;
* the status of traditional healers;
* the disbursement of donor funds and food aid; and
* the inheritance rights of widows and children.

Governments need to look carefully at how existing legislations and policies affect the operation of AIDS care programmes, and how they might be modified to make the work of carers easier and more secure.

Advice

When it comes to caring for people with HIV/AIDS, the richest resource a country has is, without question, the compassion of its people. As these examples from Uganda and South Africa demonstrate the level of funding is not the most important predictor of the quality of care. It is an extraordinary reality that some of the most effective programmes are found in the poorest communities, where care is delivered by people who not only earn nothing for their services but risk sliding deeper into poverty themselves due to the time they devote to this noble cause. Even for staff members of AIDS care organisations, the pay they receive is almost never the motivating factor for participation in this field — like the volunteers, it is most often the desire to help others who are suffering.

Drawing attention to the rich pool of compassion that sustains the care effort in so many places is by no means to downplay the importance of money — nor the pressing need for a much greater allocation of funds, nationally and internationally, to the care of people with AIDS. It is simply to highlight a resource that is too often taken for granted, and to underline the case made by this report: that carers deserve greater recognition for their extraordinary and selfless contribution to the encounter against AIDS, and that concern for their well-being should have the highest priority.

Five

Opening up the Epidemic

Introduction

HIV/AIDS is an unprecedented epidemic and public health emergency. Presently, it is approximated that more than 33 million people are infected with HIV, and over 16 million have died of AIDS-associated illnesses globally. In many underdeveloped countries and among marginalised groups of people in developed countries, the number of new HIV infections continues to rise. In some countries in Africa, AIDS-associated morbidity and mortality are decelerating the development, childhood mortality, and survival and life expectancy.[1] Due to this, and sometimes with a sense of desperation, many governments and communities are reviewing the effectiveness of their HIV/AIDS programmes. This review has taken place against the backdrop of a deepening realisation of the severe impact that HIV/AIDS is having on the well-being of individuals, families and communities. It evidences a growing political commitment to HIV prevention and care.

In the context of this review, some governments have considered whether the principles of *confidentiality* and *informed consent* contribute to the rapid spread of HIV. It is a matter of concern that these principles allow a person who is HIV-positive to keep his or her status confidential, and refuse to share it with sexual (or drug-injecting) partners, family members or the community. Governments and others have asked whether these principles hinder efforts to prevent the spread of HIV and deny protection to the sexual and drug-injecting partners of those infected. There is also concern that the principle of confidentiality contributes to the 'invisible' status of the epidemic and to the general denial of HIV/AIDS within communities and nations. Thus, policy-makers have begun to consider legislation and practice that would allow breaches in confidentiality, mandatory partner notification and named HIV case-reporting for public health reasons; and would permit the criminal prosecution of individuals who are considered to have spread the virus deliberately.

To address some of the concerns, and in response to a request for WHO assistance made by Ministers of Health in Africa, WHO (AFRO) and the UNAIDS Secretariat cosponsored a regional technical consultation on *notification, confidentiality and HIV/AIDS* in August 1999 in Windhoek, Namibia. A meeting statement was produced that aimed to assist Ministers of Health and other partners in southern Africa to develop policy and guidelines.[2] In October 1999, the UNAIDS Secretariat and WHO cohosted an international consultation in Geneva, Switzerland, on *HIV reporting and disclosure*. This consultation included epidemiologists, public health professionals, national AIDS programme managers, people with HIV/AIDS, lawyers and human rights activists from over 20 countries.

The Windhoek and Geneva meetings confirmed that the principles of confidentiality and informed consent *do not* contribute to the spread of HIV/AIDS. In fact, if employed in the appropriate context and in creative and culturally sensitive manners, confidentiality and informed consent can help to decrease the spread of HIV/AIDS.

Rather, responsibility lies with the *denial, stigma and discrimination* which surround HIV/AIDS, and which result in a high level of secrecy pertaining to the epidemic. These disempower both individuals and communities in their efforts to cope with HIV/AIDS. This denial, stigma and discrimination, and the resulting privacy, must be overcome and the HIV/AIDS epidemic "normalised" into what it is — a viral infection, as well as major human, health and development crisis.

The relevance of ethical principles such as confidentiality and informed consent has been raised throughout the history of the response to the epidemic. That these come under examination again at this juncture is a necessary and welcome development. In general, it reflects the need for greater efforts to 'open up' the HIV/AIDS epidemic. In particular, it reflects the need to discover more clearly the causes and consequences of the *denial, stigma, discrimination and secrecy* that surround HIV/AIDS and hinder effective responses; and the need to identify, fund and implement strategies that will overcome them, and lead to more effective prevention, care and support.

Denial, stigma, discrimination and secrecy about HIV/AIDS continue to exist even though prevalence of HIV, and deaths from AIDS, are very high in many places. They stem from innumerable reasons. At the individual level, people do not want to acknowledge that HIV/AIDS is within their communities, that it poses a real personal danger to them and to their families, that they themselves may already be infected and that they may be transmitting the virus to their sexual or drug-injecting partners. Moreover, people do not want to get tested for HIV or to reveal their sero status because they fear that they will be rejected by their partners, that they will face stigma and discrimination, and/or that they will be blamed for infecting others. Finally, most people in the underdeveloped world know they will not have access to drugs and treatment which would decelerate the progression of the disease or alleviate its pain and suffering. Thus, denial, stigma, discrimination and lack of access to care stem from, and lead to, a sense of fear and hopelessness, and encourage secrecy about HIV/AIDS.

At the community level, many resource-poor communities are encountering with extremely difficult circumstances in which to combat HIV/AIDS. They suffer from insufficient health care and education services, including insufficient voluntary testing and counselling; insufficient public education campaigns, particularly education projected to young people, women and marginalised groups; insufficient access not only to anti-retroviral drugs but also to drugs to reduce the pain and suffering caused by AIDS-associated illnesses; and insufficient community organisation and support, including lack of a social and legal infrastructure to protect people from HIV-associated discrimination. These conditions are exacerbated among marginalised groups in communities. These barriers seriously hamper government and community efforts to prevent the spread of HIV and to provide care and support for those affected by HIV/AIDS. They also reinforce the denial, secrecy, stigma and discrimination that prevail.

Governments and communities have felt at a loss to know how to combat this denial, stigma, discrimination and secrecy. This has justified calls for "new or different" approaches to respond to the epidemic, particularly in high-prevalence settings. Mandatory HIV case-reporting and revelation of HIV status, particularly to sexual partners but also to communities, have been suggested as sound public health measures. More generally, discussions have been commenced nationally, regionally and internationally on how to:

(a) create more openness about HIV/AIDS among individuals and within families and communities;
(b) persuade more people to test for HIV, inform sexual partners about the outcomes and prevent further infections;
(c) better protect people not infected from becoming infected;
(d) increase acceptance, care and support for people and families affected by HIV/AIDS; and
(e) improve epidemiological surveillance of HIV and AIDS.

This discussion is a follow-up to the Technical Consultation on Notification, Confidentiality and HIV/AIDS in Windhoek, and the International Consultation on HIV Reporting and Disclosure (Geneva), and draws from the expertise and input made at these meetings in an effort to offer assistance in solving these technicalities. It proposes that vital and effective steps towards opening up the HIV/AIDS epidemic involve the encouragement of beneficial disclosure, ethical partner counselling and the appropriate use of HIV case-reporting.

The prominent world institutions offer guidance concerning these issues in a context that involves commitment to human rights, ethical principles, public health and community empowerment. Such a context protects the health and safety of the individual both infected and uninfected; it also protects public health. It does so by generating an environment that motivates the most people to get tested for HIV; encourages people to modify their behaviour either to prevent their own infection or that of others and, where infected, to feel able and willing to reveal their status in a way that prevents further transmission of HIV; and results in care and compassion. Such an environment will help to open up the epidemic; reduce the denial, stigma, discrimination and secrecy about HIV/AIDS; and tailor programmes that allow governments, communities and individuals to deal with the causes and consequences of HIV/AIDS in the most effective and humane ways possible.

Confidentiality and Secrecy: The Distinction

It is important at the outset to make a clear distinction between 'confidentiality' and "secrecy". Confidentiality is an ethical principle particularly relevant in the provision of health care.[3] The principle of confidentiality encompasses the opinion that a person should be entitled to privacy with regard to his or her most personal physical and psychological secrets; but it is also the basis for an effective relationship between patient/client and health care provider, and ultimately the basis for the effectiveness of many public health interventions which rest on these relationships. Only if a person feels sure that the health care provider will keep confidential any information provided will (s)he come forward and share information that may be critical to making decisions about effective clinical care and treatment.

Thus, health care professionals have long recognised and respected their duty, and the need, to protect and confidentiality of their patients. Because of the need to protect confidentiality in order to provide effective health care, health care professionals also recognise that they should normally only reveal highly personal information, such as HIV status, with the informed consent of the patient.

However, the principle of confidentiality is not absolute, and there are situations where it is not preserved. One of these occurs when necessary and relevant information is exchanged among health care professionals who are responsible for the clinical management of a person's health needs. Often a small group of professionals, generally in a hospital or clinic setting, will share personal information about a client, including HIV status, which is necessary for the effective treatment of the case, but confidentiality will be preserved within this professional group. Another situation where confidentiality may be breached without the consent of the patient occurs when there is a clear indication that a third party may be harmed by the actions of the patient. In these situations the ethical principle of confidentiality may come in encounter with the ethical principle to "do no harm", and a difficult but necessary ethical weighing of the potential harms and benefits to the parties involved should be undertaken in order to decide how to proceed.[4] In the present discussion, there is a full detail of how such relatively rare cases in the context of HIV/AIDS should be handled.

The ethical principles of confidentiality and informed consent, which have private and public health advantages, should be distinguished from "secrecy" which is a state of affairs often resulting from fear, shame and/or a sense of vulnerability. Whether secrecy is preserved depends solely on the personal motives of those who hold the secret. As stated earlier, motives to maintain secrecy in the context of HIV/AIDS involve not only fear and shame, but also denial, and fear of rejection, stigma and discrimination. To the extent that secrecy harms the infected and the uninfected, and undermines an individual's, family's or community's ability to cope positively with HIV/AIDS, it should be strongly combated. There is a serious opinion that the secrecy about HIV/AIDS, and the related stigma, denial and discrimination, can best be countered by a greatly increased commitment to *beneficial disclosure, ethical partner counselling and appropriate use of HIV case-reporting*, as narrated below.

Motivating Beneficial Disclosure

'Disclosure' is a neutral term. In the context of HIV/AIDS, it refers to the act of informing any individual or organisation (e.g., health authority, employer, school) of the HIV status of an infected person, or it refers to the fact that such information has been transmitted, by any means, by the person him or herself, or by a third party, with or without consent[5]. However, the objectives and the consequences of disclosure may be beneficial or harmful. Examples of beneficial disclosure involve instances where an HIV-positive person informs a sexual partner of his/her status for prevention purposes, or informs family, community members or health care professionals in order to share vital personal information and obtain support. Or disclosure may include a health care professional providing information regarding an HIV/AIDS case on a confidential basis to other health care professionals involved in the management of the patient; to a health authority for surveillance purposes; or, where necessary, to a partner of an HIV-positive person to prevent further transmission of HIV (to be discussed later).

Examples of harmful disclosure involves cases where disclosure is made without the consent of person who is HIV-positive and has grave consequences for that person, such as stigma, abandonment, physical violence, imprisonment, loss of employment or housing, or other forms of discrimination. Harmful disclosure may also impair prevention and care programmes. Where people fear forced testing, or disclosure involving lack of confidentiality, they will avoid HIV counselling, testing, treatment and support, because these are likely to mean that their HIV status will become known against their will and they will face stigma, discrimination, lack of privacy and other negative effects. Thus, fear of lack of confidentiality and forced disclosure drives people away from HIV services, reducing opportunities to motivate and empower people to change their behaviour in order either to avoid getting infected or to avoid passing on their infection. It may also drive people away from other health care services, such as antenatal care or blood donation.

UNAIDS and WHO encourage beneficial disclosure. This is disclosure that is voluntary; respects the autonomy and dignity of the affected individuals; maintains confidentiality as appropriate; leads to beneficial results for those individuals, and for their families and sexual and drug-injecting partners; leads to greater openness in the community about HIV/AIDS; and meets the ethical imperatives of the situation where there is need to prevent further transmission of HIV.[6]

Such beneficial disclosure, with its elements of voluntariness and confidentiality, not only maintains ethical principles but also serves a direct public health function, because it motivates people to access HIV prevention and care services. It does this by setting up a climate of trust between health care providers and those who need HIV services, allaying their fears and respecting them as people who can and will make the right decisions regarding their behaviour. Beneficial disclosure also serves the objective of opening up the HIV/AIDS epidemic. As more people feel able and willing to disclose their status, there grows a critical mass of individuals and families within a community, and status, there grows a critical mass of individuals and families within a community, and indeed within a nation, who are openly involved in dealing with the epidemic in positive and supportive manners. As a consequence, discrimination, stigma and secrecy are reduced.

Nevertheless, preconditions are necessary to promote beneficial disclosure and to motivate people to access prevention and care activities. People must have access to voluntary counselling and testing (VCT) services in which they can learn their HIV status and receive support and referral in dealing with the news. Moreover, they must have an incentive to find out their status such that it will mean greater social support access to health care options and an increased ability to live a rewarding life irrespective of a negative or positive status. Finally, they must not fear stigma and discrimination if identified to be HIV-positive.

Revelation Incentives

It is approximated that up to 90 per cent of HIV-positive people in underdeveloped countries are not aware of their sero status.[7] In large part, this is due to the fact that there are few VCT facilities available to the populations most affected by HIV/AIDS. However, even where testing is available, many people do not want to be tested due to a perception that 'nothing is to be gained' by knowing an HIV-positive status. For the poor there will be little access to HIV/AIDS treatment and care. Moreover, there will likely be stigma and discrimination to be encountered if found to be HIV-positive.

However, even in resource-poor settings much can be done to improve access to voluntary counselling, HIV testing, treatment and care, though this many involve a shift of resources from 'traditional' HIV programmes and activities. Primarily, there must be greater investment in setting up VCT services in communities. Secondly, incentives must be created to motivate people to undergo testing. These should take the form of community services providing support, treatment and care. Finally, disincentives to test, such as stigma and discrimination, should be removed.

There are insufficient VCT services in the communities most in need of them.[8] More resources from national AIDS programmes should be devoted to set up such services,[9] which can take various forms. Most important are that VCT services are integrated into existing services where applicable (e.g., antenatal care, sexually transmitted infection (STI) clinics, family health clinics); they are user friendly (particularly to youth and women); are accessible to marginalised groups (e.g., the poor, rural populations, commercial sex workers, drug injectors, migrants); and are tailored to tie the individual using them into other support and care options (e.g., referral to STI services, support groups, family outreach programmes).[10] The creation and availability of such services is a prerequisite if people are to learn about their HIV status and discover ways of dealing with it constructively, including through disclosure.

However, the existence of VCT services is not in itself ample to get people to come forward for HIV testing. There must be incentives, and these should take the form of greater availability and affordability of care, treatment and support. In resource-poor settings, treatment, in the form of drugs, and care options are very limited. However, these barriers can in part be overcome by innovative and far-reaching community-based programmes. Such programmes offer outreach to affected families, voluntary and confidential counselling and testing, support groups, home visits, follow-up and participation of people living with HIV/AIDS in prevention and care programmes. They may also offer models of how to 'live positively' With HIV/AIDS, through which people maximise their personal and social resources, live as best as possible in the present and plan realistically for the future.

Examples of such effective community-based programmes can be witnessed in Uganda, Tanzania and Thailand, where campaigns of non-governmental organisations (NGOs) to motivate testing have created more openness and discussion about HIV.[11] [12] [13] In the parts of these countries where HIV testing has been made reasonably accessible to affected communities, the synergistic bond between reducing stigma, increasing voluntary testing and encouraging disclosure has been confirmed. Each of these activities reinforces the others and leads to greater numbers of people taking advantage of voluntary counselling, testing and support.[14 15] This leads to more voluntary disclosure (to spouses, lovers, family members, friends and health care professionals), the adoption of low-risk behaviour and a movement toward positive living.[16 17]

When such programmes are well integrated into the community and are responding to its needs, they can have a profound influence on how HIV/AIDS is perceived at the individual, family and community levels. Positive-living models, as well as the active participation of people living with and affected by HIV/AIDS, help to change attitudes from stigma and discrimination to respect and support. Affected families and communities are able to embrace their situation, are given support in how to best deal with it, while the family member who is HIV-positive is still able to contribute to family and community efforts. This helps to reduce the stigma and to change public perceptions of HIV and people living with HIV/AIDS. It also helps to encourage more people who are not aware of their new status to come forward voluntarily for counselling and testing.

Thus, there needs to be greater investment in creating the facilities for HIV testing, as well as in backing, community-based programmes which generate a supportive environment and motivate people to come forward for HIV testing, counselling, care, treatment and support. Then beneficial disclosure will increase and lead to more prevention (protection of those not yet infected), and more care and support for those already infected.

Removal of Disincentives

Despite the fact that millions of people globally are infected with HIV, there is still considerable shame, secrecy and fear about HIV; people living with HIV and AIDS are highly stigmatised. HIV is also the cause of human rights violations and acts of discrimination. As a result of the stigma and discrimination surrounding HIV/AIDS, those who *do know* their HIV status are afraid to disclose it due to the risk of loss of employment, social ostracism, violence and threats to their lives, and other adverse consequences. Those who *do not know* their status are feared to get tested if they fear that the results will be made known against their will and they will face stigma and discrimination.

Thus, to persuade voluntary testing, beneficial disclosure and use of HIV services, the disincentives of stigma and discrimination, and lack of confidentiality, must be overcome. Many steps can be taken to reduce stigma and discrimination. One of the most under-utilised has been public information campaigns which concentrate *specifically* on the promotion of tolerance, compassion and non-discrimination. Though the world has been inundated with public information about the reality that HIV cannot be transmitted casually, this information has not done enough to alleviate fear of HIV and AIDS and of people living with them. Public information campaigns should be carried out which involve creative, attractive, powerful messages against discrimination and stigma. Public forums on HIV/AIDS and/or community discussion groups, which concentrate on compassion, tolerance and support, should also be held.

Where there is protection against violence and discrimination, prominent public figures, (actors, politicians, athletes), alongwith those living with HIV, should participate in these public campaigns. The participation of people living with HIV/AIDS in public campaigns, and in policy, programmatic and community activities, is crucial to give a human face to the epidemic, to reaffirm the value of people with HIV/AIDS and to change attitudes of stigma. It also ensures that policies and programmes will be sensitive to the actual needs and realities of those affected by HIV/AIDS.[18]

Other measures can be undertaken at a national level, such as the enactment of legislations and policies against HIV-associated discrimination[19] and against breaches in confidentiality and informed consent. One essential step is the training and sensitisation of professionals who work with people affected by HIV/AIDS. It is often at the hands of such professionals that people affected by HIV/AIDS suffer the worst discrimination, despite the professional and ethical responsibility to treat people who are HIV-positive with dignity and compassion, and to protect their confidentiality in appropriate manners. Key professionals who might benefit from training in non-discrimination, confidentiality and informed consent are health care professionals, police, social service professionals, advocates and judges.

Health care professionals should be more empowered to

handle the medical, as well as psychosocial, management of clients with HIV/AIDS.[20] This should include training and empowerment about global precautions against transmission of infectious diseases, as it is the fear of transmission of HIV among health care professionals that often leads to stigma and discrimination against people with HIV/AIDS. Experience has demonstrated that the impact of this training in health settings needs regular monitoring and staff updating to ensure that infection control procedures are maintained.[21]

Recommendations for Motivating Beneficial Disclosure

(a) Conduct public information campaigns and community forums proposed at promoting tolerance, compassion and understanding, and reducing fear, stigma and discrimination.

(b) Encourage participation of people living with HIV/AIDS in public information campaigns and in HIV programmes and policy formulation.

(c) Set up more VCT services, including in rural areas and for marginalised groups.

(d) Support governmental agencies, NGOs and community-based organisations (CBOs) to make community-based services, including VCT, family outreach, community support, positive living, support groups and care options more broadly available.

(e) Encourage the media to report on HIV/AIDS in a responsible, non-discriminatory and non-sensational way.[22]

(f) Train health care professionals in the management of HIV and global precautions, in attitudes of non-discrimination, acceptance and compassion, and in the principles of confidentiality and informed consent.

(g) Train other professionals (social workers, police, advocates, judges) in attitudes of non-discrimination, acceptance and compassion, and in the principles of confidentiality and informed consent.

(h) Train key personnel in non-health employment settings, including human resource management in industry, in promoting non-discriminatory practices in the workplace.[23]

(i) Enact or reform legislations, administrative guidelines and professional codes of conduct to prohibit discrimination and breaches of confidentiality associated with HIV status.

(j) Generate legal support services for those who have encountered discrimination based on HIV status.

Motivating Ethical Partner Counselling (Partner Notification)

Partner counselling or partner notification[24] consists the process of contacting sexual and/or injecting partners of an HIV-positive person (in this context often called the "source" or "index" client or patient) in order to advise these partners that they may have been exposed to HIV and to motivate them to attend for HIV counselling, testing and, where applicable, treatment,[25] The objectives of this kind of revelation are to:

(a) prevent HIV transmission to people who may be exposed either sexually or through needle-sharing; and

(b) improve care and support for people living with HIV or AIDS.[26]

Partner counselling can be undertaken by the source client or patient him/herself, by the health care provider or through the combined efforts of both.

Source referral. HIV-positive people are encouraged to counsel partners concerning their possible exposure to HIV. This takes place without the direct involvement of health care providers. In this theory the health care provider works with the HIV-positive person regarding the nature of the information to be passed on to their partner(s) and manners of doing it.

Provider referral. An HIV-positive person gives the name(s) of his/her partner(s) to a health care provider who then confidentially counsels the partner(s) directly. In this theory, the health care provider does not reveal the name of the HIV-positive person to the partner, but only provides the information that the partner is likely to have been exposed to HIV infection. This is done with the consent of the source client or patient.

Conditional referral. The health care provider of the source client or patient obtains the names of his/her sexual/drug-injecting partner(s), but permits the source client a period of time to counsel the partner(s) him/herself. If partners are not counselled within this time period, the health care provider counsels the partners, without naming the source patient or client concerned. (Partner counselling without the consent of the source client to be discussed later in this chapter.)

Partner counselling/notification has a long history as one possible aspect of the public health response to STIs other than HIV, such as syphilis and gonorrhoea. As discussed earlier, there is current debate whether, in the context of the transmission of HIV, the status and/or name of an HIV-positive person should be disclosed mandatorily to his or her sexual or drug-injecting partners. This is a particular concern in Africa and Asia where many women are being infected by their husbands or regular partners who do not disclose their sero status or practise safe sex.

However, in the history of partner counselling, there are no clear statistics implying that the mandatory counselling of partners is more effective in preventing transmission than the voluntary counselling of partners. As said earlier, it seems that when people think that they will be forced to notify their partners, or that their status will be revealed without their consent, they choose not to attend for STI testing, counselling or other prevention and care services. This has been true in the case of syphilis and gonorrhoea even though, unlike HIV, these are curable and attract much less stigma and discrimination than HIV/AIDS. It is even more likely that a policy of mandatory partner counselling will deter people from using HIV testing and counselling services, because there is greater incentive to fear testing and revelation due to serious stigma and discrimination about HIV/AIDS.[27]

The reality is that, in several hospital and clinics in underdeveloped countries, revelation of HIV status to sexual partners and others, such as family members, often takes place without consent. This happens because there are not ample resources and personnel to store information in a way that respects privacy and/or because health care providers do not understand the professional obligations of confidentiality and informed consent and their importance in the management of HIV/AIDS. This failure of health authorities to protect the privacy and autonomy of patients deters many people in these countries from seeking HIV counselling, testing and care.

Moreover, it is not possible or practical to implement a large-scale scheme of mandatory partner counselling. It is virtually impossible to emphasise people to test mandatorily for HIV, to retest periodically and to continue to inform partners, as would be necessary. Nor do people always know, or remember, the names of their sexual partners. Nor is it possible to force them to reveal them. Finally, it is very costly to train and employ staff to trace and counsel all those whose names are given.

It appears that mandatory partner counselling schemes are not necessary because *voluntary* partner counselling schemes can accomplish the critical objectives. Voluntary partner counselling schemes can help to generate a climate of confidence which will attract people to HIV testing and counselling services so that more people learn of their HIV status. Among those who do attend health care facilities and are encountered with a decision whether to notify partners or not, it seems that *most* people *agree* to do so, on a voluntary basis, after counselling. In the context of a generally voluntary partner counselling programme, the small number of cases where persons refuse to notify their partners can be taken care of on an individual basis, as narrated below.

Thus, for reasons of principle and because it is more feasible and capable of success, UNAIDS and WHO encourage ethical partner counselling. Ethical partner counselling is based on the informed consent of the source client or patient and, where possible, maintains the confidentiality of the source client or patient: that is, his/her name is not disclosed to the partners being counselled. This will often be extremely difficult to maintain in the context of marital relationships, and necessitates the provision of counselling and support to both spouses to ensure the prospect of abuse and discrimination is minimised or eliminated. Ethical partner counselling also takes into consideration the grave consequence of *not* counselling partners - possible HIV infection. This consequence requires an ethical weighing of the advantages and disadvantages that are likely occur if and when there is refusal on the part of an HIV-positive person to counsel partners. Because of this, UNAIDS and WHO encourage ethical partner counselling programmes which:

(a) employ serious counselling and motivation towards counselling of partners;

(b) empower the health care provider, when the source client refuses to notify his/her partner, to make ethical decisions based on the potential harm and benefits to the parties, and decide whether to counsel the partner(s) without the consent of the source client, in the conditions outlined below;

(c) provide social and legal support for the source client and other relevant parties (spouses, partners, family members) to protect them from physical abuse, discrimination and stigma which may result from partner counselling.

Moreover, UNAIDS and WHO advocate that there be greater exploration of concepts and practices concerning partner counselling which are culturally appropriate, ethically sound and effective in achieving prevention and care objectives. One example is the concept of "shared confidentiality". In Uganda and some other African countries, this notion of shared confidentiality has been developed by communities, NGOs and health care providers. A person affected by HIV is encouraged, and voluntarily chooses, to reveal his/her status to a range of people from whom (s)he can get support. In the words of a former counsellor from Uganda:

The person with HIV is assured that the responsibility to share is mine; the advantage of sharing is that there is another human being that accompanies me; and I decide what components I share with whom and when. In the process of encouraging disclosure, the health provider recognises that the person with HIV retains his or her autonomy over decisions. But where there is fear of disclosure you try to change that by persuasion.[28]

The objective of shared confidentiality is to promote better support, care and prevention for individuals, families and communities affected by HIV/AIDS. In communities where shared confidentiality has been a practice of community-based organisations, there has been an increase in community discussion of HIV/AIDS and a decrease in the stigma and discriminate about HIV/AIDS. It has therefore assisted to open up the HIV/AIDS epidemic in positive and supportive ways.[29]

Partner Counselling without Consent

There will be some cases where an HIV-positive person (source client) does not wish to, and may refuse to, notify his/her partner(s) or allow them to be counselled by the health care provider. It is important to bear in mind that such refusal is most often because of a fear of rejection by partners and family, to fears of stigma and discrimination and/or to a fear of being blamed for the infection of others. It may also consist of feelings of despair, remorse and guilt. Refusal to notify partners is very *seldom* because of a desire by the HIV-positive person to place another person deliberately at risk of HIV infection.

For some, the consequences of their HIV status becoming known by their partners are severe. This is particularly the case for women who live in societies where women suffer social, monetary and legal disadvantages because they are women. In such places, a woman is often blamed for her own infection, as well as for the infection of her husband/partner, even though it is likely that she was infected by him. The reaction to revelation of her status may also include physical violence and abandonment, in which she (and her children) may be thrown out of the home and given no monetary or social support. Thus, women may have very valid reasons for fearing to reveal their status to husbands/partners.[30]

Given the possible grave consequences of counselling partners (discrimination, abandonment, violence) and of not counselling partners (transmission of HIV infection), counsellors and health care professionals must be trained to handle the difficult ethical decisions to be made. In each case, all the potential disadvantages and advantages of counselling or not counselling partners should be weighed. In most cases, with counselling and with a display of support, the HIV-positive person will agree to notify partners. Initial support may take the form of notification in the presence of the counsellor and/or in the presence of another family member who will provide support, and protection if necessary. Moreover, there should be follow-up and referral to other support services to ensure that the couple or family can cope with the HIV among them.

In cases where the source client refuses to notify, following repeated efforts to motivate him/her to do so, and where the failure to notify creates a danger to a partner whose identity is known to the counsellor (in legal language an identifiable risk to an identifiable third party) the counsellor should be authorised to counsel the partner(s) without the consent of the source client. In making this decision, the counsellor should ensure that the following factors are present:

(a) The HIV-positive person (source client) has been thoroughly counselled as to the necessity for partner notification/counselling.
(b) The counselling has failed to achieve the appropriate behavioural changes, alongwith the practice of safe sex.
(c) The HIV-positive person has refused to notify, or consent to the counselling, of his/her partner(s).
(d) A real risk of HIV transmission to the identifiable partner(s) exists.
(e) The HIV-positive person is given reasonable prior notice of the intention to counsel by the health care professional.
(f) The identity of the source client is kept latent from the partner(s) if this is probable in practice.
(g) Follow-up is provided to ensure support to those involved as necessary and to prevent violence, family disruption etc.[31]

Recommendations for Motivating Ethical Partner Counselling

Below are listed recommendations to create the enabling conditions to motivate the use of ethical partner counselling. Very important is the creation of a social and legal environment which promotes and protects the principles of non-discrimination, confidentiality, tolerance and compassion, as narrated earlier on beneficial disclosure. More specifically, to encourage ethical partner counselling, UNAIDS and WHO recommend the following:

(a) Develop national policies and public health legislation on partner counselling that safeguard the principles of confidentiality and informed consent, and provide for the limited and clearly defined conditions under which partner counselling may take place without consent.
(b) Develop public health legislation that authorises health care providers to decide, on the basis of each individual case and ethical considerations, whether to counsel partners without the consent of the source client, under certain conditions.[32]

(c) Hold consultations among health care providers, government and affected communities about how to persuade ethical partner counselling and protect people who reveal their status through such counselling.

(d) Provide training and guidelines for health care providers and counsellors about how to protect confidentiality and informed consent in the context of partner counselling; how to encourage and assist voluntary partner counselling; how to make difficult ethical decisions in cases where there is refusal to counsel partners; and how to counsel partners in manners that harm is minimised and support is provided.

(e) Promote the setting up of professional ethical codes among health care and social service providers which require respect for confidentiality and informed consent in the context of partner counselling, and provide penalties for unethical conduct.

(f) Set up techniques for accountability and ways of making complaints in health care institutions and in communities when partners are counselled unethically by health care providers and other professionals.

(g) Support practical legal and social measures that address the vulnerability of people, particularly that of women, to stigma, physical violence and abandonment, including projects in the community which will assist in providing treatment, care, emotional support and protection from discrimination to those participating in partner counselling.

(h) Promote and support community projects about people's responsibility to protect themselves and others from HIV infection, particularly among men and boys.

Appropriate Use of HIV Case-reporting

Some countries have recently considered whether they should implement a policy of *named HIV case-reporting*. Under such a policy, health care providers would be required to report by name all HIV cases diagnosed by them to a health authority. (Other forms of case-reporting include the use of a *code*, sometimes called a "unique identifier", for each case; or provide information on cases *anonymously.*)[33]. This has been promoted as a means to open up the HIV/AIDS epidemic; decrease denial; improve access to prevention and care services for those affected by HIV/AIDS; and obtain more accurate information on the prevalence and incidence of HIV/AIDS for surveillance purposes.

While *AIDS* case-reporting has been implemented in most countries, implementation of *HIV* case-reporting has been much more limited. Many countries commenced to collect statistics on HIV cases at the beginning of the epidemic but later dropped the practice when the infection became widespread. The reasons were the high cost and technicality of maintaining the system, the lack of effective treatment or preventive options once people were identified to be HIV-positive, and the small additional advantage for surveillance purposes.

However, there has been a recent trend in *high-income* countries to employ HIV, as well as AIDS, case-reporting. This trend is based on the reality that, where anti-retroviral therapies are available, the access to, and use of, these drugs has dramatically decreased the incidence of AIDS. As a result, AIDS cases are no longer an accurate base for calculating back to HIV incidence and prevalence. Moreover, in these countries, case-reporting of HIV assists to monitor the access of those who are HIV-positive to appropriate services and treatment, alongwith the use of anti-retrovirals.

Neither the reporting of HIV cases nor the reporting of AIDS cases, for the objectives listed above, has been useful in underdeveloped countries. For surveillance purposes, statistics collected on the basis of case-reporting of HIV/AIDS have been problematic. Generally, HIV/AIDS surveillance involves the routine collection, analysis and dissemination of accurate epidemiological information regarding the spread and distribution of HIV infection. Surveillance is an essential part of the response to the epidemic entailing several important objectives:

(a) to monitor trends in prevalence and incidence of HIV in populations;
(b) to evaluate disease burden in terms of morbidity and mortality due to HIV/AIDS;

(c) to be able to plan HIV prevention and care programme aimed at the particular epidemiological situation;

(d) to provide statistics for estimates and reflections of the number of people with HIV/AIDS and AIDS-associated mortality;

(e) to monitor the impact of the national response of the HIV/AIDS epidemic;

(f) to reinforce commitment to AIDS prevention and care through awareness of the numbers affected and their needs.

But the statistics collected from HIV/AIDS case-reporting in many countries have not been advantageous for the stated objectives of surveillance largely for the following reasons.

(a) Less than 10 per cent of HIV-positive people have been tested for HIV, so most are unaware of their status.

(b) Many people do not want to know their status, given the stigma and discrimination related to a positive result and the fact that they will not have access to treatment or care.

(c) Among health care providers, there are problems with under-diagnosis and under-reporting of HIV/AIDS, including the fact that health care providers may be reluctant to report cases by name of reasons of confidentiality and privacy.

(d) In comparison, where the information is provided anonymously to avoid breaches in confidentiality, there is potential for multiple reporting of the same case.

(e) There is insufficient capacity and infrastructure to maintain confidentiality for either named or coded reporting, which further deters people presenting for tests.

These conditions make HIV case-reporting in underdeveloped countries unreliable.

Advocates of HIV case-reporting point to potential advantages in terms of prevention and increased access to care. However, reporting HIV cases to health authorities does not necessarily lead to any additional benefit for either the client or the community, and may divert resources from more effective prevention and care strategies. Thus, where resources are limited, the appropriate equilibrium must be found in the use of various prevention and care strategies that have different levels of costs and impact. Strategies such as public information campaigns, youth education and distribution of condoms are comparatively cost-effective methods of reaching innumerable people for prevention and care purposes. Case-reporting, however, is expensive, and does not increase access to prevention and care services in itself. To be effective in prevention and care terms, case-reporting must be meaningfully integrated into various HIV associated services, such as VCT, health and social support services for those HIV-positive and/or presenting with AIDS-associated, and greater access to HIV-associated drugs and treatments. Resources should be put into developing these services before they are largely diverted to case-reporting. Because of these concerns, UNAIDS and WHO recommend HIV case-reporting only where certain conditions exist. These are:

(a) widespread access to, and use of, HIV testing;
(b) protection against breaches of confidentiality so as not to deter testing and reporting;
(c) access to effective care, alongwith anti-retrovirals;
(d) capacity within the health system to collect accurate statistics, and to compile, analyse, and act upon them, including follow-up of cases.

However, even when these circumstances exist, HIV case-reporting needs to be related to HIV prevalence studies in sentinel population groups and behavioural statistics to provide information of sufficient quality to monitor trends in the epidemic and the burden of disease.

In general, UNAIDS and WHO recommend that a country chooses appropriate HIV/AIDS surveillance due to its needs and resources. This means surveillance that is cost-effective given the financial and human resources available; refines as well as reinforces prevention and care efforts; maintains confidentiality; optimises access to available treatment options, where this is probable; and results in regular and widespread dissemination of information on HIV/AIDS to the population in non-stigmatising manners that help to open up the epidemic, decrease denial and discrimination, and increase commitment to prevention and care strategies. In resource-poor countries, depending on the state of the epidemic, this is likely to involve a form of sentinel surveillance.

The WHO/UNAIDS *Guidelines for 2nd Generation HIV Surveillance* provide a comprehensive framework for consideration of surveillance options.[34]

Recommendations

(a) In underdeveloped countries access to HIV testing and effective treatment is limited and where there is not ample infrastructure to maintain confidentiality, avoid case-based reporting of HIV and employ sentinel surveillance within the framework of second-generation HIV surveillance.

(b) Where there is broad access to and use of HIV tests, established surveillance systems for communicable diseases, security and confidentiality of statistics and access to anti-retroviral treatment, consider the use of HIV case-reporting to provide information to monitor HIV incidence and prevalence, and to increase access to treatment, patient compliance and long-term follow-up.

(c) Ensure that the surveillance methodology employed does not interfere with prevention of care programmes, for example, by allowing breaches of confidentiality that would make people afraid to take advantage of voluntary counselling and HIV-testing services.

(d) Ensure confidentiality and security of information through the development of policy, infrastructure (e.g., data storage and transmission systems that ensure the physical security of data and electronic security of computer files), increased capacity of health professionals to receive, report and use data, and legislation that protects against breaches of confidentiality.

(e) Increase public confidence in surveillance and protect the right to privacy through the enactment of laws, policies and legislations that preclude the non-public health use of statistics.

(f) Where name-based or coded reporting is employed, evaluate periodically the extent to which incomplete reporting, incomplete diagnosis or duplication of cases is compromising the utility of the received statistics.

(g) In the use of sentinel surveillance that is unlinked, ensure that personal identifiers are removed from blood specimens in a manner that does not permit relinkage.

(h) Strengthen the means and frequency by which the results of surveillance are disseminated in ways that open up the epidemic; reinforce prevention and care strategies; reduce fear, stigma and denial; and avoid the further stigmatisation of certain groups of people, e.g., migrants, refugees, commercial sex workers, men having sex with men.

Conclusion

People everywhere have great difficulty in openly facing issues involving sex, disease and death. In many countries, the stigma and discrimination about HIV/AIDS adds to the fears that many people who are HIV positive or have AIDS feel about informing spouses, lovers, family, friends, colleagues — and even health care providers — about their serostatus. There is every incentive to keep HIV health status secret. In underdeveloped countries, particularly, the fear of stigma, lack of treatment options, and the very limited access to voluntary counselling and HIV testing have led only a small number of people voluntarily to test for HIV and then reveal their HIV status for prevention of transmission or for care and support purposes. The fact that only a small number of people know they have HIV, and an even smaller number disclose that they are HIV positive, has added to the difficulty encountered by governments and communities in generating greater awareness of the HIV/AIDS epidemic, encouraging people to come forward for testing, preventing further HIV infections and accurately monitoring HIV/AIDS on an ongoing basis.

It is clear that much more needs to be done to open up the epidemic so that conditions are created where HIV/AIDS become what they are — a viral infection and associated illnesses that deserve, like any similar condition, a response involving compassion, support, respect and access to effective prevention, care and support options — for both the infected and the uninfected. This discussion has proposed some steps that can be taken to empower individuals and communities to engage in these programmes — beneficial disclosure, ethical partner notification and the appropriate use of HIV case-reporting.

These steps adhere to the principles of confidentiality and informed consent, not only as valid ethical principles but also as pragmatic means by which to engage people in effective prevention and care strategies. Human rights and ethics have always been related to equity and with protecting both private and public interests. In the context of HIV/AIDS, human rights (right to privacy) and ethical principles (confidentiality and informed consent) are the basis to protect individuals and communities, first by creating an environment in which a large majority of people will come forward for testing, counselling, prevention and care; and second by dealing in an ethical and effective manner with cases where people choose not to, or are unable to, inform partners about their infection. Mandatory measures are neither right, nor are they feasible or effective. They only serve to drive the epidemic further underground.

At this late, but crucial, juncture of the epidemic, it becomes ever more important for communities, health authorities, governments and international agencies to function in partnership to encourage HIV testing and counselling, revelation of status, notification of partners, and reporting on the epidemic in appropriate manners. This will involve a significant assessment of the use of resources, and may involve reorientation from traditional HIV programmes. A serious shift must now be taken towards creating a social environment where people can feel confident and safe to test for HIV and inform others that they have HIV. This will mean different sorts of activities, such as public education campaigns on tolerance and non-discrimination, training of health care professionals or ethics, implementation of more voluntary counselling and testing services, enactment of legislation and policies protecting against discrimination, support for community-based services that motivate VCT and follow-up support, and promotion of innovative concepts such as shared confidentiality and 'positive living'. Many communities are already engaged in these activities and are demonstrating a prevention and care success which involves the full community and permits the individuals in it to be able openly and positively to deal with HIV/AIDS. It is time now for countries and communities everywhere to move out from the darkness of secrecy into the light of effective individual and community action.

Terminology

Confidentiality

Confidentiality refers to the ethical and/or legal duty of the health care professional, and other professionals such as lawyers and social service providers, not reveal to anybody else, without authorisation, information that was given to, or obtained by, the professional in the context of his/her professional relationship with an HIV-positive person. It embraces intimate matters, which include sexual relationships, health status and illicit drug use. In the context of HIV/AIDS:

(a) Confidentiality applies to a person's HIV/AIDS status and necessitates that health authorities should seek the consent of the person infected for the revelation of his/her HIV/AIDS status to others.

(b) Confidentiality also involves the expectation by a person with HIV/AIDS that his/her status will not be disclosed, without his/her consent, by other person with whom that information may be exchanged.

The ethical duty of confidentiality is reinforced by the individual's right to secrecy (discussed later).

Disclosure

In the context of HIV/AIDS, disclosure refers to the act of informing any individual or organisation (such as a health authority, an employer or a school), of the serostatus of an infected person, or it refers to the fact that such information has been transmitted, by any means, by the person him or herself, or by a third party, with or without consent.[35] Except in exceptional conditions, when disclosure to another person is required by law or ethical considerations, the person with HIV has the right to secrecy and to exercise informed consent in all decisions about disclosure of his/her status.[36]

HIV/AIDS Counselling

HIV/AIDS counselling is a confidential dialogue between a client and a care provider which is aimed at enabling the client to cope with stress and take personal decisions, including those related to prevention and care, associated with HIV/AIDS. The counselling process involves an assessment of personal risk of HIV transmission and facilitates preventive behaviour.

> **Pre-test HIV/AIDS counselling** is a dialogue between a client and a health care provider aimed at discussing the HIV test and the possible implication for the client of knowing his/her serostatus, which leads to an informed decision to take, or not to take, the test.
>
> **Post-test HIV/AIDS counselling** is a dialogue between a client and a health care provider aimed at discussing the HIV test result and providing appropriate information support and referral, and at motivating behaviour that lessens risk of becoming infected, if the test is negative, or reduces the risk of transmitting HIV to others, if the test is positive.[37]

Incidence

The number of new cases discovered in a given period in a specified population.

Informed Consent

Informed consent is based on the theory that competent individuals are entitled to make informed decisions regarding their participation in, or acquiesence to, certain events in the context of a professional relationship between health care provider and patient/client. Informed consent safeguards the person's freedom of option and respects his/her autonomy, particularly with respect to decisions affecting his or her body and health. In the HIV/AIDS arena, health care professionals have an ethical duty to obtain informed consent in order to administer HIV tests and other HIV/AIDS-associated health care interventions, and before revealing to others only HIV-associated information concerning a patient/client, including HIV status.

Notifiable Disease

A disease that by legislation must be reported to the public health authority, or other designed authority in the pertinent jurisdiction, when a diagnosis is made.

Partner Counselling (Partner Notification, Partner Management, Contact Tracing)

Partner counselling or notification is the process of contacting the sexual partners (or drug-injecting partners) of an individual (source or index client or patient) who has a sexually transmitted infection (STI) alongwith HIV, and advising the partners that they have been exposed to infection. By this means, people who are at high risk of STI/HIV, many of whom are unaware that they have been exposed, are contacted and motivated to attend counselling, testing and other prevention and treatment services. Where probable, confidentiality is maintained by not providing the name of the HIV-infected person to partners.

In most cases, partner counselling is conducted with the informed consent of the HIV-infected person or provider. A situation where partner counselling might be allowed without consent arises when a health care provider is aware that a person with HIV is behaving in a manner that is placing another person at direct risk and refuses, after extensive counselling, to permit partners to be contacted. It then becomes an ethical duty of the health care provider to decide how to prevent the greatest amount of probable harm to the parties concerned, given the individual circumstances of the case.

Partner counselling can be undertaken by the HIV-infected partner him or herself, by the health care provider, or through the combined efforts of both.

Source referral: the source client or patient is encouraged to contact his or her sexual (or drug-injecting) partners and advise them to seek appropriate medical care. This process can be assisted by health care professionals who spend time educating the HIV-infected person or patient about the importance of contact tracing, give out contact cards, or by using telephone or mail reminders.

Provider referral: the health care provider involved in the HIV-infected person's or patient's care can counsel the sexual partners without naming the source concerned.

Conditional referral: the health care provider of the HIV-infected person or patient obtains names of sexual partners but permits the client a period of time to counsel partners him/herself. If the partners are not counselled within this time frame, the health care provider counsels the partners without naming the source patient or client concerned.[38]

People Living with HIV/AIDS (PLWHs)

Often this term has been used to refer to people actually infected with HIV and/or experiencing AIDS-associated illnesses or infections. More recently there has been a move to widen this term to include those also *affected* by HIV/AIDS, but not necessarily infected. Thus, the term would involve infected people, people with the symptoms of AIDS and also HIV-negative partners, family members and close friends. [39] In this discussion, when there has been a need to refer only to those who are infected with HIV, the term "HIV-positive" has been used.

Prevalence

The number of cases in a given population at a specified point in time.

Public Health Surveillance

Public health surveillance is the collection of statistics on the distribution and spread of infection of sufficient accuracy and completeness to be pertinent to the design, implementation and/or monitoring of prevention and control programmes and activities. There are several methods of surveillance of HIV. [40] These include:

(a) **Population-based surveillance**. This form of surveillance includes the collection and testing for HIV of blood specimens from a random sample of the population being studied. It also permits the collection of more detailed information, particularly on risk behaviours. Unlike sentinel surveillance studies, discussed later, population-based studies normally require that health authorities obtain the informed consent of all the people whose blood is used. This increases the cost of this form of surveillance and creates a potential for participation bias. Though population-based surveillance may be the best method to evaluate HIV prevalence, this form of surveillance is expensive and complicated and has so far been implemented in only some countries.

(b) **Sentinel surveillance.** Sentinel surveillance is the systematic collection of statistics on incidence or prevalence of HIV infection in selected populations. It may include the use of the blood of people in a particular hospital, geographic area or population group (e.g., commercial sex workers or migrant workers). Some sentinel groups (e.g., pregnant women, military recruits) may be either linked (traceable by a code to an individual) or unlinked (untraceable and anonymous). If statistics are linked, then informed consent is required. Unlinked anonymous testing includes the testing for HIV of blood collected routinely for other purposes (e.g., blood donation, antenatal attendance) on a regular basis. In this case, there is no need for individual informed consent, and participation bias is minimised. This is the most commonly used form of HIV surveillance.

(c) **Case-based surveillance**. This form of surveillance is based on an often legal requirement that health care providers report to health authorities every case of HIV/AIDS that they have diagnosed. Information is provided using a standard reporting form. The report may consist the *name* of the case (named reporting); or may use a *code* (sometimes called a 'unique identifier') for each case; or may provide information on cases anonymously. Health care providers may sometimes be reluctant to report cases identified by name due to confidentiality and to protect patient privacy. On the other hand, where the information is provided anonymously, there is potential for multiple reporting of the same case.

Reporting

Refers to the procedure through which health providers systematically inform health authorities of each individual case of HIV infection and AIDS presenting in consultation, or otherwise known to them. Where HIV and AIDS are notifiable diseases, this is required by law.

(a) **Named case-reporting.** The name of individuals with HIV infection and/or AIDS are provided. The information is confidential and is intended only for the health system to ensure that appropriate measures are taken.

(b) **Unnamed case-reporting.** Names of individuals with HIV infection and/or AIDS are removed, and health authorities are provided only with information that is useful for disease surveillance and analysis (for example, age, gender, risk factors, occupation). When possible, an identifying code is used in order to avoid duplicate reports (reporting as separate cases of HIV infection and/or AIDS each time the same individual presents for care).[41]

Right to Privacy

The right to privacy is projected in several international human rights instruments, as well as in some rational bills of rights. For example, Article 17 of the International Covenant on Civil and Political Rights provides: "No one shall be subjected to arbitrary and unlawful interference with his privacy, home or correspondence, nor to unlawful attack on his honour and reputation. Everyone has the right to protection of the law against such interference or attacks".[42] This right generates an obligation on states to promote, protect and fulfil it by ensuring that the state does not arbitrarily interfere with private matters; that others do not infringe this right; and that the state takes necessary legal or other measures to protect people's right to privacy.

General Guidelines

UNAIDS and WHO are UN-system agencies dedicated to the promotion of health, human rights and ethical principles. As such, they work with and call upon governments to promote, protect and implement the international human rights obligations found in international human rights instruments,[43] and the ethical principles found in innumerable texts on ethical principles.[44] In the context of the subjects of this paper — disclosure, partner counselling, and HIV case-reporting — UNAIDS and WHO developed the following general principles when governments and policy-makers plan appropriate national strategies.

(a) People living with HIV/AIDS and affected communities should be consulted and included in decision-making, policy formulation, programme planning, implementation and assessment.

(b) Respect and protection of human rights and ethical principles (e.g., the right to privacy, confidentiality, informed consent, the duty to do no harm) will directly facilitate the acceptance, implementation and success of HIV prevention and care strategies — particularly if they necessitate the active participation of the community. On the other hand, strategies that erode human rights and ethics and create an environment of fear, intolerance and coercion will undermine public health interventions that aim to encourage disclosure, partner counselling and appropriate use of HIV case surveillance.

(c) Human rights and ethical principles should be upheld in every policy. If limitations of human rights are to be justifiable, these limitations should be prescribed by law and not be arbitrary. They should be strictly necessary for the attainment of a legitimate objective, and be the least restrictive measure to achieve this purpose.

(d) Policies and programmes should be evaluated on the basis of the following parameters:
   (i) whether the proposed policy or programme can be effectively implemented;
   (ii) whether it is a rational allocation of resources because of other competing needs;
   (iii) the benefits and possible adverse consequences of a policy both for individuals and for wider public health and social objection;
   (iv) whether the benefits outweigh the harm;
   (v) whether the longer-term consequences of policy decisions are advantageous;

(e) Data collection, collation, analysis and dissemination should be undertaken for a specific and valid purpose, namely to enable appropriate and constructive measure for the prevention and control of the epidemic and provision of care for and support of people infected, affected and vulnerable to HIV/AIDS.

Recommendations

To encourage beneficial disclosure

(i) Conduct public information campaigns and community forums targeted at promoting tolerance, compassion and understanding, and lessening fear, stigma and discrimination.

(ii) Motivate participation of people living with HIV/AIDS in public information campaigns and in HIV programmes and policy formulation.

(iii) Set up more voluntary counselling and testing (VCT) services, including services in countryside areas and for marginalised groups.

(iv) Support governmental agencies, non-governmental organisations and community-based organisations to make community-based services, alongwith VCT, family outreach, community support, positive living, support groups and care options broadly available.

(v) Encourage the media to offer a reasonable coverage to HIV/AIDS in a responsible, non-discriminatory and non-sensational manner.

(vi) Train health care professionals in the management of HIV and global precautions, in attitudes of non-discrimination, acceptance and compassion, and in the principles of confidentiality and informed consent.

(vii) Train other professionals (social workers, policy, advocates judges) in attitudes of non-discrimination, acceptance and compassion, and in the principles of confidentiality and informed consent.

(viii) Train key personnel in non-health employment settings, including human resource management in industry in promoting non-discriminatory practices in the workplace.

(ix) Enact or reform legislations, administrative guidelines and professional codes of conduct to prohibit discrimination and breaches of confidentiality associated with HIV status.

(x) Generate legal support services for those who have suffered discrimination based on HIV status.

Encouragement of Ethical Partner Counselling

(i) Develop national policies and public health legislation on partner counselling that protect the principles of confidentiality and informed consent, and provide for the limited and clearly defined circumstances under which partner counselling may take place without consent.

(ii) Develop public health legislation that authorises health care providers to decide, on the basis of each individual case and ethical considerations, whether to counsel partners without the consent of the HIV-infected person, under certain conditions.

(iii) Hold consultations among health care providers, government and affected communities about how to encourage ethical partner counselling and protect people who reveal their status through such counselling.

(iv) Provide training and guidelines for health care providers and counsellors about how to protect confidentiality and informed consent in the context of partner counselling; how to encourage and assist voluntary partner counselling; how to make difficult ethical decisions in cases where there is refusal to counsel partners; and how to counsel partners in the manners that harm is minimised and support is provided.

(v) Promote the setting up of professional ethical codes among health care and social service providers which necessitate respect for confidentiality and informed consent in the context of partner counselling, and provide penalties for unethical conduct.

(vi) Establish techniques for accountability and manners of making complaints in health care institutions and in communities when partners are counselled unethically by health care providers and other professionals.

(vii) Support practical legal and social measures that address the vulnerability of people, particularly that of women, to stigma, physical violence and abandonment, involving projects in the community which will assist in providing treatment, care, emotional support and protection from discrimination to those involved in partner counselling.

(viii) Promote and support community projects about people's responsibility to protect themselves and others from HIV infection, particularly among men and boys.

Encouragement of the Appropriate use of HIV Case-reporting

(i) In underdeveloped countries where access to HIV testing and effective treatment is limited and where there is no ample infrastructure to maintain confidentiality, avoid case-based reporting of HIV and employ sentinel surveillance within the framework of second-generation HIV surveillance.

(ii) Where there is broad access to, and use of, HIV tests, established surveillance systems for communicable diseases, security and confidentiality of statistics and access to anti-retroviral treatment, consider the use of HIV case-reporting to provide information to monitor HIV incidence and prevalence, and to increase access to treatment, patient compliance and long-term follow-up.

(iii) Ensure that the surveillance methodology employed does not interfere with prevention of care programmes for example by allowing breaches of confidentiality that would make people afraid to take advantage of voluntary counselling and HIV testing services.

(iv) Ensure confidentiality and security of information through the development of policy, infrastructure (e.g., data storage and transmission systems that ensure the physical security of statistics, and electronic security of computer files), increased capacity of health professionals to receive, report and use statistics and legislation that protects against breaches of confidentiality.

(v) Increase public confidence in surveillance and protect the right to privacy through the enactment of regulations, policies and legislation that preclude the non-public health use of statistics.

(vi) Where name-based or coded reporting is employed, evaluate periodically the extent to which incomplete reporting, incomplete diagnosis or duplication of cases is compromising the utility of the received statistics.

(vii) In the use of sentinel surveillance that is unlinked, ensure that personal identifiers are removed from blood specimens in a manner that does not allow relinkage.

(viii) Strengthen the means and frequency by which the results of surveillance are disseminated in ways that open up the epidemic; reinforce prevention and care programmes; reduce fear, stigma and denial; and avoid the further stigmatisation of certain groups of people, e.g. migrants, refugees, commercial sex workers, men having sex with men.

References

1. See UNAIDS/WHO AIDS Epidemic Update, December 1999, pp. 5, 16-17.
2. Entitled "Technical Consultation on Notification, Confidentiality and HIV/AIDS, Windhoek, Namibia, 4-6 August 1999, Meeting Statement", available from WHO or UNAIDS, Geneva.
3. In addition to the doctor/patient relationship and the clinical setting confidentiality is also an ethical duty in other professional fields, such as social work, psychiatry, psychotherapy and the practice of law, and in research involving human participants.
4. For more on these issues in the context of HIV, see Jurgens R. *HIV Testing and Confidentiality: Final Report*. Montreal, Canadian HIV/AIDS Legal Network and Canadian AIDS Society, 1998, pp. 209-224; *Confidentiality*, Number 17 of a series of 19 Info Sheets on HIV Testing. Montreal, Canadian HIV/AIDS Legal Network, 2000.
5. From *Questions and Answers on Reporting, Partner Notification and Disclosure of HIV Serostatus and/or AIDS, Public Health and Human Rights Implications*. Geneva, WHO/UNAIDS, June 1999 (UNAIDS/00.26E).
6. For discussion of cases where it may be appropriate to disclose someone's status without their consent in order to prevent onward transmission of HIV, see section on ethical partner counselling at page 18.
7. See Zambia sexual behaviour survey 1998. Republic of Zambia, Measure and Central Statistical Office, 45; Tyndall et al., Evaluation of AIDS control strategies in women attending a family planning clinic in Nairobi, Kenya International Conference on AIDS, 1996 (abstract no. We. D. 3760).
8. For more on the availability of VCT, see *Report on the Global HIV/AIDS Epidemic*. Geneva, June 2000 (UNAIDS/00.13E).
9. See Report of the Meeting on Theme Groups on International Partnership against HIV/AIDS (IPAA) in Africa, Nairobi, 24-27 January 2000, p. 8, where there was a cell to accelerate operation research on VCT and mother-to-child transmission prevention "in order to make these interventions central in the implementation of the IPAA", available from UNAIDS, Geneva.
10. See *Voluntary Counselling and Testing Technical Update*, Geneva, UNAIDS, May 2000 (WC 503.6).
11. UNAIDS Case Study, Knowledge is Power: Voluntary HIV Counselling and Testing in Uganda. Geneva, June 1999, (UNAIDS/99.8E).
12. Vollmer N, Valadez J. A psychological epidemiology of people seeking

HIV/AIDS counselling in Kenya: an approach for improving counselling training. *AIDS*, 1999, 13:1557-1567.

13. Kalldjian L, Jekel J, Friedland G. End-of-life decisions in HIV positive patients: the role of spiritual beliefs. *AIDS*, 1998, 12:103-107.
14. Meursing K, Sibindi F. Condoms, family planning and living with HIV in Zimbabwe. *Reproductive Health Matters*, 1995, 5:56-62.
15. Meursing K. *A World of Silence, Living with HIV in Matabeleland, Zimbabwe.* The Netherlands, Royal Tropical Institute, 1997.
16. Lie G, Biswalo P. Positive patient's choice of a significant other to be informed about the HIV test result: findings from an HIV/AIDS counselling programme in the regional hospitals of Arusha and Kilimanjaro, Tanzania. *AIDS Care*, 1996, 8(3):285-296.
17. TASO Uganda. *The Inside Story. Participatory evaluation of the HIV/AIDS Counselling, Medical and Social Services* 1993-94 (WHO/GPA/TCO/HCS/95.1).
18. For more on the involvement of people living with HIV/AIDS, see *From Principle to Practice, The Greater Involvement of People Living with HIV/AIDS.* Geneva, 1999 (UNAIDS/99.43E).
19. See *Handbook for Legislators on HIV/AIDS*. Geneva, UNAIDS/IPU, 1999 (UNAIDS/99.48E).
20. For examples and more discussion, see Bharat Shalini, *HIV/AIDS Related Discrimination, Stigmatisation and Denial in India - A study in Mumbai and Bangalore*, 1999, available from UNAIDS, Geneva.
21. See Miller, D. *Dying to Care?: Work, Stress and Burnout in HIV/AIDS*. London, Routledge, 2000.
22. Adam G, Harford N. *Radio and HIV/AIDS: Making a Difference. A Guide for Radio Practitioners, Health Workers and Donors*. Geneva, UNAIDS/Media Action International, 1999.
23. For an example of this type of activity, see the Intersectoral Committee on AIDS and Employment/OATUU: Labour Relations Regulations on HIV/AIDS and Employment. Zimbabwe, ICAE/OATUU, January 1999 (Sl 202 1998).
24. The UNAIDS/WHO Consultation on HIV Reporting and Disclosure, Geneva, 20-22 October 1999, recommended that the term "partner counselling" should be substituted for the term "partner notification" because, in some contexts, partner notification is associated with coercion and pressure. The Centers for Disease Control, Atlanta, Georgia, USA, now uses the term "partner counselling". In this document, the term "partner counselling" will generally be used.
25. See also Bayer R, Fairchild A. *The Role of Name-based Notification in Public Health and Surveillance.* Geneva, 2000 (UNAIDS/0028E).
26. See also "partner counselling" in Annex 1, Definitions of important terms.
27. See also Rothenberg RB. Ptterate JJ. Partner notification for sexually transmitted disease and HIV infection, in *Sexually Transmitted Disease*, 3rd edition, NY, McGraw-Hill, 1999; Nuwaha et al., Psychological determinants for sexual partner referral in Uganda, qualitative results. *International Journal of STD and AIDS 2000*, 11:156-161.
28. Statement by Noreen Kaleeba, Founder TASO Uganda, presently UNAIDS Community Mobilisation Adviser, Geneva.
29. For further examples of community-based activities where the concept of

shared confidentiality is exemplified, see *Comfort and Hop: Six Case Studies on Mobilising Family and Community Care for and by People with HIV/AIDS.* UNAIDS, June 1999 (UNAIDS/99.10E); and Linkkhoff P, Bukanga E, Syamalevwe B, Williams G. *Under the Mupundu Tree.* Actionaid Strategies for Hope (No. 14), 1999.

30. For more on these points, see Gielen AC, O'Campo P, et al. A women's disclosure of HIV status: Experiences of mistreatment and violence in an urban setting. *Women's Health,* 1997, 25(3):19-31; Van de Straten A, et al. Couple communication, sexual coercion and HIV risk reduction in Kigali, Rwanda. AIDS, 1995, 9:935-944; Temmerman M, Ndinya-Achola J, Ambani J, Piot P. The right not to know HIV-test results. Lancet, 1995, 345(8955): 969-970.
31. Taken in large part from *HIV/AIDS and Human Rights, International Guidelines,* New York and Geneva, United Nations,. 1998 (HR/PUB/98/1): 13, para.28(g).
32. *Ibid.*
33. For more, see Annex 1, Definitions of important terms.
34. WHO/UNAIDS, 2000 (WHO/CDS/CSR/EDC/2000.5 and UNAIDS/ 00.03E/F/R).
35. From *Questions and Answers on Reporting, Partner Notification and Disclosure of HIV Serostatus and/or AIDS, Public Health and Human Rights Implications,* Geneva, WHO/UNAIDS, June 1999 (UNAIDS/00.26E).
36. An example of disclosure that might be permitted or required by law is disclosure where people accused and/or found guilty of sexual offences are required to disclose their HIV status to victims of their (presumed) offences.
37. See *Voluntary Counselling and Testing Technical Update,* Geneva, UNAIDS, May 2000, (WC 503.6).
38. Largely taken from *Questions and Answers on Reporting, Partner Notification and Disclosure of HIV Serostatus and/or AIDS, Public Health and Human Rights Implications,* Geneva, WHO/UNAIDS, June 1999 (UNAIDS/00.26E). See also *Report of the Consultation on Partner Notification for Preventing HIV Infection.* WHO, 1989 (WHO/GPA/ESR/89.2).
39. For more on this, *see Greater Involvement of People Living with or Affected by HIV/AIDS* (GIPA). September 1999, (UNAIDS/99.43E).
40. For full description of HIV surveillance, see *Guidelines for 2nd Generation HIV Surveillance,* Geneva, WHO/AIDS, 2000 (WHO/CDS/CSR/EDC/ 2000.5 and UNAIDS/00.03E/F/R).
41. *Ibid.* See Reference 5.
42. Adopted by the General Assembly under GA resolution 2200 (XXI), UN GAOR, 21st session, Supplement No. 16, UN Doc. A/6316 (1966). Entered into force 23 March, 1976.
43. For a full explanation of relevant human rights in the context of *HIV/AIDS,* see United Nations, *HIV/AIDS and Human Rights, International Guidelines,* New York and Geneva, 1998 (HR/PUB/98/1).
44. There are many relevant ethical codes. For example, see International Code of Medical Ethics, World Medical Association, 1949, 1963, 1983; The Hippocratic Oath; The World Medical Association Declaration of Helsinki, adopted in 1964 and most recently amended in 1989; the International Ethical Guidelines for Biomedical Research Involving Human Subjects, CIOMS, Geneva, 1993; Ethical Considerations in HIV Preventive Vaccine Research UNAIDS, 2000 (UNAIDS/00.07E).

Six

Voluntary Counselling and Testing (VCT)

VCT Implementation

Whether VCT is witnessed as a priority for the health system will depend on the HIV seroprevalence in the community, the resources available for HIV prevention and care, and the perceptions of politicians, service planners and managers and health care professionals. In lower-prevalence low-and middle-income countries, such as those in North Africa, Eastern Europe and some countries in Asia, it may be appropriate to target services at more affected groups, but in so doing it will be important to protect against increasing stigma and blame.

In high-prevalence areas it will be more appropriate to promote services for the general population. It is important not to provide VCT services in isolation, but develop them in association with support services for those who test seropositive and HIV prevention services.

VCT should not only be developed in association with adequate support services. There should also be a bond between the type and quality of HIV education in the community and offering VCT. If the predominant opinions in the community are that "HIV = AIDS = death", that "you can do nothing about it" and that HIV is a disease of "promiscuous" people, interest in VCT will be low. People base their decision on having an HIV test on the equilibrium of advantages and disadvantages of knowing their status. If community attitudes are unfavourable, interest in VCT will be low. If, however, the community has received education and information on the advantages of VCT for individuals and their families, people are more likely to accept it. VCT services need to be built on the fact that HIV is a discussible disease and that HIV risk is discussible too. This is the case in Uganda, and this has been achieved by the long-term commitment of its leaders in openness about AIDS. A community that feels helpless against HIV and defends itself by stigma may not be "ready" for VCT, although promoting VCT will assist achieve community openness.

For the advantages of VCT to be understood and hence used, services must be endorsed by and included in the National AIDS Programme plan. The success of VCT in Uganda, compared with other countries in sub-Saharan Africa, is thought to be in part due to the political commitment to VCT as part of the overall HIV prevention and care programme. Some underdeveloped high-prevalence countries will continue to consider VCT a low priority, and others may consider developing VCT in a phased manner. This will be particularly appropriate if support services for people living with HIV/AIDS are not well developed and resources are very limited, or when the infrastructure is not amply developed to support VCT services.

However, even if political commitment to VCT does not exist, NGOs can advocate the concept and establish projects to display the need for and advantages of VCT. The Thai Red Cross set up the "Anonymous Clinic" VCT service in Bangkok in July 1991 when HIV was a notifiable disease and mandatory HIV testing was widely practised. The success of the Anonymous Clinics succeeded in motivating the government to change the law on mandatory reporting. This was followed six months later by a policy to establish VCT centres in every province of Thailand.

Tool 1: For Assessment of the National Preparedness for VCT Implementation

Methodology

respondents = programme planners

This group would include National AIDS Programme (NAP) managers, counselling service coordinators, and NGO coordinators involved in VCT activities. It may be appropriate to interview other policy-makers in, for example, associated ministries such as education. As these will be few in number an effort should be made to interview them all. Sampling will therefore not be necessary. The interviews should be carried out individually and the respondents encouraged to elaborate on any of the items, qualify statements and provide additional comments where appropriate.

Country background

Per capita GNP ....

Per capita spending on health ....

HIV sentinel survey figures

Urban antenatal ....

Rural antenatal ....

Other available seroprevalence statistics, please specify

....

How is VCT seen by the NAP?

- Major priority ❑
- Priority in a few settings ❑
- Not a priority ❑

Have VCT services been developed in your country?

- Comprehensive country-wide service ❑
- Limited service (capital and selected large cities) ❑
- Limited service provided by NGOs ❑
- Other ❑

Please describe the VCT services in detail

....

Please describe any barriers to implementation

....

Does a national policy on VCT exist?

Yes ❑ In preparation ❑ No ❑

Have national guidelines for implementing HIV counselling been developed?

Yes ❑ In preparation ❑ No ❑

Please describe how these were developed and state whether there have been any difficulties in their implementation.

....

Is VCT promoted as part of HIV prevention and care services?

Yes ❑ In preparation ❑ No ❑

Is HIV testing a legal requirement under any circumstances?

Pre-marital	❑
Migrant workers	❑
Other (specify)	❑

Is HIV testing frequently performed in:

Pre-operative screening	❑
Pre-employment	❑
General antenatal care	❑
As part of MTCT intervention	❑
Prisons	❑
Military recruitment	❑
IDU treatment	❑
STI clinic	❑
TB clinic	❑

Are VCT services available?

General services	Yes ❑	Being considered ❑	No ❑
Services for young people	Yes ❑	Being considered ❑	No ❑

Services for special groups

MSM	Yes ❑	Being considered ❑	No ❑
Commercial sex workers	Yes ❑	Being considered ❑	No ❑
IDUs	Yes ❑	Being considered ❑	No ❑
Refugees	Yes ❑	Being considered ❑	No ❑
Prisoners	Yes ❑	Being considered ❑	No ❑
Others (please specify below)	Yes ❑	Being considered ❑	No ❑

....

Are associated services available for people living with HIV or AIDS?

Ongoing medical care	Yes ❑	In preparation ❑	No ❑
Ongoing social support	Yes ❑	In preparation ❑	No ❑
Support group for people living with HIV/AIDS	Yes ❑	In preparation ❑	No ❑
Ongoing counselling support	Yes ❑	In preparation ❑	No ❑
Liaison with NGOs	Yes ❑	In preparation ❑	No ❑
Family planning	Yes ❑	In preparation ❑	No ❑
MTCT interventions	Yes ❑	In preparation ❑	No ❑

TBPT Yes ❑ In preparation ❑ No ❑
ARV interventions Yes ❑ In preparation ❑ No ❑
Other preventive therapies[2] Yes ❑ In preparation ❑ No ❑
(Please specify) ....

Are HIV preventive services available?
Condom supplies
Yes, country-wide programme ❑ Yes, some sites ❑ No ❑
Services for IDUs
Yes, country-wide programme ❑ Yes, some sites ❑ No ❑
Ongoing counselling
Yes, country-wide programme ❑ Yes, some sites ❑ No ❑
Other (Please specify)
Yes, country-wide programme ❑ Yes, some sites ❑ No ❑
....

Are HIV counselling training courses being run? Yes ❑ No ❑
If YES, at what level National ❑
Provincial ❑
District ❑
Testing site ❑

How many counsellors have been trained? ....

What are the backgrounds of the people being trained as counsellors?
Nurses ❑
Clinical officers ❑
Social workers ❑
People living with HIV/AIDS ❑
Others (Please specify) ❑
....

What training is offered?
Basic counselling training Yes ❑ In preparation ❑ No ❑
Advanced training Yes ❑ In preparation ❑ No ❑
Follow-up supervision Yes ❑ In preparation ❑ No ❑
Follow-up evaluation of counsellors Yes, countrywide programme ❑
Yes, some sites ❑
No ❑

Number of training courses held ....

How long is the training? ....

Please describe in detail the training offered[3]

....

If counsellors are evaluated for the quality of their counselling how this is achieved?[4]

....

Are statistical data about the counselling service regularly compiled? Yes ❑ No ❑

If YES, by whom ....

The Sites and Services

Site

Accessibility and convenience

VCT services need to be accessible for the population they are serving. Opening hours need to take into consideration the needs of the clients. To allow easy access for working people, lunchtime, early evening and weekend services should be considered.

In services used by women, or families, providing a supervised space where children can play would enable less interrupted counselling.

Privacy

For VCT to be conducted correctly and effectively, privacy must be ensured. Discussion of risk factors and sexual relationships is part of VCT for HIV infection, and key information essential to the process will not be elicited unless people can discuss these problems in private. Private space will be necessitated.

Waiting area

Besides, a well-ventilated waiting area is important. TB infection is commonly related to HIV and people with reduced immunity are particularly vulnerable nosocomial tuberculosis infection.

Confidentiality

For VCT services to be acceptable, confidentiality must be guaranteed. HIV remains a stigmatising condition in most countries and uptake of services will be low if it is not known that confidentiality will be respected. Therefore a system must be in place to avoid breaches of confidentiality at all stages in the VCT process. In some settings it has been demonstrated that people feel more comfortable about attending VCT services if they can give a pseudonym[5], and anonymous testing is commonly available in many developed countries.

Linkages

VCT has been displayed to be more effective when it is developed in conjunction with support services (medical, social and emotional, family planning services, STI services, antenatal services, home-based care services and palliative care services), spiritual services and traditional healers, support groups for people living with HIV/AIDS, community groups and NGOs.

In high-prevalence areas a wide range of care and support programmes may already be in place in the community. It will be important for counsellors to be aware of these resources and to be able to make appropriate referrals. Counsellors must also be aware of the special medical requirements of people living with HIV/AIDS. The package of TB (including TB screening and TB preventive therapy) may be available; in some countries ARV therapy is available, though often only for a minority. The spiritual needs of people living with HIV/AIDS have been demonstrated to be important in many countries[6], and counsellors should be aware of these for referral.

HIV testing methods (including quality control)

Although HIV testing methods have become much more sensitive and specific (especially for sera from Africa), assessment have displayed that without rigorous quality control high numbers of false positive and negative results are common. Not only can this be extremely damaging for individuals, but it can undermine the credibility of the service. If the WHO/UNAIDS testing strategies[7] are conducted for all tests, whatever method is used, laboratory errors can be reduced to a minimum. It is particularly important when setting up an HIV testing service, or when changing an HIV testing method, that tests are cross-checked at a reference centre. Even when these are used, large numbers of clerical errors are often reported. Therefore a cross-checking system for results is important.

Cost and Sustainability

Many developing countries are undergoing health reforms that include a degree of cost-sharing of medical services. However, for services to be affordable for the majority of people, they will generally have to be provided at low cost. In some countries the services are provided free to a limited number of people, or "free days" are built into the system to ensure that people who cannot afford to pay even a small amount are not barred from the services[8].

It is also important to have a medium-term plan for the service. If a service has to be shut, or scaled down after an initial period, confidence will be lost and the community will feel let down after expectations have been raised.

Services for special and vulnerable groups

VCT services may be considered for groups of people particularly affected by HIV. For example, there is experience from working with commercial sex workers in southern Africa[9] demonstrating that VCT services must be conducted sensitively.

Tool 2: For VCT Site Assessment: Logistic Considerations and Coverage

Methodology

respondents-VCT managers

In some countries several VCT sites exist. Where a small number exist an effort should be made to interview managers from all sites. Where there are numerous sites a representative sample of managers from the various categories of VCT sites should be made — for example, one each from a blood transfusion site, free-standing VCT site, hospital clinical setting, private sector, research site, etc. The sample should also contain examples of both rural and urban sites where appropriate.

Which services do you offer?

- Pre-test counselling ❑
- Post-test counselling ❑
- Ongoing counselling ❑
- HIV testing ❑
- HIV diagnostic counselling (without testing) ❑

If pre-and post-test counselling are undertaken, do carefully defined procedures exist? Yes ❑ No ❑

Please describe these[10]

....

Opening hours

Are you open at any of the following times?

- Early evening (after 17:00) No ❑ Yes ❑
  (specify how many evenings)
- Lunch hour No ❑ Yes ❑
- Weekends No ❑ Yes ❑
  (specify Sat. or Sun. or both)

Do you have an appointment system? Yes ❑ No ❑

If YES, what happens if someone comes without an appointment?

- They are asked to make a future appointment Yes ❑ No ❑
- They will always be seen the same day Yes ❑ No ❑
- They will generally be seen the same day Yes ❑ No ❑

Privacy

Do you have adequate space to ensure counselling sessions can be private?

- Yes, there is adequate space ❑
- There is some private space, but not enough ❑
- No ❑

Specify,

private office	❑	cubicle	❑
curtained-off area	❑	other (describe)	❑

Waiting area

Describe the waiting area ....

Confidentiality

Does the site have a written policy on confidentiality?

Yes ❑ No ❑

Describe the steps that have been taken to ensure confidentiality[11]

....

Have any of the following staff received specific guidance about the role of counselling and confidentiality?

Counsellors	Yes ❑	No ❑
Laboratory staff	Yes ❑	No ❑
Non-counselling medical staff	Yes ❑	No ❑
Ward attendants	Yes ❑	No ❑
Receptionists	Yes ❑	No ❑
Ancillary staff (e.g., cleaners)	Yes ❑	No ❑
Others (specify)	....	

Linkages

Do you receive referrals from any of the following?

Medical services (e.g., clinics/hospitals)	Yes ❑	Occasionally ❑	No ❑
Social services	Yes ❑	Occasionally ❑	No ❑
Other counselling services	Yes ❑	Occasionally ❑	No ❑
NGOs	Yes ❑	Occasionally ❑	No ❑
Family planning services	Yes ❑	Occasionally ❑	No ❑
MCH services	Yes ❑	Occasionally ❑	No ❑
TB/chest clinic	Yes ❑	Occasionally ❑	No ❑
STI services	Yes ❑	Occasionally ❑	No ❑
Traditional healers	Yes ❑	Occasionally ❑	No ❑
Spiritual/religious groups	Yes ❑	Occasionally ❑	No ❑
Others (specify)	....		

Do you refer to any of the following?

Medical services (e.g., clinics/hospitals)	Yes ❑	Occasionally ❑	No ❑
Social services	Yes ❑	Occasionally ❑	No ❑
Other counselling services	Yes ❑	Occasionally ❑	No ❑
NGOs	Yes ❑	Occasionally ❑	No ❑
Family planning services	Yes ❑	Occasionally ❑	No ❑
MCH services	Yes ❑	Occasionally ❑	No ❑

TB/chest clinic	Yes ❑	Occasionally ❑	No ❑
STI services	Yes ❑	Occasionally ❑	No ❑
Traditional healers	Yes ❑	Occasionally ❑	No ❑
Spiritual/religious groups	Yes ❑	Occasionally ❑	No ❑
Others (specify)	....		

Describe how the referral systems function and any problems and successes

....

Do you feel there are ample referral services available, particularly for the needs of people who test positive?

....

HIV testing methods

Where do you conduct HIV tests?

All testing done on site ❑

Preliminary tests done on site, confirmations sent to other laboratory ❑

All testing conducted in other laboratory ❑

What is the time interval between taking blood and results being available?

....

Describe the HIV testing schedule employed[12]

....

Do you have external quality control for HIV testing?

Yes ❑ No ❑

If YES, describe

....

Cost and sustainability

Do you charge for services?

Counselling only	No ❑	Yes ❑	amount ....
Testing	No ❑	Yes ❑	amount ....
Ongoing counselling	No ❑	Yes ❑	amount ....

If YES:

Are there any people who do not pay?

Yes ❑ No ❑ % who do not pay ....

How is the service funded? ....

How long is the funding of the services ensured? ....

Are any inducements given to people attending the site?

(e.g., transport costs, refreshments, etc.) No ❑ Yes ❑

If YES, specify ....

Services for special and vulnerable groups

Do you have special services for any of the following groups?

Pregnant women	Yes ❑	No ❑
Young people	Yes ❑	No ❑
Children and families	Yes ❑	No ❑
Commercial sex workers	Yes ❑	No ❑
Refugees	Yes ❑	No ❑
MSM	Yes ❑	No ❑
IDUs	Yes ❑	No ❑

Level of service provision and utilisation

In the last 3 months:

How many people have presented at the site?

....

What per cent of people have had pre-test counselling?

....

What per cent of people have been tested for HIV?

....

What per cent of people have returned for their result?[13]

....

What per cent of people have been given post-test counselling?

....

What per cent of people have received ongoing counselling?

....

What per cent of people have been referred to other services?

....

List the services to which most referrals have been made:

....

Describe any problems and successes you have observed in people returning for test results

....

Outreach counselling (counselling in non-clinical settings)
Is outreach counselling conducted? Yes ❑ No ❑
If YES,
How many people, on average, per group? ....
How many outreach sessions in the past 3 months? ....
Where are outreach sessions carried out? ....

Advertising and promotion of the VCT service
Do you advertise or promote your service in any way?
Yes ❑ No ❑
If YES, describe ....

Group counselling
Is group pre-test counselling conducted? Yes ❑ No ❑
If YES,
How many people, on average, per group? ....
How many group counselling sessions in the past 3 months? ....
How long, on average is each session? ....

Counsellors' Necessities and Satisfaction

Counsellor Selection

Reports of counsellor selection have indicated that this process is often inadequate[14]. Counsellors are often selected by managers who have little understanding of the needs and responsibilities of counsellors. It has, however, been demonstrated that health care professionals who are encouraged to counsel are more likely to be empathetic and proficient counsellors[15]. Therefore counselling training should not be a mandatory part of work, but rather assigned to health care professionals who feel committed to counselling. In order to avoid over-commitment or the imposition of the counsellor's own personal programme, regular supervision of counsellors is important. Counsellors may not necessarily have a health background, and lay counsellors, people living with HIV/AIDS and people from other professions, such as teachers[16], have been trained as counsellors in many developing countries.

Counsellor Attitudes

Counsellors will often have clients from different backgrounds and with different health and social beliefs. If they are dealing with groups such as commercial sex workers, drug users, or young people, they may require training in special communication skills. Welcoming, friendly, sensitive and non-judgemental attitudes from counsellors are essential.

Counsellor Training (Alongwith Counsellor Training Materials)

Counsellors in VCT services will need training which should consist of primary information on HIV, transmission routes, risk factors, and possible and available interventions, as well as the role and processes of pre-test, post-test and ongoing counselling. For the latter they will often need to acquire new skills. There are various theories of counselling training. A short course (generally 1-2 weeks) followed by practical work, then a further 1-2 weeks, is a common time-scale[17]. Some centres offer longer, more in-depth training. The need for refresher courses and ongoing training and support is broadly recognised.

Counsellor Recognition

Many people in high HIV-prevalence areas have received training in HIV counselling, but are often unable to use their skills because counselling is not recognised by their fellow workers as being important. Moreover, other routine activities often take precedence over counselling or counselling-trained professionals are transferred to other posts where they cannot perform their duties. If counsellors are trained and given additional duties in HIV counselling, this role must be recognised and appreciated, and they must be allowed sufficient time to perform these duties.

Counsellor Support and Follow-up

Many counsellors encounter severe stress because of full-time counselling for HIV [18, 19]. In order to minimise 'burnout', and avoid using valuable and experienced staff, regular support and supervision should be planned and provided. This has been demonstrated to be effective and feasible, even in busy hospitals providing care in high HIV prevalence communities[20]. The questions on burnout have been adapted from previous studies[21]. Counsellors may be able to work more effectively if they alternate their counselling with other activities. It must also be recognised that many health care professionals even those working in high-prevalence areas, may have had little formula training in HIV and may have identical prejudices to those held by others in the community. These prejudices may have to be challenged during training. Moreover, some of the issues they will be expected to discuss (such as condom use, or safer sex practices for young girls) may go against their own religious sentiments, or what they have been advising previously. It has also been reported that when health care professionals commence to discuss HIV issues with their patients, their own anxieties and vulnerabilities to HIV may surface[22]. Counsellors who are themselves living with HIV/AIDS report particular need for support as, when they give seropositive results, they may relive their own experiences and empathise too closely with their clients who test seropositive. These counsellors also reported the advantages of alternating counselling with other activities. In some countries counsellors have formed groups to provide inter-group support and to discuss complex cases. Counsellors, many of whom may have limited training or work in isolated situations, need a structure for supervision and referral of difficult cases.

Tool 3: For Evaluation of Counsellor Selection, Training and Support: How to use

Methodology

This technique is not tailored to evaluate the individual counsellor's counselling skills and counsellor competence, which will be covered in the section on counselling evaluation. Rather it is to reflect the counsellor's perceived adequacy of his/her selection, training support and work satisfaction.

Respondents = Counsellors

This tool is a semi-structured interview that should be conducted individually by a trained researcher. As it will necessitate a little time to perform, a small random sample of counsellors should be used. The interviewee must be assured of his/her anonymity. The interviewer should be trained to be non-judgmental and allow the interviewee to express his/her anxieties. Additional points and comments may be recorded where necessary.

What is your background?

Nurse ❑
Clinical officer ❑
Social worker ❑
Person living with HIV or AIDS ❑
Other (specify) ....

Selection

How were you selected to be a counsellor?

Proposed by senior colleague ❑
Self-motivated (expand)[23] ❑

....

Do you feel that you have been pressurised into doing counselling? (explain)[24]

....

Training

Describe the counselling training have you received?[25]

....

How would you rate your counselling training?

very good ❑ good ❑ adequate ❑ inadequate ❑

What were the good things and poor things in your training?

....

Are they any areas in which you feel you need more training?

....

Have you had follow-up or ongoing training? Yes ❑ No ❑

If YES, describe it,

....

If NO, do you think ongoing training would be a good idea?

Yes ❑ No ❑

If YES, describe how it might, or might not, help.

....

Support and supervision

How many hours a week do you spend in counselling activities?

....

What proportion of your working life is spent counselling?

....

Do you attend a counsellor support group? Yes ❑ No ❑

If YES, in what way is the group helpful or not helpful?

....

If NO, in what ways do you think you would benefit (or not benefit) from a support group?

....

Do you have support for counselling from other sources?

Yes ❑ No ❑

If YES, explain whom and how does it help

....

Do you have access to a designated counselling supervisor to provide you with support and technical back up? Yes ❑ No ❑

If YES, who provides:

support ....

supervision ....

"Burnout"

How do you feel about your job?

....

Do you feel valued or undervalued by HIV-positive people (explain in what ways)?

....

Do you feel valued or undervalued by other health care professionals (explain in what ways)?

....

Do you feel valued or undervalued by your superiors (explain in what ways)?

....

Are you given adequate time in your job to conduct your counselling duties?

....

Please indicate how you feel about the following statements:

"I feel emotionally drained by my work"

always ❑ often ❑ occasionally ❑ never ❑

"My work is very stressful"

always ❑ often ❑ occasionally ❑ never ❑

"My work is very rewarding"

always ❑ often ❑ occasionally ❑ never ❑

"My work environment is very stressful"

always ❑ often ❑ occasionally ❑ never ❑

"I learn something new in my work every day"

always ❑ often ❑ occasionally ❑ never ❑

"I feel isolated in my work"

always ❑ often ❑ occasionally ❑ never ❑

"I have problems communicating with my colleages"

always ❑ often ❑ occasionally ❑ never ❑

"I can help my clients"

always ❑ often ❑ occasionally ❑ never ❑

"I have no confidence in my clinical skills"

always ❑ often ❑ occasionally ❑ never ❑

Please elaborate on any of the above statements

....

How many years have you been counselling?

....

How many hours per day do you do counselling?

....

If your daily schedule varies, please give an approximate indication of the number of hours you spend, for each day of the week:

Counselling about HIV-associated problems .... hours

Counselling about other issues .... hours

Other work (specify) .... hours

How many days per week do you do counselling?

....

How many clients do you see per day?

....

If your daily schedule varies, please give an approximate indication of the number of HIV-positive persons you see for each day of the week:

Clients with HIV-associated problems ....
Clients with other problems ....

How do you see your future in counselling[26]?

....

Evaluation of Counselling Quality and Content

The objective of this discussion is to make assessment of the process, content and quality of the counselling sessions and the client-counsellor interaction. The innumerable tools that have been developed have been tailored to evaluate counselling that takes place in various clinical and non-clinical settings. The tools can also be used to help in the training and assessment of individual counsellors during their training or follow-up review.

HIV-associated counselling can be divided into pre-test, post-test, follow-up counselling diagnostic HIV counselling (where testing is not available or desired) and counselling related to specific interventions such as tuberculosis preventive therapy (TBPT) and interventions to prevent mother-to-child transmission (MTCT). Counselling assessment will also have to be adapted as per the types of counselling (including individual, couple, family and children) and may vary considerably with several groups, such as counselling for young people, gay men, drug users or commercial sex workers.

The counselling evaluation has been divided into common elements (content and competency/counselling quality) which are important for all counselling sessions, and additional content elements which are important when counselling in specific conditions and when specific interventions, such as TBPT and MTCT interventions, are available. These tools may need to be adapted to correspond with VCT guidelines used in the particular setting. Although the elements contained in the tools are fairly inclusive, the particular guidelines used by a specific site may differ. The counsellor may be evaluated on the protocol (s)he has been trained to follow, rather than other external tools that may or may not correspond to that protocol. In field-testing, however, the tools were found to be compatible with the counselling service protocols.

Competency-based Elements

Interpersonal Relationship

Interpersonal interactions are governed by gender, cultural and socio-economic elements. Other factors such as workload, resources and referral opportunities will also be important. These factors should be taken into consideration when setting standards.

(a) Sensitivity to and discretion of the fact that the client may be nervous of embarrassed
(b) Appropriate physical environment for comfort, privacy and confidentiality
(c) Good client reception, greeting and introduction
(d) Rapport, respect, interest and empathy
(e) Non-judgemental attitude
(f) Engagement of the client in conversion
(g) Active listening (non-verbal and verbal)
(h) Emotional warmth and support

Establishing good rapport by demonstrating respect and understanding will make problem-solving easier in difficult conditions.

Gathering Information

(a) The use of an appropriate equilibrium of open and closed questions
(b) The appropriate use of silence to allow for self-expression, dealing with impact, thinking through implications
(c) The clarification about client expectations; information heard to avoid premature conclusions
(d) Summarising the main issues discussed

Giving Information

(a) Acceptable knowledge about HIV on the part of the counsellor

(b) Counsellor's ability to provide simple and clear information about HIV-associated issues
(c) Reception and reinforcement of important information
(d) Checking for understanding/misunderstandings
(e) Summarising

Dealing with Special Circumstances

(a) Sensitivity to and accommodation of language difficulties
(b) Talking about sensitive issues, plainly and appropriate to the culture, educational level and beliefs (spiritual and traditional) of the client
(c) Prioritising issues to cope with the limited time and short contacts
(d) Innovations for overcoming constraints, such as time and privacy
(e) Appropriate management of the client's distress or emotional reactions
(f) Flexibility to involve partner or significant other, when appropriate or requested

Content-based Elements

(a) Pre-test
(b) Post-test
(c) In HIV diagnostic counselling
(d) For special services/interventions
  TBPT
  MTCT
(e) For special and vulnerable groups

Tool 4.1: For Evaluation of Counselling Skills

Methodology

Respondents = Observers of Counselling Sessions

This section should be completed by an external assessor, counselling supervisor or counsellors who have had training. It is aimed at assessing the standards of the counselling of individuals taking place in several contexts of HIV testing, care and support services. The standards assessed are based on the performance skills of the counsellors and these are best assessed through the observation of real counselling situations. Not more than three to five sessions need to be observed at each counselling site. Where there are many counsellors, a random sample (three to five) should be selected from among them. For each selected counsellor an observation could be made on the first counselling session conducted on the day of monitoring. When only one or two counsellors exist, three to five counselling sessions could be selected at random. Before the observer sits in, the client is informed about the observation and its purpose. Consent is sought. The observer must ensure that (s)he is as unobtrusive as possible and does not disrupt the counselling session. Assurance of confidentiality must also be given. Immediate feedback to the counsellor by the trained supervisor is advised, with an opportunity for the counsellor to express his/her opinions and concerns.

Occasionally counsellors feel unhappy about a supervisor observing their session. Where there are irreconcilable concerns about observations by supervisors, alternative evaluation methods include using peer counsellors as observers, role play or audio-taped consultations (see Introduction for a discussion of alternative methods).

Function	*Skills*	*Score*	*Comments*
Interpersonal relationship	• Greets clients	3 2 1*	....
	• Introduces self	3 2 1	....
	• Engage client in conversation	3 2 1	....
	• Listen actively (both verbally and non-verbally)	3 2 1	....
	• Is supportive and non-judgemental	3 2 1	....
Gathering information	• Users appropriate equilibrium of open and closed questions	3 2 1	....
	• Uses silence well to allow for self-expression	3 2 1	....
	• Seeks clarification about information given	3 2 1	....
	• Avoids premature conclusions	3 2 1	....
	• Probes appropriately		
	• Summarises main issues discussed	3 2 1	....

Giving information	• Gives information in clear and simple terms	3 2 1	....
		3 2 1	....
	• Gives client time to absorb information and to respond	3 2 1	....
	• Has up-to-date knowledge about HIV	3 2 1	....
	• Repeats and reinforces important information	3 2 1	....
	• Checks for understanding/ misunderstanding	3 2 1	....
	• Summarises main issues	3 2 1	....
Handling special circumstances	• Accommodate language difficulty	3 2 1	....
	• Talks about sensitive issues plainly and appropriately to the culture	3 2 1	....
	• Prioritises issues to cope with limited time to short contacts	3 2 1	....
	• Uses silences well to deal with difficult emotions	3 2 1	....
	• Is innovative in overcoming constraints (e.g., space for privacy)	3 2 1	....
	• Manages client's distress	3 2 1	....
	• Flexible in involving partner or significant other	3 2 1	....
		***3-best**	

This tool is tailored to evaluate the standards of HIV counselling by monitoring the content of the counselling session. The content of the counselling session will vary, depending on its purpose and the needs of the HIV-positive person.

For counselling in relation to testing, and for counselling around an HIV diagnosis in clinical settings (where an HIV test may not always be possible), the dialogue needs to cover certain minimum ground.

This observation needs to be completed by an experienced and trained external assessor, counselling supervisor or counsellor colleague who can either sit in on a counselling session, or review audio or video recordings of the session.

Tool 4.2 For Evaluation of Pre-test Counselling

During the session have the following occurred?

Reason for attending discussed	Yes ❑	No ❑
Knowledge about HIV and modes of transmission discovered	Yes ❑	No ❑
Misconceptions corrected	Yes ❑	No ❑
Assessment of personal risk profile conducted	Yes ❑	No ❑
Information concerning the HIV test given (e.g., process of testing, meaning of possible test results, window period)	Yes ❑	No ❑
Understanding checked for	Yes ❑	No ❑
Discussion of meaning of HIV-positive and HIV-negative results and possible implications	Yes ❑	No ❑
Capacity to cope with HIV-positive results	Yes ❑	No ❑
Discussion of potential needs and available support	Yes ❑	No ❑
Discussion of a personal risk-reduction plan	Yes ❑	No ❑
Time allowed to think through issues	Yes ❑	No ❑
Informed consent/dissent given freely	Yes ❑	No ❑
Follow-up arrangements discussed	Yes ❑	No ❑
Adequate time for questions and clarifications	Yes ❑	No ❑

Tool 4.3 For Evaluation of Post-test Counselling

During the session have the following occurred?

Results given simply and clearly	Yes ❑	No ❑
Time allowed for the result to sink in	Yes ❑	No ❑
Checking for understanding	Yes ❑	No ❑
Discussion of the meaning of the result for the client	Yes ❑	No ❑
Discussion of the personal, family and social implications including who, if any, to tell	Yes ❑	No ❑
Discussion of a personal risk-reduction plan	Yes ❑	No ❑
Dealing with immediate risk-reduction plan	Yes ❑	No ❑
Dealing with immediate emotional reactions	Yes ❑	No ❑
Checking availability of ample immediate support	Yes ❑	No ❑
Discussion of follow-up care and support	Yes ❑	No ❑
Options and resources explored	Yes ❑	No ❑
Immediate plans, intentions and actions reviewed	Yes ❑	No ❑
Follow-up plans discussed and referrals where necessary	Yes ❑	No ❑

Tool 4.4 For Evaluation of Counselling where HIV Testing is not Available

During the session have the following occurred?

Symptoms and duration of illness reviewed and discussed	Yes ❑	No ❑
Investigations and treatments reviewed and discussed	Yes ❑	No ❑
Possibility/certainty of HIV-associated diagnosis based on clinical presentation	Yes ❑	No ❑
Review of knowledge about HIV including transmission and prevention	Yes ❑	No ❑
Misconceptions corrected and information given	Yes ❑	No ❑
Personal risk assessment conducted, with respect to sexual and drug-injecting behaviour, and history of blood contact	Yes ❑	No ❑
Further discussion of probability/certainty of HIV-associated diagnosis combining risk profile, symptoms and clinical state	Yes ❑	No ❑
Time allowed for news to sink in	Yes ❑	No ❑
Understanding checked for	Yes ❑	No ❑
Discussion of the meaning of the diagnosis for the client	Yes ❑	No ❑
Discussion of a personal risk-reduction plan	Yes ❑	No ❑
Discussion of the personal, family and social implications of the diagnosis for the client	Yes ❑	No ❑
Dealing with emotional reactions	Yes ❑	No ❑
Discussion of strategies, options and referral for further support and care	Yes ❑	No ❑

Counselling for Special Interventions

Tuberculosis (TB) is the leading cause of death in people with HIV in many countries. In countries where TB is common many people will have been infected, sub-clinically, during childhood and adolescence. If they then become infected with HIV a reactivation of this hidden TB infection can occur causing clinical disease. It has been demonstrated that by giving tuberculosis preventive therapy (TBPT), isoniazid 300 mg daily for 6 months, the incidence of clinical TB in people with HIV can be reduced to half[27]. It is, however, important to screen people for active TB before TBPT is given. It has been proposed that TBPT could be offered to seropositive people following VCT[28]. Specific information needs to be discussed with clients during the post-test counselling session. Besides this, the following areas would have to be covered during the post-test counselling session.

Tool 5.1 For Evaluation of Counselling Content for TBPT

Methodology

Respondents = Observers of Counselling Sessions

This section should be an external assessor, counselling supervisor or counsellors who have training. Its main aim is to assess the standards of the counselling of individuals taking place in several different contexts of HIV testing, care and support services. The standards assessed are based on the performance skills of the counsellors and these are best evaluated through the observation of real counselling situations. Not more than three to five sessions need to be observed at each counselling site. Where there are many counsellors, a random sample (three to five), should be selected from among them. For each selected counsellor an observation could be made on the first counselling session carried out on the day of monitoring. When only one or two counsellors, exist, three to five counselling sessions could be selected at random. Before the observer sits in, the client is informed about the observation and its objective. Consent is sought. The observer must ensure that (s)he is as unobtrusive as possible and does not disrupt the counselling session. Assurance of confidentiality must also be given. Immediate feedback to the counsellor by the trained supervisor is advised, with an opportunity for the counsellor to express his/her opinions and concerns.

Occasionally counsellors feel unhappy about a supervisor observing their session. Where there are irreconcilable concerns about observations by supervisors, alternative evaluation mechanisms include using peer counsellors as observers, role play or audio-taped consultation (see Introduction).

During the session have the following occurred?
Have specific questions about TB and TB treatment been covered?
Questions for TB screening (symptoms discovered)

Cough	Yes ❑	No ❑
Productive	Yes ❑	No ❑
Fever	Yes ❑	No ❑
Weight loss	Yes ❑	No ❑
Family contact with TB	Yes ❑	No ❑

Contraindications and cautions to TBPT discussed

Drug reactions	Yes ❑	No ❑
Other medicines being taken	Yes ❑	No ❑
Pregnancy	Yes ❑	No ❑
Past history of TB	Yes ❑	No ❑
Past history of TB medication	Yes ❑	No ❑

Explanation of TBPT adequately given including

The regimen explained	Yes ❑	No ❑
The need to take medicines continually as per regimen and the dangers of taking TBPT erratically	Yes ❑	No ❑
The probable side-effects and when to seek medical assistance	Yes ❑	No ❑
Understanding checked for	Yes ❑	No ❑

The risk of HIV transmission from an infected mother to her child can be halved by giving short-course zidovudine from 36 weeks of pregnancy and during labour, and by avoiding breast-feeding. Preliminary results from trials of single-dose intrapartum and postpartum (to the infant) Nevirapine have also demonstrated significant reductions in MTCT[29]. To be able to make informed decisions about infant feeding and access to antiretroviral (ARV) therapy, where this is available, a pregnant woman needs to know and understand her HIV status.

Pregnant women will necessitate the same information as other people in pre-and post-test counselling sessions but additional areas will need to be identified. An area which will require sensitive counselling is sharing results with the baby's father/her partner and close family members, as interventions to reduce MTCT may involve decisions to change infant feeding methods and to take ARVs both of which will make it difficult to outcomes a seropositive status. Moreover, there may be considerable benefits of sharing HIV outcomes in pregnancy so that women may have adequate emotional support. Even in areas of high HIV prevalence the majority of women tested during pregnancy will be seronegative and it is important to use this opportunity to reinforce safer sex messages. Women who become infected with HIV during pregnancy or during breastfeeding are at increased risk of transmitting HIV to their babies because of the high viral load related to acute infection.[30]

Studies have indicated that, for women testing in the antenatal setting, there is a big advantage for women of being tested together with their partners[31, 32]. If women are tested alone, or their partners refuse to participate in the VCT process, or if they feel unable to reveal their status to their sexual partner, it is difficult for women to take full advantage of the benefits of VCT. They will have difficulties in making decisions about using safer sex practices, planning for their and their families' future, accessing care and support, and making infant feeding choices. Despite the problems of women testing alone, in pilot projects on MTCT prevention it is usual for this to occur, and revelation to partners may only happen in a minority of cases. Where interventions to prevent MTCT are available, antenatal testing should always be provided to couples. Testing women individually should be exception (at the women's request) and not the rule.

Tool 5.2 For Evaluation of Counselling Content for MTCT Interventions

Methodology

Respondents = Observers of Counselling Sessions

An external assessor, counselling supervisor or counsellor who has had training should complete this section. It is aimed at assessing the standards of the counselling of individuals taking place in the various contexts of HIV testing, care and support services. The standards assessed are based on the performance skills of the counsellors and these are best assessed through the observation of real counselling situations. Not more than three to five sessions need to be observed at each counselling site. Where there are many counsellors, a random sample (three to five) should be selected from among them. For each selected counsellor an observation could be made on the first counselling session carried out on the day of monitoring. When only one or two counsellors exist, three to five counselling sessions could be selected at random. Before the observer sits in, the client is informed about the observation and its objective. Consent is sought. The observer must ensure that (s)he is as unobtrusive as possible and does not disrupt the counselling session. Assurance of confidentiality must also be given. Immediate feedback to the counsellor by the trained supervisor is advised, with an opportunity for the counsellor to express his/her opinions and concerns.

Occasionally counsellors feel unhappy about a supervisor observing their session. Where there are irreconcilable concerns about observations by supervisors, alternative evaluation methods include using peer counsellors as observers, role play or audio-taped consultations (see **Introduction**).

During the session have the following occurred?

In early pregnancy:

Have the following areas been adequately covered?

Client's opinions on pregnancy discovered	Yes ❑	No ❑
Full information about HIV in pregnancy and the risk of transmission to the infant given	Yes ❑	No ❑
Possible benefits of knowing her status and interventions available if the result is positive (including making it clear that ARV therapy cannot be given to women whose status is not known)	Yes ❑	No ❑
Implications of a HIV-positive result for her baby	Yes ❑	No ❑
Implications of a HIV-positive result for future children	Yes ❑	No ❑
Implications of a HIV-positive result for decisions about infant feeding	Yes ❑	No ❑
Implications of a HIV-positive result for her relationship with the baby's father	Yes ❑	No ❑

Discussions around the advantages of testing together with her partner/her baby's father Yes ❑ No ❑

Implications and advantages of sharing a HIV-positive result with her partner/her baby's father Yes ❑ No ❑

Explaining that testing is not mandatory and that she will not be denied access to antenatal care or other services if she chooses not to be tested Yes ❑ No ❑

Options for termination of pregnancy (TOP) (if available by legislation and safely) Yes ❑ No ❑

Post-test counselling for HIV-positive women attending maternity services

Besides the general issues that should be covered in post-test counselling, counselling for pregnant women who are HIV seropositive should include:

Information on ARVs, if available Yes ❑ No ❑

Information on infant feeding options and the advantages and risks of breast-feeding Yes ❑ No ❑

Information on family planning Yes ❑ No ❑

Information about treatment, care and support services available and referral Yes ❑ No ❑

Discussion of potential advantages and risks of sharing information about their HIV status with partner, family Yes ❑ No ❑

Information about safer sex and using condoms to prevent transmission of HIV and STIs Yes ❑ No ❑

Information about care of the child (including nutritional advice and seeking early treatment for illnesses) Yes ❑ No ❑

Planning for the future (including emotional, spiritual and legal support) Yes ❑ No ❑

Options for referral if required Yes ❑ No ❑

Have specific questions about MTCT and ARV treatment been covered?

Previous ARV use Yes ❑ No ❑

Not a cure Yes ❑ No ❑

Need to attend maternity services Yes ❑ No ❑

Need to take ARVs as prescribed Yes ❑ No ❑

Understanding checked for Yes ❑ No ❑

Contraindications and cautions to ZDV discussed

Drug reactions Yes ❑ No ❑

Other medicines being taken Yes ❑ No ❑

Explanation of ZDV therapy for prevention of MTCT adequately given including:

The regimen explained Yes ❑ No ❑

The need to take medicines continually according to the regimen and the dangers of taking ZDV erratically Yes ❑ No ❑

The possible side-effects and when to seek medical help Yes ❑ No ❑

Understanding checked for Yes ❑ No ❑

Post-test counselling for HIV-negative women attending maternity services

Information about safer sex and using condoms to prevent infection (especially during pregnancy and breast-feeding) Yes ❑ No ❑

Explain about discordancy Yes ❑ No ❑

References

1. Describe what services are available, e.g., CD4, viral load monitoring. Are these services available for all people living with HIV or AIDS or only available for a minority of people who can pay?
2. For example, cotrimoxazole prophylaxis, specify intervention.
3. For example, give an indication of the teaching methods, course content, curriculum if available), etc.
4. For example, are counsellors subject to regular supervision?
5. Baggaley R, Kelly M, Weinreich S, Kayawe I, Phiri G, Mulongo W, Phiri M., HIV counselling and testing in Zambia: The Kara counselling experience. *SAfAIDS News*, 1998, 6(2):1-9
6. WHO. *TASO Uganda, the inside story: Participatory evaluation of the HIV/AIDS counselling, medical and social services.* Geneva, World Health Organization, 1995.
7. UNAIDS/WHO. Recommendations for the selection and usage of HIV antibody tests. *Weekly Epidemiological Record*, 1997, 72:81-83.
8. *Knowledge is power: voluntary HIV counselling and testing in Uganda.* UNAIDS Best Practice Collection Case Study, Geneva, UNAIDS, 1999.

9. Wilson D. Provisional rapid assessment guidelines for prostitute interventions in sub-Saharan Africa and Plummer F, Ngugi E, Moses S. The Pumwani experience: Evolution of a partnership in disease control, Published in *Focusing interventions among vulnerable groups for HIV infection: experiences from Eastern and Southern Africa* NARESA Monograph No. 2, 1994.
10. For example, do written policies, checklists, data management systems, etc., exist?
11. For example, are files kept in a locked filing cabinet, is a system in place to protect confidential computerized information?
12. For example, schedule for confirmation of test results, policy about testing in the window period.
13. It is noteworthy here that 'return rates' to collect HIV test result may be very dependent on the HIV testing mechanism. Where simple/rapid testing strategies are used it may be virtually impossible for clients not to get their test results as they are available shortly after the sample is taken and the client may be asked to remain in the clinic to receive the test result. If, however, ELISA testing is used and blood samples are sent to a central laboratory, a delay of 2-3 weeks is general between taking the blood test and the results being available to the client. This may result in fewer clients receiving their test result for logistic reasons or due to people changing their minds.
14. Miller D, Casey K. Draft report on a consultancy on strategic counselling development in Thailand, Chang Mai, UNAIDS, July 1997.
15. Lie G, Biswalo P. Perception of appropriate HIV/AIDS counsellors in Arusha and Kilimanjaro regions of Tanzania: Implications for hospital counselling, *AIDS Care,* 1994, 6(2):139-151.
16. Baggaley R et al. HIV stress in the classroom and at home as identified by primary school teachers in Lusaka, Zambia. *International Journal of Public Health,* 1999, 77(3):284-288.
17. Regional AIDS Training Network, Nairobi, Kenya, 1999.
18. Baggaley R et al. HIV counsellors' knowledge and attitudes and vulnerabilities to HIV. *AIDS Care,* 1996, 8:155-166.
19. Kalibala S. Research, interventions and current issues in burnout and response, in *Health Workers and AIDS,* Ed. Bennett L, Miller D, Ross M, Hardwood Academic Publishers, Switzerland, 1995.
20. van Dis H, van Dongen E. *Burnout in HIV/AIDS health care and support,* Amsterdam University Press, 1993.
21. Questions adapted from Miller D. *Dying to care? Work, stress and burnout in HIV/AIDS. Social aspects of AIDS,* London, Routledge, 2000; Bennett, Kelaher & Ross, AIDS impact scale, 1992; Maslach & Jackson, Maslach Burnout Inventor, 1982.
22. WHO. *TASO Uganda, the inside story: Participatory evaluation of the HIV/AIDS counselling, medical and social services.* Geneva, World Health Organization, 1995.
23. For example, give reasons why you decided to train as a counsellor, e.g., "concerned about the impact of HIV in the community", "following personal experience" - e.g., have friend, relative with HIV, etc.

24. For example, is counselling something you feel comfortable doing, or do you feel it is a strain, or that you have to do it as part of your job?
25. For example, number of courses and duration of courses attended.
26. For example, "...will go on with my counselling job for the foreseeable future", "...find counselling too stressful/difficult and want to find a new job".
27. Mwingwa A, Hosp M, Godfrey-Faussett P. Twice weekly tuberculosis preventive therapy in HIV infection in Zambia, *AIDS, 1998,* 12:2447-2457.
28. WHO/UNAIDS *Policy statement on preventive therapy against tuberculosis in people living with HIV,* document WHO/TB/98.255 UNAIDS/98.34, 1998.
29. Guay L, Musoke P, Fleming T, et al. Intrapartum and neonatal single-dose nevirapine compared with zidovudine for prevention of mother-to-child transmission of HIV-1 in Kampala, Uganda: HIVNET 012 randomised trial, *Lancet,* 1999, 354:795-802.
30. UNICEF/UNAIDS/WHO. *A review of HIV transmission through breast-feeding in HIV and Infant feeding,* 1999, CHD/98.3
31. Meursing K. *A world of silence. Living with HIV in Matabeleland, Zimbabwe,* doctoral thesis, Royal Tropical Institute, The Netherlands, 1997.
32. Allen S, Tice J, Van der Perre P. Effect of serotesting with counselling on condom use and seroconversion among HIV discordant couples in Africa, *BMJ,* 1992, 304:1605-9.

Seven

Migrants' Right to Health

International Treaties and States' Rights in Equilibrium

Relevant Declarations

The HIV/AIDS epidemic has demonstrated a consistent pattern through which discrimination, marginalisation, stigmatisation, and a lack of respect for the human rights and dignity of affected and at-risk individuals and groups widen their vulnerability to HIV/AIDS. It is thus essential to understand and utilise the preliminary human rights instruments that set up international standards in order to address this issue. Most developed countries also have national anti-discrimination law.

The Commission on Global Governance[1] expressed in *Our Global Neighbourhood:* "Comparatively recent in origin, international law includes the body of legal rules and principles that apply among states and also between them and other actors, including those of worldwide civil society and other international organisations. Scholars once argued that international law was not law in the true sense, as there was no international police force to enforce it, no sanctions if it were disobeyed, and no international legislature. But with the growth in use of international law, these arguments are heard less often today. [...] Although states are sovereign, they are not free individually to do whatever they want... global rules of custom constrain the freedoms of sovereign states."[2]

International law and human rights declarations establish the principles of non-discrimination, equality before the law, freedom of movement, the right to seek and enjoy asylum and other humanitarian theories (discussed later in this chapter).

The Universal Declaration of Human Rights was adopted in 1948.[3] The Universal Declaration is built on the fundamental principle that human rights are based on the 'inherent dignity' of every person. This dignity, and the rights to freedom and equality, which flow from that, witnessed as undeniable.

Although the Declaration does not have the binding force of a treaty, it has acquired global acceptability. Many countries have cited the Declaration or included its provisions in their basic legislations or constitutions. And many human rights covenants, conventions and treaties concluded since 1948 have been built on its theories.

The International Covenant on Civil and Political Rights and the International Covenant on Economic, Social and Cultural Rights came into force in 1976. They take the Universal Declaration a step further by making provisions legally binding. A majority of the world's countries are parties to the two Conventions, thereby opening the vista to international monitoring of their human rights practices.

Specifically, the International Covenant on Economic, Social and Cultural Rights explicitly recognises the right of everyone to the enjoyment of the highest attainable standard of physical and mental health. In addition, Article 2 (1) provides that each State Party to the Covenant undertake to take steps, individually and through international assistance and cooperation, to achieve progressively the rights in the Covenant. Since 1948, some 60 human rights treaties and declarations have been negotiated at the United Nations. Additional examples are:

(a) International Convention on the Elimination of All forms of Racial Discrimination (1965)
(b) Convention on the Elimination of All Forms of Discrimination against Women (1979)
(c) Convention on the Rights of the Child (1989)
(d) International Convention on the Protection of the Rights of All Migrant Workers and Members of Their Families (1990)

However, the last-named treaty has not yet come into force because it needs ratification by at least 20 governments and as of May 2000 only some twelve countries were recorded as fully or partly through the process: Azerbaijan, Bonsia and Herzegovina, Cape Verde, Colombia, Egypt, Mexico, Morocco, Philippines,

Senegal, Seychelles, Sri Lanka, and Uganda. Unfortunately, none of these countries are members of the G7 group,[4] major developed countries or major recruiters of migrant labour, and thus even if they all complete the process the overall impact will not be great.

It should be noted that the right to enter a state is confined to nationals of that state, and states have wide discretion to choose the grounds by which to exclude and expel aliens. Nevertheless, the international treaties do impose some limitations (albeit often only implicitly) on states' prerogatives. In addition, as *Our Global Neighbourhood* expresses: The norms of international law — particularly on human rights — are already guiding judges in cases in individual countries as they rightly seek to ensure, to the extent allowed by their legal system, that universally recognised norms and values are protected domestically."[5]

In fact, it has been argued by Somerville and Wilson that there should be a presumption that all visitors to a country should have a right of entry, unless the state can show justification for excluding them; that while the state may exclude immigrants, including on medical bases, such exclusion should comply with principles of human rights and justice; and that refugees should never be excluded on the bases of medical inadmissibility.[6]

Similarly, Ngwena argues that "despite the inclination of governments to treat access to medical treatment as a privilege rather [than] a right, it is no less a right than other rights such as the right to life, human dignity and freedom which are unambiguously inscribed in national constitutions".[7] He notes that Tomasevski[8] (among others) has demonstrated that the recognition and acceptance of a universal right to health care in international human rights instruments is not in question. What is in the equilibrium are the parameters and enforceability of such a right. However, a forthcoming statement by the UN Committee on Economic, Social and Cultural Rights is expected to express their interpretation that health is both a fundamental human right in itself and an indispensable precondition for the exercise of other human rights.

WHO was the first international organisation to formulate health in terms of a human right. The WHO Constitution, adopted in 1946, recognise that "the enjoyment of the highest attainable standard of health is one of the fundamental rights of every human being". The WHO constitution defines health as "a state of complete physical, mental and social well-being and not merely the absence of disease or infirmity". Various human rights instruments — treaties as well as resolutions and recommendations — have been adopted since which proclaim health as a human right and include many provisions referring to the wide description of health as set forth in the WHO constitution. The latter does not indicate that everyone has a right to be healthy, but above all imposes a duty upon states to respect, protect and fulfil the aspirations enshrined in WHO's definition of health.[9]

The right to healthy working and living conditions, the right to health education, and the right to affordable and accessible health care are three examples of rights that governments should guarantee for their migrant populations.[10]

When discussing cross-border movement barriers in general it should be noted that: restrictions projected at reducing or regulating in-migration are mainly imposed by countries that are either developed countries or at an intermediate stage of development, but may bear heavily upon the nationals of developing countries who are affected by them. It should also be noted that obstacles that discriminate against people with HIV infection or AIDS, or people from countries with high rates of reported AIDS cases violate various provisions of international law (and in many cases also national law) prohibiting discrimination.[11]

In 1996, UNAIDS and the Office of the United Nations High Commissioner for Human Rights formulated International Guidelines on HIV/AIDS and Human Rights. With UNAIDS funding, in 1997 the International Council of AIDS Service Organisations (ICASO) prepared and distributed (in English, French and Spanish) an NGO Summary and an Advocate's Guide to the Guidelines,[12] which consisted tips on how to use the Guidelines to upgrade the response to the epidemic and lessen the vulnerability of affected communities.

The International Guidelines on HIV/AIDS and Human Rights were reflected at the UN Commission on Human Rights at its 53rd session, in April 1997. At its 55th session, in April 1999, the

Commission adopted a resolution calling on governments to report back to the Commission at its 57th session, in 2001, on the measures they have taken on promote and implement the Guidelines.[13] Within the International Guidelines, reference is made to the Vienna Declaration and Programme of Action, which was adopted at the World Conference on Human Rights in June 1993. This Declaration 'affirmed that all human rights are universal, indivisible, interdependent and interrelated. While the significance of national and regional particularities and various historical, cultural and religious backgrounds must be borne in mind, states have the duty, regardless of their political, economic and cultural systems to promote and protect universal human rights standards and fundamental freedoms.[14]

Beyond the formal legal system, as noted by *Our Global Neighbourhood,* the technical, organisational, and lobbying skills of some NGOs are an efficient means of achieving enhanced compliance. We motivate these groups to continue lobbying and pressuring governments, multilateral institutions, transnational corporations, and other topics of international law to comply with their international legal obligations.[15] This discussion would add, and to comply with implicit worldwide ethical and monetary needs.

International Spread of Disease

The use of restrictive measures as a response to infectious diseases has been discouraged since the mid-19th Century and especially since the inception of WHO.[16] The International Health Regulations require WHO member states to refrain from enforcing restrictions for non-regulations diseases: HIV infection and AIDS are not included in the regulations.

As Wahdan has stated: One of the main purposes for which the International Health Regulations (IHR) were adopted is to bring some order to a chaotic situation that could develop in which every country will be imposing regulations in a way it chooses — regulations that it considers will protect its population from the occurrence of the diseases already happening in other countries. IHR are meant to be a universal code of practice to standardise the mechanisms to be followed by all countries in controlling diseases. [...] It specifies what should be done by whom and for what purpose — whether it is notification or measures for prevention and control.

The policing sense of the old regulations projected in the emphasis on quarantining of cases and contacts have given way to sensible public health measures. The amendments to the IHR reflected the fact that main effective strategy and defence mechanism against international spread of disease is better surveillance through which foci of infection are detected early and dealt with.[17] The advent of HIV and the emergence (or re-emergence) of other key infectious diseases has caused a substantial review of the role of instruments such as the IHR in the protection of global public health, and in how such international instruments are mandated.

For example, Fidler[18] states: "The HIV/AIDS crisis dramatically illustrated the weaknesses of the health regulations. Since AIDS was not originally (or subsequently) made subject to the regulations, states had, and continue to have, no notification requirements pertaining to this new disease. Further, as HIV/AIDS spread worldwide, many states adopted exclusively policies that, according to experts, violated provisions of the health regulations. In relation to one of the biggest disease crises of this century, parts of the International Health Regulations were irrelevant, and other parts were openly violated.[19] Fidler, however, does not feel there are inherent problems in international law, rather a previous lack of attention to its application. He notes, "In connection with emerging infections, WHO is advocating an international legal strategy by recommending revision of the International Health Regulations. This recommendation suggests that WHO acknowledges the need for international legal agreement in dealing with emerging infections. The global threat posed by these infections represents in many ways a test case for international public health law.[20] Fidler suggests a number of possible strategies for the way forward, including learning from progress in the international environment area.

Effect of Globalisation

Increasing globalisation of all human societies is causing some reconsideration of the concept of total State sovereignty within a country's borders. Of course, major human rights betrayals such as genocide have always attracted outside attention, but there is growing acknowledgement and understanding that 'what goes around comes around'. The 'Global Village' is much more than a global market — in a global village there is a global public health. Tuberculosis (TB) provides an example of this: in Australia, Hong Kong (China), Malaysia and Singapore, the numbers of tuberculosis cases have not decreased for several years due to the incidence of tuberculosis among new immigrants.[21]

Unfortunately, HIV is causing an associated and increasing epidemic of TB in many of the most severely affected countries — and, while active TB can easily be detected in a clinical examination, it can also comparatively easily be transmitted in a work or social situation, unlike HIV. In a plenary address at the XI-ICASA in September 1999, Dr. Okware from the Ministry of Health in Uganda noted that "in some parts of Africa, the incidence of tuberculosis is increasing at an alarming rate — sometimes as high as 8 per cent every year". While people undermined by HIV infection are more easily infected with the TB bacillus, many already harbour it from childhood. Globally, millions of people are already infected with both HIV and the tuberculosis bacillus, and the potential for accelerated growth of co-infection in the developing countries is vast, given the crushing prevalence of TB carriers in the general population (some 30 per cent) and the almost 6 million new HIV infections every year. The expected skyrocketing of TB incidence worldwide[22] is also expected to be related to the emergence of a significant number of drug-resistant strains of TB. And perhaps the further spread of multidrug resistant (MDR) strains of TB throughout developed countries, as well as developing countries.

Thus delay in tackling the dual HIV/TB epidemics in developing countries by stronger TB case-detection and treatment—tuberculosis can be cured with antibiotics irrespective of whether the person is HIV-infected or not—may directly lead to major problems in the health care sector for all countries. *Our Global Neighbourhood* notes that "Sovereignty has been the cornerstone of the interstate system. In an increasingly interdependent world, however, the notions of territoriality, independence, and non-intervention have lost some of their meaning. In some areas, sovereignty must be exercised collectively, particularly in relation to the global commons. Moreover, the most serious threats to national sovereignty and territorial integrity now often have internal roots. The principles of sovereignty and non-intervention must be adapted in ways that recognise the need to bring in the rights of states with the rights of people, and the interests of nations with the interests of the global neighbourhood".[23]

Similarly, Christakis argues that there are some problems that are not global problems but international problems: he cites pollution, ozone depletion, arms proliferation, hunger, and AIDS as examples of problems based on 'the direct interrelatedness of the problem in one country with the problem in another'.[24] Much of the past policy concern about migrants has focussed on whether they are likely to become a burden on health and social services in receiving countries — thus, there are a number of countries that require HIV negative status at entry or at renewal of work permits.[25, 26, 27] (Restrictions are reported in, or by, both countries with very high, and countries with very low, numbers of reported cases).[28] It is noteworthy that restrictions may ultimately increase migrants' vulnerability to infection by HIV by undermining trust, increasing hostility, and discouraging individuals who may be affected from coming forward for counselling and support.[29]

Restrictions provide very little benefit to any country. Gilmore states "more than sixty countries prohibit one or more classes of HIV-infected foreigners from entering their countries. Often this is done in a misguided attempt to prevent transmission of HIV, or to avoid public expenditures involved in HIV care. The former situation might be less of a problem if people already residing in the country did not expose themselves to HIV; excluding infected foreigners does nothing to change behaviours of those who are not foreigners. The monetary burden attributed to HIV infected individuals fails to recognise that infected foreigners often work, contribute to their new society, and enrich it by bringing new values and skills to the country.[30] In general, comparatively little attention has been paid to the economic (and ethical) dangers of ignoring the health needs of these workers.

Since the majority of migrants are adults in the prime of their earning potential as well as their reproductive life, HIV could have devastating social and economic impacts, should a large number of this sizeable earning population cease contributing to society. This scenario is already the case in many African countries, and now increasing in importance in other parts of the world with large migrant populations. The 1998 UNAIDS background paper states, "As long as illegal and undocumented migration continues to be witnessed only in relation to security and national interests, public health will be neglected.[31] However, the present discussion takes a broader view, and would argue that as long as any segment of a population (whether or not they are present illegally) is neglected in public health terms, the global response to AIDS will be limited and there will be concomitant cost and suffering.

The Alma Ata Conference (1978) undertook a major examination of the underlying principles and focus of health care systems, and led to a re-commitment to a Primary Health Care strategy as the first step in major health improvements for any nation.[32] However, the health impacts of a global recession and of globalisation were not considered at Alma Ata, nor the need for human-centred sustainable development. Nevertheless, the Alma Ata declaration did state that 'the attainment of health by people in any one country directly concerns and benefits every other country'.

The future will require stronger global action to protect and improve local and national health, by recognising the interdependence of health among nations.

Access to Health

Financing of Health Care

Financing of health care may be predominantly government funded, predominantly privately funded or a mixture. Governments also find out the priorities for available funds: in Zambia, for instance, only 0.8 per cent of the gross national product (GNP) is spent on health care, compared with about 7-10 per cent in most developed countries.

It should be noted that monetary resources for health are overwhelmingly provided within countries. This situation does not change even in those countries which are the recipients of significant international development assistance from sources such as development banks, bilateral development agencies, international nongovernmental organisations, foundations and UN agencies. For example, in 1994 health spending in low and middle income countries totalled about US$250 billion, of which only US$2 or 3 billion was from development assistance.

Substantial reforms in the health systems of many countries in the past few decades have led in many cases to substantial privatisation or significant increases in co-payments by patients. Dr Gro Harlem Brundtland, Director-General of WHO, states in her introduction to the *World Health Report for 1999* that "Active government participation in providing universal health care has contributed to the great achievements of recent years — but many governments have overextended themselves. Efforts to provide all services to all people have led to arbitrary rationing, inequities, non-responsiveness and inadequate finance for essential services." She notes that governments cannot 'provide and finance everything for everybody' but also rejects the approach of rationing health services to those with the ability to pay: 'Not only do market-oriented approaches lead to intolerable inequity with respect to a fundamental human right, but growing bodies of theory and evidence indicate markets in health to be inefficient as well. ... But the very countries that have relied heavily on market mechanisms to achieve the high incomes they enjoy today are the same countries that rely most heavily on governments to finance health systems.[33] She calls for changes in all countries to ensure participatory, fair and efficient regulation of the health sector.

In many developing countries and because of many factors, health services are often poorly equipped, drugs are not always available and in particular, STD/HIV prevention and care is poor. A recent WHO paper commented on the use of resources within poor countries: "National health systems tend to spend money on poor quality and low-impact interventions.[34] And of course, in some developing countries, the increased mortality of health sector staff because of HIV has begun to directly affect the delivery of health services.

Most developed countries provide universal or widespread health insurance for all nationals and legal permanent residents: thus, the burden of health care is rarely substantial for any individual, and in particular drug costs are comparatively cheap— in marked comparison to the situation in most developing countries.[35]

Even between neighbouring developing countries, there may be disparate health care provision: Burkina Faso, Ghana and Togo have large numbers of cross-border workers — migrant patients mainly attend clinics in Ghana (sometimes crossing over specifically for this purpose), because health services cost the least among the three countries. Given that, due to global migration health risks cannot be addressed adequately if they are only dealt with inside national parameters, many developed countries provide direct funding assistance to health care in targeted developing countries. For example, the New Zealand (NZODA) South Pacific Regional Health Programme was set up in 1997 as a direct result of the concern in New Zealand about the adverse health trends in neighbouring Pacific Island countries, especially those with the closest connections with New Zealand.[36]

Another issue is that of differential cost for access to health care for nationals/legal residents and others: many developed countries permit free access to health care services for legal migrants but require full-cost recovery for non-residents. In some countries, health care provision may also be regulated by bilateral or multilateral agreements, thus providing full health care access to a national of a country with whom, such agreements are in force. For example, Australia has bilateral agreements with Finland, Italy, Malta, Netherlands, New Zealand, Sweden and the United Kingdom.

The 'New' Public Health

One of the fundamental public health principles is that major achievements in health require the development of preventive and early intervention strategies. The improvements in population health status of this century have exemplified this principle. Environmental, social and personal changes that promote health and prevent the onset and development of disease hold the most promise for the future, as there is general acknowledgement that therapy and rehabilitation have always been insufficient by themselves to conquer disease. Active prevention is required to achieve such an outcome.

These insights have led in the last two decades to the development of a 'new' public health: one that relies less on exclusion and screening and moves more to inclusion and cooperation with the relevant sub-population. With an increasing emphasis on illness prevention, aimed mainly at reducing smoking and cardiovascular risks, there has been a substantial change in the public health approach to population associated behaviour modification-because coercive models were proving to be ineffective.

The new model, as described by Haour-Knipe:[37] This model, one of social learning, of inclusion and cooperation, involves harm reduction, motivation to change lifestyles linked to disease, education, voluntary testing and counselling, protecting privacy and social interests. When emphasis is transferred away from control and towards information, and primary assumptions are transformed in a critical epistemological shift:fruitless and potentially harmful calculation of risks is sidestepped, and all segments of the population are put on an equal footing. The assumption underlying obligatory measures, that people will necessarily behave irresponsibly, is replaced by the opposite, that enabled, they will behave responsibly. The ground rules are first and foremost to protect lives and keep the disease from spreading and second to work in collaboration with those who are to be protected to develop and utilise their own possibilities to avoid risk. Much of this 'new' approach is summarised in the five principles of the Ottawa Charter:[38]

(a) build healthy public policy;
(b) create environments that support health and health-improving choices;
(c) strengthen community action;
(d) help people develop necessary skills for health-improving choices; and
(e) reorient health services to prevention and early intervention.

Unfortunately, although there has generally been a philosophical change in approach among public health specialists in the last twenty years, in many countries legislation and regulations still reflect old approaches and attitudes. Innumerable barriers are in place in both developed and developing countries (generally based on the traditional infectious disease/public health legislation approach of the 19th century). Many of these provisions are not enforced (and, in the case of the developing world generally minimal inward mobility makes the application there limited), but nevertheless, the restrictions are there and can legally be used.

Fluss[39] refers to "Incorporating principles of objective risk assessment, evaluation of efficacy, minimisation of human rights burdens into communicable diseases legislations encourages decisions based on rational, scientific findings rather than public fear or ignorance".

Levels of Access

Migrants tend to occupy a comparatively vulnerable position in terms of access to health in the receiving society, because of general factors such as language obstacles, different, concepts of health and disease, and racism among service providers and the general society. In addition, undocumented migrants in particular will often be operating in unsafe working conditions and accommodation, and may be exploited for pigmy wages. Many migrants may lack the money to purchase health services or be unable to access local services because of their legal status. These general problems are often compounded in relation to HIV/AIDS, and to a lesser extent to STD matters.

Sometimes, governments may directly add extra obstacles to health care access even for legal migrants. For example, as noted by Bronfman: The US Congress, presumably motivated by the belief that authorised and non-authorised migrants participate 'excessively' in public assistance programmes, approved migrant-associated provisions as a part of the Illegal Immigration Reform and Immigrant Responsibility Act of 1996. This law restricts access to social assistance programmes even to the authorised migrants.[40] However, the obstacles to health care may vary greatly between countries. Decosas notes that in the African context, 'some migrant labourers and their families in fact receive health services superior to those available to their communities of origin, and sometimes even superior to those available to their host communities'.[41]

There have been a number of specific projects aimed at

improving access. Some of these approaches are narrated later in the present discussion. Unfortunately, few address the issues of access to prevention and care at the origin, transit places and final destination of migrants. All points on the moving continuum need to be addressed if migrants are to achieve full access to their right to health.

As Gilmore[42] notes, "When non-nationals are deprived of opportunities to be healthy this not only endangers their own health, but also promotes denial and discrimination. It hampers public health efforts, in particular prevention efforts, thereby threatening the public's health".

Speakers at a session on *Mobile Populations and HIV: vulnerability, risk and human rights* at the 12th World AIDS Conference presented a crystal clear picture that the health of migrant populations has often not fared very well when the matter is left to national instances in either the country they have left or that to which they have gone.[43] It will be essential for more countries to acknowledge that mobility is a process that affects two (or more) communities, not just one, and adjust their policies accordingly.

Early Intervention is Cheapest

Despite the widespread acknowledgement of the importance of prevention and early intervention, innumerable personal, social and monetary forces have generated obstacles to the widespread development and implementation of prevention and early intervention programmes.

Traditionally, health only becomes of personal significant concern to people when they are in danger of losing it through injury or disease.

Secondly, as noted by Barlinguer,[44] "the notion of health as a cornerstone of economic advancement, as a multiplier of human resources, and most importantly as a primary objective of such advancement, has been replaced far and wide by an opposing notion. Public health services and health care for all are now perceived as a barrier, often as the hardest barrier, threatening public finance and the wealth of nations; reduction in health expenditure (not rationalisation, which is the imperative everywhere) has become one of the top priorities for all governments.

The model of primary health care as fundamental for the prevention and treatment of diseases has been almost abandoned. The trend is now towards dismantling the whole machinery of public health. Even in countries with minimal resources, priority is given to costly technologies".

Some of the past change in the understanding of the importance to economic growth of health has been perceived to arise out of the policies and approach of the World Bank and the International Monetary Fund. The World Bank is now committed to highlighting that health sector reform is a means rather than an end in itself, and to ensure that there is a focus again on the determinants of health (education, poverty, environment, gender) and on tangible health outcomes.

Ngwena recently noted[45] that, in Africa, "the state health care sectors are over-burdened, ill-equipped and badly managed. Declining health budgets as a result of reduced government expenditure on public services have seen many public health services collapsing in several African countries. Drugs for common diseases are either unavailable or of poor quality and so is the medical equipment. The structural adjustment programmes that have been imposed by the Bretton Woods institutions to assist Africa in economic reform, are simultaneously leaving little by way of adequate resources for health care".

The World Bank announced in July 1999 that it planned in future to take more stringent action against AIDS. A Bank official noted that AIDS is no longer solely a health problem, but a development crisis that is particularly affecting Africa. Working with governments and other groups, the World Bank has stated it will review its existing efforts in Africa and plans to redirect funding, if needed.

Discussing the World Bank's new emphasis on the African AIDS epidemic, Mr Callisto Madavo, Vice President, Africa Region said: "With ferocious speed, AIDS has wiped out many of the development achievements Africa has achieved over the last decades. It has reduced life expectancy in the most-affected areas and now threatens businesses and economies", he said. "Africa is in urgent need of resources and support to turn around this major disaster. For this reason we are putting the epidemic at the centre of our development front, mainstreaming AIDS into all aspects of our work in Africa".[46]

A similar review of the interaction between economic development and AIDS may shortly occur in Asia: the Malaysian Prime Minister called in October 1999 for regional leadership, including "all heads of governments in the Asia-Pacific region to hold a summit on AIDS so that we may better co-ordinate our efforts .. underline the gravity of the AIDS pandemic and the need for urgent action to combat it." Dr Mahathir also talked about the rights of migrant workers, emphasising 'the transborder nature of the epidemic'.[47]

An additional major obstacle to appropriate emphasis on prevention or early intervention has been that in almost all countries, health care systems have been structured in accordance with acute care models of disease and illness. Health professionals are trained to operate within the general parameters of the system—and preventive health is rarely where the 'best and brightest' concentrate their time and energy.

In general, for most countries massive commitments of public monies have been dedicated to supporting acute health care delivery systems. Many decision-makers tend to be oriented toward after-the-fact treatment of disease rather than prevention, perhaps because the advantages of prevention are more long-term and therefore not immediately obvious.

Lomas[48] has taken the problem of heart disease as a tool to examine the effectiveness of possible interventions: the points on an intervention continuum of probable responses to premature death from heart disease comprised:

(a) rescue, e.g., coronary artery bypass surgery, thrombolysis
(b) routine medical care, e.g., cholesterol-lowering drugs, hypertension control
(c) improved access to health care, e.g., 'free' care, increased supply of care
(d) traditional public health, e.g., lifestyle variation programmes
(e) family and support services, e.g., home visitors, social support
(f) social cohesion, e.g., subsidised clubs, reduced income inequality.

The last intervention, social cohesion, is rarely mentioned in health policy discourse. As Lomas states "these are measures to ensure and advance social cohesion". This involves preservation and advancement of social structures such as meeting places, sports leagues, clubs, associations and all the other elements of a community that permit for the exchange of views and values and engender confidence".[49] Lomas identified, using a cost-effectiveness approach, that interventions to increase social support and/or social cohesion in a community are at least as effective in preventing premature death from heart disease as improved health care access or routine medical care.

If Lomas' work is able to be extrapolated to HIV/AIDS, which is likely, then greater attention to support services and social cohesion (well within the reach of even the poorest developing country), may result in improved access for migrants (and others) to prevention and care, at no more and possibly less cost than currently. Similarly, if the formation of support groups for people living with HIV/AIDS is advantageous not only for psychological support of group members, but also understood as part of a necessary strategy in HIV/AIDS cost-effective prevention and care, greater attention and support for such support groups may eventuate from government and other key players. It should be noted that at the XIth International Conference on AIDS and STDs in Africa (Lusaka Conference), a Satellite conference on the 'Principle of Greater Involvement of People Living with HIV/AIDS' reported that though less than 1 per cent of those who are HIV-positive in Africa have come out in the open declaring their sero-status, they have become powerful change agents in the sub-continent.

Besides this, an approach focusing on social support and social cohesion would also imply the need for a greater concentration on 'community-level' interventions rather than merely 'community-based'. (Community-level interventions attempt to change the entire community through community organisation and activation, while community-based interventions attempt to change individual health behaviours.)

Decosas has also expressed that small improvements in the physical and social environment of migrants and of their communities may in fact reap greater benefits than targeted service provision. He narrates the example of some plantations in Côte d'Ivoire, where employers have commenced improving social infrastructure by providing schools, family housing, and recreational facilities.[50]

The account of a session on 'What Works?' in the HIV/AIDS/STDs and the Community Track at the September 1999 Lusaka Conference reported that the major achievements of the session were:

(a) It is important not to impose programmes on the community but to go in on their invitation
(b) Communities are able to use their resources and expertise to run effective and sustainable prevention programmes
(c) It is necessary to involve community mobilisers and facilitators in planning and implementation of programmes
(d) Linking care to prevention and sustaining volunteer service is indispensable to a successful prevention strategy
(e) It is important to integrate care of HIV-infected and affected in existing structures.[51]

These basic premises should also inform specific programmes aimed at migrant populations.

Necessity of Specific HIV/AIDS Interventions

There is a strong bond between sexually transmitted diseases (STDs)[52] and the sexual transmission of HIV infection. The presence of an untreated STD can enhance both the acquisition and transmission of HIV by a factor of up to 10. Thus, STD treatment is an important HIV prevention strategy in any population. Treatment of STDs, which is comparatively cheap, is highly cost-effective in its own right. It becomes even more cost-effective when the advantages of reduced HIV transmission are added.[53,54] In addition, in developing countries STDs are a major public health hazard making up the second cause of healthy life lost in women between 15 and 45 years of age after maternal morbidity and mortality.

UNAIDS has stated that "the magnitude of the problem of STDs, and the strong association with HIV transmission, reflect the need to explore new and innovative approaches to prevent and control their transmission. One such approach is the adoption of the `public health package'. This package for STD control includes the following components:

(a) promoting safer sex behaviour
(b) strengthening condom programming
(c) promoting health-care-seeking behaviour
(d) integrating STD control into basic health care and other health care services
(e) providing specific services for populations at increased risk
(f) comprehensive case management
(g) prevention and care of congenital syphilis and neonatal conjunctivitis
(h) early detection of asymptomatic and symptomatic infections.[55]

A complementary approach is to widen family planning programmes so that all people can realise their right to reproductive health. Several countries with significant migrant populations have developed targeted family planning services for their migrant communities—these migrant-specific services could be further promoted in line with worldwide changes in family planning. Since the 1994 International Conference on Population and Development, most governments and major funding agencies have pledged a commitment to implementing an agenda which emphasises:

(a) the need to develop better quality services for reproductive and sexual health care
(b) the need for gender equality and, therefore, the empowerment of women
(c) greater male responsibility for their sexual and reproductive behaviour and their social and family functions
(d) greater attentions to the sexual and reproductive needs of adolescents
(e) elimination of violence against women
(f) special efforts to counter the spread of sexually transmitted infections, including HIV

(g) wider participation in reproductive health and family planning activities

Policy-makers may need to examine their existing reproductive health and STD services and expand the scope and/ or target populations for these activities. There are extensive and clear bonds between the general objective of safeguarding sexual and reproductive health, and the specific objective to check STD and HIV.

In practice for most countries, migrant and mobile populations have tended to have less access to reproductive health and STD services than non-mobile nationals. Planning and implementing appropriate programmes for migrant and mobile populations thus necessitates urgent attention worldwide.

Promising Approaches: Future Exploration and Expansion

Promising approaches to HIV/AIDS/STD prevention and care for migrants cover a variety of interventions including assuring access to condoms, media campaigns to promote HIV/AIDS awareness and knowledge, theatre and small group education sessions, peer education, outreach and mobile health services, and specialised care and support activities. The most effective are those that consist of several different strategies.

Many countries have found that it is frequently both cost-effective and less threatening to integrate HIV/AIDS/STD into more general health services which address other health concerns of migrants. It should be noted that health services aimed at migrants need elasticity and commitment from staff, in conjunction with the involvement of target group representatives in the design and delivery of the services. Specialised training and continuous education are also often necessary for all staff and associated personnel.

One particular problem (not only in the migrants and HIV/ AIDS/STD arena) is the tendency for some successful programmes to be curtailed due to the belief that a target population has been well informed regarding prevention methods and access to care. It should be noted that successful programmes need to be continued (although perhaps modified), even in situations where saturation is approximated to have been reached. New recruits are constantly joining any target population (becoming sexually active, initiating drug use, entering sex trade, etc.), while others need to have their knowledge and understanding increased or reinforced. Similarly, sometimes recommendations, guidelines and programmes are not necessarily fully implemented in the field,[56] thus regular assessment and follow-up is required.

Outlined below are a number of projects: they are included as illustrative of some of the promising interventions underway in different parts of the world. It should be noted that successful interventions can rarely be transferred intact to another setting: these selected projects are mentioned both to demonstrate the scope of probable interventions and as a potential prompt for considering modifications of these projects for other settings. The one characteristic that all these projects have in common is that they all target policy-makers at one or multiple levels, in addition to any service delivery aspects of the project.

UNAIDS and UN System Projects

West Africa

In Africa, projects aimed at reducing HIV vulnerability from mobility, migration and sex trade (often accompanying migration) are being conducted by the West Africa, Initiative, for which the UNAIDS Intercountry Team based in Abidjan serves as the secretariat.

Covering 17 countries and networks of NGOs and people living with HIV/AIDS, and funded (with contributions from the Canadian and German governments) by the World Bank, the West African Initiative has produced a practical manual for organisations implementing HIV prevention projects with commercial sex workers and their clients, and has generated a strong network of technical experts to assist countries in project development and implementation.[57] The action-research programme has involved seven countries: Burkina Faso, Côte d'Ivoire, Ghana, Mali, Niger, Senegal and Togo. While a few of these projects are located in important market towns along international trade routes, others have been elaborated in frontier regions characterised by a high intensity of border crossings.

The success of these projects in West Africa has stimulated interested in Central African countries, which are now initiating similar programmes. The West African Initiative, in collaboration with the United Nations Development Programme (UNDP), is also helping to strengthen associations of people living with HIV.

The Chad government has commenced a project in association with the Swiss Institute of Tropical Medicine to develop a 'One Medicine' approach, grouping together attention to human and veterinary services for nomadic peoples in Chad. The important objective of the project is to ensure that access to services encompasses the particular needs of women and children, alongwith nutritional attention, and will address both health care and health education (including STI) in active association with the participating groups.

East Africa

The "Great Lakes Initiative on HIV/AIDS" concentrates on mobile populations and HIV/AIDS, and includes Burundi, Democratic Republic of Congo, Kenya, Rwanda, Uganda and United Republic of Tanzania. Activities include information exchange, care support, integration of the response to HIV/AIDS into socio-economic and development agendas, promotion of operational research, development of techniques of coordination and collaboration between countries, and resource mobilisation.[58]

Central America and Mexico

Mobility and sex trade are the centre of a sub-regional initiative in Central America and Mexico involving governments, bilateral agencies, NGOs and the UN system. The initiative, commenced in 1999, will prioritise the prevention of HIV and sexually transmitted diseases among mobile populations, including commercial sex workers and their clients living in border and port communities.[59]

South and South-East Asia

In South and South-East Asia, an identical initiative is under way for truck drivers, whose lengthy absences from home increase their risk of acquiring and transmitting HIV in both casual partners and spouses. The initiative is intended to increase HIV awareness and condom use among drivers. UNAIDS provided some seed funding: as at mid-1999, the Asian Development Bank and the German technical aid agency, GTZ, had pledged substantial funding.[60]

UNAIDS Intercountry Teams

The UNAIDS Intercountry Teams (ICTs) have, for the last few years, focussed their efforts on facilitating and strengthening collaboration between intercountry and regional bodies on cross-border problems, migration and mobility. For example, the Asia-Pacific Intercountry Team in Bangkok is facilitating intercountry collaboration and regional dialogue on migration and drug use, two issues with particular relevance for the region. The Asia-Pacific ICT is also supporting rapid applied research on HIV vulnerability and migrant labour in the region. The Cluster Team for the Caribbean intends to address the issue of mobility in the Caribbean—this programme will include research on immigrants, sex trade and tourism.

Working with Seafarers in the Pacific

A major proportion of the populations of most Pacific Island countries are seafarers (or wives of seafarers). The Secretariat of the South Pacific (SPC) is working through the regional maritime training schools and colleges to ensure they provide quality HIV/AIDS and STD training. Some of the main activities include:

Curriculum development — in consultation with the Regional Maritime Training Programme a module has been developed and included in the regional maritime training curriculum to be implemented by 14 colleges in 12 Pacific Island countries.

Train the trainer workshops — for maritime, health department and NGO trainers who are responsible for implementing the module, or who have an on-going role in providing information and/or support to students and seafarers.

Resource support — through in-country assistance by a member of the SPC team in partnership with college trainers. Provisions of a training guide, videos, and other training and information materials for students and trainers.

Peer education training — offered through sub-regional

workshops for young seafarers who are prepared to assume a role as a peer educator.

Small grants — for each participating country to develop their own materials or to translate other materials into local languages.

Condom supply — in consultation with the college principals, condoms will be supplied to colleges.

The project is being implemented in Vanuatu, Fiji, Tuvalu, Solomon Islands, Tonga, Kiribati, Samoa, Federated States of Micronesia, Marshall Islands, and to a lesser extent, in Papua New Guinea.[61]

European Projects

European AIDS & Mobility Project

The European Project AIDS & Mobility was commenced at the request of the (then) Global Programme on AIDS of the World Health Organisation. Set up in 1991, it has predominantly concentrated on HIV/AIDS prevention, targeting travellers and migrants in Europe. In recent years, it has increased its coverage to care and support services.[62, 63]

The Project brings together National Focal Points representing 14 European Union member states, and operates by stimulating collaboration and exchange of information on AIDS Programmes aimed at ethnic minority and migrant communities. The EU member states represented include Austria, Belgium, Denmark, Finland, France, Germany, Greece, Italy, Ireland, The Netherlands, Portugal, Spain, and the United Kingdom.

During 1999, each of the National Focal Points organised a national seminar with themes based on priorities set at country level with respect to HIV/AIDS and STD prevention and migrant and ethnic minority communities and other mobile groups. Network activities have included regional training programmes, aimed at NGOs and CBOs, and addressing peer education among migrant populations, migrants living with HIV/AIDS, and culturally and linguistically appropriate services.

In addition, the Project provides an information and documentation centre, with material and literature databases bonded to the internet.[64] The project regularly publishes an updated bibliography of relevant books, articles and reports, as well as providing a reference service to other organisations in Europe that are active in the field of migration and health.

In their Athens Declaration of November 1999, the Project noted that access of migrants living with HIV/AIDS in Europe to health care, and specifically to HIV treatment, was frequently very limited. They noted that this was due to such factors as legal and administrative barriers, socio-economic problems, lack of culturally and linguistically appropriate information and services, and stigmatisation.

The Project has acknowledged the general need to make health services more accessible for migrants. The collaborating parties have noted that they need to work for strengthening of the services that already work with migrants, improved collaboration between various services, increased involvement by migrant workers, and sensitisation of health social professionals to cultural and linguistic issues and needs of migrants.

The AIDS & Mobility Project noted that although EU member states in theory are not permitted to expel migrants with serious health problems to countries where their health needs cannot be met, there are many examples of such people being deported. The Project has called for access to new treatments to be guaranteed for all people with HIV infection and AIDS, living in the member states of the European Union, whatever their residency status. A recent Project report makes reference to each National Focal Point having drawn up a plan of action to provide a basis for future programmes in their country to specifically improve migrants' access to treatments for HIV infection and AIDS.[65]

Transnational AIDS/STD Prevention among Migrant Prostitutes in Europe Project (TAMPEP)

TAMPEP[66] started in 1993, with the objective of developing models of health promotion for women and transvestites/ transsexuals (men to women) from Eastern Europe, Latin America, Africa and South-East Asia who were working in the prostitution centres of Western, Northern and Southern Europe. The main concern of the project is HIV/STD prevention, but the project notes that, in order to support safe behaviour they have needed to address health in general for the target populations, as well as the entire social position and the working conditions of the migrant commercial sex workers.

In general, migrant commercial sex workers in Europe have extremely limited access to health care services.[67] The specialised TAMPEP project had been effective in reaching migrant commercial sex workers: from 1995 to 1997, the TAMPEP national teams had contacted more than 30,000 migrant commercial sex workers in Italy, Austria, Germany and the Netherlands.[68]

> About 30,000 persons work in prostitution in the Netherlands. Official authorities approximate that 50-60 per cent of all sex workers originate from non-EU countries and are residing illegally in the Netherlands. TAMPEP notes that its outreach activities find that 80-90 per cent of sex workers in the windows are migrants.
>
> In 1997, there were between 200,000 and 400,000 women working in Germany in the sex trade: the percentage of migrant commercial sex workers varied between 60 and 70 per cent in towns and border areas.

From 1994 to 1997, TAMPEP had noted an increase in both the numbers of female/transsexual commercial sex workers and in their originating countries: in 1997, 25 nationalities were recorded in the four participating countries. The socio-cultural characteristics of the workers had also been widening. Besides this, by 1997, TAMPEP was noting an increased mobility within and between countries by migrant commercial sex workers in Europe. The majority of women contacted by TAMPEP teams worked in at least two different European countries in any given year, with many working in three or more countries.[69]

TAMPEP has increasingly linked its own prevention strategy with an international network of service providers and basic projects in the countries of origin, transition and final destination, linking, for example, with EUROPAP, a project which targets all commercial sex workers in Europe. They have been developing as a centre of expertise for training, consultation and advice on migrant commercial sex work for service providers and policy-makers (government and non-government) in all EU member countries, and to some extent more broadly.

TAMPEP has mediated some increased access to health and social services for migrant commercial sex workers in the original four participating countries. However, the majority of migrant commercial sex workers even in these countries have very little access to health and social services.[70] It should be noted that most EU countries provide HIV and STD testing (and some treatments) generally free of charge, and in many cases anonymously. Unfortunately, many migrant commercial sex workers are unaware of this, or distrust government services.

North America

Whitman Walker Clinic, Washington, DC, USA

The Whitman Walker Clinic (WWC) in Washington, DC, is one of the largest AIDS service organisations in the United States: it offers services for people living with HIV/AIDS[71] in the United States regardless of their immigration status.[72] Consequently, they provide care and support to probably more undocumented than legally documented migrants. The clinic has a broad range of services available to persons living with HIV, ranging from anonymous testing and counselling to medical and dental care, legal services, case management services, mental health and addiction treatment services, and day treatment services. Besides these, they have a food bank and housing services for clients who have been diagnosed with AIDS. All of the Clinic's services are available irrespective of a client's income, insurance status or 'documented' status.[73]

Asia

Coordination of Action Research on AIDS and Migration (CARAM)

CARAM, set up in March 1997, is a regional network of NGOs from South and South-East Asia engaged in a major action research programme on Mobility and HIV/AIDS.[74] The organisations involved in CARAM as of mid-1999 included Tenaganita (Malaysia), CCDB (Bangladesh), Kalayaan (Philippines) CARE Thailand, CARE Vietnam, CARE Cambodia and UCM (Indonesia). It is probable that the network will soon expand to more countries of the region. The network is technically supported by the staff of Health Care and Culture of the Vrije Universiteit, the Netherlands. The objectives of CARAM are:

(a) production of information on vulnerability and health status of migrant workers in general and HIV/AIDS in particular

(b) advocacy work to improve the living conditions of migrants and to demonstrate how migration contributes to increased vulnerability to HIV infection

(c) development of grass-roots interventions in the field of health, especially STD/HIV/AIDS education for migrants and the improvement of access to facilities

(d) development of action research theories to do the above and to collect the statistics that are needed for CARAMs advocacy work

(e) protection of the human rights of migrants.

The partner organisations of CARAM are primarily responsible for the production of information and the development and stimulation of local/national interventions (ranging from provision of health services at the grassroots level to advocacy at local and national levels). CARAM-Asia leads in regional advocacy and international coordination and information exchange.

CARAM-Asia and its partner organisations try to ensure that migrants within the region are accessed at both point of origin and destination. For example, if the Ministry of Labour in Cambodia announced that a significant number of women will be going as housemaids to Malaysia, then CARAM-Cambodia would commence developing pre-departure programmes, CARAM-Malaysia would develop interventions for Cambodian women on arrival, and CARAM-Asia would react at policy level concerning issues such as HIV testing for these women.[75]

Members of CARAM-Asia have noted that multiple-country and multiple-level mobility interventions and studies are rare. They advise, however, that "experience with participatory action research from the CARAM programme has demonstrated that participation of the people themselves in learning what the problems are, the collection of information that is needed, and the analysis, contributes greatly to the feasibility of interventions that result from the research. The nature of the research in the field of

HIV/AIDS (sexual behaviour, hidden prejudices against foreigners, people with other sexual preferences, etc.) makes the cooperation of those involved very significant. People that are stigmatised and fear discrimination (if not worse) are in no way likely to be willing to share information with people from outside.[76]

CARAM-Asia has now developed a matrix framework for intervention involving the concepts of "vulnerability (leading to community interventions and empowerment), risk (associated with a more personalised intervention and making individual choices) and human rights (associated with advocacy work) and opportunities in time, place and conditions for implementation of interventions. The intervention framework also encompasses explicit attention to gender issues. The dimensions of time and place that are important include the pre-departure process, the migration itself, the initial period of adaptation, successful adaptation, return migration, and re-integration into the original community.[77]

Australian Multicultural AIDS Projects

Within a context of ample government/NGO attention to ethnic communities, particularly new arrivals, both national and state governments in Australia have funded a range of HIV/AIDS education projects targeting ethnic communities, especially those with large populations of people who speak English poorly or not at all. A video (in 6 language versions plus English) on HIV/AIDS-associated issues, produced for new arrivals by the New South Wales Multicultural AIDS Project, won the 1999 Australian Multicultural Marketing Award. All national and state HIV/AIDS media campaigns have at least one component in multiple languages, and in most cases printed information is translated into more than 16 languages. In addition, there are specialised HIV and ethnic group health care professionals in most part of Australia, alongwith specialised targeted sex worker and IDU projects.

> Siren's story is a booklet in Tagalog for Filipina sex workers in Australia. It contains information about how to work and manage money as well as health information and tips for negotiating protected sex. There are different versions

of the booklet for commercial sex workers from different countries.

While government-funded health care is officially only available to legal residents, sometimes unofficial arrangements are possible. Undocumented migrants with HIV/AIDS in Australia have been treated through the Sexual Health Centre network. Sexual Health Centres operate confidential services and do not ask for identification, whereas most other health services have to ask for the national health insurance card which is only available to legal residents. This means that people with HIV/AIDS without legal residence in Australia can obtain outpatient care and treatment at comparatively little or no personal cost, including antiretrovirals, other relevant drugs and health monitoring. The situation becomes more complicated if patients have to be admitted to hospital since they need to show a health insurance card, have private health insurance or pay for the care themselves.

Australia provides a (free access) national translating and interpretation service, 24 hours a day, seven days a week in over 100 languages.

Implications for Policy-makers

One of the overall problems in the area of migrant health, in particular in respect of STI/HIV and reproductive health, is that attention has for the most part been limited, patchy and sporadic.

This discussion has argued for a more comprehensive, and worldwide, approach, with clear leadership requirements from several international agencies. However, whatever the influence of an 'international' or 'global' agenda, the centre of decision-making will remain the nation state. The challenge will be to ensure that nation states understand that their self-interest requires attention to STI/HIV among all people globally. In addition, policy-makers will need to consider the spectrum of decision-making and ensure that migrant health does not continue to fall off the agenda at most points along the spectrum. As Parsons[78] has expressed, "If we define decision-making as a process in which choices are made or a preferred option is selected, the notion of decision consists of a point or series of points in time and space when policy-makers allocate values. Decision-making in this sense extends throughout the policy cycle; for example:

(a) decisions about what to make into a 'problem'
(b) what information to choose
(c) choices about strategies to influence the policy agenda
(d) choices about what policy options to consider
(e) choices about what option to select
(f) choices about ends and means
(g) choices in how a policy is implemented
(h) choices about how policies may be assessed.

At each of these points decision-making is taking place. Some of these decisions consist of the allocation of values and the distribution of resources by the formulation of a policy, or through the ongoing conduct of a programme. Decision-making thus takes place in different arenas and at different levels. At one level, there is a decision by high policy actors to make 'national' health or monetary policy, at another there are the decisions of other actors who are involved in 'health' policy at the level of a hospital or local service.

International agencies may be able to assist countries by developing best practice policies and arrangements addressing all points on the decision-making continuum in relation to migrants' right to health, particularly in relation to HIV/AIDS/STD reproductive health matters. In addition, the numerous research publications in the area need to be 'translated' so that policy- and decision-makers have better access to the research and the policy implications of the research.

It must be acknowledged by policy-makers and planners that parity of access to information and to health service delivery often necessitates a number of different and additional strategies to ensure that all parts of a population, especially the hard-to-reach such as illegal immigrants, have real access. Too often, in developed countries in particular, statements are made that health care access is available for all, without reference or attention to practical and psychological obstacles for sub-populations such as females, people speaking a different languages, people from different cultural backgrounds, people from rural areas or outlying regions, people with limited monetary resources in generally affluent settings, or people ashamed of having contracted to sexually transmitted infection. This discussion has argued for a number of changes to improve migrant's health (particularly associated with HIV/AIDS, other sexually transmitted infections and reproductive health), at global, national and local levels. In summary, these include:

(a) acknowledgement of the right to the highest attainable standard of physical and mental health. In relation to migrant populations, this might necessitate attention to the right to affordable and accessible health services, the right to healthy working and living conditions, and the right to appropriate health education;

(b) attention to, and compliance by all countries with international treaties and agreements to which they are a party, and to relevant international customary legislation. It seems that many countries sign international treaties agreements but do not necessarily put in place the measures required for compliance with the letter and spirit of such agreements;

(c) general application of, and compliance with, the international health regulations;

(d) measures to ensure that major sending, transit and receiving countries have joint/tripartite health access programmes in place to address all time and place points on the moving continuum for citizens, migrant workers. Such points include pre-departure, the migration itself, the initial period of adaptation, successful adaptation, return migration, and re-integration into the original community;

(e) health care access programmes for travellers and migrant populations that move beyond emergency are, and address physical, mental and social well-being, particularly associated with HIV/AIDS/STD and reproductive health;

(f) greater attention to prevention in health service policy and delivery for migrant/mobile populations, including widespread development and implementation of community-level interventions;

(g) for migrants and for mobile populations within countries, measures to ensure good access to health-associated HIV/

AIDS/STD reproductive health prevention and care for all members of such populations. For example, appropriate health education may require the production of highly specific material in a range of languages;

(h) attention to the gender disparities often involved in migrant worker movements, both within countries and across borders, and to gender power relationships which frequently govern women's access to information and health care;

(i) understanding by major sending countries that contributions to the Gross National Product by migrant workers sending money back to their families may be brought in equilibrium by emphasis placed on health and social services, if migrant workers return to their home country ill or disabled.

Conclusion

Migrants can be especially vulnerable to HIV/AIDS/STD, but are often excluded or simply missed in many prevention and care programmes. The effects of globalisation would appear to require governments, if only for self-interest, to ensure that this state of affairs does not continue. In addition, there is evidence of human rights, and other ethical violations occurring that need to be urgently addressed at local, national and international levels. Changing this state of affairs will necessitate consideration of innumerable socio-economic and political issues.

Successful HIV/AIDS/STD prevention and care programmes for migrant populations tend to be those promoted with and guided by migrant communities, and involving substantial community mobilisation. Programmes must ensure access to care and be integrated with other local and national AIDS-associated activities. Peer educators often may play a prominent role, but flexibility and committed staff are necessary to supervise and support peer educators.

It is particularly difficult for government agencies to address HIV/AIDS/STD issues as they concern undocumented migrants. However, non-government organisations in several countries and settings have demonstrated that they can readily access and work effectively with people without legal status in the countries in which they are living.

Progress has been made in preventing the transmission of HIV to and from migrants, and in ameliorating the impact of the disease upon HIV-infected migrants. Projects addressing other sexually transmitted infections and reproductive health for migrants and mobile populations are available in several countries and settings. The challenge now is to address more comprehensively the complex issues involved, in all countries and at all levels.

Recommendations

Guidelines and policy recommendations must be issued and implemented in regard to migrant health, especially concerning HIV/AIDS/STD and reproductive health. It is international organisations with either migration or health within their mandate that must take leadership in such policy recommendations, and as a matter of urgency. The IOM may assist this process by providing a clearinghouse support regarding status and progress for improvements in (migrant) health in major sending and receiving countries. Worldwide attention must be drawn to the health access needs of migrants, particularly in relation to HIV/AIDS/STD. Strategic action will need to be undertaken at global, regional, national, and local levels. Policies, activities, and information exchange must be coordinated between countries where migrants originate, transit and settle. It is UN agencies, and relevant international organisations and international NGOs that should organise to ensure that this happens. Countries that receive migrants need to adopt health policies and practices that will remove economic, administrative and linguistic obstacles to their access to health. Such policies and practices should specifically encompass all types of migrant, including the most vulnerable, such as seasonal workers and undocumented migrants. Gender issues will need to be integrated within policies and programmes.

STD and reproductive health services for mobile migrant populations must be strengthened, in addition to and as part of HIV/AIDS prevention and care programmes. Where appropriate, such programmes should address cross-border traffic and zones.

Prevention and care interventions addressing HIV/AIDS/STD and reproductive health should consist community mobilisers and facilitators. Members of the target community must participate at all stages, from planning then delivering to make assessment of health promotion and services delivery programmes.

International Instruments alongwith Relevant Clauses

This discussion seeks to provide some of the prominent clauses in international instruments of relevance for this chapter.

Charter of the United Nations (1945)

Art 2. The Organisation and its members, in pursuit of the Purposes stated in Article 1, shall act in accordance with the following principles.

(1) The Organisation based on the principle of the sovereign equality of all its members.

(2) All members shall refrain in their international relations from the threat or use of force against the territorial integrity or political independence of any state, or in any other manner inconsistent with the purpose of the United Nations.

Art 10. The General Assembly may discuss any questions or any matters within the scope of the present Charter or relating to the powers and functions of any organs provided for in the present Charter, and except as provided in Article 12, may make recommendations to the Members of the United Nations or to the Security Council or to both on any such questions or matters.

Art 55. With a view to the creation of conditions of stability and well being which are necessary for peaceful and friendly relations among nations based on respect for the principle of equal rights and self-determination of peoples, the United Nations shall promote:

(a) higher standards of living, full employment, and conditions of economic and social progress and development;

(b) solutions of international economic, social, health, and related problems; and international cultural and educational cooperation; and

(c) universal respect for, and observance of, human rights and fundamental freedoms for all without distinction as to race, sex, language, or religion.

Art 56. All Members pledge themselves to take joint and separate action in cooperation with the Organisation for the achievement of the purposes set forth in Article 55.

World Health Organisation Statute (1946)

Preamble: The enjoyment of the highest attainable standard of health is one of the fundamental rights of every human being without distinction of race, religion, political belief, economic or social conditions.

Universal Declaration of Human Rights (1948)

Art. 25.1. Everyone has the right to a standard of living adequate for the health and well-being of himself and of his family, including food, clothing, housing and medical care and necessary social services, and the right to security in the event of unemployment, sickness, disability, widowhood, old age or other lack of livelihood in circumstances beyond his control.

International Covenant on Economic, Social and Cultural Rights (1966)

Art 12.1. The States Parties to the present Covenant recognise the right of every one to the enjoyment of the highest attainable standard of physical and mental health.

2. The steps to be taken by the States Parties to the present Covenant to achieve the full realisation of this right shall include those necessary for;

(a) The provision for the reduction of the stillbirth-rate and of infant mortality and for the healthy development of the child;

(b) The improvement of all aspects of environmental and industrial hygiene;

(c) The prevention, treatment and control of epidemic, endemic, occupational and other diseases;

(d) The creation of conditions which would assure access to all medical service and attention in the event of sickness.

Art 2.1. Each State Party to the present Covenant undertakes to take steps, individually and through international assistance and cooperation, especially economic and technical, to the maximum of its available resources, with a view to achieving progressively the full realisation of the rights recognised in the present Covenant by all appropriate means, including particularly the adoption of legislative measures.

2. The States Parties to the present Covenant undertake to guarantee that the rights enunciated in the present Covenant will be exercised without discrimination of any kind as to race, colour, sex, language, religion, political or other opinion, national or social origin, property, birth or other status.

3. Developing countries, with due regard to human rights and their national economy, may determine to what extent they would guarantee the economic rights recognised in the present Covenant to non-nationals.

International Covenant on Civil and Political Rights (1966)

Art. 6. Every human has the inherent right to live. This right shall be protected by law. No one shall be arbitrarily deprived of his life.

Art. 7. No one shall be subjected to torture or to cruel, inhuman or degrading treatment or punishment. In particular, no one shall be subjected without his free consent to medical or scientific experimentation.

Art. 17.1. No one shall be subjected to arbitrary or unlawful interference with his privacy, family, home or correspondence, nor to unlawful attacks on his honour and reputation.

2. Everyone has the right to protection of the law against such interference or attacks.

International Covenant on the Elimination of all Forms of Racial Discrimination (1965)

Art. 5. In compliance with the fundamental obligations laid down in Article 2 of this Convention, States Parties undertake to prohibit and to eliminate racial discrimination in all its forms and to guarantee the right of everyone, without distinction as to race, colour, or national or ethnic origin, to equality before the law, notably in the enjoyment of the following rights (...)

(e) Economic, social and cultural rights, in particular (...)

(iv) The right to public health, medical care, social security and social services.

References

1. The Commission on Global Governance was set up in 1992 in the hope that international developments had created a unique opportunity for strengthening global cooperation to meet the challenge of securing peace, achieving sustainable development, and universalizing democracy. It involved an independent group of 28 world leaders with diverse experience and responsibilities. They proposed a 'global civil ethic' based on the notion of bringing in equilibrium the rights and responsibilities and involving seven core values that must guide global governance: respect for life; liberty; justice; equity; mutual respect; caring; and integrity.
2. *Our Global Neighbourhood: The Report of The Commission on Global Governance.* Oxford University Press, 1995, p. 305.
3. After thorough scrutiny and 1,400 rounds of voting on practically every word and every clause.
4. Seven countries acknowledged as major international economic powers.
5. *Our Global Neighbourhood,* op. cit., p. 325.
6. Somerville MA and Wilson S. "Crossing Boundaries: Travel, Immigration, Human rights and AIDS", *McGill Law Journal,* 1998, Vol. 43, p. 782.
7. Ngwena C. *AIDS and Rights of Access to Treatment: The Scope and Limits,* Paper presented at the XIth International Conference on AIDS and STDs in Africa, Lusaka (Zambia), 12-16 September 1999. p. 2.
8. Tomasevski, K. 1995. Health rights. In Eide, A., Krause, C & Rosas, A. (eds.) 1995. *Economic, social and cultural rights: A textbook.* Dordrecht, Boston, London, Martinus Nijhoff Publishers, pp. 125-142; Montgomery, J. 1992. Recognising a right to health. In Beddard, R. & Dilys, DM (eds.). 1992. *Economic, social and cultural rights: Progress and achievement.* New York, St. Martin's Press, pp. 184-203 at 184-186.
9. Hendriks A. "The Right to Health and Access to New Treatments" in European Project AIDS & Mobility: *Access to New Treatments for Migrants Living with HIV and AIDS* — Second *Annual Seminar, National Focal Points, European Project AIDS & Mobility.* Clarke K and Bröring G (eds) October 1999, p. 8.
10. CARAM-Asia.
11. Somerville MA and Orkin AJ. "Human rights, discrimination and AIDS: concepts and issues", AIDS 1989, 3 (suppl. 1): S283-287.
12. International Council of AIDS Service Organizations. *An Advocate's Guide to the International Guidelines on HIV/AIDS and Human Rights* and NGO *Summary of the International Guidelines on HIV/AIDS and Human Rights.* October 1997.

13. Resolution 1999/49.
14. Office of the United Nations High Commissioner for Human Rights/ UNAIDS. *HIV/AIDS and Human Rights. International Guidelines.* United Nations, New York and Geneva, 1998, p. 40.
15. *Our Global Neighbourhood, op. cit.*, p. 327.
16. Allin NE. "The AIDS Pandemic: international travel and immigration restrictions and the World Health Organization's Response", *Virginia J Int Law* 1988, 28: 1043-1063.
17. Wahdan MH. "Shortcomings in the Current Version of the International Health Regulations and Difficulties in their Implementation", *WHO Informal Consultation to review the International Response to Epidemics and Application of the International Health Regulations,* December 1995, EMC/IHR/GEN/ 95.4.
18. Fidler D.P. *Globalization,* "International Law, and Emerging Infectious Diseases", *Emerging Infectious Diseases,* Vol. 2, No. 2, April-June 1996.
19. *Ibid,* p. 80.
20. *Ibid,* p. 80.
21. *Tuberculosis in the Western Pacific,* 'WHO Regional Office for the Western Pacific, 1999.
22. In developed countries, one-quarter of all TB cases occur in the over-65s, compared with only 10 per cent in developing countries of Africa, Asia and Latin America. In the developing world, TB is predominantly a disease of young adults: 60 per cent of all cases are young men and women of reproductive age. There are also major gender implications with TB; Tuberculosis is at present the single biggest infectious killer of women in the world, and the single leading cause of deaths among women of reproductive age.
23. *Our Global Neighbourhood, op. cit.*, p. 337.
24. Christakis NA. "Responding to a Pandemic: International Interests in AIDS Control", in Graubard, SR (Ed.) *Living with AIDS,* Cambridge, MA, MIT Press. p. 330.
25. Duckett M and Orkin AJ. "HIV/AIDS-related migration and travel policies and restrictions: a global study". *AIDS* 1989:3 (Suppl. 1); S231-252.
26. Archiv für Sozialpolitik AIDS Archiv. "Restrictions of entry and residence for people with HIV/AIDS: a global survey". Frankfurt am Main, 1991.
27. Laboratory Centre for Disease Control, Health Canada: *Countries with HIV-Related Entry Restrictions.* December 1996.
28. Many countries adopt a double standard: compassionate policies and practices relating to HIV/AIDS in regard to their own citizens, but an approach encompassing economic death in relation to migrants.
29. *Technical Update on Migration and HIV/AIDS,* op. cit.
30. Gilmore N. *Human Rights Issues and Migration,* presentation at the 12th World AIDS Conference, Geneva, Switzerland, July 1998.
31. UNAIDS. *Migration and HIV/AIDS.* Paper prepared for UNAIDS Programme Coordinating Board meeting, December 1998, p. 5.
32. World Health Organization. 1978. *Primary Health Care. Report of the International Conference on Primary Health Care,* Alma Ata, USSR, 6-12 September 1978.

33. WHO. *The World Health Report 1999: Making a Difference*. World Health Organization, 1999, p. xiv.
34. WHO. "The Global Health Priority. Reducing the burden on the poor", *World Health Opportunity: Developing Health, Reducing Poverty. Meeting Report*, May 1999, p. 36.
35. "The inequities are striking', says Dr Jonathan Quick, Director of Essential Drugs and Other Medicines at WHO. "In developed countries a course of antibiotics can be bought for the equivalent of two or three hours' wages. One year's treatment for HIV infection costs the equivalent of four to six months' salary. And the majority of drug costs are reimbursed. In developing countries, a full course of antibiotics to cure simple pneumonia may cost one month's wages. In many of these countries one year's HIV treatment—if it were purchased — would consume 30 years' income. And the majority of households must buy medicines with money from their own pockets." Quote taken from Press Release WHA/13 - 22 May 1999 *WHO to Address Trade and Pharmaceuticals*.
36. New Zealand Ministry of Foreign Affairs and Trade. *NZODA Regional Health Programme Initiatives, 1997-1999*.
37. Haour-Knipe M. Social enquiry and HIV/AIDS, Background paper prepared for the XIV International Conference on the Social Sciences and Medicine, Peebles, Scotland, 2-6 September 1996.
38. Ottawa Charter, WHO/HPR/HEP/95.1. Charter adopted at an International Conference on Health Promotion, November 1986.
39. Fluss S., *Some recent patterns and trends in communicable disease legislation in selected European countries* presentation at the May 1996 meeting of the Biomed 2 Project on Communicable Diseases, Lifestyles and Personal Responsibility: Ethics and Rights.
40. Bronfman M. "Mexico and Central America" in Appleyard R and Wilson A (eds.). "Migration and HIV/AIDS", *International Migration Quarterly Review*, Vol. 36 (4), 1998, p. 614.
41. Decosas J. *Labour Migration and HIV Epidemics in Africa*, presentation at the 12th World AIDS Conference, Geneva, Switzerland, July 1998.
42. Gilmore N. *Human Rights Issues and Migration*, presentation at the 12th World AIDS Conference, Geneva, Switzerland, July 1998.
43. Haour-Knipe M. *In conclusion*, presentation at the 12th World AIDS Conference, Geneva, Switzerland, July 1998.
44. Berlinguer G. "Indivisibility and Globalisation of Health" in *The Effects of Globalisation on Health*, Report from a Symposium held at the Annual Meeting of the NGO Forum for Health, Geneva, May 1998.
45. Ngwena C. *AIDS and Right of Access to Treatment: The Scope and Limits, op. cit*, p. 10.
46. UNAIDS Press Release: *UN Officials in Lusaka Commit to Increased Action against AIDS in Africa.* Lusaka, 15 September 1999.
47. Report posted on 25 October 1999 on Sea-aids, an independent electronic forum provided by the Fondation du Présent http://www.fdp.org
48. Lomas J. "Social Capital and Health: Implications for Public Health and Epidemiology", *Soc. Sci. Med.* Vol. 47, No. 9, pp. 1181-1188, 1998.

49. *Ibid*, p. 1183.
50. Decosas J. *Labour Migration and HIV Epidemics in Africa*, op. cit.
51. AF-AIDS listing no. 408 *Community initiatives — what works?* XIth International Conference on AIDS and STDs in Africa, Lusaka (Zambia) 12-16 September 1999, September 22, 1999.
52. Increasingly being referred to as Sexually transmitted infections (STIs).
53. UNAIDS: *Technical Update: The public health approach to STD control.* May 1998.
54. Piot R "Sexually transmitted diseases in the 1990s. Global epidemiology and challenges for control". *Sex Transm Dis* 1994 Mar-Apr, 21 (2 Suppl.): S7-13.
55. *Ibid*, p. 2.
56. See, for example, an EC-funded Project Report from the Merchant Navy Welfare Board, UK: *Seafarers: EC Co-ordination of Information on HIV and STDs. Final Report* 1998.
57. For full discussion, see UNAIDS Inter-country Team for West and Central Africa, *Findings of the Research-Action 'Migration and AIDS' Project*, available from UNAIDS, Geneva and Abidjan, and from the World Bank, Washington.
58. Meeting of national programme managers of GLIA countries, Kampala, Uganda, March 1998.
59. Bronfman M. *Diagnostic, Intervention and Evaluation of AIDS and Migration in Central America and Mexico*, project proposal, 1999.
60. See http://www.hivundp.apdiap.net
61. Armstrong W. Pacific Islands HIV/AIDS and STD project final report, 1998.
62. AIDS and Mobility Project. *AIDS & STDs and Migrants, Ethnic Minorities and other Mobile Groups; the State of Affairs in Europe*, de Putter J (ed.). June 1998.
63. European Project AIDS & Mobility: *Access to New Treatments for Migrants Living with HIV and AIDS - conclusions and recommendations.* August 1999; European Project AIDS & Mobility: Access to New *Treatments for Migrants Living with HIV and AIDS - Second Annual Seminar, National Focal Points, European Project AIDS & Mobility.* Clarke K and Broring G (eds) October 1999; *Athens Declaration*, November 1999.
64. http://www.nigz.nl/aidsmob/
65. European Project AIDS & Mobility: *Access to New Treatment for Migrants Living with HIV and AIDS - Second Annual Seminar*, op. cit. p. 5.
66. Transnational AIDS/STD Prevention among migrant prostitutes in Europe Project (TAMPEP) *October 96/September 97 Final Report*, 1997.
67. EUROPAP/ TAMPEP: *1996 - 1997 Final Report*, October 1997.
68. *TAMPEP Final Report, op. cit.*, p. 1.
69. *Ibid*, p. 3.
70. Access to specialized health care for (illegal) migrant commercial sex workers is reasonably easy and cheap or free in most areas of The Netherlands. Germany allows non-insured people to have anonymous and free HIV tests, butthey cannot obtain any kind of treatment or have preventive therapy. Official institutions (apparently also German commercial sex

worker groups) tend to be unwilling to adapt services to better meet the needs of migrants, and some migrant commercial sex workers use any health care service. For Austria, where free medical check-ups are only available for legal residents, a network providing cheap or free medical care for migrant commercial sex workers has been started in Vienna and Linz. In Italy, officially, free-of-charge emergency outpatient treatment is available to anyone, including temporarily-resident foreigners - however, TAMPEP notes that in practice many regions do not provide these services (regions cite budget barriers), and migrant commercial sex workers rarely use any health care service.

71. Persons living with HIV/AIDS.
72. Personal communication, Glenn Clark, Director, Fleming-Morgan Access Center, Whitman-Walker Clinic, 17 September 1999.
73. At the point of intake, Clinic personnel evaluate a client's situation and need for services, including their eligibility for public benefits. Legal services, available in-house, can assist a client in applying for public benefits. Although undocumented immigrants are ineligible for many public benefits programmes in the United States, they are eligible for the AIDS Drug Assistance Program, which provides free HIV medications to low-income clients. All information gathered about a client is kept confidential. Language obstacles are addressed by providing access to staff who speak the language, if available, or by providing an interpreter to ensure the client is actively involved in their service provision. For Latino/Latina clients, the Clinic has developed a Latino Services department. The Access Center, specifically, is funded by a private donor, which thus allows WWC leeway in how intake services are provided. The funding sources for other HIV services (which include federal, local and private funding) also allow the Clinic to provide services to clients irrespective of their migrant status.
74. CARAM-Asia: *Coordination of Action Research on AIDS and Migration. The vulnerability of migrants to HIV/ AIDS.* June 1998
75. ibid, p. 28.
76. Wolffers I, Fernandez I, Verghis S and Painter T. A *Model for Evaluating HIV/AIDS Interventions For Mobile Populations,* Paper presented at the Fifth International Congress on AIDS in Asia and the Pacific, Kuala Lumpur, 23-27 October 1999
77. ibid, p. 8.
78. Parsons W: *Public Policy. An Introduction to the Theory and Practice of Policy Analysis.* Edward Elgar Publishing Ltd, UK 1997, p. 245.

Index

D

E

W

Y

Z